# Small Animal Clinical Oncology

# Small Animal Clinical Oncology

## SECOND EDITION

**Stephen J. Withrow, D.V.M.**
Professor of Surgery and Oncology
Chief, Clinical Oncology Service
Comparative Oncology Unit
College of Veterinary Medicine
Colorado State University
Fort Collins, Colorado

**E. Gregory MacEwen, V.M.D.**
Professor of Medicine and Oncology
Department of Medical Sciences
School of Veterinary Medicine
Member, Wisconsin Comprehensive Cancer
  Center
School of Medicine
University of Wisconsin–Madison
Madison, Wisconsin

W.B. Saunders Company
*A Division of Harcourt Brace & Company*
Philadelphia   London   Toronto   Montreal   Sydney   Tokyo

W. B. SAUNDERS COMPANY

*A Division of Harcourt Brace & Company*

The Curtis Center
Independence Square West
Philadelphia, Pennsylvania 19106

**Library of Congress Cataloging-in-Publication Data**

Small animal clinical oncology / edited by Stephen J. Withrow, E.
   Gregory MacEwen.—2nd ed.
      p.   cm.
      Rev. ed. of: Clinical veterinary oncology / edited by Stephen J.
   Withrow. 1989.
      Includes bibliographical references (p.    ) and index.
      ISBN 0-7216-5592-0
      1. Dogs—Diseases.   2. Cats—Diseases.   3. Veterinary oncology.
   I. Withrow, Stephen J.   II. MacEwen, E. Gregory.   III. Clinical
   veterinary oncology.
   SF991.S5915   1996
   636.089'6994—dc20                                        95-23427

SMALL ANIMAL CLINICAL ONCOLOGY          ISBN  0–7216–5592–0

Printed in the United States of America

Last digit is the print number:     9    8    7    6    5    4    3    2    1

# Dr. Robert S. Brodey
## 1927–1979

A leader in veterinary oncology. We will
always remember him for his tireless effort
to advance the field of oncology, to teach
principles of surgery, and, most important, to
preserve nature.

We dedicate this book to this fine man.

# CONTRIBUTORS

**CAROLYN BUTLER, M.A.**
Instructor, Department of Clinical Sciences, Colorado State University; Co-Director, Changes: The Support for People and Pets Program, Colorado State University, Veterinary Teaching Hospital, Fort Collins, Colorado.
*Companion Animal Death and Pet Owner Grief*

**RICHARD R. DUBIELZIG, D.V.M.**
Diplomate, American College of Veterinary Pathologists; Associate Professor of Pathology, Department of Pathobiological Sciences, School of Veterinary Medicine, University of Wisconsin–Madison, Madison, Wisconsin.
*Ocular Tumors; Mesothelioma*

**EDWARD L. GILLETTE, D.V.M., Ph.D.**
Diplomate, American College of Veterinary Radiation (Diagnostic and Radiation Oncology); American College of Veterinary Internal Medicine (Oncology); Professor and Chairman, Department of Radiological Health Sciences, Director of Comparative Oncology Unit, College of Veterinary Medicine and Biomedical Sciences, Colorado State University, Fort Collins, Colorado.
*Radiation Therapy*

**STUART C. HELFAND, D.V.M.**
Diplomate, American College of Veterinary Internal Medicine (Medicine and Oncology); Assistant Professor, Oncology/Internal Medicine, Department of Medical Sciences, School of Veterinary Medicine; Member, University of Wisconsin Comprehensive Cancer Center, School of Medicine, University of Wisconsin–Madison, Madison, Wisconsin.
*Immunology and Biologic Therapy of Cancer*

**EVAN T. KELLER, D.V.M., M.S.**
Diplomate, American College of Veterinary Internal Medicine (Oncology); Postdoctoral Fellow, The Institute on Aging, University of Wisconsin–Madison, Madison, Wisconsin.
*New Developments in Cancer Therapy*

**WILLIAM C. KISSEBERTH, D.V.M., M.S.**
Assistant Scientist, Department of Pathobiological Sciences, School of Veterinary Medicine, University of Wisconsin–Madison, Madison, Wisconsin.
*Complications of Cancer and Its Treatment; Neoplasia of the Heart*

**MARY KAY KLEIN, D.V.M., M.S.**
Diplomate, American College of Veterinary Internal Medicine (Oncology); Clinical Lecturer, Arizona Cancer Center, University of Arizona; Southwest Veterinary Specialty Center, Tucson, Arizona.
*Tumors of the Female Reproductive System*

**LAURA D. KRAVIS, D.V.M.**
Resident, Clinical Oncology, Department of Medical Sciences, School of Veterinary Medicine, University of Wisconsin–Madison, Madison, Wisconsin.
*Mesothelioma*

**ILENE D. KURZMAN, Ph.D. M.S., Ed.D.**
Associate Scientist, Department of Medical Sciences, School of Veterinary Medicine, University of Wisconsin–Madison, Madison, Wisconsin.
*New Developments in Cancer Therapy*

## LAUREL LAGONI, M.S.

Instructor, Department of Clinical Sciences, College of Veterinary Medicine, Colorado State University; Co-Director, Changes: The Support for People and Pets Program, Colorado State University Veterinary Teaching Hospital, Fort Collins, Colorado.
*Companion Animal Death and Pet Owner Grief*

## SUSAN M. LaRUE, D.V.M., Ph.D.

Diplomate, American College of Veterinary Surgery; Diplomate, American College of Veterinary Radiation (Radiation Oncology); Assistant Professor of Radiation Oncology, Department of Radiological Health Sciences, College of Veterinary Medicine and Biomedical Sciences, Colorado State University, Fort Collins, Colorado.
*Radiation Therapy*

## RICHARD A. LeCOUTEUR, B.V.Sc., Ph.D.

Diplomate, American College of Veterinary Internal Medicine (Neurology); Professor of Neurology, Department of Surgical and Radiological Sciences, School of Veterinary Medicine, University of California, Davis, Davis, California.
*Tumors of the Nervous System*

## CHERYL A. LONDON, D.V.M.

Clinical Instructor, Tufts University School of Veterinary Medicine, North Grafton, Massachusetts. Ph.D. candidate, Department of Immunology, Harvard University, Cambridge, Massachusetts.
*Tumor Biology*

## E. GREGORY MacEWEN, V.M.D.

Diplomate, American College of Veterinary Internal Medicine (Internal Medicine and Oncology; Professor of Medicine and Oncology, Department of Medical Sciences, School of Veterinary Medicine, University of Wisconsin–Madison; Affiliate Professor, Department of Animal Health Biomedical Sciences; Member, Wisconsin Comprehensive Cancer Center, School of Medicine, University of Wisconsin–Madison, Madison, Wisconsin.
*Immunology and Biologic Therapy of Cancer; Complications of Cancer and Its Treatment; New Developments in Cancer Therapy; Soft Tissue Sarcomas; Tumors of the Mammary Gland; Canine Lymphoma and Lymphoid Leukemias; Feline Lymphoma and Leukemias; Canine Myeloproliferative Disorders and Malignant Histiocytosis; Hemangiosarcoma; Transmissible Venereal Tumors; Mesothelioma*

## DENNIS W. MACY, D.V.M, M.S.

Diplomate, American College of Veterinary Internal Medicine (Internal Medicine and Oncology); Professor of Medicine and Oncology, College of Veterinary Medicine, and Biomedical Sciences, Colorado State University, Fort Collins, Colorado.
*Feline Retroviruses*

## D. J. MEYER, D.V.M.

Diplomate, American College of Veterinary Pathology (Clinical Pathology) and American College of Veterinary Internal Medicine; Senior Research Pathologist, Sanofi-Winthrop Pharmaceuticals, Collegeville, Pennsylvania.
*Diagnostic Cytology in Clinical Oncology*

## PAUL E. MILLER, D.V.M.

Diplomate, American College of Veterinary Opthalmologists; Clinical Assistant Professor of Opthalmology, Department of Surgical Sciences, School of Veterinary Medicine, University of Wisconsin–Madison, Madison, Wisconsin.
*Ocular Tumors*

## GREGORY K. OGILVIE, D.V.M.

Diplomate, American College of Veterinary Internal Medicine (Internal Medicine and Oncology); Associate Professor of Oncology and Internal Medicine, Comparative Oncology Unit, Department of Clinical Sciences, College of Veterinary Medicine and Biomedical Sciences, Colorado State University, Fort Collins, Colorado.
*Paraneoplastic Syndromes; Chemotherapy; Metabolic Alterations and Nutritional Therapy for the Veterinary Cancer Patient; Tumors of the Endocrine System*

## BARBARA E. POWERS, D.V.M., Ph.D.

Diplomate, American College of Veterinary Pathologists; Associate Professsor, Department of Radiological Health Sciences, College of Veterinary Medicine and Biomedical Sciences, Colorado State University, Fort Collins, Colorado.
*The Pathology of Neoplasia*

## NANCY P. REEVES, D.V.M., M.S.

Diplomate, American College of Veterinary Internal Medicine (Internal Medicine); Senior Veterinarian, Pfizer Animal Health, West Chester, Pennsylvania.
*Tumors of the Male Reproductive Tract*

## RODNEY C. STRAW, B.V.Sc.

Diplomate, American College of Veterinary Surgeons; Associate Professor, Oncology, College of Veterinary Medicine and Biomedical Sciences, Colorado State University, Fort Collins, Colorado.
*Hepatic Tumors; Tumors of the Skeletal System*

## DAVID M. VAIL, D.V.M., M.S.,

Diplomate, American College of Veterinary Internal Medicine (Oncology); Assistant Professor of Oncology, Department of Medical Sciences, School of Veterinary Medicine; Associate Member, Comprehensive Cancer Center, School of Medicine, University of Wisconsin–Madison, Madison, Wisconsin.
*Tumor Biology; Metabolic Alterations and Nutritional Therapy for the Veterinary Cancer Patient; Tumors of the Skin and Subcutaneous Tissues; Mast Cell Tumors; Plasma Cell Neoplasms*

## STEPHEN J. WITHROW, D.V.M.

Diplomate, American College of Veterinary Surgeons and American College of Veterinary Internal Medicine (Oncology); Professor of Surgery and Oncology; Chief, Clinical Oncology, Comparative Oncology Unit, College of Veterinary Medicine and Biomedical Sciences, Colorado State University, Fort Collins, Colorado.
*Why Worry About Cancer in Pet Animals?; Biopsy Principles; Surgical Oncology; Cryosurgery; Tumors of the Skin and Subcutaneous Tissues; Soft Tissue Sarcomas; Cancer of the Oral Cavity; Cancer of the Salivary Glands; Esophageal Cancer; Exocrine Pancreas; Gastric Cancer; Tumors of the Intestinal Tract; Perianal Tumors; Tumors of the Respiratory System; Tumors of the Mammary Gland; Tumors of the Urinary System; Thymoma; Companion Animal Death and Pet Owner Grief*

## KAREN M. YOUNG, V.M.D., Ph.D.

Clinical Associate Professor, Clinical Pathology, Department of Pathobiological Sciences, School of Veterinary Medicine, University of Wisconsin–Madison, Madison, Wisconsin.
*Canine Lymphoma and Lymphoid Leukemias; Canine Myeloproliferative Disorders and Malignant Histiocytosis.*

# PREFACE

The field of clinical veterinary oncology has grown remarkably in the last 15 years, as evidenced by increased coverage in journals, a proliferation of textbooks, expansion of training programs in the field, and by the establishment and growth of the Veterinary Cancer Society and sanction of the discipline by board certification under the American College of Veterinary Internal Medicine in 1988. In 1994, the American College of Veterinary Radiology established board certification in radiation oncology.

Historically, clinical veterinary oncology was characterized by strong opinions based on weak data. Unusual case reports and small anecdotal case series predominated the literature, as did pathologic descriptions with an emphasis on morphology and metastatic distribution. In recent years, more attention to controlled and randomized therapeutic trials that are stratified for histologic grade, clinical stage, and other prognostic variables has enhanced the understanding of this complex disease. It is clear that cancer is no more "one disease" than is kidney disease or heart failure. A given histologic type of cancer is likely to have different natural behavior and response to treatment depending on anatomic location and species differences. Because tumors may be biologically or therapeutically heterogenous, careful analysis of all variables is required in management of the patient with cancer and interpretation of end results.

During the planning of our first edition, we made the decision to produce a book that was clinically relevant for the general practitioner and veterinary medical student and a helpful reference for the veterinary oncologist. In the development of the second edition, we have followed the same objective; however, we also want this text to be a state of the art book with an emphasis on biologic behavior and treatment of cancer in small animals.

The second edition follows the same basic format as the first edition. We begin with introductory chapters on pathology, cancer biology, and paraneoplastic syndromes. The next section of the book covers principles of diagnosis and cancer treatment, including chapters on nutrition and complications of tumor and treatment. All of these chapters have been extensively rewritten and most are entirely new.

The major portion of the text is devoted to specific tumor types and follows a consistent format of incidence and risk factors, pathology and natural behavior, history and clinical signs, diagnostic techniques and workup, treatment, and prognosis. As in the first edition, at the end of each chapter a section of comparative aspects (human cancer–related) has been included. All of these chapters have been extensively reworked and revised. Great care has been taken to include chemotherapy protocols that have been evaluated with sufficient case material to allow a determination of efficacy. Due to the increase and importance of the human companion animal bond, we end the book with a chapter on pet loss, grief, and support.

We are delighted at the exceptional quality of the chapters our invited authors produced. We are particularly pleased with our new publisher, W. B. Saunders Co. We especially want to thank Ray Kersey, our editor, and David H. Kilmer, Senior Developmental Editor of the W. B. Saunders staff. We also want to thank Fran Bartlett of G & H Soho Inc. for her detail in editing the typed manuscript.

It is our desire to provide the reader with the most current information in clinical oncology and a better understanding of cancer biology, diagnostic approaches, therapeutic interventions, and prognostic variables. Cancer is not always curable, but in most cases the patient can be helped to an improved quality and quantity of life.

Stephen J. Withrow, D.V.M
E. Gregory MacEwen, V.M.D

# CONTENTS

# NOTICE

Companion animal practice is an ever-changing field. Standard safety precautions must be followed, but as new research and clinical experience grow, changes in treatment and drug therapy become necessary or appropriate. The authors and editors of this work have carefully checked the generic and trade drug names and verified drug dosages to assure that dosage information is precise and in accord with standards accepted at the time of publication. Readers are advised, however, to check the product information currently provided by the manufacturer of each drug to be administered to be certain that changes have not been made in the recommended dose or in the contraindications for administration. This is of particular importance in regard to new or infrequently used drugs. Recommended dosages for animals are sometimes in regard to new or infrequently used drugs. Recommended dosages for animals are sometimes based on adjustments in the dosage that would be suitable for humans. Some of the drugs mentioned here have been given experimentally by the authors. Others have been used in dosages greater than those recommended by the manufacturer. It is the responsibility of those administering a drug, relying on their professional skill and experience, to determine the dosages, the best treatment for the patient, and whether the benefits of giving a drug justify the attendant risk. The editors cannot be responsible for misuse or misapplication of the material in this work.

# 1

# Why Worry About Cancer in Pet Animals?

## Stephen J. Withrow

Why should veterinarians be concerned about cancer in pet animals? Whether we like it or not, the prevalence of cancer in pet animals is increasing.[1] Prevalence simply implies an increased number of diagnosed cancer cases per year without documenting number versus population at risk (incidence). This prevalence is increasing for a variety of reasons but is at least in part related to animals living to older and older ages. Since cancer is generally a disease of the older animal, the price these animals pay for living longer is an increased likelihood of developing cancer. The greater life span is a result of better nutrition, vaccinations (preventing many previously fatal contagious diseases), better preventative and therapeutic medical practices, leash laws, and possibly a deeper devotion (human-animal bond) to pet animals within the last 10 to 20 years. With this increasing prevalence, veterinarians will be called upon more frequently to diagnose and manage the pet with cancer.

Cancer is a major cause of pet animal death.[2,3] This is a difficult statement to document but is supported by a study that determined the cause of death in a series of over 2,000 autopsy cases. In that study, 45% of dogs that lived to 10 years or older died of cancer.[3] With no age adjustment, 23% of patients presented for autopsy died of cancer. Regardless of the exact numbers, cancer is one of the leading killers of pet animals.

Breakthroughs in treatment of human cancer have received a great deal of exposure through the news media. Although this progress is slow, it does expose pet owners to what can be done and promotes an atmosphere of optimism. With this increased and optimistic media coverage, pet owners are becoming more knowledgeable and more demanding in seeking care for the animal with cancer. The veterinary profession needs to be prepared for these demands rather than saying nothing can be done.

More open acknowledgment of the human-animal bond has elevated the importance of pet animals to the level of human beings in many owners' eyes. Some owners consider their pet more important than any human contact.[4] Proper care of these animals will be of increasing importance to many owners.

Cancer is a common and serious disease for human beings. Many owners have had or will have a personal experience with cancer in themselves, a family member, or a close friend. Keeping this in mind, the veterinarian should approach the pet with cancer in a positive, compassionate, and knowledgeable manner. Frequently the veterinary profession has taken a negative approach ("test and slaughter") to cancer. This attitude will not only be a detriment to the pet but may also negatively bias the owner, creating unfounded fears about the disease in humans. We owe it to our pet animal patients and their owners to be well informed and up-to-date on current treatment methods for the cancer patient to prevent imparting feelings of hopelessness unnecessarily.

Pet animals with spontaneously developing cancer provide an excellent opportunity to study many aspects of cancer from etiology to treatment. Provided these studies are done in a humane fashion, they may unlock clues to improving the outlook for this disease in animals and human beings.[5–7] Some of the aspects of animal cancer that make pets attractive comparative models are:

1. Pet dogs and cats are outbred animals (like humans), as opposed to some strains of rats, mice, and other experimental animals.
2. The cancers seen in practice are spontaneously developing, as opposed to experimental carcinogen induced. Spontaneous cancers may behave in a significantly different fashion than induced or transplanted cancers.
3. Pets share the same environment as their owners and may serve as sentinels for the changing patterns of cancer development in humans.
4. Pets have a higher incidence of some cancers (e.g., osteosarcoma and non-Hodgkin's lymphoma) than humans, allowing more cases to be studied.
5. Most animal cancers will progress at a more rapid rate than their counterparts in humans. This allows more rapid determination of end points such as the length of time to metastasis, local recurrence, and survival.
6. Because fewer established "gold standard" treatments exist in veterinary medicine compared to human medicine, it is easier and morally acceptable to attempt new forms of therapy on an untreated cancer rather than wait until all "known" treatments have failed, as is common in the treatment of humans. Unfortunately, this latitude in clinical trials can be abused to allow diverse and unethical treatments to be attempted as well. We have an obligation not to deny our patients known effective treatment while at the same time planning well-designed clinical trials of prospective treatment methods.

   Investigations of new treatment methods are becoming more and more difficult to perform on normal laboratory animals because of the animal rights movement. This development makes spontaneously occurring pet animal cancer a more attractive and morally acceptable research tool but should not imply that poorly conceived and executed research is permissible on any animal.
7. Pet animal cancers are more akin to human cancers than are rodent tumors in terms of size and cell kinetics. Dogs and cats also share similar characteristics of physiology and metabolism for most organ systems and drugs. This similarity allows better comparison of treatment modalities such as surgery, radiation, and chemotherapy between animals and humans to be made.

Owners who seek treatment for their pet animals with cancer are a devoted and compassionate subset of the population. Working with these owners can be a very satisfying aspect of a sometimes frustrating specialty. These owners are almost always satisfied with an honest and aggressive attempt to cure or palliate the disease of their pet, making the experience rewarding for the veterinarian, owner, and, most important, the pet.

Oncology also offers the inquisitive veterinarian a complex and challenging area for both clinical and bench research. Without being condescending to other specialties in our profession, the challenges and accomplishments in oncology are very impressive. For the veterinarian who has become bored with the day-to-day routine of the profession, oncology offers unlimited opportunity for the pursuit of knowledge for the benefit of animals and humankind. *"Cancer, unlike politics and religion, is not a topic of controversy. No one is for it. Cancer is not another word for death. Neither is it a single disease for which there is one cure. Instead, it takes many forms, and each form responds differently to treatment."*[8]

Clinical and comparative oncology is a rapidly growing field of study. More training programs are being developed each year that will allow a wider distribution of experienced veterinarians into practice, research, and the university setting. Through study and treatment of pet animal cancer, it is to be hoped that the veterinarian can have an impact on both cancer as it manifests itself in pets and the same disease in humans.

## REFERENCES

1. Dorn CR: Epidemiology of canine and feline tumors. Compend Contin Educ Pract Vet 12:307–312, 1976.
2. Animal Health Survey. *In* Companion Animal News. Englewood, CO, Morris Animal Foundation, August 1986.
3. Bronson RT: Variation in age at death of dogs of different sexes and breeds. Am J Vet Res 43:2057–2059, 1982.
4. Lagoni L, Butler C, Hetts S: The Human–Animal

Bond and Grief. Philadelphia, PA, WB Saunders, 1994.

5. Richardson RC: Spontaneous canine and feline neoplasms as models for cancer in man. Kal Kan Forum 2:89–94, 1983.

6. Gillette EL: Spontaneous canine neoplasms as models for therapeutic agents. *In* Figler IJ, White RJ (eds): Design of Models for Testing Cancer Therapeutic Agents. New York, Van Nostrand Reinhold, 1982, pp. 185–192.

7. MacEwen EG: Spontaneous tumors in dogs and cats: Models for the study of cancer biology and treatment. Cancer Metastasis Rev 9:125–136, 1990.

8. Mooney S: A Snowflake in my Hand. New York, Bantam Doubleday Dell, 1989.

# 2

# The Pathology of Neoplasia

Barbara E. Powers

Veterinary pathologists play a critical role in the treatment of neoplasia of pet animals by providing accurate diagnostic information to clinical oncologists so that a prognosis can be determined and adequate treatment provided. The clinical oncologist needs to have knowledge of the pathology of neoplasia to understand neoplastic conditions and understand the limitations of histopathologic assessment in the diagnosis of neoplasia. Both the pathologist and the clinical oncologist must work together to determine optimal treatment for the patient because the diagnosis and treatment of neoplasia in veterinary medicine have become more complex. No longer is it adequate simply to determine if the tumor is benign or malignant. The tumor type needs to be identified as accurately as possible, and tumor subtypes should be identified if prognostically significant. Grading of tumors is becoming of increasing importance because the behavior of some tumors has been shown to be dependent on grade. In addition, the assessment of margins for completeness of surgical removal is very important. In some cases, the histologic assessment of preoperative treatment is of importance in predicting treatment outcome. Special procedures such as immunohistochemistry, electron microscopy, or flow cytometry may be advantageous in some cases to correctly identify tumor type or subtype or to predict clinical behavior of certain tumors. Classification of neoplasia in veterinary medicine is not as advanced as in human medicine, but rapid strides in this direction are continuously occurring. As more is learned about the diagnosis and treatment of neoplasia in veterinary medicine, new classifications and grading schemes will continue to develop.

## SAMPLE HANDLING

The biopsy sample should be visually inspected by the oncologist to determine that the appropriate tissue was obtained. If the biopsy was a needle core or incisional specimen, the sample should be of sufficient size and consistency so that it does not fall apart in formalin or become lost in processing. Samples less than $1 \times 1$ mm are usually inadequate, although a needle core sample 1 mm wide but at least 5 mm long can be sufficient. If the biopsy samples are needle core samples, more than one core of tissue should be obtained, if possible. Samples containing excessive blood, mucous, or necrotic material may not be diagnostic and may need to be repeated. If the specimen was an excisional sample, the entire sample should be submitted if feasible, and margins of concern should be identified with suture or painted with ink. For very large samples, such as large splenic tumors, representative sections can be submitted. Usually it is best to submit at least three sections in case some portions of the tumor have excessive distortion, necrosis, or inflammation. When taking representative samples, the tumor and normal tissue interface should be included so that tumor invasiveness into normal tissue can be assessed. Tissue samples should be handled gently because compression during biopsy sampling or excessive use of electrocautery or cryosurgery can cause specimen artifact, which can prevent a definitive diagnosis from being made.[1]

The sample needs to be preserved in fixative. The most widely used fixative is 10% neutral buffered formalin, which is readily available and frequently supplied in individual specimen containers by most laboratories. Prior to immersion in fixative, larger samples may need to be sliced to facilitate adequate fixation; however, one side, such as the deep edge, should be left intact rather than slicing all the way through the sample so that orientation is not lost. Slices less than 1 cm thick should be avoided because this sometimes causes curling and distortion of the tissue during fixation. The volume of tissue to fixative should approximate 1 to 10. In cases where this volume ratio is not feasible, because of large tumor size, multiple representative sections can be obtained. When mailing large samples, use of smaller volumes of fixative is acceptable if the specimen has been in the recommended volume for at least 12 hours.[2]

Sample containers must always be properly labeled (on the container, not the lid) prior to submission to the laboratory. During unpacking at the laboratory, paperwork can be inadvertently separated from the sample container, and unless the container is properly labeled, samples could become mixed. Most important, adequate history, including signalment, pertinent clinical findings, radiographic findings, and pertinent treatment should be provided to the pathologist. A drawing of the sample, indicating the position of the tissue in the animal, is helpful in some situations, especially when margin determination is needed. A proper history is crucial for accurate diagnosis; without this the pathologist can be severely handicapped. The end result might be an inaccurate diagnosis, culminating in an inaccurate prognosis and improper treatment.[1,2]

After arrival at the laboratory the specimens are catalogued and assigned an identification number, visually examined, trimmed to fit into processing cassettes, processed into paraffin blocks, sectioned, and stained. Most of these procedures are done by trained technicians and automated laboratory equipment. In most laboratories, tissues are trimmed into cassettes on the day of arrival and processed overnight, and completed slides are ready for examination by the pathologist 24 hours after receipt. In the processes of trimming in or sectioning on the microtome, margins could become distorted and orientation may be lost, in which case re-examination of the gross specimen by the pathologist may be necessary. Most laboratories will hold remnant wet tissues in formalin for variable periods of time in the event further examination or sectioning is needed. Most laboratories file paraffin blocks and glass slides indefinitely, permitting review of previously submitted tissue on a given patient or retrospective studies on a series of cases.

Frozen sections can be made during operative procedures to provide the oncologist with a more rapid diagnosis. Samples are quick-frozen, sectioned on a cryostat, fixed, stained, and examined within 10 to 15 minutes. However, these tissue sections are inferior to those processed routinely into paraffin, and as a result diagnostic accuracy suffers. Furthermore, only a few veterinary institutions provide this service and few veterinary pathologists are experienced in the interpretation of frozen sections. This procedure may be helpful in establishing the identity of the tissue, adequacy of surgical margins, or adequacy of the tissue for more routine processing. Occasionally a provisional diagnosis can be made. It must be stressed, however, that this technique is less accurate than examination of tissues processed with routine methods.[2]

## TERMINOLOGY

Numerous terms associated with tumors or suspected tumors often are encountered in the description of the features of a tissue sample. *Hyperplasia* is an increase in the number of cells present and is not a neoplastic condition. *Metaplasia* is the abnormal transformation of a differentiated tissue of one kind into a differentiated tissue of another kind and is not a neoplastic condition. An example is squamous metaplasia in the lung bronchi, where normally cuboidal to columnar epithelium becomes squamous. *Dysplasia* is abnormal tissue development and can be a feature of neoplasia but is not necessarily a neoplastic condition, although tissue dysplasia can be a preneoplastic condition. *Anaplasia* is a loss of differentiation and is a feature of many, but not all, malignancies. *Neoplasia* is the abnormal growth of a tissue into a tumor that is not responsive to normal control mechanisms and may be benign or malignant (cancer).[3]

Terms associated with cellular or growth features are frequently encountered in descriptions of tumors. *Pleomorphism* is the occurrence of multiple forms, shapes, and sizes of cells and nuclei. *Anisocytosis* and *anisokaryosis* are greater than normal variations in cell and nuclear size, respectively. Round or polygonal cell shapes are usually associated with epithelial or hematologic tumors, whereas spindloid cell shapes are usually associated with mesenchymal tumors. A *scirrhous* or *desmoplastic* response is an abundant fibroblastic proliferation with collagen formation that occurs in some malignant invasive cancers.

**Table 2–1**   Nomenclature of Common Tumor Types in Veterinary Medicine

| Tissue or Cell of Origin | Benign | Malignant |
|---|---|---|
| Epithelial | | |
| Squamous | Squamous papilloma | Squamous cell carcinoma |
| Transitional | Transitional papilloma | Transitional cell carcinoma |
| Glandular | Adenoma, cystadenoma | Adenocarcinoma |
| Nonglandular | Adenoma | Carcinoma |
| Mesenchymal | | |
| Fibrous tissue | Fibroma | Fibrosarcoma |
| Fat | Lipoma, infiltrative lipoma | Liposarcoma |
| Cartilage | Chondroma | Chondrosarcoma |
| Bone | Osteoma | Osteosarcoma, multilobular osteochondrosarcoma |
| Muscle (smooth) | Leiomyoma | Leiomyosarcoma |
| (skeletal) | Rhabdomyoma | Rhabdomyosarcoma |
| Endothelial cells | Hemangioma | Hemangiosarcoma |
| Synovium | — | Synovial cell sarcoma |
| Mesothelium | — | Mesothelioma |
| Melanocytes | Benign melanoma, melanocytoma | Malignant melanoma, melanosarcoma |
| Peripheral nerve | Schwannoma, neurofibroma | Malignant schwannoma, neurofibrosarcoma |
| Meninges | Meningioma | Malignant meningioma |
| Uncertain origin[a] | — | Malignant fibrous histiocytoma, hemangiopericytoma |
| Hematopoietic and lymphoreticular | | |
| Lymphocytes | — | Lymphoma, lymphocytic leukemia |
| Plasma cells | Cutaneous plasmacytoma | Multiple myeloma |
| Granulocytes | — | Myeloid leukemia |
| Red blood cells | — | Erythroid leukemia |
| Macrophages | Histiocytoma | Malignant histiocytosis |
| Mast cells | — | Mast cell tumor[b] |
| Thymus | Thymoma, encapsulated | Invasive thymoma |
| Gonadal | | |
| Germ cells[c] | Seminoma, dysgerminoma | Seminoma, dysgerminoma |
| Supportive cells[c] | Sertoli cell tumor, granulosa cell tumor | Sertoli cell tumor, granulosa cell tumor |
| Interstitial cells | Interstitial (Leydig) cell tumor, thecoma, luteoma | — |

[a]Pathologists disagree about the origin of these tumors; some believe they are a class of peripheral nerve sheath tumors.
[b]Theoretically all mast cell tumors are potentially malignant, but grade 1 mast cell tumors are clinically benign.
[c]Unfortunately, the terminology of these tumors does not distinguish between benign and malignant forms.

*In situ* refers to a malignancy, usually limited to lesions of epithelial origin, that has not yet become invasive or invaded beyond the basement membrane.[1-3]

For each type of tumor, specific terminology is used to denote the origin of the tumor and whether the tumor is benign or malignant (Table 2–1). Tumors can develop from any normal tissue type; therefore there are a considerable number of different tumor types. As more is learned about certain tumors, names and subclassifications may change, creating some confusion. Benign tumors of epithelial origin are termed adenoma, papilloma, or epithelioma. Benign tumors of mesenchymal origin are designated by the suffix *-oma* after the tissue type, i.e., fibroma, osteoma, etc. Malignant tumors of epithelial origin are termed carcinoma, or adenocarcinoma if forming glands and ducts, while malignant tumors of mesenchymal origin are termed sarcoma. In some cases the *-oma* suffix is used when the tumor is malignant, as in malignant melanoma and lymphoma, which are more appropriately termed melanosarcoma and lymphosarcoma. Leukemia is a malignant neoplasia of white blood cells in hematopoietic tissues and usually in the blood and has no benign counterpart, although a leukemoid reaction is a nonmalignant condition that mimics leukemia.[1,2,4]

## HISTOLOGIC FEATURES OF NEOPLASIA

Despite recent advances in a number of areas of pathology, including molecular techniques, evaluation of tissue by light microscopy remains the most important means of diagnosing neoplasia.[2] Neoplasia has certain histologic features that distinguish it from hyperplasia or inflammation, and there are features that distinguish benign from malignant neoplasia. In some cases, these features can be difficult to observe. Definitive diagnosis of malignant versus benign versus inflammatory or hyperplasia may not always be possible. In these cases a rebiopsy, either immediately or after a period of clinical observation, may facilitate a definitive diagnosis.

When inflammation is present, the cellular features of reactive fibroblasts and reactive endothelial cells can be misleading.[1,4] However, in reactive tissue with inflammation, the fibroblasts and endothelial cells usually are oriented perpendicular to one another and usually a substantial amount of inflammation relative to reactive tissue is present. When granulomatous inflammation occurs, large reactive and epithelioid macrophages can be mistaken for tumor cells, but the pattern of tissue involvement and presence of other inflammatory cells helps to rule out neoplasia. In some tumors, especially those with surface ulceration or extensive necrosis, or some synovial cell sarcomas, an extensive amount of inflammation can obscure neoplasia.

Benign tumors may be most difficult to distinguish from hyperplasia (Table 2–2) because both have a proliferation of well-differentiated cells that are easy to identify. There is a loss of normal tissue orientation or architecture in benign neoplasia, and usually the tumor is growing in an expansive manner, causing compression rather than invasion of adjacent tissue. Hyperplasia tends to retain normal tissue orientation and does not compress adjacent tissue. In general, if allowed to grow, benign neoplasia will attain a larger size than a hyperplastic lesion.[4] In some instances, such as thyroid gland adenoma versus adenomatous hyperplasia of the thyroid gland in cats, or sebaceous gland adenoma versus sebaceous hyperplasia, the distinction between benign tumor or hyperplasia is not clinically important.

Features that distinguish malignant from benign neoplasia include increased anisocytosis and anisokaryosis; increased nuclear and cellular pleomorphism; increased and variable nuclear to cytoplasmic ratio; abnormal nuclear chromatin; increased mitotic figures; abnormal mitotic figures; abnormal large or multiple nucleoli, or both; increased necrosis; and invasiveness of malignant tumors (Table 2–2). With invasion, individual cells or groups of cells infiltrate extensively into surrounding tissue, may invade into vascular or lymphatic spaces, and may invoke a scirrhous or desmoplastic response characterized by an excessive fibrous reaction. A further feature of malignancy is destruction of the normal tissue or obliteration of normal tissue architecture. Evidence of lymph node or more widespread metastasis obviously distinguishes malignant from benign

**Table 2–2**   Histologic Features of Hyperplasia and of Benign and Malignant Neoplasia

| Histologic Feature | Hyperplasia | Benign Neoplasia | Malignant Neoplasia |
|---|---|---|---|
| Overall differentiation | Normal | Disorganized, but well differentiated | Disorganized, well to poorly differentiated |
| Cell and nuclear pleomorphism | None | Minimal | Moderate to marked |
| Mitotic index | Variable, usually low | Usually low | Often high |
| Nucleoli | Normal | Normal | Large and/or multiple |
| Amount of necrosis | None | Usually minimal | Minimal to abundant |
| Tissue demarcation | Blends with normal tissue | Expansive and/or compressive | Invasive |

tumors.[1,2,4] However, in certain tumors histologic features do not correlate with behavior, for example, canine histiocytoma and benign plasmacytoma. Both have most of the histologic features of malignancy but are clinically benign. Histologically low-grade, yet biologically high-grade fibrosarcomas of the canine head have histologic features of a benign condition but are clinically malignant.[5] In these instances, knowledge of clinical behavior is needed to distinguish benign from malignant neoplasia.

Generally a pathologist makes the diagnosis of tumor versus reactive tissue and sometimes tumor type at relatively low magnification to assess the overall tissue pattern and behavior with respect to adjacent normal tissue. Higher magnification is then used to confirm the low-magnification impression, to classify tumor type if not already done, and to assess nuclear features and mitotic index. Immediate use of high magnification is a mistake because very reactive tissue and inflammation, especially when macrophages are present, may be mistaken for neoplasia. For this reason, a definitive diagnosis may be difficult to establish with small samples or with samples that lack some normal tissue. There are numerous instances, such as in osteosarcoma, mast cell tumor, prostatic carcinoma, some soft tissue sarcomas, and squamous cell carcinoma, in which histologic features are sufficiently distinct to make a definitive diagnosis on a small sample if the tumor was sampled correctly and the diagnosis fits the clinical situation. In other cases, such as in lymphosarcoma or granulomatous inflammation, small samples may be inadequate to establish a final diagnosis because the overall cellular pattern and interaction with normal tissue is an important diagnostic feature.

## GRADING AND STAGING OF NEOPLASIA

In certain tumors, grading the degree of malignancy is predictive of biologic behavior[1,2,4] and, in the future, quite likely the behavior of more tumors will be shown to be related to histologic grade. Grading of tumors is somewhat subjective and reproducibility between pathologists can be low. Another difficulty is that tumors are heterogeneous and patterns as well as features of increased malignancy may vary from area to area. If there are variabilities present, the most malignant areas are usually assessed for grading purposes. However, if the sample is small, the more malignant areas may not be included in the sample. When this occurs, accurate grading is not possible; therefore grading should not be attempted on small samples.

Features of tumors that are often evaluated to assess grade include (1) degree of differentiation, (2) mitotic index (number of mitotic figures per 1 or 10 high-magnification—400×—fields), (3) degree of cellular or nuclear pleomorphism, (4) amount of necrosis, (5) invasiveness, (6) stromal reaction, and (7) lymphoid response. Of these features, only mitotic index and perhaps the amount of necrosis are objective.[1,2,4] Often, in determining a grade, these individual features are scored, and then each score is added to obtain a total tumor score and a grade is assigned to a small range of total tumor scores.

Tumor grade may correlate with survival; metastatic rate; disease-free interval; or with frequency or speed of local recurrence, or both. Tumors in which grade or histologic features are predictive of biologic behavior in dogs include mast cell tumor,[6,7] lymphoma,[8,9] dermal and ocular melanoma,[10,11] mammary gland carcinoma,[12] synovial cell sarcoma,[13] multilobular osteochondrosarcoma,[14] nonlymphoid nonhematogenous splenic sarcomas,[15] transitional cell carcinoma of the urinary bladder,[16] squamous cell carcinoma of the tongue,[17] and soft tissue sarcoma[18,19] (Table 2–3). In humans with soft tissue sarcoma, the histologic grade is more important than the tumor type,[1,20] and this also may be true in dogs. Tumors in which grade or histologic features are predictive of biologic behavior in cats include mast cell tumors[21] and mammary gland carcinomas[22] (Table 2–3).

Grading systems have not been well established for some malignant tumors, yet the pathologist can make an assessment of presumed biologic behavior based on the overall degree of tumor differentiation. In these cases the terms *well differentiated, moderately differentiated,* or *poorly differentiated* may be suggestive of a low-grade, medium-grade, and high-grade malignancy, respectively.[1] This type of assessment is most commonly done for squamous cell carcinomas, some sarcomas, and carcinomas of the lung, thyroid gland, mammary gland, lymphoma, mast cell tumor, salivary gland, gastrointestinal tract, liver, exocrine pancreas, urinary bladder, and perianal gland. Tumor grading probably will become even more widespread and important in the future. Not only can a prognosis be determined based on tumor grade, and differentiation, but treatment may be modified to apply more aggressive therapies to tumors of higher grade.

**Table 2–3** Neoplasia with Grades or Histologic Features Having Prognostic Significance

| Tumor Type | Grades Given | Features of Importance | Reference |
|---|---|---|---|
| Mast cell tumor (dog) | 1, 2, 3 | Cellularity, nuclear to cytoplasmic ratio, cell morphology, mitotic index, extent, stromal reaction | 6, 7 |
| Mast cell tumor (cat) | Well differentiated, poorly differentiated, histiocytic | Cellular and nuclear pleomorphism, mitotic index | 21 |
| Lymphoma | Low, intermediate, high | Architecture, mitotic index, nuclear size and morphology | 8, 9 |
| Dermal melanoma | Well differentiated, poorly differentiated | Mitotic index | 10 |
| Ocular melanoma | Benign, potentially malignant | Mitotic index | 11 |
| Soft tissue sarcoma | 1, 2, 3 or mitotic index > 9[a], mitotic index < 9 | Overall differentiation, mitotic index, necrosis | 18, 19 |
| Mammary gland carcinoma (dog) | Well, moderate, poorly differentiated | Invasiveness, nuclear differentiation, lymphoid response | 12 |
| Mammary gland carcinoma (cat) | Well, moderate, poorly differentiated | Differentiation, cellular pleomorphism, mitotic index | 22 |
| Synovial cell sarcoma | 1, 2, 3 | Nuclear pleomorphism, mitotic index, necrosis | 13 |
| Multilobular osteochondrosarcoma | 1, 2, 3 | Borders, lobule size, organization, mitotic index, nuclear pleomorphism, necrosis | 14 |
| Nonlymphoid, nonangiomatous spleen sarcomas | Mitotic index > 9[a], mitotic index < 9 | Mitotic index | 15 |
| Transitional cell carcinoma | 1, 2, 3 | Overall differentiation, stromal reaction | 16 |
| Squamous cell carcinoma, tongue | 1, 2, 3 | Overall differentiation, mitotic index, nuclear pleomorphism, invasion, stromal reaction | 17 |

[a]Sum of mitoses in ten 400× fields.

The pathologist also may assist in the staging of cancer by assessing tumor size, depth of tumor invasion, and the presence of tumor in regional lymph nodes, and by identifying tumors in distant sites. This information is needed to stage tumors into the T (tumor size and/or invasion), N (nodal involvement), and M (distant metastasis) system. For some tumors, such as bladder cancer in humans, tumor staging is based largely on the depth of tumor invasion into the bladder wall.[1,2,4] This may prove to be useful in cases of bladder cancer in pets and has been shown to correlate with tumor grade in dogs.[16] In both processes of tumor grading or tumor staging, these procedures are useful only if they have been shown to correlate with clinical behavior.

## ASSESSMENT OF TUMOR MARGINS

The tumor margin assessment is an essential part of the pathology report whenever curative-intent surgical excision of neoplasia is to be attempted.[2,4] Completeness of removal needs to be assessed regardless of whether the tumor is benign or malignant. Benign tumors are usually well demarcated and often surrounded by a connective tissue capsule. The margin of normal tissue around a benign, well-demarcated tumor may be less than 1 cm thick for removal to be considered complete. Even benign tumors can recur if tumor margins reveal incomplete removal. Malignant tumors are usually invasive and not well demarcated. Fingers and clumps of cells may extend from the main tumor mass and invade surrounding tissue. Margins need to be larger for removal to be considered complete. If tumor cells extend to the surgical edge, removal is incomplete or intracapsular and the margins are considered "dirty." In human medicine margins are considered close and probably incomplete if less than 1 cm of normal tissue is present around a malignant tumor.[23,24] Often this is not feasible in veterinary medicine because obtaining a 1 cm margin of normal tissue around a mass in some locations, such as on the distal extremities, is very difficult. If tumor cells do not extend to the margin, yet are within 1 cm of the margin or just outside of or on the tumor pseudocapsule, tumor margins can be called "clean, but close" or "marginal." These cases must be monitored closely for recurrence, or immediate, more aggressive removal or adjuvant therapy can be considered. Margins are considered "wide" if there is 1 to 3 cm of normal tissue around the tumor or if the tumor and its capsule are not entered. Margins are radical if there is greater than 3 cm around the tumor or if the entire compartment or structure is removed, as in amputation[23,24]

When the surgeon excises a tumor, the margins may not be marked, marked with a suture, or marked with India ink or commercially available dyes. If the tumor is not marked, the sample is usually taken in one complete plane, including tumor and surrounding normal tissue. Two samples are then taken perpendicular to the original section, one on either side. Any margins that appear to be close to the tumor also may be sampled. This method allows assessment of four lateral margins; the deep margins; and the superficial margin, if relevant.[25] Margins of special concern also may be marked by the surgeon with either suture or ink.[2,26] A disadvantage of the suture method is that sutures need to be removed prior to sectioning on the microtome to prevent sectioning artifacts. The retention of ink through processing of the tissue permits the pathologist to visualize the margin through the microscope. An inked margin also prevents the pathologist from mistaking false margins resulting from tissue trimming or caused by retraction of fatty or loose connective tissue from the tumor mass, with true surgical margins. Furthermore, the inked margin allows distinction from artifactually created margins that may occur during sectioning on the microtome if the tissue section tears or fragments. Inks come in a variety of colors, permitting more than one margin to be inked for proper orientation into cranial, caudal, superficial, deep, medial, or lateral planes.[26]

Margins around mast cell tumors are of special concern in veterinary medicine. These tumors frequently have clumps of cells separated from the main mass by normal tissue. These clumps of cells cannot be seen without the aid of a microscope, and resection of the main mass, even with the microscopic appearance of a clean, but close margin, may in reality leave a clump of tumor cells behind. For mast cell tumors, a 3 cm margin of grossly normal-appearing tissue is usually recommended.[27] This usually results in clean margins, although there may be some clumps of cells within the grossly normal-appearing 3 cm margin of normal tissue. Mast cell tumors pose another problem for the pathologist in that it is difficult to impossible to distinguish a resident, non-neoplastic mast cell from a well-differentiated neoplastic cell.

In veterinary medicine soft tissue sarcomas are another common tumor requiring special attention. To the inexperienced surgeon these tumors often appear well demarcated and easily "shell out." However, fine strands and fingers of neoplastic cells often extend to the margins of grossly normal-appearing tissue. At least 3 cm of grossly normal-appearing tissue should be included in the resection, if possible.[28] Microscopic examination has shown that when adequate margins are obtained, an artifactually created space can be seen around the outer portion of the tumor, giving the impression of a well-demarcated tumor. Neoplastic cells frequently are present in the normal tissue around this space.

If the margins are not complete, the surgical oncologist may wish to resect the suture line and wound bed to prevent tumor recurrence. In these resected samples, small foci of tumor may be obscured within the granulation tissue and inflammation resulting from the first surgery. However, the deep and lateral margins adjacent to the suture line usually can be assessed for the presence of residual tumor and the effectiveness of surgical resection. The inability to identify tumor cells in resected suture areas should not be interpreted to indicate that the second surgery was unnecessary but rather how difficult it is to distinguish reactive tissue from the small foci of neoplastic tissue.

If surgical resection is determined to be complete by microscopic evaluation, this lessens the chance of local recurrence but by no means guarantees local tumor control. Recurrence of soft tissue sarcomas in humans has been shown to occur in about 10% of cases in which margins were deemed to be complete by the pathologist;[29] a similar situation likely occurs in veterinary medicine. Serial sections through every margin of a tumor is not feasible; consequently tumor extension to the cut edge may be missed. However, if the surgical margin is incomplete, local recurrence is almost guaranteed unless further treatment is initiated.

## ASSESSMENT OF TREATMENT RESPONSE

Sometimes histologic assessment of preoperative treatment response may help predict outcome and can even affect subsequent therapy. Assessment of preoperative therapy is most common with osteosarcoma and soft tissue sarcoma. Percent tumor necrosis is the most commonly used parameter to quantify the impact of presurgical chemotherapy or radiation therapy. In dogs with osteosarcoma, percent tumor necrosis is a good predictor for local recurrence following limb-sparing surgery subsequent to preoperative radiation therapy or chemotherapy or both. A 90% or greater percent tumor necrosis had a local control rate of 91%, an 80% to 90% tumor necrosis had a control rate of 78%, while a less than 80% tumor necrosis had a control rate of only 28%.[30,31] In humans, the percent tumor necrosis in osteosarcoma following preoperative chemotherapy is also predictive for survival and poor responders may be treated with alternative chemotherapeutic regimes.[32] In soft tissue sarcomas, percent tumor necrosis has been used to assess presurgical therapy in humans[33] and could be done in pet animals.

The effect of previous treatment also may be evaluated histologically when there is progressive growth of tissue in an area treated previously with radiation, surgery, chemotherapy, or photodynamic therapy. In these cases, distinguishing between reactive tissue and neoplasia is important but also may be extremely difficult. Inflammation, fibrovascular proliferation (granulation tissue), or epithelial hyperplasia (if applicable) is usually present in the area. Furthermore, especially after radiation therapy, the area may have some bizarre reactive cells, including fibroblasts (called radiation fibroblasts), with many features of malignancy although these cells are not neoplastic.[34] If tumor cells are identified, the oncologist may wish to know if these cells are viable or dead, or viable but sterilized by radiation or chemotherapy. Distinction between a viable and dead cell is often possible, but determining if a cell is viable but sterilized, or nonclonogenic, is not possible microscopically. However, the presence of numerous mitotic figures in a viable-appearing tumor is suggestive of an active regrowth.

## SPECIAL PROCEDURES

Approximately 90% of oncologic cases in humans can be diagnosed by light microscopy using hematoxylin and eosin stains.[2] This percentage is probably a close estimation of the situation in veterinary medicine as well. In the remaining 10% of cases, special stains or special procedures such as immunohistochemistry or electron microscopy may help. Flow cytometry may also be of use in predicting tumor behavior and may help in distinguishing benign from malignant tumors.

### Special Stains

Special stains are commonly used to assist in the diagnosis of certain poorly differentiated tumors.[4] The special stains most frequently used are toluidine blue or giemsa to identify granules in poorly differentiated mast cell tumors. Giemsa also may stain plasma cells, but these can be differentiated from mast cells by the lack of granularity to the cytoplasm. Some feline and ferret mast cell tumors stain better with periodic acid Schiffs than toluidine blue.

Masson's trichrome or other trichrome stains may be used to identify collagen fibrils as an aid in the differentiation of certain mesenchymal tumors such as those derived from muscle (leiomyomas, leiomyosarcomas, rhabdomyoma, rhabdomyosarcomas) versus those that produce matrix (fibroma, fibrosarcoma). It should be realized, however, that muscle-derived tumors may have a small amount of collagen and fibrosarcomas can be so undifferentiated that little collagen is produced. Alcian blue stain may help identify ground substance glycosaminoglycans that may be seen in some neurofibrosarcomas or myxosarcomas. Another useful stain is mucicarmine or periodic acid Schiffs for mucous to identify poorly differentiated carcinomas. A melanin bleach or iron stain may help distinguish between hemosiderin and melanin in suspected cases of melanoma. Other less frequently used special stains such as reticulum fiber stain may also be available.

## Immunohistochemistry

Immunohistochemistry has been used as an aid in the classification of numerous tumors in veterinary medicine but is not used as routinely as in human medicine. Immunohistochemistry is a staining procedure using antibodies to identify specific intermediate filaments, secretory substances, or proteins. Immunohistochemistry can be done on specimens fixed in formalin and processed into paraffin blocks or on frozen tissue. Primary antibodies to specific cell components (the antigens) are exposed to secondary antibodies directed against the primary antibody. The secondary antibody is linked to peroxidase or avidin biotin peroxidase complexes. The peroxidase catalyzes a reaction in the presence of dye, which precipitates on the complex.[2] Commonly used immunohistochemical stains are those for intermediate filaments, such as vimentin for mesenchymal cells, cytokeratin for epithelial cells, and desmin for muscle cells.[2,35,36] Immunohistochemistry also can be used to identify certain hormonal secretory products such as insulin, glucagon, thyroglobulin, and calcitonin to identify endocrine tumors accurately.[2,37,38] Other proteins and secretory products that may be stained include s-100 protein and HMB-45 for melanomas, chromogranin for neurosecretory granules in neuroendocrine tumors, neuron-specific enolase for nervous tissue or neuroendocrine tumors, and glial fibrillary acidic protein for astrocytic tumors. Immunohistochemical stains for macrophages or histiocytes include alpha-1-antitrypsin or lysozyme. Leukocyte common antigen is used to identify tumors of white blood cell origin, including lymphoma in humans; unfortunately this stain does not appear to work well in dogs and cats.[2,36] The availability of specific stains for canine and feline white blood cell antigens are currently limited.

Immunohistochemistry can be a valuable tool for identifying certain tumors, but there are some complicating factors. A negative stain does not exclude a certain cell type, because technical difficulties or poor tumor cell differentiation may result in a negative stain. The most common technical problem causing negative staining is overlong fixation resulting in excessive cross-linking of the antigenic components. However, if this is a suspected problem, antigens can be unmasked by pretreatment of sections with trypsin or pepsin. Areas of tissue necrosis, autolysis, section drying, hemorrhage, and sometimes collagenous matrix components can cause excessive background nonspecific staining. Immunohistochemistry does not distinguish between neoplastic and non-neoplastic tissue, as reactive tissue and tumor cells will have the same normal components of the specific cell of origin. For example, immunohistochemistry will not distinguish between epithelial hyperplasia and carcinoma because both may be positive for cytokeratin. Finally, there may be considerable cross-reactivity of staining in different tumor types because some markers, such as s-100, may be found in a variety of cells or tumors, including melanomas, cartilage, and certain epithelial cells.[2,39] Immunohistochemistry can be tedious, difficult to perform on a routine basis, and expensive; consequently, although the procedure is available, it is not used in all diagnostic veterinary laboratories.

## Electron Microscopy

Electron microscopy involves preserving very small representative tumor samples (1 × 1 mm) in special fixatives such as glutaraldehyde, processing tissue into epoxy-based plastic blocks, and sectioning at 1 μm for thick sections to determine the adequacy of the sample and inclusion of appropriate tumor cells. Subsequently sectioning is done at about 600 Å, stained with heavy metal-based stains, and examined with the aid of the electron microscope. Samples fixed in formalin can be used, although the quality of the subsequent sections is less than ideal. Electron microscopy may help identify certain specific features, such as intercellular junctions or basal lamina in epithelial cells, melanosomes in melanocytic cells, mast cell granules in mast cells, neurosecretory granules in neuroendocrine cells, or mucin droplets in certain glandular cells. These features are useful in distinguishing carcinomas from lymphomas and identifying melanomas, mast cell tumors, and neuroendocrine tumors. Unless a specific feature is sought, however, electron microscopy will be no more useful than a higher magnification of a tumor that could not be diagnosed with the light microscope. Furthermore, electron microscopy is not useful for distinguishing benign from malignant cells in many cases because the magnification is too high and the tumor pattern in the tissue is not evident.[2,4] Many veterinary diagnostic laboratories do not have the technical support and equipment needed for electron microscopy.

## Flow Cytometry

Flow cytometry is an analytic procedure that can be used to evaluate cell suspensions obtained from suspected neoplastic masses. In human medicine this procedure is frequently used to diagnose and occasionally to monitor for recurrence of various tumors such as bladder carcinoma. Use of flow cytometry for humans is especially useful for detecting neoplastic cells in the urine of bladder cancer patients and in evaluation of leukemia and lymphoma. In solid tumors the cells must first be disassociated to create a single cell suspension. Cell suspensions are stained with specific fluorochromes, passed through the flow cytometer chamber, and analyzed and sorted by use of a focused laser beam. The most routine analysis is to determine DNA content or ploidy of the cells. Malignant cells may be diploid (normal DNA content) or aneuploid (nondiploid), but normal tissue, benign tumors, and reactive tissues are usually diploid. Occasionally, however, benign tumors and reactive tissue can be aneuploid. In some instances, aneuploidy may be prognostically significant and can be predictive of survival time. Flow cytometry also can be used to evaluate S-phase distribution or cell cycle time if the tumor is sampled at appropriate times after injecting the patient with bromo-oxyuridine, which labels the cycling cells. Cell cycle time also may be of prognostic significance in some cancers.[2,4]

Flow cytometry has been used to evaluate tumors in dogs, although it has yet to become a routine procedure. In the earliest report, various canine tumors were characterized for DNA ploidy.[40] In subsequent studies, tumor cell heterogeneity, comparisons of primary and metastatic tumors, and the positive predictive value of kinetic parameters in canine osteosarcomas were assessed.[41,42] Other studies have indicated the value of flow cytometry in predicting the behavior of various canine tumors, including mammary gland tumors,[43] melanomas,[44] and plasmacytomas.[45] As samples to be evaluated by flow cytometry are cell suspensions derived from tumor masses, a correlate sample from the same site or same specimen should always be taken for histopathologic assessment. Histologic correlation is necessary because flow cytometry cannot distinguish a benign from a diploid malignant tumor, nor can it identify tumor type.[2] Currently the use of flow cytometry in the analysis of cancer in veterinary medicine is mostly investigational, but it may become more routine in certain laboratories and institutions as more is learned about its potential as a predictive assay in pet animals.

## CLINICAL-PATHOLOGIC CORRELATION AND SECOND OPINIONS

Sometimes the pathologist cannot make an accurate diagnosis without clinical correlations.[1,2,4] This is especially true for some primary bone tumors or secondary tumors involving bone. Diagnosis of a surface or juxtacortical osteosarcoma is based on both radiographic and histologic features. An osteoma may be difficult to distinguish from reactive bone without a corroborative radiograph. A synovial cell sarcoma may be difficult to distinguish from other sarcomas or even inflammatory or immune mediated joint disease unless there is radiographic or gross evidence of joint involvement and bone invasion. An acanthomatous epulis may be difficult to distinguish from a fibrous epulis unless there is bone invasion in the former. The best example of the need for clinical and pathologic correlation is with histologically low-grade yet biologically high-grade fibrosarcomas of the canine head in which the histologic appearance is of benign fibrous tissue but the clinical presentation is an aggressive invasive mass, often recurrent after conservative surgery, causing bone destruction. These examples demonstrate the necessity for an accurate history with pertinent clinical results being provided to the pathologist along with the biopsy sample. In some cases photographs of the tumor site or inclusion of radiographs is most helpful.

Before any major treatment is undertaken or *if a pathology diagnosis is not consistent with clinical presentation*, a second opinion should be requested from the pathologist. The two major categories of mistakes that may occur at the pathology laboratory are technical mistakes and mistakes in interpretation of the tissue.[1] Technical mistakes may occur if the histotechnologist improperly labels specimens, tissue blocks, or slides, or fails to process all the critical tissue submitted by the clinician. If tissue is improperly processed because of equipment malfunction or poorly sectioned because of inadequate skill of the histotechnologist, artifacts can occur that make the tissue specimen impossible to interpret. Mistakes in interpretation by the pathologist may occur in difficult cases. If a pathology service staffed by physicians is used, certain tumors such as histiocytoma, mast cell tumor, or perianal gland adenoma may be misdiagnosed because these do not have a human counterpart. Many pathologists will obtain opinions from other pathologists when confronted with difficult cases, just as clinicians will seek second opinions on difficult radiographs or clinical problems. *The clinician should never hesitate to ask for a second opinion, nor should the pathologist be offended by the request.* Pathologists are human, and every pathologist has made at least one major misdiagnosis in his or her career and potentially can make more. A second or even third pathologist can offer a different perspective on a difficult case, offer an alternative diagnosis, confirm the primary pathologist's diagnosis, or confirm that an accurate diagnosis is not possible. As the patient's treatment or decisions regarding euthanasia are often based on the final pathology diagnosis, it is not at all unreasonable for the clinician to request a second opinion. A misdiagnosis can result in unnecessary major surgery, unnecessary chemotherapy, unnecessary radiation therapy, insufficient treatment resulting in cancer progression, and, worst of all, unwarranted euthanasia. Considering these possible scenarios, not to mention the clinician's time, the owner's expense, and the pet's health, a second opinion not only would be prudent but highly recommended.

The clinical oncologist needs to have knowledge of the pathology of neoplasia to understand neoplastic conditions and understand the limitations of histopathologic assessment in the diagnosis of neoplasia. In the case of tumor diagnosis, histopathologic assessment of a thin slice of tissue may not always be an exact science. The pathologist and the clinical oncologist must work together to establish the most appropriate diagnosis so that proper treatment can be initiated.

## REFERENCES

1. Bonfiglio TA, Terry R: The pathology of cancer. *In* Rubin P (ed): Clinical Oncology, 6th ed. Rochester, NY, American Cancer Society, 1983, p. 20.
2. Pfeifer JD, Wick MR: The pathologic evaluation of neoplastic diseases. *In* Holleb AL, Fink DJ, Murphy GP (eds): Clinical Oncology. Atlanta, GA, American Cancer Society, 1991, p. 7.
3. Stedman's Medical Dictionary, 23rd ed. Baltimore, MD, Williams & Wilkins, 1976.
4. Misdorp W: General considerations. *In* Moulton JE (ed): Tumors in Domestic Animals, 3rd ed. Berkeley, University of California Press, 1990, p .1.
5. Ciekot, PA, Powers, BE, Withrow, SJ, et al: Histologically low-grade, yet biologically high-grade, fibrosarcomas of the mandible and maxilla in dogs: 25 cases (1982–1991). J Am Vet Med Assoc *204*(4):610, 1994.
6. Patniak AK, Ehler WJ, MacEwen EG: Canine cutaneous mast cell tumor: Morphologic grading and survival time in 83 dogs. Vet Pathol *21*(5):469, 1984,
7. Bostock, DE: The prognosis following surgical removal of mastocytomas in dogs. J Small Anim Pract *14*:27, 1973.
8. Carter RF, Harris CK, Withrow SJ, et al: Chemotherapy of canine lymphoma with histopathological correlation: Doxorubicin alone compared to COP as first treatment regimen. J Am Anim Hosp Assoc *23*(6):587, 1987.
9. Carter RF, Valli VEO, Lumsden JH: The cytology, histology and prevalence of cell types in canine lymphoma classified according to the National Cancer Institute working formulation. Can J Vet Res *50*:154, 1986.
10. Bostock DE: Prognosis after surgical excision of canine melanomas. Vet Pathol *16*:32, 1979.
11. Wilcox BP, Peiffer RL: Morphology and behavior of primary ocular melanomas in 91 dogs. Vet Pathol *23*(4):418, 1986.
12. Kurzman ID, Gilbertson SR: Prognostic factors in canine mammary tumors. Sem Vet Med Surg *1*(1):25, 1986.
13. Vail DM, Powers BE, Getzy DM, et al: Evaluation of prognostic factors for dogs with synovial sarcoma: 36 cases (1986–1991). J Am Vet Med Assoc *205*(9):1300, 1994.
14. Straw RC, LeCouteur RA, Powers BE, Withrow SJ: Multilobular osteochondrosarcoma of the canine skull: 16 cases (1978–1988). J Am Vet Med Assoc *195*(12):1764, 1989.
15. Sprangler WL, Culbertson MR, Kass PH: Primary mesenchymal (nonangiomatous/nonlymphomatous) neoplasms occurring in the canine spleen: Anatomic classification, immunohistochemistry, and mitotic activity correlated with patient survival. Vet Pathol *31*(1):37, 1994.
16. Valli, VE, Norris, A, Laing, E, et al: Pathology of canine bladder and urethral cancer and correlation with tumor progression and survival. Vet Pathol 1994; submitted.
17. Carpenter LG, Withrow SJ, Powers BE, et al: Squamous cell carcinoma of the tongue in 10 dogs. J Am Anim Hosp Assoc *29*:17, 1993.
18. Gillette SM, Dewhirst MW, Gillette EL, et al: Response of canine soft tissue sarcomas to radiation or radiation plus hyperthermia: A randomized phase II study. Int J Hyperthermia *8*(3):309, 1992.
19. Bostock DE, Dye MT: Prognosis after surgical excision of canine fibrous connective tissue sarcomas. Vet Pathol *17*:581, 1980.
20. Coindre J, Binh BN, Bonichon F, et al: Histopatho-

logic grading in spindle cell soft tissue sarcomas. Cancer *61*:2305, 1988.

21. Wilcox BP, Yager JA, Zink MC: The morphology and behavior of feline cutaneous mastocytomas. Vet Pathol *23*(3):320, 1986.

22. Weijer K, Head KW, Misdorp W: Feline malignant mammary tumors I. Morphology and biology: Some comparisons with human and canine mammary carcinomas. J Natl Cancer Inst *49*:1697, 1972.

23. Bell RS, O'Sullivan B, Liu FF, et al: The surgical margin in soft-tissue sarcoma. J Bone and Joint Surg *71*-A(3):370, 1989.

24. Enneking, WF: Musculo-skeletal Tumor Surgery. New York, Churchill-Livingstone, 1983.

25. Abide JM, Nahai F, Bennett RG: The meaning of surgical margins. Plast Reconstr Surg *73*(3):492, 1984.

26. Rochat MC, Mann FA, Pace LW, Henderson RA: Identification of surgical biopsy borders by use of India ink. J Am Vet Med Assoc *201*(6):873, 1992.

27. Macy DW, MacEwen EG: Mast cell tumors. *In* Withrow SJ, MacEwen EG (eds): Clinical Veterinary Oncology. Philadelphia, JB Lippincott, 1989, p. 156

28. MacEwen EG, Withrow SJ: Soft tissue sarcomas. *In* Withrow SJ, MacEwen EG (eds): Clinical Veterinary Oncology. Philadelphia, JB Lippincott, 1989, p. 167.

29. Mandard AM, Petiot JF, Marnay J, et al: Prognostic factors in soft tissue sarcomas; A multivariate analysis of 109 cases. Cancer *63*:1437, 1989.

30. Powers BE, Withrow SJ, Thrall DE, et al: Percent tumor necrosis as a predictor of treatment response in canine osteosarcoma. Cancer *67*(1):126, 1991.

31. Withrow SJ, Thrall DE, Straw RC, et al: Intra-arterial cisplatin with or without radiation in limb-sparing for canine osteosarcoma. Cancer *71*(8):2484, 1993.

32. Rosen G, Caparros B, Huvos AG, et al: Preoperative chemotherapy for osteogenic sarcoma: Selection of postoperative adjuvant chemotherapy based on the response of the primary tumor to preoperative chemotherapy. Cancer *49*:1221, 1982.

33. Willett CG, Schiller AL, Suit HD, et al: The histologic response of soft tissue sarcoma to radiation therapy. Cancer *60*:1500, 1987.

34. Fajardo LF: Morphologic changes in irradiated tumors. *In* Fajardo LF (ed): Pathology of Radiation Injury. New York, Masson, 1982, p. 244.

35. Andreasen CB, Mahaffey EA, Duncan JR: Intermediate filament staining in the cytologic and histologic diagnosis of canine skin and soft tissue tumors. Vet Pathol *25*(5):343, 1988.

36. Sandusky GE, Carlton WW, Wightman KA: Diagnostic immunohistochemistry of canine round cell tumors. Vet Pathol *24*(6):495, 1987.

37. Hawkins KL, Summers BA, Kuhajda FP, Smith CA: Immunocytochemistry of normal pancreatic islets and spontaneous islet cell tumors in dogs. Vet Pathol *24*(2):170, 1987.

38. Leblanc B, Parodi AL, Lagadic M, et al: Immunocytochemistry of canine thyroid tumors. Vet Pathol *28*(5):370, 1991.

39. Lewis RE, Johnson WW, Cruse JM: Pitfalls and caveats in the methodology for immunoperoxidase staining in surgical pathologic diagnosis. Surv Synth Path Res *1*:134, 1983.

40. Johnson TS, Raju MR, Giltinan RK, Gillette EL: Ploidy and DNA distribution analysis of spontaneous dog tumors by flow cytometry. Cancer Res *41*:3005, 1981.

41. Fox MH, Armstrong LW, Withrow SJ, et al: Comparison of DNA aneuploidy of primary and metastatic spontaneous canine osteosarcomas. Cancer Res *50*:6176, 1990.

42. LaRue SM, Fox MH, Withrow SJ, et al: Impact of heterogeneity in the predictive value of kinetic parameters in canine osteosarcoma. Cancer Res *54*:3916, 1994.

43. Hellmen E, Bergstrom R, Holmberg L, et al: Prognostic factors in canine mammary tumors: A multivariate study of 202 consecutive cases. Vet Pathol *30*(1):20, 1993.

44. Bolon B, Calderwood Mays MB, Hall BJ: Characteristics of canine melanomas and comparison of histology and DNA ploidy to their biologic behavior. Vet Pathol *27*(2):96, 1990.

45. Frazier KS, Hines ME, Hurvitz AL, et al: Analysis of DNA aneuploidy and c-myc oncoprotein content of canine plasma cell tumors using flow cytometry. Vet Pathol *30*(6):505, 1993.

# 3

# Tumor Biology

Cheryl A. London and David M. Vail

Much of what we know about the diagnosis, prognosis, and therapy of clinically relevant tumors has resulted directly from our understanding of basic tumor biology. Future strides, especially in the area of specifically targeted therapies, are even more likely to result from an expansion of our knowledge base in this area.

Our intent is to provide a basic understanding of the terms encountered in the field of tumor biology and to build a framework for understanding the biology of neoplastic disease. This chapter is organized so as to begin discussion at the level of the genome, then progress to the cellular level, and finally reach the level of the tumor itself.

The process by which a normal functioning cell is transformed into a malignant unregulated cell has long perplexed the scientific community. Much research has focused on attempts to unravel the mechanisms of carcinogenesis with the hope that greater understanding will lead to more efficacious therapies for cancer patients. With the advent of molecular biology and DNA cloning techniques, many of the complicated events that occur during malignant transformation have been successfully elucidated.

It is now known that malignant transformation is associated with a series of genetic changes that take place within the cell. Many different chromosomal abnormalities have been identified within several different tumor types. Recently, the exact nature of some of these genetic perturbations has been uncovered. Two of the most important discoveries include the existence of oncogenes and tumor suppressor genes.

## PROTO-ONCOGENES, ONCOGENES, AND TUMOR SUPPRESSOR GENES

*Proto-oncogenes* are normal cellular sequences of DNA whose function is to regulate cellular responses to external signals that stimulate cell growth and differentiation.[1,2] These genes do not initiate malignant transformation in their normal state; rather they function to affect gene expression, DNA synthesis, cellular metabolism, cytoskeletal architecture, and cell-cell contact and communication. They accomplish this by tightly regulating cell activity through both positive and negative signaling pathways. In the normal cell, the expression of proto-oncogene products is extremely well regulated, allowing for normal growth, development, and function of the cell. Proto-oncogenes are referred to as *oncogenes* if their level of expression or their gene product is altered so that the cell gains the potential for malignant transformation. The products of proto-oncogenes fall into several categories which are listed in Table 3–1.[1–7]

Several mechanisms exist through which individual oncogenes may become activated in an aberrant fashion. Furthermore, any given oncogene may be altered in more than one way, causing a number of abnormalities in the resultant protein product. Point mutations, deletions, or both, may occur spontaneously, or as the result of chemical or radiation injury to the DNA. A single point mutation or deletion can significantly alter the biologic behavior of the normal gene. A large body of evidence indicates that amplification of oncogenes within a given tumor cell may play a

**Table 3–1** Categories of Proto-Oncogene Products

| Category | Function | Effect of Aberrant Product |
|---|---|---|
| Growth factors | Protein/peptides that act at cell surfaces by binding specific receptors. Initiate cellular signals that maintain cell viability or stimulate cell proliferation and/or differentiation. | Excessive production may impart cells with a growth advantage, predisposing to further genetic change. |
| Growth factor receptors | When stimulated, possess tyrosine kinase activity that activates intracellular signaling pathways. | Blockage of signals or, conversely, excessive signaling, can result in diminished control of normal growth. |
| Cytoplasmic tyrosine kinase family | Function in signal transduction within the cell. | Signal control of normal cell growth disrupted. |
| Guanine-binding (ras) family | Intermediate signal transduction between growth factor receptors and the nucleus. | Results in constant signal activation of the nucleus. |
| Serine-threonine kinase family | Act directly to regulate transcriptional and translational control of gene expression. Role in control of cell cycle. | Abrogate normal control of cell cycle. |
| Nuclear proteins | Regulate transcription of mRNA from DNA. Essential control of proliferation and self-renewal. | When overexpressed, can induce transformation and decrease control of proliferation. |

role in the process of transformation. The vast majority of oncogenes alter the processing of signals by subverting the normal function of membrane, cytoplasmic, or nuclear proteins constituting the signal transduction pathways. Thus, they may affect whether a cell enters a new cycle of cell division (and whether this will lead to a differentiated cell), but they do not directly control cell division. The possible consequences of such an event include the production of new proteins, loss of control of regulation of differentiation or proliferation, and constitutive production of a gene product secondary to loss of appropriate regulation.[1,2] The prevalence of oncogenes in veterinary patients is presently under study.[8–11]

Recently, a different class of cancer genes has been identified, termed *tumor suppressor genes*, also known as antioncogenes or recessive oncogenes. The products of such genes act to restrict or inhibit cell proliferation. When tumor suppressor genes are lost, cell proliferation may occur in an uncontrolled fashion, leading to the development of cancer. It has become increasingly clear that expression of a single oncogene is not sufficient to cause a tumor. Rather, at least two and more mutated (or deleted) dominant and recessive oncogenes have to cooperate to cause a

full-blown malignance.[12,13] Unlike oncogenes, which are usually activated through somatic mutations, suppressor gene mutations may be found in germ cells, allowing the defect to be passed from one generation to the next. Offspring acquiring the mutated suppressor gene are more likely to develop cancer because of preexisting defect in cell growth regulation.[14] The classic example of a tumor suppressor gene is the p53 gene, which has been found to be mutated in as many as 60% of human tumors.[15] The p53 gene product plays an important role in both cell viability and cell death.

## PRINCIPLES OF CARCINOGENESIS

### The Multistep Carcinogenesis Model

With the exception of acutely transforming retroviruses, most cancers are believed to arise through the process of *multistep carcinogenesis*. This theory is based on the fact that in the majority of cancers, at least two genetic changes have occurred prior to the induction of the malignant phenotype.[16, 17] There are three basic steps involved in multistep carcinogenesis that ultimately lead to the generation of a cancer cell from a normal cell (Fig. 3–1). (1) *Initiation:* Initiating agents induce a permanent and irreversible change in the DNA of the affected cell. DNA synthesis is required for fixation (irreversibility) of the initiated state. In and of itself, the initiating event is not sufficient to induce neoplastic trans-

formation. Initiated cells cannot be distinguished from other cells in the surrounding environment.[16–18] (2) *Promotion:* Promoting agents cause reversible tissue and cellular changes. Promoting agents are not capable of inducing neoplastic transformation unless they act on previously initiated cells. Promoting action is reversible up to

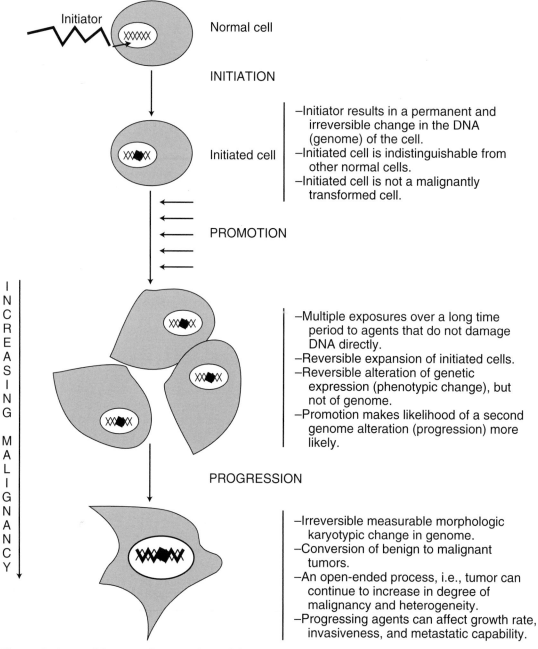

**Figure 3–1.** Multistep carcinogenesis model.

the development of the first autonomous tumor cell and generally takes place over a long latency period requiring near continuous exposure of the promoting agent (e.g., cigarette smoke). Promoting agents can induce changes in cellular morphology, mitotic rate, and degree of terminal differentiation; however, they do not alter the genome itself. They may enhance the outgrowth of initiated cells or the expression of other cellular genes previously altered by the initiating event.[1,16,17] More simply, promotion serves to expand the initiated cell population and alter its phenotype in such a way as to increase the likelihood of another irreversible genome change occurring (i.e., progression). (3) *Progression:* Progressing agents (e.g., benzene, hepatitis B virus) are able to convert an initiated cell, or a cell undergoing promotion, into a cell exhibiting the malignant phenotype, capable of developing into a mature neoplasm. These agents do so in a stepwise fashion, progressively increasing the malignant potential of a cell. Progressing agents induce alterations in the genome, affecting growth rate, invasiveness, and metastatic capability. Whereas initiation usually results from a more subtle genomic alteration, progression typically involves a genetic alteration of major proportion such as chromosomal translocation. The process of progression is irreversible.[16–18] An analogy to the multistep carcinogenesis model would be a "two-hit" theory of DNA damage. Simply, in order for a tumor to result, the genome must be irreversibly altered ("hit") at least twice. The promotion phase increases the likelihood that cells hit once (i.e., initiation) will be in a position to be hit a second time (i.e., progression).

Multistep carcinogenesis can occur through five basic pathways. More than one pathway may be involved in the generation of a particular tumor:

### 1. Heritable Carcinogenesis

There are a select number of neoplastic diseases in humans that have been demonstrated to be the result of an inherited genetic defect. Most of these tend to exhibit recessive inheritance and involve tumor suppressor genes. The most well-described heritable cancer is retinoblastoma, a tumor of the eye found in young children. The disease occurs in a hereditary form approximately 40% of the time because of a germ line mutation of the long arm of chromosome 13 (the RB1 locus).[14,19] In addition to retinoblastoma, those individuals with the RB1 germ line mutation are at a high risk for developing other primary tumors, particularly osteosarcoma. The RB1 gene has recently been identified as a tumor suppressor gene. When the initial mutation occurs in a germ line, every cell in that line is essentially initiated. As there are such a large number of target cells, it is almost inevitable that one or more cells will experience a second mutation and go on to develop into a malignancy. Loss of RB1 function has been shown to occur frequently in bladder carcinoma, acute myelogenous leukemia, and non-small-cell lung carcinoma, and also appears to be associated with overall survival.[20–22]

Although no breed-specific genetic alterations have been found in domestic animals that may lead to a predisposition to develop neoplastic disease, certain breeds of dogs have been identified as having a higher incidence of cancer than others and are referred to throughout the chapters of this book. These include the boxer, German shepard, Scottish terrier, and golden retriever.[23] It is possible that intensive breeding practices may have inadvertently selected for traits such as deficient immune surveillance or defective tumor suppressor genes.

### 2. Passive Carcinogenesis

Point mutations, chromosomal translocations, and gene amplification may occur as spontaneous events in any dividing (and some nondividing) cell populations. Cellular DNA repair mechanisms are usually quite efficient at recognizing the resultant defect and affecting appropriate repair. However, inadequate or inefficient repair may result in permanent heritable DNA changes. Within the dividing cell population, the number of affected cells may be greatly expanded.[24] It is likely that spontaneous mutations are accumulated over a lifetime and may provide some explanation as to why many cancers arise in the mature or aged individual.

### 3. Biological Carcinogenesis

The most common biologic agents capable of inducing cancer are viruses (e.g., RNA retroviruses and DNA tumor viruses), some parasites *(Spirocerca lupi, Clonorchis sinensis)*, and certain hormones.

*RNA retroviruses* have been studied extensively and the manner in which some of them induce neoplasia is relatively well understood.[25–27] Retroviruses enter the cell, convert their single-stranded RNA to DNA, and then integrate into the host chromosome, creating a provirus. Transcription of the provirus then occurs, resulting in the production of new virus particles. Two forms of transforming retroviruses exist: (1) *Acutely transforming* (transducing) retroviruses contain an oncogene that has been obtained through the process of transduction. At some point in their evolution, they integrated into a host genome at or close to the location of an oncogene. During subsequent viral replication, new virus particles incorporate the host-derived oncogene into the resultant viral RNA. In the process, the virus loses a portion of its own RNA and becomes replication deficient. Therefore, all acutely transforming retroviruses (with the exception of the Rous sarcoma virus) are replication deficient and require the presence of a replication-competent helper virus to aid in replication and assembly. The viral oncogene is expressed at inappropriately high levels in any subsequently infected cell. These viruses tend to transform cells very quickly, and every cell that expresses the viral oncogene has the potential to become transformed. The feline sarcoma virus is an example of a replication-deficient acutely transforming retrovirus, requiring the help of the feline leukemia virus to complete replication. Some other examples include simian sarcoma virus and Ableson murine leukemia virus. (2) *Slow-acting* (cis-activating) retroviruses are replication competent and tend to induce tumors after a long latency period. In these instances, proviral insertion leads to aberrant activation of adjacent cellular genes (i.e., oncogenes). It is also possible for these viruses to integrate within the normal oncogene, resulting in an altered protein product.[25] Some examples include the feline leukemia virus, mouse mammary tumor virus, and avian leukosis virus.

*DNA tumor viruses* have been identified that appear to have a role in the induction of certain cancers, although the link between virus and malignancy is often indirect.[25–27] For instance, the exact role the Epstein-Barr virus plays in the induction of Burkitt's lymphoma has not been elucidated, but viral particles and products have been consistently identified in these tumors. Some researchers believe that the products of these DNA viruses affect cellular DNA transcription, especially that involving cellular oncogenes. It has also been suggested that viral proteins may bind to cellular tumor suppressor genes or their gene products, thereby affecting normal cell growth regulation.[25] Some examples of suspected tumor-inducing DNA viruses include simian virus 40, human papilloma virus, and polyoma virus. Additionally, transformation of virally induced papillomas to squamous cell carcinoma has been rarely noted in the dog.[28,29]

*Hormones* can also act as promoting or pro-

gressing agents. Diethylstilbestrol can induce mutation and neoplastic transformation in tissue culture.[30] Hormones have been demonstrated to be involved in certain malignancies in the animal population. For instance, it is clear that female dogs allowed to progress through at least two heat cycles develop mammary tumors seven times more frequently than dogs spayed at 2 years or less.[31] Additionally, perianal gland adenomas occur almost exclusively in intact male dogs, demonstrating a potential role for testosterone in the development of these neoplasms.[32]

Parasitic infection has occasionally been associated with the development of malignant neoplasia. *Spirocerca lupi* has been demonstrated within esophageal fibrosarcomas and osteosarcomas of dogs.[33] It is hypothesized that the adult worms may induce tumors in the esophagus, stomach, or aorta by secreting a chemical carcinogen.

**4. Chemical Carcinogenesis**   Many different chemical compounds, some naturally occurring and some synthetic, have been identified that are capable of inducing malignant neoplasia. In most instances, chemical carcinogens require repeated administration to demonstrate an effect. These effects are usually additive over the lifetime of that person or animal. Although a few potent carcinogens are capable of inducing tumors after a single exposure, a long latency period between exposure and tumor development is more common. The carcinogenic potential of a chemical can be influenced by a number of different factors, including species, age, sex, and duration of exposure.[34]

Traditionally, individual chemicals have been tested for potential carcinogenic activity by repeated administration to laboratory rats. A more recent approach has been the Ames test, which utilizes the mutagenic activity in bacteria after chemical exposure as a gauge of carcinogenic potential.[34, 35] A number of different chemicals have been identified as carcinogens through this methodology. Pyrrolizidine alkaloids, derived from nonedible plants that may contaminate grains and other foods, have been shown to induce liver cancer in rodents. Many different food additives, either intentionally utilized as preservatives or indirectly added through processing or packaging of foods, have demonstrated carcinogenic activity in laboratory animals. A partial list includes nitrate and nitrite, used as preservatives in many foods, and polyvinylchloride, a contaminant from packaging material. Environmental contaminants such as pesticides (chlordane, toxaphene), polychlorobiphenyls (PCBs), and various air pollutants, have also been demonstrated to present carcinogenic risk to humans and animals.[36]

**5. Physical Carcinogenesis**   This category of carcinogens includes ultraviolet and ionizing radiation, as well as foreign bodies and fibers (i.e., asbestos).

*Ultraviolet radiation* deposits energy in selected molecules, resulting in pyrimidine dimer formation, ultimately conferring point mutations to the DNA.[37] Ultraviolet radiation has long been recognized as a cause of squamous cell carcinoma in animals.[38–40] Lack of pigmentation, along with prolonged sunlight exposure, has been associated with the development of squamous cell carcinoma on the pinnae and nasal planum of cats, ocular region in cattle, ventral abdomen of Dalmatians, and nasal region of collies and Shetland sheepdogs.

*Ionizing radiation* includes electromagnetic radiation (X rays, gamma rays), particulate radiation (electrons, protons, neutrons, alpha particles), and heavy ions. Direct and indirect effects of ionizing energy on DNA can result in damage to nucleotides and may induce strand breaks, eventually leading to point mutations, deletions, and actual chromosome fragmentation. Although most cells are capable of repairing the damage, the repair process may be incomplete, disrupted, or rendered incorrect by a second dose of radiation. Alternatively, the radiation-induced damage may be too great for the cell to repair completely.[41] Studies in humans have demonstrated a higher incidence of chronic leukemias, thyroid tumors, and breast cancer secondary to radiation exposure. Additionally, radon ($^{222}$Rn), which can emit from the ground into homes, has been associated with increased lung cancer risk.[42] In humans, there is a 1% incidence of second primary cancers after therapeutic radiation. This phenomenon has also been recognized in dogs, where radiation-induced tumors have been reported to occur from 30 to 78 months after radiation therapy.[43, 44]

## CELL VIABILITY, PROLIFERATION, AND DEATH

Armed with a basic understanding of carcinogenesis, oncogenes, and tumor suppressor genes, a discussion of how cells, including neoplastic cells, live and die can be undertaken. In the last few years, a literal explosion of information on the control of cell viability and ultimate death has taken place. Such knowledge is extremely important to the field of oncology, as alterations in these control mechanisms are intimately involved in tumor production and progression. Furthermore, a greater understanding of these phenomena may lead to intriguing methods of therapy.

## Programmed Cell Death, or Apoptosis

In a normal organism, a balance must exist between cell renewal and cell death such that the population size remains relatively constant. Oncologists have traditionally been concerned more with cell proliferation because that is the process that typically brings the patient to our clinics. More recently, we have been turning our attention to an understanding of how normal and abnormal cells die in the hope of manipulating this process. Life would not be possible without some mechanism of deleting individual cells that have developed an abnormal function or that are no longer necessary to the community of cells as a whole. Such a mechanism has been termed *programmed cell death*, or *apoptosis*. Several recent reviews have been written on the subject of apoptosis.[45–55] To the purist, the two terms are not mutually inclusive and apoptosis should be used only to describe the actual event of cell death resulting from various well-regulated programmed pathways. However, for the sake of clarity, we will use the term interchangeably with programmed cell death.

Apoptosis is very different from the process of necrosis (accidental cell death) both morphologically and biochemically.[46,50,51] No homeostatic function is attributable to necrosis, which is always pathologic, a relatively rare event, and due to some catastrophic injury (e.g., ischemia, physical trauma). There is nothing accidental about apoptosis. It is a highly regulated homeostatic phenomenon that can be both inhibited and activated. It requires energy, an mRNA product, and protein synthesis in order to occur. The terminal event involves cell condensation, a highly specific cleavage of DNA into fragments, and the formation of membrane-enclosed apoptotic bodies, which are phagocytosed and digested by nearby resident cells. Apoptosis is not associated with inflammation or leakage of cellular contents into surrounding tissues.

Apoptosis functions as an equal and opposite

force to mitosis, and indeed the two processes share similar control points (i.e., growth factors and trophic hormones) that regulate in a reciprocal fashion. Examples of apoptotic death in normal tissues include (1) loss of the epithelial lining of intestinal crypt, (2) deletion of autoreactive T-cells in the thymus necessary for self-tolerance, (3) regression of postlactation mammary tissue, (4) death of mature neutrophils, and (5) regression of the prostate in a dog following castration. Apoptosis not only functions to delete cells in normal tissues, it also eradicates cells whose survival might be harmful to the host, such as those with acquired DNA damage. This "suicide" of abnormal cells is essential because persistence of a stem cell with unrepaired DNA damage could result in immortalization of genetic abnormalities, leading to tumorigenesis.

Apoptosis is not exclusive to normal cells, it also occurs in neoplastic cells.[48] The comparative rates of cell division and cell death determine how quickly a tumor grows. Some cancer cells grow more slowly than normal cells but can still expand because of an increased life span resulting from decreased apoptotic activity.

## Control of Apoptosis

A key question is, are cancer cells immortal or do they maintain the program for cell death? If the latter is true, it may be possible to manipulate this to favor increased tumor cell death. While it is recognized that multiple pathways can lead to apoptosis, we will concentrate on the most well known of these, that involving the tumor suppressor gene p53.[15,56–59] The primary hope of oncologists through the years has been to discover a single aberrant pathway that controls growth in all cancer cells despite the inherent heterogeneity of the various cancer types. Such a "common pathway" would ultimately lead to the proverbial "silver bullet" therapy for all neoplastic disease. The p53 control pathway of apoptosis, known to be defective in approximately 60% of human cancers, is as close to such a common pathway as has been found so far.[14]

The p53 gene is responsible for the cellular response to DNA injury and as such has been referred to as the "genome police."[15,46,56–59] Following DNA damage, expression of p53 increases dramatically. It functions in the simplest sense to arrest the damaged cell in the G1 phase of the cell cycle by blocking cyclin-dependent kinases and to prevent progression into S-phase. Two possibilities are then available to the arrested cell. It

can repair its DNA damage, if this is desirable, and reenter the cell cycle. Conversely, if the damage is too severe, it can undergo p53-driven apoptosis, the so-called "better-dead-than-wrong phenomenon." Which of the two pathways is taken depends on the degree of DNA damage and the presence or absence of a variety of external growth factors and trophic stimuli. If p53 were not present, or mutated to an abnormal state, the abnormal cell could not arrest and would continue to proliferate, resulting in accumulation of damage-induced mutations that may ultimately result in tumorigenesis. Figure 3–2 summarizes the p53 control phenomenon.

Not only will abnormal p53 function lead to a hypermutatable state, it can also result in tumor resistance to DNA-damaging therapy.[46,48,56,57] Radiation and many forms of chemotherapy (e.g., alkylators) confer their antineoplastic effect by creating DNA damage that ultimately results in apoptotic death rather than necrosis. Normally functioning p53 is an absolute requirement of DNA-damage-related apoptosis. Cancers curable by chemotherapy execute signal transduction pathways culminating in apoptosis in response to DNA damage. Tumor cells with defective p53 are unable to undergo apoptosis following exposure to therapy and can continue to be viable. To illustrate, consider three situations: (1) tumors containing p53 mutations (abnormal p53) are typically chemoresistant from the outset (e.g., malignant melanoma);[58] (2) tumors with normal p53 function are typically chemosensitive (e.g., testicular tumors, lymphoma);[53] (3) tumors that develop p53 mutations at some point eventually become resistant to chemotherapy (e.g., relapsed lymphoma).[53] The p53 tumor suppressor gene is not alone in its genetic control of apoptosis. A proto-oncogene, bcl-2, functions to inhibit apoptosis and can act as an oncogene in a fashion opposite to p53.[46,48,50,52] Ultimately, knowledge of such basic biologic processes as apoptosis should lead to more efficacious antineoplastic therapies. Gene therapy, aimed at replacing wild-type p53 into mutant tumor cells could allow for restoration of apoptosis and therapy sensitivity.

## Tumor Proliferation

We now move from the single-cell level to the developing tumor cell population. Tumor proliferation rates have long been considered to reflect biologic behavior with respect to metastatic potential, recurrence following therapy, and overall survival.[60–62] Information now exists to sug-

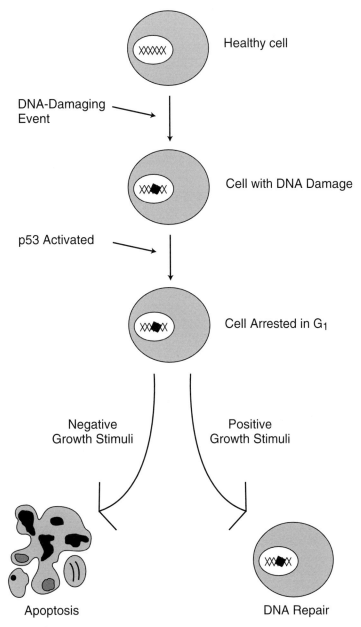

Healthy cell

DNA-Damaging Event

Cell with DNA Damage

p53 Activated

Cell Arrested in $G_1$

Negative Growth Stimuli

Positive Growth Stimuli

Apoptosis

DNA Repair

**Figure 3–2.** Role of p53 following DNA damage.

gest that tumor growth rate before and during a course of cytotoxic treatment might also impact outcome. That is, tumors with the capacity to proliferate rapidly between treatment cycles or intervals may be able to overcome or lessen the efficacy of such a treatment. In fact, cytotoxic therapy appears to accelerate tumor growth during therapy and after therapy has been instituted. Local control rates for rapidly proliferating experimental and clinical human tumors under-

going radiation therapy at a given dose decrease when the overall treatment time is increased, likely because of accelerated tumor cell repopulation during treatment. While less data exist to support accelerated repopulation in tumors undergoing chemotherapy, intuitively speaking, it probably does occur. Radiotherapy and chemotherapy are often spread out over weeks or months to permit normal tissues to repopulate. If the particular tumor in question has a very slow doubling time (i.e., growth rate), protractment of therapy permits normal tissue recovery and should enhance the therapeutic differential. However, in tumors with rapid doubling times, protracting therapy allows the tumor to repopulate, often at an accelerated level, subsequently diminishing the therapeutic differential. Clinicians are currently evaluating various means to compress treatment time through intensified therapeutic strategies such as accelerated fractionated dose regimens in radiotherapy and intensive chemotherapy with subsequent marrow stimulation or rescue. Tumor proliferation also has important implications when combining different modalities of therapy. For example, if a combination of radiotherapy and chemotherapy is contemplated, accelerated tumor growth will contribute to failure if the duration of combined therapy is protracted to accommodate both modalities. Neoadjuvant therapy (chemotherapy administered weeks prior to radiation therapy) is probably a poor strategy in light of this phenomenon. Rather, the two agents should either be given simultaneously or sequenced as close together as acute toxicities will permit. Theoretically, chemotherapy should be most effective given late in the course of radiotherapy when accelerated tumor regrowth is occurring and cells are actively cycling. It is important to bear in mind that not all patients would benefit from intensified treatment protocols and may indeed be disadvantaged by them. Those individuals with inherently slow proliferating tumors may be better served by protracted treatments that produce less toxicity on normal tissues, resulting in an enhanced therapeutic differential. Therefore, the key to such strategies appears to lie in our ability to predict (i.e., measure) which tumors are rapidly proliferating and which are not.

## Measures of Tumor Proliferation

There exist three primary levels at which we can contemplate the rate of tumor growth:[63] (1) Volume doubling time (Tvol) is defined as the time required for the tumor to double in size based on clinically observable growth (e.g., caliper measurements, radiographic size). This is the longest measurable parameter because it accounts for the length of the cell cycle (Tc), the number of cells actively participating in the growth fraction (i.e. percentage of tumor cells actively dividing within the tumor mass), as well as ongoing cell loss. (2) Potential doubling time (Tpot) is the shortest period of time a tumor could potentially double if

no cell loss were occurring while still taking into account the growth fraction. (3) Cell cycle time (Tc) is the time it takes for the tumor cell to pass through the cell cycle. Figure 3–3 illustrates the relationship between these three measures of tumor proliferation.

A clinically relevant technique for measuring the length of the cell cycle (Tc) at present eludes us. Furthermore, measurement of tumor doubling time in patients usually does not provide us with clinically useful information until after the tumor has reached late stages of development beyond our ability to intervene meaningfully. We do, however, have methods of measuring the potential doubling time (Tpot) of tumors in a way that provides information prior to initiating therapy. Several reviews on determining Tpot in patients have recently been published.[64–66] The authors have used this technique in dogs with lymphoma and found Tpot to be predictive of treatment response and overall survival. Another approach for the indirect measurement of tumor proliferation is the quantification of nuclear antigens that are associated with proliferation using monoclonal antibodies. These so-called proliferation antigens include Ki-67, DNA polymerase alpha, PCNA/cyclin, ribonuclease reductase, and p105.[67–69] These antigens are present in the nuclear matrix of proliferating cells but absent in nonproliferating cells. Monoclonal antibodies developed against these proliferation antigens are applied to tissue sections or cytological preps (i.e., fine-needle aspirates) and the percentage of cells reacting with the antibody is determined either visually or by flow cytometric analysis. Several reports have demonstrated a correlation between proliferation antigen labeling and cell proliferation and therapy outcome. This technique (using the PCNA antigen) has been applied to cats with nasal planum squamous cell carcinoma and found to be predictive of treatment outcome following radiation therapy.[70] Another indirect marker of proliferation, agrophillic nuclear organizer regions (AgNOR), has been correlated with histologic grade and postsurgical outcome in dogs with mast cell tumors.[71] Silver staining of paraffin-embedded tissues or cytology preps allows visualization of AgNORs, as black dots within the nucleus and relative counts correlate with proliferative activity.

Quantitative proliferation assays may offer several potential benefits to the clinical oncologist of the future. They may prove to have clinical significance independent of that provided by most qualitative prognostic variables, allowing a

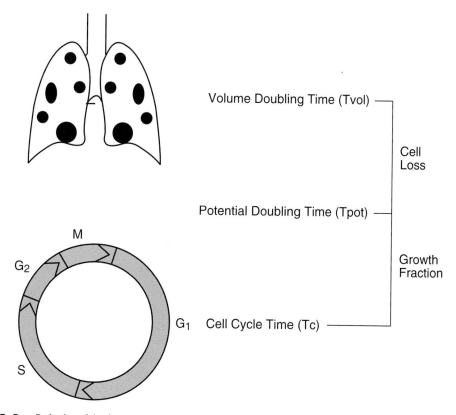

**Figure 3–3.** Relationship between measurable levels of tumor growth. Volume doubling time (Tvol) is the time required for the tumor to double in size clinically (e.g., radiographic size). Potential doubling time (Tpot) is the shortest period of time a tumor could double if no cell loss were occurring while still taking into account the growth fraction. Cell cycle time (Tc) is the time it takes for the tumor cell to pass through the cell cycle.

more accurate prediction of treatment response and long-term survival. They may also allow more individual tailoring of treatment protocols based on the growth rates of a particular tumor. Finally, they may permit the identification of tumors most likely to respond to pharmacologic alteration of cell cycles.

## TUMOR HETEROGENEITY

The concept that a tumor may be heterogeneous with respect to such characteristics as cytologic appearance, content of growth hormone receptors, immunogenicity, cell surface antigens, susceptibility to therapy, and metastatic potential is defined as *tumor heterogeneity*.[17,72,73] Furthermore, because malignant neoplasms are in a state of unregulated, uncontrolled growth, tumor cells inherently possess karyotypic instability. There-

fore, individual tumor cells may gain or lose specific characteristics, such as metastatic potential or chemotherapy resistance, as the tumor grows. That the heterogeneous nature of a given tumor may also be in a constant state of change provides tumors with a tremendous growth advantage, allowing them to be more efficient at avoiding immune recognition and developing resistance to different treatment modalities. This characteristic of tumors may also explain why metastatic disease may exhibit a different response from that of the primary tumor to such therapeutics as chemotherapy or radiation therapy. Evidence suggests that tumor heterogeneity is an acquired trait. Initially, cancer cells in a given tumor demonstrate common features. However, by the time tumors become clinically overt, their constituent cells are already endowed with diverse biologic characteristics. Diversity among tumor cells becomes increasingly more evident as the malignant process progresses. Essentially, we have many different tumors within a single mass.

## METASTASIS

Although the treatment of primary tumors has improved dramatically, metastatic disease remains responsible for the majority of cancer-related deaths. It is the ability of cancer cells to metastasize and form new centers of growth that has long frustrated clinical oncologists. Much of recent oncologic research has focused on dissecting the mechanisms of metastasis in an effort to address more effectively this aspect of malignant neoplasia. One of the most important discoveries has been that metastasis is an active process, not necessarily the result of random events. Furthermore, several steps must be completed before a cancer cell can grow into a metastatic focus.

In general, two major routes for metastatic spread exist: via the lymphatic system or through vascular channels (some types of cancer can also spread along or through tissue planes, tissue spaces, and body cavities). Although it was initially believed that these two pathways were separate and specific to an individual tumor type (i.e., carcinomas spread via lymphatics and sarcomas via blood vessels), it cannot be ignored that the lymphatic and vascular channels are intimately connected. It is true, however, that different tumor types exhibit different patterns of metastasis, especially to specific target organs. For example, in the dog, metastatic osteosarcoma is almost always first recognized in the lungs, while apocrine gland adenocarcinoma generally spreads to the sublumbar lymph nodes before lung metastasis is noted.

Two hypotheses have been generated to explain the specific patterns of metastasis that are recognized to occur with different tumor types. The first is that proposed in 1889 by Paget, known as the *seed-and-soil hypothesis*. That is, very specific interactions occur between metastatic cells and the target organ, which may or may not possess conditions favorable for the growth of these cells.[74–76] The second hypothesis maintains that the likelihood of metastasis to a particular organ is related to the vascular interconnections that exist between it and the primary tumor. Tumor cells would become trapped in the first capillary bed they encountered and would therefore be more likely to develop into a metastatic focus at that site. These two concepts

are not necessarily mutually exclusive. While it does appear that the circulatory anatomy relative to the primary tumor plays an important role in the resultant metastasis, it cannot fully explain the metastatic patterns of certain tumors.

The process of metastasis is complex and multistep in nature. A tumor cell must survive and complete several events before it can develop into a secondary tumor. However, metastatic events are extremely inefficient. Experiments that have introduced tumor cells directly into the vascular system of mice and rats have demonstrated that only 1% or less of these cells actually survive to develop into tumor nodules.[77] In fact, fewer that 1 in 10,000 of the tumor cells that leave the primary tumor survive to grow into new tumor colonies.[76] Additionally, there is substantial evidence that only a subpopulation of the primary tumor cells possess the specific cellular properties that enable them to complete the metastatic process.[76–78]

The sequence of events that occur in the development of metastatic disease is sometimes termed the *metastatic cascade*. These events appear to be similar for metastasis through either the lymphatic or vascular routes. For this process to succeed, the metastatic tumor cells must complete *all* of the necessary steps (Fig. 3–4).

**1. Detachment**   The first step in the metastatic cascade is detachment of a tumor cell from the primary tumor mass. In some instances, tumor cells may shed directly into the bloodstream if they happen to be adjacent to a vessel wall or actually lining the vessel. Detachment may be facilitated by rapid tumor growth, necrosis of the tumor, or mechanical stresses.[77] Additionally, decreased levels of cellular adhesion molecules (integrins, etc.) may enhance the likelihood of detachment. Some tumor cells actually secrete proteases, aiding in the separation of a cell from the primary mass. Tumor cells may also produce motility factors that promote movement of cells away from the primary mass.[76–79] It is probable that a combination of several alterations, in addition to local environmental changes, confers the ability to detach and begin the process of metastasis.

**2. Invasion**   Once detached, the tumor cell must enter either the vascular or lymphatic system. Many of the newly formed blood vessels within the tumor are relatively "leaky" and malignant cells appear to cross into them easily. However, tumors do not induce their own lymphatic supply, and lymphatic vessels are not present within the tumor itself. Therefore, neoplastic cells can only enter the lymphatics at the host-tumor interface.[76,77] It appears that tumor cells can readily penetrate small lymphatic vessels and be transported passively in lymph to the lymph nodes.

Tumor cell invasion into lymphatics and blood vessels is often aided by the production of several enzymes (e.g., plasminogen activator and cathepsin B) in addition to a wide variety of collagenases that can lyse basement membrane components and connective tissues.[76,77,80] The tumor cell may not have to do all the work itself. Some tumor cells can induce the local accumulation of macrophages, which secrete large amounts of plasminogen activator, allowing these cells to penetrate blood vessel walls.[77]

**3. Evasion of Host Defenses** Within the vascular or lymphatic channels, tumor cells must withstand challenge by cells of the immune system. Mechanisms of cell death in the vascular compartment may include mechanical stresses, poor nutrition, or toxicity due to high oxygen levels in the blood. Specific and nonspecific immune cells, including T-lymphocytes, neutrophils, macrophages, and natural killer (NK) cells, are all capable of killing tumor cells free in the bloodstream. It appears as if NK cells and macrophages are the most effective at this task.[79] Tumors that metastasize via lymphatics encounter challenge by the immune system at the level of the lymph node. Lymph nodes may represent a temporary barrier to tumor spread through

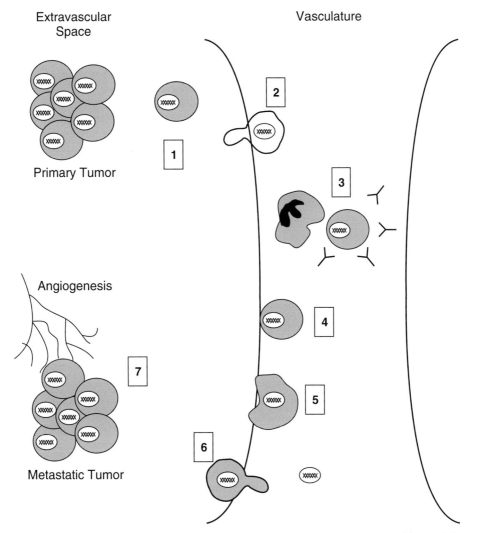

**Figure 3–4.** The metastatic cascade. *1,* Detachment. *2,* Invasion. *3,* Evasion of host defenses. *4,* Arrest. *5,* Attachment. *6,* Extravasation. *7,* Establishment of new growth.

the activation of cytotoxic T-lymphocytes, NK cells, as well as monocytes and macrophages.[81]

**4. Arrest**   Having evaded the immune system, metastatic tumor cells come to rest in the small blood vessels and capillaries of various organs. Often this involves the interaction of these cells with platelets. Thrombus formation has been noted around tumor cells that have arrested. In most instances, these remain only for a short period of time as they are broken down by various fibrinolytic enzymes. Thrombus formation has been hypothesized to provide protection for metastatic cells against mechanical trauma and also against attack by the immune system.[82,83] It may also be true that adhesions between the tumor cells themselves may facilitate cell arrest. In the mouse model, metastatic efficiency increases greatly when injections of small clumps of tumor cells are given as an intravenous injection as opposed to single-cell suspensions.[77]

Cancer cells have been demonstrated in loose aggregates of platelets and some have been shown to induce platelet aggregation. This may be through the release of procoagulant activity or prostaglandins.[84] Aspirin and dipyridamole, both known to inhibit platelet aggregation, have minimal effects on the formation of metastatic disease. However, drugs that modify prostaglandin synthesis have been shown to decrease the number of metastases in experimental models. Newer inhibitors of platelet aggregation that appear to be more potent have recently been tested. These include calcium channel blockers, antiplatelet antibodies, prostacyclin, nafazatrom, forskolin, and the protease inhibitor leupeptide, which inhibits thrombus formation.[77,85]

**5. Attachment**   There is evidence that individual tumor types may selectively adhere to organ-specific vascular endothelial cells.[86–90] Experiments in vitro have demonstrated that liver metastatic tumor cells adhere preferentially to liver-conditioned endothelial cells in culture. Conversely, lung metastatic tumor cells prefer adhesion to endothelial cells grown on lung-derived factors. It is hypothesized that target specificity may involve chemoattractants, growth factors, extracellular matrix components, and perhaps specific endothelial cell surface adhesion molecules. These cellular adhesion molecules (CAMs) include the cahedrins, cell surface lectins, and lectin-binding glycoproteins expressed by endothelial cells. Different levels of CAMs are present on endothelial cells derived from different organs.[77,88]

**6. Extravasation**   Once arrested and attached, tumor cells must begin the process of invasion through the vascular or lymphatic endothelium and into the extracellular matrix. This process, which involves several steps, is similar to the early metastatic event of invasion but in the reverse direction. Tumor cells can induce retraction of endothelial cells to expose the basement membrane and extracellular matrix. The tumor cell may extend cellular pseudopodia between endothelial cells (i.e., directly into endothelial cell junctions).[76,77] Digestion of the basement membrane and extracellular matrix is then accomplished by various proteolytic enzymes/released by tumor cells, including plasminogen activator, metalloproteinases, and cathepsins.[76–78,91] In the normal situation, proteolysis is tightly regulated, with proteases and inhibitors in balance. However, malignant cells disturb the balance, leading to uncontrolled invasion. Once digestion of the extracellular matrix has occurred, the tumor cell's pseudopodia protrude into the zone of lysis, and the cell gradually migrates forward. This process is tightly controlled: the advancing front activates proteolytic enzymes to break down the matrix while the "rear" of the tumor cell remains fixed. Once a path has been cleared, the cell must turn off these proteases so it can advance.

**7.  Establishment of New Growth**   Once in the interstitial space, tumor cells must survive to proliferate into a clinically detectable colony. The ability of cells to grow depends on various intrinsic properties of the cells themselves, and specific factors present within the surrounding environment (the seed-and-soil hypothesis).

It is believed that tumor cells may be less dependent on growth factors than normal cells. This could be the result of *autocrine* growth stimulation, whereby the tumor cell produces a growth factor that can autostimulate itself. The ability of tumor cells to grow in an autocrine fashion may be an important determination of the metastatic phenotype.[88,92] Conversely, metastatic foci may be dependent on paracrine growth, whereby the local microenvironment of the target organ contains specific growth factors necessary for the survival of metastatic tumor cells.[88,92] Several investigations have shown that in vitro growth of metastatic tumor cell lines can be stimulated by extracts derived from target organs. Furthermore, their growth may actually be inhibited by extracts from nontarget organs.[86,89] If a metastatic tumor cell is incapable of producing sufficient autocrine growth factors to support the development of a secondary tumor, specific growth factors in the cell's microenvironment may be the essential determining factor in the ultimate localization of metastatic colonies. That is, cells capable of autocrine growth will develop into secondary tumors in the first capillary bed in which they arrest, whereas tumor cells with minimal autocrine growth capacity will be more likely to develop in a favorable environmental setting. Furthermore, both of these subpopulations may exist within any given primary tumor.

In order to fully develop into a metastatic focus, tumor cells must be capable of inducing the growth of new blood vessels, a process known as *angiogenesis*. Several different growth factors, including basic fibroblast growth factors (b-FGF), angiogenin, prostaglandins, heparin fragments, laminin peptides, and transforming growth factors (TGF-α, TGF-β), have been found to stimulate endothelial cell growth and morphologic differentiation.[92,93] Tumor cells release these growth factors or stimulate the surrounding normal tissue to do so. This process generates proliferation of vascular endothelium and growth of blood vessels into the tumor. Neovascularization is an essential component of growth of the primary tumor and helps firmly establish the metastatic focus.

Because the process of angiogenesis is necessary for tumor growth, several researchers have been attempting to develop agents that inhibit the activity or release of endothelial growth factors. The inhibition of angiogenesis would prevent recently metastasized tumor cells from developing their own blood supply. It may also prevent further growth of the primary tumor or of metastatic disease that is already well established.

# REFERENCES

1. Minden MD, Pawson AJ: Oncogenes. *In* Tannok IF, Hill RP (eds): The Basic Science of Oncology. New York, McGraw-Hill, 1992, pp. 61–87.
2. Cross M, Dexter TM: Growth factors in development, transformation, and tumorigenesis. Cell *64*:271–280, 1991.
3. Hunter T: A thousand and one protein kinases. Cell *50*:823–829, 1987.
4. Cantley LC, Auger KR, Carpenter C, et al: Oncogenes and signal transduction. Cell *64*:281–302, 1991.
5. Linder ME, Gilman AG: G proteins. Scientific American *267*:56–65, 1992.
6. Edelman AM, Blumenthal DK, Krebs EG: Protein serine/threonine kinases. Ann Rev Biochem *56*:567–613, 1987.
7. Lewin B: Oncogenic conversion by regulatory changes in transcription factors. Cell *64*:303–312, 1991.
8. Saunders KA, Madewell BR, Oreffo VIC, et al: Nucleotide sequence of canine c-N-ras: Codons 1 to 71. Am J Vet Res *53*:600–603, 1992.
9. Miyoshi N, Tateyama S, Ogawa K, et al: Abnormal structure of the canine oncogene, related to the human c-yes-1 oncogene, in canine mammary tumor tissue. Am J Vet Res *52*:2046–2049, 1991.
10. Miyoshi N, Tateyama S, Ogawa K, et al: Proto-oncogenes of genomic DNA in clinically normal animals of various species. Am J Vet Res *52*:940–944, 1991.
11. Ahern TE, Bird RC, Bird AEC, Wolfe LG: Overexpression of c-erbB-2 and c-myc but not c-ras, in canine melanoma cell lines, is associated with metastatic potential in nude mice. Anticancer Res *13*:1365–1372, 1993.
12. Weinberg RA: Oncogenes, antioncogenes and the molecular basis of multistep carcinogenesis. Cancer Res *49*:3713–3721, 1989.
13. Fearon ER, Vogelstein B: A genetic model for colorectal tumorigenesis. Cell *61*:759–767, 1990.
14. Weinberg RA: Finding the anti-oncogene. Scientific American *259*:44–51, 1988.
15. Levine AJ, Perry ME, Chang A, et al: The 1993 Walter Hubert Lecture: The role of the p53 tumour-suppressor gene in tumorigenesis. Br J Cancer *69*:409–416, 1994.
16. Pitot HC, Dragon YP: Facts and theories concerning the mechanisms of carcinogenesis. FASEB *5*:2280–2285, 1991.
17. Farber E: The multistep nature of cancer development. Cancer Res *44*:4217–4223, 1984.
18. Weinstein IB: The origins of human cancer: Molecular mechanisms of carcinogenesis and their implications for cancer prevention and treatment. Cancer Res *48*:4135–4143, 1988.
19. Couture J, Hansen MF: Recessive oncogenes in tumorigenesis. Cancer Bull *43*:41–50, 1991.
20. Cordon-Cardo C, Waringer D, Petrylak D, et al: Altered expression of the retinoblastoma gene product; prognostic indicator in bladder cancer. J Natl Cancer Inst *84*:1251–1256, 1992.
21. Kornblau SM, Xu H-J, delGiglio A, et al: Clinical implication of decreased retinoblastoma protein expression in acute myelogenous leukemia. Cancer Res *52*:4587–4590, 1992.
22. Xu H-J, Quinlan DC, Davidson AG, et al: Altered retinoblastoma protein expression in early-stage non-small cell lung carcinoma. J Natl Cancer Inst *86*:695–699, 1994.
23. Priester WA, McKay FW: The Occurrence of Tumors in Domestic Animals. National Cancer

Institute Monograph No. 54, Washington, DC, U.S. Govt. Printing Office, 1980, p. 152.

24. Loeb LA: Endogenous carcinogenesis: Molecular oncology into the twenty-first century—Presidential address. Cancer Res 49:5489–5496, 1989.

25. Benchimol S: Viruses and cancer. In Tannok IF, Hill RP (eds): The Basic Science of Oncology. New York, McGraw-Hill, 1992, pp. 88–101.

26. Varmus H: Retroviruses. Science 240:1427–1435, 1988.

27. Bishop JM: Cellular oncogenes and retroviruses. Ann Rev Biochem 52:301, 1983.

28. Allison AC: Viruses inducing skin tumors in animals. In Rook AJ, Walton CS (eds): Comparative Physiology and Pathology of the Skin. Oxford, Blackwell, 1965, pp. 665–684.

29. Shimada A, Shinya K, Awakura T, et al: Cutaneous papillomatosis associated with papillomavirus infection in a dog. J Comp Pathol 108:103–107, 1993.

30. Jaggi W, Lutz WK, Schlatter C: Covalent binding of ethinylestradiol and estrone to rat liver DNA in vivo. Chem Biol Interact 23:13–18, 1978.

31. Schnieder R, Dorn CR, Taylor DON: Factors influencing canine mammary cancer development and post-surgical survival. J Natl Cancer Inst 43:1249–1261, 1969.

32. Nielson SW, Aftomsis J: Canine perianal gland tumors. J Am Vet Med Assoc 144:127–135, 1964.

33. Bailey WS: Parasites and cancer: Sarcomas in dogs associated with Spirocerca lupi. Ann NY Acad Sci 108:890–923, 1963.

34. Farber E: Chemical carcinogenesis. N Engl J Med 305:1379–1389, 1981.

35. Archer MA: Chemical carcinogens. In Tannok IF, Hill RP (eds): The Basic Science of Oncology. New York, McGraw-Hill, 1992, pp. 102–118.

36. MacEwen EG: Cancer overview: Epidemiology, etiology, and prevention. In MacEwen EG, Withrow SJ (eds): Clinical Veterinary Oncology. Philadelphia, JB Lippincott, 1989, pp. 3–13.

37. Rauth AM: The induction and repair of ultraviolet light damage in mammalian cells. In Burns FJ, Upton AC, Silini G (eds): Radiation Carcinogenesis and DNA Alterations. New York, Plenum Press, 1986, pp. 212–226.

38. Dorn CR, Taylor D, Schneider R: Sunlight exposure and the risk of developing cutaneous and oral squamous cell carcinoma in white cats. J Natl Cancer Inst 46:1073–1078, 1971.

39. Madewell BR, Conroy JD, Hodgkins EM: Sunlight skin cancer association in the dog: A report of 3 cases. J Cutan Pathol 8:434–443, 1981.

40. Nikula KJ, Benjamin SA, Angleton GM, et al: Ultraviolet radiation, solar dermatosis, and cutaneous meoplasia in beagle dogs. Radiat Res 129:11–18, 1992.

41. Hall EJ: Principles of carcinogenesis: Physical. In Devita VT Jr, Hellman S, Rosenberg SA (eds): Cancer: Principles and Practice. Philadelphia, JB Lippincott, 1993.

42. Upton AC: Physical carcinogenesis: Radiation—history and sources. In Becker FF (ed): A Comprehensive Treatise, Vol. I. New York, Plenum Press, 1978, pp. 387–403.

43. Thrall DE, Goldschmidt MH, Evans SM, et al: Bone sarcoma following orthovoltage radiotherapy in two dogs. Vet Rad 24:169–173, 1983.

44. Thrall DE, Goldschmidt MH, Biery DN: Malignant tumor formation at the site of previously irradiated acanthomatous epulides in four dogs. J Am Vet Med Assoc 178:127–132, 1981.

45. Williams GT, Smith CA: Molecular regulation of apoptosis: Genetic controls on cell death. Cell 74:777–779, 1993.

46. Kerr JFR, Winterford CM, Harmon BV: Apoptosis. Cancer 73:2013–2026, 1994.

47. Schimke RT, Mihich E: Fifth annual Pezcoller symposium: Apoptosis. Cancer Res 54:302–305, 1994.

48. Carson DA, Ribeiro JM: Apoptosis and disease. Lancet 341:1251–1254, 1993.

49. Eastman A: Apoptosis: A product of programmed and unprogrammed cell death. Toxical Appl Pharmacol 121:160–164, 1993.

50. McDonnell TJ, Marin MC, Hsu B, et al: Symposium: Apoptosis/programmed cell death. Radiat Res 136:307–312, 1993.

51. Cohen JJ: Apoptosis. Immunol Today 14:126–130, 1993.

52. Schwartzman RA, Cidlowski JA: Apoptosis: The biochemistry and molecular biology of programmed cell death. Endocr Rev 14:133–151, 1993.

53. Wyllie AH: Apoptosis [the 1992 Frank Rose memorial lecture]. Br J Cancer 67:205–208, 1993.

54. Bowen ID: Apoptosis or programmed cell death. Cell Biol Int Rep 17:365–380, 1993.

55. Evans VG: Multiple pathways to apoptosis. Cell Biol Int Rep 17:461–476, 1993.

56. Vogelstein B, Kinzler KW: p53 Function and dysfunction. Cell 70:523–526, 1992.

57. Sachs L, Lotem J: Control of programmed cell death in normal and leukemic cells: New implications for therapy. Blood 82:15–21, 1993.

58. Lowe SW, Ruley HE, Jacks T, Housman DE: p53-Dependent apoptosis modulates the cytotoxicity of anticancer agents. Cell 74:957–967, 1993.

59. Harris CC, Hollstein M: Clinical implications of the p53 tumor supressor gene. N Engl J Med 329:1318–1327, 1993.

60. Mitchell JB: Potential applicability of nonclonogenic measurements to clinical oncology. Radiat Res 114:401–414, 1988.

61. Wither HR: Clinical implications of accelerated tumor growth during cytotoxic therapies. In Fortner JG, Rhoads JE (eds.): Accomplishments in Cancer Research 1991. Philadelphia, JB Lippincott, 1992, pp. 301–310..

62. McNally NJ: Can cell kinetic parameters predict the response of tumors to radiotherapy. Int J Radiat Biol 56:777–786, 1989.

63. Fowler JF: Rapid repopulation in radiotherapy: A debate on mechanism. The phantom of tumor treatment—continually rapid proliferation unmasked. Radiother Oncol 22:156–167, 1991.

64. Ritter MA, Fowler JF, Kim Y, et al: Single biopsy, tumor kinetic analyses: A comparison of methods and an extension to shorter sampling intervals. Int J Radiat Oncol Biol Phys 23: 811–820, 1992.

65. Wilson GD: Assessment of human tumor proliferation using bromodeoxyuridine—Current status. Acta Oncol 30:903–910, 1991.

66. White RA, Terry NH, Meistrich ML, Calkins DP: Improved methods for computing potential doubling time from flow cytometric data. Cytometry 11:314–317, 1990.

67. Henry MJ, Stanley MW, Swenson B, et al: Cytologic assessment of tumor cell kinetics: Applications of monoclonal antibody Ki-67 to fine needle aspiration smears. Diagn Cytopathol 7:591–596, 1991.

68. Linden MD, Ma CK, Kubus J, et al: Ki-67 and proliferating cell nuclear antigen tumor proliferative indices in DNA diploid colorectal adenocarcinomas. Am J Clin Pathol 100:206–212, 1993.

69. Inada T, Imura J, Ichikawa A, et al: Proliferative activity of gastric cancer assessed by immunostaining for proliferating cell nuclear antigen. J Surg Oncol 54:146–152, 1993.

70. Theon AP, Madewell BR, Shearn V, Moulton JE: Irradiation of squamous cell carcinomas of the nasal planum in 90 cats. Proc Annu Conf Vet Cancer Soc 13:147–148, 1993.

71. Bostock DE, Crocker J, Harris K, Smith P: Nuclear organiser regions as indicators of post-surgical prognosis in canine spontaneous mast cell tumors. Br J Cancer 59:915–918, 1989.

72. Arvan DA: Tumor cell heterogeneity: An overview. Clin Chim Acta 206:3–7, 1992.

73. Heppner GH: Cancer cell societies and tumor progression. Stem Cells 11:199–203, 1993.

74. Paget S: The distribution of secondary growths in cancer of the breast. Lancet 1:571–573, 1889.

75. Fidler IJ: Metastasis as a consequence of aberrant homeostasis. Clin Exp/Metastasis 10:5–7, 1992.

76. Liotta LA: Cancer cell invasion and metastasis. Scientific American 266:54–63, 1992.

77. Hill RP: Metastasis. In Tannok IF, Hill RP (eds): The Basic Science of Oncology. New York, McGraw-Hill, 1992, pp. 178–195.

78. Killion JJ, Fideler IJ: The biology of tumor metastasis. Semin Oncol 16:106–115, 1989.

79. Feldman M, Eisenbach L: What makes a tumor cell metastatic? Scientific American 259:60–85, 1988.

80. Liotta LA: Mechanisms of cancer invasion and metastasis. In Liotta LA (ed): Influence of Tumor Development on the Host. Dordrecht, Netherlands, Kluwer, 1989, pp. 58–71.

81. Fisher B, Saffer E, Fisher ER: Studies concerning the regional lymph node in cancer: IV-tumor inhibition by regional lymph node cells. Cancer 33:631–636, 1974.

82. Hamilton HB, Withrow SJ: Antiplatelet therapy: A possible new therapeutic modality for controlling metastasis. Comp Cont Ed 7:907–912, 1985.

83. Zacharski LR, Rickles RF, Henderson WG, et al: Platelets and malignancy. Am J Clin Oncol 5:593–609, 1982.

84. Gasic GJ: Role of plasma, platelets and endothelial cells in tumor metastasis. Cancer Metastasis Rev 3:99–114, 1984.

85. Honn KV, Menter DG, Onoda JM, et al: Role of prostacyclin as a natural deterrent to hematogenous tumor metastasis. In Nicolson GL, Milas L (eds): Cancer Invasion and Metastasis: Biologic and Therapeutic Aspects. New York, Raven Press, 1984, pp. 361–388.

86. Cavanaugh PG, Nicolson GL: Organ preference of metastasis: Role of organ paracrine growth factors. Cancer Bull 43:9–16, 1991.

87. Sher BT, Bargatze R, Holzmann B, et al: Homing receptors and metastasis. Adv Cancer Res 51:361–390, 1988.

88. Rusciano D, Burger MM: Why do cancer cells metastasize into particular organs? BioEssays 14:185–195, 1992.

89. Nicolson GL, Dulski KM: Organ specificity of metastatic tumor colonization is related to organ-selective growth properties of malignant cells. Int J Cancer 38:289–294, 1986.

90. Pauli BU, Lee CL: Organ preference of metastasis: The role of organ-specifically modulated endothelial cells. Lab Invest 58:379–385, 1988.

91. Aznavoorian S, Murphy AN, Stetler-Stevenson WG, Liotta LA: Molecular aspects of tumor cell invasion and metastasis. Cancer 71:1368–1383, 1993.

92. Bicknell R, Harris AL: Novel growth regulatory factors and tumor angiogenesis. Eur J Cancer 27:781–785, 1991.

93. Tannok IF: Cell Proliferation. In Tannok IF, Hill RP (eds): The Basic Science of Oncology. New York, McGraw-Hill, 1992, pp. 178–195.

# 4

# Paraneoplastic Syndromes

Gregory K. Ogilvie

The symptoms produced by cancer are often manifestations of direct or metastatic involvement of any part of an animal's body. Tumors can also cause distant alterations in the structure and function of the body that are unrelated to the malignancy. These distant systemic effects of cancer are known as paraneoplastic syndromes. Paraneoplastic syndromes are usually caused by the production of unusual amounts of micromolecules and their release into the circulation. The best characterized paraneoplastic syndromes are those produced by a tumor that secretes a polypeptide hormone that is distributed by the circulation to act at distant sites. There are many nonendocrine organ-associated paraneoplastic syndromes with no known etiologic substance or macromolecule. Indeed, in veterinary medicine, the cause of most paraneoplastic syndromes is unknown. Although not rare, few paraneoplastic syndromes develop in veterinary cancer patients. As the awareness of paraneoplastic syndromes expands, these syndromes will be recognized in more cancer-bearing animals. A partial list of paraneoplastic syndromes and associated malignant conditions seen in animals is listed in Table 4–1.

The importance of paraneoplastic syndromes is often underestimated. Clinically, paraneoplastic syndromes can cause greater morbidity than the actual physical presence of the malignant tumor. Their appearance may be the first sign of a malignancy and they may be so severe that appropriate therapy for the underlying cancer is not initiated.

This chapter reviews some of the most common paraneoplastic syndromes in veterinary medicine. Several other excellent reviews are available for the interested reader.[1–3]

## CANCER CACHEXIA

A profound state of malnutrition and wasting is a frequent and important systemic effect of cancer in animals.[4–15] Weight loss and all metabolic alterations that are observed in cancer patients when adequate nutritional intake is present is termed cancer cachexia (Fig. 4–1). Cancer cachexia occurs frequently, with an estimated incidence of 45 to 87% in hospitalized human patients.[16,17] Because the annual incidence rate of cancer is higher in dogs than in people,[18] cancer cachexia is potentially a more significant problem in dogs.[19] Alterations in carbohydrate, protein[20–31] and lipid metabolism associated with this paraneoplastic syndrome usually occur before weight loss is observed and they last for some time after the animal is rendered free of the tumor.[20–31] A more complete discussion of this paraneoplastic syndrome is found elsewhere in this book (Chap. 12).

## ECTOPIC HORMONE PRODUCTION

### Hypercalcemia

Cancer is the most common cause of hypercalcemia in the dog and cat. Tumors that are associated with hypercalcemia in dogs and cats are lymphoma, apocrine gland adenocarcinoma of the anal sac, multiple myeloma, thyroid carcinoma, mammary adenocarcinoma, tumors infiltrating bone, and neoplasia of the parathyroid gland.[32] Lymphoma is the most common cause of tumor-associated hypercalcemia (pseudohypoparathyroidism); many dogs with hypercalcemia secondary to lymphoma have the medi-

**Table 4–1**   Paraneoplastic Syndromes and Associated Tumors

*Cancer Cachexia*
  Multiple tumors

*Ectopic Hormone Production*
  *Hypercalcemia-producing factors*

| | |
|---|---|
| Lymphoma | Parathyroid tumors |
| Mammary | Gastric carcinoma |
|   adenocarcinoma | Thyroid carcinoma |
| Multiple myeloma | Nasal carcinoma |
| Epidermoid carcinoma | Thymoma |
| Anal sac apocrine gland | |
|   adenocarcinoma | |

  *Hypoglycemia-producing factors*

| | |
|---|---|
| Hepatocellular carcinoma | Hepatoma |
| Oral melanoma | Plasmacytoid tumor |
| Hemangiosarcoma | Lymphoma |
| Salivary gland | Leiomyosarcoma |
|   adenocarcinoma | |

  *Erythropoietin*

| | |
|---|---|
| Primary or metastatic | Hepatic tumor |
|   renal tumors | Nasal fibrosarcoma |
| Lymphoma | TVT |

  *ACTH*
    Primary lung tumor

*Hypertrophic Osteopathy*

| | |
|---|---|
| Primary lung tumor | Lung metastases |
| Rhabdomyosarcoma | Esophageal sarcomas |
|   (bladder) | |

*Hematologic-Hemostatic Abnormalities*
  *Anemia*
    Multiple tumors

*Disseminated intravascular coagulation*

| | |
|---|---|
| Hemangiosarcoma | Inflammatory |
| Thyroid carcinoma | carcinoma |
| | Multiple other tumors |

*Leukocytosis*

| | |
|---|---|
| Lymphoma | Multiple other |
| | tumors |

*Thrombocytopenia*

| | |
|---|---|
| Lymphoma | Mast cell tumor |
| Mammary | Hemangiosarcoma |
|   adenocarcinoma | Fibrosarcoma |
| Nasal adenocarcinoma | |

*Hyperproteinemia*

| | |
|---|---|
| Multiple myeloma | Lymphoma |

*Renal Manifestations*
  *Nephrotic syndrome*
    Multiple myeloma
  *Renal disease due to hypercalcemia, amyloid,*
    *paraproteins*
    Multiple tumors

*Fever*
  Multiple tumors

*Neurologic Abnormalities*

| | |
|---|---|
| Lymphoma | Beta cell tumor |
| Myelomonocytic neoplasia | Primary lung tumor |
| Thymoma | |

astinal form of the disease. The incidence of hypercalcemia in veterinary patients is unknown; however, up to 30% of human cancer patients develop this paraneoplastic syndrome sometime during the course of their disease.[33, 34]

There are several mechanisms associated with the development of hypercalcemia in human and animal cancer patients: lytic bone metastases, true hyperparathyroidism that occurs simultaneously with the malignant disease, ectopic tumor-produced parathormone (PTH) or the PTH-related peptide (PTH-rp), tumor-produced prostaglandins ($PGE_1$, $PGE_2$), and tumor-produced osteoclast activating factor (OAF).[2,3,32,33,35,36] PTHrP is a common cause of hypercalcemia in tumors such as lymphoma and anal sac adenocarcinoma.[35,36] The cDNA of PTHrP has been cloned and found to encode a 16,000-Dalton protein in which 8 of 13 amino acids are identical to PTH. Despite identification of the etiopathogenesis of

hypercalcemia in select cases, the cause of the electrolyte abnormality in most animals is unknown. Other differentials that must be considered when an animal is presented for true hypercalcemia (Ca++ > 12 mg/dl) include laboratory error, error in interpretation (e.g. young growing dogs), hyperproteinemia from dehydration, acute renal failure, vitamin D and calcium toxicosis, granulomatous disorders, non-neoplastic disorders of bone, and hypoadrenocorticism.[37]

When an elevated calcium is identified one must first ensure the parameter is not a laboratory error. Then it is important to interpret calcium in relation to serum albumin and the blood pH. A correction formula that takes the albumin into account is as follows:

Adjusted calcium (mg/dl) =
[calcium (mg/dl) − albumin (g/dl)] + 3.5

Acidosis results in an increase in the free, ionized

**Figure 4–1.** Cancer cachexia is a common paraneoplastic syndrome that results in involuntary weight loss despite adequate nutritional intake. Although some dogs become overtly cachectic, most are affected biochemically long before clinical signs are obvious.

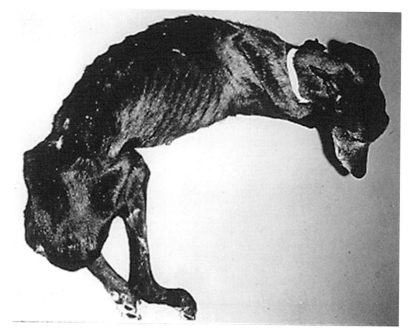

fraction of calcium and can magnify the observed clinical signs associated with hypocalcemia.

The predominant clinical manifestations of hypercalcemia from malignant disease are usually a result of alterations in renal function.[37] The effects of hypercalcemia on the kidney are the most clinically significant, with an inability to concentrate urine noted first. There is decreased sensitivity of the distal convoluted tubules and collecting ducts to pH. The vasoconstrictive properties of calcium decrease renal blood flow and glomerular filtration rate. The epithelium undergoes degenerative changes, necrosis, and calcification. Progressive renal disease is noted clinically as polyuria, polydipsia, vomiting, hyposthenuria, and dehydration. Calcium can also affect the gastrointestinal, cardiovascular, and neurologic systems directly by causing anorexia, vomiting, constipation, bradycardia, hypertension, skeletal muscle weakness, depression, stupor, coma, and seizures.

It may be difficult to diagnose the cause of hypercalcemia that results from malignant disease. Frequently associated laboratory findings include azotemia, normo- or hypophosphatemia, hypercalciuria, hyperphosphaturia, hypernaturia, and decreased glomerular filtration rate as noted during a creatinine clearance study. Table 4–2 reviews the laboratory findings in the more common causes of hypercalcemia.

In each case the primary objective should be identification and specific treatment of the underlying cause of hypercalcemia. Premature and inappropriate administration of symptomatic therapy may interfere with identification of the source of the electrolyte abnormality. This is especially true with premature use of glucocorticoids. The treatment of hypercalcemia that results from neoplastic diseases involves appropriate use of surgery, chemotherapy, radiation therapy, and biologic response modifiers.

Symptomatic therapy is often necessary while searching for the underlying cause or during the time when specific therapy is administered. The overall goals of symptomatic therapy are to increase renal excretion of calcium, inhibit bone reabsorption, promote calcium deposition in soft tissues, and promote external loss of calcium.[37] The severity of the hypercalcemia and the resultant clinical signs dictate the choice of treatment agents and their dosages. The administration of 0.9% NaCl (45–80 ml/kg/24 hrs) intravenously is effective in expanding extracellular fluid volume, increasing glomerular filtration rate, decreasing renal tubular calcium reabsorption, and enhancing calcium and sodium excretion. The loop diuretic furosemide (1–4 mg/kg BID, IV or PO) is often administered concurrently to well-hydrated hypercalcemic patients; the drug inhibits calcium resorption at the level of the ascending loop of Henle. Prednisone (0.5–1 mg/kg BID PO) is very effective in treating hypercalcemia because it inhibits osteoclast activating factor, prostaglandins, vitamin D, and the absorption of calcium across the intestinal tract. The glucocorticoid is also cytotoxic to some tumor cells, notably lymphoma, the most common malignant cause of hypercalcemia. Therefore, caution is indicated when prednisone is administered because the drug may obscure the extent of the tumor and thereby may delay a diagnosis of lymphoma and appropriate therapy. Other treatments that may be considered in unusual cases include:

*Calcitonin.* A dosage of 4 to 8 MRC units/kg SQ can cause a dramatic, rapid reduction in calcium levels that may remain low for days.

*Mithramycin.* This drug can be used at 25 $\mu$/kg IV, once or twice weekly. At higher dosages it has anticancer properties.

*Diphosphonate.* This class of agents is currently being explored as a therapeutic agent for hypercalcemia of malignancy. The drug most commonly used in human medicine is didronel. Early work in human patients with this condition suggests that this class of drug is effective in long-term control of chronic hypercalcemia. Unlike phosphates that bind calcium in the gastrointestinal tract, biphosphonates bind to hydroxyapatite in bone and inhibit the dissolution of crystals.[2]

*Gallium nitrate.* This agent has recently been approved in human medicine for the treatment of hypercalcemia; it appears to inhibit bone resorption by adsorbing to and reducing the solubility of hydroxyapatite crystals.[2] If the hypercalcemia results in renal failure, appropriate steps (aggressive fluid therapy, dopamine, furosemide, dextrose) should be taken to treat that condition.

## Hypoglycemia

Insulinoma is one of the most common causes of hypoglycemia (blood glucose < 70 mg/dl) in the dog. In addition, nonislet cell tumors that are sources of ectopic hormone production also cause hypoglycemia in man and dogs.[38–41] Most nonislet cell tumors associated with the paraneoplastic syndrome of hypoglycemia in the dog are hepatocellular carcinomas; other reported tumors include hepatoma, plasmacytoid tumor, lymphoma, leiomyosarcoma, oral melanoma, hemangiosarcoma, and salivary gland adenocarcinoma.[39–47] In contrast to insulinomas that produce excessive quantities of insulin, hypoglycemia of extrapancreatic tumors in the dog has been associated with low to low normal insulin levels.[39] Possible mechanisms of hypoglycemia in cases of extrapancreatic tumors include secretion of insulin or an insulinlike substance, accelerated utilization of glucose by the tumor, and failure of gluconeogenesis or glycogenolysis by the liver. The most common differential diagnoses of hypoglycemia include hyperinsulinism, hepatic dysfunction, adrenocortical insufficiency, hypopituitarism, extrapancreatic tumors, starvation, sepsis, and laboratory error.

Clinical signs associated with hypoglycemia in companion animals are generally seen when the blood glucose falls below 45 mg/dl. Neurologic signs (weakness, disorientation, seizures that may progress to convulsions, coma, death) predominate because carbohydrate reserve is limited in neural tissue and brain function depends on an adequate quantity of glucose. Hypoglycemia is a potent stimulus for the release of catecholamines, growth hormone, glucocorticoids, and glucagon. These substances tend to compensate for hypoglycemia by promoting glucogenolysis. It is impossible to identify the cause of hypoglycemia in many extrapancreatic tumors. Insulin-producing tumors may be diagnosed by identifying elevated insulin levels in association with low blood glucose concentrations. Periodic sampling during a 72-hour fast may be necessary to identify times when the blood glucose is dramatically reduced with elevated insulin levels. Although controversial, the amended insulin-glucose ratio (AIGR), the glucose-insulin ratio, and the insulin-glucose ratio have been advocated as a method to help

**Table 4–2** Hypercalcemia: Differential Diagnoses

| Disease (Tissue) | Serum CA++ | Serum PO$_4$ | Bone Lesion | Mineralization |
|---|---|---|---|---|
| Primary hyperparathyroidism (parathyroid tumors) | High | Low | ++++ | +++ |
| Vitamin D intoxication | High | High | ± | ++++ |
| Bone metastases (mammary, prostatic tumors, etc.) | High | Normal-elevated | ++++ | − |
| Pseudohyperparathyroidism (lymphoma, nasal tumors, etc.) | High | Low | ± | +++ |

diagnose insulin-producing tumors in domestic animals.[43] The following is the AIGR:

$$\frac{\text{Serum insulin } (\mu U/ml \times 100) = (AIGR)}{\text{Serum glucose (mg/dl)} - 30}$$

AIGR values above 30 suggest a diagnosis of an insulinoma or other insulin-producing tumor. Higher insulin values have been linked to a shorter survival time.

Surgical extirpation is the treatment of choice for tumors that produce hypoglycemia. In the case of insulinomas, a partial pancreatectomy may be indicated; iatrogenic pancreatitis and diabetes mellitus are recognized complications. Advanced stage of disease, high serum insulin concentrations, and younger age are associated with a poor response to therapy. Medical management is often necessary before, during, and after definitive therapy, especially in cases of insulinomas in which the metastatic rate is high. Prednisone (0.5–2 mg/kg divided BID PO) is often effective in elevating blood glucose levels by inducing hepatic gluconeogenesis and decreasing peripheral utilization of glucose.[44] Diazoxide (10–40 mg/kg divided BID PO) is effective in elevating blood glucose levels by directly inhibiting pancreatic insulin secretion and glucose uptake by tissues, enhancing epinephrine-induced glycogenolysis, and increasing the rate of mobilization of free fatty acids.[44,47] Diazoxide's hyperglycemic effects can be potentiated by concurrent administration of hydrochlorothiazide (2–4 mg/kg daily PO). Propranolol (10–40 mg/kg TID PO), a beta-adrenergic blocking agent, may also be effective in increasing blood glucose levels by blocking insulin release through the blockade of beta-adrenergic receptors at the level of the pancreatic beta cell, inhibition of insulin release by membrane stabilization, and by alteration of peripheral insulin receptor affinity.[46] Combined surgical and medical management of pancreatic tumors has been associated with remission times of one year or more.

## Erythropoietin

The glycoprotein hormone erythropoietin is normally produced by the kidney in dogs and cats, and from the carotid bodies of cats. Excessive erythropoietin levels result in increased red cell production by increasing the differentiation of the early stages of red blood cells. Tumors that infrequently induce a pathologic increase in the red blood cell mass by direct or indirect means include renal cell tumors, lymphoma, TVT,

hepatic tumors, and nasal fibrosarcoma.[48–50] A renal tumor mass may cause local kidney hypoxia and induce excess erythropoietin production, which leads to a secondary inappropriate erythrocytosis. Tumors of the kidney may produce erythropoietin directly.[48,49] Other causes of polycythemia include dehydration, pulmonary and cardiac disorders, arteriovenous shunts, Cushing's disease, the chronic administration of adrenocortical steroids, and polycythemia vera.[49] Polycythemia vera is thought to be a myeloproliferative disorder that results from a clonal proliferation of red blood cell precursors.

Erythrocytosis of paraneoplastic origin can be distinguished from polycythemia vera by the absence of pancytosis or splenomegaly and from secondary polycythemia by the absence of decreased arterial oxygen saturation.[1–3,50] Surgical removal of the erythropoietin-producing tumor is the treatment of choice. Phlebotomies may assist in temporary reduction of the red blood cell load. This can be accomplished by withdrawing blood from the patient and readministering the plasma while giving fluids to combat volume depletion. The chemotherapeutic agent hydroxyurea (40–50 mg/kg divided BID PO) can be used to induce reversible bone marrow suppression by inhibiting DNA synthesis without inhibiting RNA or protein synthesis.[1–3,50]

## Other Syndromes of Ectopic Hormone Production

One of the best characterized and most frequently encountered ectopic hormone syndromes in human medicine is the syndrome of inappropriate secretion of antidiuretic hormone (SIADH).[1–3] Although recognized in a variety of cancers in man, it is largely unrecognized in veterinary oncology. The diagnostic criteria for the syndrome of inappropriate secretion of antidiuretic hormone include hypo-osmolality and hyponatremia of extracellular fluids, urine that is less than maximally dilute, absence of volume depletion, sustained renal excretion of sodium, and normal renal and adrenal function.[1–3,5] The clinical signs result from the excess retention of water. Clinical manifestations of this water retention include weakness and lethargy that may progress to seizures, coma, and death. The treatment of choice for SIADH is to eliminate the underlying cause. If clinical signs warrant treatment before or after the tumor is identified or eliminated, the following may be helpful:

*Water restriction.* This procedure is effective

in mild cases when the animal can be watched carefully for over- or underhydration. The objective is to raise the serum sodium while restricting water intake to approximately 66 ml/kg/day.

*Demeclocycline.* This drug antagonizes the actions of ADH on the kidney and therefore causes a reversible nephrogenic diabetes insipidus. In people, nausea, vomiting, skin rashes, and hypersensitivity reactions are potential side effects. Demeclocycline is effective for mild to moderate cases of SIADH. Other drugs such as lithium carbonate and phenytoin are not as effective as demeclocycline.

*Hypertonic sodium chloride.* This intravenous solution is generally reserved for patients that are treated for significant clinical signs related to hyponatremia. The hypertonic solution draws fluid from extravascular sources to dilute the serum sodium. Prolonged use of hypertonic saline can cause clinical manifestations due to lack of water in the extravascular tissues or due to volume expansion of the circulating blood.

The ectopic production of adrenocorticotropic hormone (ACTH) or related polypeptides has been described for a variety of human cancers, including small cell lung cancer, bronchial carcinoids, islet cell tumors of the pancreas, medullary cancer, and pheochromocytoma.[1-3,5] This condition occurs in primary lung tumors in the dog.[51] The syndrome results from excessive production of steroids from normal adrenal glands that are under the influence of the ectopic production of ACTH or ACTH-like substances. Clinical signs seen are similar to those of Cushing's disease; in addition, muscle weakness, lethargy, weight loss, pronounced hypokalemia, metabolic alkalosis, glucose intolerance, and mild hypertension may be identified. The tumors are rarely suppressible with dexamethasone.[1-3,5]

## HYPERTROPHIC OSTEOPATHY

Hypertrophic osteopathy (Fig. 4–2) is a bony disease of dogs and cats, often associated with primary and metastatic lung tumors. Other extrathoracic tumors such as the esophageal sarcoma and rhabdomyosarcoma of the urinary bladder have also been identified with this paraneoplastic syndrome.[5,51-54] Pneumonia, heartworm disease, congenital and acquired heart disease, and focal lung atelectasis have also been implicated in this condition.[52] The disease results in increased peripheral blood flow and periosteal proliferation of new bone along the shafts of long

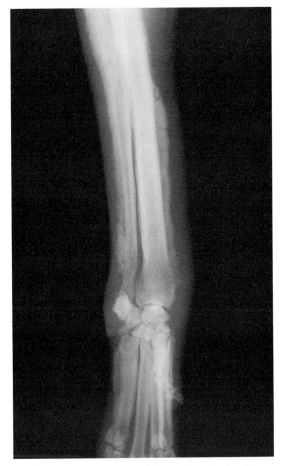

**Figure 4–2.** Hypertrophic osteopathy is a bony disease that results from periosteal proliferation and lameness. The condition is seen with a wide variety of neoplastic and non-neoplastic diseases, including primarily lung tumors.

bones, often beginning with the digits and extending as far proximally as the femur and humerus; occasionally the pelvis and ribs will be affected. Initially there is soft tissue proliferation followed by production of osteophytes that tend to radiate from the cortices at 90 degrees (see Fig. 4–1).[52] The cause of this unique syndrome is unknown; however, successful treatment by vagotomy suggests a neurovascular mechanism that may involve a reflex emanating from the tumor and the nearby pleura that is carried through afferent vagal fibers.[55] Other factors incriminated include hyperestrogenism, deficient oxygenation, and increased blood flow.[56] Prednisone can be used and offers temporary improvement in clinical signs; the glucocorticoid may also reduce the extent of swelling. Removal of the tumor may result in resolution of clinical signs and regression of bony changes. Other treatments such as unilateral vagotomy on the side of the lung lesion, incision through the parietal pleura, subperiosteal rib resection, or bilateral cervical vagotomy, and the use of analgesics have been suggested.[57]

## HEMATOLOGIC-HEMOSTATIC ABNORMALITIES

### Anemia

One of the most common hematologic abnormalities associated with cancer is anemia. It is found in at least 20% of human cancer patients and is a significant problem in cancer-bearing companion animals.[58] The mechanisms associated with the development of anemia are numerous (Table 4–3).[59]

Anemia of chronic inflammatory disease is common in animals with metastatic or disseminated tumors. A shortened erythrocyte life span, disordered iron metabolism, depressed bone marrow response, and disordered iron storage characterize this type of anemia.[58] Anemia of chronic inflammatory disease is recognized clinically as normocytic, normochromic, normal bone marrow cellularity, depressed iron metabolism, and reticuloendothelial iron sequestration. Treatment is directed at elimination of the neoplastic condition.

Blood loss anemia is often seen in many types of cancer and may be recognized when the red blood cells are microcytic and hypochromic because of decreased hemoglobin synthesis. Poikilocytosis, microleptocytosis, inadequate reticulocytosis, increased total iron-binding capacity, decreased serum iron concentrations, and ele-

vated platelet counts may also be seen in this condition.[59,60] The blood loss may be obvious (bleeding superficial tumors) or inapparent (bladder or gastrointestinal tumors). The marked decrease in serum iron concentration may be treated with ferrous sulfate (10–20 mg daily PO) along with appropriate steps to eliminate the tumor.[60] Clinically significant blood loss is treated with blood transfusions.

Microangiopathic hemolytic anemia occurs secondary to hemolysis in the arteriolar circulation and may be a result of damage to arteriolar endothelium or from fibrin deposition within the artery.[58] An important cause of this type of anemia is cancer-induced disseminated intravascular coagulation. Hemolysis and schistocytosis is the hallmark of microangiopathic hemolytic anemia. A variety of tumors, including hemangiosarcoma, have been associated with this condition. Removal of the tumor, transfusions, and appropriate supportive care (intravenous fluids) may be useful for this type of anemia.

Immune-mediated hemolytic anemia is sometimes triggered by the tumors of animals. It results in the premature destruction of red blood cells by immune mechanisms.[61,62] The diagnosis is based on finding antibody or complement on the surface of the patient's red blood cells through a Coomb's test or slide agglutination test, spherocytosis, and a regenerative anemia. Medical management with prednisone ($\leq$ 2 mg/kg daily PO) and azathioprine (2 mg/kg daily for 4 days, then 0.5–1 mg/kg every other day PO) may be indicated if a rapid resolution of the underlying neoplastic condition is not possible.[61] Cyclosporin may also be of value in refractory cases. Contrary to some reports, cyclophosphamide may be of limited value in treating immune-mediated hemolytic anemia and associated conditions in the dog.[63]

Chemotherapy-induced aregenerative anemia is seen in animals with bone marrow hypoplasia of the erythroid or other cell lines and results in a decreased red cell mass, normal erythrocytic indices, and an inadequate reticulocytosis.[58] Chemotherapeutic agents frequently cause a reduction of white blood cells and platelets. The degree of anemia associated with the administration of chemotherapeutic agents is generally mild and not associated with clinical signs.

Other less likely causes of cancer-induced anemia include leukoerythroblastic anemia, hematopoietic dysplasia, hypersplenism, erythrophagocytosis, megaloblastic anemia, and red cell aplasia.[58] Many of the mentioned mechanisms work alone or in concert to induce a

**Table 4–3   Types of Anemias in Cancer-Bearing Small Animals**

Anemia of chronic inflammatory disease
Blood loss anemia
Leukoerythroblastic anemia
Microangiopathic hemolytic anemia
Immune-mediated hemolytic anemia
Hematopoietic dysplasia
Chemotherapy-induced aregenerative anemia
Hypersplenism
Histiocytic medullary reticulosis
Megaloblastic anemia
Red cell aplasia

decrease in red blood cell numbers. Clinical signs related to the anemia can limit the quality of life of the cancer-bearing animal, but they may be overshadowed by the manifestations of the underlying neoplastic condition.

## Leukocytosis

An elevation in the white blood cell count has been seen in people with cancer and in dogs with lymphoma.[64,65] The mechanism of the elevated white blood cell count is obscure but may involve a hematopoietic factor of the tumor or result from tissue necrosis and granulocyte breakdown with positive feedback that initiates an increase in the production of neutrophils or other cell lines.[65] Generally, the condition is not clinically significant.

## Thrombocytopenia

The incidence of thrombocytopenia in tumor-bearing dogs has been reported to be as high as 36%.[62] Mechanisms associated with the decrease in platelet numbers in dogs with cancer include decreased platelet production from the bone marrow, sequestration of platelets in capillaries, increased platelet consumption such as in disseminated intravascular coagulation (DIC), and increased platelet destruction. One investigator reported that platelet consumption was the most significant hemostatic abnormality in tumor-bearing dogs.[66] In addition, decreased platelet numbers and elevated plasma fibrinogen concentrations were most often seen in animals that had extensive tumors of the spleen or marrow.[66] DIC, a common cause of platelet consumption, is seen in 39% of all dogs with the condition.[62] If DIC is suspected, prolongation of clotting times (ACT, OSPT, APTT) and an elevated fibrinogen may be identified along with the thrombocytopenia. Elimination of the neoplastic condition, intravenous fluids, and heparin may be of therapeutic value in these cases.

Immune-mediated thrombocytopenia is also a significant cause of decreased platelet numbers in the dog.[67] The diagnosis of this condition is made by demonstration of antibodies against bone marrow megakaryocytes. Immune-mediated thrombocytopenia has been resolved successfully in the dog by elimination of the tumor and by treatment with immunosuppressive drugs such as prednisone ≥ 2 mg/kg daily) and azathioprine (2 mg/kg daily for 4 days, then 0.5–1 mg/kg every other day).[61]

## Hypergammaglobulinemia

M-component disorders, also known as monoclonal gammopathies, are common in animals with cancer.[68–71] These diseases result from excessive secretion of a single monoclonal line of immuno-globulin-producing cells. IgG, IgA, IgM, and light chain protein classes are produced in large quantities and may be identified by performing a protein electrophoresis on serum.[68] In addition, Bence Jones proteins (light chains) may be identified in the urine.[68] Approximately 75% of the plasma cell tumors in the dog have M-component disorders; other tumors associated with this condition include lymphoma, lymphocytic leukemia, and primary macroglobulinemia.[68] A more complete discussion of this important paraneoplastic syndrome is found in Chapter 28E on multiple myeloma.

## FEVER

Fever that is not associated with infection may be a manifestation of malignant disease. The increased body temperature may be mediated by a tumor-produced lymphokine (e.g., interleukin 1) or reactive macrophages that release lymphokines (IL-6) in response to the tumor. Although the incidence of cancer-associated fever is unknown in animals, up to 40% of people who presented with fever of unknown origin are found to have cancer.[1,5] Fever that is directly related to malignant disease can be treated symptomatically with antipyretics or nonsteroidal anti-inflammatory agents. A resolution of the underlying malignant condition usually results in disappearance of the fever.

## NEUROLOGIC ABNORMALITIES

The remote effects of cancer on the nervous system result in a wide variety of clinical signs. To be a true paraneoplastic syndrome, these conditions must not result from tumors that directly involve the nervous system. The cause of these neurologic syndromes is not well understood. There are several reports in the veterinary literature of cancer-induced peripheral neuropathies, including a case of trigeminal nerve paralysis and Horner's syndrome in the dog.[72–80] Animals also exhibit neurologic signs secondary to endocrine, fluid, and electrolyte disturbances that result from neoplasia. Hypercalcemia, hyperviscosity syndrome, and hepatoencephalopathy are common examples.

The neurologic syndromes of myasthenia gravis (e.g. megaesophagus, acetyl cholinesterase-responsive neuropathy) secondary to thymoma are well described in the literature. Elimination of the neoplastic condition may result in the resolution of these neurologic syndromes.

## REFERENCES

1. Hall TC: Paraneoplastic syndromes. Ann NY Acad Sci 230:1–577, 1974.
2. Odell WD, Wolfsen AR: Hormonal syndromes associated with cancer. Ann Rev Med 29:379–406, 1978.
3. Blackman MR, Rosen SW, Weintraub BD: Ectopic hormones. Ann Intern Med 23:85–113, 1978.
4. Ogilvie GK, Vail DM: Nutrition and cancer: Recent developments. In Couto GM (ed): Clinical Management of the Cancer Patient. Vet Clin North Am, Small Anim Pract 20:1–15, 1990.
5. Ogilvie GK: Paraneoplastic syndromes. In Withrow SJ, MacEwen EG (eds): Clinical Veterinary Oncology. Philadelphia, JB Lippincott, 1989, pp. 29–40.
6. Vail DM, Ogilvie GK, Wheeler SL: Metabolic alterations in patients with cancer cachexia. Compend Contin Educ Pract Vet 12:381–387, 1990.
7. Ogilvie GK: Alterations in metabolism and nutritional support for veterinary cancer patients: Recent advances. Compend Contin Educ Pract Vet 15:925–937, 1993.
8. Ogilvie GK, Vail DM, Wheeler SL, Fettman MJ, Salman MD, Johnston DS, et al: Effects of chemotherapy and remission on carbohydrate metabolism in dogs with lymphoma. Cancer 69:233–238, 1992.
9. Vail DM, Ogilvie GK, Fettman MJ, et al: Exacerbation of hyperlactatemia by infusion of LRS in dogs with lymphoma. J Vet Intern Med 4:228, 1990.
10. Vail DM, Ogilvie GK, Wheeler SL, et al: Alterations in carbohydrate metabolism in canine lymphoma. J Vet Intern Med 4:8–11, 1990.
11. Ogilvie, GK, Ford RD, Vail DM, et al: Alterations in lipoprotein profiles in dogs with lymphoma. J Vet Intern Med 8:62–66, 1994.
12. Ogilvie GK, Walters LM, Fettman MJ, et al: Energy expenditure in dogs with lymphoma fed two specialized diets. Cancer 71:3146–3152, 1993.
13. Walters LM, Ogilvie GK, Fettman MJ, et al: Repeatability of energy expenditure measurements in normal dogs by calorimetry. Am J Vet Res 54:1881–1885, 1993.
14. Ogilvie GK, Vail DM: Unique metabolic alterations associated with cancer cachexia in the dog. In Kirk RW (ed): Current Veterinary Therapy XI. Philadelphia, WB Saunders, 1992, pp. 433–438.
15. Ogilvie GK: Paraneoplastic syndromes. In Withrow SJ, McEwen EG (eds): Clinical Veterinary Oncology. Philadelphia, JB Lippincott, 1989, pp. 29–40.
16. Landel AM, Hammond WG, Megiud MM: Aspects of amino acid and protein metabolism in cancer-bearing states. Cancer 55:230–237, 1985.
17. Chory ET, Mullen JL: Nutritional support of the cancer patient: Delivery systems and formulations. Surg Clin North Am 66:1105–1120, 1986.
18. Dorn CR: Epidemiology of canine and feline tumors. J Am Anim Hosp Assoc 12:307–312, 1976.
19. Crowe SE, Oliver J: Cancer cachexia. Compend Contin Educ Pract Vet 3:681–690, 1981.
20. DeWys WD, Begg C, et al: The impact of malnutrition on treatment results in breast cancer. Cancer Treat Rep (suppl) 65:87–91, 1981.
21. Harvey KB, Moldawer LL, et al: Biological measures for the formulation of a hospital prognostic index. Am J Clin Nutr 34:2013–2022, 1981.
22. Herber D, Byerly LO, et al: Pathophysiology of malnutrition in the adult cancer patient. Cancer 58:1867–1873, 1986.
23. Fields ALA, Cheema-Dhadli S, et al: Theoretical aspects of weight loss in patients with cancer. Cancer 50:2183–2188, 1982.
24. Daly JM, Copeland EM, Dudrick SJ: Effects of intravenous nutrition on tumor growth and host immunocompetence in malnourished animals. Surgery 44:655–659, 1978.
25. Chlebowski RT, Herber D: Metabolic abnormalities in cancer patients: Carbohydrate metabolism. Surg Clin North Am 66:957–968, 1986.
26. Landel AM, Hammond WG, Meguid MM: Aspects of amino acid and protein metabolism in cancer-bearing states. Cancer 55:230–237, 1985.
27. Tayek JA, Bistrain BR, et al: Improved protein kinetics and albumin synthesis by branched chain amino acid-enriched total parenteral nutrition in cancer cachexia. Cancer 58:147–157, 1986.
28. Dempsey DT, Mullen JL: Macronutrient requirements in the malnourished cancer patient. Cancer 55:290–294, 1985.
29. McAndrew PF: Fat metabolism and cancer. Surg Clin North Am 66:1003–1012, 1986.
30. Crowe DT: Enteral nutrition for critically ill or injured patients. Part II. Compend Contin Educ Pract Vet 10:719–732, 1986.
31. Hodgkins E: Metabolic alternations and nutritional support in the small animal cancer patient. Monograph, Hill's Pet Products, Topeka, KS, 1987, pp. 1–24.
32. Weller RE, Hoffman WE: Renal function in dogs with lymphoma and associated hypercalcemia. J Small Anim Pract 33:61–66, 1992.
33. Forrester SD, Fallin EA: Diagnosing and managing the hypercalcemia of malignancy. Vet Med 1:26–39, 1992.
34. Cryer PE, Kissane JM: Clinicopathologic conference: Malignant hypercalcemia. Am J Med 65:486–494, 1979.
35. Weir EC, Norrdin RW, Matus RE, et al: Humoral

hypercalcemia of malignancy in canine lymphosarcoma. Endocrinology 122:602–612, 1988.

36. Weir EC, Burtis WJ, Morris CA, et al: Isolation of a 16,000-dalton parathyroid hormone-like protein from two animal tumors causing humoral hypercalcemia of malignancy. Endocrinology 123:2744–2754, 1988.

37. Kruger JM, Osborne CA, Polzin DJ: Treatment of hypercalcemia. In Kirk RW (ed): Current Veterinary Therapy IX. Philadelphia, WB Saunders, pp. 75–90, 1986.

38. Brennan MD: Hypoglycemia in association with non-islet cell tumors. In Service FJ (ed): Hypoglycemic disorders: Pathogenesis, Diagnosis, and Treatment. GK Hall, Boston, 1983, pp. 143–151.

39. Leifer CE, Peterson ME, Matus RE, Patnaik AK: Hypoglycemia associated with nonislet cell tumors in 13 dogs. J Am Vet Med Assoc 186:53–55, 1985.

40. Strombeck DR, Krum S, Meyer D, et al: Hypoglycemia and hypoinsulinemia associated with hepatoma in the dog. J Am Vet Med Assoc 169:811–812, 1976.

41. DiBartola SP, Reynolds HA: Hypoglycemia and polyclonal gammopathy in a dog with plasma cell dyscrasia. J Am Vet Med Assoc 180:1345–1349, 1982.

42. Dunn JK, Bostock DE, Herrtage ME, et al: Insulin-secreting tumours of the canine pancreas. Clinical and pathological features of 11 cases. J Small Anim Pract 34:325–331, 1993.

43. Dyer KR: Hypoglycemia: A common metabolic manifestation of cancer. Vet Med 1:40–47, 1992.

44. Feldman EC: Disease of the endocrine pancreas. In Ettinger SJ (ed): Textbook of Veterinary Internal Medicine. Philadelphia, WB Saunders, 1983, pp. 1615–1649.

45. Hammer AS, Couto CG: Complications of multiple myeloma. J Am Anim Hosp Assoc 30:9–14, 1994.

46. Scandellari C, Zaccaria M, de Palo C, et al: The effect of propranolol on hypoglycemia: Observations in five insulinoma patients. Diabetologia 15:279–302, 1978.

47. Leifer CE, Peterson ME: Hypoglycemia. Vet Clin North Am 14:873–889, 1984.

48. Giger U, Gorman NT: Acute complications of cancer and cancer therapy. In Gorman NT (ed): Oncology. New York, Churchill-Livingstone, 1986, pp. 147–168.

49. Peterson ME, Randolph JF: Diagnosis and treatment of polycythemia vera. In Kirk RW (ed): Current Veterinary Therapy VIII. Philadelphia, WB Saunders, 1983, pp. 406–408.

50. Couto, CG, Boudrieau RJ, Zanjani ED: Tumor-associated erythrocytosis in a dog with nasal fibrosarcoma. J Vet Intern Med 3:183–185, 1989.

51. Ogilvie GK, Haschek WM, Weigel RM, Withrow SJ, et al: Canine primary lung tumors: Prognostic factors for remission and survival after surgery. J Am Vet Med Assoc. 195:109–112, 1989.

52. Brodey RS: Hypertrophic pulmonary osteoarthropathy in the dog: A clinicopathologic survey of 60 cases. J Am Vet Med Assoc 178:1242–1256, 1971.

53. Halaliwell WH, Ackerman N: Botryoid rhabdomyosarcoma of the urinary bladder and hypertrophic osteoarthropathy in a young dog. J Am Vet Med Assoc 165:911–913, 1974.

54. Wandera JG: Further observations on canine spirocircosis in Kenya. Vet Rec 99:348–351, 1976.

55. Daly PA, Chang P, Goodman L, Wiernik PH: Hypertrophic pulmonary osteoarthropathy and metastases from a malignant fibrous histiocytoma. Cancer 45:595–598, 1980.

56. Holing HE: Hypertrophic pulmonary osteopathy. J Thorac Cardio Surg 46:310–321, 1963.

57. Brodey RS: Hypertrophic osteoarthropathy. In Spontaneous Animal Models of Human Disease. San Diego, Academic Press, 1980.

58. Madewell BR, Feldman BF: Characterization of anemias associated with neoplasia in small animals. J Am Vet Med Assoc 176:419–425, 1980.

59. Comer, KM: Anemia as a feature of primary gastrointestinal neoplasia. Compend Contin Educ Pract Vet 12:13–19, 1990.

60. Feldman BF: Management of the anemic dog. In Kirk RW (ed): Current Veterinary Therapy VIII, Philadelphia, WB Saunders, 1983, pp. 395–400.

61. Dodds WJ: Autoimmune hemolytic disease and other causes of immune-mediated anemia: An overview. J Am Anim Hosp Assoc 13:437–441, 1977.

62. Madewell BR, Feldman BR, O'Neil S: Coagulation abnormalities in dogs with neoplastic disease. Thrombo Haemostas 44:35–38, 1980.

63. Ogilvie GK, Felsberg PJ, Harris SW: Short term effect of cyclophosphamide and azathioprine on the selected aspects of the canine immune system. J Vet Immunol Immunopathol 18:119–127, 1988.

64. Crinn D, Meyers RK, Matthews SA: Neutrophilic leukocytosis associated with metastatic fibrosarcoma in a dog. J Am Vet Assoc 186:806–809, 1985.

65. Couto CG: Tumor-associated eosinophilia in a dog. J Am Vet Med Assoc 184:837–838, 1984.

66. Hatgis AM, Feldman, BF: Evaluation of hemostatic defect secondary to vascular tumors in dogs: 11 cases (1983–1988). J Am Vet Med Assoc 198:891–894, 1991.

67. Helfand SC, Couto CG, Madewell BR: Immune-mediated thrombocytopenia associated with solid tumors in dogs. J Am Anim Hosp Assoc 21:787–794, 1985.

68. MacEwen EG, Hurvitz AI: Diagnosis and management of monoclonal gammopathies. Vet Clin North Am 7:119–132, 1977.

69. Forrester SD, Reeford RL: Serum hyperviscosity syndrome: Its diagnosis and treatment. Vet Med 1:48–54, 1992.

70. Cotter SM, Goldstein MA: Comparison of two protocols for maintenance of remission in dogs with lymphoma. J Am Anim Hosp Assoc 23:495–499, 1987.

71. Matus RE, Leifer CE: Immunoglobulin-producing tumors. Vet Clin North Am, Small Anim Pract 15:741–753, 1985.

72. Presthus J, Teige J: Peripheral neuropathy associated with lymphoma in a dog. J Small Anim Pract 27: 463–469, 1976.

73. Carpenter JL, King NW, Abrams KL: Pheochromocytoma in dogs: 13 cases. J Am Vet Med Assoc 191:1594–1596, 1987.

74. Cardinet GH, Holliday TA: Neuromuscular diseases of domestic animals: A summary of muscle biopsies from 159 cases. Ann NY Acad Sci 317:290–313, 1979.

75. Shahar R, Rosseau C, Steiss J: Peripheral polyneuropathy in a dog with functional islet B-cell tumor and widespread metastases. J Am Vet Med Assoc 187:175–177, 1985.

76. Sorjonen DA, Braund KG, Hoff EJ: Paraplegia and subclinical neuromyopathy associated with a primary lung tumor in a dog. J Am Vet Med Assoc 180:1209–1211, 1982.

77. Carpenter JL, Knong NW, Agrams K1: Bilateral trigeminal nerve paralysis and Horner's syndrome associated with myelomonocytic neoplasia in a dog. J Am Vet Med Assoc 191:1594–1596, 1987.

78. Korn TJ, Aromondo MC, Ero HN: Horner's syndrome in dogs and cats (1975–1985). J Am Vet Med Assoc 195:369–373, 1989.

79. Krotze LT, Fix AS, Potthoff AD: Acquired myasthenia gravis and cholangiocellular carcinoma in a dog. J Am Vet Med Assoc 197:488–490, 1990.

80. Bergman PJ, Bryette DS, Coyne BE, et al: Canine clinical peripheral neuropathy associated with pancreatic islet cell carcinoma. J Compar Neurol 5:57–62, 1994.

# 5

# Diagnostic Cytology in Clinical Oncology

## D. J. Meyer

Aspiration cytology was born in this country in the 1930s[1] but was not enthusiastically adopted as it was in Europe, especially Scandinavia.[2] The lag in the clinical use of cytology in the medical profession was largely due to ignorance of its diagnostic utility and the insecurity associated with its interpretation. Veterinary medicine actively endorsed the clinical application of cytology and its incorporation into the curriculum earlier in this country than did the medical profession. The use of cytology in veterinary medicine continues to increase in popularity. This chapter will focus on the value and limitations of cytology for the differential diagnosis of neoplasia.

## THE MICROSCOPE

The microscope is one of the oldest analytic instruments in the clinical laboratory. Even the early crude versions paved the way for the advancement of medical knowledge: Van Leeuwenhoek identified microorganisms, Malpighi mapped the microanatomy of tissues, and Hooke implemented use of the term *cell* in association with his study of the microscopic structure of cork. Improvement in body design, especially binocularity, and optics has enhanced its ease of use. However, illiteracy in the maintenance and effective clinical use of the microscope is common. General suggestions for the selection and use of this critical tool in diagnostic cytology will be made. While there are a variety of "correct" options, users are encouraged to select the one that meets their needs.

It is desirable to have a minimum of two microscopes in a clinical setting. One is dedicated to the examination of "clean" specimens such as hematology and cytology, and the other is used for the evaluations of "dirty" microscopic specimens such as routine fecal parasite examinations and skin scrapings. For the latter specimens, an economical microscope with a limited number and quality of objectives is acceptable. The most frequently used in this setting are the 10× and 40×, with the latter requiring a coverslip for best resolution. In fact, many of these "dirty" specimens can be adequately examined with a 20× objective, which will identify most infectious agents without the use of coverslipping for clarity, and the distance between objective and sample precludes it from touching thick preparations.

Finally, proper alignment and adjustment of the condensing system are often overlooked basics for maximizing the optical value of the microscope. A useful, economical, and nicely illustrated booklet is recommended for this purpose.[3]

### Microscope Objectives

The brand of microscope dedicated for cytologic examinations is less important than the type of objectives. Planachromatic objectives are recommended. They are cost effective yet provide high-quality resolution. Traditionally, most microscopes have 4×-, 10×-, 40×-, and 100×-oil objectives. As mentioned earlier, in most clinical settings, the 4× has no value and the 10× has limited utility. The author finds a combination of a 20×- and 50×-oil to be very "user friendly" for most clinical applications pertaining to hematology and cytology. This combination permits scanning the slide and precludes the need for coverslipping while facilitating the use of immersion oil on all samples without concerns of the 40×-high-dry being inadvertently dragged through the oil. The addition of a 100×-oil amplifies the ability to recognize microorganisms such as bacteria, *Hemobartonella sp.,* and *Ehrlichia sp.*

## MANAGEMENT OF THE SPECIMEN

The dictum "garbage in–garbage out" is well applied to the preparation of the cytology specimen. Even the expert cytologist using the best microscope cannot observe what is not there. A detailed and well-illustrated review of sample management is available.[4] What will be emphasized here is that the quintessence of cytology can only be fully appreciated with an adequate sample that is properly prepared.

Management of the specimen is an "art" that receives minimal attention in most educational systems. Fortunately, educators are beginning to respond to this need.[5] They describe a simple yet pragmatic ex vivo instructional tool. Portions of an organ obtained at necropsy are placed in a container filled with saline. The tissue is aspirated, a slide preparation made, stained, and examined. Some organs suggested for this exercise that easily exfoliate include the liver and lymph node.

Incorporated into this approach is the concept of the "aspirator also serving as the interpreter."[6,7] This author supports this concept and, in clinical settings with a clinical pathologist, active participation for sample acquisition in collaboration with the clinician should occur whenever possible. The advent of ultrasonography has enhanced the use of cytology and, in some cases, the specimen is best obtained by the radiologist as the operator. Nonetheless, the interpreter should be a participant in order to gain as much information as possible pertinent to the sample, to participate in sample preparation, and to understand what information is expected from the examination of the specimen.

### Obtaining the Specimen and Slide Preparation

The oncology dictum "biopsy, biopsy, biopsy"[8] can be adopted for cytology as "aspirate, aspirate, aspirate." The full value of the cytologic examination of tissue cannot be realized unless it is fre-

quently used in the decision-making process instead of continually trying to decide when to use it. In general, body cavity fluids, cutaneous and subcutaneous lumps, lymph nodes, and diffuse organomegaly lend themselves to aspiration cytology. Suggestions for needle and syringe sizes vary and often reflect preference; use what works. A 22-gauge, 1-inch needle and a 6-cc syringe are useful combinations for obtaining many of these specimens. A 2.5-inch, 22-gauge spinal needle with stylet can be used for sampling internal organs. When using a spinal needle, the stylet is removed after the organ of interest is penetrated, a syringe attached, and suction applied. As with other aspiration techniques, the suction is gently relieved *before* the needle is removed from the tissue. It usually will be necessary to remove the needle from the syringe, aspirate 1 to 2 cc of air into the syringe, replace the needle (while holding the tip of the needle over the glass slide), and *gently* expel the specimen. Multiple slide preparations should be made when possible.

In fact, aspiration may not even be necessary for obtaining a diagnostic cytologic specimen from certain tissues. A technique that is based on the principle of capillarity, consequently referred to as fine-needle capillary sampling, is performed by placement of a needle into the lesion without the syringe being attached.[9] Cells are displaced into the cylinder of the needle and subsequently expelled onto a glass slide, as previously described. No statistically significant difference in diagnostic accuracy occurred when comparing this method and the conventional suction technique in human patients.[9] The author has successfully applied the technique to lymph nodes for the diagnosis of lymphoma and cutaneous mast cell tumors. One has the option of subsequently performing the suction technique if the initial specimen is nondiagnostic. One advantage is minimization of blood contamination and possibly reduced risk of cell breakage. Further comparative evaluation of the technique in veterinary medicine appears warranted.

### Dissemination of Neoplastic Cells

The dissemination, or "seeding," of neoplastic cells in the needle tract subsequent to puncture is a risk factor that must be weighed against the benefits of diagnosis and impact on the long-term outcome of the disease process. It seems reasonable to assume that cells are displaced into unaffected tissue with relative frequency during needle biopsy (including aspiration) procedures.[10]

Clinical findings suggest that neoplastic implants subsequent to these procedures are uncommon, probably as a consequence of cytotoxic mechanisms associated with the immune system or the inflammatory response.[11,12] However, despite the low risk, it is prudent to locate the needle track in the field of anticipated surgery so that it is removed along with the lesion.

## Management of Effusions and Bronchoalveolar Washings

The examination of effusions is one of the more important and useful applications of cytology. Since cellularity varies tremendously in these specimens, both direct and sedimentation preparations should be routinely made. The same recommendation is made for specimens obtained by bronchoalveolar washings and lavages. Several direct smear preparations should always accompany fluids that are submitted to an outside laboratory should the question of artifact arise. Again, only general comments are made here regarding management of these specimens.

It is paramount that when a direct slide preparation is made from a fluid specimen, *all* the fluid used for making the cytologic preparation remains on the slide. The excess fluid may contain diagnostic clumps of cells that are discarded into the garbage if dragged off the end of the slide ("edge-of-the-cliff" syndrome).[6] The spreader (pusher) slide should be stopped approximately 1 cm from the end of the specimen slide and the excess fluid allowed to flow slightly backward (toward the start point) and dried. A small hair dryer mounted on a stand facilitates the drying process, especially in geographic locations with high humidity. This technique also serves to concentrate cells in hypocellular fluids.

## Staining the Specimen

Just as making the specimen involves a certain amount of art and practice, the same applies to the staining procedure. The single most common problem observed is an understained specimen. This is especially true for the thicker preparations such as an aspirate from a lymph node. A combination of circumstances contributes to this deficiency. These include inadequate exposure to the staining solutions, dilution and weakening of the solutions over time, and cytology preparations that are too thick.

The marketing dictum "one size fits all" does not apply to the use of Romanowsky-type stains

**Table 5–1** Suggested Procedure for Staining Cytologic Specimens Using Diff-Quik Solutions[a]

| | |
|---|---|
| Fixative: | 60–120 seconds |
| Solution 1: | 30–60 seconds |
| Solution 2: | 5–60 seconds[b] |

Rinse under cold tap water: 15 seconds

Examine staining adequacy using low power; eosinophilia or basophilia can be enhanced by returning to solution 1 or solution 2, respectively, followed by a rinse.

Air dry and examine.

[a]Suggested times are based on fresh stains; with time and use the stains weaken and longer times will be required. Consistently understained specimens are an indication for replenishing with fresh stain.

[b]The shortest times are suggested for hypocellular fluids that are low in protein, such as transudates, cerebral spinal fluids, and urine sediments.

such as Diff-Quik (Baxter Scientific Products, McGraw Park, IL), i.e., five dips in each solution "fits" all cytologic specimens. This is recognized in the medical profession but has received minimal attention in veterinary medicine.[13] Modifications to their recommendations based on clinical experience are found in Table 5–1. General suggestions for successfully staining most specimens include placement in the fixative for at least 60 seconds; 120 seconds for thick preparations such as lymph node and bone marrow. Specimens cannot be overfixed. The length of time for "dipping" in each of the next solutions depends on the age of the stain and the cellularity (thickness) of the sample. The active process of "dipping" ensures exposure of the specimen to stain. Short times are adequate for hypocellular samples that have a low protein content such as transudates, while longer times are required for thick specimens. Subsequent to staining, the preparation is washed under cold tap water for at least 15 seconds to remove stain precipitate and debris. The slide is air-dried, facilitated with a hair dryer, and examined. Understained specimens can be placed in either solution 1 or 2 or both again. An overstained specimen can be tempered by dipping in the fixative several times, although the staining quality sometimes appears to be altered.

## Sample Shipment and Identification

Whether shipping by courier or mailing cytology specimens, the glass slides must be protected by rigid plastic containers or styrofoam. The flat cardboard or plastic slide containers that generally hold two slides are definitely not acceptable for mailing specimens. Cytology slide preparations should never be placed in the same shipping container as formalin-fixed tissues. In fact, making a cytology preparation in the same room as an open formalin container can violate the diagnostic integrity of the specimen. The formalin fumes will alter the staining characteristics and morphology of the cells. Nucleated cell types often stain a bland, nondiscriminate bluish color with poor cellular detail. Erythrocytes often appear greenish-blue.

Glass slides with a "frosted" end on which information pertinent to the patient, labeled with pencil, should be used for all cytologic preparations. The signalment, the aspiration site, and history associated with the lesion should be included. It is rare to hear a pathologist complain that too much information is provided with specimens. Once the results have been reviewed by the clinician, a subsequent phone conversation with the pathologist that provides missing or new information may greatly influence the impact of the findings on a definitive diagnosis, formulation of a prognosis, or direction of further diagnostic strategies.

## EXAMINATION AND CLASSIFICATION OF THE SPECIMEN

> *Dr. Watson:* And yet I believe my eyes are as good as yours.
> *Sherlock:* Quite so. You see but do not observe. The distinction is quite clear.
>
> *Scandal in Bohemia*

While the first part of Holmes' statement is quite true, the latter part requires training and experience to appreciate clearly the important findings and disregard the detractors and artifact. When examining a thoracic fluid that contains neoplastic cells, the untrained eye sees clumps of what appear to be dark-blue cellular structures of unknown identity. The trained eye observes clumps of epithelial cells forming acinar structures consisting of variably sized cells (anisocytosis) with variable nuclear to cytoplasm ratios, variable nuclear size (anisokaryosis), surrounded by basophilic cytoplasm with variable tinctorial intensity compatible with a (adeno) carcinoma. It is from the summation of all the findings present and subsequently observed that a valid conclusion is formed.

## Procedure for Examining the Specimen

The procedure for the microscopic evaluation of the cytology specimen is similar to that used for the hematology slide. The entire specimen is scanned using low-power (10× or 20×) and sample adequacy, stain quality, and unusual findings such as cell clumps or structures are noted. Emphasis is given to the "feathered" end of the slides made from fluid specimens. Once an overall impression of the specimen has been attained, high-power (40× with a coverslip or 50×-oil/100×-oil) is used to define the cell morphology.

Microscopic findings should be routinely and immediately recorded; initial impressions are important to jot down on paper. These initial findings can be expanded or tempered during the detailed examination of the specimen. There are several basic statements that should be addressed for each specimen examined. The statement that should initiate every cytologic description is, "The predominant cell type is _____." Making a commitment to the definition of cell type is a critical first step in defining the cytologic process. If definition of the prominent cell type is problematic, it may be at this point that a decision must be made to seek assistance, with the knowledge that the specimen is of adequate quality.

## Expect the Expected, Anticipate the Unexpected

When a known tissue is aspirated, it should be determined if the specimen is or is not interpreted to be compatible with the expected tissue. Defining the predominant cell type often accomplishes this responsibility. Making observations that support or deny what is cytologically expected is critical to proceeding in the interpretive process. For example, if the tissue aspirate is thought to be from a lymph node and the specimen is compatible with lymphoid tissue, then the subsequent observations are used to classify the lymph node cytologically.[14] However, if the tissue is not compatible with the expected observation of lymphoid constituents, then the specimen remains an unknown and requires additional cytologic definition.

A relatively frequent example of this process is the inadvertent aspiration of the salivary gland instead of the submandibular or retropharyngeal lymph node. The import of this example is intuitive: either the lump expected to be a lymph node has been effaced by a well-differentiated (adeno) carcinoma, or the lump represents a normal salivary gland. The diagnostic dilemma may be accentuated by the clinical setting; either the patient has a unilateral nasal discharge or an oral mass. At other times, the subcutaneous mass thought to be consistent with a lymph node is actually an unexpected nonlymphoid neoplasm or inflammatory process. Again, the involvement of the interpreter in obtaining the specimen is especially valuable when dealing with problematic specimens.

## WHAT IT IS

Figure 5–1 indicates one approach to guiding the decision-making process when examining the cytology specimen. This approach is predicated on the dictum that "common things occur commonly," i.e., inflammatory diseases occur with relative frequency in animals of all ages, while neoplasms tend to occur in older animals. An important application of cytology is for differentiating an inflammatory or reactive process from neoplasia.

## Inflammation

The segmented neutrophil is an easily recognized cell as an indicator of acute inflammation. With time and in certain types of inflammatory processes, the nonsuppurative cell component

increases. It is the *mixture* of macrophages and lymphocytes along with the neutrophil of variable numbers, with or without constituents of the tissue examined, that often defines the chronic inflammatory process. The identification of these cellular sentinels of inflammation guides the attendant differential diagnoses. At times, macrophages (histiocytes) morphologically mimic neoplastic cells. Obtaining a second opinion can be rewarding, or the histologic examination of tissue may be required for the assessment of tissue architecture.

The inflamed/infected neoplasm can be problematic. For ulcerated cutaneous lesions, a biopsy can bring an efficient resolution to any questions. The inflamed effusion that contains hyperplastic mesothelial cells, with or without neoplastic epithelial cells, is also problematic. The ability to deal with these cytologic situations is directly proportional to experience. It is emphasized that the two most important guidelines in dealing with these specimens are to make quality preparations and to obtain professional assistance when bothersome or unidentifiable cells are observed.

## Noninflammatory Lesions

The noninflammatory cytologic specimen may represent either neoplasia or nonneoplastic tissue.

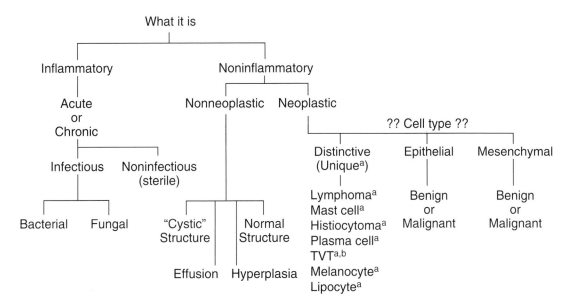

a These have been referred to as discrete or "round cell."
b TVT = transmissible venereal cell tumor.

**Figure 5–1.** Diagnostic approach to the microscopic examination of a cytologic specimen.

Epidermal cysts and adnexal (epithelial-derived) tumors, with or without cystic components, are virtually impossible to sort out with cytology, but their benign nature is usually apparent. The possibility of a normal structure is a consideration, as illustrated by the cytologic faux pas associated with the submandibular salivary gland aspirate described earlier.

**Neoplasia—Distinctive Cell Type**    When a neoplastic cell population is considered, the first goal in cytology is to place the predominant cell type into a general classification (see Fig. 5–1). The easiest group of tumors to define is predicated on their distinctive or "unique" morphologic features. Consequently, this author prefers simply to use the former term for the nomenclature of that classification. The cytoplasmic constituents or features of mast cells, plasma cells, transmissible venereal cell tumors (TVT), melanocytes, and lipocytes are denotative of the cell types in this classification. By default, lymphoma and histiocytoma are included because of their discrete appearance on preparations combined with selected morphologic features used as additional descriptors.

This author avoids the use of the histologically based term *round cell* because neoplastic cells of epithelial derivation can appear round to oval cytologically, obfuscating their classification. *Discrete* has descriptive value, since most, but not all, of those listed in the unique classification generally do not consistently show cell-to-cell cohesion on a cytologic specimen. However, epithelial- and mesenchymal-derived tumors can occasionally appear as discrete (noncohesive) cell preparations cytologically.

**Neoplasia—Epithelial and Mesenchymal Cell Types**    A neoplasm that lacks the criteria for inclusion into the distinctive classification is placed into the epithelial or mesenchymal category. Epithelial cells are generally oval to polygonal and tend to form sheets or clumps. The mesenchymal classification includes connective tissue, skeletal tissue, and vessels (blood and lymphatic). The cell types are spindle to ovoid in shape.

In contrast to the neoplasms listed in the distinctive category, definitive nomenclature of a neoplasm placed into one of these two categories is more difficult and should have lesser import. An important initial goal is to differentiate between benign and malignant tissue. The "variables" listed in Table 5–2 are supportive of this exercise. Histologic examination to assess architecture is often

**Table 5–2**    Morphologic Variables of Epithelial and Mesenchymal Neoplasms Suggestive of Malignancy[40]

Variable cell sizes (anisocytosis)
Variable cell forms (pleomorphism)
Variable cytoplasmic staining intensity
Variable nuclear sizes (anisokaryosis)
Variable nucleolar sizes and shapes (may be multiple)
Variable nuclear to cytoplasm ratio

required for a definitive diagnosis, especially for neoplasms of mesenchymal derivation.

Well-illustrated veterinary[15,16] and medical[17–21] sources, in addition to those already cited, are available for the reader to reflect upon when defining the morphologic criteria for placement into these three classifications.

## DIAGNOSTIC APPLICATION

Defining the use of cytology in oncology is, in some ways, both a pragmatic and philosophical issue. When indications are appropriate (see Chap. 6), an excisional biopsy should be pursued because it permits the assessment of tissue architecture, classification (grade) of selected neoplasms, and examination of tissue margins, and provides the appropriate substrate for immunohistochemistry, special stains, and determination of nuclear ploidy. Incisional biopsy is being increasingly utilized prior to excision, with the goal of defining the need for an aggressive or conservative surgical procedure. However, there are situations when a biopsy is not possible or not needed, or additional information is required to support or deny a surgical strategy. Table 5–3 lists some of the indications for the use of cytology.

### Effusions

Cytology plays a pivotal role in the differential approach for evaluating effusions.[22–24] Figure 5–1 can be effectively applied to this decision-making process. The cytologic findings not only identify neoplastic cells but often suggest cell type. This provides valuable information in determining therapeutic management for some of the more common neoplasms identified in effusions such as lymphoma and carcinomas.

As alluded to earlier, inherent to the examination of effusions is the cytologic incubus of the

**Table 5–3**  Indications for the Use of Cytology

Effusions—thoracic and abdominal

Urine sediments, urinary bladder washing

Vitreous/aqueous infiltrates

Prostate—direct aspirate, washing

Pulmonary/nasal lesion—direct aspirate, bronchoalveolar/nasal washing/lavage

Lymphadenopathy—focal, generalized

Cutaneous/subcutaneous mass, ulcerative lesion

Diffuse organomegaly—liver, spleen, kidney

Unidentified abdominal mass

Evaluation of a mass or lesion discovered intraoperatively

mesothelial cell. This chameleon of cells can take on a variety of morphologic appearances that mimic immature basophilic clumps of epithelial cells, pale-staining vacuolated epithelial cells, and even individual immature basophilic large lymphoblasts. When the decision-making cytologic process is obfuscated by their presence in a possible neoplastic effusion, it is always prudent to get a second opinion. There are times when even the most experienced cytopathologist must acquiesce to indecision. It is emphasized that this potentially problematic cell type in effusions should not cause one to circumvent its cytologic examination.

## Lymphoid Tissue

Aspiration cytology can be effectively applied for the evaluation of lymphadenopathy. Even in humans, the value of the procedure is receiving increased recognition.[25] In veterinary medicine, the most common use is for differentiating between lymphoid hyperplasia (reactive) and neoplasia (lymphoma). This differential diagnosis can be economically and effectively accomplished using aspiration cytology. In addition to the identification of the predominant cell type, i.e., lymphoid, it is critical to characterize the predominant type of lymphocyte. When the small lymphocyte comprises the majority ( > 50%) and variably sized lymphocytes (medium, large, blastic) constitute the remaining population, hyperplasia is defined. Observing a relatively uniform (monotonous) population of predominantly ( > 50%) medium, large, or blastic lymphocytes supports a cytologic diagnosis of lymphoma.

To semiquantitate the cell type proportions, 10 (or more) oil fields of 10 lymphocytes are counted and the percentage of small calculated. Lympho-

cyte size determination is aided by the use of other cell types that may be present in the sample as micrometers. The small lymphocyte with its visibly scant rim of cytoplasm approximates the size of an erythrocyte and is smaller than a neutrophil. Using this criteria as an example, if the majority of the lymphocytes from an aspirate from an enlarged lymph node are relatively monomorphic and larger than a neutrophil, a diagnosis of lymphoma is made.

A similar cytologic strategy can be used to define lymphoma in aspirates from other organs, such as the liver, spleen, and kidney. An additional advantage for the assessment of lymphoma in these organs is that large numbers of lymphocytes are not expected findings; in other words, "What is that cell type doing here?" While lymphomas can be classified cytologically by cell type, it does not appear to have prognostic implications at this time.[26] There are occasions in dogs when there is a sufficiently polymorphous lymphoid picture to cause indecision. The two options are to aspirate a different lymph node (if generalized lymphadenopathy is present) or submit the lymph node for the histologic examination of architecture.

In contrast to the dog, in which lymphoma is a relatively common differential consideration for generalized lymphadenopathy, a caveat must be made for the cat. A syndrome of generalized lymphadenopathy referred to as distinctive lymph node hyperplasia develops in cats, often young adults with or without other clinical signs.[27] Cytologically there can be a marked polymorphic lymphoid picture in which the small lymphocyte is in the minority and huge lymphoblasts are observed. Remarkable erythrophagocytosis usually can be found by adequate scanning.

There can be sufficient distortion of the architecture so that even the histologic examination of the lymph node can be suggestive of lymphoma.[28] The majority spontaneously resolve weeks to months later without subsequent development of neoplasia. Argyrophilic bacteria (silver stain positive), not visible with routine stains, were later identified in some of these cases.[29] Exposure to the feline immunodeficiency virus also has been proposed to be a cause of this exuberant lymphoid reaction.[30, 31]

"What is that cell type doing here?" The examination for metastatic disease can be applied to peripheral and internal lymph nodes enountered before or during surgery. Since a lymph node is cytologically comprised of lymphoid elements, it provides a useful backdrop for the identification of "alien" cells. Multiple specimens should be scanned; a 20× objective is valuable for this task.

Cytology is a useful screening, as well as diagnostic, test for neoplasia when diffuse splenomegaly is present. The more common cell types involved are those that readily exfoliate and are identifiable cytologically. These include mast cell, lymphoma, and myeloproliferative disease.[32,33] Extramedullary hematopoiesis is reported to be a relatively common nonneoplastic cause of diffuse splenomegaly in the dog.[33] Complications associated with the aspiration of a diffusely enlarged spleen are reported to be minimal.[33,34] Undoubtedly, proper presampling assessment of hemostasis and the expertise of the aspirators contributed to the safety of the procedure. The use of ultrasonography for the identification of focal, cavitational lesions is valuable for the characterization of hemangiosarcomas, which are the most common splenic neoplasia in the dog[35] and are not recommended for cytologic evaluation because of their poor exfoliation and potential for "seeding" if leakage occurs.

## Cutaneous and Subcutaneous Lesions

Cutaneous and subcutaneous lesions lend themselves well to cytologic assessment by aspiration or scraping techniques. However, a broad array of disease processes are possible, and the extent to which a decision-making "tree" (see Fig. 5–1) is pursued depends on the experience and philosophy of the aspirator. For some, the value of cytology may be limited to the differentiation of inflammatory and noninflammatory processes. When the latter is identified, an incisional or excisional biopsy is performed. For others, the identification of selected neoplastic cell types is diagnostic.

The experienced cytopathologist can identify an extensive variety of cutaneous and subcutaneous lesions.[36,37] In one study, not surprisingly, the "miscellaneous" group, the same as this author's distinctive classification, with the exception of the lipoma, was correctly diagnosed 88% of the time.[38] The histiocytoma was occasionally misdiagnosed as a malignant mesenchymal tumor, a finding that impacted on the overall diagnostic accuracy for this group. These results are similar to those previously reported.[39] A caveat highlighted in both studies pertains to the use of cytology for the examination of canine mammary gland tissue. Poor correlation with the histologic findings caused most of the false positives and false negatives for discriminating between benign and malignant tissue.[38,39] If cytology is used for the identification of neoplasia in the canine mammary gland, the absence of neoplastic cells should be interpreted with circumspection. Fortunately, the surgical procedure applied to a neoplasm of the canine mammary gland, malignant or benign, does not vary by tumor type and a preoperative diagnosis is rarely necessary (see Chap. 23).

## SUMMARY

The quality of information provided by the cytologic examination of tissues in clinical oncology is directly proportional to the appropriate application of the technique, the quality of sample management, and the expertise of the cytopathologist. The rapid availability of information for an economical investment of time and money makes cytology an attractive diagnostic adjunct for the recognition of neoplasia. The application of cytology is amplified through the use of ultrasonographic and diagnostic imaging techniques. The future appears to be exciting, as the combined talents of the clinician, radiologist, and cytopathologist are blended to maximize the clinical utility of cytology in the management of neoplasia.

## REFERENCES

1. Stewart FW: The diagnosis of tumors by aspiration. Am J Pathol 9:801–813, 1933.
2. Soderstrom N: Fine-Needle Aspiration Cytology. New York, Grune & Stratton, 1966, pp. 1–239.
3. Simpson RM, Meuten DJ: Development of a teaching laboratory aid for instruction of fine needle aspiration biopsy cytology technique. Vet Clin Pathol 21:40–44, 1992.
4. Smith RF: Microscopy and Photomicroscopy: A Working Manual. Boca Raton, FL, CRC Press, 1990, pp. 1–135.
5. Meyer DJ: The management of the cytology specimen. Compend Contin Educ Pract Vet 9:9–16, 1987.
6. Perman V, Alsaker RD, Riis RC: Cytology of the Dog and Cat. American Animal Hospital Association, Denver, CO, 1979, pp. 1–159.
7. Oertel YC: Fine needle aspiration: A personal view. Lab Med 13:343–347, 1982.
8. Withrow SJ: The three rules of good oncology: Biopsy, biopsy, biopsy. J Am Anim Hosp Assoc 27:311–314, 1991.
9. Mair S, Dunbar F, Becker PJ, Du Plessis W: Fine

needle cytology—Is aspiration suction necessary? A study of 100 masses in various sites. Acta Cytol 33:809–813, 1989.

10. Struve-Christensen E: Iatrogenic dissemination of tumor cells. Dan Med Bull 25:82–87, 1978.

11. Smith EH: The hazards of fine-needle aspiration biopsy. Ultrasound Med Biol 10:629–634, 1984.

12. Livraghi T, Damascelli B, Lombardi C, et al: Risk in fine-needle abdominal biopsy. J Clin Ultrasound 11:77–81, 1983.

13. Henry MJ, Burton LG, Stanley MW, Horwitz CA: Application of a modified Diff-Quik stain to fine needle aspiration smears: Rapid staining with improved cytologic detail. Acta Cytol 31:954–955, 1987.

14. Thrall MA: Cytology of lymphoid tissue. Comp Cont Educ Pract Vet 9:104–112, 1987.

15. Cowell RL, Tyler RD: Diagnostic Cytology of the Dog and Cat. Goleta, CA, American Veterinary Publishers, 1989, pp. 1–259.

16. French TW: The use of cytology in the diagnosis of chronic nasal disorders. Compend Contin Educ Pract Vet 9:115–121 1987.

17. Bibbo M: Comprehensive Cytopathology. Philadelphia, WB Saunders, 1991, pp. 1–1101.

18. Kjeldsberg CR, Knight JA: Body Fluids: Laboratory Examination of Amniotic, Cerebrospinal, Seminal, Serous, and Synovial Fluids, 2nd ed. Chicago, American Society of Clinical Pathologists, 1986, pp. 1–190.

19. Takeda M: Atlas of Diagnostic Gastrointestinal Cytology. New York, Igaku-Shoin, 1983, p. 229.

20. Ross DL; Neely AE: Textbook of Urinalysis and Body Fluids. Norwalk, CT, 1983, pp. 1–336.

21. Papanicolaou GN: Atlas of Exfoliative Cytology. Cambridge, MA, Harvard University Press, 1963, pp. 1–438.

22. Else RW, Simpson JW: Diagnostic value of exfoliative cytology of body fluids in dogs and cats. Vet Rec 123:70–76, 1988.

23. Meyer DJ, Franks P: Effusion: Classification and cytologic examination. Compend Contin Educ Pract Vet 9:123–128, 1987.

24. Meyer DJ, Coles EH, Rich L: Effusions. In Veterinary Laboratory Medicine: Interpretation and Diagnosis. Philadelphia, WB Saunders, 1992, pp. 125–133.

25. Gupta AK, Nayar M, Chandra M: Reliability and limitations of fine needle aspiration cytology of lymphadenopathies: An analysis of 1,261 cases. Acta Cytol 35:777–783, 1991.

26. Carter RF, Valli VEO: Advances in the cytologic diagnosis of canine lymphoma. Sem Vet Med Surg 3:167–175, 1988.

27. Moore FM, Emerson WE, Cotter SM, DeLellis RA: Distinctive peripheral lymph node hyperplasia of young cats. Vet Pathol 23:386–391, 1986.

28. Mooney SC, Patnaik AK, Hayes AA, MacEwen EG: Generalized lymphadenopathy resembling lymphoma in cats: Six cases (1972–1976). J Am Vet Med Assoc 190:897–900, 1987.

29. Kirkpatrick CE, Moore FM, Patnaik AK, Whiteley HE: Argyrophilic, intracellular bacteria in some cats with idopathic peripheral lymphadenopathy. J Comp Pathol 101:341–349, 1989.

30. Brown PH, Hopper CD, Harbour DA: Pathological features of lymphoid tissues in cats with natural feline immunodeficiency virus infection. J Comp Pathol 104:345–355, 1991.

31. Rideout BA, Lowenstine LJ, Hutson CA, et al: Characterization of morphologic changes and lymphocyte subset distribution in lymph nodes from cats with naturally acquired feline immunodeficiency virus infection. Vet Pathol 29:391–399, 1992.

32. Spangler WL, Culbertson MR: Prevalence and type of splenic diseases in cats: 455 cases (1985–1991). J Am Vet Med Assoc 201:773–776, 1992.

33. O'Keefe DA, Couto CG: Fine-needle aspiration of the spleen as an aid in the diagnosis of splenomegaly. J Vet Intern Med 1:102–109, 1987.

34. Leveille R, Partington BP, Biller DS, Miyabayashi T: Complications after ultrasound-guided biopsy of abdominal structures in dogs and cats: 246 cases (1984–1991). J Am Vet Med Assoc 203:413–415, 1993.

35. Spangler WL, Culbertson MR: Prevalence, type, and importance of splenic diseases in dogs: 1,480 cases (1985–1989). J Am Vet Med Assoc 200:829–834, 1992.

36. Barton CL: Cytologic diagnosis of cutaneous neoplasia: An algorithmic approach. Comp Contin Educ Pract Vet 9:20–33, 1987.

37. Hall RL, MacWilliams RS: The cytologic examination of cutaneous and subcutaneous masses. Sem Vet Med Surg 3:94–108, 1988.

38. Vos JH, van den Ingh TSGAM, van Mil FN: Non-exfoliative canine cytology: The value of fine needle aspiration and scrapping cytology. Vet 11:222–231, 1989.

39. Griffiths GL, Lumsden JH, Valli VEO: Fine needle aspiration cytology and histologic correlation in canine tumors. Vet Clin Pathol 13:13–17, 1984.

40. Meyer DJ, Franks P: Clinical cytology, Part 2: Cytologic characteristics of tumors. Mod Vet Pract 67:440–445, 1986.

# 6

# Biopsy Principles

Stephen J. Withrow

One of the most important steps in the management of the cancer patient is the procurement and interpretation of an accurate biopsy specimen.[1,2] Not only will the biopsy afford a diagnosis but it will help predict biologic behavior and thus aid in determining the type and extent of treatment that should be afforded. All too often the biopsy is done too casually (or not at all), which may have serious implications for patient management. Virtually all masses should be histologically evaluated before or after removal. If a mass is worth surgical removal, it is worth submitting the tissue for analysis!

Many variations in technique and equipment for biopsy procedures are described in the veterinary literature, but the common goal is to procure enough neoplastic tissue to establish an accurate diagnosis without jeopardizing local tumor control. Many biopsy techniques could be used on any given tissue mass. Which procedure to use will often be determined by your goals for the case (diagnosis and no treatment versus diagnosis and treatment), site of the mass, equipment available, general medical status of the patient, and personal preference and experience. Specific techniques unique to a specific tumor or location will be discussed in their respective chapters.

When should the clinician know what he is treating *before* the actual treatment? The answer to this question is simple but all too often overlooked. An accurate tissue diagnosis should be attained before treatment for most externally accessible masses:

1. Preoperative biopsy is indicated if the type of treatment (surgery versus radiation versus chemotherapy, etc.) or the extent of treatment (conservative versus aggressive resection) would be altered by knowing the tumor type. Certain cancers (e.g., soft tissue sarcomas, oral fibrosarcomas, or mast cell tumors) have high local recurrence rates and therefore require removal with wider margins than benign or low-grade malignant lesions. Several studies in animals and man have shown a positive correlation between permanent local disease control (preferably after the first surgery) and survival. In other words, do the resection correctly the first time. A biopsy is particularly important if the surgery is in a difficult location (e.g., distal extremity, tail, or head and neck) for reconstruction or if the proposed procedure carries significant morbidity (e.g., maxillectomy or hemipelvectomy). Virtually all externally accessible masses, beyond obviously benign skin tumors, should have a tissue biopsy prior to therapeutic operative intervention.

   On the other hand, if knowledge of the tumor type would not change the treatment (lung lobectomy for solitary lung mass, or splenectomy for localized splenic mass) or if the biopsy is as difficult or dangerous as the curative treatment (brain biopsy), then the biopsy information should be attained after the surgical removal.

2. If the owner's willingness to treat his or her pet would be altered by knowledge of the tumor type and therefore prognosis, a biopsy is desirable before major therapeutic intervention. For example, some owners would be willing to do a mandibulectomy for an acan-

thomatous epuli ("benign" but locally invasive oral tumor) with an excellent prognosis but not for a large melanoma with a poor prognosis.

## GENERAL GUIDELINES FOR TISSUE PROCUREMENT AND FIXATION

1. The proper performance of an incisional or needle biopsy does *not* negatively influence survival, even though a short-lived increase in cancer cells can be measured in draining vessels and lymphatics. The advantages of an accurate diagnosis far outweigh the theoretical disadvantage of enhancing tumor metastasis. On the other hand, cancer cells may be allowed to contaminate the tissues surrounding the mass, making resection more difficult. Careful hemostasis and obliteration of dead space will minimize local contamination of the biopsy site. Biopsy sites should not be drained, if possible, because the drain tract can become contaminated with tumor cells. Furthermore, the biopsy site should be planned so that it may be subsequently removed along with the entire mass. During a biopsy procedure care should be taken not to "spill" cancer cells within the thoracic or abdominal cavities, where they may seed pleural or peritoneal surfaces.

2. When biopsies are performed on the legs or the tail, the incision should be longitudinal and not transverse because transverse incisions are much harder to completely resect and obtain primary closure.

3. The junction of normal and abnormal tissue is frequently the best area for the pathologist to see differences in tissue as well as invasiveness. Care should be taken, however, to not incise normal tissue that cannot be resected or would be used in reconstructing the surgical defect. Avoid biopsies that contain only ulcerated or inflamed tissues.

4. The larger the sample, the more likely it is to be diagnostic. Tumors are not homogeneous and usually contain areas of necrosis, inflammation, and reactive tissue. Several samples from one mass are more likely to yield an accurate diagnosis than a single sample.

5. Biopsies should not be obtained with electrocautery because it tends to deform (autolysis or polarization) the cellular architecture. Electrocautery is better utilized for hemostasis after blade removal of a diagnostic specimen or not at all.

6. Care should be taken not to unduly deform the specimen with forceps, suction, or other handling methods prior to fixation.

7. Intraoperative diagnosis of disease states by frozen sections, although not routinely available in veterinary medicine, has enjoyed widespread use in human hospitals. Special equipment and training are required for this technique to be utilized fully. One study in veterinary medicine revealed an accurate and specific diagnosis rate of 83%.[3]

8. If evaluation of the margins of excision is desired, it is best if the surgeon marks the specimen (fine suture on questionable edges) or submits margins in a separate container. An alternate method of orienting the pathologist is the use of ink or various colored dyes.* One method is to paint or dip the lateral and deep margins of an excised mass with india ink, allow it to dry for several minutes, and place it in formalin. When the pathologist reads the slides and sees tumor cells to the black line, you can be certain tumor cells have been left in the patient.[4,5] Different-colored ink can also be used to denote different sites on the tumor, such as proximal margin or deep margin near nerve.

   It is vital that both the pathologist and the clinician communicate well what is required for the accurate assessment of margins. Of course, margin evaluation is necessary only for excisional biopsy or curative-intent surgery and does not apply to needle core biopsies or incisional biopsies, which by definition will have inadequate margins. Incomplete surgical resection of malignant disease is best detected early so that further surgery or other effective adjuvant therapies can be instituted immediately instead of waiting for inevitable local recurrence or metastasis.

9. If you have stainless steel staples in the resected specimen, it is wise to remove them before the tissue is submitted, because they can damage valuable microtomes.

10. Proper fixation is vital. Tissue is generally fixed in 10% buffered neutral formalin with one part tissue to 10 parts fixative. As the technology rapidly expands in the general area of pathology and related fields, the need for special studies on tissue will increase. The clinician may want to call and consult with the pathologist on how to submit tissue for

---

*American Histology Reagent Company, Inc., Lodi, California 95241-2539.

electron microscopy, hormone receptors, tissue culture, flow cytometry, immunohistochemistry, or cytogenetics.

11. Tissue should not be thicker than 1 cm or it will not fix deeply. Large masses can be cut into appropriate-sized pieces and representative sections submitted or sliced like a loaf of bread, leaving one edge intact, to allow fixation. A commonly asked question is how to submit large visceral and especially splenic masses in which 90% of the mass may be hematoma and only 10% is neoplastic. Ideally the entire spleen is submitted, but an alternate approach is to have the surgeon take representative smaller samples from the mass (e.g., soft and hard pieces, red and pale pieces, top and bottom pieces) in the hope that one of them is diagnostic. The rest of the mass can be saved in your clinic in case more tissue needs to be evaluated. After fixation (2–3 days), tissue can be mailed with a 1:1 ratio of tissue to formalin.

12. A detailed *history should accompany all biopsy requests!* Interpretation of surgical biopsies is a combination of art and science. Without all the vital diagnostic information (signalment, history of recurrences, invasion in bone, rate of growth, etc.), the pathologist will be significantly compromised in his or her ability to deliver accurate and clinically useful information.

13. A veterinary-trained pathologist is preferred over a pathologist trained in human diseases. Although many cancers are histologically similar across species lines, enough differences exist to result in interpretive errors.

## BIOPSY METHODS

The more commonly used methods of tissue procurement are needle punch biopsy, incisional biopsy, and excisional biopsy.

### Needle Punch Biopsy

Needle punch biopsy utilizes various types of needle core instruments (Tru-cut* or A.B.C. needle,** etc.) to obtain soft tissue.[1,2] Specialized needle core instruments are used for bone biopsies and will be covered in another section (Chap. 20). The most common instrument used in our hospi-

*Tru-cut biopsy needles, Travenol Labs Inc, Deerfield, Illinois 60015.
**A.B.C. needles, Monoject, St. Louis, Missouri 63103.

tal is the Tru-cut needle. Students practice the use of the instrument on apples prior to the biopsy of an actual tumor. If you cannot biopsy an apple, you won't have much luck on a tumor! These instruments are generally 14-gauge in diameter and procure a piece of tissue that is about the size of the lead in a lead pencil and 1 to 1.5 cm long. In spite of this small sample size, the structural relationship of the tissue and tumor cells can usually be visualized by the pathologist. Virtually any accessible mass greater than 1 cm in diameter can be sampled by this method. It may be used for externally located lesions or for deeply seated lesions (kidney, liver, prostate, etc.) via closed methods or at the time of open surgery.

The most common usage of the needle punch biopsy is for externally palpable masses. Except for highly inflamed and necrotic cancers (especially in the oral cavity) in which incisional

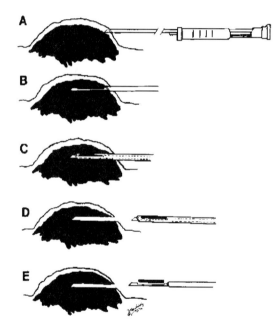

**Figure 6–1.** Mechanism of action of Tru-Cut biopsy needle for typical nodular tumor. *A,* A small skin incision is made with a Number 11 blade to allow insertion of the instrument. With the instrument closed, the outer capsule is penetrated. *B,* The outer cannula is fixed in place and the inner cannula with the specimen notch is thrust into the tumor. The tissue then protrudes into the notch. *C,* The inner cannula is now held steady while the outer cannula is moved forward to cut off the biopsy specimen. *D,* The entire instrument is removed closed with the tissue contained within it. *E,* The inner cannula is pushed ahead to expose the tissue in the specimen notch.

biopsy is preferred, most biopsies can be done on an outpatient basis with local anesthesia and only rarely sedation. The area to be biopsied is clipped and cleaned. The skin or overlying tissue is prepared as for minor surgery. If the overlying tissue (usually skin and muscle) is intact, it is blocked with local anesthetic in the region that the biopsy needle will penetrate. Tumor tissue itself is very poorly innervated and generally does not require local anesthesia.

The mass is fixed in place with one hand or by an assistant. A small 1 to 3 mm stab incision is made in the overlying skin with a scalpel blade to allow insertion of the biopsy instrument. Through the same skin hole, several needle cores are removed from different sites to a get a "cross section" of tissue types within the mass (Fig. 6–1). The tissue is then gently removed from the instrument with a scalpel blade or hypodermic needle and placed in formalin. Samples may be gently rolled on a glass slide for cytologic preparations before fixation. With experience, the operator can generally tell from the appearance of the core sample whether diagnostic material has been attained. Small bits of tissue and fluid will only rarely be diagnostic and usually imply

the need for incisional biopsy. Soft tissue sarcomas in particular may not yield good tissue cores because of necrosis and fibrous septa that often permeate the mass. Sutures are generally not required in the skin hole. Needle biopsy tracts are probably a minimal risk for tumor seeding but if possible are removed intact with the tumor at subsequent resection.

Many of these needles are "disposable" with plastic casings and therefore cannot be steam sterilized. They may, however, be gas (ethylene oxide) sterilized and used repeatedly until they become dull.

Needle core biopsies are fast, safe, easy, and cheap, and they usually can be performed as outpatient procedures. They are generally more accurate than cytology but not as accurate as incisional or excisional biopsy.

## Incisional Biopsy

Incisional biopsy (Fig. 6–2) is utilized when neither cytology nor needle core biopsy has yielded diagnostic material. Additionally, it is preferred for ulcerated and necrotic lesions, since more tissue can be obtained. Many cancers are large, exo-

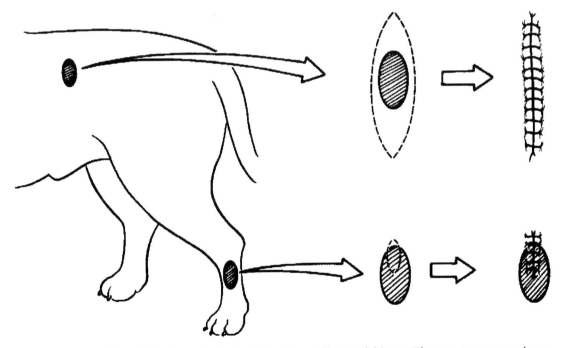

**Figure 6–2.** Excisional (*top*) contrasted with incisional (*bottom*) biopsy. The top tumor may be as easy to remove as to biopsy, and removal may not negatively influence other possible treatments (more surgery, radiation, etc.). The bottom tumor, however, requires knowledge of the tumor type prior to excision because inappropriate removal could compromise a subsequent aggressive excision (short of amputation). Note that the biopsy incision is in a plane that would be included in a subsequent resection.

phytic, and ulcerated. These tumors are very poorly innervated and may be biopsied without the need for local anesthesia or sedation. Under "sterile" conditions, a wedge of viable tumor tissue is removed from the mass. Ideally, a composite biopsy of normal and abnormal tissue is obtained from a location that will not compromise subsequent curative resection. Care should be taken not to widely open uninvolved tissue planes that could become contaminated with released tumor cells. Making small incisions through muscle bellies is preferred to contaminating intramuscular compartments. The incisional biopsy tract is always removed in continuity with the tumor at subsequent resection.

## Specialized Biopsy Techniques

Specialized biopsy techniques will generally be covered under the specific individual tumors. However, some general comments follow.

**Endoscopic Biopsies**   Endoscopic biopsies utilize flexible or occasionally rigid scopes that allow visualization of hollow lumens, especially gastrointestinal, respiratory, and occasionally urogenital systems. Although these techniques are convenient, cost effective, and generally safe, they may suffer from inadequate visualization and limited biopsy sample size when compared to other techniques. An endoscopic biopsy result of ulcerative gastritis in a dog with a firm, infiltrative mass of the lesser curvature of the stomach does not rule out gastric adenocarcinoma.

**Laparoscopy**   Laparoscopic evaluation of the abdomen and occasionally the thorax, when performed by an experienced operator, can yield important information regarding the stage of the disease and can procure tissue for biopsy. The drawbacks of laparoscopy in this author's opinion are that it can take as long as an exploratory laparotomy (both requiring general anesthesia), does not give the operator as good a visualization as open exploratory, cannot provide for excision, carries some danger of hemorrhage or leakage of fluid (bile, urine, tumor cells, or bowel content), and tissue samples will tend to be small. The best indication for laparoscopy is when all staging procedures suggest diffuse and inoperable disease. Animals staged by whatever means as having solitary and potentially resectable disease are often best served by open exploratory laparotomy or thoracotomy whereby more definitive staging and hopefully curative-intent resection can be performed.

**Image-Guided Biopsy**   Diagnostic imaging has greatly expanded the ability to stage various neoplasias and even suggest possible tumor types. In addition, the use of radiographic, ultrasonographic, and computed tomographic guided needle aspirates or core biopsies can avoid the need for more invasive diagnostic procedures. All of the limitations of laparoscopy generally apply, and a careful consideration of the pros and cons of closed guided biopsy should be considered.

"Solitary" lung masses, much like solitary abdominal masses, are best diagnosed and treated by exploratory thoracotomy. Lung masses localizable and adjacent or adherent to the chest wall can be safely aspirated or needle core biopsied with or without imaging. Transgressing the normal lung, pleura, and tumor capsule can result in problems if surgical resection is contemplated. It is generally considered for animals with diffuse inoperable disease in the hope that the diagnosis may help guide selection of chemotherapy.

## Excisional Biopsy

Excisional biopsy is utilized when the treatment would not be altered by knowledge of the tumor type (e.g., "benign" skin tumors, solitary lung mass, solitary splenic mass, retained testicle, etc.). This method is more frequently performed than indicated, but when used on properly selected cases, it can be both diagnostic and therapeutic and is cost effective as well.

## INTERPRETATION OF RESULTS

The pathologist's job is to determine (1) tumor versus no tumor, (2) benign versus malignant, (3) histologic type, (4) grade (if available clinically), and (5) margins (if excisional). Making an accurate diagnosis is not as simple as putting a piece of tissue in formalin and waiting for results. Many pitfalls can take place to render the end result inaccurate. Potential errors can take place at any level of diagnosis, and it is up to the clinician in charge of the case to interpret the full meaning of the biopsy result. As high as 10% of biopsy results may be inaccurate in a clinically significant sense. If the biopsy result does not correlate with the clinical scenario, several options are possible:

1. Call the pathologist and express your concern over the biopsy result. This exchange of information should be helpful for both parties and not looked upon as an affront to

the pathologist's authority or expertise. It may lead to:

a. Resectioning of available tissue or paraffin blocks.

b. Special stains for certain possible tumor types (e.g., toluidine blue for mast cells).

c. A second opinion by another pathologist.

2. If the tumor is still present in the patient, and particularly if widely varied options exist for therapy, a second (or third) biopsy should be performed.

A carefully performed, submitted, and interpreted biopsy may be the most important step in management and subsequent prognosis of the patient with cancer. All too often tumors are not submitted for histologic evaluation after removal because "the owner didn't want to pay for it." Biopsies should not be an elective owner decision. Instead, they should be as automatic as closing the abdomen after ovariohysterectomy (do you okay that with the owner?). The charge for submission and interpretation of the biopsy should be included in the surgery fee if need be, but the biopsy must be done. Because of increasing medicolegal concerns, it is not medical curiosity alone that mandates knowledge of tumor type.

## REFERENCES

1. Withrow SJ (ed): Symposium on Biopsy Techniques. Vet Clin North Am 4(2), W.B. Saunders, 1974.

2. Withrow SJ, Lowes N: Biopsy techniques for use in small animal oncology. J Am Anim Hosp Assoc 17:889–902, 1981.

3. Whitehair JG, Griffey SM, Olander HJ, et al: The accuracy of intraoperative diagnoses based on examination of frozen sections: A prospective comparison with paraffin-embedded sections. Vet Surg 22:255–259, 1993.

4. Rochat MC, Mann FA, Pace LW, Henderson RA: Identification of surgical biopsy borders by use of india ink. J Am Vet Med Assoc 201:873–878, 1992.

5. Parkinson AV, Cannon CR, Hayne ST: Color coding surgical margins with the Davidson marking system. J Histotechnol 13:293–295, 1990.

# 7

# SURGICAL ONCOLOGY

Stephen J. Withrow

Complete surgical removal of localized cancer cures more patients (humans and animals) than any other form of treatment.[1] Before this hope for cure can be realized, surgeons must have a thorough understanding of anatomy, physiology, resection and reconstruction options for all organs, expected tumor behavior, and the various alternatives or adjuvants to surgery. Surgical oncologists should not only be good technicians (cancer carpenters) but dedicated tumor biologists. Surgery will play a role at one point or another in the management of most cancer patients. This surgery may include any of the following: diagnosis (biopsy), resection for cure, palliation of symptoms, debulking, and a wide variety of ancillary procedures to enhance and complement other forms of treatment.

Most patients with cancer are "old." *Old* is a relative term. It is much more important to know the physiologic age of patients than their chronologic age. An "old" dog or cat with normal measurable organ function should not be denied treatment simply on the basis of age. This author is not aware of any cancer in which the older age of the patient has a direct bearing on a tumor-related prognosis. In fact, dogs with osteosarcoma that are less than two years of age do worse than dogs older than two years.[2] "Old" animals will tolerate aggressive surgical intervention as well or as poorly as "young" patients.

## SURGERY FOR DIAGNOSIS

Although biopsy principles are covered in Chapter 6, it must be emphasized that properly timed, performed, and interpreted biopsies are one of the most crucial steps in the management of the cancer patient. Not only does the surgeon need to procure adequate tissue to establish a diagnosis but the biopsy must not compromise subsequent surgical resection.

## SURGERY FOR CURE

Before a surgeon can be in a position to provide the optimal operation for the patient with cancer, the following questions need to be answered:

1. What is the type, stage, and grade (if available and clinically relevant) of cancer to be treated?
2. What are the expected local and systemic effects of this tumor type and stage?
3. Is a cure possible?
4. Is an operation indicated at all?
5. What are the options for alternative treatment?

A recurring theme in surgical management of cancer is that the first surgery has the best chance of cure. Several mechanisms for this improvement in survival have been advanced. Untreated tumors have had less chronologic time to metastasize than recurrent cancer. Untreated tumors have near normal anatomy that will facilitate operative maneuvers. Recurrent tumors may have had seeding of previously noninvolved tissue planes requiring wider resection than would have been required on the initial tumor. If one thinks about a given cancer as resembling a crab, incomplete surgery removes the body of the crab and leaves the legs behind. The "body" of most tumors is often quiescent and hypoxic, whereas the leading edge of the tumor (legs) is the most invasive and well vascularized. Subtotal removal may actually select to leave behind the most aggressive components of the tumor. Patients with recurrent cancer will often have less normal tissue for closure. An ill-defined negative aspect of recurrent cancer is reported to be related to changes in vascularity and local immune responses. Regardless of the mechanism, curative-intent surgery is best performed at the first operation.

The actual surgical technique will vary with the site, size, and stage of the tumor. Some general statements about cancer surgery that need to be emphasized are:

1. All incisional biopsy tracts should be excised in continuity with the primary tumor, since tumor cells are capable of growth in these wounds. Fine-needle aspiration cytology tracts are of minor but not zero concern, whereas punch biopsy tracts are of intermediate concern. With this in mind, all biopsies should be positioned in such a manner that they can be removed at surgery.
2. Early vascular ligation (especially venous) should be attempted to diminish the release of large tumor emboli into the systemic circulation. This is probably clinically meaningful only for those tumors with a well-defined venous supply such as splenic tumors, retained testicles, and lung tumors. Small numbers of cancer cells are constantly being released into the venous circulation by most tumors. Larger, macroscopic cell aggregates may be more dangerous, however, and these may be prevented from vascular escape with early venous ligation.
3. Local control of malignant cancer requires that

variable margins of normal tissue be removed around the tumor. Resection of the "bad from the good" can and should be classified in more detail than radical versus conservative (Table 7–1).[3] Tumors with a high probability of local recurrence (soft tissue sarcoma, high-grade mast cell tumors, feline mammary adenocarcinoma, etc.) should have 2 to 3 cm margins removed three-dimensionally (Fig. 7–1). The tumors are not flat, so wide removal in one plane does not ensure complete excision. Fixation of cancer to adjacent structures mandates the removal of the adherent area in continuity with the tumor. This is commonly seen in oral cancer that is firmly adherent to the underlying mandible or maxilla. Invasive cancer should not be peeled out, shelled out, enucleated, curetted, or whittled on if a cure is expected. Many cancers are surrounded by a pseudocapsule. This capsule is almost invariably composed of compressed and viable tumor cells, *not* healthy reactive host cells. If a malignant tumor is entered at the time of resection, that procedure is often no better than a large biopsy. One should strive for a level of dissection that is one tissue plane away from the mass. For example, invasion of cancer into the medullary cavity of a bone requires subtotal or total bone resection and not curettage.
4. Tumors should be handled gently to avoid the risk of breaking off tumor cells into the operative wound, where they may grow.[4] Copious lavage of all cancer wound beds will help mechanically remove small numbers of exfoliated tumor cells but should not replace gentle tissue handling.

The aggressiveness of resection should only rarely be tempered by fears of wound closure. It

**Table 7–1    Classification of Wound Margins in Cancer Surgery**

| Type | Plane of Dissection | Result |
|---|---|---|
| Intracapsular | Tumor removed in pieces or curetted: "debulking" | Macroscopic disease left behind |
| Marginal | Removal just outside or on pseudocapsule or reactive capsule: "shelled out" | Usually leaves microscopic disease |
| Wide | Tumor and capsule never entered; normal tissue surrounds specimen | Possible skip lesions |
| Radical | Entire compartment or structure removed (e.g., amputation) | No local residual cancer |

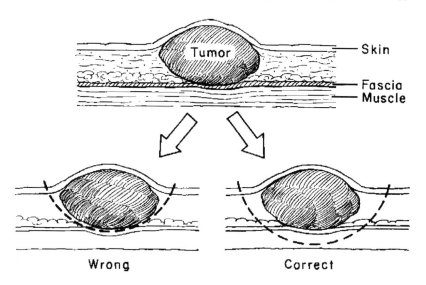

**Figure 7–1.** Typical soft tissue cancer is in proximity to skin and underlying fascia. Inappropriate removal is to "peel it off" the deeper fascia, where microscopic extension is probable. Correct removal entails wide margins three-dimensionally, including overlying skin and underlying fascia.

is better to leave a wound partially open with no cancer than closed with residual cancer. Numerous innovative reconstructive techniques are available for closure of cancer wounds, and the surgeon is only limited by his or her ingenuity.[5]

## LYMPH NODE REMOVAL

A great deal of controversy surrounds the surgical management of regional lymph nodes draining the primary tumor site.[6] As a general rule, epithelial cancers are more likely to metastasize to lymph nodes than are mesenchymal cancers. However, any enlarged regional lymph node requires investigation. Lymphadenopathy may be from metastasis of cancer (firm, irregular, and sometimes fixed to surrounding tissue) or from hyperplasia and reactivity to various tumor factors, infection, or inflammation. The former cause is a poor prognostic sign and the latter may be a beneficial host response. Enlarged lymph nodes as a result of cancer metastasis and invasion are generally uniformly effaced by tumor cells and can often be diagnosed by fine-needle aspiration. Histologically positive lymph nodes usually are a sign of impending emergence of systemic metastasis. Lymph nodes should be removed under two general circumstances:

1. If the lymph node is positive for cancer and not fixed to surrounding normal tissues, it may be possible to remove the node with some therapeutic intent. Frequently, however, many lymph nodes drain a primary tumor site

(e.g., oral cavity) and lymphadenectomy is incomplete (e.g., neck dissection). Lymph node metastasis at the time of initial diagnosis is a poor prognostic sign. However, some patients develop metastasis in a delayed fashion (1 to 2 years) after local tumor control and may benefit from lymphadenectomy. Although it is usually not practical, removal of the primary tumor, intervening lymphatic ducts, and draining lymph node has been recommended (en bloc resection). En bloc resection may be possible for a malignant toe tumor with metastasis to the popliteal lymph node, but is usually only accomplished with amputation. A mastectomy that includes the regional lymph node is another example of en bloc resection. Few other anatomic sites are routinely amenable to this therapy.

A specific instance in which local lymphadenectomy may be beneficial is in removal of sublumbar lymph nodes in patients with metastatic apocrine or sebaceous gland adenocarcinomas of the perineum. Although removal of these lymph nodes is rarely curative, it may help increase the benefit of radiation therapy and should help alleviate, at least in the short term, the paraneoplastic syndrome of hypercalcemia by reducing levels of parathormone or parathormone-like substances.

2. Normal-appearing lymph nodes that are known to drain a primary tumor site should be randomly sampled (biopsy or cytology) to gain further staging information. This is particularly important if adjuvant therapy decisions (irradiation or chemotherapy) would be

predicated on confirmation of residual cancer. Intrathoracic or intra-abdominal lymph nodes are perhaps most crucial, since they are not readily accessible to histologic or cytologic follow-up examination.

Lymph nodes are *not* removed under two general circumstances:

1. Lymph nodes in critical areas (retropharyngeal, hilar, mesenteric) that have eroded through the capsule and become adherent (fixed) to surrounding tissues cannot be curatively removed without serious harm to the patient. They are best biopsied and left in situ or treated with other modalities. The occasional exception is metastasis of limb and foot tumors to prescapular and popliteal lymph nodes, which can be removed with amputation (radical en bloc resection).
2. Prophylactic removal of "normal" draining lymph nodes or chains of lymph nodes (as opposed to sampling for stage) is of no benefit and may be harmful.[6] Regional lymph nodes may in fact be the initiator of favorable local and systemic immune responses, and elective removal has been associated with poor survival in certain human cancers.[6–8]

## PALLIATIVE SURGERY

Palliative surgery is an attempt to improve the quality of the patient's life (providing pain relief or improved function) but not necessarily the length of the patient's life. This type of surgery requires very careful consideration of the expected morbidity of the procedure versus the expected gain to the patient and the client. In essence, it comes down to a decision of when to give up. One of the most difficult decisions in surgical oncology is the decision *not* to operate. Treatment of any kind should never be worse than no treatment.

Certain situations do exist, however, in which palliative surgery may be beneficial. If an infected and draining mammary tumor in a patient with asymptomatic lung metastasis is the limiting factor in the patient's life, mastectomy may still be a logical procedure. Splenectomy for hemangiosarcoma is commonly performed but probably has little impact on survival and can be considered palliative, since it will stop the immediate threat of hemorrhage.

## DEBULKING SURGERY

Incomplete removal of a tumor (planned or unplanned) is referred to as debulking or cytoreductive surgery. It is commonly performed but rarely indicated.[9] Its theoretical indication is to enhance the efficacy of other treatment modalities. Debulking is a practical consideration prior to cryosurgery to decrease the amount of tissue to freeze and the time it will take. It may also help the treatment planning and dosimetry with certain forms of irradiation, but the improved cancer control achieved is more a result of geometric and dosimetry considerations than removal of a few logs of tumor cells. Removing 99.9% of a 1-cm tumor ($1 \times 10^9$ cells) still leaves a million cancer cells behind. Immunotherapy and chemotherapy could theoretically be helped by tumor volume reduction[10] but few well-controlled clinical trials have shown a benefit to date in veterinary medicine. Amputation or limb sparing of dogs with osteosarcoma is essentially a debulking procedure and clearly requires postoperative chemotherapy for prolongation of life. If tumors are debulked with the anticipation of postoperative radiation therapy, the margins of known tumor or the operative field should be marked with radiopaque metal clips to allow proper treatment planning from radiographs.

## SURGERY AND CHEMOTHERAPY

The combined use of chemotherapy and surgery is becoming more common in veterinary oncology. Many chemotherapy agents will impede wound healing to some extent. In spite of this risk, few clinically relevant problems occur when surgery is performed on a patient receiving chemotherapy.[11,12] General recommendations are to wait 7 to 10 days after surgery to begin chemotherapy, especially for high-risk procedures such as intestinal anastomosis.[13] The use of intraoperative or perioperative chemotherapy is receiving increased attention[14,15] and could have greater implications for wound healing.

## SURGERY AND RADIATION

Theoretical advantages can be advanced for both pre- or postoperative radiation.[16] Either way, some impairment of wound-healing potential will exist. Radiation damage to normal tissues (stem cells, blood vessels, and lymphatics) is more permanent than chemotherapy damage. As total radiation dose, dose per fraction, and field size increase, the potential complications (with or without surgery) increase. If radiation therapy is given preoperatively, surgery can be performed after acute radiation reactions have resolved. Postoperative radiation is recommended to start immediately postoperatively or after a 10-to-14-day delay. In spite of the theoretical problems, surgery can be safely performed on irradiated tissues. Complications may occur but are not prohibitive.

## PREVENTION OF CANCER

Certain common cancers in dogs and cats can be prevented. It is well known that early (< 1 year) oophorectomy will reduce the risk of mammary cancer in dogs by 200-fold compared to intact bitches (and, to a lesser degree, cats). Castration of the male dog will help prevent perianal adenomas, possibly prostatic adenocarcinoma and obviously testicular cancer. Removal of in situ squamous cell carcinoma (precancerous) from the skin of white cats or removal of in situ adenomatous polyps from the rectum of dogs may also prevent development of cancer later. Elective removal of cryptorchid testes is another example of preventative surgery.

## MISCELLANEOUS ONCOLOGIC SURGERY

With greater use of regional intra-arterial chemotherapy, surgeons may be called upon to place long-term vascular access catheters. Surgeons and radiotherapists may work together for the operative exposure of nonresectable cancer so that large doses of irradiation may be delivered to the tumor or tumor bed after the exclusion of radiosensitive tissues (Chap. 10).

## DISCUSSION

It is clear that surgery will be the mainstay of cancer treatment in veterinary medicine for many years to come. It is also clear that the mere possibility of a surgical procedure is not the best reason to do it. It was not long ago that surgical resection of the external genitalia was "routine treatment" for dogs with transmissible venereal cell tumors. It is now recognized that chemother-apy alone is curative in more than 90% of dogs and surgery is needed for biopsy only. Although rhinotomy and curettage of nasal cavity cancer can be performed, it does not improve survival over untreated patients.[17] Likewise, simple versus radical mastectomy in the dog and humans does not influence survival but it may in the cat.[18–20] More surgery is not always better surgery. Long-term follow-up of well-staged and graded tumors with defined surgical technique is necessary to demonstrate the true value of any operation. A great deal of progress in surgical technique and surgical thinking needs to take place before the use of surgery can be optimized. It is hoped that better understanding of tumor biology and more precise staging methods (ultrasound, CT scans, MRI, etc.) will enable more precise surgical operations to be performed. In spite of these anticipated advances in technology and biology, however, the most difficult aspect of surgery remains and will always remain surgical judgment.

## REFERENCES

1. Chabner BA, Curt GA, Hubbard SM: Surgical oncology research development: The perspective of the National Cancer Institute. Cancer Treat Rep 68:825–829, 1984.
2. Spodnick GJ, Berg J, Rand WM, et al: Prognosis for dogs with appendicular osteosarcoma treated by amputation alone: 162 cases (1978–1988). J Am Vet Med Assoc 200:995–999, 1992.
3. Enneking WF: Musculoskeletal Tumor Surgery. New York, Churchill-Livingstone, 1983.
4. Gilson SD, Stone EA: Surgically induced tumor seeding in eight dogs and two cats. J Am Vet Med Assoc 196:1811–1815, 1990.
5. Pavletic M: Atlas of Small Animal Reconstructive Surgery. Philadelphia, JB Lippincott, 1993.
6. Cady B: Lymph node metastases: Indicators, but not governors of survival. Arch Surg 119:1067–1072, 1984.
7. Olson RM, Woods JE, Soule EH: Regional lymph node management and outcome in 100 patients with head and neck melanoma. Am J Surg 142:470–473, 1981.
8. Veronesi U, Adamus J, Bandiera DC, Brennhovd IO, et al: Delayed regional lymph node dissection in Stage I melanoma of the skin of the lower extremities. Cancer 49:2420–2430, 1982.
9. Moore GE: Debunking debulking. Surg Gyn Obstet 150:395–396, 1980.
10. Morton DL: Changing concepts of cancer surgery: Surgery as immunotherapy. Am J Surg 135:367–371, 1978.
11. Ferguson MK: The effect of antineoplastic agents

on wound healing. Surg Gyn Obstet *154:*421–429, 1982.

12. Graves G, Cunningham P, Raaf JH: Effect of chemotherapy on the healing of surgical wounds. Clin Bull *10:*144–149, 1980.

13. Laing EJ: The effects of antineoplastic agents on wound healing: Guidelines for combined use of surgery and chemotherapy. Compend Contin Educ Pract Vet *11:*136–143, 1989.

14. Fisher B, Gunduz N, Saffer EA: Influence of the interval between primary tumor removal and chemotherapy on kinetics and growth of metastases. Cancer Res *43:*1488–1492, 1983.

15. Fisher B: Cancer surgery: A commentary. Cancer Treat Rep *68:*31–41, 1984.

16. Tepper J, Million RR: Radiation therapy and surgery. Cancer Treat Symp *1:*111–117, 1984.

17. MacEwen EG, Withrow SJ, Patnaik AK: Nasal tumors in the dog: Retrospective evaluation of diagnosis, prognosis, and treatment. J Am Vet Med Assoc *170:*45–48, 1977.

18. MacEwen EG, Hayes AA, Harvey HJ, Patnaik AK, Mooney S, Passe S: Prognostic factors for feline mammary tumors. J Am Vet Med Assoc *185:*201–204, 1984.

19. Golinger RC: Breast cancer controversies: Surgical decisions. Semin Oncol *7:*444–459, 1980.

20. Kurzman ID, Gilbertson SR: Prognostic factors in canine mammary tumors. Semin Vet Med Surg *1:*25–32, 1988.

# 8

# CRYOSURGERY

## Stephen J. Withrow

Cryosurgery is the controlled use of cold temperature to induce cellular death. After an initial intense enthusiasm for its use on a variety of neoplastic and non-neoplastic conditions, its use has settled down to more selected conditions in selected sites.[1] Cryosurgery is not absolutely essential to treat animals with cancer properly. However, it can be a useful addition to conventional therapy because of its speed, predictability, and avoidance of general anesthesia in many settings.

## SOURCE OF CRYOGEN AND EQUIPMENT

Many types of cryogen exist to induce cold temperature in tissue. The most commonly used are nitrous oxide ($N_2O$) and liquid nitrogen ($N_2$). The advantages and disadvantages of these cryogens are summarized in Table 8–1.

Liquid nitrogen is a little more difficult to work with, since it evaporates slowly and usually requires transfer from the dewar (storage container) to the applicator. Nitrous oxide utilizes the same blue tank employed for anesthesia purposes and does not evaporate between uses. Cost per procedure for each cryogen is comparable.

Nitrous oxide is suitable for small (< 1 cm) lesions but is somewhat restrictive because of its lower temperature, speed of freezing, depth of penetration, and lack of effective spray capabilities. On the other hand, it is acceptable for the more common small benign lesion that is frequently treated (skin and eyelid). If one intends to treat larger than 1 cm diameter lesions having a rich blood supply or that are invading bone, liquid nitrogen is a superior cryogen in spite of its more difficult handling properties.

Nitrous oxide machines are usually portable, on wheels, with the tank attached, and they have a variety of probe sizes and configurations. Some models have a spray orifice provided, but this is very ineffective compared to liquid nitrogen. Certain machines also have incorporated into the probe head a thermistor, which documents the

**Table 8–1** Advantages and Disadvantages of the Two Most Commonly Used Cryogens

|  | Liquid Nitrogen ($N_2$) | Nitrous Oxide ($N_2O$) |
|---|---|---|
| Lowest temperature | –196° C | –89° C |
| Availability | Welding firms, medical supply firms, artificial insemination stations | Medical supply firms |
| Storage | Requires a dewar (storage container) and evaporates at 1% per week | Contained in standard blue tank (as for anesthesia purposes) |
| Probe freezing | Yes | Yes |
| Spray freezing | Yes | Poor |
| Depth of freezing | Deep | Shallow |

probe temperature (not tumor temperature). A feature allowing rewarming of the probe tip is also available on some models to allow more rapid detachment of the probe from the tumor after freezing.

Liquid nitrogen machines may be small and portable in a briefcase* or can be purchased with a combination of a dewar and applicator.** Liquid nitrogen may be applied with various probes or with a fine mist or spray. Spray freezing is capable of faster and deeper penetration of tissue per time of application than is probe freezing. Additionally, it has advantages in treating lesions that are not spherical.

Regardless of the cryogen, it is advisable to purchase a temperature-monitoring device with thermocouple needles to monitor temperature in the tumor and normal tissues to be protected. This monitoring is especially important as one is learning the technique and is always used in monitoring the temperature of critical normal tissue (nerves, rectal mucosa, joint capsule, etc).

## MECHANISMS OF CELL DEATH

Much literature exists on the mechanisms of cell death after freezing.[2] In summary, two basic events lead to the death of a cell after freezing:

1. *Direct cellular death.* This occurs in the first few minutes after freezing and results from ice crystal disruption of cellular membranes, electrolyte changes, alteration of cellular proteins, and thermal shock.
2. *Vascular collapse.* Small blood vessels, particularly capillaries, are irreversibly damaged after freezing and subsequently collapse, inducing hypoxia and infarction of frozen tissue. Large and medium-sized arteries, and to a lesser extent veins, are resistant to permanent injury.

The most important factors that influence cell death or survival after freezing are the speed of freezing and thawing, the number of freezes applied, and the coldest temperature reached throughout the tumor.

Fast freezing and slow thawing are most lethal to mammalian cells. The time to reach the coldest temperature is influenced by many factors, including cryogen (liquid nitrogen is fastest) and tumor/host variables. Local factors that slow

*Cryogun, Brymill Corp., Vernon, Connecticut 06066.
**CS-76, Frigitronics, Shelton, Connecticut 06484.

down the freezing process are high vascularity, density (bone is harder to freeze than soft tissue), and large volume.

The number of freezes applied per treatment session is important. Most small benign tumors are treated twice at the same sitting (freeze-thaw, freeze-thaw), while malignant, vascular, dense, or large tumors are generally treated three times. Little advantage in cell kill is gained by more than three freezes to the same volume of tissue.

A general lethal temperature for most mammalian cells is stated to be –20° C. This minimum temperature is desired throughout the tumor. Colder temperatures are desirable when possible. The time that the tissue is maintained at a given temperature is not a crucial factor in cell death.

## GENERAL TECHNIQUE[1,3]

The treatment of externally accessible tumors (e.g., skin and anus) may be done under local anesthesia only. The treatment of other tumor sites may require sedation (eyelid) or general anesthesia (oral cavity) for adequate restraint of the patient.

A minimal clip of surrounding hair and application of an antiseptic are performed. The tumor is then biopsied and debulked of redundant tissue. Exposed hemorrhagic tumor tissue may be coagulated with silver nitrate or a suture ligature applied to the base of pedunculated lesions. Sterile placement of this ligature is not necessary because it will slough with the frozen tumor tissue. The ligature provides the additional advantage of providing a "tourniquet" to decrease rewarming by the host. If convenient, debulking can be performed, because it will decrease the freezing time and allow colder temperatures to reach the tumor margins. Freezing a large tumor to depth has no advantage to freezing the margins to depth after debulking.

Once the tumor has been biopsied, it can be frozen by probe or spray. Probe freezing is adequate for smaller lesions, which are more or less spherical, since the ensuing ice ball is spherical. The ratio of probe size to tumor should approach 1. This facilitates a faster freeze of tumor tissue. Warm probes should be applied to a warm moist tumor surface, and freezing is begun. A bond of the probe to the tumor (cryoadhesion) will rapidly ensue, and this bond is maintained throughout the freeze (30 seconds to a few minutes). A probe will not adhere to dry, intact epithelium. If the probe prematurely detaches from the tumor, both the probe and the tumor should be allowed to thaw and the process begun again. Once the desired depth of freezing has been achieved, active freezing is stopped. The probe may take several minutes to detach and should not be forcibly detached, because undesirable tissue injury may occur. Once the tumor surface is moist again, the tumor is refrozen.

The author prefers spray freezing with liquid nitrogen to probe freezing, since it is faster, more lethal to depth, and more easily applied to non-spherical lesions. Various-sized spray orifices are provided with most machines. Practice is required to learn how to control the fine spray of liquid nitrogen to just cover the tumor or desired tissue and prevent "run-off." Careful observation and palpation of surrounding tissue is necessary to avoid inadvertent freezing of normal tissue. Insulation (styrofoam cups, vaseline, etc.) is only rarely employed and, in fact, may be dangerous, since it may act as a "cryoprobe" when frozen and cover up frozen tissue below it. Sufficient practice with spraying will virtually eliminate the need for insulators. Practice on gelatin molds or necropsy material should be done before treating patients!

Regardless of whether probe or spray freezing is used, adequate margins of normal tissue should be frozen outside the lesion. These may encompass several millimeters of tissue for benign lesions or as much as a centimeter for malignant lesions. Although thermocouples are ideal for monitoring temperatures in tissue, visual observation and palpation of the "ice ball" are suggestive. The ice ball is anything below 0° C and since mammalian cells are only reliably killed at −20° C, the entire ice ball will not die. Approximately 70 to 80% of the frozen tissue will slough. If you "guess" correctly and freeze the entire tumor to −20° C, the lesion should not recur. If you "guess" wrong, tumor recurrence is likely.

## EXPECTED TISSUE RESPONSE

Immediately after freezing, the patient may experience mild discomfort. This rarely requires pain relief and is absent within 12 hours. The frozen tissue will swell slightly and turn a darker color because of necrosis and collapse of blood vessels. If exposed tissue is present (ulcerated tumor, or biopsy surface) it may ooze a small amount of serum or blood. This usually forms a dry scab within several days. Mucous membrane

sites (oral, eyelid, anus) may have a moist discharge for up to a week or more.

Even though the tissue may "look" infected by standard criteria, antibiotics are not necessary. In essence, the frozen and dead tissue acts like a biologic band-aid, during which time the body is producing bacteria-resistant granulation tissue at the deep junction of dead to viable cells.

Within 10 to 21 days the scab will fall off, exposing a pink bed of epithelium (small lesions) or a reddish bed of granulation tissue, which will contract or epithelialize or both (leaving a small hairless area).

Superficial layers of frozen necrotic bone will generally be adherent and may require debriding 2 or 3 months postfreezing. Hair regrowth may be white or gray on the periphery of the lesion because of the death of melanocytes and preservation of hair follicles.

Owners are instructed to leave the area alone, afford minimal general hygiene, and keep the pet from licking or rubbing the area. Most animals leave the site alone, presumably because of the death of sensory nerves. A routine recheck is requested at 2 to 3 weeks, and subsequent rechecks are determined by the histologic tumor type and its biologic behavior.

## SPECIFIC TUMOR SITES

Although many tumor types and sites have been frozen, experience has suggested four specific sites that may be treated by cryosurgery with predictably successful results (eyelid, perianal, oral, and skin). As a general rule, large, malignant cancers should be frozen only as a last resort because cryosurgery does not afford evidence of surgical margins for pathologic review, and further appropriate treatment must be delayed until recurrence. Additionally, large lesions (greater than 2.5 cm) will have a protracted healing time when compared to surgery. With this in mind, tumor types treated in the following sites are generally benign (or only locally invasive) and small (< 2.5 cm).

### Eyelid[4–6]

Benign tumors of the eyelid (meibomian gland adenoma, papilloma, etc.) are common in older dogs. Although not life-threatening, they may cause problems because of irritation or corneal ulceration. Surgical excision and reconstruction of the eyelid can be performed but often requires general anesthesia and longer treatment time than cryosurgery.

Most patients require light sedation or anesthesia prior to treatment. Local anesthesia at the base of the tumor is usually performed. A chalazion forcep is then applied around the tumor and eyelid, which allows the lid to be held steady and removes it from contact with the globe. Additionally, the forcep acts as a tourniquet, reducing blood flow to the tumor, thus speeding the freezing process.

The excised portion of the tumor is then submitted for biopsy purposes. Silver nitrate should be used with caution to prevent exposure of the conjunctiva to irritation. A cryoprobe (small lesions) or a cryospray is then applied to the tumor and a few millimeters of surrounding eyelid. This is generally a full-thickness freeze. Any length of eyelid may be frozen.

The eyelid is unique in its properties to maintain near-normal cosmetics and function after freezing. The eyelid is supported by a circumferential array of connective tissue called the tarsal plate. After freezing, the tarsal plate remains intact to allow epithelialization while adnexal structures (eyelashes, sebaceous glands, and tumor) die. Most cryosurgery sites are covered with pink epithelium by 2 weeks and have a minimal recession of the eyelid margin. The area will slowly repigment over 3 to 6 months, during which time the cilia will not regrow.

Recurrence rates are less than 5%, which is at least as good as surgery with less anesthesia and surgery time and comparable cosmetics. Large, malignant tumors or tumors fixed to the orbit should generally be excised, including enucleation and orbitectomy, if indicated.

## Perianal[7]

Perianal tumors, the most commonly seen tumors in the older intact male dog (Chapter 18H), are usually perianal adenomas. Cryosurgery can be an effective treatment for isolated and defined lesions that do not encompass more than 180 degrees of the anal circumference.

Since most dogs are under general anesthesia for castration, freezing can be performed at the same time. The superficial aspect of the tumor or a wedge of tissue is removed with a blade, and a suture at the base (ligature or mattress) is applied for hemostasis. The tumor is then frozen with care to avoid extensively freezing the anal and rectal mucosa. No more than 180 degrees of the

anal circumference should be frozen to avoid anal stenosis resulting from fibrosis. Multiple lesions may be frozen as long as they are separated by normal unfrozen tissue.

The resulting eschar may be more moist than most haired skin cryosurgery sites but still does not require antibiotics. Elizabethan collars may be utilized if perineal licking is severe (this is rare).

Local recurrence rates, when combined with castration, have been less than 5%. The advantages of cryosurgery over blade excision are speed, economy, and lack of infection. Deeply invasive cancers, 360 degrees, and malignant cancers should generally not be frozen.

## Oral[8]

Cancer of the oral cavity may invade bone. Eradication of tumor in bone can be accomplished with a variety of methods, including cryosurgery. Freezing is generally applicable to low-grade tumors that are adherent or minimally invasive into one cortex. Full-thickness freezing of the maxilla or mandible will usually result in an oronasal fistula or fracture, respectively. Freezing of normal bone will significantly reduce its breaking strength for a year or more.[9] If the bone can be protected from stress and infection (impossible in the mouth), the full-thickness frozen bone can act like an autograft and become revascularized and viable.

The advantage that cryosurgery has in minimally invasive bone lesions is the destruction of tumor cells within the bone and maintenance of a bony framework for the preservation of function. Tumors with extensive bone fixation or invasion should generally be surgically removed. Freezing of pharyngeal or tonsillar lesions may result in life-threatening edema and swelling.

Under general anesthesia, regional radiographs will help determine the extent of bony invasion. Tumors adherent to underlying bone without evidence of radiographic bone involvement must still be considered invasive into the underlying bone. If the extent of bone invasion does not preclude freezing, the tumor is aggressively debulked and biopsied. The underlying bone is frozen three times with at least a 5 mm margin. The depth of freezing can only be determined by placing a thermocouple into underlying bone through a small drill hole. The depth of freezing in bone will not be as easily accomplished as in soft tissues.

After freezing, the tissue will slough off

rapidly because of abrasion by food and the tongue. A superficial area of dead bone 2 to 3 mm in depth may become necrotic. This will often form a sequestra, which may take several months to fall off or can be electively removed when it becomes loose to the touch. Once the sequestra is removed, healing progresses rapidly.

A rare reported complication is nitrogen embolization.[10] This problem is induced when nitrogen is sprayed under pressure into exposed cancellous bone and expands intravenously. These nitrogen emboli then travel to the right atria and cause cardiovascular compromise and death. Theoretically, cardiocentesis and removal of nitrogen could be beneficial.

Control rates for oral malignancy in the published literature are generally poor. This is largely due to poor case selection (malignant, advanced stage, large), rather than inherent resistance to cryosurgery.

## Skin[11]

Benign skin tumors, particularly in the dog, are perhaps the most common tumor condition in pet animals. Most of these tumors are not life-threatening and treatment is for cosmetic, inflammatory, and occasionally functional reasons. Freezing these tumors is fast, easy, safe, and economical.

A small area around the tumor is clipped of hair to prevent it from matting on the ensuing eschar. The skin and subcutaneous tissue is then infiltrated with a local anesthetic. The top of the tumor or a wedge of tissue is removed for biopsy purposes and the tumor is frozen twice.

Healing may produce white hair on the periphery of the frozen area and small areas of hairless epithelium in the center. Most cryosurgery sites are cosmetically normal.

Large mast cell tumors should not be frozen because rapid degranulation may result in a release of histamine, heparin, and other vasoactive substances, which may induce hypotensive shock. Small mast cell tumors (< 1 cm) may be safely frozen but may have a marked local response.

## DISADVANTAGES OF CRYOSURGERY

Several factors make cryosurgery less desirable than conventional surgery.

1. *Equipment expense.* Initial equipment expense for cryosurgical instruments, thermocouples, and a dewar (if using liquid nitrogen) can run from 500 dollars to several thousand. This investment can be made up in savings from anesthesia, surgical expenses (sterilization, suture, etc.), and time.
2. *Evaporation of liquid nitrogen.* Depending on how many cases are treated per week, the evaporation of liquid nitrogen can be an inconvenience. Since most cases are elective and benign, they can be scheduled and treated every 2 to 3 weeks to coincide with the delivery of the liquid nitrogen.
3. *Aesthetics of necrotic tissue.* Cryosurgery is not as "clean" as blade excision, but if owners are advised in advance of expected responses and the advantages of cryosurgery, few owner complaints will arise.
4. *False hopes for cryosurgery.* Contrary to some published reports, a systemic immunologic response to released or altered tumor antigens killed in vivo, has not been clinically documented.

   Cryosurgery is also not a panacea for untreatable conditions. If a tumor cannot be excised and expected to granulate or epithelialize (e.g., tumors more than one third the circumference of a limb or tail), then granulation, epitheliazation, and ultimate healing will not happen after freezing.
5. *Lack of surgical margins.* Because the deeper levels of tumor invasion are left in situ, the margins of tumor destruction cannot be determined (true for hypothermia and phototherapy as well). For most conditions treated with cryosurgery (small, benign, and not life-threatening) this is not crucial but may allow an undesirable time lapse between incomplete treatment and recurrence of malignancies.

## ADVANTAGES OF CRYOSURGERY

1. *Speed.* Most lesions can be frozen faster than they can be surgically excised.
2. *Expense per treatment.* Although initial equipment expense can be substantial, cost per treatment for consumables (liquid nitrogen or nitrous oxide) is usually less than three or four dollars.
3. *Ease of treatment.* Once some experience has been gained, cryosurgery will be considered easier than surgical excision for most surgeons.
4. *Safety.* Because of the ability to avoid general anesthesia in many cases, the usual risk of general anesthesia is avoided.

## TUMORS, CONDITIONS, OR SITES THAT SHOULD NOT BE FROZEN

1. *Osteosarcoma of long bones.* Although local tumor control may be achieved, secondary fracture through further weakened bone will invariably occur when full-thickness freezing of a long bone is performed.[9]
2. *Intranasal tumors.* Aggressive freezing of intranasal tumors will frequently result in the serious loss of palatine bone and large oronasal fistulas.[12]
3. *Circumferential anus.* The anus (or any body orifice) should not be frozen 360 degrees for fear of inducing a fibrotic stricture of the lumen.[7]
4. *Large mast cell tumors.* Rapid degranulation of killed mast cells may lead to profound hypotensive shock.
5. *Large, aggressive tumors* with life-threatening potential are better treated surgically when possible.

## REFERENCES

1. Withrow SJ (ed): Symposium on Cryosurgery. Vet Clin North Am, Small Anim Pract 10(4), 1980.
2. Hoyt RF Jr, Seim HB III: Veterinary cryosurgery: Mechanisms of cell death, cryosurgical instrumentation, and cryogens. Part I. Compend Contin Educ Pract Vet 3(5):426–436, 1981.
3. Seim HB III, Hoyt RF, Jr: Veterinary cryosurgery. Part II: Principles of application. Compend Contin Educ Pract Vet 3(8):695–702, 1981.
4. Holmberg DL, Withrow SJ: Cryosurgical treatment of palpebral neoplasms: Clinical and experimental results. Vet Surg 8(3):68–73, 1979.
5. Holmberg DL: Cryosurgical treatment of canine eyelid tumors. Vet Clin North Am, Small Anim Pract 10(4):831–836, W.B. Saunders, 1980.
6. Roberts SM, Severin GA, Lavach JD: Prevalence and treatment of palpebral neoplasms in the dog: 200 cases (1975–1983). J Am Vet Med Assoc 189:1355–1359, 1986.
7. Liska WD, Withrow SJ: Cryosurgical treatment of perianal gland adenomas in the dog. J Am Anim Hosp Assoc 14(4):457–463, 1978.
8. Harvey HJ: Cryosurgery of oral tumors in dogs and cats. Vet Clin N Am, Small Anim Pract 10(4):821–830, W.B. Saunders, 1980.
9. Withrow SJ: Application of cryosurgery to primary malignant bone tumors in dogs (phase I study). J Am Anim Hosp Assoc 16:493–495, 1980.
10. Harvey HJ: Fatal air embolization associated with cryosurgery in two dogs. J Am Vet Med Assoc 173(2):175–176, 1978.
11. Krahwinkel DJ, Jr: Cryosurgical treatment of skin diseases. Vet Clin North Am, Small Anim Pract 10(4):787–801, W.B. Saunders, 1980.
12. Withrow SJ: Cryosurgical treatment for nasal tumors in the dog. J Am Anim Hosp Assoc 18:585–589, 1982.

# 9

# CHEMOTHERAPY

Gregory K. Ogilvie

Successful cancer therapy often may involve combinations of surgery, radiation therapy, biologic response modifiers, and chemotherapy. Advances in treatment of animal tumors with chemotherapy are realized virtually every year. New drugs are being explored and new combinations of these agents extend the disease-free interval and survival of many malignant conditions. The successful use of these drugs with maximal efficacy and minimal toxicity depends on the clinician's understanding of the principles and clinical application of chemotherapy. This chapter reviews some of the basic concepts of cancer chemotherapy for the veterinary practitioner.

## PRINCIPLES OF CANCER CHEMOTHERAPY

Before chemotherapy is instituted, the patient should be fully evaluated and stabilized, and the tumor identified histologically and staged to determine the extent of disease. When chemotherapeutic agents are to be employed, the owner and the veterinarian should both have a clear knowledge and understanding of the potential benefits and risks associated with this treatment approach. In addition, the veterinarian should

make a commitment to assist the animal and client if toxicoses are noted.

To utilize chemotherapeutic agents to their fullest advantage, the clinician should be knowledgeable about specific *indications and uses, dosage, timing, resistance,* and *toxicity.* [1–5] Once this crucial information is known, then the drugs should be chosen either alone (single-agent chemotherapy) or in combination (combination chemotherapy).

## Indications and Uses

Chemotherapy should be considered for treatment of a wide variety of tumors, such as in leukemia, lymphoma, pulmonary lymphomatoid granulomatosis, multiple myeloma, and other hematopoietic tumors, or highly malignant tumors that metastasize rapidly (Tables 9–1 and 9–2). [1,4,5] Recent reports document beneficial results when animals with feline and canine mammary neoplasia, canine thyroid carcinoma, squamous cell carcinoma, transmissible venereal tumor, canine hemangiosarcoma, osteosarcoma, and oral malignant melanoma are treated with antitumor compounds (see Table 9–2).

The role of chemotherapeutic agents includes *remission induction* followed by *intensive ther-*

**Table 9–1** Chemotherapeutic Agents Used in Veterinary Medicine

| Name | Brand Name (Manufacturer) | Possible Indications | Suggested Dosages | Toxicity |
|---|---|---|---|---|
| *Alkylating Agents* | | | | |
| Cyclophosphamide | Cytoxan (Mead Johnson) | Lymphoma; various sarcomas; and some carcinomas, including mammary carcinoma | 50 mg/m$^2$ PO 4 consecutive days/wk; 250 mg/m$^2$ weekly or every 3 weeks | Leukopenia, anemia, thrombocytopenia (less common), nausea, vomiting, sterile hemorrhagic cystitis |
| Chlorambucil | Leukeran (Burroughs Wellcome) | Chronic lymphocytic leukemia, lymphoma | 2–8 mg/m$^2$ PO daily | Mild leukopenia, anemia, nausea, vomiting (not common); cerebellar toxicity |
| Nitrogen mustard | Mustargen (Merck Sharp & Dohme) | Lymphoma | 5 mg/m$^2$ IV | Leukopenia, thrombocytopenia nausea, vomiting, anorexia |
| Melphalan | Alkeran (Burroughs Wellcome) | Multiple myeloma, monoclonal gammopathies, lymphoma | 1.5 mg/m$^2$ PO for 7–10 days, repeat cycle | Leukopenia, thrombocytopenia, anemia, anorexia, nausea, vomiting |
| Busulfan | Myleran (Burroughs Wellcome) | Chronic granulocytic leukemia | 4–6 mg/m$^2$ PO daily until white blood cell count approaches normal | Leukopenia, thrombocytopenia, anemia, pulmonary fibrosis (rare in animals) |
| Dacarbazine | DTIC (Dome Laboratories) | Malignant melanoma, various sarcomas | 200 mg/m$^2$ IV for 5 days every 3 weeks | Leukopenia, thrombocytopenia, anemia, nausea, vomiting, diarrhea (often decreases with later cycles) |
| N.N′, N″ triethylenethio-phosphoramide | Thiotepa | Bladder tumors | Bladder instillation: 30 mg/m$^2$ once every 3–4 weeks; remove after 1 hour | Leukopenia |
| *Antimetabolites* | | | | |
| Methotrexate | Methotrexate (Lederle) | Lymphoma, myeloproliferative disorders, various carcinomas and sarcomas | 2.5 mg/m$^2$ PO daily, or 20 mg/m$^2$ IV weekly | Leukopenia, thrombocytopenia, anemia, diarrhea, vomiting, hepatopathy, renal tubular necrosis |
| 6-Mercaptopurine | Purinethol (Burroughs Wellcome) | Lymphoma, acute lymphocytic leukemia, granulocytic leukemia | 50 mg/m$^2$ PO daily until response or toxicity | Leukopenia, nausea, vomiting, hepatopathy |
| 5-Fluorouracil | Fluorouracil (Roche Laboratories) | Various carcinomas and sarcomas | 200 mg/m$^2$ IV weekly | Leukopenia, thrombocytopenia, anemia, anorexia, nausea, vomiting, diarrhea, stomatitis, CNS (dog and cat) |
| | Efudex Cream (Roche Laboratories) | Cutaneous tumors | Apply twice daily for 2–4 weeks | DO NOT USE IN CATS BY ANY ROUTE |
| Cytosine arabinoside | Cytosar-U (Upjohn) | Lymphoma (especially renal lymphomas in the cat), myeloproliferative disorders | 100 mg/m$^2$ SQ or IV drip for 4 days, repeat q3–4 weeks; 600 mg/m$^2$ over 48 hours, repeat in 3–4 weeks; 10 mg/m$^2$ SQ daily or q12h | Leukopenia, thrombocytopenia, anemia, nausea, vomiting, anorexia, bone marrow toxicity |
| *Plant Alkaloids* | | | | |
| Vincristine | Oncovin (Eli Lilly) | Transmissible venereal tumor, lymphoma, mast cell tumor, sarcomas | 0.75 mg/m$^2$ IV weekly | Peripheral neuropathy, paresthesia, constipation, alopecia, perivascular slough |
| Vinblastine | Velban (Eli Lilly) | Lymphoma, various carcinomas | 2.0 mg/m$^2$ IV weekly | Leukopenia, nausea, vomiting, alopecia, perivascular slough |

*(continued)*

**Table 9–1** *(continued)*

| Name | Brand Name (Manufacturer) | Possible Indications | Suggested Dosages | Toxicity |
|---|---|---|---|---|
| *Antibiotics* | | | | |
| Doxorubicin | Adriamycin (Adria Laboratories), generic | Lymphoma, various sarcomas, thyroid carcinoma, mammary carcinoma, hemangiosarcoma | 30 mg/m$^2$ IV every 3 weeks (do not exceed 240 mg/m$^2$ total); 1mg/kg for small dogs, cats | Leukopenia, thrombocytopenia, nausea, vomiting, diarrhea including colitis, cardiac toxicity, reactions during administration, alopecia, perivascular slough |
| Bleomycin | Blenoxane (Bristol Laboratories) | Squamous cell carcinomas, other carcinomas | 10 units/m$^2$ IV or SQ for 3–9 days, then 10 units/m$^2$ IV weekly (do not exceed 200 units/m$^2$ total) | Allergic reactions after administration, pulmonary fibrosis, alopecia |
| Mitoxantrone | Novantrone (Lederle) | Lymphoma, squamous cell carcinoma, bladder tumors, mammary adenocarcinoma | 5.5 mg/m$^2$ (dog); 6.5 mg/m$^2$ (cat) every 3 weeks | Leukopenia, thrombocytopenia, alopecia, vomiting diarrhea |
| Actinomycin | Dactinomycin | Lymphoma, sarcomas | 0.7–1 mg/m$^2$ IV every 2–3 weeks | Bone marrow suppression, gastrointestinal toxicity alopecia, extravasation reaction |
| *Hormones* | | | | |
| Prednisolone | Many available | Lymphoma, mast cell tumors, central nervous system tumors | Vary widely depending on indication: 30–60 mg/m$^2$ PO daily to 20 mg/m$^2$ PO q48h | Hyperadrenocorticism, secondary adrenocortical insufficiency |
| *Miscellaneous* | | | | |
| L-Asparaginase | Elspar (Merck Sharp & Dohme) | Lymphoma | 10,000–12,000 units/m$^2$ IM weekly | Anaphylaxis, coagulation abnormalities, pancreatitis |
| o,p'DDD | Lysodren (Calbiochem) | Adrenocortical tumors | 50 mg/kg PO daily to effect, then 50 mg/kg PO every 7–14 days PRN | Adrenocortical insufficiency |
| cis-platinum | Platinol (Bristol) | Squamous cell carcinoma, osteosarcoma, other carcinomas, germinal cell tumors, transitional cell carcinoma of bladder, nasal adenocarcinoma | 70 mg/m$^2$ IV drip q3wk, 2mg/kg small dogs; saline diuresis before and after treatment required DO NOT USE IV IN CATS | Nausea, vomiting, bone marrow, renal |
| Carboplatin | Paraplatin (Bristol) | Osteosarcoma, squamous cell carcinoma | 300 mg/m$^2$; 135 mg/m$^2$ with caution in cats | Bone marrow, vomiting, diarrhea, alopecia (caution in cats) |
| Hydroxyurea | Hydrea (Squibb) | Chronic myelogenous leukemia | 40–50 mg/kg PO divided BID until white blood cell count returns to normal | Anemia, leukemia, altered nail growth |
| Taxol | Taxol (Bristol) | Mammary carcinoma | Dogs 165 mg/m$^2$ q9.3 weeks to be administered slowly (24 hours) after pretreatment with diphenkydramine, cimetidine, and dexamethasone | Bone marrow, suppression vomiting, diarrhea, alopecia; pruritis during administration |

**Table 9–2**

| Drug | Species | No. of Animals | Overall Response Rate (%) | Complete Response Rate (%) | Median Response Duration (days) | Reference |
|------|---------|----------------|---------------------------|----------------------------|---------------------------------|-----------|
| *Lymphoma* | | | | | | |
| Single Agent Therapy | | | | | | |
| Mitoxantrone | Dogs, cats | 44 | 41 | 30 | 127 | 53–57 |
| Epirubicin | Dogs | 35 | 82 | 74 | 143 | 2, 97 |
| Idarubicin | Cats | 13 | — | — | — | 58 |
| Actinomycin D | Dogs, cats | 12 | 85 | 70 | 42 | 59, 78 |
| Doxorubicin | Dogs | 21 | 85 | 76 | 190 | 50 |
| Combination Therapy | | | | | | |
| LVPCD[a] | Dogs | 55 | 91 | 84 | 252 | 79 |
| CVP | Dogs | 77 | 89 | 75 | 180 | 80 |
| CVPD | Dogs | 46 | 87 | 83 | 210 | 35 |
| VLCM | Dogs | 147 | 94 | 77 | 140 | 36 |
| VLCMP | Cats | 103 | 82 | 62 | — | 81 |
| CVP | Cats | 38 | 94 | 79 | 321 | 34 |
| VCM | Cats | 62 | — | 52 | 112 | 40 |
| *Chronic Lymphocytic Leukemia* | | | | | | |
| Vincristine, chlorambucil, prednisone | Dogs | 20 | 85 | 70 | 340 | 82 |
| *Multiple Myeloma* | | | | | | |
| Melphalan, prednisone | Dogs | 37 | 92 | 42 | 540 | 83 |
| *Transmissible Venereal Tumor* | | | | | | |
| Vincristine | Dogs | 42 | 96 | 96 | Cure | 84 |
| *Thyroid Carcinoma* | | | | | | |
| Cisplatin | Dogs | 10 | 60 | 0 | 143 | 87 |
| Doxorubicin | Dogs | 16 | 18 | 0 | — | 45 |
| *Transitional Cell Carcinoma of Bladder or Urethra* | | | | | | |
| Cisplatin | Dogs | 15 | 20 | 0 | 147 | 90 |
| Doxorubicin, cyclophosphamide | Dogs | 41 | | | 259 | 92 |
| *Mammary Adenocarcinoma* | | | | | | |
| Doxorubicin | Cats | 14 | 64 | | | 51 |
| Doxorubicin, cyclophosphamide | Cats | 14 | 50 | 14 | | 43 |
| *Hemangiosarcoma (Adjuvant)* | | | | | | |
| Doxorubicin, cyclophosphamide, vincristine | Dogs | 15 | | | 172 | 41 |
| Doxorubicin | Dogs | 46 | | | 267 | 98 |
| *Osteosarcoma (Adjuvant)* | | | | | | |
| Cisplatin | Dogs | 5–162 | | | 134–413 | 11, 85–94 |
| Cisplatin doxorubicin | Dogs | 19 | | | 300 days | 62 |
| Carboplatin | Dogs | 48 | | | 257 | 95 |
| Doxorubicin | Dogs | 16 | | | 200 | 96 |

[a]L=L-asparaginase; V=vincristine; P=prednisone; C=cyclophosphamide; D=doxorubicin; M=methotrexate.

*apy* and *maintenance therapy*. Consolidation (treatment to solidify a remission) and maintenance therapies are not commonly used in the treatment of solid tumors. Chemotherapeutic agents can also be used as *adjuvant therapy* to delay recurrence, treat micrometastatic disease, and increase survival time. *Neoadjuvant therapy* is used to decrease the bulk of primary tumors before surgery or radiation. The beneficial effects of chemotherapy are inversely proportional to the amount of tumor to be treated; therefore, for best results (when anticancer drugs are not used neoadjuvantly) the tumor should be reduced to its smallest volume and number of cells before chemotherapy is initiated.

The benefits of single-drug treatment regimens versus multiple-drug regimens include less toxicity and less expenses.[1-4] The disadvantages of a single-drug regimen are decreased efficacy and rapid development of tumor resistance. Multiple-drug treatment protocols in humans are generally more effective and the development of tumor resistance is generally slower than with single-drug treatment regimens. The disadvantages of multiple antineoplastic protocols or approaches are increased cost and toxicity. Chemotherapy was not curative in human oncology until effective combinations were employed. When drugs are used in combination, several important points must be kept in mind.[1-4]

1. Each drug in a combination must be effective when used alone to treat a specific malignancy.
2. To prevent unacceptable toxicity, drugs with overlapping toxicities should be avoided unless they are arranged in a protocol to prevent superimposition of their toxicoses. For example, doxorubicin and cyclophosphamide are both myelosuppressive, with the nadir (lowest portion of the white blood cell count) occurring on approximately the same day when these drugs are given simultaneously. To reduce unacceptable toxicity and myelosuppression when used in combination, the drugs can be used together by altering the dosage or timing of administration.
3. Drugs should be used with an intermittent treatment schedule for maximum efficacy.
4. Maximal acceptable doses of the drugs should be used.
5. Combined chemotherapeutic regimens are most effective when they have different mechanisms of action and act at different

stages of the cell cycle. Examples of treatment and their relationship to the cell cycle include:

a. The plant alkaloids (e.g., vincristine) and taxol inhibit formation of the mitotic spindle and arrest cells in mitosis. Purine and pyrimidine analogs (e.g., cytosine arabinoside) work by inserting a faulty nucleotide sequence into the DNA of the dividing tumor cell during the "s" phase of the cell cycle. These agents work on only one part of the cell cycle and are termed *cell cycle specific.*
b. Alkylating agents (e.g., cyclophosphamide, chlorambucil, melphalan) and antitumor antibiotics (doxorubicin, daunorubicin) affect the cell cycle in a variety of locations and are generally considered *cell cycle nonspecific.*

## Dosage

For maximum therapeutic efficacy, a drug should be used with a dosage that causes minimal toxicity with maximal effectiveness.[1-7] The most effective dose of chemotherapeutic agents is often very close to the toxic dose. In addition, a given dose of drug kills a constant fraction of cells regardless of the number of cells present at the initiation of therapy. Doses of chemotherapeutic agents are often given on the basis of body surface area in square meters ($m^2$ or $m^2$/body surface area, Table 9–3). Three possible exceptions to the dosing of chemotherapeutic agents on a meter-squared basis are melphalan, doxorubicin, and cisplatin. Melphalan is best dosed intravenously on a mg/kg basis because it is not excreted or metabolized in a complex fashion.[8] Doxorubicin is more toxic for small animals (< 10 kg);[9] the metabolism and elimination of this antitumor antibiotic appears to be delayed in small animals when compared to larger animals dosed on a per-meter-squared basis. Finally, small dogs that receive cisplatin are more likely to vomit than large animals.[10] When chemotherapy is dosed on a mg/$m^2$ method, small animals ultimately receive more melphalan, doxorubicin, and cisplatin per pound than large dogs and exhibit more toxicity; it is unknown whether their tumors respond better.

Dosages are modified only when the efficacy of the chemotherapeutic agent can be enhanced or the toxicity diminished. When organ dysfunction delays metabolism or elimination of a drug, alter-

**Table 9–3** Conversion Table to Convert Body Weight (kg) to Body Surface Area (m²) for Dogs[a]

| kg | m² | kg | m² |
|------|------|------|------|
| 0.5 | 0.06 | 26.0 | 0.88 |
| 1.0 | 0.1 | 27.0 | 0.90 |
| 2.0 | 0.15 | 28.0 | 0.92 |
| 3.0 | 0.20 | 29.0 | 0.94 |
| 4.0 | 0.25 | 30.0 | 0.96 |
| 5.0 | 0.29 | 31.0 | 0.99 |
| 6.0 | 0.33 | 32.0 | 1.01 |
| 7.0 | 0.36 | 33.0 | 1.03 |
| 8.0 | 0.40 | 34.0 | 1.05 |
| 9.0 | 0.43 | 35.0 | 1.07 |
| 10.0 | 0.46 | 36.0 | 1.09 |
| 11.0 | 0.49 | 37.0 | 1.11 |
| 12.0 | 0.52 | 38.0 | 1.13 |
| 13.0 | 0.55 | 39.0 | 1.15 |
| 14.0 | 0.58 | 40.0 | 1.17 |
| 15.0 | 0.60 | 41.0 | 1.19 |
| 16.0 | 0.63 | 42.0 | 1.21 |
| 17.0 | 0.66 | 43.0 | 1.23 |
| 18.0 | 0.69 | 44.0 | 1.25 |
| 19.0 | 0.71 | 45.0 | 1.26 |
| 20.0 | 0.74 | 46.0 | 1.28 |
| 21.0 | 0.76 | 47.0 | 1.30 |
| 22.0 | 0.78 | 48.0 | 1.32 |
| 23.0 | 0.81 | 49.0 | 1.34 |
| 24.0 | 0.83 | 50.0 | 1.36 |
| 25.0 | 0.85 | 51.0 | 1.38 |

[a]Most, but not all, chemotherapeutic agents are dosed on a body-surface-area basis.

ations in the dosage should be considered. Table 9–4 reviews some circumstances in which dosage modifications may be indicated for veterinary patients with altered liver or kidney function.[1–7]

## Timing

The timing of the administration of antitumor drugs is critical.[1–7] Unlikely many tumor cells, normal cells have better repair mechanisms that better enable them to correct cellular damage. Therefore, cytotoxic drugs must be given at proper intervals to allow the tumor cells to die while normal cells recover. If the drug dose is not properly timed, excess toxicity or lack of antitumor activity results.

The therapeutic ratio (efficacy : toxicity) can be enhanced by altering either the dosage of the drug or the length of time the malignant cell is exposed to the drug (efficacy = dosage × time).[1–7] As mentioned earlier, the efficacy of a drug is directly related to the time the tumor cell is exposed to the drug. In addition, the acute and short-term toxicoses of a drug are often directly related to the peak serum concentration of that agent. Sustained release of a drug increases the time the tumor is exposed to a drug and also reduces the peak serum concentration of that drug. This important concept is applied clinically with many chemotherapeutic agents that are being formulated in a wide array of sustained-release products. The concept has merit because the active agent can be released over a prolonged period of time to induce very high concentrations locally at the site of injection, which subsequently is released systemically over a prolonged period of time.

One sustained-release formulation that has been used to reduce local recurrence of osteosarcoma in the dog is OPLA-pt (polylactic acid impregnated with cisplatin).[11] Preliminary evidence suggests that this polymer reduces local

**Table 9–4** Effect of Organ Dysfunction on Dosing of Select Chemotherapeutic Agents

| Drug | Organ Failure | Potential Dose Change |
|------|---------------|----------------------|
| Doxorubicin Vincristine Vinblastine | Liver | Consider initial dosage reductions of 50% when bilirubin > 1.5 mg/100 ml; escalate subsequent dosages if acceptable toxicity |
| Carboplatin VP-16 | Kidney | Dosage reduction directly proportional to creatinine clearance; note that the carrier in VP-16 can cause profound hypotension and cutaneous reactions |
| Bleomycin | Kidney | Decrease initial dosage 50–75% if creatinine clearance < 25 ml/min/m² |
| Cyclophosphamide | Kidney (Liver) | Decrease initial dosage 50–75% if creatinine clearance < 25 ml/min/m² (activation of the drug in the liver may decrease efficacy) |
| Cisplatin | Kidney | Do not use with clinically evident renal failure; caution with any renal problems |
| Methotrexate | Kidney | Dosage reduction directly proportional to creatinine clearance |

recurrence of osteosarcoma after limb sparing and delays metastases with minimal toxicity. In other studies, a wide variety of chemotherapeutic agents have been implanted into a protein carrier matrix and a vasoactive drug to treat dogs with oral melanomas.[12] The dogs treated this way developed a complete response (55%) and a partial response (20%). A similar but unrelated method for delivering chemotherapeutic agents over a sustained period of time is by intracavitary therapy. For example, dogs with mesotheliomas can be treated in the thoracic or abdominal cavities by administering cisplatin in saline.[13] The cisplatin is applied as therapy for the tumor lining the body cavity using very high concentrations of drug. In addition, the cisplatin becomes protein bound within the body cavity for later slow release locally and systemically over a prolonged period of time (days to weeks). In contrast, when administered systemically, almost all of the cisplatin is eliminated within 1 day.

## Resistance

The development of resistance to chemotherapeutic agents is, without a doubt, one of the most important challenges facing oncology.[14–17] Biochemical mechanisms of resistance that have been identified include:

1. Decreased drug uptake from the site of administration (e.g., intestinal tract).
2. Decreased drug-activating enzymes for those drugs that require biotransformation (e.g., decreased deoxycytidine kinase that is required to activate cytosine arabinoside).
3. Increased drug-inactivating enzymes (e.g., doxorubicin and alkylating agents are inactivated by glutathione in resistant cancer cells).
4. Increased concentrations of the inhibited target enzyme (e.g., asparagine in the case of L-asparaginase therapy).
5. Altered affinity of the target for the drug (e.g., altered tubulin results in resistance to vincristine).
6. Increased DNA repair (reported for doxorubicin, cisplatin, and alkylating agents).
7. Increase in an alternative metabolic pathway, bypassing the drug inhibition, as with methotrexate.
8. Increase in drug removal from the cell that is seen with the p-glycoprotein pump or altered drug binding to topoisomerase II, which both contribute to the phenomenon known as multiple-drug resistance (MDR).

The use of multiple agents, each with cytotoxic activity for the treatment of a malignancy and each with a different mechanism of action that allows independent cell killing by each drug, will minimize drug resistance.[1–4] The most important of the aforementioned mechanisms is that of MDR resistance. This is mediated in one situation by increased expression of the P-170 membrane glycoprotein, which mediates the efflux of vinca alkaloids, anthracycline antibiotics, actinomycin D, and epipodophyllotoxins such as VP-16 from the cell. This cell membrane pump occurs in many normal tissues, including the kidney, liver, adrenal gland, and large intestine and is induced in many malignant tissues. The all-membrane pump, also known as gp 170, mediates resistance, which results in decreased levels of the chemotherapeutic agent within the cell. This pump may be blocked by various agents, including calcium channel blockers, amiodarone, and tamoxifen. The use of these agents and many others may be invaluable clinically.

MDR can also be mediated by altered drug binding to topoisomerase II, an enzyme that promotes DNA strand breaks in the presence of anthracyclines, epipodophyllotoxins, and amsacrine (m-AMSA).[1–4, 14–18] The clinical relevance of any mediator of MDR is that chemotherapeutic agents should be used optimally to prevent induction of MDR regardless how it is mediated. It is important to note that normal cells do not develop resistance to antitumor drugs.

## Toxicity[1–7, 18–24]

Several chemotherapeutic agents and their toxicities are noted in Table 9–5. Identification and treatment of some of the more common side effects are listed below.

**Bone Marrow Toxicity**   Neutropenia and thrombocytopenia are early signs of bone marrow suppression. Anemia may develop later because of the longer life span of the red blood cell. This anemia is secondary to the anemia of chronic disease and also results from the drug's impact on the red cell precursors. Many antitumor drugs decrease blood cell numbers days to weeks after they are given. Before a myelosuppressive chemotherapeutic agent is administered, a complete blood count should be performed to ensure there are at least 3,000 neutrophils/$\mu$l and 100,000 platelets/$\mu$l. The nadir (lowest neutrophil and platelet counts) should be above 1,500 and 60,000 neutrophils and platelets/$\mu$l, respectively. Tables 9–5 and 9–6 give

**Table 9–5** Myelosuppressive Effects of Chemotherapeutic Agents Commonly Used in Veterinary Medicine[1–7, 18–24]

| Highly Myelosuppressive | Moderately Myelosuppressive | Mildly Myelosuppressive |
|---|---|---|
| Doxorubicin | Melphalan | L-Asparaginase[a] |
| Vinblastine | Chlorambucil | Vincristine[a] |
| Cyclophosphamide | 5-Fluorouracil | Bleomycin |
| Actinomycin D | Methotrexate | Corticosteroids |
| Carboplatin | Cisplatin | |

[a]Categorization of chemotherapeutic agents based on the severity of myelosuppression that may be noted after administration of therapeutic dosages of each drug alone.

examples of drugs with different myelosuppressive capabilities and different times when myelosuppression is noted to occur.

Clinical signs secondary to bone marrow suppression may include those related to sepsis, petechial and ecchymotic hemorrhages, pallor, and weakness. Because many animals do quite well with low white blood cell and platelet counts, only patients that show clinical signs should be treated. Some treat animals with prophylactic antibiotics if neutrophils are less than 1,000/μl. The treatment of clinically significant bone marrow toxicity includes the use of aseptic techniques when placing catheters, etc.; minimization of trauma; control of any bleeding with prolonged application of direct pressure or cold packs; and if the animal develops a fever or becomes septic, culture of the urine, blood, and, if indicated, any material obtained with a transtracheal wash. The affected animal should be treated with appropriate bactericidal antibiotics (cephalosporins, trimethoprim sulfa, and, when appropriate, aminoglycosides (in a well-hydrated patient with adequate renal function); supported with fluids, warmth, and nutritional therapy; and transfused with individual cell lines or fresh whole blood collected in plastic containers. The drug(s) that induced the bone marrow supression should be discontinued until the blood counts have recovered and subsequent administration of marrow-suppressant drugs should be done at a reduced dose (e.g., decrease cyclophosphamide dose by 25%).

**Gastrointestinal Toxicity** The clinical signs of this relatively common side effect include vomiting and diarrhea. Treatment includes the use of antiemetics (e.g., metoclopramide, propulsid, chlorpromazine); motility modifiers (e.g., diphenoxylate in dogs); protectants and absorbants (e.g., kaolin and pectin); broad-spectrum antibiotics if indicated; sulfasalazine to alter the colonic flora and decrease inflammation within the colon for patients with colitis; and, finally, support with fluids, warmth, and nutritional therapy. Doxorubicin is commonly associated with development of colitis. These patients may benefit from a high-fiber diet and early treatment if signs of colitis (fresh blood and mucus in the stool, straining to defecate, passing small amounts of stool frequently) are noted.[9]

**Allergic Reactions** Signs of L-asparaginase hypersensitivity include urticaria, vomiting, diarrhea, hypotension, and loss of consciousness.[25] Animals with doxorubicin-induced allergic reactions develop cutaneous hyperemia, intense pruritus, head shaking, and vomiting.[9] Other drugs that may induce allergic reaction include bleomycin, cytosine arabinoside, and procar-

**Table 9–6** Drugs with Myelosuppressive Capabilities[a]

| Delayed Myelosuppression (3–4 Weeks) | Mid range Myelosuppression (7–10 Days) | Early Myelosuppression (< 7 Days) |
|---|---|---|
| BCNU | Cyclophosphamide | Taxol |
| CCNU | Doxorubicin | |
| Mitomycin C | Mitoxantrone | |
| Melphalan | | |

[a]Drugs cause myelosuppression at different times and therefore may be associated with the development of pyrexia and sepsis at different times after treatment.[1–7, 18–24]

bazine. The treatment for allergic reactions includes discontinuing drug administration and giving epinephrine and glucocorticoids for acute allergic reactions. (*Note:* Some veterinarians continue to give doxorubicin despite cutaneous reactions. The signs abate soon after the drug is administered.) Other drugs, such as VP-16 (etoposide), which contains polysorbate 80 as a carrier and taxol, which is formulated with the carrier Cremophor EL, can cause potentially life-threatening side effects.[26,27] The adverse effects are induced by the carriers, which cause massive degranulation of canine mast cells when either etoposide or taxol are administered intravenously. This can result in a severe drop in blood pressure and whole-body edema and hyperemia. Because of the potential allergic reaction, these drugs should be administered with extreme caution. Premedication with diphenhydramine, cimetidine, and glucocorticoids may prevent or reduce doxorubicin-, etoposide-, and taxol-induced allergic reactions.

**Cardiac Toxicity**   Doxorubicin may induce a dose-dependent dilatative (congestive) cardiomyopathy and non-dose-dependent dysrhythmias in dogs.[9,28–32] Some clinicians limit the cumulative dose of doxorubicin to 150 to 250 mg/m$^2$ during the dog's lifetime to reduce the number of drug-induced cardiomyopathies. The treatment for dysrhythmias includes discontinuing the drug and use of antiarrhythmic agents if necessary. Doxorubicin should be discontinued if cardiomyopathy is detected. In addition, milrinone or digoxin, diuretics, a low-salt diet, and vasodilators may be employed.

**Cystitis**   Cyclophosphamide may induce a sterile chemical cystitis and, in rare cases, transitional cell carcinoma of the bladder.[33] Clinical signs include stranguria, hematuria, and dysuria. The treatment of this problem includes replacing the cyclophosphamide with a different alkylating agent (e.g., chlorambucil). Appropriate antibiotics may be used if cystitis becomes septic. Palliative therapy consists of intravesicular instillation of dilute 1% formalin or a formulation of dimethyl sulfoxide (DMSO) specifically designed for instillation into the bladder for severe cases. Most cases resolve with time (4–6 weeks).

**Local Dermatologic Toxicity**   Doxorubicin, actinomycin D, vincristine, and vinblastine are some of the drugs known to cause a severe localized cellulitis if they are extravasated perivascu-

larly.[1–4,9] Treatment for this problem includes stopping the injection, aspirating the drug and 5 ml of blood back into the syringe, then withdrawing the syringe. For vincristine, and vinblastine perivascular injections, infiltrating the area with 4 to 6 ml of 8.4% sodium bicarbonate and approximately 8 mg of dexamethasone may be helpful, followed by the application of warm compresses. Cold compresses or ice should be applied to the site of a doxorubicin perivascular injection. The use of topical DMSO is controversial. For deep ulcerative lesions secondary to extravasation, aggressive surgical debridement and skin grafts may be necessary.

**Alopecia**   Dogs and cats can lose hair as a result of the administration of chemotherapeutic agents, although this is rare except for those animals with constantly growing haircoats (e.g., poodles, schnauzers, Old English sheepdogs, etc.). Cats may lose whiskers and occasionally may develop generalized alopecia.

**Neuropathy**   The vinca alkaloids and cisplatin have been shown to induce various types of neuropathies. Vincristine and vinblastine may cause a peripheral neuropathy, whereas cisplatin may cause ototoxicity and result in hearing loss.

## DRUGS USED IN VETERINARY CHEMOTHERAPY

Drugs used in chemotherapy are classified as alkylating agents, antimetabolites, antibiotics, enzymes, hormones, plant alkaloids, nitrosoureas, and synthetic anticancer drugs.

### Alkylating Agents

Alkylating agents act by cross-linking DNA and are considered cell cycle nonspecific.[1–4] Examples of this cell-cycle-nonspecific family of drugs include cyclophosphamide, chlorambucil, melphalan, and thiotepa.

**Cyclophosphamide**   Cyclophosphamide is one of the most common and effective antineoplastic agents used in veterinary medicine. This alkylating agent is used alone or in combination with other drugs to treat lymphoma (when combined with drugs such as vincristine, prednisone, doxorubicin, mitoxantrone, cytosine arabinoside, methotrexate, and L-asparaginase),[34–40] soft tissue sarcomas (when combined with vincristine and doxorubicin),[41] feline mammary neoplasia,[43] synovial cell sarcoma,[2] hemangiosarcoma,[41,42] oral tumors in cats (when combined with doxorubicin),[44] thyroid carcinoma,[45] and transmissible venereal tumors.[1-4] The drug commonly causes decreased white blood cell count in 7 to 10 days and is periodically associated with vomiting, diarrhea, hair loss, and occasionally sterile hemorrhagic cystitis. A rare toxicity is development of bladder tumors secondary to the metabolites excreted in the urine. The development of sterile hemorrhagic cystitis occurs more commonly when the drug is administered intravenously and, when compared to the dog, is rare in the cat. The prevention of cyclophosphamide-induced sterile hemorrhagic cystitis and subsequent clinical and clinicopathologic evidence of cystitis should include:[1-4,33]

1. Exclusion of patients with cystitis because they may be predisposed to the development of cyclophosphamide-induced sterile hemorrhagic cystitis.
2. Administration of cyclophosphamide in the morning and provision of easy access to fresh clean water to ensure adequate hydration.
3. Allowing the patient to urinate just before owners retire for the night to prevent prolonged contact of cyclophosphamide metabolites with bladder mucosa.
4. Lightly salting food, administering furosemide, or, when medically appropriate, prescribing prednisone, because these procedures enhance water consumption and subsequent urination.

The drug does not decrease platelet numbers as markedly as other myelosuppressive agents such as doxorubicin, taxol, and cytosine arabinoside. Cyclophosphamide also requires metabolism and subsequent activation in the liver, which should be considered when treating patients with advanced liver disease and an elevated total bilirubin. Because of this need for hepatic activation, cyclophosphamide must be given intravenously or orally.

*Administration:* Orally (25, 50 mg tablets), intravenously (100, 200, 500, 1 gm and 2 gm/vial) at a dosage of 50 mg/m² orally daily for 4 days every 3 weeks at 250 mg/m² orally once every 3 weeks.

**Chlorambucil**  Chlorambucil is used in cases of lymphoma (especially when substituted for cyclophosphamide in those patients with an induced sterile hemorrhagic cystitis) and chronic lymphocytic leukemia.[1-4] Remissions of longer than a year are frequently reported in cases of chronic lymphocytic leukemia treated with chlorambucil.[46] The most common dosage employed ranges from 2 to 8 mg/m² administered orally on a daily basis. Studies done in the 1950s showed that chlorambucil may induce a unique cerebellar toxicity at very high doses.[3,4] Bone marrow suppression has been reported.

*Administration:* Orally (2 mg tablets) at a dosage of 2 to 8 mg/m² daily.

**Melphalan**  Melphalan has been used for several years to treat multiple myeloma (also known as plasma cell myeloma).[1-4] Remissions that exceed 1 year are frequently reported. Melphalan has been used with limited success to treat oral malignant melanoma. Toxicities are similar to those found with cyclophosphamide.

*Administration:* Orally (2 mg tablets), intravenously (500 mg vials); several dosing schemes are recommended. A dosage of 7 mg/m² daily, administered for 5 days, then no therapy for 3 weeks, has been recommended. Another dosing scheme uses a dosage of 0.05 to 0.1 mg/kg orally, once daily, until remission is obtained, and then 0.05 to 0.1 every other day thereafter.

### N.N', N" Triethylenethiophosphoramide (Thiotepa)

Thiotepa has been used to treat bladder tumors and intrathoracic masses,[1-4] with drug instillation into these cavities. The drug must be removed after 1 hour to prevent toxicity. Myelosuppression is reported in some patients.

*Administration:* Bladder instillation (15 mg vial). The dose most commonly recommended for instillation in the bladder is 30 mg/m² once every 3 to 4 weeks.

## Antimetabolites

Antimetabolites interfere with biosynthesis of nucleic acids by substituting them for normal metabolites and inhibiting normal enzymatic reactions. The dosage of each drug differs with the different protocols.

**Methotrexate**  Methotrexate has been used with variable results in combination with other drugs to treat lymphoma, myeloproliferative syndromes, transmissible venereal tumors, Sertoli cell tumors, and osteosarcoma.[1-4,36,37,39,40] Methotrexate, an inhibitor of dihydrofolate reductase that interferes with purine and pyrimidine synthesis, is given to human patients at a very high dosage and then reversed with leucovorin; this is rarely done in veterinary medicine. The drug has many toxicities, including myelosuppression, renal and hepatic damage, vomiting, diarrhea, and hair loss.

*Administration:* Orally (2.5 mg tablets) intravenously (5, 20, 50, 100, 200, 250 mg, and 1 gm vials). The most common dosage used in veterinary medicine is 2.5 mg/m$^2$ daily, a relatively low dosage that does not require leucovorin rescue.

### 6-Mercaptopurine

Six-mercaptopurine is mentioned in the literature as a treatment for leukemia and lymphoma.[1-4] Results are varied.

*Administration:* Oral (50 mg tablets). Dosages of 50 mg/m$^2$ PO daily until the desired effect has been reached followed by 50 mg/m$^2$ PO every 48 hours as needed has been recommended.

### 5-Fluorouracil

This drug should *never* be used in cats because it can cause severe, potentially fatal neurotoxicity that is less commonly seen in dogs.[1-4,47,48] The antineoplastic agent has been used to treat canine carcinomas with variable success. In addition, it comes in a topical cream and has been used with variable results to treat superficial malignances, including cutaneous lymphoma.

*Administration:* Intravenously (500 mg, 5 gm ampules or vials) or topically (1% or 2% topical ointment or solution). One dosage that has been used is 150 mg/m$^2$ IV or intracavitarily weekly.

### Cytosine Arabinoside

This drug has been used alone or in combination with other drugs to treat lymphoma and myeloproliferative disorders.[1-4,49] Some doubt its efficacy for treatment of lymphoma.[49] Cytosine arabinoside has been innovatively administered intrathecally for treatment of dogs with lymphoma of the central nervous system and effectively reduces the development of central nervous system metastases when administered systemically to cats with renal lymphoma.

*Administration:* There are two philosophies for the systemic administration of cytosine arabinoside. One is that the drug should be administered at high doses and infrequent intervals (e.g., 600 mg/m$^2$ once every 3 weeks); the other is that the drug be administered at a low-dose constant schedule (e.g., 10 mg/m$^2$ daily or q12h SQ). The drug has a very short half-life in the dog; therefore, some investigators choose to administer 100 mg of the drug over a 3-day period, with slow constant infusion to ensure the availability of aberrant nucleotide to the tumor cells at all times. Toxicities may include vomiting, diarrhea, myelosuppression, hair loss, etc.

## Antibiotics

Antibiotics form stable complexes with DNA and therefore inhibit DNA or RNA synthesis. Examples include doxorubicin, bleomycin, and actinomycin D. These drugs are cell cycle nonspecific and may cause bone marrow suppression, gastrointestinal toxicity, and alopecia.

### Doxorubicin

Doxorubicin has been used to treat lymphoma, thyroid carcinomas, sarcomas, and feline mammary neoplasia.[1-4,9,35-40,50-52] This antineoplastic agent has a broad spectrum of activity against a variety of tumors. The drug may cause a unique renal toxicity in the cat at a total cumulative dose above 80 mg/m$^2$ body surface area. The most common dosage used in the dog is 30 mg/m$^2$ IV, in the cat 20 to 25 mg/m$^2$, once every 3 weeks, with the total dosage not to exceed 180 to 250 mg/m$^2$. Toxicities seen with doxorubicin include those of most cytotoxic drugs, including a unique colitis and dose-dependent cardiomyopathy (> 250 mg/m$^2$) and development of clinically significant renal toxicity. The cardiomyopathy is dose dependent and cannot be successfully predicted in advance with standard clinical procedures other than with serial endomyocardial biopsies and gaited nuclear imaging studies. A variety of arrhythmias, especially supraventricular tachyarrhythmias, are often noted after cardiac damage occurs.[32] An allergic reaction (erythema of the skin, head shaking, or pruritis noted at or around the time the drug is administered) to the release of histamine can be reduced by pretreatment with diphenhydramine and glucocorticoids. Doxorubicin can induce a severe perivascular slough if given perivascularly.

*Administration:* Slow intravenous infusion (30 mg/m$^2$ in dogs and 1 mg/kg in cats or small dogs < 10 kg over at least 15 minutes; 10 mg, 20 mg, 50 mg, 150 mg, and 200 mg vials); avoid heparin flushes because this drug will precipitate the doxorubicin.

### Mitoxantrone

Mitoxantrone has been used for the treatment of lymphoma, squamous cell carcinoma, transitional cell carcinoma, mammary gland tumors, and a number of other neoplastic conditions.[53-57] Unlike doxorubicin, this drug does not commonly cause allergic reactions, cardiomyopathy, cardiac arrhythmias, colitis, and tissue damage at the site of extravasation. It is more myelosuppressive than doxorubicin and can cause alopecia and gastrointestinal disturbances.

*Administration:* Intravenous infusion (20, 25, and 30 mg multidose vial). The effective dosage is 6.0 mg/m$^2$ every 2 to 3 weeks in the dog, and 6.5 mg/m$^2$ IV every 2 to 3 weeks in the cat.

**Idarubicin**   Idarubicin is an expensive oral drug that may be effective for the treatment of lymphoma in cats.[58] The drug causes bone marrow suppression, gastrointestinal disturbances, and whisker loss in cats.

*Administration:* Intravenous infusion (FDA approval pending). The intravenous product has been administered at a dosage of 0.20 mg/kg IV on days 1, 2, and 3 every 3 weeks.

**Bleomycin**   Bleomycin has been mentioned as a treatment for squamous cell carcinoma but can cause a unique pulmonary fibrosis and currently is cost prohibitive for most cases.[1-4]

*Administration:* Intravenous infusion (15 unit vial).

**Actinomycin D**   This drug has been used to treat bone or soft tissue sarcomas and lymphoreticular neoplasms, including lymphoma and malignant melanoma.[59]

*Administration:* Slow intravenous infusion (0.5 mg vial) at a dosage of 0.7–1 mg/m$^2$ every 2 to 3 weeks.

## Enzymes

The enzyme most commonly used in veterinary and human medicine is L-asparaginase.

**L-asparaginase**   L-asparaginase inhibits the enzyme asparaginase synthetase and depletes asparagine in tumor cells. The drug is used to treat lymphoma and lymphoblastic leukemia and may be combined with other neoplastic agents.[25,36,37] Asparaginase does not induce a sustained remission when it is used alone to treat lymphoma. The most frequently used dosage is 10,000 U/m$^2$ IM weekly. If the drug is administered intramuscularly, the incidence of anaphylaxis is minimal. If the drug is administered intravenously, the potential for inducing an acute anaphylactic reaction is quite high. PEG-asparaginase* is a relatively new product that has equal efficacy to native L-asparaginase; it is administered at a dosage of 30 U/kg IV.[60]

*Enzon, Inc.

*Administration:* Intramuscularly (10,000 unit vial) at a dosage of 10,000 units/m$^2$.

## Hormones

Hormones are thought to interfere with cell receptors that stimulate growth. The most common example of hormones used for cancer treatment are the corticosteroids used to treat lymphoma and mast cell tumors.[1-4] The dose of prednisolone that is used most frequently in veterinary oncology is 30 mg/m$^2$ daily for 4 weeks then 15 mg/m$^2$ daily for another 3 weeks, followed by an every-other-day dosage at 15 mg/m$^2$. Another dosage regimen is 1 mg/kg daily for 4 weeks, then 1 mg/kg every other day thereafter.

## Plant Alkaloids

Plant alkaloids bind to the microtubules to prevent the normal formation and function of the mitotic spindle, thus arresting the cell division in metaphase (e.g., vincristine).

**Vincristine**   Vincristine is most commonly used in combination with other chemotherapeutic agents to treat lymphoma and various sarcomas, including hemangiosarcomas and as a single agent to treat mast cell tumors.[1-4,34-41,59,61] It is the drug of choice for treatment of transmissible venereal tumors (TVT).[1-4,61] Treatment of TVT results in a greater than 90% cure rate with an average of 3.3 doses. The drug can also cause premature release of platelets from megakaryocytes and therefore is a treatment for thrombocytopenia. Vincristine can be bound to platelets and reinfused to patients for treatment of immune-mediated thrombocytopenia; this latter methodology is effective for reducing the platelet destruction by the reticuloendothelial system.

*Administration:* Intravenous infusion (1 mg, 2 mg, and 5 mg vials). The dosage most commonly used in 0.5 to 0.75 mg/m$^2$ IV once weekly.

**Vinblastine**   Vinblastine has been used to treat lymphoma and mastocytoma.[1-4] Unlike vincristine, vinblastine results in myelosuppression. The most common dosage used in veterinary medicine is 2 mg/m$^2$ body surface area (BSA) administered weekly. Both vincristine and vinblastine are potent vesicants when administered outside the vein.

*Administration:* Intravenous infusion (10 mg vial) at a dosage of 2 mg/m$^2$.

## Miscellaneous

**Cisplatin**   Cisplatin is a heavy metal compound that is effective for the treatment of osteosarcoma adjuvantly, squamous cell carcinoma, bladder tumors, and mesotheliomas.[1–4, 62–71] The drug may cause myelosuppression (double nadir on days 5 and 16), alopecia, gastrointestinal toxicity, neurotoxicity (rare), and nephrotoxicity. Small dogs are more likely to develop toxicity than large ones. An aggressive fluid diuresis and eliminating dogs with pre-existing renal disease are essential to prevent nephrotoxicity. Although several saline diuresis protocols exist,[72–75] a 4-hour diuresis protocol appears to be relatively safe. In that protocol, saline is administered intravenously to the dog at 25 ml/kg/hr for 3 hours. Cisplatin is then given at a dosage of 70 mg/m$^2$ IV every 3 weeks over approximately 20 minutes, using a slow intravenous administration schedule followed by saline administered at 25 ml/kg/hr for one more hour.[75] Vomiting that occurs secondary to cisplatin therapy usually resolves within hours after therapy is complete. This may be prevented by pretreatment with butorphanol or serotonin antagonists.

*Administration:* Slow intravenous infusion during aggressive diuresis (10 mg, 50 mg, 100 mg vials) at a dosage of 70 mg/m$^2$ every 3 weeks. The drug may cause less toxicity in small dogs if dosed at 2 mg/kg.

**Carboplatin**   Carboplatin is a relatively new chemotherapeutic agent that is similar to cisplatin except that nephrotoxicity and emesis are rare toxicoses.[11] The drug is thought to have a spectrum of activity similar to cisplatin, but may be more bone marrow suppressive. It may be most effective when used to treat osteosarcoma.[95]

*Administration:* Intravenous infusion (50 mg, 150 mg, 450 mg vials) at a dosage of 300 mg/m$^2$. In cats, an effective dosge has not been determined.

## GENERAL GUIDELINES FOR HANDLING CHEMOTHERAPEUTIC AGENTS[76,77]

Chemotherapeutic agents are being utilized more frequently in private practice. The benefits of these drugs are being proven in a number of clinical studies. When any drug is utilized, there are risks to the patient and also to the individual administering the agent. The potential risks often are unknown; therefore it is essential that exposure to these drugs is minimized. Awareness of the risks of chemotherapeutic agents began in 1970, and this concern has resulted in several recommendations, which will be briefly reviewed below.

Because of many unanswered questions regarding the risks of chemotherapeutic agents and the exposure to workers, the Occupational Safety and Health Administration (OSHA) has issued guidelines for proper handling of chemotherapeutic agents. They do not constitute mandatory standards. The OSHA does suggest that potential risks exist and that the risks are minimized by compliance with these guidelines. Chemotherapeutic agents can be handled safely by decreasing exposure. The most common situations in which exposure is likely to occur are:[76,77]

1. Withdrawal of a needle from a pressurized drug vial.
2. Drug transfers between various sorts of equipment.
3. Opening of glass ampules.
4. Expulsion of air from drug-filled syringes.
5. Failure of equipment or improperly set-up equipment.
6. Exposure to excreta from patients that have received certain cytotoxic drugs.
7. Crushing or breaking tablets of cytotoxic drugs.

## Personnel

Individuals who work with chemotherapeutic agents should have specialized training to enhance a thorough understanding of the potential risks of chemotherapeutic agents.[76,77] Any exposure to chemotherapeutic agents must be documented, and the workers who administer these drugs should have routine health examinations to ensure there are no adverse effects that are inapparent to that individual. Women of childbearing age should exercise caution when handling chemotherapeutic agents. In addition, women who are breast-feeding should be cognizant that these agents may be present in the milk of exposed women.

## Equipment[76,77]

All chemotherapeutic agents should be mixed in a Class II biologic safety cabinet or by a method that minimizes exposure. When syringes and IV sets are utilized, a Luer-lok fitting should be used. Latex surgical gloves and a low permeability gown should also be worn. Hands should be washed frequently. IV tubing should be primed with a noncytotoxic agent when administering drugs by intravenous drip. Sterile gauze should be wrapped around all chemotherapy needles and syringes when they are removed from the injection ports. This gauze and all other disposables should be discarded with local, state, or national guidelines in mind. No eating, drinking, or smoking in the drug preparation area should be allowed. When a chemotherapeutic agent is utilized, it should have a chemotherapy hazard label on it. Also, when a veterinary patient has recently received chemotherapeutic agents, latex gloves and a gown should be worn when cleaning up or handling body fluids.

## Disposal Procedures[76,77]

All equipment used for compounding and administering chemotherapeutic agents should be placed in a sealable, leak-proof, puncture-proof plastic container. All personnel handling patients or the disposal of material should be instructed on the appropriate handling of chemotherapeutic agents. Owners should be advised when they take their animals home that all body fluids may be a risk, especially to children and pregnant women. Therefore, urination and defecation of exposed pets should be encouraged outside the area of potential human exposure.

## Client Information

Clients should be made aware of the potential risks of handling chemotherapeutic agents and the body fluids of pets that are given these drugs. This is best done by recommending safe handling procedures in oral and written form. Following are some recommendations:

1. Wear latex gloves when handling chemotherapeutic agents.
2. Never break tablets.
3. Make sure the animal swallows the medication.
4. Store medication in an area separate from other drugs and food.
5. Dispose of latex gloves in a closed plastic container.
6. Wash hands after removing gloves.

## Disposal of Body Waste

1. Wear latex gloves when handling the pet's feces, urine, or vomit.
2. Flush feces down the toilet.
3. Clean household areas that have been soiled with vomit, feces, or urine with household cleaners, and dispose of soiled paper towels in a closed plastic container.
4. Soiled rags or towels, cloths, bedding, etc., should be laundered separately from other laundry.
5. For cats, clean litter box frequently. Remove feces and flush down the toilet. Dispose of litter in closed plastic containers.
6. For dogs, leash-walk in restricted areas to minimize the exposure of the pet's yard to body excreta for 1 to 3 days after therapy.

## REFERENCES

1. Rosenthal RC: Chemotherapy. In Withrow SJ, MacEwen EG (eds): Clinical Veterinary Oncology. Philadelphia, WB Saunders, 1989.
2. Haskell CM: Principles of cancer chemotherapy. In Haskell CM (ed): Cancer Treatment. Philadelphia, WB Saunders, 1980, pp. 27–52.
3. Ogilvie GK, Moore AS: Chemotherapy: Properties, uses and patient management. In Managing the Veterinary Cancer Patient: A Practice Manual. Trenton, NJ, Veterinary Learning Systems, 1995, pp. 64–86.
4. Ogilvie GK: Principles of oncology. In Morgan RV (ed): Handbook of Small Animal Internal Medicine. Philadelphia, Churchill-Livingstone, 1992, pp. 799–812.
5. MacEwen EG: Cancer chemotherapy. In Kirk RW (ed): Current Veterinary Therapy VII. Philadelphia, WB Saunders, 1980.
6. Harris JB: Nausea, vomiting and cancer treatment. Cancer 28:194, 1987.
7. Sulkes A, Collins JM: Reappraisal of some dosage adjustment guidelines. Cancer Treat Rep 71:229–233, 1987.
8. Page RL, Thrall DF, Dewhirst MW, et al: Phase I study of melphalan and whole body hyperthermia in dogs with malignant melanoma. Int J Hyperthermia 7:559–566, 1991.
9. Ogilvie GK, Curtis C, Richardson RC, Withrow SJ, et al: Acute short term toxicity associated with the administration of doxorubicin to dogs with malignant tumors. J Am Vet Med Assoc 195:1584–1587, 1989.
10. Ogilvie GK, Moore T: Cisplatin induced emesis in the dog. J Am Vet Med Assoc 195:1399–1403, 1989.
11. O'Brien MG, Straw RC, Withrow SJ: Recent advances in the treatment of canine appendicular osteosarcoma. Compend Contin Educ Pract Vet 15:939–947, 1993.
12. Kitchell BE, Brown DM, Luck EE, et al: Intralesional implant for treatment of primary malignant melanoma in dogs. J Am Vet Med Assoc 204:204, 1994.
13. Moore AS, Cardona A, Shapiro W, Madewell BR:

Cisplatin (cisdiaminedichloroplatinum) for treatment of transitional cell carcinoma of the urinary bladder or urethra: A retrospective study of 15 dogs. J Vet Intern Med 4:148–152, 1990.

14. Bergman PJ, Ogilvie GK: Drug resistance and cancer therapy: Recent advances and future prospects. Compend Contin Educ Pract Vet, in press.

15. Curt GA, Clendeninn NJ, Chabner BA: Drug and resistance in cancer. Cancer Treat 68:87–98, 1984.

16. DeVita VT: The relationship between tumor mass and resistance to chemotherapy. Cancer 51:1209–1220, 1983.

17. Myers C, Cowan K, Sinha B, et al: The phenomenon of pleiotropic drug resistance. In DeVita VT, Hellman S, Rosenberg SA (eds): Important Advances in Oncology. Philadelphia, JB Lippincott, 1987, pp. 27–38.

18. Crow SE, Theilen GH, Madewell BR, et al: Cyclophosphamide-induced cystitis in the dog and cat. J Am Vet Med Assoc 171:259, 1977.

19. Giger U, Gorman NT: Acute complications of cancer and cancer therapy. In Gorman NT (ed): Oncology. New York, Churchill-Livingstone, 1986, pp. 147–168.

20. Rosenthal RC: Chemotherapy. In Slater D (ed): Textbook of Small Animal Surgery, 2nd ed. Philadelphia, WB Saunders, 1993, pp. 2067–2074.

21. Carter SK, Livingston RB: Drugs available to treat cancer. In Carter SK, Glatstein E, Livingston RB (eds): Principles of Cancer Treatment. New York, McGraw-Hill, 1981, pp. 111–145.

22. Freireich EJ, Gehan EA, Rall DP, et al: Quantitative comparison of toxicity of anticancer agents in mouse, rat, hamster, dog, monkey and man. Cancer Chemother Rep 50:219–244, 1966.

23. Henness AM, Theilen GH, Madewell BR, et al: Use of drugs based on square meters of body surface area. J Am Vet Med Assoc 171:1076, 1977.

24. Vriesendorp HM: Optimal prescription method for cancer chemotherapy. Exp Hematol 13:57–63, 1985.

25. Ogilvie GK, Atwater SW, Ciekot PA, et al: Prevalence of anaphylaxis associated with the intramuscular administration of L-asparaginase to 81 dogs with cancer: 1989–1991. J Am Anim Hosp Assoc 30:62–65, 1994.

26. Ogilvie GK, Cockburn CA, Tranquilli WJ, Reschke RW: Hypotension and cutaneous reactions associated with etoposide administration in the dog. Am J Vet Res 49:1367–1370, 1988.

27. Ogilvie GK, Powers BE, Meyer DM, et al: Organ toxicity of NBT taxol in the dog. Am J Vet Res, in press.

28. Susaneck SJ: Doxorubicin therapy in the dog. J Am Vet Med Assoc 182:70–73, 1983.

29. Cotter SM, Kanki PJ, Simon M: Renal disease in five tumor-bearing cats treated with adriamycin. J Am Anim Hosp Assoc 21:405–409, 1985.

30. Calvert CA, Leifer CE: Doxorubicin for treatment of canine lymphosarcoma after development of resistance to combination chemotherapy. J Am Vet Med Assoc 179:1011–1012, 1981.

31. Postorino NC, Susaneck SJ, Withrow SJ, et al: Single agent therapy with adriamycin for canine lymphosarcoma. Proc Vet Cancer Soc 7:37, 1987.

32. Mauldin GE, Fox PE, Patnaik AK, et al: Doxorubicin-induced cardiotoxicosis: Clinical features in 32 dogs. J Vet Intern Med 6:82–88, 1992.

33. Weller RE: Intravesical instillation of dilute formation for treatment of cyclophosphamide-induced hemorrhagic cystitis in two dogs. J Am Vet Med Assoc 172:1206, 1978.

34. Cotter SM: Treatment of lymphoma and leukemia with cyclophosphamide, vincristine, prednisone: II. Treatment of cats. J Am Anim Hosp Assoc 19:166–172, 1983.

35. Cotter SM, Goldstein MA: Comparison of two protocols for maintenance of remission in dogs with lymphoma. J Am Anim Hosp Assoc 23:495–499, 1987.

36. MacEwen EG, Brown NO, Patnaik AK, et al: Cyclic combination chemotherapy for canine lymphosarcoma. J Am Vet Med Assoc 178:564–568, 1987.

37. MacEwen EG, Hayes AA, Matus RE, et al: Evaluation of some prognostic factors for advanced multicentric lymphosarcoma in the dog: 147 cases (1978–1981). J Am Vet Med Assoc 190:564–568, 1987.

38. Carter RF, Harris CK, Withrow SJ, et al: Chemotherapy of canine lymphoma with histopathological correlation: Doxorubicin alone compared to COP as first treatment regimen. J Am Anim Hosp Assoc 23:587–596, 1987.

39. Mooney SC, Hayes AA, MacEwen EG: Treatment and prognostic factors in lymphoma in cats: 103 cases (1977–1981). J Am Vet Med Assoc 194:696–699, 1989.

40. Jeglum KA, Whereat A, Young K: Chemotherapy of lymphoma in 75 cats. J Am Vet Med Assoc 190:174–178, 1987.

41. Hammer AS, Couto CG, Filppi J, et al: Efficacy and toxicity of VAC chemotherapy (vincristine, doxorubicin and cyclophosphamide) in dogs with hemangiosarcoma. J Vet Intern Med 5:160–166, 1991.

42. deMadron E, Helfand SC, Stebbins KE: Use of chemotherapy for treatment of cardiac hemangiosarcoma in a dog. J Am Vet Med Assoc 190:887–891, 1987.

43. Jeglum KA, deGusman E, Young KM: Chemotherapy of advanced mammary adenocarcinoma in 14 cats. J Am Vet Med Assoc 187:157–160, 1985.

44. Mauldin GN, Matus RE, Patnaik AK, et al: Efficacy and toxicity of doxorubicin and cyclophosphamide used in the treatment of selected malignant tumors in 23 cats. J Vet Intern Med 2:60–65, 1988.

45. Jeglum KA, Whereat A: Chemotherapy of canine thyroid carcinoma. Compend Contin Educ Pract Vet 5:96–98, 1983.

46. Leifer CE, Matus RE: Chronic lymphocytic leukemia in the dog: 22 cases (1974–1984). J Am Vet Med Assoc 198:214–217, 1986.

47. Harvey HJ, MacEwen EG, Hayes AA: Neurotoxi-

cosis associated with use of 5-fluorouracil in five dogs and one cat. J Am Vet Med Assoc *171*:277–278, 1977.

48. Hennes AM, Theilen GH, Madewell BR, et al: Neurotoxicosis associated with use of 5-fluorouracil. J Am Vet Med Assoc *171*:692, 1977.

49. Ruslander D, Moore AS, Cotter SM, L'Heureux D: Cytosine arabinoside in the treatment of canine lymphoma. Proc 11th Annu Conf Vet Cancer Soc, 1991, pp. 61–62.

50. Postorino NC, Susaneck SJ, Withrow SJ, et al: Single agent therapy with adriamycin for canine lymphosarcoma. J Am Anim Hosp Assoc *25*:221–225, 1989.

51. Ogilvie GK, Reynolds HA, Richardson RC, Withrow SJ et al: Treatment of malignant neoplasia in the dog with doxorubicin: Initial response. J Am Vet Med Assoc *195*:1580–1583, 1989.

52. Ogilvie GK, Vail DM, Klein MK, et al: Weekly administration of low-dose doxorubicin for treatment of malignant lymphoma in dogs. J Am Vet Med Assoc *198*:1762–1764, 1991.

53. Ogilvie GK, Moore AS, Obradovich JE, et al: Toxicoses and efficacy associated with the administration of mitoxantrone to cats with malignant tumors. J Am Vet Med Assoc, *202*:1839–1844, 1993.

54. Ogilvie GK, Obradovich JE, Elmslie RE, et al: Efficacy of mitoxantrone against various neoplasms in dogs. J Am Vet Med Assoc *198*:1618–1621, 1991.

55. Ogilvie GK, Obradovich JE, Elmslie RE, et al: Toxicoses associated with administration of mitoxantrone to dogs with malignant tumors. J Am Vet Med Assoc *198*:1613–1617, 1991.

56. Ogilvie GK, Moore AS, Obradovich JE, et al: Toxicoses and efficacy associated with the administration of mitoxantrone to cats with malignant tumors. J Am Vet Med Assoc *202*:(11):1839–1844, 1993.

57. Moore AS, Ogilvie GK, Ruslander D, et al: Mitoxantrone for the therapy of canine lymphoma. Proc 11th Annu Conf Vet Cancer Soc, 1991, pp. 304.

58. Moore AS, Cotter SM, Ruslander D, et al: Interim analysis of the toxicoses and efficacy associated with idarubicin administration in cats with malignant tumors. Proc 11th Annu Conf Vet Cancer Soc 1991, pp. 102–103.

59. Hammer A, Couto G, Ayl R, et al: Treatment of tumor-bearing dogs and cats with actinomycin D. J Vet Intern Med *8*:236–239, 1994.

60. MacEwen EG, Rosenthal RC, Fox LE, et al: Evaluation of L-asparaginase:polyethylene glycol conjugate versus natrol combined with chemotherapy: A randomized double-blind study in canine lymphoma. J Vet Intern Med *6*:230–234, 1992..

61. Calvert CA, Leifer CE, MacEwen EG: Vincristine for treatment of transmissible venereal tumor. J Am Vet Med Assoc *181*:163–164, 1982.

62. Mauldin GN, Matus RE, Withrow SJ, Patnaik AK: Canine osteosarcoma. Treatment by amputation versus amputation and adjuvant chemotherapy

using doxorubicin and cisplatin. J Vet Intern Med *2*:177–180, 1988.

63. Withrow SJ, Powers BE, Straw RC, et al: Comparative aspects of osteosarcoma: Dog versus man. Clin Orthop *270*:159–168, 1991.

64. LaRue SM, Withrow SJ, Powers BE, et al: Limb sparing treatment for osteosarcoma in dogs. J Am Vet Med Assoc *195*:1734–1743, 1989.

65. Shapiro W, Fossum TW, Kitchell BE, et al: Use of cisplatin for treatment of appendicular osteosarcoma in dogs. J Am Vet Med Assoc *192*:507–511, 1988.

66. Straw RC, Withrow SJ, Richter SL, et al: Amputation and cisplatin for treatment of canine osteosarcoma. J Vet Intern Med *5*:205–210, 1991.

67. Kraegel SA, Madewell BR, Simonsen E: Osteogenic sarcoma and cisplatin chemotherapy in dogs: 16 cases (1986–1989). J Am Vet Med Assoc *199*:1057–1059, 1991.

68. Withrow SJ, Thrall DE, Straw RC, et al: Intra-arterial cisplatin with or without radiation in limb sparing for canine osteosarcoma. Cancer *71*:2484–2490, 1993.

69. Moore AS, Kirk C, Cardona A: Intracavitary cisplatin chemotherapy experience with six dogs. J Vet Intern Med *5*:227–231, 1991.

70. Straw RC, Withrow SJ, Cooper MF, et al: Local slow release cisplatin therapy after marginal local tumor resection (Abstract). Proc 11th Ann Conf Vet Cancer Soc, 1991.

71. Ogilvie GK, Straw RC, Jameson FJ, et al: Evaluation of single-agent chemotherapy for treatment of clinically evident osteosarcoma metastases in dogs: 45 cases (1987–1991). J Am Vet Med Assoc *202*:304–306, 1993.

72. Ogilvie GK, Krawiec DR, Gelberg HB, Twardock AR, Reschke RW: Short-term diuresis protocol for the administration of cisplatin. Am J Vet Res *49*:1076–1078, 1988.

73. Ogilvie GK, Straw RC, Powers BE, et al: Prevalence of nephrotoxicity associated with a short-term saline diuresis protocol for the administration of cisplatin in 61 dogs with malignant tumors (1987– 1989). J Am Vet Med Assoc *199*:613–616, 1991.

74. Ogilvie GK, Fettman MJ, Jameson VJ, et al: Evaluation of a one hour saline diuresis protocol for the administration of cisplatin to dogs. Am J Vet Res *53*:1666–1669, 1992.

75. Ogilvie GK, Straw RG, Jameson VJ, et al: Prevalence of nephrotoxicosis associated with a four hour saline diuresis protocol for the administration of cisplatin to dogs with malignant tumors: 64 cases (1989–1991). J Am Vet Med Assoc *202*:1845–1848, 1993.

76. OSHA Work Practice Guidelines for Personnel: Dealing with Cytotoxic Drugs. OSHA Instructional Publication 8–1.1. Washington, DC, Office of Occupational Medicine, 1986.

77. Ogilvie GK, Moore AS: Safe handling of chemotherapeutic agents. *In* Managing the Veterinary

Cancer Patient: A Practice Manual. Trenton, NJ Veterinary Learning Systems, 1995, pp. 53–57.

78. Ogilvie GK, Vail DM: Actinomycin D for remission in resistant canine lymphoma. J Vet Intern Med 8:343–344, 1994.

79. Keller ET, MacEwen EG, Rosenthal RC, et al: Evaluation of prognostic factors and sequential combination chemotherapy for canine lymphoma. J Am Vet Med Assoc, in press, 1992.

80. Cotter SM: Treatment of lymphoma and leukemia with cyclophosphamide, vincristine, and prednisone: I. Treatment of dogs. J Am Anim Hosp Assoc 19:159–165, 1983.

81. Mooney SC, Hayes AA, MacEwen EG: Treatment and prognostic factors in lymphoma in cats: 103 cases (1977–1981). J Am Vet Med Assoc 194:696–699, 1989.

82. Leifer CE, Matus RE: Lymphoid leukemia in the dog. Vet Clin North Am [Small Anim Pract] 16:723–739, 1985.

83. Matus RE, Leifer CE, MacEwen EG, Hurvitz AL: Prognostic factors for multiple myeloma in the dog. J Vet Intern Med 180:1288–1292, 1986.

84. Amber EL, Henderson RA: Canine transmissible venereal tumors: Evaluation of primary and metastatic lesions in Zaire-Nigeria. J Am Anim Hosp Assoc 31:350–352, 1982.

85. Shapiro W, Fossum TW, Kitchell BE, et al: Use of cisplatin for treatment of appendicular osteosarcoma in dogs. J Am Vet Med Assoc 192:507–511, 1988.

86. Knapp DW, Richardson RC, Bonney PL, Hahn K: Cisplatin therapy in 41 dogs with malignant tumors. J Vet Intern Med 2:41–46, 1988.

87. Hamilton TA, Morrison WB, Vonderhaar MA, et al: Cisplatin chemotherapy for canine thyroid carcinoma. Proc 11th Annu Conf Vet Cancer Soc, 1991.

88. Straw RC, Withrow SJ, Richter SL, et al: Amputation and cisplatin for treatment of canine osteosarcoma. J Vet Intern Med 5:205–210, 1991.

89. Shapiro W, Kitchell BL, Fossum TW, et al: Cisplatin for treatment of transitional cell and squamous cell carcinomas in dogs. J Am Vet Med Assoc 193:1530–1533, 1988.

90. Thompson JP, Fugent MJ: Evaluation of survival times after limb amputation, with and without subsequent administration of cisplatin for treatment of appendicular osteosarcoma in dogs: 30 cases (1979–1990). J Am Vet Med Assoc 200:531–533, 1992.

91. Kraegel SA, Madewell BR, Simonson E, Gregory CR: Osteogenic sarcoma and cisplatin chemotherapy in dogs: 16 cases (1986–1989). J Am Vet Med Assoc 199:1057–1059, 1991.

92. Helfand SC, Hamilton TA, Hungerford LL, et al: Comparison of three treatments for transitional cell carcinoma of the bladder in the dog. J Am Anim Hosp Assoc 30:270–275, 1994.

93. Berg J, Weinstein J, Schelling SH, Rand WM: Treatment of dogs with osteosarcoma by administration of cisplatin after amputation or limb-sparing surgery: 22 cases (1987–1990). J Am Vet Med Assoc 200:2005–2008, 1992.

94. Spodnick GJ, Berg J, Rand WM, et al: Prognosis for dogs with appendicular osteosarcoma treated by amputation alone: 162 cases (1978–1988). J Am Vet Med Assoc 200:995–999, 1992.

95. Bergman PJ, MacEwen EG, Kurzman ID, et al: Amputation and carboplatin for treatment of dogs with osteosarcoma: 48 cases (1991–1993). J Vet Intern Med, in press.

96. Berg J, Weinstein MJ, Springfield DS, Rand WM: Response of osteosarcoma in dogs to surgery and chemotherapy with doxorubicin. J Am Vet Med Assoc, in press.

97. Hahn K, Hahn E: Epirubicin (4'-epi-doxorubicin) chemotherapy. In Kirk RW, Bonagura JD (eds): Current Veterinary Therapy XI. Philadelphia, WB Saunders, 1992, pp. 393–395.

98. Ogilvie GK, Powers BE, Mallinckrodt, et al: Doxorubicin in chemotherapy and surgery for hemangiosarcoma in the dog. Proc Vet Cancer Soc, 1994, pp. 39–41.

# 10

# Radiation Therapy

## Susan M. LaRue and Edward L. Gillette

Radiation therapy has been used in veterinary medicine since shortly after the discovery of X rays by Roentgen near the turn of the twentieth century. Alois Pommer, an Austrian veterinarian, published extensively on the irradiation of benign and malignant diseases and established a radiation therapy protocol widely used for many years.[1] Through randomized clinical trials and retrospective studies the efficacy of radiation therapy for many tumors occurring in animals has been established. Newer imaging technology such as computerized tomography scanning (CT), magnetic resonance imaging (MRI), and nuclear scanning have dramatically improved the localization and staging of tumors, allowing radiotherapy to be administered to a wide variety of tumors. Advances in radiation therapy and equipment, including isocentrically mounted megavoltage radiotherapy units and computerized treatment planning, allow for greater sparing of normal tissues during radiotherapy and delivery of effective doses to deeper tumors. This should both improve the probability of tumor control as well as make the patient more comfortable during treatment. Finally, a better understanding of the underlying radiation biology of normal and tumor tissues has allowed the development of improved radiotherapy protocols. Radiotherapy is an effective treatment modality for animal cancer patients, just as it is for human cancer patients with serious cancers, almost half of whom undergo radiotherapy treatment.

Unfortunately in veterinary medicine, this useful treatment has been unavailable to many patients because of the limited number of veterinary radiotherapy centers. In the past decade, however, the number of centers has increased, and clients remote from centers have been more willing to transport their animals for therapy. At least 25 facilities in North America are actively treating animals with radiotherapy.[2] Most veterinarians will never have a radiation unit in their practice, but it is extremely important that the veterinarian become familiar with the following:

1. The basic principles of radiation oncology.
2. The equipment used in radiation therapy.
3. Decision making: the factors involved in selecting patients for radiotherapy.
4. The types of tumors commonly treated with radiotherapy.
5. The use of palliative radiotherapy.
6. The effects of radiotherapy on normal tissues.

## BASIC PRINCIPLES OF RADIATION ONCOLOGY

Ionizing radiation kills cells by the discreet deposition of energy on or near DNA, a process that eventually leads to cellular death. Proliferating cells are by definition radiation sensitive. Proliferating cells include tumors as well as renewing cell populations, such as epithelial cells. The effects of irradiation on normal rapidly proliferating tissue systems occur during the course of or shortly after radiotherapy. These types of tissues are referred to as acutely or early-responding normal tissues. More slowly dividing or nondividing cells, such as bone and cells of the nervous system, are also affected by irradiation, although the changes may take longer to become apparent.

These types of tissues are referred to as late-responding normal tissues. A certain amount of damage to normal acutely responding tissues occurs in every patient during radiotherapy, and the total dose of irradiation administered is dependent on the probability of damage to the late-responding tissues. The goal of radiotherapy is to destroy the reproductive capacity of the tumor without excessive damage to normal surrounding tissues. This goal is best achieved by the use of fractionation, or dividing the *total dose* into a number of smaller *fractions,* administered over a period of *time.* The relationship between these three parameters must be carefully considered in the development of radiotherapy protocols. These parameters are impacted by what is commonly referred to as the four R's of radiobiology: repair, redistribution, repopulation, and reoxygenation.

## Fractionation

Dividing the total radiation dose into fractions is important for a number of reasons. The first reason is to exploit potential differences in *repair* capabilities between tumors and normal tissues. Mammalian cells have been shown to repair a portion of the damage caused by radiation. This repair proceeds rapidly in most tissues and is complete within 24 hours after a fraction is administered. Early- and late-responding tissues differ in their response to irradiation. Although slowly dividing cells appear to be somewhat less sensitive to small doses of radiation than more rapidly dividing cells, they appear to become relatively more sensitive if radiation is delivered in larger doses per fraction. If smaller doses per fraction are used, late-responding tissues can be spared relative to tumor and acutely responding tissues.

Another event that occurs between radiation fractions is cell *redistribution.* Tumors and replicating normal tissues proliferate by mitosis. After an interval of time has elapsed, cells divide again. The interval from mitosis to the next mitosis is known as the cell cycle time. Between mitotic events the DNA must replicate in order to undergo subsequent mitosis. The period of the cell cycle when DNA is undergoing synthesis is known as the S-phase. Before and after the S-phase are periods without overt activity by the DNA, called $G_1$ and $G_2$. Cells are distributed throughout the cell cycle. The sensitivity to irradiation varies depending on the phase of the cell cycle the cells are in at the time of irradiation. Cells in late S-phase are most resistant to irradiation, while cells in mitosis are most sensitive. When a fraction of radiation therapy is administered, many of the cells in the sensitive portions of the cell cycle are killed. During the interval between fractions, cells from the late S-phase, which are more likely to be alive than other cells, redistribute to more sensitive parts of the cell cycle. This is known as *redistribution.*

Tumors, because of rapid growth and abnormal vasculature, will often become partially hypoxic. This is an important factor in the response to irradiation, because lack of oxygen results in a decrease in the damage to the DNA from irradiation. Fortunately, during the interval between radiation fractions many of the hypoxic tumor cells become aerobic, and thus more sensitive to irradiation. This is known as tumor *reoxygenation.*

## Time

The duration of time over which the course of radiation therapy is administered is important primarily because of tumor *repopulation.* Tumor cells that have not been destroyed by irradiation will continue to replicate during the course of therapy. This process is exacerbated by a phenomenon known as accelerated repopulation. After approximately 4 weeks of therapy the tumor repopulates more rapidly than under normal conditions. It is not clearly understood how this occurs, but it could be related to (1) a decrease in cell cycle time, (2) an increase in the fraction of tumor cells that are actively dividing, or (3) a decrease in the number of tumor cells that normally die (cell loss factor). Whatever the cause, the result is that when treatment extends longer than 4 weeks, repopulation *may* impact outcome. Accelerated repopulation may have more impact in rapidly dividing tumors than in slowly dividing tumors.

Acutely responding normal tissues are also impacted by time. These tissues also try to repopulate during radiotherapy. The same total dose of irradiation administered in a short period of time will result in more severe acute effects than if administered over a longer time course. However, although acute effects may cause discomfort to the patient, the effects are generally self-limiting and can be managed with supportive care.

Late-responding normal tissues are not significantly impacted by the duration of time over which therapy is administered. Fraction size is a far more important consideration. The time *between* treatment fractions is important. Some treatment protocols advocate multiple fractions per day in order to administer the total dose in a short period of time to prevent repopulation, but in smaller fraction sizes to minimize damage to late-responding tissues. Fractions should be separated by at least 6 hours to allow repair of normal tissues. The brain and spinal cord may require additional time for complete repair, and the impact of multiple fractions per day on these late-responding tissues is not clearly understood.

## Total Dose

Radiation doses are delivered in units known as Gray or Gy. A Gy is 1 Joule/kg, and is equal to 100 rad, the previously used measure of radiation dose. The total dose administered to a patient should have a low probability for causing significant late normal tissue reactions in the region of therapy. However, as mentioned above, the response of these tissues is dependent on the fraction size. Forty-eight Gy administered in 4 Gy fractions will have a much higher probability of causing late effects than 48 Gy administered in 3 Gy fractions (Figure 10–1). The probability of tumor control is thought to be fairly similar, because acutely responding tissues, like tumor, are not as sensitive to the fraction size in which the dose is administered. It is clear that the benefit of protocols that use small doses per fraction is

that a higher total dose can be administered without increasing the probability of damage to normal late-responding tissues. This higher dose translates into a better probability of tumor control. However, gains from this can be lost if the radiation protocol is spread over such a length of time that tumor repopulation begins to impact tumor control adversely. The total dose tolerated is also dependent on the type of late-responding normal tissue in the radiotherapy field. For example, the brain and spinal cord are less tolerant to the effects of irradiation than muscle or bone. Another factor that must be considered when selecting the appropriate dose is the volume of tissue in the field. Large volumes of normal tissues are more susceptible to damage from irradiation than smaller volumes.

There is no perfect radiation therapy protocol, and there are advantages and disadvantages to all protocols commonly used in veterinary and human medicine. It is not within the scope of this chapter to prescribe specific radiation doses or fractionation schedules, because many factors must be considered. Rather, it is important that the referring veterinarian know what to expect when sending patients to a radiotherapy center and be able to explain some of the fundamental principles to clients. The radiation oncologist should communicate to the referring veterinarian and owner the probabilities of late effects and tumor control as well as an idea of the degree of acute effects expected in the patient when treated with a specific protocol.

## EQUIPMENT

Ionizing radiation can be administered by an external source (teletherapy), through placement of radioactive isotopes interstitially (brachytherapy), or by systemic or cavitary injection of radioisotopes such as $^{131}$Iodine. Teletherapy, also referred to as external beam radiotherapy, is the most common method of radiotherapy employed. External beam radiotherapy is commonly classified as orthovoltage or megavoltage, based on the energy of the photon. Orthovoltage machines produce X rays with an energy of 150 to 400 kVp, while megavoltage radiotherapy implies photons with an average energy greater than 1 million electron volts (1MeV). Although some veterinary radiation oncology centers continue to treat with orthovoltage machines, megavoltage radiation, which is used almost exclusively at

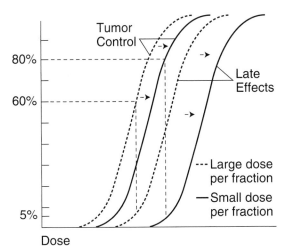

**Figure 10–1.** Radiotherapy delivered in small fractions (solid lines) can result in a higher probability of tumor control with the same level of late effects as radiotherapy delivered in large fractions (broken lines).

human centers, is becoming more accessible. Megavoltage radiation for therapy can be obtained from linear accelerators or, more commonly, from cobalt machines. Megavoltage radiation has excellent penetrating capabilities, so radiation therapy can be performed on deeply seated tumors for which orthovoltage therapy would not be an option. Radiation therapy is still performed at some centers with Cesium machines. Cesium emits photons with an energy of 662 KeV. This energy photon has limited skin-sparing effect; however, the distribution of dose throughout the tissues is more uniform than with orthovoltage.

Orthovoltage X rays, which are of low energy, distribute the maximum dose of radiation to the skin surface. Acute effects to the skin can be quite severe, causing discomfort to the patient, and the late effects to the skin and subcutaneous tissues can be dose limiting. Megavoltage radiation has higher energy than orthovoltage, and the photons must interact with tissues, allowing the dose to *build up* before the maximum dose can be achieved. Therefore, the skin can receive a significantly lesser dose than the underlying tumor. This *skin-sparing* effect of megavoltage radiation allows the optimal dose to be administered to the more deeply seated tumor without causing severe reactions to the skin. When tumor involves the skin, megavoltage radiation can be used successfully by placing a sheet of tissue-equivalent material, termed *bolus*, over the tumor. This allows dose buildup to occur prior to reaching the skin, so that the skin and associated tumor can receive the maximum dose.

The absorption of megavoltage radiation, unlike that of orthovoltage radiation, is minimally dependent on the density of the tissue. This permits an even distribution of dose throughout the tissues in the field. Orthovoltage radiation is preferentially absorbed by bone. If a tumor adjacent to or overlying bone is administered a meaningful dose of orthovoltage radiation, the probability of developing late effects to the bone is quite high.

The interaction of megavoltage radiation with tissues is quite predictable, allowing for the development of computerized treatment planning systems. These planning systems allow treatment of the tumor with multiple beams administered from different angles. Beam modifiers, such as wedges, can be incorporated into the treatment plan. Wedges are triangular-shaped pieces of lead that can be placed between the beam and the patient. Less radiation penetrates through the thick side of the wedge, thus modifying the dose distribution. The goal of computerized treatment planning is to ensure a desired minimum tumor dose to a region specified by the radiation oncologist, and to spare normal tissue structures when possible. The use of treatment planning systems in veterinary medicine may be responsible for improvement in tumor control.[3]

The availability of CT scans and MRI has also impacted radiation oncology by providing better data on the extent of disease. Images from the CT scan can be used by the treatment planning system to help formulate the optimal treatment plan. Although improved imaging has improved treatment quality in general, it has revolutionized the treatment of brain tumors in animals by confirming and locating masses that can then be treated.

## DECISION MAKING

After a tumor is diagnosed, determining the best treatment modality for the patient can be challenging. For the treatment of solid tumors there are always two issues that must be addressed: local tumor control and control of potential metastatic disease. For local tumor control, treatment options generally include surgery or radiotherapy or both. Chemotherapy can cure transmissible venereal tumor but is not considered curative for other solid tumors. However, chemotherapy has a definite adjuvant role in eliminating metastatic spread of some tumor types. The following discussion will focus on the principles used to determine whether surgery, radiotherapy, or a combination, is the most appropriate method of gaining local tumor control for solid tumors. If a tumor is likely to metastasize, then chemotherapy must also be considered.

The following factors must be considered in every patient when making the decision whether to treat with surgery alone, radiation alone, or a combination of radiotherapy and surgery.

1. Probability of local tumor control.
2. Predicted functional outcome.
3. Predicted cosmetic outcome.
4. Salvage potential.
5. Cost.
6. Other patient factors (concomitant disease, etc.).
7. Owner's desire.

If a tumor can be excised with a very good to excellent probability of tumor control, good function of remaining organs or tissues, and good cosmetic outcome, then surgery should be the treatment method selected. Local tumor control can be obtained with surgery alone in many types of animal cancers, including mammary tumors, some oral tumors, some soft tissue sarcomas of the body and extremities, and some mast cell tumors.

Sometimes local tumor control can be achieved with surgery alone, but with significant impairment of function or cosmetic outcome. For example, a dog presenting with a large bilateral acanthomatous epulis of the maxilla that extends from the incisors caudally to the level of the second premolar would have an excellent probability of tumor control with en bloc surgical resection; however, the functional and cosmetic outcome would be compromised. Radiation therapy alone has an excellent probability of tumor control with this type of tumor, and the functional and cosmetic outcome should be improved over that of en bloc surgical excision.

Cosmetic outcome is not important to the patient, yet the patient's life can be adversely affected by an owner who is uncomfortable with the cosmetic outcome. With a tumor such as an acanthomatous epulis, there is no known benefit of combining aggressive surgical excision and radiotherapy. Tumor control is excellent with either modality alone. Combining aggressive surgical excision and radiotherapy offers the worst of both modalities: the dysfunction and poor cosmesis of surgery alone with the expense and acute effects of radiotherapy.

*Salvage potential* is a term used to describe the options available should the primary method of treatment fail. As a rule, the salvage potential is better if a patient fails radiotherapy than if a patient fails following aggressive surgery, because the same surgery can be performed as would have been performed had surgery been the primary treatment modality. If tumor recurs locally following an aggressive surgical excision, the radiotherapy field is quite different and more extensive. Radiation therapy cannot be repeated to an area because of the tolerance of normal tissue structures.

Cost is another factor that must be addressed. Most of the time the cost of a surgical excision would be less than that of radiotherapy. Other factors that must be considered are the patient's overall health and any concurrent diseases. Anesthetic risk is sometimes cited as a disadvantage when considering radiation therapy. However, the risk of prolonged anesthesia associated with major surgery, combined with other events such as blood loss, may be riskier than multiple short, light anesthetic episodes. Severe concurrent diseases that drastically reduce the patient's life expectancy may also impact treatment considerations. Finally, the owner's wishes must ultimately be followed. It is the obligation of the veterinarian to inform the owner of the alternatives and the positives and negatives of those alternatives. The owner must make a decision he or she is comfortable with, and that decision must be respected.

The decision to combine radiotherapy and surgery is based on improving tumor control or improving the functional or cosmetic outcome, or both. Extensive soft tissue sarcomas of the extremity, for example, often cannot be controlled with surgical excision alone, nor with radiotherapy alone. Tumor control can be achieved with amputation, and if local tumor control were the only issue, amputation would be the best treatment alternative. Functionally, many dogs maneuver well with amputation, and this procedure has extended life in many patients with a wide variety of conditions. It is certainly more desirable to spare the limb if possible, especially if there is minimal risk to the survival of the patient. In some dogs concurrent orthopedic or neurologic problems eliminate amputation as a treatment alternative. Cosmetically, most owners can accept amputation in their pets, but there is a small but real subset who cannot. Also, many owners who would be receptive to amputation in a situation in which the life of the patient is at stake are reluctant to pursue such a drastic approach if other alternatives are available. Surgical excision to subclinical disease along with radiotherapy offers excellent tumor control plus improved function and cosmetic appearance over amputation. The salvage potential is excellent because, should the tumor recur, amputation could be performed and tumor control regained.

## TUMORS COMMONLY TREATED WITH RADIOTHERAPY

### Oral Tumors

Radiation therapy is beneficial in the treatment of many oral tumors. The oral region is anatomically complex, and aggressive surgery can often leave functional and cosmetic abnormalities.

Additionally, many of the oral tumors are known to be responsive to radiation.

Acanthomatous epulides, previously called adamantinomas, are very radiation responsive. Tumor control with radiotherapy is close to 90%.[4] If the tumor is inoperable, radiotherapy is the treatment of choice. If the tumor is felt to be operable, the functional and cosmetic outcome of surgery versus radiation therapy must be considered.

Oral squamous cell carcinomas in dogs have been frequently studied. Coarsely fractionated (10–11 fractions of 4 Gy each) radiation offers a tumor control at 1 year of about 65%.[5] Use of more radiobiologically sound fractionation schedules, as suggested above, should result in better tumor control. The prognosis is site dependent, with rostral tumors having a better probability of control.[6] Tumors of the base of the tongue and tonsil are highly metastatic and are likely to recur locally or regionally. In these cases radiation therapy has the advantage of including associated lymphatic structures in the treatment field.

Oral fibrosarcomas are unlikely to metastasize but can be difficult to control locally. The histologic appearance can be deceptive; tumors diagnosed as fibromas or low-grade fibrosarcomas can be extremely locally malignant in biologic behavior.[7] If clinical evidence of rapid growth, invasion into bone, or tumor recurrence exists, the tumor should be treated aggressively in spite of bland pathology. En bloc complete surgical resection is often curative but is difficult to accomplish because of the invasive nature of the tumor. Oral fibrosarcomas are less radioresponsive than epulides and squamous cell carcinomas, although tumor control probabilities ranging from 33 to 67% at 1 year have been reported.[8,9]

Surgical resection followed by radiotherapy is currently felt to offer the best probability of tumor control. Surgical cytoreduction improves the probability of tumor control by radiotherapy by reducing the number of tumor clonogenic cells. It is advantageous that the decision to follow surgery with irradiation be made prior to surgery. The surgeon can then focus on removing clinical disease and obtaining a tension-free closure. The surgery can be less aggressive and disfiguring when subclinical disease is to be managed with radiation; however, it is extremely important that all macroscopic tumor be removed. The optimal time to begin irradiation after surgery has not been determined. If it appears that there may be difficulty in obtaining primary wound healing, radiation can be delayed. However, any therapeutic gain obtained from combining modalities will be lost if the tumor recurs in the interim. Initiating radiation therapy any time in the immediate days following surgery does not appear to be a problem if the suture line is tension free. In tumors too large to be surgically resected to a level of microscopic disease, radiation therapy alone is indicated but is more likely to be palliative rather than curative.

In cats, oral squamous cell carcinomas have a very poor prognosis.[10] A treatment regimen at Colorado State University improved median survival to 6 months in seven cats by combining the chemotherapeutic agent mitoxantrone with an aggressive radiotherapy protocol. A shrinking-field technique was used to achieve a total dose of nearly 60 Gy to the tumor volume.[11] The probability of late effects due to radiation were predictably high; however, the improvement in local tumor control was encouraging. Further sparing of normal tissues, by administering the same total dose in smaller fractions, may be worthwhile for this tumor.

## Nasal Tumors

Nasal tumors in dogs are difficult to control locally, and surgery alone does not appear to improve survival over no therapy. Radiation therapy, with or without surgery, is indicated for these tumors. Surgical cytoreduction followed by orthovoltage radiation offers the best prognosis (median survival 16–23 months).[4] Megavoltage radiotherapy offers a median survival of close to a year.[3] It can be administered with or without prior surgery, although the addition of surgery does not appear to enhance survival.[12] The role of chemotherapy combined with radiotherapy in nasal tumors is not clear.

Intranasal tumors in cats have a good prognosis when treated with radiotherapy.[13] Tumors of the nasal planum can be treated with radiotherapy.[14] If squamous cell carcinomas of the planum are excised surgically the margins should be checked for tumor infiltration. If margins are tumor infiltrated, radiation therapy is indicated.[15]

## Brain Tumors

Brain tumors can be treated successfully with radiotherapy. Studies of primary brain tumors have indicated median survival times near or greater than 1 year.[16,17] Preliminary data analysis of 65 animals with brain tumors at Colorado State University indicated a median survival of 13.5 months for all brain tumors treated with radiotherapy with or without surgery. Meningiomas and pituitary macroadenomas were most responsive to radiotherapy, but survival was enhanced in dogs with gliomas, granulomatous meningoencephalitis (GME), and metastatic brain tumors.

Surgery is clearly indicated when necessary to relieve life-threatening clinical signs. In dogs with meningiomas, surgery alone is unlikely to result in tumor control[18] and radiation therapy should always be performed adjuvantly. Radiotherapy alone should be performed in dogs with surgically inaccessible meningiomas. It is currently not clear whether the addition of surgery to irradiation enhances survival in dogs with meningiomas. The decision to proceed with surgery should be weighed against the potential morbidity and mortality to the patient. Unlike dogs, meningiomas in cats can often be controlled with surgery alone. Surgical margins should be closely evaluated for tumor infiltration. If residual tumor is suspected, radiotherapy should be recommended. The data for other types of brain tumors are limited. Current recommendations for other types of brain tumors include radiation therapy for inoperable tumors, and adjuvant radiation therapy following surgery in operable tumors. In surgically accessible tumors, the morbidity of surgery needs to be weighed against the potential therapeutic gain that could be achieved by reducing the tumor volume.

Radiation alone is advocated for dogs and cats with pituitary macroadenomas. Dogs with pituitary tumors were reported to have a median survival of 743 days.[19] The tumors are generally responsive to radiation, and surgical access is limited. Therapy for signs of Cushing's disease may need to be continued after therapy, but the patient should have pre- and post-ACTH cortisol levels monitored at regular intervals so medications can be modified or discontinued, if indicated.

Brain tissue is extremely sensitive to the late effects of irradiation. *Early delayed* effects, which can occur from 2 weeks to 3 months after treatment, may be due to transient demyelination. Animals with early delayed effects may present with signs similar to those of the initial presentation, or may be generally stuporous. These signs are often transient and respond to systemic cortisone. *Late delayed* effects generally occur at least 6 months after treatment but can also occur years later. Late delayed effects are associated with brain necrosis. The signs are like those associated with early delayed effects; however, response to steroids is limited. It can often be difficult to distinguish clinically between late effects and tumor recurrence. In order to reduce the probability of late effects to less than 5%, the total dose should be limited to 48 Gy or less in 3 Gy fractions, and if surgical biopsy or excision was performed first, the dose should be limited to 45 Gy in 3 Gy fractions.

## Tumors of the Body and Extremities

Many tumors involving the body or extremities are amenable to treatment by radiotherapy. Small tumors generally respond the best; however, surgical excision is generally the treatment of choice in small skin tumors. Hemangiopericytomas, fibrosarcomas, neurofibrosarcomas, and nerve sheath tumors are classified together as soft tissue sarcomas because of similar biologic behavior. Metastasis is unlikely, but local tumor control can be difficult to achieve. These tumors are locally invasive, and tumor cells may extend far beyond the bulk of the tumor. Radiation therapy can be successfully combined with surgery to gain local tumor control. Radiation therapy can be administered first, making an inoperable tumor into an operable one. Surgical excision can also be performed first as a cytoreductive procedure, to be followed by radiation therapy to kill the remaining subclinical disease. Surgery alone can be curative *if* the tumor can be completely removed. If en bloc surgical resection is attempted, margins should be closely examined by a histopathologist for evidence of tumor infiltration. If tumor cells extend out to the margin, radiotherapy should be recommended. The likelihood of success is much greater if the tumor is irradiated while still microscopic. Soft tissue sarcomas can be treated with radiation therapy alone; however, tumor control is less than satisfactory.[9] Combining radiotherapy with surgery should provide excellent tumor control and cosmetic results.[20,21]

Cutaneous mast cell tumors (Grades I and II) can be successfully treated with radiotherapy. The obvious advantage is that greater margins can be obtained with radiation than with surgery. The probability of control may be improved if surgical cytoreduction is performed first. In a study involving 40 dogs with Grade II tumors treated with cytoreduction and radiotherapy, tumor control at 1 and 2 years was close to 90%.[22]

Soft tissue sarcomas, believed to be related to prior vaccination, have been identified in cats. These tumors are challenging to control locally and seem unresponsive to aggressive radiotherapy or surgery alone. Some combination of radiotherapy and surgery seems indicated. Early results from investigators at North Carolina State University show tumor control in 17 of 24 cats irradiated to 48 Gy in 3 Gy fractions, followed by surgical excision of the lesion. The median follow-up time for patients included was 470 days.[23] In cats from which the tumor had already been surgically excised, the incision and tumor bed were removed following surgery.

## Other Tumors

Radiation therapy is being used for a variety of tumors of the colon and urinary tract. Radiation therapy can follow surgery to help control microscopic tumor spread. This allows for a more conservative surgery, and better postsurgical function can be maintained. Limited information is available on the response of urinary tract and colon cancers to external beam radiotherapy; however, based on information from human patients, combining surgery and irradiation may be worthwhile. A summary of commonly treated tumors is presented in Table 10–1.

## PALLIATIVE RADIOTHERAPY

Palliative radiotherapy is commonly used in human medicine but has only recently been employed in veterinary medicine. The goal of palliative radiotherapy is not to provide long-term or definitive tumor control. Rather, it is used to provide relief of pain or improve dysfunction associated with the tumor in patients in whom other factors such as advanced metasta- tic disease or a severe concurrent condition are likely to lead to the demise of the patient. Palliative radiotherapy has been used most often for metastatic bone tumors, primarily osteosar-coma. Although this relief is not indefinite, the dog can live a relatively normal life until metastatic disease advances. The procedure is relatively uncomplicated for the owner, and costs are modest compared to traditional radiotherapy because the number of fractions administered is minimized.

The mechanism associated with the amelioration of pain associated with bony neoplasia is not completely understood. The relief of pain often occurs shortly after the first fraction of therapy. Since long-term tumor control is not the goal, a full course of radiotherapy is not necessary. A number of different fractionation schemes have been developed. At some radiotherapy centers 7 to 10 Gy fractions are administered on days 1, 8, and 22.[24,25] Twelve of 15 dogs with appendicular bone tumors treated with palliative radiotherapy experienced improvement of limb function, with a median survival of 130 days.[25] At Colorado State University, to which many clients are traveling long distances, completion of the protocol in a short period of time, rather than returning for weekly treatments, was more convenient for many owners. Fractions of 4.5 Gy are administered daily for 5 treatment days. This allows the therapy to be completed in a week, and the smaller fraction size is more amenable to retreatment should the patient respond well to the first course of palliative radiotherapy and live long enough to warrant a second treatment course.

Palliative radiotherapy is used primarily for animals with osteosarcoma presented with advanced disease, such as lesions already present in other bones or the lungs or in dogs who have failed conventional treatment (amputation or limb sparing followed by high-dose cisplatin) and present with local relapse or bone metastasis. Palliative radiotherapy is also an option for the treatment of primary osteosarcoma when the owner has severe financial constraints and cannot afford conventional treatment. Palliative therapy has also been reported in dogs with oral melanomas.[26] Traditional radiotherapy has not been effective on melanoma in dogs, primarily because the animals die of metastatic spread.[27] The reported median survival for dogs with oral melanoma treated with palliative radiotherapy was approximately 8 months, and 83% of patients had some response to treatment.[26]

## EFFECTS OF IRRADIATION TO NORMAL TISSUES

Reactions from radiation therapy are classified as early or late. Late effects involve more slowly proliferating tissues, such as bone, lung, heart, kidneys, and spinal cord. When late effects occur they may be quite severe and can result in necrosis, loss of function, or even death. The dose of radiation administered is limited by the tolerance of the normal tissue structures in the field. Late reactions can be expensive and difficult to treat. Severe late reactions should be treated under the guidance of or referred to a surgeon experienced in dealing with radiation injury.

Early effects will occur during or shortly after radiation therapy. Early effects involve tissues that are rapidly proliferating, such as oral mucosa, intestinal epithelium, and skin. These effects are generally self-limiting and have a rapid recovery. However, early effects can be unpleasant for the animal and owner and in rare instances can result in the demise of the patient if not cared for properly. The referring veterinarian is often called upon to treat recently irradiated patients. Treatment is based on common sense, supportive care, and the knowledge that the signs will resolve within a few weeks!

## Mucositis

Mucositis of the oral cavity, pharynx, or esophagus can occur when tumors of the head and neck region are irradiated, and always occurs to some degree in patients that have received irradiation for oral tumors. The mucositis begins to develop during the second week of therapy and reaches a maximum severity during the last week of therapy. The clinical signs include increased salivation and tenderness of the mouth. The animal may become reluctant to eat or drink and thus without treatment can become dehydrated and debilitated. Low-salt foods are more palatable and less irritating to the oral mucosa than regular commercial diets. Hand-feeding and pampering by the owner aid in maintaining caloric intake. The owners should be instructed on the specific caloric and fluid requirements of their animals and assisted in developing a diet that meets those needs. Administration of fluids, usually subcutaneously, may be necessary. In some animals, placement of a gastrostomy tube may be necessary to facilitate feeding. *Oral mucositis should subside 2 to 3 weeks following therapy.* Mucositis can also occur whenever any portion of the alimentary system receives radiation therapy. Colitis is a common acute effect during radiation therapy for bladder or colorectal tumors. Severe large-bowel diarrhea can be observed. Anusitis from irradiation will be worsened by the diarrhea, and the patient can be quite uncomfortable. High-bulk diets are recommended along with good hygiene to the region. Steroid enemas seem beneficial in some patients.

## Skin

Early effects to the skin are restricted to the radiation field. The severity of effect is dose related, and the patient may have a variety of lesions. Epilation is common and in some cases may be permanent. Several months may be required for fur to return, and the amount of regrowth varies depending on the dose administered to the skin and the individual patient's sensitivity. Damage to the melanocytes may result in hypo- or hyperpigmentation of skin or alteration of coat color when regrowth occurs. Dry desquamation may accompany epilation. It generally does not cause any problem or discomfort to the dog and usually is not treated. Moist desquamation usually appears 1 to 2 weeks after the end of treatment, and the severity is variable. It is associated with pruritus, and self-inflicted mutilation exacerbates the problem. If moist desquamation develops, the area should be cleansed with warm water. Petroleum-based products over the wound are contraindicated. Drying agents can be used, but no evidence of efficacy exists. Preventing self-mutilation and promoting good general hygiene are of paramount importance. Elizabethan collars, side braces, or padded bandages on the paws may be indicated, depending on the location of the field. *Moist desquamation should subside 2 to 4 weeks after it first appears.*

## Eyes

The effects to the eye are dose related and vary in severity.[28] The eye is avoided if at all possible, but sometimes the location of the tumor prohibits exclusion of the eye from the radiation field. Acute effects include blepharitis, blepharospasm, conjunctivitis, and the development of keratoconjunctivitis sicca (KCS). KCS is treated with artificial tears and steroids to prevent corneal ulceration. If corneal ulceration is present, healing may be delayed because of damage of the corneal stem cells by the radiation. The KCS may be temporary or permanent, depending on the dose administered and the sensitivity of the patient. Late effects include vascular changes that may have subtle effects on vision but in most cases do not result in blindness. Radiation-induced cataracts may occur but take years to develop fully and are generally not of clinical importance.

**Table 10–1**    Response to Irradiation of Commonly Treated Tumors

| Tumor Location/Type | Modality | Control or Survival Data | Comments | References |
|---|---|---|---|---|
| *Brain Tumors—Dogs* | | | | |
| Meningiomas | Radiation ± surgery | 16 months survival | Unclear whether addition of surgery improves survival. | 16 |
| Pituitary macroadenomas/carcinomas | Radiation only | 24 months median survival | For control of neurologic signs. Necessary to continue treating for Cushing's indefinitely. | 19 |
| *Ceruminous Gland—Dogs and Cats* | | | | |
| | Surgery plus radiation | 56% 1 year control | 39.5 months mean control | 29 |
| *Extremity and Body—Dogs* | | | | |
| Soft tissue sarcomas | Radiation only | 67% 1 year, 33% 2 years tumor control | Conservative surgery followed by radiation. | 20, 21 |
| | Surgery plus radiation | 75% control | | |
| Mast cell tumor | Radiation only | 44–78% 1 year tumor control | Control at 1 year similar to control at greater times. | 22, 30, 31 |
| | Surgery plus radiotherapy | ≈90% 1 year tumor control | For grade II tumors. | |
| *Extremity and Body—Cats* | | | | |
| Vaccine-associated sarcomas | Radiation followed by surgery | ≈70% control at 1 year | Study not yet complete | 23 |
| *Lymphoma—Cats (localized)* | | | | |
| | Radiation ± chemotheraphy | 28 months median | Non-nodal, localized forms. | 32 |
| *Nasal Tumors—Dogs* | | | | |
| All types | Orthovoltage plus surgery | 23 months control | Surgery must be performed for cytoreduction when using orthovoltage. | 12, 33 |
| Carcinomas (all) | Megavoltage | 8–12.8 months median control | The role of adjuvant chemotheraphy has not been determined. Addition of surgery does not appear to improve tumor control. | 3, 12. 34, 35 |
| Adenocarcinoma | | 10–12.8 | | |
| Squamous cell | | 6.1–12.8 | | |
| Sarcomas (all) | | 8–12.8 | | |
| Chondrosarcomas | | 12–15 | | |
| *Nasal Tumors—Cats* | | | | |
| All types | Ortho or mega | 20.8 months median | | 13, 36 |
| *Oral—Dogs* | | | | |
| Acanthomatous epulis | Radiation ony | 85% 1 year control | | 37 |
| Squamous cell carcinoma | Radiation only | 65% 1 year control | | 5, 6 |
| Fibrosarcoma | Radiation only | 4 months median control | Surgical cytoreduction followed by radiotherapy may improve tumor control. | 8, 9 |

| Tumor Location/Type | Modality | Control or Survival Data | Comments | References |
|---|---|---|---|---|
| Melanoma | Radiation (palliative) | 8 months median survival | Coarse fractions used palliatively. Traditional fractionation not beneficial. | 26, 27 |
| *Osteosarcoma—Dogs* | | | | |
| Extremities | Palliative | 4 months median control | Provides pain relief. | 24 |
| Axial skeleton | Radiation ± surgery and chemotherapy | 4.5 months median control | Surgery for cytoreduction if paralysis and/or severe pain, and cisplatin as radiosensitizer. | 25 |

## REFERENCES

1. Gillette EL: Principles of radiation therapy. *In* Theilen GH, Madewell BR (eds.): Veterinary Cancer Medicine, 2nd ed. Philadelphia, Lea & Febiger, 1987, pp. 137–143.
2. Adams WM: Veterinary Radiation Therapy. Compend Contin Educ Pract Vet 13:262–266, 1991.
3. McEntee MC, Page RL, Heidner GL, et al: A retrospective study of 27 dogs with intranasal neoplasms treated with cobalt radiation. Vet Radio 32:(3):135–139, 1991.
4. Thrall DE: Orthovoltage radiotherapy of acanthomatous epulides in 39 dogs. Amer Vet Med Assoc 184:(7):826–829, 1984.
5. Gillette EL, McChesney SL, Dewhirst MW, et al: Response of canine oral carcinomas to heat and radiation. Int J Radiat Oncol Biol Phys 13:1861–1867, 1987.
6. Evans SM, Shofer F: Canine oral nontonsillar squamous cell carcinomas: Prognostic factors for recurrence and survival following orthovoltage radiation therapy. Vet Radio 29:133–137, 1988.
7. Ciekot PA, Powers BE, Withrow SJ, et al: Histologically low-grade, yet biologically high-grade, fibrosarcomas of the mandible and maxilla in dogs: 25 cases (1982–1991). Amer Vet Med Assoc 204(4):610–615, 1994.
8. Gillette SM, Dewhirst MW, Gillette EL, et al: Response of canine soft tissue sarcomas to radiation or radiation plus hyperthermia: A randomized phase II study. Int J Hyperthermia 8:309–320, 1992.
9. McChesney SL, Withrow SJ, Gillette EL, et al: Radiotherapy of soft tissue sarcomas in dogs. J Am Vet Med Assoc 194(1):60–63, 1989.
10. Postorino-Reeves NC, Turrel JM, Withrow SJ: Oral squamous cell carcinoma in the cat. Amer Anim Hosp Assoc 29:1–4, 1993.
11. LaRue SM, Vail DM, Ogilvie GK, et al: Shrinking-field radiation therapy plus mitoxantrone for the treatment of oral squamous cell carcinoma in the cat. Proc Amer Coll Vet Radio, 1991 (Abstract).
12. Adams WM, Withrow SJ, Walshaw R, et al: Radiotherapy of malignant nasal tumors in 67 dogs. Amer Vet Med Assoc 191(3):311–315, 1987.
13. Straw RC, Withrow SJ, Gillette EL, et al: Use of radiotherapy for the treatment of intranasal tumors in cats: Six cases (1980–1985). Amer Vet Med Assoc 189(8):927–929, 1986.
14. Carlisle CH, Gould S: Response of squamous cell carcinoma of the nose of the cat to treatment with X rays. Vet Radio 23:186–192, 1982.
15. Withrow SJ, Straw RC: Resection of the nasal planum in nine cats and five dogs. Amer Anim Hosp Assoc 26(2):219–222, 1982.
16. Evans SM, Dayrell-Hart B, Powlis W, et al: Radiation therapy of canine brain masses. Vet Intern Med 7:216–219, 1993.
17. Turrel JM, Fike JR, LeCouteur RA, et al: Radiotherapy of brain tumors in dogs. J Am Vet Med Assoc 184:82–86, 1984.
18. Niebauer GW, Dayrell-Hart BL, Speciale J: Evaluation of craniotomy in dogs and cats. J Am Vet Med Assoc 198:89–95, 1991.
19. Dow SW, LeCouteur RA, Rosychuk RAW, et al: Response of dogs with functional pituitary macroadenomas and macrocarcinomas to radiation. J Small Anim Pract 31:287–294, 1990.
20. Atwater SW, LaRue SM, Powers BE, et al: Adjuvant radiotherapy for soft tissue sarcomas. Proc Vet Cancer Soc, 1992 (Abstract).
21. Mauldin GN, Meleo KA, Burk RL: Radiation therapy for the treatment of incompletely resected soft tissue sarcomas in dogs: 21 cases. Vet Cancer Soc 13th Annu Conf, Colombus, OH, 1993 (Abstract).
22. Frimberger AE, Moore AS, LaRue SM, et al: Radiotherapy of incompletely resected, intermediately differentiated mast cell tumors in dogs. Proceed Vet Cancer Soc, 1994 (Abstract).
23. Cronin KL, Page RL, Thrall DE: Radiation and surgery for treatment of feline fibrosarcomas. 1994. (Unpublished data).
24. McEntee MC, Page RL, Novotney CA, Thrall DE: Palliative radiotherapy for canine appendicular osteosarcoma. Vet Radio Ultrasound 34:367–370, 1993.
25. Van Vechten BJ, Withrow SJ, Straw RC, et al: Vertebral tumors in 20 dogs. Proc Vet Cancer Soc, 1994 (Abstract).
26. Bateman KE, Catton PA, Pennock PW, et al: 0-7-21

radiation therapy for the treatment of canine oral melanoma. Vet Intern Med 8:267–272, 1994.

27. Dewhirst MW, Sim DA, Forsyth K: Local control and distant metastases in primary canine malignant melanomas treated with hyperthermia and/or radiotherapy. Int J Hyperthermia 1:219–234, 1983.

28. Roberts SM, Lavach JD, Severin GA, et al: Ophthalmic complications following megavoltage irradiation of the nasal and paranasal cavities in dogs. Amer Vet Med Assoc 190(1):43–47, 1987.

29. Theon AP, Barthez PY, Madewell BR, Griffey SM: Radiation therapy of ceruminous gland carcinomas in dogs and cats. J Am Vet Med Assoc 205:566–569, 1994.

30. Turrel JM: Prognostic factors for radiation treatment of mast cell tumor in 85 dogs. J Am Vet Med Assoc 193:936–940, 1988.

31. Allan GS, Gillette EL: Response of canine mast cell tumors to radiation. J Natl Cancer Inst 63:69, 1979.

32. Elmslie RE, Ogilvie GK, Gillette EL, et al: Radiotherapy with and without chemotherapy for localized lymphoma in 10 cats. Vet Radio 32:277–280, 1991.

33. Thrall DE, Harvey CE: Radiotherapy of malignant nasal tumors in 21 dogs. Amer Vet Med Assoc 183(6):663–666, 1983.

34. Mauldin GN, Meleo KA: Combination carboplatin and radiotherapy for nasal tumors in dogs. Proc Vet Cancer Soc, 1994 (Abstract).

35. LaRue SM, Gillette EL, Ogilvie GK, McChesney-Gillette S, Powers BK, Withrow SJ: Irradiation plus mitoxantrone for treatment of canine nasal tumors. Vet Radio 31, 1990 (Abstract).

36. Evans SM, Hendrick M: Radiotherapy of feline nasal tumors: A retrospective study of nine cases. Vet Radio 30:128–132, 1989.

37. Thrall DE, Adams WM: Radiotherapy of squamous cell carcinomas of the canine nasal plane. Vet Radio 23(5):193–196, 1982.

# 11

# Immunology and Biologic Therapy of Cancer

E. Gregory MacEwen and Stuart C. Helfand

It has long been conjectured that the immune system could play a major role in treating cancer. Observations supporting this hypothesis include (1) spontaneous remissions of cancer without treatment; (2) increased incidence of cancer in immunosuppressed patients; (3) the presence of lymphoid cellular infiltrates in solid tumors; and (4) rare documented remission with immuno-modulators. The earliest efforts using an immunologic approach to treat (human) cancer, which are nearly 100 years old, utilized heteroimmune sera obtained from animals inoculated with human cancer tissues.[1] This approach, continually used in humans until the 1960s, was based on the idea that tumor cells express unique antigens that could induce a specific antibody response that would, in turn, cause tumor lysis.[1] In general, this approach has uniformly failed to produce convincing antitumor effects. Indeed, the presentation of asymptomatic patients with widely disseminated cancer would suggest tumor-specific antigens do not exist or do not elicit an immune response. To this day, antigens uniquely and solely expressed by cancer cells have yet to be described.

Another pioneering effort to activate the cancer patient's immune system was described by W.B. Coley in 1909.[2,3] Based on the observation that some cancer patients with incidental bacterial infections survived longer than those without sepsis, he used mixtures of bacteria as "vaccines" (referred to as Coley toxins) to try to stimulate the immune system nonspecifically. Some patients did remarkably well, surviving more than 2 decades following treatment, their cases forming the basis of further research.

The lack of understanding for the biologic basis of these antitumor responses and the seemingly risky nature of therapy relegated Coley toxins to the back burner as more attention was given to development of anticancer drugs throughout much of this century. However, the vision of successful treatment of cancer by immunologic approaches has been revitalized over the last 20 years, because of an increased understanding of the immune system, the identification of cytokines, the molecular methods designed to engineer genetically their production, and the advent of monoclonal antibody (Mab) technology.

Antibodies (especially Mabs) that recognize so-called differentiation antigens expressed both on normal and neoplastic cells but to a greater degree by cancer cells, are highly relevant to modern approaches to immunotherapy. Coley toxins also have been shown to have a valid biologic basis for therapy in that they likely elicited cytokine responses involving interferons, tumor necrosis factor (TNF), and interleukin-1 (IL-1), all proteins of great interest for their antitumor properties.[4,5]

The modern expanded field of "immunotherapy," based on the newer technologies, is often referred to as a biologic therapy, biotherapy, or biologic response modification. *Biotherapy* or *biologic response modifiers* refers to natural or synthetically produced substances or methods that alter the tumor-host relationship, with resultant therapeutic benefits. The methods or agents used may act via the host's immune system or may involve direct effects on the tumor cell itself or the microenvironment of tumors, altering the metastatic process or tumor angiogenesis. Some approaches used under the classification of biologic therapy are summarized in Table 11–1.

## TUMOR IMMUNOLOGY OVERVIEW

### Antigens on Tumors

With the exception of tumors caused by oncogenic viruses, the antigens expressed on tumors are differentiation antigens and are not specific for cancer cells.[6] Several virally induced tumors express antigens that *are* unique to those tumors. In humans, Burkitt's lymphoma, caused by the Epstein-Barr (herpesvirus) is such an example, and in veterinary medicine, Marek's disease of chickens (caused by a herpesvirus) and feline leukemia virus (FeLV)–induced tumors of cats both express tumor specific antigens. The advent of Mab technology changed the focus from searching for unique tumor antigens to identifying antigens shared by tumor cells recognized by a specific Mab. The antigens recognized on tumor cells by a particular Mab may in fact be expressed on more than one histologic type of tissue. To be a useful Mab for immunotherapy, the antigen it recognizes must be more highly expressed on tumor cells than normal cells. The greater the difference in antigen expression (as measured by Mab binding) between malignant and normal cells, the more likely such a Mab can be used clinically.

Hundreds of Mab-defined human tumor antigens have been described. Examples of antigens recognized by Mabs include mucins (on carcinomas of the breast, colon, and ovary),[7,8] proteins (colorectal carcinoma),[9] and disialogangliosides (neuroblastoma, melanoma, and osteosarcoma).[10–12] The present authors recently investigated Mab 14.G2a, a murine Mab developed against $GD_2$ gangliosides expressed by human neuroblastoma and melanoma. It is of interest to us because it recognizes fresh and cultured canine melanoma, indicating these same gangliosides are present on canine melanoma.[13]

Another group of tumor antigens are the abnormal protein products (quantitatively or qualitatively) expressed through the transcription of oncogenes in malignant cells.[6,14] These often include growth factor receptors and growth factors.[15,16] Some of these proteins are normally present only during fetal development.[16]

Although cell surface molecules are likely to be the targets for immunotherapy, cytosolic and nuclear proteins are also important because they may be processed into peptides and expressed on the cell surface with major histocompatibility proteins. Here, these peptides serve as antigenic targets for cytotoxic T-lymphocytes.

### Antibodies

Mabs are the most important type of antibody for immunotherapy. The technique for their production was described by Kohler and Milstein in 1975, by which normal immunoglobulin-producing spleen cells are fused with malignant plasma cells, resulting in immortalization of the spleen cells.[17]

There are multiple uses for Mabs in cancer therapy, including the targeting of radioisotopes, chemotherapy, and immunotoxins directly to tumor cells when these compounds are coupled to the Mab.[18–20] By themselves, tumor-reactive Mabs do not usually destroy tumor targets. However, after binding to an antigen on a tumor cell, the Fc (fragment, crystalline) end of the antibody can be engaged by immune effector cells that have Fc receptors. These include natural killer (NK) cells, monocytes and macrophages, and neutrophils. When the Fc end of the Mab is engaged, lytic mechanisms can be activated within the effector cell, resulting in lysis of the tumor target. This form of tumor killing, specifically mediated by the interaction of the Mab and immune effector cell, is called antibody-depen-

**Table 11–1**   Biography of Cancer

| Approach | Agents |
| --- | --- |
| Nonspecific immunomodulation | Bacterial agents, IL-2, IFNs, TNF, L-MTP-PE, Acemannan |
| Specific immunomodulation | Tumor antigen vaccines |
| Adoptive cellular therapy | T-cells, macrophages, LAK cells, TIL cells |
| Adoptive antibody therapy | Monoclonal antibodies |
| Growth regulators | Colony-stimulating factors, IFNs, retinoids, IL-6, IL-4 |
| Genetic modification | Gene therapy |

dent cellular cytotoxicity (ADCC).[21] It is an important mechanism for promoting tumor cytotoxicity by cell-mediated pathways. In ADCC, Mabs add a high level of specificity to the tumoricidal properties of immune effector cells, specifically helping to identify appropriate targets for destruction by immune cells. The most effective Mabs for mediating ADCC belong to the immunoglobulin subclasses IgG2a and IgG3.[22,23]

Some antibodies are also able to fix and activate the complement cascade after having bound to a tumor antigen.[24–27] This results in membrane damage to the target bringing about cellular death or enhanced phagocytosis.

Because Mabs are made in murine cells, these immunoglobulins are eventually "seen" as foreign proteins in any species receiving them except mice. Antimurine Mab responses are a well-known disadvantage in humans receiving Mab immunotherapy. This results in more rapid clearance and lower concentrations of Mab to bind to tumor targets. The "second generation" of Mabs for human immunotherapy has attempted to circumvent this problem by genetically engineering chimeric Mabs.[28] These antibodies have a fragment, antigen-binding (Fab) gene sequence that is murine spliced to the Fc gene sequence for human immunoglobulin. In man, chimeric antibodies are more potent than murine Mabs in mediating ADCC.[26] Other genetically engineered Mabs in development are known as bispecific Mabs.[29] These antibodies are designed so that one Fab site recognizes an antigen on a tumor cell and the other recognizes a surface molecule associated with the antigen receptor on a cytotoxic T-lymphocyte (CTL). The interaction of the Mab with the surface molecule of the CTL is enough to trigger killing by the lymphocyte that is held in close proximity to the tumor target by the other Fab site.[29] In this system, the Mab not only acts to add specificity but serves as a trigger for tumor killing by immune cells. These Mabs have shown promise in treating cancer in murine tumor models.

## Effector Cells

There are multiple effector cell subsets within the immune system that are capable of killing tumor cells. These include T-lymphocytes, NK cells, monocytes, macrophages, and neutrophils. The level of tumor cytotoxicity mediated by effector cells is generally greater than that of antibodies alone and of longer duration.

**T-Lymphocytes**    T-lymphocytes recognize antigen specifically through the T-cell antigen receptor (TCR).[30] This receptor "sees" antigen only when the antigen is "presented" to it by another cell in association with a specialized membrane protein called a major histocompatibility complex (MHC) protein.[31] MHC proteins are either of Class I or Class II. Thus, antigen recognition by a T-cell is restricted by the ability of its unique TCR not only to bind the antigen but also to bind the MHC protein presenting the antigen.

Different T-cell subsets recognize either MHC Class I or Class II proteins. In particular, T-helper ($T_h$; CD4) cells are restricted to antigen recognition only when presented in association with Class II MHC proteins. Cytotoxic T-lymphocytes ($T_c$; CD8; CTLs) can only recognize antigen presented by self MHC Class I proteins. For cancer immunotherapy, the most important function of $T_h$ cells is the production and secretion of cytokines that foster cell-mediated antitumor responses. Interleukin-2 (IL-2) is the best known and most studied of these cytokines. Besides IL-2, interferon gamma (IFN-γ) is released by activated $T_h$ cells.[32] IFN-γ enhances the tumoricidal activities of monocytes/macrophages. $T_h$ cells have recently been further subdivided into $T_{h1}$ subsets, principally responsible for providing cytokine "help" (e.g., IL-2, IFN-γ) for cell-mediated responses, while $T_{h2}$ cells produce cytokines (e.g., IL-4, IL-5, IL-10) that enhance humoral responses.[33] CTLs require IL-2 to enhance their antitumor cytotoxic functions. These cells contain several lytic proteins (e.g., perforin, granzyme, and lymphotoxin [tumor necrosis factor β]) that are used to kill tumor targets.

**NK Cells**    NK cells are lymphocytes and unlike T-cells they lack an antigen receptor and are cytolytically active in a nonspecific manner.[34] Their killing is not restricted by MHC determinants, and memory response does not develop in NK cells upon re-exposure to a sensitizing antigen. Another difference between NK cells and T-cells is the presence of Fc receptors on the NK cell.[35] This characteristic allows NK cells to engage in ADCC. NK activation via the Fc receptor causes NK cells to release cytolytic mediators (similar to those released by CTLs). It is not known how an NK cell "sees" its target, since it lacks an antigen receptor, but the evidence to date suggests target cells are recognized and bound by NK cells via surface adhesion molecules.[36] Morphologically, NK cells appear as large granular lymphocytes on a blood smear.

For cancer immunotherapy, one of the most important features of NK cells is their ability to be stimulated by IL-2 to become more potent killers of tumor targets.[37] The term *lymphokine-activated killer (LAK)* cell has been coined to indicate IL-2 activation of resting NK cells to this heightened state of tumoricidal capacity.

**Monocytes/Macrophages**    Monocytes and macrophages are able to recognize, bind, and destroy malignant cells in vitro and in vivo while sparing non-neoplastic cells.[38–40] The mechanisms by which tumor cells are preferentially recognized are not yet certain. Nevertheless, the ability of macrophages to distinguish quantitatively between malignant and nonmalignant phenotypes makes them an ideal effector cell for increasing antitumor specificity when using an immunologic approach to treat cancer. Macrophages can also kill tumor cells known to be resistant to chemotherapy.[41]

A variety of mechanisms are responsible for macrophage-mediated tumor cytotoxicity. These include the production and secretion of several effector molecules, including TNF-α, IL-1, cytolytic proteases, reactive nitrogen intermediates, and reactive oxygen intermediates.[42–44] Although cells of the monocyte/macrophage pool can selectively destroy neoplastic cells, Fc receptors on their cell membranes allow them to kill tumor targets by ADCC mechanisms when the appropriate antitumor Mab is present.[23]

**Neutrophils**    Neutrophils are the major phagocytic cell involved in the firstline defense against micro-organisms. They also function in acute inflammation and autoimmune processes. Recently, human neutrophils have been shown to participate in the potent killing of human tumor cells such as neuroblastoma and melanoma, in the presence of tumor-specific Mabs.[45] We recently reported that canine neutrophils kill canine melanoma cells in vitro in the presence of tumor-specific antiganglioside Mabs.[13] Because the molecular mechanism of neutrophil ADCC against tumor targets is distinct from that of either T-lymphocytes, NK cells, or monocytes, the activation of neutrophils with lymphocytes and monocytes in concert to kill tumor cells would likely be additive or possibly synergistic.

## Cytokine Cellular Activators

In addition to the effector cells, a number of cytokines are produced by a variety of leukocytes and other cells that play a very important role in the regulation, activation, growth, and functional activity of the immune system. Over the last decade, recombinant DNA technology has contributed to the rapid development and production of these cytokines in vitro for research and therapy. Because these cellular products act as messengers for other leukocytes, they are called interleukins (ILs).

**IL-1**    Antigen-stimulated macrophages are the major source of IL-1.[46] IL-1, in conjunction with a presented antigen, directly activates T-cells to produce IL-2.[47] Also, IL-1 can directly activate macrophages and monocytes to produce TNF α and IL-6 and become cytotoxic to tumor cells.[48,49]

IL-1 has a profound effect on the hematopoietic system.[50] IL-1 will induce the production of hematopoietic growth factors granulocyte/monocyte-colony-stimulating factor (GM-CSF), granulocyte-colony-stimulating factor (G-CSF), monocyte-colony-stimulating factor (M-CSF), IL-6, and IL-3. In vivo administration of IL-1 has produced significant antitumor activity in a number of murine tumors. Clinical studies in humans have shown that IL-1 is extremely toxic, but it is still being investigated to ameliorate drug-induced myelosuppression.[51]

**IL-2**    IL-2 is a 15 kD glycoprotein secreted by activated helper T-lymphocytes. It is a major regulatory hormone of the immune system, inducing proliferation and differentiation of lymphocytes (and other cells) and modifying their function. The potential use of IL-2 for cancer therapy is based on the augmentation of the direct cell-mediated lysis it confers on lymphocytes and the associated release of other cytokines that can play a direct or indirect role in tumor cell destruction.[37]

There are several lymphocyte subsets that acquire potentiated tumor-killing functions following culture with IL-2. These include NK cells and cytotoxic T-cells. The enhanced tumor-killing ability imparted by IL-2 on these immune effectors has been termed lymphokine-activated killer (LAK) cell activity. In a population of peripheral blood lymphocytes (PBLs), most lytic activity is derived from the NK cells and the term *LAK cell* has come to imply IL-2-activated NK cells and not a distinct lineage of lymphocytes.[52] NK cells comprise less than 15% of the circulating lymphocyte pool. The biologic effects of IL-2 are mediated through binding to a specific cell membrane receptor complex (IL-2R).[53–55]

**IL-3**    IL-3 (multicolony stimulating factor) is produced by activated T-cells. In vivo administration in mice of IL-3 results in a multilineage response in the peripheral blood, with a 10-fold increase of eosinophil counts and 3-fold expansion of neutrophils and monocytes. Interestingly, there is a 100-fold increase in splenic mast cells. IL-3 may be used with other hematopoietic growth factors to correct primary or secondary hematopoietic insufficiencies.[56,57]

**IL-4**   IL-4 is a pleiotropic cytokine first identified as a B-cell growth factor (B-CGF). IL-4 enhances IgG and IgE production. In clinical trials in humans, IL-4 it has been shown to have some antitumor activity against Hodgkin's and non-Hodgkin's lymphoma.[58] No antitumor effects have been observed against solid tumors. Combination therapy involving IL-4 gene transfer into tumor cells along with genes for other cytokines (e.g., IL-2, IFNα IFNβ, and TNFα) may prove promising in the future.[58]

**IL-5**   IL-5 has profound proliferative effects on eosinophil precursors, eosinophil activation, and survival.[59] The association of eosinophilia and neoplasia has been noted for many years in humans and its presence has been associated with a favorable prognosis in some cancers, notably bladder carcinomas, cervical carcinoma, and head and neck carcinomas.[60] Eosinophilia has also been noted in dogs and cats with mast cell tumors. IL-5 is also associated with tissue-dwelling parasitic infections. The potential of IL-5 to be useful for the treatment of neoplasms is doubtful.[60]

**IL-6**   IL-6 is produced and released from monocytes and macrophages after activation.[61] IL-6 plays an important role in promoting the differentiation of B-lymphocytes into antibody-secretory cells and increases the production of IgM, IgA, and IgG. IL-6 stimulates the release of acute-phase proteins from the liver and stimulates thrombocytopoieses, resulting in increased platelet counts.[62] IL-6 causes fever through a prostaglandin $E_2$-dependent mechanism.

IL-6 also will cause bone resorption and is produced by osteoblasts. IL-6 has been shown to increase with age and may play a role in osteoporosis because estrogens will inhibit the production of IL-6.[63]

In malignancy, IL-6 may act as an autocrine factor for multiple myeloma. In tumor model systems in mice, IL-6 has been shown to reduce the metastasis and tumor growth of melanoma, fibrosarcoma, and lung carcinoma. The role of IL-6 in treating spontaneous tumors needs further study.[64]

**IL-7**   IL-7 is important in inducing early B- and T-lymphoid growth. Few studies have been done to evaluate the biologic effects of IL-7 given in vivo in humans. Because IL-7 acts to induce differentiation of early lymphoid progenitors, IL-7 may play a role in lymphocyte recovery after chemotherapy.[65]

**IL-8**   IL-8 is a chemotactic factor for neutrophils, and in vivo administration results in profound granulocytopenia, followed by a granulocytosis. IL-8 will inhibit the migration of neutrophils to inflammatory sites. IL-8 seems to be important in the pathophysiology of inflammation but may play a minimal role in tumor control.[66]

**IL-9**   IL-9 is a growth factor for mast cells as well as B-cells, resulting in a modulation of IgE to increase production. IL-9 will also regulate the maturation of erythroid progenitors in the presence of erythropoietin.[67]

It has been reported that the lymph nodes from patients with Hodgkin's disease and large cell anaplastic lymphomas express large amounts of IL-9 and thus this cytokine may act as a growth factor in an autocrine loop.[68]

**IL-10**   IL-10 may function as a natural anti-inflammatory agent in vivo. The injection of IL-10 to simultaneously LPS-treated (lethal dose) mice, protects animals from septic shock, presumably by preventing the synthesis of proinflammatory monokines (e.g., TNFα and IL-1).[69]

IL-10 cooperates with other cytokines to augment the growth of pluripotent stem cells, megakaryocyte progenitors, erythroid progenitor, mast cell progenitors, and lymphoid progenitors.[70]

IL-10 may play a role in HIV-AIDS lymphoma because of the increased expression of IL-10 in these lymphomas.[71] In humans with non-Hodgkin's lymphoma, increased levels of IL-10 have been associated with reduced survival time.[72]

**IL-12**   IL-12 is a newly identified cytokine that may serve a role as a "Th switch" to stimulate uncommitted T-helper cells toward the type 1 helper cells ($T_{h1}$). This may be especially important in HIV-infected patients in which there appears to be a shift toward a $T_{h2}$-like cytokine profile that seems to lead to clinical AIDS. IL-12 is being tested for its ability to restore T-cell function and increase $T_{h1}$ activity. IL-12 will also induce the secretion of a large amount of IFN-γ from $T_{h1}$ cells and NK cells. IL-12 in many ways may mimic the immunologic effects of IL-2 without the toxicity. Studies in rodent models have demonstrated very significant antitumor activity. Clinical trials are now under way in humans.[73]

**Tumor Necrosis Factor**   Tumor necrosis factor (TNFα) is secreted from macrophages after activation by lipopolysaccharides (LPSs) and other lymphokines such as IL-2.[74] TNFα, as well as IL-1, are important mediators of the pathophysiologic sequelae of a diverse array of diseases, infections, and inflammatory states. When TNF∝, as is produced acutely and released in large quantities into the circulation during a serious septic condition, it triggers a state of shock and tissue injury (septic shock syndrome) that has a high mortality rate. When produced during chronic disease states, TNFα is capable of mediating alterations in homeostasis. This syndrome can be characterized by accelerated catabolism, weight loss, anemia, and loss of lean body mass, as well as lipid stores. This has been termed *cachexia*. TNF α has also been called cachectin.[74]

Most cells have TNFα receptors and respond to TNFα. Resistant cells appear to express protective cytoplasmic proteins that prevent TNFα cytotoxicity.[75] These include manganous superoxide dismutase (MnSOD), and glutathione (GSH), proteins involved in free-radical (superoxide radicals) scavengers. TNFα will up-regulate the expression of MnSOD and GSH and this may partially explain the observation that TNFα will protect mice from lethal doses of radiation and chemotherapy. A single dose of IV TNFα induces MnSOD in bone marrow and protects hematopoietic progenitor cells from radiation.[76] TNFα-induced MnSOD and GSH may also render tumor cells resistant to subsequent treatment with TNFα.

The tumoricidal effects of TNFα are not clearly understood. However, it is known that TNFα can induce changes on the cell membrane, especially those having a strong effect on lipids, leading to lysosomal damage.[77] TNFα will also cause the formation of pores to develop within the cell membrane, thus leading to cytopathic effects.

TNFα has also been shown to induce apoptosis in tumor cells.[78] Apoptosis is characterized by an active biochemical alteration within cells, resulting in DNA degradation and fragmentation, possibly related to the induction of oxygen-free radicals. TNFα exerts some of its antitumor activity through its effects on the endothelial cells.[79] TNFα is able to suppress anticoagulant mechanisms, increasing the procoagulant cofactor tissue factor and reduce the barrier function, leading to vascular leakage. This leads to hemorrhage and necrosis of tumors.

The results of clinical trials using rhTNFα have been disappointing.[80] Little antitumor activity has been documented and excessive toxicity has been noted. Most likely, recombinant TNFα will be effective when used in combination with other treatments such as radiation, chemotherapy, and hyperthermia.

## CURRENT APPROACHES TO IMMUNOTHERAPY

### Nonspecific Immunomodulators

Historically, bacterial agents have been used for many years as vaccines against cancer. As previously mentioned, in the early 1900s, W.B. Coley, a surgeon at the New York Cancer Hospital, developed a vaccine using extracts of *Streptococcus pyogenes* and *Serratia marcescens* ("Coley's toxins"), which resulted in sporadic tumor responses in very advanced cancers.[2,3] These observations led to studies by Shear and collegues in 1943, showing that *S. marcescens* extracts would induce necrosis and hemorrhage in mouse sarcomas.[4] The polysaccharide they isolated is now known as endotoxin. In 1978, the first reports of using a killed vaccine of *S. pyogenes* and *S. marcescens* in dogs and cats with spontaneous tumors were published.[81–82] Although this vaccine resulted in antitumor activity, the toxicity and lack of consistent activity limited its clinical usefulness. Table 11–2 provides a summary of nonspecific immunomodulators.

An agent that is still used today for immunotherapy is the bacillus Calmette-Guérin (BCG), an attenuated *mycobacterium*. BCG, as well as other bacterial vaccines, such as *Corynebacterium parvum* (also called *Propionibacter acnes*) received a great amount of attention in preclinical and clinical trials the past 20 years.[83] BCG has been shown to have activity when directly injected into cutaneous melanomas in humans and by instillation in the bladder for the treatment of superficial transitional carcinomas. In addition, BCG and *C. parvum* have shown some activity in canine mammary tumors. *C. parvum* was shown to have antitumor activity in human[84] and canine[85] melanomas, when combined with surgery.

The principles of therapy using nonspecific bacterial vaccines are as follows:[86]

**Table 11–2** Nonspecific Immunomodulators

| Category | Agent |
|----------|-------|
| Intact organisms | Viable: BCG<br>Nonviable: *C. parvum*<br>Mixed bacterial<br>    vaccine: *S. marcescens*<br>    and *S. pyogenes* |
| Microbial cell wall | BCG-cell wall<br>Methanol extract, BCG<br>    (MER) |
| Galactomannans | Acemannan |
| Synthetic compounds | Muramyl dipeptide (MDP)<br>Muramyl tripeptide (MTP)<br>Lipopolysaccharide (LPS)<br>Modified endotoxin<br>    (detoxified LPS)<br>Staphage lysate (SpL) |
| Natural hormones | Thymic hormone extracts<br>Dehydroepiandrosterone<br>    (DHEA) |
| Chemical agents | Levamisole<br>Piroxicam (PGE$_2$ inhibitor)<br>H$_2$ receptor antagonists:<br>    Cimetidine |
| Vitamims/Minerals | Retinoids<br>Vitamin C<br>Folic acid<br>Zinc<br>Selenium<br>Vitamin E |

1. These agents are most effective against minimal residue tumor and when used in conjunction with cytoreductive surgery or following radiation or chemotherapy.
2. An immunocompetent host is most desirable or, at least, a host capable of immunorestoration. Patients who have been heavily immunosuppressed with chemotherapy are unlikely to respond.
3. Immunosuppressive therapy such as corticosteroids must be avoided.
4. Immunotherapy, may, depending on the chemotherapy drug, be given concurrently with chemotherapy.
5. The effectiveness of the vaccine may be improved if administered in close proximity to the tumor via intratumor, intracavity, or regional lymph node drainage by injection.

## Liposome-Encapsulated Muramyl Tripeptide

Liposome-encapsulated muramyl tripeptide-phosphatidylethanolamine (L-MTP-PE) is a nonspecific activator of monocytes and macrophages.[87] MTP-PE is a lipophilic derivative of muramyl dipeptide (MDP). MDP is the minimal structural unit of mycobacterium cell walls and is a potent monocyte-macrophage activator in vitro. In vivo MDP has limited clinical usefulness because it is cleared from the circulation within 60 minutes after parenteral administration and can induce nephrotoxicity and vasculitis. Encapsulation of MDP into multilamellar phospholipid vesicles or liposomes results in effective delivery of the MDP to monocytes and macrophages, resulting in activation and in situ antitumor activity.[87,88]

Lipophilic L-MTP-PE has been shown to be more effective in in situ monocyte-macrophage tumoricidal activity in both rodents and humans.[87,89] In humans, phase I and II studies have been completed and L-MTP-PE has been shown to result in significant cytokine release, such as IL-1β, TNFα, IL-6, as well as neoptrin, C-reactive protein, and β 2-microglobulin.[90,91] Clinical antitumor activity has been documented in human metastatic osteosarcoma, melanoma and, renal cell carcinoma.

The present authors have been evaluating L-MTP-PE in dogs with osteosarcoma treated with amputation.[92,93] In the first study, following amputation, dogs were randomized to either L-MTP-PE or empty liposomes (control). Dogs receiving the L-MTP-PE had a median survival time of 7.4 months versus those dogs treated by surgery alone (empty liposomes), which had a median survival time of 3 months. (Fig. 11–1). This study in dogs clearly demonstrated that L-MTP-PE has significant activity for the prevention or treatment of metastasis.[92] However, since 70% of the dogs still died of metastasis, we further expanded this study, using cisplatin chemotherapy to reduce the extent of micrometastatic disease. Briefly, dogs with osteosarcoma of the extremities, without evidence of distant metastases, were treated with amputation, followed by four courses of cisplatin (70 mg/M$^2$ IV q 28 days) and then randomized to either saline liposomes (placebo) or L-MTP-PE. This was a double-blind trial. Forty dogs were entered into this clinical study. Thirteen dogs developed metastasis during the chemotherapy and 2 died of other causes. Twenty-five dogs were randomized after the completion of the chemotherapy. Eleven dogs were randomized into the L-MTP-PE group and 14 were randomized into the placebo group. Of the 14 dogs in the placebo group, 13 have died of metastasis and 1 of an unrelated death. The median survival time for

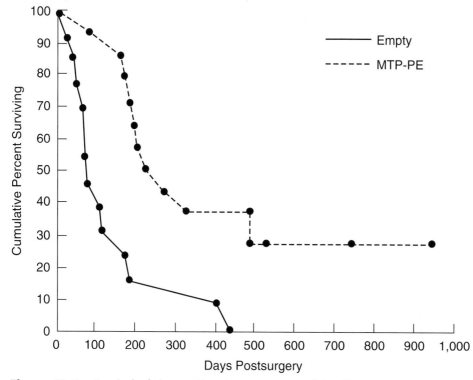

**Figure 11–1.**   Survival of dogs with osteosarcoma receiving liposome-MTP-PE versus those receiving empty liposomes, $p = 0.002$.

the dogs in the placebo group was 10 months and the median disease-free interval was 7.2 months ($P<.05$). In the L-MTP-PE group, 8 of 11 dogs developed metastases. Two died of unrelated causes and 3 are still alive. The median survival time for the L-MTP-PE group was 14.6 months, and the median disease-free interval was 12 months ($P<.05$)[93] (Fig. 11–2). These two studies clearly indicate that L-MTP-PE is an effective agent for the treatment of micrometastases in dogs with osteosarcoma. With the addition of the chemotherapy, the survival time of dogs with osteosarcoma can be greatly enhance.

L-MTP-PE has also been shown to induce canine monocytes to become tumoricidal,[94,95] and release TNFα and IL-6 into the serum.[96] More recently, we have been evaluating the combined effectiveness of L-MTP-PE and doxorubicin on the induction of in vivo monocyte cytotoxicity and cytokine release in dogs. We have found that combining L-MTP-PE and doxorubicin together results in enhanced serum TNFα levels of monocyte cytotoxicity following doxorubicin.[95] This finding has prompted us now to evaluate doxorubicin and L-MTP-PE combined with surgery in dogs with splenic hemangiosar-

coma, in a randomized, double-blind clinical trial.[97] (See Chap. 29).

**Acemannan**   Acemannan is a water-soluble, long-chain, polydispersedβ[(1,4)]-linked mannan polymer, synthesized from the aloe vera plant.[98] Acemannan has been shown to enhance macrophage release of IL-1β, TNFα, IL-2, IL-6, IFNγ and GM-CSF.[98] Acemannan has been found to enhance T-cell function, as demonstrated by the allogeneic response in mixed lymphocyte cultures.[98] It also has been shown to inhibit the replication of HIV-1 in vitro[99] and may retard the development of clinical signs in cats infected with the feline leukemia virus.[100] In addition, acemannan has been shown to have synergistic antiviral effects in combination with azidothymidine (AZT) and acyclovir in vitro.[101] Acemannan has been shown to have antitumor activity in a murine sarcoma model.[102]

In clinical trials in solid tumors in dogs and cats, acemannan has been reported to have therapeutic activity against fibrosarcoma.[103] Treated tumors develop necrosis, edema, and lymphocytic infiltration. More studies are needed to determine the optimal route and dose of administra-

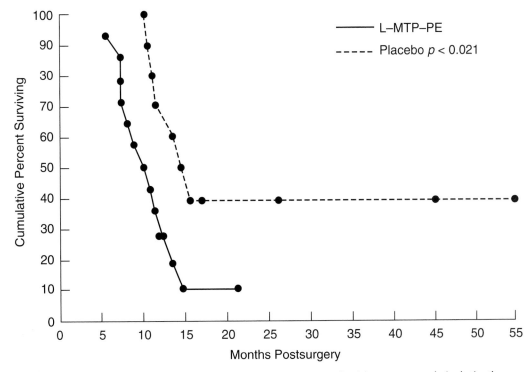

**Figure 11–2.** Survival time of dogs with osteosarcoma treated with surgery and cisplatin then randomized to liposome-MTP-PE or empty liposomes, $p = 0.021$.

tion, as well as other possible tumor types that may be responsive.

**Levamisole**   Levamisole is an orally active synthetic phenylimidazole, and is the Levo isomer of tetramisole, a potent, broad-spectrum antihelmintic agent. Levamisole has been shown to increase both T-cell numbers and proliferative responses, if initially depressed. Levamisole also enhances phagocytic and chemotactic activities of polymorphonuclear leukocytes and monocytes.[104]

Two recently reported large-scale clinical trials have now demonstrated that postoperative adjuvant therapy with levamisole plus 5-fluorouracil significantly improves survival in colon cancer patients.[105,106]

Randomized studies using levamisole, in combination with surgery in canine and feline mammary adenocarcinoma, failed to demonstrate any beneficial effects.[107,108] In addition, levamisole combined with combination chemotherapy in canine lymphoma showed no significant beneficial clinical activity over chemotherapy alone.[109]

**Prostaglandin Antagonists**   Prostaglandins (PGs) are local hormones with an important role

in the regulation of cell functions and cell interactions.[110] Activated monocytes and macrophages are major sources of $PGE_2$. $PGE_2$ inhibits several lymphocyte functions: proliferation, lymphokine production, cytotoxic activity, and suppressor activity. $PGE_2$ has also been shown to down-regulate gene expression of TNFα in activated monocytes.

The nonsteroidal anti-inflammatory drug (NSAID) piroxicam (Feldene), a $PGE_2$ antagonist, has been shown to have antitumor activity in canine bladder carcinoma.[111] Thirty-four dogs with histopathologically confirmed, nonresectable transitional cell carcinoma of the bladder were treated with piroxicam (0.3 mg/kg daily PO) and evaluated at 1 and 2 months after the initiation of the drug. Two of the 34 had a complete regression, 4 had partial responses, 18 had stable disease, and 10 had progressive disease. The median survival time for all dogs treated was 181 days. These response rates compare favorably to response rates reported with cisplatin chemotherapy. Another NSAID, oxyphenbutazone, has been shown to improve survival in humans with stage 3 cervical cancer, when administered during radiation therapy.[112]

**Cimetidine**   This histamine-2 ($H_2$ receptor antagonist) has been shown to have immunomodulating activity.[113,114] Because T-suppressor cells express $H_2$ receptors, cimetidine may modulate T-suppressor activity. Histamine has been shown to inhibit cell-mediated immune function in vivo and in vitro. Cimetidine has been found to increase responsiveness to skin test antigens and increase lymphocyte response to antigens.

There are also studies reporting on the synergistic effects of interferon and cimetidine in melanoma, acute myeloid leukemia, and myelodysplastic syndrome.[115] Recently, a study in women with ovarian cancer showed that cimetidine improved CD4 cell counts and IL-2 production undergoing chemotherapy.[116] Cimetidine has also been reported to cause the regression of equine cutaneous melanoma.[117] However, its use as a therapeutic immunomodulator is still unproven.

## Lymphokines/Monokines

**IL-2**   Following the initial report in 1982 by Grimm et al that described in vitro lysis of NK-resistant tumor cells by IL-2-activated autologous human PBLs, there was great enthusiasm for IL-2 as an antitumor agent.[37] Initially, it was thought that LAK cells would be "cancer specific" and spare non-neoplastic tissue. This, however, has not turned out to be true because some normal tissues are destroyed by IL-2-activated lymphocytes, but to a lesser degree than tumor cells. The greatly publicized toxicity of IL-2 in human patients is probably due (in part) to this nonselective cellular injury, but the magnitude of destruction between tumor and normal tissue provides a therapeutic window for cancer treatment.

The mechanisms underlying the LAK phenomenon are not completely understood, although much is known. IL-2 stimulates "resting" NK cells to produce and store cytoplasmic lytic molecules (e.g., perforin, granzymes, and tumor necrosis factor β that can induce pore formation and DNA fragmentation in target cells.[118] NK-derived LAK cells, which lack a T-cell antigen receptor, must next bind to a target, an event accomplished via adhesion molecules located on the cell membrane. Up-regulation of these molecules on LAK cells is also an IL-2-dependent effect. Once a target cell is "engaged," the LAK cell delivers a "kiss of death," with the subsequent death of the target occurring within hours. The LAK cells are not destroyed in this process and are able to engage in another round of killing. In this regard, some have likened LAK cells to "mass murderers."

Advances in the immunotherapy of human cancer patients with IL-2 have been slow, despite the extraordinary tumoricidal properties of LAK cells and convincing data from rodent models showing the clinical effectiveness of IL-2 immunotherapy.[119] To date, only a minority of human patients (e.g., 20% of patients with renal cell carcinoma or metastatic melanoma) show measurable antitumor responses, but, for many, the remissions have been prolonged.[120]

Some of the questions in the preclinical and early clinical testing of IL-2 related to optimal treatment schedule, dose, route, decreased toxicity (e.g., fever, pulmonary edema secondary to capillary leakage, dermatitis, hepatocellular injury, renal dysfunction), and the need to add the patient's own NK cells, activated exogenously with IL-2. Data from murine studies, which have been confirmed in human IL-2 cancer trials, indicate the greatest antitumor effects were seen when (1) IL-2 was given when the tumor burden had been reduced; (2) treatment was prolonged over several days to weeks; (3) serum levels of IL-2 were maintained in vivo during the treatment period; and (4) the highest (nontoxic) doses of IL-2 were used.

A number of observations in veterinary medicine with human recombinant (hr)IL-2 indicate that cancer immunotherapy with this cytokine may prove effective in several species. Canine PBLs bind hrIL-2 with high affinity, comparable to that observed for human PBL[53] In addition, hrIL-2 stimulates a proliferative response in canine PBLs, indicating that this recombinant cytokine induces signal transduction through the canine IL-2R.[53] In vitro induction of the LAK phenomenon in canine lymphocytes has been reported with high and very high doses of hrIL-2[121,122] and data from our laboratory indicate that low doses of hrIL-2 are effective in inducing canine LAK cell activity in vitro.[123] We also studied the clinical and immunologic effects of in vivo infusions of hrIL-2 in dogs.[124] The data indicate that these infusions induce the LAK phenomenon in vivo in dogs when measured by an in vitro tumor-killing assay. IL-2 also induced lymphocyte proliferation in vivo, as indicated by progressive lymphocytosis (Fig. 11–3).

The major limiting toxicity in dogs given hrIL-2 combined with hrTNF was gastrointestinal.[125] In that study, objective antitumor responses were seen in dogs with oral melanoma and mast cell tumors. Another report using hrIL-2 and hrTNF in dogs did not indicate appreciable side effects other than transient gastrointestinal dysfunction.[126]

Human recombinant IL-2 was reported to augment the tumor cytotoxicity of lymphocytes obtained from biopsies of bovine ocular squamous cell carcinoma.[127] These cells proliferated in response to culture with hrIL-2. Several cows were injected intratumorally with hrIL-2 in an effort to induce LAK activity in situ within the tumor-infiltrating lymphocytes. Three out of 5 cows showed tumor regression.

It is clear that augmenting the tumor-destructive abilities of NK and cytotoxic T-lymphocytes is feasible with IL-2. However, the optimal dose, route, and schedule for IL-2 administration have yet to be determined in any species. Because the physiologic role of IL-2 is involved with a cascade of cytokines, it is likely that as more is learned, an optimum combination of cytokines, including IL-2, will be determined that are synergistic in the cancer patient. It will be important, however, to increase the specificity of this immune approach to potentiate specific tumor killing and decrease normal tissue toxicity. One approach is to combine tumor-specific Mab with IL-2.[128] LAK cells express Fc receptors on the cell membranes. This enables LAK cell killing to become antibody directed, because antibodies bound to the tumor cell can serve as a bridge to link the LAK cell (by its Fc receptor) specifically to the tumor target. This approach becomes even more appealing in light of data indicating that in vivo infusion of IL-2 enhances ADCC by patients' PBLs in vitro.[129] When PBLs from the IL-2 treated patients are used as the effector cells in vitro (against several different human tumor cell lines), in the presence of Mab, the magnitude of cytolysis increases as much as 1,000-fold.

Additional enthusiasm for combining Mab with IL-2 (and other leukocyte activators) resides in the expression of Fc receptors on macrophages and neutrophils that could also participate in antitumor ADCC.[45,130] Furthermore, IL-2 can directly enhance the tumoricidal activity of human monocytes,[131] extending the possibilities of positive, multiplicative interactions. We have shown that in vitro, canine peripheral blood lymphocytes and neutrophils can mediate specific lysis of canine tumor cells in the presence of antitumor Mabs.[13] These preliminary results are encouraging.

**Interferons—α, β, γ** Interferons (IFNs) are a family of naturally occurring glycoproteins elaborated from cells in response to virus, double-

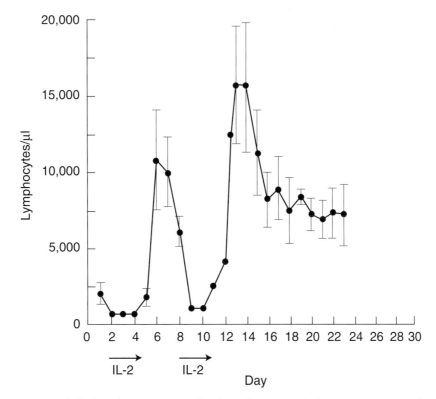

**Figure 11–3.** Mean daily lymphocyte counts for four dogs completing two weekly cycles of interleukin-2 (IL-2).

stranded ribonucleic acid (RNA), antigens, and mitogens. Interferons have both direct and indirect cytoxic, cytostatic, antiangiogenic, and immunomodulatory properties. Gamma (γ) IFN is a more potent immune system modulator than is alpha (α) or beta (γ) IFN. IFNα is a more powerful antitumor agent. IFNγ plays an extremely important role in the function of CD4 ($T_{h1}$) cells, NK cells, B-cells, and macrophages. IFN γ is needed for the production of nitric oxide by macrophages, and for the killing of intracellular parasites, such as *Listeria* and *Mycobacteria*. The recombinantly synthesized IFNs (human, mouse, bovine, feline) are generally species specific for γ and β and not for α.[132]

Clinically, IFNα has been studied in cats infected with FeLV.[133,134] Experimental and clinical studies in cats infected with FeLV have reported that low doses of human IFNα (0.5 to 5.0 U) will prevent disease development in cats experimentally infected with FeLV. The mean survival time for cats given HuIFNα was significantly longer than those given no treatment (control). The average survival time for the control cats ($n = 7$) was 73 days versus 500 days for the 0.5 U group ($n = 9$) and 313 days for the high-dose 5.0 U group ($n = 5$).[133] In a follow-up clinical study using IFNα in 31 FeLV(+) "clinically ill" cats and bovine IFNβ in 36 cats, survival at 12 months was 19/31 (61%) for the HuIFNα group versus 13/36 (36%) for the IFNβ group. The differences between these groups was reported as statistically significant ($p<.05$).[134] This was not a controlled or randomized study, and the cause of death was not reported. Despite treatment, almost all cats remained FeLV (+). The authors recommend 30 U/cat given orally once daily for seven days, on a week-off schedule. Further details are available as published.[134]

IFNα has been shown to have antitumor activity in Kaposi's sarcoma, renal carcinoma, lymphoma, and hairy cell leukemia.[135] More recently, IFNα has been reported to have significant antiangiogenic activity in human hemangiomas.[136] The clinical responses reported with IFNβ and IFNγ in human cancers have been minimal. Additional studies are necessary, especially evaluating the IFNs in early stages of disease and combined with other immunomodulators.

## HEMATOPOIETIC GROWTH FACTORS

The hematopoietic colony-stimulating factors (CSFs) are regulatory molecules that control the differentiation and proliferation of hematopoietic progenitors. In some cases, the CSFs may also enhance the function and release of other biologically active molecules from mature cells. The CSFs act through their own specific receptors but may also interact through other cell-surface components.[137,138] The CSFs and the target cells are presented in Table 11–3.

These CSFs have been evaluated in humans,[137,138] dogs,[139–142] and cats.[143] A recombinant canine G-CSF (rcG-CSF) has been developed and studies have been reported regarding its use in dogs.[139–141] Recombinant human (rh) GM-CSF and rhG-CSF have been used to treat dogs with cyclic neutropenia.[142,144] Both CSFs induced an increase in granulocytic production; however, only G-CSF altered the cyclic phenomenon. It has potential therapeutic value to reduce the duration of neutropenia following chemotherapy and total body radiation therapy. Studies in our laboratory, as well as others, have shown that rcG-CSF can be administered safely to dogs for as long as 69 days.[140,141] We were able to increase the total leukocyte count to 80,000 to 100,000 cells/μl without any adverse reaction in normal dogs. The monocyte count was also increased 4.5-fold during the treatment period.[140]

In one study, (rhG-CSF) was administered to normal dogs for 30 days.[144] Initially, a neutrophilia developed; however, this was followed by a prolonged period of chronic neutropenia. It was determined that serum from the dogs taken during the neutropenia period contained antibody to rhG-CSF, which neutralized the stimulatory effects of both rhG-CSF and endogenous cG-CSF. The investigators were able to transfer this neutropenia effect to another dog, using plasma from a neutropenic dog given rhG-CSF. Caution must be exercised when using the rhG-CSF in dogs. Unfortunately, the rcG-CSF is not yet available commercially.

GM-CSF supports the growth of multipotential hematopoietic progenitor cells, as well as cells already committed to myeloid, erythroid, or megakaryocytic lineages.[138] GM-CSF also enhances the multiple functions of mature cells, including oxidative metabolism, phagocytosis, lysozyme secretion, and ADCC. In humans, GM-CSF is useful in overcoming neutropenia in patients with myelodysplastic syndromes and aplastic anemia.[145] Studies have also shown that rhGM-CSF has been useful in stimulating neutrophil recovery after chemotherapy for acute leukemias and seems to improve the therapeutic outcome in a high-risk group.[142] rhGM-CSF also

**Table 11–3**  Hematopoietic Colony-Stimulating Factors and Related Molecules

| Factor | Abbreviation | Target Cells |
|---|---|---|
| Granulocyte— Colony-stimulating factor | G-CSF | Granulocytes Monocytes |
| Granulocyte— Macrophage colony- stimulating factor | GM-CSF | Monocytes Granulocytes Eosinophils |
| Macrophage colony-stimulating factor | M-CSF | Monocytes/macrophages |
| Multipotential colony-stimulating factor (interleukin 3) | Multi-CSF or IL-3 | Multipotent stem cells and progenitors from granulocytes, monocytes, erythroids, megakaryocytes, eosinophils, basophils, and mast cells |
| Erythropoietin | EPO | Erythroid progenitors |
| Stem cell factor, C-kit ligand, or mast cell growth factor | SCF | Primitive multilineage blood cell progenitors, and mast cells |

has been shown to lessen the duration and severity of granulocytopenia after autologous bone marrow transplant.[145] Current studies are in progress using IL-3 combined with GM-CSF. A very significant improvement using the IL-3 is the stimulation of thrombopoiesis, because of the stimulation of megakaryocytic progenitors.[146]

We have studied rhGM-CSF in normal dogs.[140] The rhGM-CSF resulted in elevated neutrophil counts within 1 week (40,000 cells/$\mu$l), but counts declined by the end of week 2. We suspect that antibodies to rhGM-CSF developed and resulted in the inactivation of the rhGM-CSF.

The clinical activity of CSFs as regulators for the formation and function of granulocytes and monocytes will be very important to reduce the bone marrow suppression associated with chemotherapy and radiation. In addition, these regulators hold some potential as a method to enhance ADCC, as well as increasing the effector cell population for immunotherapy trials.

## MONOCLONAL ANTIBODIES

Conceptually, antibodies directed against a tumor-associated antigen (TAA) offer potential specificity that is directly related to the degree to which that antigen is found on the tumor cell, and the success of that antibody attaching to that cell.

A number of factors will influence the effectiveness of Mab therapy. These include the number of antigen molecules per cell surface, number of cells expressing the antigen, size of the tumor mass, degree of tumor vascularization, presence and reactivity of circulating antigen in the blood, presence of antigen on non-neoplastic (normal) tissues, clearance of Mab from blood, dose and route of administration, and development of an antimonoclonal antibody immune response.[147]

A monoclonal antibody has been developed that recognizes canine lymphoma cells (Mab 231).[148] This monoclonal antibody has been reported to mediate ADCC against a canine lymphoma cell line. More important, this antibody has been reported to prolong remission duration when used following chemotherapy in dogs with lymphoma. In studies performed at the University of Pennsylvania, comparing chemotherapy alone to chemotherapy plus Mab 231, the median survival time of dogs treated with chemotherapy plus the antibody was 591 days. Compared to a historical control group of dogs treated with a similar chemotherapeutic protocol, the median survival time was only 184 days.[149] The results of this study are encouraging and warrant further, more controlled, clinical trials. Currently, this monoclonal antibody is available commercially and is being actively evaluated in additional clinical studies.

## REFERENCES

1. Oettgen HG, Old LJ: The history of cancer immunotherapy. *In* De Vita VT, Hellman S, Rosenberg SA (eds): Biologic Therapy of Cancer. Philadelphia, JB Lippincott, 1991, pp. 87–119.

2. Coley WB: Treatment of inoperable malignant tumors with the toxins of erysipelas and the *Bacillus prodigiosus*. Trans Am Surg Assoc 12:183–212, 1894.

3. Coley WB: The treatment of inoperable sarcoma by bacterial toxins (the mixed toxins of *Streptococcus erysipelatis* and the *Bacillus prodigiosus*). Proc R Soc Med, Surg Sect 3:1, 1909.

4. Shear MJ, Turner FC, Perrault A, et al: Chemical treatment of tumors V. isolation of the hemorrhage producing fraction from *Serratia marcescens* culture filtrate. J Natl Cancer Inst 4:81–97, 1943.

5. Carswell EA, Old LJ, Kassel RL, et al. An endotoxin induced serum factor which causes necrosis of tumors. Proc Natl Acad Sci USA 72:3666–3670, 1975.

6. Hellström KE, Hellström I: Principles of tumor immunity: Tumor antigens. *In* DeVita VT, Hellman S, Rosenberg SA (eds): Biologic Therapy of Cancer. Philadelphia, JB Lippincott, 1991, pp. 35–52.

7. Girling A, Bartkova J, Burchell J, et al: A core protein epitope of the polymorphic epithelial mucin detected by the monoclonal antibody SM-3 is selectively exposed in a range of primary carcinomas. Int J Cancer 15:1072–1076, 1989.

8. Schlom J, Colcher D, Roselli M, et al: Tumor targeting with monoclonal antibody B72.3. Int J Radiol Appl Instrum 16:137–142, 1989.

9. Koprowski H, Steplewski Z: Human solid tumor antigens defined by monoclonal antibodies. *In* Hammerling GJ, Hammerling U, Kearnes JF (eds): Monoclonal Antibodies and T-cell Hybridomas. Amsterdam, Elsevier/North-Holland Biomedical Press, 1981, p. 161.

10. Mujoo K, Kipps TJ, Yang HM, et al: Functional properties and effect on growth suppression of human neuroblastoma tumors by isotype switch variants of monoclonal antiganglioside GD2 antibody 14.18. Cancer Res 49:2857–2861, 1989.

11. Helfand SC, Surfus J, Kleinerman ES, et al: Monoclonal antibodies 14.G2a and CH14.18 mediate cytotoxicity of human osteosarcoma cells by human lymphocytes. Proc Am Assoc Cancer Res 33:40, 1991.

12. Hamilton WB, Helling F, Lloyd KO, et al: Ganglioside expression on human melanoma assessed by quantitative immune thin-layer chromatography. Int J Cancer 53:566–573, 1993.

13. Helfand SC, Soergel SA, Donner RL, et al: Potential to involve multiple effector cells with human recombinant IL-2 and antiganglioside monoclonal antibodies in a canine malignant melanoma immunotherapy model. J. Immunother 16:188–197, 1994.

14. Sell, S. Cancer markers of the 1990s. Comparison of the new generation of markers defined by monoclonal antibodies and oncogene probes to prototypic markers. Clin. Lab. Med. 10:1–37, 1990.

15. Heldin CH, Johansson A, Wennergren S, et al: A human osteosarcoma cell line secrets a growth factor structurally related to a homodimer of PDGF A-chains. Nature 319:511–514, 1986.

16. Drebin JA, Link VC, Greene MI: Monoclonal antibodies specific for the new oncogene product directly mediate antitumor effects *in vivo*. Oncogene 2:387–394, 1988.

17. Kohler G, Milstein C: Continuous culture of fused cells secreting antibodies of predefined specificity. Nature 256:495–497, 1975.

18. Bacha P, Williams DP, Waters C, et al: Interleukin-2 receptor-targeted cytotoxicity: Interleukin-2 receptor-mediated action of a diphtheria toxin-related interleukin-2 fusion protein. J Exp Med 167:612–622, 1988.

19. Larson SM, Cheung NKV, et al: Radioisotope conjugates. *In* DeVita VT, Hellman S, Rosenberg SA (eds): Biologic Therapy of Cancer. Philadelphia, JB Lippincott, 1991, pp. 496–511.

20. Trail PA, Willner D, Lasch SJ, et al: Cure of xenografted human carcinomas by BR96-doxorubicin immunoconjugates. Science 261:212–215, 1993.

21. Duffus WPH: Immunity to infection. *In* Halliwell REW, Gormans NT (eds): Veterinary Clinical Immunology. Philadelphia, WB Saunders, 1989, pp. 143–148.

22. Johnson WJ, Steplewski Z, Matthews TJ, et al: Cytolytic interactions between murine macrophages, tumor cells, and monoclonal antibodies: Characterization of lytic conditions and requirements for effector activation. J Immunol 136:4704–4713, 1986.

23. Lubeck MD, Kimoto Y, Steplewski Z, et al: Killing of human tumor cell lines by human monocytes and murine monoclonal antibodies. Cell Immunol 111:107–117, 1988.

24. Cheresh DA, Honsik CJ, Staffileno LK, et al: Disialoganglioside GD3 on human melanoma serves as a relevant target antigen for monoclonal antibody-mediated tumor cytolysis. Proc Natl Acad Sci USA 82:5155–5159, 1985.

25. Bajorin DF, Chapman PB, Wong G, et al: Phase I evaluation of a combination of monoclonal antibody R24 and interleukin 2 in patients with metastatic melanoma. Cancer Res 50:7490–7495, 1990.

26. Mueller BM, Romerdahl CA, Gillies SD, et al: Enhancement of antibody-dependent cytotoxicity with a chimeric anti-GD2 antibody. J Immunol 144:1382–1386, 1990.

27. Ohta S, Honda A, Tokutake Y, et al: Antitumor effects of a novel monoclonal antibody with high affinity to ganglioside GD3. Cancer Immunol Immunother 36:260–266, 1993.

28. Morrison SL, Oi VT: Genetically engineered antibody molecules. Adv Immunol 44:65–92, 1989.

29. Fanger MW, Segal D, Wunderlich JR: Going both ways: Bispecific antibodies and targeted cellular cytotoxicity. FASEB J 4:2846–2849, 1990.

30. Allison JP, Lanier LL: Structure, function, and

serology of the T-cell antigen receptor complex. Annu Rev Immunol 5:503–540, 1987.

31. Moss PAH, Rosenberg WMC, Bell JI: The human T cell receptor in health and disease. Annu Rev Immunol 10:71–96, 1992.

32. Reem GH, Yeh N-H: Interleukin-2 regulates expression of its receptor and synthesis of gamma interferon by human T lymphocytes. Science 225:429–430, 1985.

33. Mosmann TR, Coffman RL: TH1 and TH2 cells: Different patterns of lymphokine secretion lead to different functional properties. Annu Rev Immunol 7:145–173, 1989.

34. Trinchieri G: Biology of natural killer cells. Adv Immunol 47:187–376, 1989.

35. Lanier LL, My Le A, Civin CI, et al: The relationship of CD16 (Leu-11) and Leu-19 (NKH-1) antigen expression on human peripheral blood NK cells and cytotoxic T lymphocytes. J Immunol 136:4480–4485, 1986.

36. Zarcone D, Cerruti G, Tenca C, et al: Human NK cell adhesion molecules (CAMs). In Lotzová E, Herbermans RB (eds): NK cell mediated cytotoxicity: receptors, signaling and mechanisms. CRC Press, Boca Raton, FL, 1992, pp. 77–83.

37. Grimm EA, Mazumder A, Zhang HZ, et al: The lymphokine activated killer cell phenomenon: Lysis of NK resistant fresh solid tumor cells by IL-2 activated autologous human peripheral blood lymphocytes. J Exp Med 155:1823–1841, 1982.

38. Fidler IJ: The in situ induction of tumoricidal activity in alveolar macrophages by liposomes containing muramyl dipeptide is a thymus-independent process. J Immunol 127:1719–1720, 1981.

39. Kleinerman ES, Erickson KL, Schroit AJ, et al: Activation of tumoricidal properties in human monocytes by liposomes containing lipophilic muramyl tripeptide. Cancer Res 43:2010–2014, 1983.

40. Fidler IJ, Kleinerman ES: Lymphokine-activated human monocytes destroy tumor cells but not normal cells under cocultivation conditions. J Clin Oncol 2:937–943. 1984.

41. Giavazzi R, Bucana CD, Hart IR: Correlation of tumor growth inhibitory activity of macrophages exposed to Adriamycin and Adriamycin sensitivity of the target tumor cells. J Natl Cancer Inst 73:447–455, 1984.

42. Hibbs JM, Taintor RR, Vavrin Z, et al: Nitric oxide: A cytotoxic activated macrophages effector molecule. Biochem Biophys Res Comm 157:87–94, 1988.

43. Ichinose Y, Bakouche O, Tsao JY, et al: Tumor necrosis factor and IL-1 associated with plasma membranes of activated human monocytes lyse monokine-sensitive but not monokine-resistant tumor cells, whereas viable activated monocytes lyse both. J Immunol 141:512–518, 1988.

44. Martin JHJ, Edwards SW: Changes in mechanisms of monocyte/macrophage-mediated cytotoxicity during culture. J Immunol 15:3478–3486, 1993.

45. Barker E, Mueller BM, Handgreitinger R, et al: Effect of chimeric anti-ganglioside $G_{D2}$ antibody on cell-mediated lysis of human neuroblastoma cells. Cancer Res 51:144–149, 1991.

46. Matusushima K, Taguchi M, Kovas EJ, et al: Intracellular localization of human monocyte associated interleukin-1 (IL-1) activity and release of biologically active IL-1 by trypsin and plasmin. J Immunol 136:2883–2891, 1986.

47. Larsson EL, Iscove NN, Coutinho A: Two distinct factors are required for induction of T-cell growth. Nature 283:664–666, 1980.

48. Kishimoto T: The biology of interleukin 6. Blood 74:1–10, 1989.

49. Philip R, Epstein LB: Tumor necrosis factor as immunomodulator and mediator of monocyte cytotoxicity induced by itself, gamma-interferon and interleukin 1. Nature 323:86–89, 1986.

50. Mochizuki DY, Eisenman JR, Conlon PG, et al: Interleukin 1 regulates hematopoietic activity, a role previously ascribed to hemopoietin 1. Proc Natl Acad Sci USA 84:5267–5271, 1987.

51. Johnson CJ: Interleukin-1: Therapeutic potential for solid tumors. Cancer Invest 11:600–608, 1993.

52. Ortaldo JR, Longo DL: Human natural lymphocyte effector cells: Definition, analysis of activity and clinical effectiveness. J Natl Cancer Inst 80:999–1010, 1988.

53. Helfand SC, Modiano JF, Nowell PC: Immunophysiological studies of interleukin-2 and canine lymphocytes. Vet Immunol Immunopathol 33:1–16, 1992.

54. MacEwen EG, Helfand SC: Recent advances in the biologic therapy of cancer. Compend Contin Ed Pract Vet 15:909–922, 1993.

55. Voss SD, Hong R, Sondel PM: Severe combined immunodeficiency, interleukin-2 (IL-2), and the IL-2 receptor: Experiments of nature continue to point the way. Blood 83:626–635, 1994.

56. Oster W, Schulz G: Interleukin 3: Biological and clinical effects. Int J Cell Cloning 9:5–23, 1991.

57. Lindemann A, Mertelsman R: Interleukin-3: Structure and function. Cancer Invest 11:609–623, 1993.

58. Puri RK, Siegel JP: Interleukin-4 and cancer therapy. Cancer Invest 11:473–486, 1993.

59. Sanderson CJ: The biological roles of interleukin-5. Int J Cell Cloning 1:147–153, 1990.

60. Mahanty S, Nutman TR: The biology of interleukin-5 and its receptor. Cancer Invest 11:624–634, 1993.

61. Kishimoto T: The biology of interleukin-6. Blood 74:1–10, 1989.

62. Ishibash T, Kimura H, Shikama Y, et al: Interleukin-6 is a potent thrombopoietic factor in vivo in mice. Blood 74:1241–1244, 1989.

63. Ishimi Y, Miyaura C, Jin CH, et al: IL-6 is produced by osteoblasts and induces bone resorption. J Immunol 145:3297–3303, 1990.

64. Lotz M: Interleukin-6. Cancer Invest 11:732–742, 1993.

65. Appasamy PM: Interleukin-7: Biology and potential clinical applications. Cancer Invest *11*:482–499, 1993.

66. Herbert CA, Baker JB: Interleukin-8: A review. Cancer Invest *11*:743–750, 1993.

67. Renauld JC, Houssiau F, VyHenhove C, et al: Interleukin-9: A T-cell growth factor with a potential oncogenic activity. Cancer Invest *11*:635–640, 1993.

68. Merz H, Houssiau F, Orscheschk K, et al: Interleukin-9 expression in human malignant lymphoma: Unique association with Hodgkin's disease and large cell anaplastic lymphoma. Blood *78*:1311–1317, 1991.

69. Howard M, Muchamuel T, Androde S, et al: IL-10 protects mice from lethal endotoxemia. J Exp Med *177*:1205–1213, 1993.

70. Holland G, Zlothnik A: Interleukin-10 and cancer. Cancer Invest *11*:751–758, 1993.

71. Emilie D, Touitou R, Raphael M, et al: *In vivo* production of interleukin-10 by malignant cells in AIDS lymphoma. Eur J Immunol *22*:2937–2942, 1992.

72. Blay TY, Burdin N, Rousset F, et al: Prognostic value of IL-10 in non-Hodgkin's lymphoma. Blood *80* (Suppl. 1):38a, 1992 (Abstract).

73. Gately MK: Interleukin-12: A recently discovered cytokine with potential for enhancing cell-mediated immune responses to tumors. Cancer Invest *11*:500–506. 1993.

74. Old LJ: Antitumor activity of microbial products and tumor necrosis factor. *In* Bonavida B, Gifford GE, Kirchner H, Old LJ (eds): Tumor Necrosis Factor/Cachectin and Related Cytokines. Basel, Karger, 1988, pp. 7–19.

75. Tracey KJ: The acute and chronic pathophysiologic effects of TNF: Mediation of septic shock and wasting (cachexia). *In* Beutler B (ed): Tumor Necrosis Factors: The Molecules and Their Emerging Role in Medicine. New York, Raven Press, 1992, pp. 255–273.

76. Slordal L, Muench MO, Warren DJ, et al: Radioprotection by murine and human tumor-necrosis factor: Dose-dependent effects on hematopoiesis in the mouse. Eur J Haematol *43*:428–434, 1989.

77. Fitzgerald-Knauer M, et al: Mechanism of human lymphotoxin and tumor necrosis factor induced destruction of cells *in vitro:* Phospholipase activation and deacylation of specific-membrane phospholipids. J Cell Physiol *142*:469, 1990.

78. Kinebuchi T, Yoshida T: Mechanism of cellular apoptosis induced by tumor necrosis factor. *In* Osawa T , Bonavida B (eds): Tumor Necrosis Factor: Structure-Function, Relationship, and Clinical Application. Basel, Karger, 1992, pp. 125–134.

79. Nawroth P, Stern D: Modulation of endothelial cell hemostatic properties by tumor necrosis factor. J Exp Med *163*:740, 1986.

80. Alexander RB, Rosenberg SA: Tumor necrosis factor: Clinical applications. *In* DeVita VT, Hellman S, Rosenberg SA (eds): Biologic Therapy of Cancer. Philadelphia, JB Lippincott, 1991, pp. 378–392.

81. Brown NO, Patnaik AK, Mooney S, et al: Soft tissue sarcomas in the cat. JAVMA *173*:744–749, 1978.

82. MacEwen EG, Hess PW, Hayes AA, et al: A clinical evaluation of the effectiveness of immunotherapy combined with chemotherapy for the treatment of canine lymphosarcoma. *In* Bentvelzen P, Hilgers J, Yohn DS (eds): Advances in Comparative Leukemia Research. New York, Elsevier/North Holland, 1978, pp. 395–399.

83. Oettgen HF, Old LT: The history of cancer immunotherapy. *In* DeVita VT Jr, Hellman S, Rosenberg SA (eds): Biologic Therapy of Cancer. Philadelphia, JB Lippincott, 1991, pp. 87–119.

84. Balch CM, Smalley RV, Bartolucci AA, et al: A randomized prospective clinical trial of adjuvant *C. parvum* immunotherapy in 260 patients with clinical localized melanoma (Stage I). Cancer *49*:1079–1084, 1982.

85. MacEwen EG, Patnaik AK, Harvey HJ, et al: Canine oral melanoma: Comparison of surgery versus surgery plus *Corynebacterium parvum.* Cancer Invest *4*:397–402, 1986.

86. Hersh EM, Taylor CW: Immunotherapy by active immunization: Use of nonspecific stimulants and immunomodulators. *In* DeVita VT, Hellman S, Rosenberg SA (eds): Biologic Therapy of Cancer. Philadelphia, JB Lippincott, 1991, pp. 612–626.

87. Whitworth PW, Pak CC, Esgro JJ, et al: Macrophages and cancer. Cancer Metastasis Rev *8*:319–351, 1990.

88. Sone S, Fidler IJ: *In vitro* activation of tumoricidal properties in rat alveolar macrophages by synthetic muramyl dipeptide encapsulated in liposomes. Cell Immunol *57*:42–50, 1981.

89. Kleinerman ES, Murray JL, Snyder JS, et al: Activation of tumoricidal properties in monocytes from cancer patients following intravenous administration of liposomes containing muramyl tripeptide phosphatidylethanolamine. Cancer Res *49*:4655–4670, 1989.

90. Kleinerman ES, Jia SF, Griffin J, et al: Phase II study of liposomal muramyl tripeptide in osteosarcoma: The cytokine cascade and monocyte activation following administration. J Clin Oncol *10*:1310–1316, 1992.

91. Liebes L, Walsh CM, Chachoua A, et al: Modulation of monocyte functions by muramyl tripeptide phosphatidylethanolamine in a Phase II study in patients with metastatic melanoma. J Natl Cancer Inst *84*:694–699, 1992.

92. MacEwen EG, Kurzman ID, Rosenthal RD, et al: Therapy for osteosarcoma in dogs with intravenous injection of liposome-encapsulated muramyl tripeptide. J Natl Cancer Inst *81*:935–938, 1989.

93. MacEwen EG, Kurzman ID, Rosenthal RC, et al: Combined liposome-encapsulated muramyl

tripeptide and cisplatin in dogs with osteosarcoma. *In* Novak JF, McMaster JH: Frontiers of Osteosarcoma Research. Toronto, Hogrefe and Huber, 1993, pp. 117–119.

94. Smith BW, Kurzman, ID, Schultz KT, et al: Muramyl peptides augment the *in vitro* and *in vivo* cytostatic activity of canine plastic-adherent mononuclear cells against canine osteosarcoma cells. Cancer Biother 2:137–144, 1993.

95. Shi F, MacEwen EG, Kurzman ID, et al: *In vitro* and *in vivo* effects of doxorubicin combined with liposome-encapsulated muramyl tripeptide on canine monocyte activation. Cancer Res 53:3986–3991, 1993.

96. Kurzman ID, Shi F, MacEwen EG: *In vitro* and *in vivo* canine mononuclear cell production of tumor necrosis factor induced by muramyl peptides and lipopolysaccharide. J Vet Immunol Immunopath 38:45–56, 1993.

97. MacEwen EG, Kurzman ID, Helfand S, et al: Current studies of liposome muramyl tripeptide (CGP 19835 A lipid) therapy for metastasis in spontaneous tumors: A progress review. J Drug Targeting, 2:391–396, 1994.

98. Womble D, Helderman JH: The impact of acemannan on the generation and function of cytotoxic T-lymphocytes. Immunopharamacol Immunotoxicol 14:63–77, 1992.

99. Kahlon JB, Kemp MC, Carpenter RH, et al: Inhibition of AIDS virus replication by acemannan *in vitro*. Mol Biother 3:127–135, 1991.

100. Sheets MA, Unger BA, Giggleman GF, et al: Studies of the effect of acemannan on retrovirus infections: Clinical stabilization of feline leukemia virus-infected cats. Mol Biother 3:41–45, 1991.

101. Kahlon JB, Kemp MC, Yawei N, et al: *In vitro* evaluation of the synergistic antiviral effects of acemannan in combination with azidothymidine and acyclovir. Mol Biother 3:214–223, 1991.

102. Peng SY, Norman J, Curtin G, et al: Decreased mortality of normal murine sarcoma in mice treated with the immunomodulator acemannan. Mol Biother 3:179–187, 1991.

103. Harris C, Pierce K, King G, et al: Efficacy of acemannan in treatment of canine and feline spontaneous neoplasms. Mol Biother 3:207–213, 1991.

104. Symoens J: Levamisole, an antianergic chemotherapeutic agent: An overview. *In* Chirigos MA (ed): Control of Neoplasia by Modulation of the Immune System. New York, Raven Press, pp. 1–24, 1977.

105. Laurie JA, Moertel CG, Fleming TR, et al: Surgical adjuvant therapy of poor prognosis colorectal cancer with levamisole alone or combined levamisole with 5-fluorouracil. J Clin Oncol 7:1447–1456, 1989.

106. Moertel CG, Fleming TR, Macdonald JS, et al: Levamisole and fluorouracil for adjuvant therapy of resected colon carcinoma. N Engl J Med 322:352–358, 1990.

107. MacEwen EG, Harvey HJ, Patnaik AK, et al: Eval-uation of effect of levamisole and surgery on canine mammary cancer. J Biol Resp Modif 4:418–426, 1985.

108. MacEwen EG, Hayes AA, Mooney S, et al: Evaluation of effect of levamisole on feline mammary cancer. J Biol Resp Modif 5:541–546, 1984.

109. MacEwen EG, Hayes AA, Mooney S, et al: Levamisole as adjuvant to chemotherapy for canine lymphosarcoma. J Biol Resp Modif 4:427–433, 1985.

110. Chang J, Lewis AJ: Prostaglandins and cyclyoxygenase inhibitors. *In* Fenichel RL, Chirigos MA (eds): Immune Modulation Agents and Their Mechanisms. New York, Marcel Dekker, 1984, pp. 649–667.

111. Knapp DW, Richardson RC, Chan TCK, et al: Piroxicam therapy in 34 dogs with transitional cell carcinoma of the urinary bladder. J Vet Intern Med. 8:273–278, 1994.

112. Weppelmann B, Monkemeir D: The influence of prostaglandin antagonists on radiation therapy of carcinoma of the cervix. Gynecol Oncol 17:196–199, 1984.

113. Ershler WB, et al: Pharmacologic modulation of the immune response in mice by cimetidine. Intern J Immunopharmacol 4:359, 1982.

114. Ershler WB, et al: Inhibition of suppressor cell function by cimetidine in a murine model. Clin Immunother Immunopathol 38:350, 1986.

115. Ershler WB, Hacker MP, Burroughs BJ, et al: Cimetidine and the immune response. I. In vivo augmentation of nonspecific and specific immune response. Clin Immunol Immunopath 26:10–17, 1983.

116. Kituchi Y, et al: Effects of cimetidine on interleukin-2 production by peripheral blood lymphocytes in advanced ovarian carcinoma. Eur J Cancer Clin Oncol 24:7, 1988.

117. Goetz TE, Ogilvie GK, Keegan KG, et al: Cimetidine treatment of melanomas in three horses. JAVMA 196:499–452, 1990.

118. Young JDE, Cohn ZA: How do killer cells kill? Sci Am 258:28–44, 1988.

119. Mule JJ, Shu S, Rosenberg SA: The antitumor efficacy of lymphokine-activated killer cells and recombinant interleukin 2 *in vivo*. J Immunol 135:646–652, 1985.

120. Rosenberg SA, Yang JC, Topalian SL, et al: Treatment of 283 consecutive patients with metastatic melanoma or renal cell cancer with high-dose bolus interleukin 2. J Am Med Assoc 271:907–913, 1994.

121. Jardine JH, Jackson HJ, Lotzova E, et al: Tumoricidal effect of interleukin-2-activated killer cells in canines. Vet Immunol Immunopathol 21:53–160, 1989.

122. Raskin RE, Holcomb CS, Maxwell AK: Effects of human recombinant interleukin 2 on *in vitro* tumor cytotoxicity in dogs. Am J Vet Res 52:2029–2032.

123. Helfand SC, Soergel SA, Hank JA, et al: Induc-

tion of lymphokine-activated killer (LAK) activity in canine lymphocytes with low-dose human recombinant interleukin-2 *in vitro*. Cancer Biother 9:237–244, 1994.

124. Helfand SC, Soergel SA, MacWilliams PS, et al: Clinical and immunological effects of human recombinant interleukin-2 given by repetitive weekly infusion in normal dogs. Cancer Immunol Immunother 39:84–92, 1994.

125. Jeglum KA, Sorenmo K, Nannos J, et al: Sequential administration of recombinant tumor necrosis factor and the continuous infusion of recombinant interleukin-2 in canine patients with advanced malignancies. Proc Annu Mtg Am Assoc Cancer Res 31:294, 1990.

126. Moore AS, Theilen GH, Newell AD, et al: Preclinical study of sequential tumor necrosis factor and interleukin 2 in the treatment of spontaneous canine neoplasms. Cancer Res 51:233–238, 1991.

127. Rutten VPMG, Klein WR, deJong MA, et al: Immunotherapy of bovine ocular squamous cell carcinoma: The potential role of tumor infiltrating lymphocytes. J Cell Biochem Suppl 14B:102, 1990.

128. Munn DH, Cheung NK: Interleukin-2 enhancement of monoclonal antibody mediated cellular cytotoxicity against human melanoma. Cancer Res 47:6600–6605, 1987.

129. Hank JA, Robinson RR, Surfus J, et al: Augmentation of antibody-dependent cell-mediated cytotoxicity following *in vivo* therapy with recombinant interleukin 2. Cancer Res 50:5234–5239, 1990.

130. Liesveld J, Frediani K, Winslow J, et al: Cytokine effects and role of adhesive proteins and Fc receptors in human macrophage-mediated antibody dependent cellular cytotoxicity. J Cell Biochem 45:381–390, 1991.

131. Malkovsky M, Loveland B, North M, et al: Recombinant interleukin-2 directly augments the cytotoxicity of human monocytes. Nature 325:262–265, 1987.

132. Kurzrock R, Gutterman JU, Talpaz M: Interferons- α, β, γ: Basic principles and preclinical studies. *In* DeVita VT, Hellman S, Rosenberg SA (eds): Biologic Therapy of Cancer. Philadelphia, JB Lippincott, 1991, pp. 242–274.

133. Cummins JM, Tompkins MB, Olsen RG, et al: Oral use of human alpha interferon in cats. J Biol Resp Modif 7:513–523, 1988.

134. Weiss RC, Cummins JM, Richards AB, et al: Low dose orally administered alpha interferon treatment for feline leukemia virus infection. JAVMA 199:1477–1481, 1991.

135. Goldstein D, Laszlo J, Rudnick SA, et al: Interferon therapy in Cancer. *In* Oldham RK (ed): Principles of Cancer Biotherapy, 2nd ed. New York, Marcel Dekker, 1991, pp. 363–393.

136. White CW, Sondheimer HM, Crouch EC, et al: Treatment of pulmonary hemangiomatosis with recombinant interferon alpha. N Eng J Med 320:1197–1200, 1989.

137. Metcalf D: *In vivo* effects of recombinant colony-stimulating factors. ISI Atlas of Science: Immunol 1:238, 1988.

138. Groopman JE, Molina JM, Scadden DT, et al. Hematopoietic growth factors. N Engl J Med 321:1449–1459, 1989.

139. Ogilvie GK, Obradovich JE, Cooper MF, et al: Use of recombinant canine granulocyte colony-stimulating factor to decrease myelosuppression associated with administration of mitoxantrone in the dog. J Vet Intern Med 6:44–47, 1992.

140. Kurzman ID, MacEwen EG, Broderick C, et al: Effect of colony-stimulating factors on number and function of circulating monocytes in normal dogs. Mol Biother 4:29–33, 1992.

141. Obradovich JE, Ogilvie GK, Powers BE, et al: Evaluation of recombinant canine granulocyte colony-stimulating factor as an inducer of granulopoiesis. J Vet Intern Med 5:75–79, 1991.

142. Hammond WP, et al: Purified recombinant human granulocytes-macrophage colony-stimulating factor stimulates granulocytopoiesis in canine cyclic hematopoiesis. Blood 68 (Suppl.), 1:165a, 1986 (Abstract).

143. Obradovich JE, Ogilvie GK, Stadler-Morris S, et al: Effect of recombinant canine granulocyte colony-stimulating factor on peripheral blood neutrophil counts in normal cats. J Vet Intern Med 7:65–67, 1993.

144. Hammond WP, Csiba E, Canin A, et al: Chronic neutropenia: A new canine model induced by human granulocyte colony-stimulating factor. J Clin Invest 87:704–710. 1991.

145. Gabrilove JL: Colony-stimulating factors: Clinical status. *In* DeVita VT, Hellman S, Rosenberg SA (eds): Biologic Therapy of Cancer. Philadelphia, JB Lippincott 1991, pp. 445–463.

146. Lindemann A, Herrman F, Mertelsman R, et al: Human recombinant interleukin-3: A phage I/II clinical trial. *In* Mertelsman R, Herrmann F (eds): Hematopoietic Growth Factors in Clinical Application. New York, Marcel Dekker, 1990, pp. 149–159.

147. Schlom H: Monoclonal antibodies: They're more or less than you think. *In* Broder S: Molecular Foundations of Oncology. Baltimore, Williams & Wilkins, 1991, pp. 95–134.

148. Rosales C, Jeglum KA, Obrocka M, et al: Cytolytic activity of murine anti-dog lymphoma monoclonal antibodies with canine effector cells and complement. Cell Immunol 115:420–428, 1988.

149. Jeglum AK: Monoclonal antibody treatment of canine lymphoma. Proc Eastern States Vet Conf, 1992, p. 222.

# 12

# Metabolic Alterations and Nutritional Therapy for the Veterinary Cancer Patient

Gregory K. Ogilvie and David M. Vail

More thorough attention to the nutritional well-being and application of nutritional support modalities have substantially improved the quality of life of many veterinary cancer patients. Weight loss, often encountered in the tumor-bearing individual, may be due to the primary effects of the tumor (e.g., compression or infiltration of the alimentary tract), effects related to therapy (e.g., chemotherapy-induced anorexia, nausea, or vomiting), or the alteration of metabolic pathways comprising the paraneoplastic syndrome of cancer cachexia.[1-3] The results of recent research suggest that many tumor-bearing animals have alterations in metabolism necessitating not only special methods for delivering nutrients but also specific types of fluid and nutrient support.[1-12] Cancer cachexia is a complex paraneoplastic syndrome of progressive involuntary weight loss that occurs even in the face of adequate nutritional intake.[1-3,8,13-17] People with cancer cachexia have a decreased quality of life, decreased response to treatment, and a shortened survival time when compared to those with similar diseases who do not exhibit the clinical or biochemical signs associated with this condition.[18,19,20] The purpose of this article is to review briefly what is known about some of the metabolic alterations that occur with cancer and how this knowledge can be used to meet the unique dietary and parenteral fluid needs of veterinary cancer patients.

## METABOLIC ALTERATIONS IN CANCER

### Carbohydrate Metabolism

Perhaps the most dramatic alterations in the metabolism of animals with cancer occur in carbohydrate metabolism. Abnormalities have been documented in peripheral glucose disposal, hepatic gluconeogenesis, insulin effects, and whole-body glucose oxidation and turnover.[21-23] These abnormalities exist often before clinical evidence of cachexia are present. For example, when dogs with lymphoma without clinical evidence of cachexia were evaluated with a 90-minute intravenous glucose tolerance test, lactate and insulin concentrations were significantly higher when compared to controls.[4] (Figs. 12-1 and 12-2). The hyperlactatemia and hyperinsulinemia did not improve when these dogs achieved remission with doxorubicin chemotherapy.[6] Metabolic alterations result in part because tumors preferentially metabolize glucose for energy by anaerobic glycolysis forming lactate as an end product.[23-25] The host must then expend the necessary energy to convert lactate to glucose by the Cori cycle, which results in a net energy gain by the tumor and a net energy loss by the host.[14,24,26]

The clinical significance of the alterations in carbohydrate metabolism are just now becoming understood. A recent report documented the

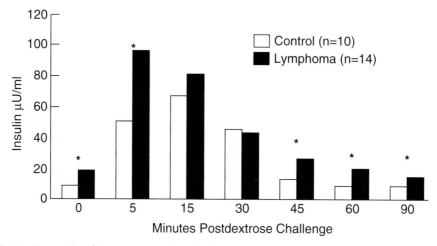

**Figure 12–1.** Serum insulin concentrations in dogs with and without lymphoma before and after IV administration of 500 mg/kg dextrose. Asterisks (*) indicate values from dogs with lymphoma that differ significantly ($p < 0.001$) from control dogs at the same time. (From Vail DM, Ogilvie GK, Wheeler SL, et al: Alterations in carbohydrate metabolism in canine lymphoma. J Vet Intern Med 4:11, 1990; with permission.)

exacerbation of hyperlactatemia by infusion of lactated Ringer's solution (LRS) in dogs with lymphoma[5] (Figure 12–3). During that study, blood lactate concentrations of relatively healthy, well-hydrated dogs with lymphoma were compared to control dogs and determined to be significantly elevated before, during, and after LRS was infused at a relatively modest rate (4.125 ml/kg/hr). This LRS-induced increase in lactate concentration may place a metabolic burden on the host to convert lactate back to glucose, further exacerbating the energy demands on the host. This may be even more important for septic, critically ill patients with cancer that require more intensive fluid therapy. It is also logical to assume that glucose-containing fluids would likely increase hyperlactatemia, as evidenced by glucose tolerance tests. Therefore, until further

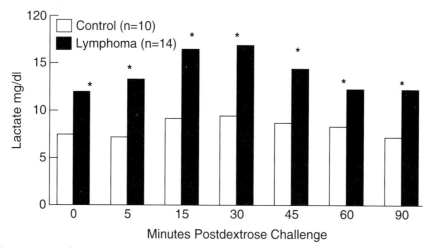

**Figure 12–2.** Serum lactate concentrations in dogs with and without lymphoma before and after IV administration of 500 mg/kg dextrose. Asterisks (*) indicate values from dogs with lymphoma that differ significantly ($p < 0.001$) from control dogs at the same time. (From Vail DM, Ogilvie GK, Wheeler SL, et al: Alterations in carbohydrate metabolism in canine lymphoma. J Vet Intern Med 4:11, 1990; with permission.)

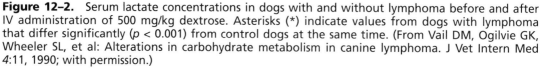

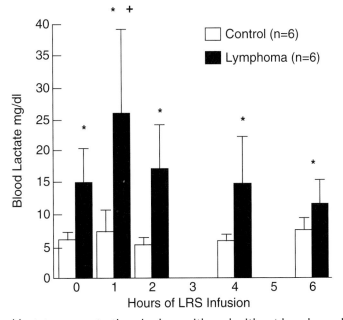

**Figure 12–3.** Blood lactate concentrations in dogs with and without lymphoma before and during IV infusion of lactated Ringer's solution. Asterisks (*) indicate values from dogs with lymphoma that differ significantly ($p < 0.05$) from controls at the same time. Plus sign (+) indicates values differ significantly ($p < 0.05$) from preinfusion baseline values within the same test group. (From Vail DM, Ogilvie GK, Fettman MJ, et al: Exacerbation of hyperlactatemia by infusion of lactated Ringer's solution in dogs with lymphoma. J Vet Intern Med 4:228–232, 1990; with permission.)

information is known about the effects of hyperlactatemia on critically ill animals with cancer, glucose- or lactate-containing fluids should be avoided.

The inability of some tumor-bearing animals to tolerate glucose parenterally may have some bearing on the dietary management of the cancer patient. Logically it can be concluded that diets high in simple carbohydrates may increase the total amount of lactate produced and the need for the host to utilize energy unwisely for conversion of lactate. This may have long-term detrimental effects on animals with cancer. Others have published data to support this hypothesis.[27,28]

## Protein Metabolism

Cancer has been shown to result in decreased body muscle mass and skeletal protein synthesis and to alter nitrogen balance while concurrently increasing skeletal protein breakdown, liver protein synthesis, and whole-body protein synthesis.[29] Tumors preferentially use energy stores at the expense of the host. For example, tumors often preferentially use amino acids for energy via gluconeogenesis.[19,30,31] The use of amino acids by the tumor for energy becomes clinically significant for the host when protein degradation and loss exceed synthesis. This can result in alterations in many important bodily functions such as immune response, gastrointestinal function, and surgical healing.[32]

In one study, amino acid analyses were performed on the plasma of 32 dogs with cancer and 8 normal control dogs.[3,12] Of the 25 amino acids evaluated, tumor-bearing dogs had significantly lower plasma concentrations of threonine, glutamine, glycine, valine, cystine, and arginine and significantly higher levels of isoleucine and phenylalanine. The results did not differ between the different types of tumors represented.

Providing high-quality amino acids or protein dietarily may be of critical importance for the veterinary cancer patient. A quality protein diet that is highly bioavailable may be ideal. Arginine and glutamine may be of specific value for therapeutic purposes.[33,34] Arginine will stimulate lymphocyte blastogenesis, and its addition to total parenteral nutrition solutions has been shown to decrease tumor growth and metastatic rate in some rodent systems.[33,34] Some amino acids may decrease toxicity associated with chemotherapy. For example, glycine has been shown to reduce cisplatin-induced nephrotoxicity.[35]

## Lipid Metabolism

Fat loss accounts for the majority of weight loss occurring in cancer cachexia; therefore, it is not surprising that human beings and animals with cancer have dramatic abnormalities in lipid metabolism.[25,36–38] The decreased lipogenesis and increased lipolysis observed in humans and rodents with cancer cachexia result in increased levels of free fatty acids, very low density lipoproteins, triglycerides, plasma lipoproteins, and hormone-dependent lipoprotein lipase activity, while levels of endothelial-derived lipoprotein lipase decrease.[14,23,36,37,39] Recently lipid profiles in dogs with lymphoma were studied to determine if alterations similar to those reported in other species were present.[9] When compared to healthy controls, dogs with lymphoma had significantly higher concentrations of the cholesterol concentrations associated with very low density lipoprotein (VLDL-CH), total triglyceride (T-TG), as well as the triglyceride concentrations associated with very low density lipoprotein (VLDL-TG), low density lipoprotein (LDL-TG), and high density lipoprotein (HDL-TG). Significantly lower levels of cholesterol concentrations associated with high density lipoprotein (HDL-CH) were also noted. HDL-TG and VLDL-TG concentrations from dogs with lymphoma were significantly increased above pretreatment values after remission was lost and the dogs had developed overt signs of cancer cachexia. These abnormalities did not normalize when clinical remission was obtained.

The clinical significance of the previously mentioned lipid parameters in dogs with lymphoma is not known; however, abnormalities in lipid metabolism have been linked to a number of clinical problems, including immunosuppression, which correlates with decreased survival in affected humans.[14] The clinical impact of the abnormalities in lipid metabolism may be lessened with dietary therapy. In contrast to carbohydrates and proteins, some tumor cells have difficulty utilizing lipid as a fuel source while host tissues continue to oxidize lipids for energy.[27,36,40,41] This has led to the hypothesis that diets relatively high in fat may be of benefit to the animal with cancer when compared to a diet high in simple carbohydrates. Further research

may reveal that the type of fat, rather than the amount, may be of greater importance.[42] Mean nitrogen intake, nitrogen balance, in vitro lymphocyte mitogenesis, time for wound healing, the prevalence of wound complications, and the duration of hospitalization were significantly better in 85 surgical patients fed an omega-3 fatty acid supplement when compared to controls.

## Energy Expenditure

Cancer cachexia may in part be due to a negative energy balance secondary to decreased energy intake or altered energy expenditure.[43,44] Alterations in basal metabolic rate (BMR) and resting energy expenditure (REE) have been observed in human patients with cancer cachexia, and these changes are associated with derangements in carbohydrate, protein, and lipid metabolism.[36–44] This is in contrast to the adaptive decrease in metabolic rate observed to occur in healthy fasted individuals. This attenuation of adaptive response may be responsible in part for the increased energy demand and subsequent weight loss occurring in the cancer-bearing host. Because the thyroid gland and its constitutive hormones are intimately involved in the control of energy homeostasis,[45,46] it is not unreasonable to speculate that perturbations in thyroid function or thyroid hormone concentrations may play a role in altering energy states in tumor-bearing cachectic individuals. It is plausible that abnormally high concentrations of active thyroid hormone may play a significant role in the hypermetabolic state often encountered in individuals suffering from cancer cachexia. This hypothesis did not hold true in a recent investigation of thyroid function in tumor-bearing dogs. In this study of 83 dogs, serum concentrations of thyroxine ($T_4$),3,5,3'-triiodothyronine ($T_3$), free thyroxine ($fT_4$), and free 3,5,3'-triiodothyronine ($fT_3$) were compared among tumor-bearing dogs[47] with and without chronic weight loss and non-tumor-bearing dogs with and without chronic weight loss. Diminished serum concentrations of $T_4$, $T_3$, and $fT_3$ occurred in dogs under study in proportion to the degree of weight loss associated with their disease state, regardless of their tumor-bearing status. It appears that these declines are related to abnormal nutritional state or severity of illness rather than to a tumor-related phenomenon.

Indirect calorimetry, a method by which REE is estimated from measurements of oxygen consumption and carbon dioxide production, is evaluated to understand more about nutrient assimilation, substrate utilization, thermogenesis, the energetics of physical exercise, and the pathogenesis of diseases such as cancer.[48,49–54] Indirect calorimetry was performed on 22 dogs with lymphoma that were randomized into a blind study and fed isocaloric amounts of either a high-fat diet or a high-carbohydrate diet before and after chemotherapy.[10] Surprisingly, during the initial evaluation period, resting energy expenditure (REE/kg$^{0.75}$) was significantly lower than 30 tumor-free controls. Six weeks after the start of the study, REE/kg$^{0.75}$ was significantly lower in both groups of dogs with lymphoma when compared to the controls and the pretreatment values from the dogs with lymphoma. The dogs fed the diet relatively high in fat maintained a more normal energy expenditure than the dogs fed a diet relatively high in carbohydrates.

## NUTRITIONAL SUPPORT FOR THE VETERINARY CANCER PATIENT

The ideal method of addressing cancer cachexia is to eliminate the underlying neoplastic condition; however, this is often not possible, and efforts to provide nutritional support become important. Specific recommendations for nutritional support of patients with neoplastic disease should be based on estimates of caloric requirements, the patients' current and past nutritional status, and a knowledge of the underlying disease. Not all cancer patients are candidates for nutritional support. Clinical judgment based on historical information regarding past, present, and anticipated nutrient intake and needs; on physical examination with attention to body condition; and on a working knowledge of underlying disease mechanisms has proven superior as a measure of nutritional status and the need for nutritional support in people.[55–57] Consequently, this seems the simplest, most reliable method of assessment in veterinary patients and would also be clinically judicious. Additionally, as with any treatment modality, serial assessment of nutritional status and subsequent modifications in nutritional support are indicated as the patient's status changes.

Enteral feeding has been shown to be a practical, cost-effective, physiologic, and safe modality that may abate or eliminate cancer cachexia.[2,58,59] Several studies have failed to document the possibility of increasing tumor growth by enhancing the nutritional status of the host.[60–63] Enteral dietary support of the cancer patient can result in weight gain as well as increased response to and

tolerance of radiation, surgery, and chemotherapy.[19,62] Other factors that improve with enteral nutritional support include thymic weight, immune responsiveness, immunoglobulin and complement levels, as well as the phagocytic ability of white blood cells.[60] Although the optimum diet formulation is still unknown, the following guidelines may apply.

As a general rule, mature dogs and cats with a functional gastrointestinal tract that have a history of inadequate nutritional intake for 3 to 7 days or have lost at least 10% of their body weight over a 1- to 2-week period of time are candidates for enteral nutritional therapy.[3,59,64,65] A note of caution: the present dogma of allowing 2 or more days of inappetence to pass before considering nutritional support may not be appropriate for the feline patient who has a relatively higher metabolic rate. For example, daily adenosine triphosphate (ATP) turnover in an 80 kg man at rest is roughly 60% of body weight versus 136% in a 3.5 kg cat, and humans have approximately twice the energy storage capabilities per unit of metabolic body size.[66] In light of this, we feel it is prudent to implement nutritional support earlier in those feline patients where it is clearly indicated.

All methods to encourage food consumption, including the use of chemical stimulants, should be attempted first[3,59,64,65] (Fig. 12–4). Enhancing the palatability of food is the simplest means of increasing voluntary intake. Offering a variety of freshly opened food and warming it to body temperature may help. Appetite stimulants of the benzodiazepam family (diazepam, oxazepam) used at low doses orally or intravenously while presenting a variety of foods may result in the consumption of nearly 25% of daily requirements in responsive cats.[67] This is usually reserved for short-term appetite stimulation to "kick-start" a patient likely to recover quickly. Many other pharmacologic compounds have or are undergoing scientific scrutiny for reversing or abating the metabolic alterations occurring in cancer-bearing patients. Carefully controlled studies with human cancer patients suggest that cyproheptadine, corticosteroids, and nandrolone decanoate have little or no impact on objective indices of nutritional status or clinical outcome.[68–70] Megestrol acetate has been shown to be of benefit in patients with significant gastrointestinal morbidity.[71] Several studies recently reviewed by Chlebowski[72] have shown that the clinical use of megestrol acetate has resulted in substantial increases in weight gain in people

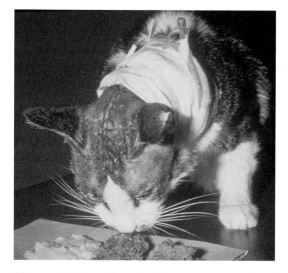

**Figure 12–4.** All methods to encourage food consumption, including feeding the patient a variety of highly palatable aromatic foods, uniformly warming the food to just below body temperature, and administering chemical stimulants, should be tried before starting enteral support. The optimum pharmacologic agent for use in the veterinary cancer patient is unknown; however, megestrol acetate has been shown to result in substantial weight gain in humans with cancer. (From Ogilvie GK: Alterations in metabolism and nutritional support for veterinary cancer patients: Recent advances. Compend Contin Educ Pract Vet *15*:925–937, 1993; with permission.)

with cancer; the clinical utility of this drug for the treatment of cancer cachexia in veterinary patients remains to be determined.

## Routes of Enteral Feeding

Once the decision to provide nutritional support has been made, an appropriate method of feeding must be chosen. Enteral feeding should always be considered over total parenteral nutrition unless it is contraindicated because of an inability of the gastrointestinal tract to digest or assimilate nutrients in adequate quantities. A vast body of basic and clinical literature exists that supports the adage "If the gut works use it!"[73–76] While parenteral nutrition is certainly a useful tool, maintenance of gut mucosal integrity and the complex neuroendocrine network that orchestrates nutrient digestion, absorption, and metabolism is paramount and best served by enteral nutrition. Additionally, enteral feeding tends to be more cost effective and associated with fewer complications. A number of enteral feeding

routes are commonly used in veterinary patients. Simply put, the gastrointestinal tract should be accessed with a feeding tube as far proximal as possible in order to maximize normal digestion, thus minimizing complications associated with bypassing normal digestive processes. The anticipated duration of nutritional support, patient tolerance, overall expense, and familiarity of hospital staff with a specific tube type should be considered as well when choosing a feeding site.

Nasogastric tube feeding is one of the most common methods used for short-term nutri-

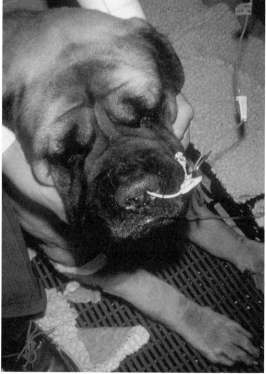

**Figure 12–5.** Nasogastric tube feeding is one of the most common methods used for short-term nutritional support of dogs and cats. The use of small-bore silastic or polyurethane catheters have minimized complications associated with this delivery system. Lidocaine is instilled into the nasal cavity, and the tube is lubricated and passed to the level of the thirteenth rib in dogs and the ninth rib in cats. In dogs, permanent adhesive or a suture should be used to secure the tube to the side of the face that is ipsilateral to the intubated nostril. (From Ogilvie GK: Alterations in metabolism and nutritional support for veterinary cancer patients: Recent advances. Compend Contin Educ Pract Vet *15*:925–937, 1993; with permission.)

tional support of dogs and cats.[3,28,59,64,65] (Fig. 12–5). The use of small-bore, silastic, or polyurethane catheters have minimized complications associated with this delivery system. To decrease any discomfort associated with the initial placement of the catheter, tranquilization may be indicated and lidocaine is instilled into the nasal cavity, with the nose pointing up. The tube is lubricated and passed to the level of the thirteenth rib in dogs and the ninth rib in cats.[60] In cats, the tube should be bent dorsally over the bridge of the nose and secured to the frontal region of the head with a permanent adhesive.* In dogs, the permanent adhesive or a suture should be used to secure the tube to the side of the face that is ipsilateral to the intubated nostril.

Gastrostomy tubes are being used more and more in veterinary practice for those animals that need nutritional support for longer than 7 days[3,58,59,64,65] (Fig. 12–6). These tubes can be placed surgically or with endoscopic guidance.[3,58,59,65] If surgery is used, a 5 ml balloon-tipped urethral catheter **is usually inserted, or a "mushroom"-tipped pezzer proportionate head urological catheter+. The reader is referred to other sources for a detailed description of this surgical procedure.[3,59,64,65] In this author's practice, endoscopically placed gastrostomy tubes are considered ideal for many cancer patients and are described later.

The percutaneous placement of a gastrostomy tube by endoscopic guidance is quick, safe, and effective.[3,59,64,65] A specialized 20 French tube‡ is used for placement in both dogs and cats. First, the stomach is distended with air from an endoscope that is placed into the stomach. Once the stomach is distended, an area just caudal to the last left rib below the transverse processes of the lumbar vertebrae is depressed and then located by the person viewing the stomach lining by endoscopy. A polyvinylchloride over-the-needle IV catheter is then placed through the skin and into the stomach in the area previously located by the endoscopist. The first portion of a 5-foot-long piece of 8-pound test, nylon filament, or suture is introduced through the catheter into the stomach and then grabbed by a biopsy snare passed through the endoscope. The attached

nylon and endoscope is then pulled up the esophagus and out the oral cavity. The end of the gastrostomy tube opposite the "mushroom" tip is trimmed so that it has a pointed end that will fit inside another polyvinylchloride catheter, after the stylet has been removed and discarded. This second polyvinylchloride IV catheter is then placed over the nylon suture so that the narrow end points toward the stomach. The free end of the nylon that has just been pulled out of the animal's mouth is then sutured to the end of the tube. The catheter-tube combination is then pulled from the end of the suture located outside the abdominal wall until the pointed end of the IV catheter comes down the esophagus and out the abdominal wall. The tube is then grasped and pulled until the mushroom tip is adjacent to the stomach wall as viewed by endoscopy. To prevent slippage, the middle of a 3- to 4-inch piece of tubing is pierced completely through both sides and passed over the feeding tube so that it is adjacent to the body wall and then glued or sutured securely in place. The tube is capped and bandaged in place. An Elizabethan collar is recommended. Once the tube has been in place for 7 to 10 days, the tube just below the bumper is severed to allow the mushroom tip to fall into the

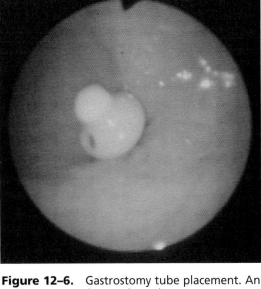

**Figure 12–6.** Gastrostomy tube placement. An endoscope can be used to place a gastrostomy tube into the stomach. A mushroom-tip catheter is ideal; it allows the stomach to be snugged up to the body wall. Blenderized food is put through the tube frequently throughout the day.

*Superglue, Loctite Corp., Cleveland, Ohio.
**E.g., Foley Catheter, Bardex, Murray Hill, New Jersey.
+Bard Urological Catheter, Bard Urological Division, Covington, Georgia.
‡E.g., Dubhoff PEG, Biosearch, Summerville, New Jersey, and Bard Urological Catheter, Bard Urological Division, Covington, Georgia.

stomach. This piece may need to be removed by endoscopy in all but very large dogs.

Needle catheter jejunostomy tubes should be considered for dogs and cats with functional lower intestinal tracts that will not tolerate nasogastric or gastrostomy tube feeding.[3,59,64,65] This method is especially valuable in cancer patients following surgery to the upper gastrointestinal tract. In this procedure,[3,59,64,65] the distal duodenum or proximal jejunum is located and isolated by surgery (Fig. 12–7). A purse-string suture of 3-0 nonabsorbable suture is placed in the antimesenteric border of the isolated piece of bowel. A number 5 French polyvinyl infant nasogastric infant feeding tube is passed through a small incision in the skin and abdominal wall, through a piece of omentum (referred to as an omental patch) and then into

the lumen of the bowel through a small stab incision in the center of the area encircled by the purse-string suture. An ideal placement site is in the bowel 20 to 30 cm from the enterostomy site or neoplastic lesion. The purse string is tightened and secured around the tube. The loop of bowel with the enterostomy site is then secured to the abdominal wall with four sutures that later will be cut after the tube is removed when feeding is complete in 7 to 10 days. Complications with this method, as with the gastrostomy tubes, include peritonitis, diarrhea, and cramping.

## Enteral Feeding Formulations

The type of nutrients to be used depends largely on the enteral tube that will be used and on the

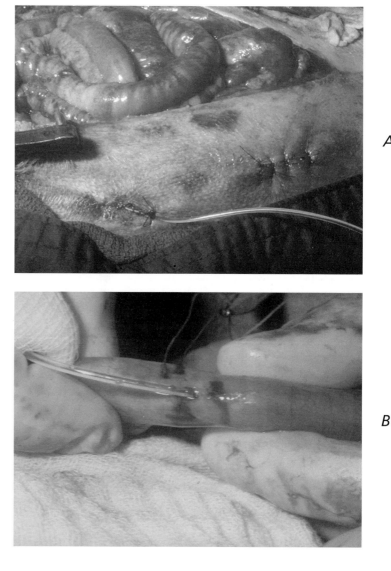

**Figure 12–7.** *A,* A jejunostomy tube is surgically placed through a stab incision in the antimesenteric side of the jejunum. The other end of the tube is then placed through the abdominal wall, whereupon, *B,* the jejunum is securely sutured to the abdominal wall. Jejunostomy tubes are ideal for supporting cancer patients with alterations in the upper GI tract. (From Ogilvie GK: Alterations in metabolism and nutritional support for veterinary cancer patients: Recent advances. Compend Contin Educ Pract Vet *15:*925–937, 1993; with permission.)

*A*

*B*

status of the patient. Blended canned pet foods may be adequate for feeding by gastrostomy tubes while human enteral feeding products are easily administered though nasogastric and jejunostomy tubes.[3,59,64,65] In any case, feeding usually is not started for 24 hours after the tube is placed. Once feeding is started, the amount of nutrients is gradually increased over several days and administered frequently in small amounts or continuously to allow the animal to adapt to this method of feeding. Either way, the tube should be aspirated 3 to 4 times a day to ensure there is not excessive residual volume in the gastrointestinal tract and should be flushed periodically with warm water to prevent clogging.

Additional research is necessary to determine if recent studies are correct in determining that standard texts overestimate the caloric requirements of normal dogs, including those with cancer.[10,11] Until that time, the recommendation for determining the amount of enteral nutrients should be followed.[3,58,59,64,65] Briefly, the basal energy requirement (BER, Kcal/day) is calculated by multiplying 70 times the animal's weight in $kg^{0.75}$ and then multiplying by a factor to derive the illness energy requirement (IER, Kcal/day as nonprotein calories). For normal dogs that are at rest in a cage, the BER is multiplied by 1.25. For those that have undergone recent surgery or that are recovering from trauma, the BER is multiplied by 1.2 to 1.6. If the dog is septic or has major burns, the BER is multiplied by 1.5 to 2.0. The IER has not been determined for dogs with cancer; however it may be high even in the absence of sepsis, burns, trauma, or surgery.[2] The protein requirement for dogs is 4 gm/kg/day for normal dogs and 6 gm/kg/day in dogs that have heavy protein losses. Dogs and cats with renal or hepatic insufficiency should not be given high-protein loads ($\leq$ 3 gm/100 Kcal in the dog; $\leq$ 4 gm per 100 Kcal in the cat). Since most high-quality pet foods can be put through a blender to form a gruel that can be passed through a large-bore catheter, the IER of the animal is divided by the caloric density of the canned pet food to determine the amount of food to feed. The same calculation can be done with human enteral feeding products; the volume fed may need to be increased if the enteral feeding product is diluted to ensure it is approximately iso-osmolar before it is administered.

## Total Parenteral Nutrition

Indications for total parenteral nutrition (TPN) include those previously discussed for enteral nutrition in conjunction with an inability of the gastrointestinal tract to retain, digest, or absorb adequate quantities to meet the animal's nutritional needs. The benefit of *long-term* TPN in cancer patients is questionable at best. While the theoretical gains of TPN are similar to those espoused for enteral support, few have been realized to date in the scientific literature. Meta-analysis of large numbers of clinical trials for TPN in tumor-bearing people has revealed no significant benefit with respect to nutritional parameters, survival, treatment tolerance, or tumor response.[77–79] Bone marrow transplant recipients are one important exception to the rule, as they appear to enjoy significant improvement with TPN. At the same time, tumor-bearing patients receiving TPN are much more likely to develop serious systemic infections and are slightly less likely to achieve a response to their antineoplastic therapy. The authors recommend TPN in our cancer patients only when we anticipate recovery from the underlying circumstances. This includes postoperative gastrointestinal surgery patients, those with chemother- apy-induced anorexia, and patients with tumors for whom remission or cure is likely. The reader is directed to several excellent reviews of TPN principles and procedures in the veterinary literature.[80–82]

## CONCLUSION

As mentioned earlier, cancer cachexia is a common paraneoplastic syndrome that is associated with many of the alterations in metabolism noted in dogs with this condition.[13–17] Cancer cachexia may have more clinical significance than the underlying malignancy. The clinical manifestations of cancer cachexia can impact a patient's quality of life, response to therapy, and overall survival time. Nutritional support is of paramount concern for the patient with cancer; the considerations are essentially the same, regardless of species.

## REFERENCES

1. Vail DM, Ogilvie GK, Wheeler SL: Metabolic alterations in patients with cancer cachexia. Compend Contin Educ Pract Vet 12:381–387, 1990.
2. Ogilvie GK, Moore AS: Nutritional Support. Managing the Veterinary Cancer Patient: A Practice Manual. Trenton, NJ, Veterinary Learning Systems, 1995, pp. 124–136.
3. Ogilvie GK, Vail DM: Advances in nutritional therapy for the cancer patient. Vet Clin North Am [Small Anim Pract] 20:4, 1990.
4. Vail DM, Ogilvie GK, Wheeler SL, Fettman MJ, et

al: Alterations in carbohydrate metabolism in canine lymphoma. J Vet Intern Med 4:8–11, 1990.

5. Vail DM, Ogilvie GK, Fettman MJ, Wheeler SL: Exacerbation of hyperlactatemia by infusion of lactated Ringer's solution in dogs with lymphoma. J Vet Intern Med 4:228–232, 1990.

6. Ogilvie GK, Vail DM, Wheeler SJ: Effect of chemotherapy and remission on carbohydrate metabolism in dogs with lymphoma. Cancer 69:233–238, 1992.

7. Ogilvie GK: Paraneoplastic syndromes. In Withrow SJ, MacEwen EG (eds): Clinical Oncology. Philadelphia, JB Lippincott, 1989, pp. 29–40.

8. Ogilvie GK, Vail DM: Unique metabolic alterations associated with cancer cachexia in the dog. In Kirk RW (ed): Current Veterinary Therapy XI. Philadelphia WB Saunders, 1992, pp. 433–438.

9. Ogilvie GK, Ford RD, Vail DM: Alterations in lipoprotein profiles in dogs with lymphoma. J Vet Intern Med 8:62–66, 1994.

10. Ogilvie GK, Walters LM, Fettman MJ, et al: Energy expenditure in dogs with lymphoma fed two specialized diets. Cancer 71:3146–3152, 1993.

11. Walters LM, Ogilvie GK, Fettman MJ, et al: Repeatability of energy expenditure measurements in normal dogs by indirect calorimetry. AM J Vet Res 54:1881–1885, 1993.

12. Ogilvie GK, Vail D, Ford R, Garnecke G: Lipoprotein, free fatty acids, amino acid levels in dogs with cancer. Proc Vet Cancer Soc, 1988.

13. Heber D, Byerley LO, Chlebowski RT: Metabolic abnormalities in the cancer patient. Cancer 55:225–229, 1958.

14. Kern KA, Norton JA. Cancer cachexia. J Parenteral Enteral Nutr 12:286–298, 1988.

15. DeWys WD: Pathophysiology of cancer cachexia: Current understanding and areas of future research. Cancer Res 42:721–726, 1982.

16. Shein PS, Kisner D, Haller D, et al: Cachexia of malignancy. Cancer 43:2070–2076, 1976.

17. Theologides A: Cancer cachexia. Cancer 43:2004–2012, 1979.

18. Buzby GP, Steinberg JJ: Nutrition in cancer patients. Symp Surg Nutr 61:691–699, 1981.

19. Landel AM, Hammond WG, Mequid MM: Aspects of amino acid and protein metabolism in cancer-bearing states. Cancer 55:230–237, 1985.

20. Bray GA, Campfield LA: Metabolic factors in the control of energy stores. Metabolism 24:99–117, 1975.

21. Burt ME, Lowry SF, Gorschboth C, et al: Metabolic alterations in a non-cachectic animal tumor system. Cancer 47:2138–2146, 1981.

22. Norton JA, Maher M, Wesley R, et al: Glucose intolerance in sarcoma patients. Cancer 54:3022–3027, 1984.

23. Richtsmeier WJ, Dauchy R, Sauer LA: In vivo nutrient uptake by head and neck cancers. Cancer Res 47:5230–5233, 1987.

24. Holroyde CP, Reichard GA: Carbohydrate metabolism in cancer cachexia. Cancer Treat Rep 65:55–59, 1981.

25. Heber D, Byerley LO, Chi J, et al: Pathophysiology of malnutrition in the adult cancer patient. Cancer 58:1867–1873, 1986.

26. Bozzetti F, Pagnoni AM, Del Vecchio M: Excessive caloric expenditure as a cause of malnutrition in patients with cancer. Surg Gynecol Obstet 150:229–234, 1980.

27. Dempsey DT, Mullen JL: Macronutrient requirements in the malnourished cancer patient. Cancer 55:290–294, 1985.

28. Chory ET, Mullen JL: Nutritional support of the cancer patient: Delivery systems and formulations. Surg Clin North Am 66:1105–1120, 1986.

29. Langstein HN, Norton JA: Mechanisms of cancer cachexia. Hematol/Oncol Clin North Am 5:103–123, 1991.

30. Kurzer M, Meguid MM: Cancer and protein metabolism. Surg Clin North Am 66:969–1001, 1986.

31. Teyek JA, Bistrian BR, HehirDJ, et al: Improved protein kinetics and albumin synthesis by branched chain amino acid-enriched total parenteral nutrition in cancer cachexia. Cancer 58:147–157, 1986.

32. Oram-Smith JC, Stein TP: Intravenous nutrition and tumor host protein metabolism. J Surg Res 22:499–503, 1977.

33. Barbul A, Sisto DA, Wasserkrug HL, et al: Arginine stimulates lymphocyte immune response in healthy human beings. Surgery 90:244–251, 1981.

34. Tachibana K, Mukai K, Hirauka I, et al: Evaluation of the effect of arginine enriched amino acid solution on tumor growth. J Parenteral Enteral Nutr 9:428–434, 1985.

35. Heyman SN, Rosen S, Silva P, et al: Protective action of glycine in cisplatin nephrotoxicity. Kidney Int 40(2):273–279, 1991.

36. Brennan NF: Uncomplicated starvation versus cancer cachexia. Cancer Res 37:2359–2364, 1977.

37. Chlebowski RT, Heber D: Metabolic abnormalities in cancer patients: Carbohydrate metabolism. Surg Clin North Am 66:957–968, 1986.

38. Dewys WD: Pathophysiology of cancer cachexia: Current understanding and areas of future research. Cancer Res 42:722–726, 1982.

39. McAndrew PF: Fat metabolism and cancer. Surg Clin North Am 66:1003–1012, 1986.

40. Shein PS, Kisner D, Haller D, et al: The oxidation of body fuel stores in cancer patients. Ann Surg 204:637–642, 1986.

41. Tisdale MJ, Brennan RA, Fearon KC: Reduction of weight loss and tumour size in a cachexia model by a high fat diet. Br J Cancer 56:39–43, 1987.

42. Daly JM, Lieberman M, Goldfine J, et al: Enteral nutrition with supplemental arginine, RNA and omega-3 fatty acids: A prospective clinical trial. Abstract, 15th Clinical Congress, American Soci-

ety for Parenteral and Enteral Nutrition, J Parenteral Enteral Nutr 15:19S, 1991.

43. Lawson DH, Richmond A, Nixon DW, et al: Metabolic approaches to cancer cachexia. Ann Rev Nutr 1982 2:277–301.

44. Dempsy DT, Feurer ID, Knox LS, et al: Energy expenditure in malnourished gastrointestinal cancer patients. Cancer 53:1265–1273, 1984.

45. Premachandra BN, Perlstein IB, Williams K: Circulating and tissue thyroid hormones in relation to hormone action: Pathophysiologic significance. In Fatherby K, Palde Druyter SB (eds): Hormones in Normal and Abnormal Human Tissues, Vol 2. Berlin, New York, W. deGruyter, 1981, pp. 287–282.

46. Sestoft L: Metabolic aspects of the calorigenic effect of thyroid hormone in mammals. Clin Endocrinol 13:489–506, 1980.

47. Vail DM, Panciera DL, Ogilvie GK: Thyroid hormone concentrations in conditions of chronic weight loss in dogs with special reference to cancer cachexia. J Vet Intern Med 1994, 8:122–127.

48. Ferrannini E: The theoretical basis of indirect calorimetry: A review. Metabolism 37:287–301, 1988.

49. Dempsey DT, Knox LS, Mullen JL, et al: Energy expenditure in malnourished patients with colorectal cancer. Arch Surg 121:789–795, 1986.

50. Hansell DT, Davies JWL, Burns HJG: The relationship between resting energy expenditure and weight loss in benign and malignant disease. Ann Surg 203:240–245, 1986.

51. Fredrix EWHM, Wouters EFM, Soeters PB, et al: Resting energy expenditure in patients with non-small cell lung cancer. Cancer 68:1616–1621, 1991.

52. Quebbeman EJ, Ausman RK, Schneider TC: A Re-evaluation of energy expenditure during parenteral nutrition. Ann Surg 195:282–286, 1982.

53. Zyliez Z, Schwantje O, Wagener DJT, Folgering HTM: Metabolic response to enteral food in different phases of cancer cachexia in rats. Oncology 47:87–91, 1990.

54. Delarue J, Lerebours E, Tilly H, et al: Effect of chemotherapy on resting energy expenditure in patients with non-Hodgkin's lymphoma. Cancer 65:2455–2459, 1990.

55. Ament ME: Enteral and parenteral nutrition. In Brown M (ed): Present Knowledge in Nutrition. Washington, DC, International Life Sciences Institute, 1990, pp. 444–450.

56. Detsky AS, Baker JP, Mendelson RA, et al: Evaluating the accuracy of nutritional assessment techniques applied to hospitalized patients: Methodology and comparisons. J Parenteral Enteral Nutr 8:153–159, 1984.

57. Jeejeebhoy KN, Detsky AS, Baker JP: Assessment of nutritional status. J Parenteral Enteral Nutr 14:193S–196S, 1990.

58. Fields ALA, Chemma-Dhadli S, Wolman SL, et al:

Theoretical aspects of weight loss in patients with cancer. Cancer 50:2183–2188, 1982.

59. Wheeler SL, McGuire BM: Enteral nutritional support. In Kirk RW (ed): Current Veterinary Therapy X. Philadelphia, WB Saunders, 1989, pp. 30–36.

60. Copeland EM, Daly JM, Dudrick SJ: Nutrition as an adjunct to cancer treatment in the adult. Cancer Res 37:2451–2456, 1977.

61. Dempsy DT, Mullen JL: Macronutrient requirements in the malnourished cancer patient. Ann Surg 55:290–294, 1985.

62. Lawson DH, Nixon DW, Kutner MJ, et al: Enteral versus parenteral nutritional support in cancer patients. Cancer Treat Rep 65:101–105, 1981.

63. Serrau B, Cupissol D: Nutritional support and the immune system in cancer management: A critical review. Cancer Treat Rep 65:101–105, 1981.

64. Donohue S: Nutritional support of hospitalized patients. Kallfelz FA (ed). Vet Clin North Am [Small Anim Pract] 19(3):475–495, 1989.

65. Allen TA: Specialized nutritional support. In Ettinger SJ (ed): Textbook of Veterinary Internal Medicine, 3rd ed. Philadelphia, WB Saunders, 1989, pp. 450–455.

66. Kleiber M: The Fire of Life: An Introduction to Animal Energetics. Malabar, FL, Robert E. Krieger, 1987, pp. 179–221.

67. Macy DW, Gasper PW: Diazepam-induced eating in anorexic cats. J Am Anim Hosp Assoc 21:17–20, 1985.

68. Kardinal CG, Loprinzi CL, Schaid DJ, et al: A controlled trial of cyproheptadine in cancer patients with anorexia and/or cachexia. A Mayo Clinic/North Central Cancer Group trial. Proc Am Soc Clin Oncol 9:325, 1990.

69. Willox JC, Cou J, Shaw J, et al: Prednisolone as an appetite stimulant in patients with cancer. Br Med J 288:27–31, 1984.

70. Chlebowski RT, Herrold J, Ali I, et al: Influence of nandrolone decanoate on weight loss in advanced non-small cell lung cancer. Cancer 58:183–186, 1986.

71. Shivshanker K, Bennett RW, Haynie TP: Tumor associated gastroparesis: Connection with meteclopramide. Am J Surg 145:221–225, 1983.

72. Chlebowski RT: Nutritional support of the medical oncology patient. Hematol/Oncol Clin N Am 5(1): 147–160, 1991.

73. Alexander JW, Gottschlich MM: Nutritional immunomodulation of burn patients. Crit Care Med 18:S149–153, 1990.

74. Gosche JR, Garrison RN, Harris PD, et al: Absorptive hyperemia restores intestinal blood flow during Escherichia coli sepsis in the rat. Arch Surg 125:1573–1576, 1990.

75. Nussbaum MS, Shujun L, Cora KO, et al: Lipid-free total parenteral nutrition and macrophage function in rats. Arch Surg 126:84–88, 1991.

76. Saito H, Trocki O, Alexander J, et al: The effect of

nutrient administration on the nutritional state, catabolic hormone secretion, and gut mucosal integrity after burn injury. J Parenteral Enteral Nutr 11:1–7, 1987.

77. Lipman TO: Clinical trials of nutritional support in cancer. Hematol/Oncol Clin North Am 5:91–102, 1991.

78. Chlebowski RT: Nutritional support of the medical oncology patient. Hematol/Oncol Clin North Am 5:147–160, 1991.

79. McGeer AJ, Detsky AS, O'Rourke K: Parenteral nutrition in cancer patients undergoing chemo-

therapy: A meta-analysis. Nutrition 6:478–483, 1990.

80. Remillard RL, Thatcher CD: Parenteral nutritional support in the small animal patient. Vet Clin North Am [Small Anim Pract] 19:1287–1305, 1989.

81. Lippert AC, Fulton RB, Parr AM: A retrospective study of the use of total parenteral nutrition in dogs and cats. J Vet Intern Med 7:52–64, 1993.

82. Jackson MW, Vail DM: Nutritional management of cats with infectious disease. Vet Clin North Am [Small Anim Pract] 23:155–171, 1993.

# 13

# Complications of Cancer and Its Treatment

William C. Kisseberth and E. Gregory MacEwen

Many animals will present to the veterinarian because of complications of the underlying malignancy or the treatment itself. In many situations it is difficult to determine if the presenting problem is due to the tumor or the treatment. It is very important that the natural history of the tumor be known and potential complications be considered. In many situations the presenting problem may not be associated with the primary tumor or its location, but due to metastatic spread or paraneoplastic syndromes. It is important to know the status of the metastatic sites as well as the state of control of the primary tumor. Likewise, the clinician must be aware of the treatment and potential side effects, both acute and late. The goal of therapy must be carefully considered *before* therapeutic intervention is initiated. Some severe metabolic disturbances associated with the treatment may lead the clinician to believe that the tumor has irreversibly progressed. The major goal of an attending clinician is to determine if the underlying complication is associated with the treatment or tumor, whether it is reversible, and how this information fits into the overall prognosis of the patient. Restoration of the patient to a normal or reasonable functional status, with good potential of a satisfactory quality of life, is often the goal of treatment. If the tumor is widespread and considered terminal, then no treatment is justified.

This chapter will review the common local and systemic complications associated with the malignant process. In addition, special consideration will be given to complications associated with treatment. Paraneoplastic syndromes are covered in Chapter 4.

## HEMATOLOGIC COMPLICATIONS OF TUMOR AND TREATMENT

Hematologic abnormalities are common in the cancer patient. These abnormalities may be related to the underlying disease or may be a consequence of its treatment. Hematologic toxicity is the most common toxicity seen in patients receiving chemotherapy. The bone marrow is particularly susceptible to the toxic effects of chemotherapy because of its high mitotic rate and growth fraction.

The temporal sequence of cytopenias as a result of chemotherapy can be anticipated with a knowledge of the bone marrow transit times and circulating half-lives of the different cell lineages. In the dog the bone marrow transit time and circulating half-life for granulocytes is 6 days and 4 to 8 hours, respectively; for platelets 3 days and 4 to 6 days, respectively; and for red blood cells 7 days and 120 days, respectively.[1] Similar bone marrow transit times and circulating half-lives are seen in the feline hematopoietic cell lineages, with the exception of a significantly shorter red blood cell circulating half-life of 60 to 80 days.[1] Therefore, neutropenia will typically precede thrombocytopenia, with clinically significant anemias being a rare event in cats and dogs.

### Pancytopenia

Pancytopenia in the cancer patient is due to a decreased production of hematopoietic elements or to an accelerated destruction or sequestration of mature blood cells. Table 13–1 lists the causes of marrow failure seen in cancer patients. Myelo-

**Table 13–1**   Causes of Bone Marrow Failure in the Cancer Patient

Myelosuppression secondary to:
    Chemotherapy
    Radiation therapy
Myelophthisis
    Marrow replacement by tumor
    Marrow replacement by reticulum (myelofibrosis)
Bone Marrow Necrosis
Infection

suppression due to chemotherapy affects all cell lines; however, only granulocytopenia is normally of clinical significance with the cytotoxic chemotherapeutic drugs and schedules used most commonly in veterinary medicine. The hematologic consequences of radiation therapy depend on the volume of exposed marrow, the dose and schedule of treatment, and the use of any concurrent therapies[2]. Significant marrow toxicity may be seen with total-body or large-volume regional irradiation but is not seen as a consequence of irradiation of solitary tumors. The combination of systemic chemotherapy with local radiotherapy may result in more severe cytopenias.

Myelophthisis (replacement of marrow by tumor or fibrosis) is an occasional cause of pancytopenia and subsequent marrow failure. Hematologic malignancies, including lymphoma, and rarely a variety of solid tumors, may invade the bone marrow, resulting in cytopenias. Minimally infiltrated marrows typically do not result in cytopenias. Bone marrow aspiration or biopsy is indicated in all patients with significant cytopenias that cannot be explained by concurrent chemotherapy treatment. Myelofibrosis (replacement of bone marrow with fibrous connective tissue) is poorly described in veterinary medicine. It may be the final result of tumor infiltration or chronic chemotherapy administration. Melphalan therapy in particular has been associated with myelofibrosis with long-term use.

Myelosuppression associated with a variety of infections, including those due to bacterial, viral, fungal, mycobacterial, and rickettsial pathogens, may be seen in the cancer patient. Most commonly this suppression is superimposed on that produced by the tumor or treatment. FeLV has been associated with myelosuppression in the cat.

## Granulocyte Abnormalities

Granulocytopenia (neutropenia) is the dose-limiting toxicity of most cytotoxic chemotherapeutic drugs. Severe neutropenia often leads to life-threatening sepsis. Mild neutropenias are common in patients receiving cytotoxic chemotherapy. The neutropenic nadir (the lowest neutrophil count) usually occurs 5 to 8 days following treatment with most drugs (Fig. 13–1). The neutropenic nadir will vary with the particular chemotherapeutic agent. For example, doxorubicin's nadir occurs at 7 to 10 days and cisplatin has a unique double nadir occurring at 6 and 15 days.[3]

A complete blood count (CBC) should be obtained prior to the administration of each bone marrow suppressive chemotherapy treatment. Treatment should be delayed or the drug dose reduced if the neutrophil count is less than 3,000 to 3,500/µl. Most patients with a treatment delay can be treated 3 to 5 days later, at which time their neutrophil counts typically will have risen to above 3,500/µl. Patients with neutrophil counts above 1,500/µ are usually afebrile and otherwise asymptomatic for their neutropenia. Animals with counts of less than 1,500/µl and are afebrile should be monitored closely for sepsis (e.g., temperature monitored at home by the owner) and be placed on bactericidal prophylactic antibiotics such as trimethoprim/sulfa (13–15 mg/kg, PO, BID). Life-threatening sepsis as a consequence of neutropenia rarely occurs with neutrophil counts of greater than 1,000/µl[4] though it is more common at counts of 500/µl or less.

It is recommended that patients who have had a significant neutropenic episode in response to a particular chemotherapy agent receive a reduced dose the next time the drug is administered. Typically the dose is reduced by 20 to 25% of the initial dose. If this is well tolerated, escalation of the dose is subsequently attempted.

Granulocytosis is commonly seen associated with myeloproliferative disorders as well as chronic myelogenous leukemia. In humans, granulocytosis associated with the apparent release of factors with colony-stimulating activity has been observed in patients with a variety of carcinomas.[2] Granulocytosis may also accompany infection.

Resurgent granulopoiesis characterized by a mild to moderate leukocytosis, a left shift, and no toxic changes is commonly observed during the time of marrow recovery following treatment-induced myelosuppression. These patients are afebrile and show no other signs of infection. Antibiotic therapy is not indicated.

## Management of the Septic Neutropenic Patient

As stated previously, patients with neutrophil counts of less than 1,000/µl are at high risk for the

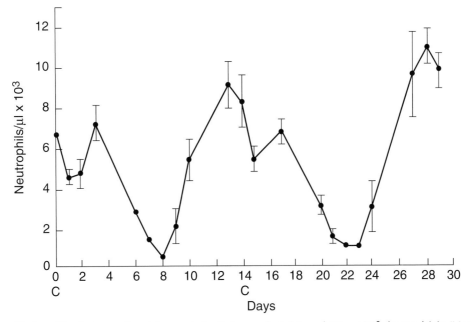

**Figure 13–1.** Absolute neutrophil counts in 5 dogs administered 30 mg/M² doxorubicin IV and 200 mg/M² cyclophosphamide IV days 0 and 14. Note nadir day 7 to 8 postchemotherapy. C = chemotherapy administration.

development of sepsis. Chemotherapy-induced death of gastrointestinal crypt cells combined with concurrent neutropenia allows for the entry of gastrointestinal pathogens through mucosal barriers and into the systemic circulation. Neutrophil numbers are insufficient to clear the infection, and microbial colonization of multiple organs occurs.

Severely neutropenic patients may not show all of the classic signs of infection due to insufficient neutrophil numbers to produce an adequate inflammatory response. Febrile or hypothermic neutropenic patients, or clinically ill, afebrile, severely neutropenic patients should be treated aggressively for sepsis. These patients should be considered as a medical emergency.

Neutropenic patients should receive antimicrobial therapy as soon as fever or other signs of sepsis are documented. An intravenous catheter should be placed sterilely and a balanced electrolyte fluid administered as required. Blood samples should be drawn to determine the CBC, platelet count, serum glucose, serum electrolytes, and serum chemistries. Two or three aseptically obtained blood samples should be collected at at least 30-minute intervals for aerobic and anaerobic culture and sensitivity. The likelihood of obtaining a positive culture is increased with the culture of larger blood volumes.[5,6] A urine sample for urinalysis and bacterial culture and sensitivity should be obtained. The patient should be care-

fully evaluated for any other septic focus (e.g., pneumonia, pyoderma, surgical incision, radiation treatment site, previously placed intravenous or urinary catheters, surgical implants). If a likely focus is found, it should be cultured as well.

Empiric broad-spectrum antibiotic therapy is initiated as soon as the last blood culture sample is drawn. Most animals are septic with *Streptococcus spp., Staphylococcus spp.,* or gram-negative enteric bacteria *(Enterobacter spp., Klebsiella spp., Pseudomonas spp.,* and *E. coli).*[4,7] Combinations of a penicillin or cephalosporin plus an aminoglycoside antibiotic are commonly effective against the most common isolates. A combination of cephalothin (30–40 mg/kg, IV, TID) or ampicillin (10–20 mg/kg, IV, TID) and gentamicin (2 mg/kg, IV, TID) or amikacin (5–10 mg/kg, IV, TID) provides good antibacterial coverage in most patients.[4,8] Renal function must be monitored closely, especially with aminoglycoside use and the use of potentially nephrotoxic chemotherapeutic drugs, in particular cisplatin. More recently four-quadrant antibiotic coverage using a second-generation cephalosporin such as cefotetan (30 mg/kg, IV, TID) or one of the fluoroquinolones (enrofloxacin 5 mg/kg or ciprofloxacin 10 mg/kg, BID) with either clindamycin (10 mg/kg, BID) or metronidazole (15 mg/kg, IV, BID)[8] has been used by the authors with success in selected cases.

Aggressive monitoring is imperative in the septic patient. It will take 24 to 72 hours for the appropriate antibiotics to achieve their desired effects. It is during this period that intensive monitoring is the most critical. The following parameters must be monitored in the septic patient: fluid balance, oncotic pull, serum glucose concentration, serum electrolytes, acid-base balance, oxygenation, mentation, blood pressure, cardiac function, serum albumin concentration, coagulation parameters, hematocrit, renal function, white blood cell count, gastrointestinal motility and integrity, nutritional status, pain control, and nursing and bandage care.[9] It may take several days to begin to observe an upward trend in the neutrophil count, particularly if the few leukocytes that are present are being consumed as part of an inflammatory process.

Human recombinant hematopoietic growth factors or colony-stimulating factors (CSFs) have become commercially available. Granulocyte-CSF (G-CSF) and granulocyte-monocyte-CSF (GM-CSF) are particularly effective at stimulating early granulocytic and monocytic precursor cells to proliferate, and have a profound effect on enhancing the bone marrow recovery from the myelosuppressive effects of chemotherapy and radiation.[10,11] Human recombinant G-CSF (5–10 µg/kg, SC, SID) can be used in dogs and cats,  but is of limited usefulness because of anti-CSF antibody production when used repeatedly in nonhuman species.[12,13] However, canine recombinant G-CSF has been available for clinical investigation.[14,15]

The septic neutropenic patient is a therapeutic challenge that must be treated aggressively. With intensive monitoring and treatment most of these patients can be treated successfully.

## Platelet Abnormalities

Thrombocytopenia in the cancer patient may be the result of decreased platelet production or increased peripheral destruction (Table 13–2). Although absolute platelet numbers commonly decrease subsequent to chemotherapy (Fig. 13–2), the decrease is rarely of clinical significance. Treatment should be delayed with chemotherapy-induced thrombocytopenia if the platelet count drops below 50,000/µl. Spontaneous bleeding usually does not occur in dogs until the platelet counts fall below 10,000/µl.

Other causes of thrombocytopenia due to decreased platelet production in the cancer patient include myelophthisis, most commonly associated

**Table 13–2   Neoplastic Conditions Associated with Thrombocytopenia**

Decreased Platelet Production
    Myelophthisis
    Myelodysplasia
    Estrogen-secreting tumors
    Feline leukemia virus
    Antineoplastic drugs
Increased Platelet Destruction
    Immume-mediated thrombocytopenia
    Shortened platelet survival
    Microangiopathy
Increased Platelet Utilization
    Disseminated intravascular coagulation
    Tumor-associated hemorrhage
Increased Platelet Sequestration

with hematologic malignancies (lymphoma, acute leukemias);[16] myelodysplastic syndromes;[17,18] estrogen-secreting tumors;[19] feline leukemia virus; and feline immunodeficiency virus.

Thrombocytopenia may be due to shortened platelet survival associated with malignancy,[20] microangiopathy, disseminated intravascular coagulation (DIC), and tumor-associated hemorrhage. DIC is most commonly seen in patients with disseminated malignancies, including carcinomas; hematopoietic malignancy including lymphoma and acute lymphoblastic leukemia (ALL); and hemangiosarcoma in the dog.

Immune-mediated destruction of platelets may occur as a paraneoplastic syndrome and has been reported in association with hematopoietic malignancy as well as solid tumors.[21,22] Specific treatment is directed toward the underlying malignancy. Treatment with immunosuppressive agents may be necessary in severely affected patients if they are not already being used to treat the primary disease. Corticosteroids (prednisone 1 to 4 mg/kg, PO, BID) are used initially during the first 24 to 48 hours of treatment, and if a significant response is not seen within a week vincristine (0.5–0.7 mg/m², IV) or cyclophosphamide (200 mg/m², IV) is given with corticosteroids. Maintenance immunosuppression can be accomplished with oral corticosteroids (prednisone 1–2 mg/kg, PO, BID) and cyclophosphamide (50 mg/m², PO, day 1–4 every week) or azathioprine (50 mg/m², PO, SID).

Thrombocytosis (peripheral platelet count greater than 400,000/µl) induced by unknown mechanisms has been reported in animals with osteosarcoma, gingival carcinoma, chronic myelogenous leukemia, and metastatic squamous cell

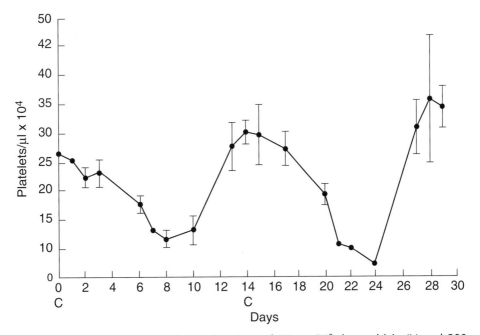

**Figure 13–2.** Platelet counts in 5 dogs administered 30 mg/M² doxorubicin IV and 200 mg/M² cyclophosphamide IV days 0 and 14. Note nadir days 8 to 10 postchemotherapy. C = chemotherapy administration.

carcinoma.[1,23,24] Thrombocytosis may be observed in association with myelodysplastic disorders and megakaryoblastic leukemia.[25,26] Rebound thrombocytosis can occur in overcompensated states in response to previous thrombocytopenia; these include chronic DIC, chemotherapy-induced bone marrow rebound, and acute tumor hemorrhage.[2] The vinca alkaloids, vincristine and vinblastine, have been shown to produce thrombocytosis in dogs and cats as well as other species. These drugs increase the number of megakaryocyte precursor cells and stimulate megakaryocyte endomitosis, thus resulting in early platelet release from the bone marrow. Other causes of thrombocytosis include that which is associated with iron deficiency anemia. Bleeding tumors of the gastrointestinal tract such as adenocarcinoma, fibrosarcoma, and leiomyoma have been reported to result in an iron-deficient state.[27]

## Erythrocyte Abnormalities

Anemia is a common finding in the cancer patient.[28] However, anemia induced by chemotherapeutic agents is rare in cats and dogs.[4] The majority of cases of anemia in the cancer patient without other concurrent cytopenias are probably due to the syndrome of anemia of chronic disease (ACD). ACD is characterized by a mild, typically normocytic, normochromic anemia with decreased serum iron concentrations, normal or elevated serum ferritin levels, and abundant marrow stores of iron. In humans with ACD, decreased erythropoietin concentrations have been reported.[29] This anemia is usually mild and of little clinical significance. Therapy is directed at treating the underlying malignancy.

Blood loss may result in anemia in the cancer patient. Tumors most often associated with blood loss include gastrointestinal and urinary tract neoplasms, mast cell tumors, as well as hemangiosarcoma in the dog. Immune-mediated hemolytic anemia may be observed as a paraneoplastic syndrome in the cancer patient.[28] Diagnosis and treatment are discussed elsewhere in this volume (Chap. 4). Microangiopathic hemolytic anemia (MAHA) is characterized by red blood cell fragmentation (acanthocytosis) due to alterations of the microvascular endothelium. This results in the production of schistocytes in the peripheral blood, indirect hyperbilirubinemia, thrombocytopenia, and anemia. Large tumor burdens and tumors associated with bone marrow and hepatic or splenic infiltration are malignancies in which MAHA has been seen in dogs. Other possible causes of cancer-related anemia include myelophthisis, myelodysplastic syndromes, pure red cell aplasia, and hypersplenism.

Polycythemia has been reported as a paraneoplastic syndrome in association with renal cell carcinoma, lymphoma, and hepatic tumors.[30] The mechanism of production of polycythemia is likely due to the ectopic secretion of erythropoietin or erythropoietin-like substances by the neoplasm or the release of endogenous erythropoietin due to renal ischemia. Most patients with polycythemia vera have splenomegaly, thrombocytosis, and leukocytosis. Patients with secondary polycythemia, not due to paraneoplastic causes, have decreased arterial oxygen saturation.[2] Temporary treatment with phlebotomy is generally indicated in patients with a hematocrit of 65% or more. The removed blood should be replaced with an equivalent amount of a balanced electrolyte solution.[31]

## GASTROINTESTINAL TOXICITY

Gastrointestinal toxicity from cancer chemotherapy is the toxicity most commonly noted by pet owners. Nausea and vomiting may be seen immediately during the administration of the drug, or shortly thereafter. Drugs reported to be associated with nausea and vomiting in the dog and cat include dacarbazine (DTIC), cisplatin, doxorubicin, methotrexate, actinomycin-D, cyclophosphamide, and 5-fluorouracil, although vomiting can be seen with any drug.[4,32]

Cisplatin is the one drug that is a consistently potent emetic in the dog, especially during the first 24 hours postadministration. Butorphanol (0.4 mg/kg, IM) and metoclopramide (0.2 to 0.5 mg/kg, IV or SC, TID) are commonly used to try to manage cisplatin-induced emesis. Preliminary studies with the 5-HT3 receptor antagonist ondansetron (0.1 mg/kg, IV) suggest that this may be a useful agent for managing acute cisplatin-induced emesis in the dog.[33]

Gastrointestinal toxicity with signs varying from decreased appetite, occasional vomiting, and loose stool with normal activity to anorexia with persistent vomiting and diarrhea and severe depression may be seen. Clinical signs are generally first noticed 48 to 72 hours after treatment. Virtually all anticancer chemotherapeutics may produce gastrointestinal signs of toxicity.

The treatment of gastrointestinal toxicity is usually symptomatic. Patients with mild signs may need no treatment. Animals with intermittent vomiting may benefit from antiemetic treatment. Those with enterocolitis may respond to withholding food for 24 to 48 hours and treatment with a gastrointestinal protectant such as a bismuth subsalicylate-containing product. Animals with severe signs and dehydration may require hospitalization for fluid and additional therapy. A CBC should be evaluated on all animals with more severe signs, particularly if they are febrile. Concurrent loss of mucosal barrier integrity and neutropenia is a potentially lethal combination.

Methotrexate, 5-fluorouracil, and doxorubicin occasionally cause mucositis. Mucositis as a complication of chemotherapy is uncommonly seen in animals but is a common problem in people. Radiation-induced mucositis is an expected early effect of radiation therapy of the oral cavity, esophagus, rectum, and urogenital area. Mucositis begins to develop during the second to third week of therapy and will gradually subside over three to four weeks.[34] Most dogs will continue to eat in spite of their mucositis, but may do better with soft, low-salt foods, or if hand-fed. Anorexia tends to be more of a problem with cats. If anorexia is persistent, the use of a nasogastric or gastrostomy tube is indicated.

## PANCREATITIS

Pancreatitis is an occasional complication of cytotoxic chemotherapy in veterinary medicine. The true incidence of pancreatitis is likely underreported because signs of vomiting in chemotherapy patients are commonly attributed to other causes, such as gastrointestinal toxicity, direct emetic effects on the brain, or anaphylactic reactions. L-asparaginase, doxorubicin, cisplatin, azathioprine, various chemotherapy combinations, and glucocorticoids have all been associated with pancreatitis in the dog.[4,35-38] In one study pancreatitis was associated with 10 of 1,977 (0.5%) chemotherapy treatments given. In 6 of the patients anthracycline drugs (doxorubicin or epirubicin) were given.[38] The mechanism of chemotherapy-induced pancreatitis is unknown. Treatment is symptomatic, as for most other causes of pancreatitis.

## UROTOXICITY

Although several potentially nephrotoxic drugs are used in the treatment of neoplasia in cats and dogs, the nephrotoxic effects of cisplatin and intermediate- or high-dose methotrexate in the dog and doxorubicin (primarily in the cat) are of the most concern. Nephrotoxicity has been reported in doxorubicin-treated tumor-bearing cats.[39] Azotemia and decreasing urine specific gravity was seen in 2 of 6 cats that received a cumulative dose of 300 mg/m$^2$ doxorubicin.[40]

Cisplatin, a platinum coordination compound, is the most nephrotoxic cytotoxic drug used in the treatment of canine neoplasms. In the dog 80 to 90% of the drug is eliminated in the urine within 48 hours.[41] Cisplatin-induced nephrotoxicosis is characterized by reduced glomerular filtration rate and tubular injury. Because cisplatin is much less toxic in a high-chloride environment, a number of saline diuresis protocols have been developed to limit nephrotoxicity.[42]

A minimum data base prior to the administration of cisplatin should include a CBC, creatinine/BUN, and urinalysis. If there is any question regarding the patient's renal function, an exogenous creatinine clearance test should be considered. An increased incidence of clinically evident cisplatin-induced nephrotoxicity occurs in patients with any preexisting urinary tract disease.

Other methods of preventing cisplatin-induced nephrotoxicity have been studied experimentally, including administration of cisplatin in hypertonic saline[43] and with the concomitant use of methimazole.[44] The safety of these protocols in clinical patients remains to be determined.

Sterile hemorrhagic cystitis is a potential complication of cyclophosphamide therapy in the dog (Fig. 13–3), and is occasionally seen in the cat. This toxicity is more common during chronic cyclophosphamide therapy, but may be seen acutely as well.[45] Sterile hemorrhagic cystitis was seen in 14 of 203 dogs (7%) and 1 of 32 cats (3%) treated with oral cyclophosphamide in one study.[46]

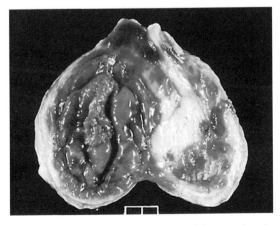

**Figure 13–3.** Gross specimen of hemorrhagic cystitis from a dog induced by cyclophosphamide.

Sterile hemorrhagic cystitis results from the toxic effects of one of cyclophosphamide's metabolites, acrolein, on the bladder mucosa. Strategies to decrease the potential of developing toxicity have focused on promoting diuresis. One method that has been suggested for decreasing signs of cystitis is to administer cyclophosphamide in the morning (allowing the patient to urinate frequently during the day rather than having metabolites accumulate in the bladder overnight), salting the food, and administering prednisone, at a dose of 0.5 to 1.0 mg/kg PO, SID, for both its diuretic and anti-inflammatory effects.[4] Another method that has shown some benefit is to administer furosemide, at a dose of 2 mg/kg PO, BID, concomitantly with the cyclophosphamide.[47]

The clinical signs of sterile hemorrhagic cystitis include hematuria, dysuria, and pollakiuria. Urinalysis typically reveals red blood cells with mild to moderate numbers of white blood cells and the absence of bacteruria. Urine cultures, at least initially, are negative. The most important therapeutic measure that can be taken in the event of development of sterile hemorrhagic cystitis is to discontinue the drug. Any therapies beyond this are of questionable benefit, but in spite of this they are commonly employed. Promoting diuresis by either prednisone or furosemide therapy may be useful in speeding the elimination of any remaining cyclophosphamide metabolites and decreasing their contact with the bladder mucosa. Prophylactic antibiotics are commonly given to prevent or treat secondary bacterial cystitis. Favorable results have been reported in a few dogs with the use of intravesical 1% formalin or 25 to 50% dimethyl sulfoxide.[48,49] Studies in a large number of dogs are lacking. Mesna (2-mercaptoethanesulfonate) and prostaglandin E2 have been reported to be beneficial in the treatment of sterile hemorrhagic cystitis in humans. Their efficacy in veterinary patients has not been investigated.

Although rarely reported, transitional cell carcinomas of the urinary bladder have been seen in association with long-term cyclophosphamide administration. Signs of cystitis do not necessarily need to precede the development of carcinoma.[50]

## CARDIOTOXICITY

Cumulative cardiac toxicity is the unique dose-limiting toxicity of doxorubicin and the related anthracycline antitumor antibiotic daunorubicin.

The precise mechanism of doxorubicin-induced myocardial damage remains unclear; however, experimental evidence suggests that cardiac toxicity is at least in part the result of drug-stimulated reactive oxygen metabolism. A drug-induced free-radical cascade is produced that may overwhelm the heart's antioxidant defenses, leading to the oxidation of critical cardiac proteins and membrane components.[51] Histologically, degeneration and atrophy of cardiac myocytes with myofibrillar loss, cytoplasmic vacuolization, and cell lysis is seen.

Doxorubicin-induced cardiomyopathy is a consistent histologic finding in experimental dogs receiving cumulative doses of > 240 mg/m$^2$ (8 doses).[52] In a retrospective study of 175 dogs treated with doxorubicin, 7 dogs (4%) developed congestive heart failure. The median total dose of doxorubicin before the development of congestive heart failure was 150 mg/m$^2$ (range, 90–210 mg/m$^2$).[53] In a study of the short-term toxicoses associated with the administration of doxorubicin, 2 of 185 dogs (1%) receiving one or two doses of doxorubicin (30 mg/m$^2$ IV) developed cardiomyopathy.[54] These studies suggest that even though the myocardial damage is cumulative and in humans is dose dependent, cardiomyopathy may be seen in individual dogs at relatively low cumulative doses.[53,54]

Acute atrial and ventricular dysrhythmias are well described in human patients. Similar findings were reported in 31 of 175 clinical canine patients[53] and experimental normal dogs[55] receiving doxorubicin. The most commonly reported electocardiograph (ECG) abnormalities are ventricular premature complexes, supraventricular arrhythmias, and R-wave amplitude changes. Experimentally, no ECG abnormalities were noted in 6 cats that were given a cumulative dose of 300 mg/m$^2$ doxorubicin.[40] It is unclear whether the mechanism of the dysrhythmia production is the same as that for the cumulative myocardial damage.

ECGs and ultrasonography are relatively insensitive indicators of cardiotoxicity. In one study of 52 dogs receiving doxorubicin, 4 dogs (8%)[56] developed clinical signs of heart failure despite normal ECG and echocardiographic parameters at the time of each treatment. Another 7 dogs developed signs of toxicity based on echocardiographic (reduced left ventricular fractional shortening) and ECG (e.g., ventricular/supraventricular premature complexes, atrioventricular block) changes. None of these dogs developed clinical evidence of failure after treatment

was discontinued. The guidelines for the use of doxorubicin in dogs include:

1. Breeds with an increased risk of cardiomyopathy and dogs with underlying cardiac abnormalities should be considered at greater risk for cardiotoxicity.
2. Serial ECGs and echocardiography should be performed on those patients at greater risk for cardiotoxicity. However, neither technique is a particularly sensitive indicator of cardiotoxicity.
3. Cumulative doses of doxorubicin exceeding 180 mg/m$^2$ are to be avoided. Consider the substitution of other potentially effective drugs (e.g., mitoxantrone or actinomycin-D) in patients that are still responding to doxorubicin.
4. If tumor response can be maintained only with the use of doxorubicin at a cumulative dose of greater than 180 mg/m$^2$, then clinical judgment regarding risk versus benefit must be considered. Close monitoring of these patients is imperative.

Radionuclide angiography and endomyocardial biopsy are currently the most sensitive means of monitoring cardiac toxicity in man. The predictive value of endomyocardial biopsy for the identification of doxorubicin-induced cardiotoxicity is being prospectively evaluated in dogs.[56]

A variety of anthracycline analogs (e.g., mitoxantrone, epirubicin, idarubicin) have been developed with reduced cardiotoxicity. The efficacies of these compounds are being evaluated in cats and dogs with neoplasia. Doxorubicin encapsulated in a liposome is significantly less cardiotoxic than free doxorubicin.[57] Cumulative doses of 240 mg/m$^2$ have been given to normal dogs with no clinical and minimal histologic evidence of cardiotoxicity.[57]

## DERMATOLOGIC TOXICITY

Alopecia or delayed hair growth may be seen in dogs and cats receiving chemotherapy. This is more commonly a problem in breeds such as poodles and terriers in which a greater percentage of the hair follicles are in the anagen (growth) phase of the hair cycle (Fig. 13–4). Alopecia usually resolves after discontinuation of treatment, or with a prolongation of the interval between treatments. In some cases the hair may regrow in a different color and consistency. Most

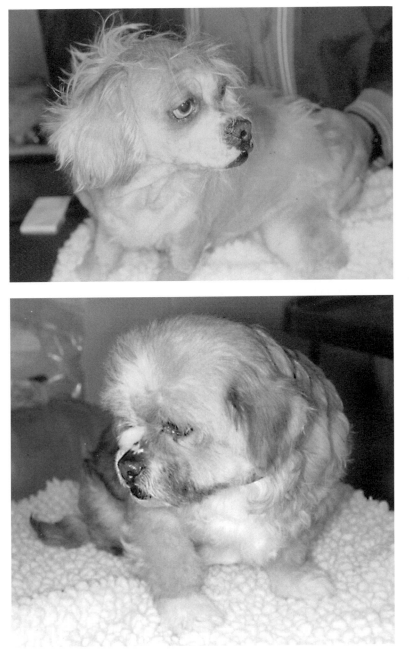

**Figure 13–4.** *A*, Alopecia during chemotherapy and, *B*, following completion of chemotherapy.

*A*

*B*

dogs and cats will lose their tactile hairs around the muzzle and will have a generalized thinning of the haircoat. Any areas that are shaved at this time may be slow to regrow hair. Hyperpigmentation is occasionally associated with the use of antineoplastic agents. Usually this is in association with doxorubicin-containing protocols. Altered toenail growth or loss has been seen by the authors in dogs treated with hydroxyurea.

Extravasation of vincristine, vinblastine, actin-omycin-D, and doxorubicin results in local tissue necrosis (Fig. 13–5). The mechanism of this toxicity is poorly understood. Clinical signs, including pain, pruritus, erythema, moist dermatitis, and necrosis of the affected area, may occur 1 to 7 days following perivascular injection of the vinca alkaloids, and 7 to 10 days following extravasation of doxorubicin.[58] More severe reactions are typically seen with doxorubicin, probably because greater volumes of doxorubicin may be

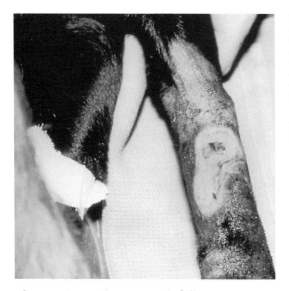

**Figure 13–5.**   Tissue necrosis following perivascular injection of vincristine.

extravasated. In the event of perivascular injection of these drugs, some authors advocate the administration of sterile saline through the catheter in an attempt to dilute the drug, as well as subcutaneous infiltration of the affected area with more saline and dexamethasone sodium phosphate (1–4 mg). The application of warm and cold compresses to the area has been suggested. It is doubtful whether any of these measures results in less severe reactions, and some argue that infiltration of the area with additional fluid only serves to distribute the offending agent to a greater area with resultant necrosis. If tissue reactions occur, significant tissue sloughing is common. Topical antibiotic ointments, bandages, local corticosteroid injections (methylprednisolone, 10–20 mg SC), and Elizabethan collars may be needed to manage reactions. For more severe reactions surgical debridement and reconstruction may be necessary.

## ALLERGIC AND HYPERSENSITIVITY REACTIONS

Allergic reactions occur with anticancer chemotherapeutic agents as with other drugs. The chemotherapy agent most frequently associated with acute type I hypersensitivity reactions is L-asparaginase.[36,59,60] Allergic reactions to intravenous etoposide has been reported in the dog[4,61] and to intravenous taxol in the dog and cat.[62] For the latter two drugs the allergic reactions have been attributed to reactions to the solvents that have been added to the intravenous formulations of these drugs in order to improve solubility. Doxorubicin can induce direct mast cell degranulation, particularly when infused at rapid rates, that mimics a true hypersensitivity reaction.[63]

The clinical signs of hypersensitivity reactions in dogs are primarily cutaneous or gastrointestinal in nature. The signs may include urticaria, erythema, restlessness, vomiting, head shaking, edema of the head, especially the eyelids and lips, and rarely collapse due to hypotension. The clinical signs in cats may be similar; however, they commonly show respiratory signs, including dyspnea and open-mouth breathing.

Anaphylactic reactions can be prevented to some extent by pretreatment with H-1 blockers such as diphenhydramine (1–2 mg/kg, IM, 30 minutes prior to administration of the drug). In patients that are receiving L-asparaginase therapy, the risk of having a reaction is greater if they have received the drug anytime previously. The likelihood of having anaphylactic reactions is decreased if the intramuscular route of administration is used.[60] Studies with polyethylene glycol-conjugated L-asparaginase in dogs with lymphoma suggest that this formulation of the drug may be less allergenic.[59,64]

Therapy for acute hypersensitivity reactions are the same as those for any other drug, including the discontinuation of the infusion of the offending drug if still in progress and then the administration of H$_1$ blockers (diphenhydramine 0.2 to 0.5 mg/kg, slowly IV), corticosteroids (dexamethasone sodium phosphate, 1.0–2.0 mg/kg, IV), intravenous fluids, and epinephrine (0.1 to 0.3 ml of a 1 : 1000 solution, IV).

## NEUROTOXICITY

Neurotoxicity is rarely observed in small animal patients receiving chemotherapy treatment. In humans neurotoxicity is most frequently associated with the vinca alkaloids and cisplatin. Profound motor weakness, characterized by foot and wrist drop, is completely reversible within several months. The earliest manifestation of autonomic nervous system disorder is usually abdominal pain and constipation. The authors have observed rear leg weakness in large-breed dogs on high and frequent doses of vincristine. Vincristine has also been reported to cause a peripheral neuropathy in a dog.[65] Constipation has also been seen in dogs.

Neurotoxicity has also been seen in dogs treated with cisplatin. Cortical blindness was seen in two dogs given high doses of cisplatin (90 and 120 mg/m²). In humans ototoxicity and cranial nerve palsies have been reported. By far the drug associated with the highest incidence of neurotoxicity is 5-fluorouracil (5-FU). 5-FU produces a rapid, profound neurotoxic reaction in cats.[66] Cats treated with 5-FU show cerebellar ataxia and gross dysmetria. *Do not use 5-FU in cats.* 5-FU has also been shown to cause neurotoxic reactions in dogs, although less commonly.[66–68] Dogs develop hyperexcitation, seizures, ataxia, and death.[66–68] Caution must be used in dogs undergoing 5-FU administration.

## HEPATOTOXICITY

Hepatotoxicity associated with chemotherapy is very rare. In man, liver damage is most frequently associated with the use of methotrexate and 6-mercaptopurine (6-MP). Azathioprine, which is frequently used to treat autoimmune disorders in dogs, is metabolized in vivo to 6-MP and can produce hepatic toxicity similar to that of 6-MP. The authors have seen severe hepatic dysfunction in dogs on azathioprine. Dogs on long-term methotrexate, 6-MP, or azathioprine should have periodic monitoring of serum transaminase and alkaline phosphatase concentrations.

## MALIGNANT EFFUSIONS

Development of malignant pleural, peritoneal, or pericardial effusions is an occasional consequence of neoplastic disease in the cat and dog. Malignant pleural effusions are most commonly associated with tumors of the cranial mediastinum, including thymoma, lymphoma, and chemodectoma, as well as with malignant mesothelioma, hemangiosarcoma, and carcinomatosis. Pericardial effusions are most commonly associated with hemangiosarcoma, mesothelioma, and chemodectoma. Malignant abdominal effusions are seen most commonly with hemangiosarcoma, lymphoma, and carcinomatosis.

Malignant effusions affect performance status and quality of life, and are associated with shortened life expectancy in human patients. In a retrospective study of radiographically diagnosed simultaneous pleural and peritoneal effusion, double effusions were observed most frequently in dogs and cats with neoplastic disease, and was suggestive of a poor prognosis, with a greater risk of death when compared to case controls.[69]

Neoplasia may cause effusion by any mechanism that interferes with the formation and absorption of pleural/peritoneal fluid, including invasion of lymph nodes, obstruction or erosion of lymphatic or blood vessels, increased capillary permeability, secondary pleuritis and atelectasis, and hypoalbuminemia.

Initial diagnosis of malignant pleural effusion is based on clinical history, physical exam, and confirmatory thoracic radiographs. Ultrasonography of the thorax can be performed at this time if there is enough fluid present and the patient is sufficiently stable. Pleural fluid provides an "acoustic window" that allows ultrasonic evaluation of the thorax, which is otherwise impossible.

Thoracentesis is generally done in a sternal or standing position below the fluid line at the seventh or eighth intercostal space using an 18- or 20-gauge needle or catheter, extension set, and three-way stopcock. If a malignant etiology for the effusion has not already been determined, fluid samples are collected for cytologic and fluid analysis, as well as aerobic and anaerobic culture and sensitivity. Therapeutic thoracentesis is continued as long as fluid can be readily aspirated. Repositioning of the needle or catheter or aspiration from the opposite side may be helpful. Response to thoracentesis can be assessed by alleviation of the patient's respiratory distress, blood gas analysis if available, and repeat thoracic radiography. At this time better evaluation of the thorax can be made and any signs of an iatrogenically induced pneumothorax checked for as well.

The recommended treatment of malignant pleural effusions is dependent on the underlying disease and the patient's clinical signs. Effusions due to lymphoma will generally respond well to combination chemotherapy. Initial, and possibly intermittent, thoracentesis may be needed for some patients until a remission is achieved. Effusions due to some solid tumors such as thymoma or chemodectoma are best treated surgically, with or without adjuvant therapy. In the immediate postoperative period, tube thoracostomy with continuous suction may be needed to control the effusion.

Refractory effusions caused by tumors for which there is no good primary treatment (e.g., mesothelioma, carcinomatosis) may be treated in a palliative manner. Thoracic tube drainage followed by instillation of a sclerosing agent to create a chemical pleuritis and subsequent pleurodesis is the standard of care in human medicine.

The most commonly used sclerosing agents have been tetracycline, bleomycin, and talc. Evidence for the clear superiority of any one of these agents is lacking. The most important factors in achieving a successful pleurodesis appear to be adequate removal of the pleural effusion by tube thoracoscopy prior to the instillation of the sclerosing agent, and maximal expansion of the lungs. Experience with pleurodesis in veterinary medicine is limited. Tetracycline failed to produce significant pleurodesis in dogs in one experimental study.[70] Temporary resolution of pleural effusion was seen in two dogs treated with intrapleural oxytetracycline; however, significant pleurodesis was not seen at necropsy.[71]

Intracavitary chemotherapy is being investigated with renewed interest. It has the potential of decreasing the effusion, as well as treating the tumor. Intracavitary therapy has the theoretical advantage of delivering increased concentrations of drug locally. In humans cisplatin, carboplatin, mitoxantrone, liposome-encapsulated doxorubicin, methylprednisolone, IL-2, and alpha-2 interferon, among others, have been reported to produce objective responses in selected cases.[72–76] In one study intracavitary chemotherapy with cisplatin was associated with palliation and control of malignant and/or peritoneal effusion associated with pleural mesothelioma or carcinoma in five of six dogs treated.[77] Toxicity was minimal. Intracavitary chemotherapy is a therapeutic option that should be considered more often for malignant effusions when other forms of primary treatment are not clearly superior.

Cancer patients with pericardial effusions may present with cardiac tamponade and clinical signs of right heart failure, or they may be asymptomatic with an effusion detected during the course of diagnostic workup or at necropsy. Pericardial effusions are a rare finding in the cat. Pericardial effusions in the dog of neoplastic cause are most often due to right atrial hemangiosarcoma or chemodectomas. Mesothelioma, metastatic adenocarcinoma, lymphoma, ectopic thyroid and thymoma have been reported in association with pericardial effusions as well.[78] Thoracic radiographs may demonstrate the classic cardiac silhouette that is enlarged and spherical, or "globoid." A pleural effusion is commonly observed, as well as caudal vena cava distention. ECG abnormalities are not always present, but may include diminished QRS voltages and P-mitrale.[78] Echocardiography is the most sensitive and specific diagnostic technique for the detection of pericardial effusion. Demonstration of an echo-free space between the parietal pericardium and the epicardial surface is diagnostic of effusion.

Pericardiocentesis, generally on the right side at the sixth intercostal space, is a useful and simple therapeutic technique. Unfortunately, pericardial fluid analysis does not reliably distinguish neoplastic from non-neoplastic disorders.[79] Diagnosis of a neoplastic disorder associated with the pericardium usually requires additional diagnostic procedures, such as two-dimensional echocardiography or exploratory thoracotomy. Masses within the pericardial sac can rarely be removed in their entirety, but removal of the pericardium (subphrenic) is often palliative for a long time.

## ACUTE TUMOR LYSIS SYNDROME

Acute tumor lysis syndrome (ATLS) is described as a distinct clinical entity in humans. It is caused by rapid lysis of tumor cells shortly after chemotherapy. ATLS is most commonly reported in humans with tumors that are particularly sensitive to treatment with chemotherapy agents, including lymphomas, leukemias, and small cell lung cancer.[80] ATLS has been sporadically reported in the veterinary literature, and only in association with lymphomas treated with chemotherapy and/or radiation therapy. ATLS in the dog is characterized by hyperphosphatemia, hyperkalemia, hypocalcemia, metabolic acidosis, hyperuricemia, with or without azotemia. These biochemical findings are thought to be secondary to the acute release of large quantities of intracellular phosphate, uric acid, potassium, calcium, and nucleic acid metabolites from rapidly dying bulky tumors. Clinical signs that occur include depression, vomiting, and diarrhea that may be hemorrhagic. The clinical course of this syndrome is acute. Successful treatment of this syndrome has been reported with aggressive fluid therapy and correction of electrolyte and acid-base disturbances.[4]

## SUPERIOR (CRANIAL) VENA CAVA SYNDROME

Superior (cranial) vena cava syndrome is a well-recognized oncologic emergency in humans, but is not well documented in small animals. This syndrome is associated with tumors in the mediastinum that obstruct venous return from the head and neck, forelimbs, and cranial thorax. In humans superior vena cava syndrome is most commonly caused by neoplastic compression by bronchogenic carcinoma, lymphoma, thymoma, and mediastinal metastases.[80] The authors have seen this syndrome most commonly with thyroid tumors and lymphoma. Rapid resolution of clinical signs is imperative if significant dyspnea is present. Mediastinal lymphoma typically responds rapidly to standard chemotherapy protocols or radiation therapy. Other mediastinal masses may require surgical intervention.

## METASTATIC DISEASE

Metastatic disease is one of the major causes of cancer mortality in veterinary patients. The mechanisms of cancer metastasis are discussed elsewhere in this volume. For many tumors therapy must take into account not only the primary tumor, but also microscopic or macroscopic metastasis. The veterinary literature regarding the management of metastatic disease is limited.[81] Many of the basic principles discussed here are extrapolated from human studies.

Different tumors metastasize to different organs preferentially. Overall, the most common sites of metastasis are the lymph nodes, lung, bone, liver, and brain. The treatment of metastatic disease must take into account the anatomic location of the metastasis, the extent of metastasis, primary tumor control, and the overall condition and prognosis of the patient.

### Skeletal Metastases

The most common sites for skeletal metastasis are the vertebral column, humerus, and femur. The tumors most commonly associated with skeletal metastasis are mammary, prostate, and thyroid carcinomas, osteosarcoma, and hemangiosarcoma. Diagnosis of suspected metastatic sites may be obtained by the use of radiography or nuclear scintigraphy.

Most therapy for bone metastasis is palliative in intent. Surgical resection of metastatic sites has limited usefulness because the vast majority of dogs have multiple sites. Surgical procedures for control of solitary metastatic lesions include limb amputation and segmental resection of bone with prosthetic replacement of bone. Limb salvage procedures performed with a curative intent are generally reserved for primary tumors.[82]

Radiation therapy for the palliation of the pain associated with bone metastasis is commonly done in humans. The results of palliative radiotherapy for the treatment of primary canine osteosarcoma are good. Treatment with three 10 Gy fractions (= 30 Gy) delivered over a 3-week period on days 0, 7, and 21 results in improvement in limb function within 1 to 3 weeks in most patients. The average duration of response is for several months.[83] Similar responses are seen using a protocol of five 4 Gy fractions (= 20 Gy) given Monday through Friday. Metastatic bone tumors have been successively managed with these protocols as well.

### Pulmonary Metastases

Pulmonary metastases are commonly seen in a variety of tumor types. Radiographically detectable pulmonary metastases are detected at initial presentation most commonly in dogs with thyroid cell carcinoma, hemangiosarcoma, melanoma, and osteosarcoma.

There are limited studies in the veterinary literature evaluating chemotherapy for the treatment of established, non-micrometastatic disease. Combination doxorubicin and cyclophosphamide chemotherapy produced complete and partial responses in some cats with pulmonary metastases secondary to mammary adenocarcinoma.[84] Clinically evident osteosarcoma metastases failed to respond to single-agent (cisplatin, doxorubicin, or mitoxantrone) chemotherapy in a retrospective study of 45 dogs.[85]

Small numbers of pulmonary metastases with relatively long tumor doubling times are potential candidates for surgical metastasectomy. General guidelines for this treatment have been developed for canine osteosarcoma. Similar criteria are probably appropriate for other tumor types as well. Guidelines for treatment include (1) primary tumor under control, (2) less than three radiographically visible nodules, (3) no tumor known to be present outside the thorax, and (4) tumor diameter doubling time of greater than 40 days.[86]

### Brain Metastases

The incidence of metastatic brain tumors in animals is unknown. The goal of therapy for brain metastases is to control elevated intracranial pressure and other secondary tumor effects. For many patients symptomatic palliative treatment to reduce elevated intracranial pressure and control seizures is most appropriate. Corticosteroids (dexamethasone, prednisone) and anticonvulsants (phenobarbital), respectively, are commonly used for these purposes.

Surgical removal of brain metastases is offered to human patients with a single brain metastasis if they have an accessible lesion, limited or no systemic cancer, and a life expectancy greater than 2 months.[87] Similar criteria can probably be extrapolated for veterinary species. Performance status and survival are improved in appropriately selected patients, probably by delaying the onset of fatal complications such as intracranial hemorrhage or other causes of increased intracranial pressure.[88] Similar results are seen in human patients with multiple brain metastases as long as all known metastases are removed at surgery.[87] The median survival time after metastasectomy of a single brain metastasis is 9 to 14 months[87] versus 3 to 6 months with corticosteroids and whole-brain radiation therapy.

Radiation therapy has been used to treat primary brain tumors in cats and dogs. Doses of 40 to 48 Gy given in 10 to 12 fractions over 22 to 26 days have produced encouraging results, including tumor regression and clinical improvement after radiation therapy.[89] Results in the treatment of brain metastases have not been reported.

The use of cytotoxic drug therapy for the treatment of canine brain tumors has been limited. Part of the reason for the limited use of cytotoxic chemotherapy in humans and dogs is because of the theoretical concern of delivering adequate drug concentrations to the tumor because of the blood-brain barrier. New evidence based on drug concentrations in brain tumor biopsy specimens suggests that significant drug levels are achieved in brain tumors with drugs that were not thought to pass the blood-brain barrier, such as cisplatin.[90] These findings would suggest that the choice of chemotherapeutic agent for the treatment of brain metastases might be better based on the anticipated responsiveness of the primary tumor, rather than on the theoretical ability to pass the blood-brain barrier.

The nitrosoureas and cytosine arabinoside have most commonly been used to treat brain tumors because of their ability to cross the blood-brain barrier and achieve a reasonable drug concentration in the cerebral spinal fluid.[91,92] Carmustine (BCNU) has been used successfully to reduce tumor size and improve clinical signs in a dog.[92]

Experimental therapies for the treatment of clinical veterinary patients with brain tumors include adoptive immunotherapy utilizing autologous lymphokine-activated killer (LAK) cells combined with surgery[93] and photodynamic therapy combined with surgery.

## CANCER PAIN

The pain associated with cancer and its treatment has been a poorly addressed problem in veterinary medicine. Pain may result from tumor infiltration of pain-sensitive structures; from injury to nerves, bone, and soft tissue as a result of chemotherapy, radiotherapy, or surgery; and from tumor- or radiation-induced vascular occlusion.[94]

In humans three different types of pain are recognized in the cancer patient: somatic, visceral, and deafferentation. Somatic pain may be caused by bone metastasis, postsurgical pain, or musculoskeletal pain. Somatic pain occurs as a result of the activation of the nociceptive receptors in cutaneous and deep tissues. Typically this type of pain is well localized and in humans is described as aching or gnawing. Visceral pain results from infiltration, compression, distention, or stretching of viscera as a result of tumor growth. Patients describe this pain as "squeezing" or "pressure" and it is often associated with nausea and vomiting. Deafferentation pain results from injury to the peripheral or central nervous systems or both because of tumor compression or infiltration, or from injury caused by surgery, radiation, or chemotherapy. Human patients describe this as a constant dull ache with pressure, and paroxysms of a burning sensation.[94]

Assessment and recognition of pain can be difficult in veterinary species. The existence of pain in an animal is dependent on the observation of behavioral changes that could reasonably be attributed to pain. Behavioral changes might include decreased appetite, weight loss, decreased energy, being unable to rest comfortably, less tolerance in being handled, fearfulness, or aggressiveness. The animal may move stiffly or infrequently, or tense and cry when the painful area is touched.[95]

The degree of pain may be characterized as mild, moderate, or severe. Mild pain does not alter behavior, is easily tolerated, and often goes unnoticed. Severe pain is pain that is intolerable. Unprovoked crying and whimpering, along with decreased movements, or thrashing about are commonly seen. Some degree of moderate pain should be considered as the cause of altered behavior, appetite, or activity in the cancer patient.[95]

The World Health Organization advocates a so-called three-step ladder approach to the management of cancer pain.[96] This approach is applicable to the needs of the veterinary patient as well. This approach advocates the use of non-narcotic, narcotic, and adjuvant analgesics, alone or in combination, titrated to the needs of the individual patient.[97]

The antiprostaglandins, agonist opioids, and agonist-antagonist opioids are the mainstays of analgesic therapy in the patient with cancer pain. The antiprostaglandin drugs may be effective agents for the alleviation of mild to moderate somatic pain in dogs. Aspirin (10 mg/kg, PO, BID in dogs; every 48 to 72 hours in cats) is probably the safest of the nonsteroidal anti-inflammatory drugs (NSAIDs) to use. The disadvantage of this class of drugs is the associated gastrointestinal effects including ulceration, hemorrhage, and perforation.[98]

Corticosteriods have specific and nonspecific benefits in the management of acute and chronic pain. In humans steroids are reported to reduce metastatic bone pain.[98] Improvement in limb function and clinical signs of discomfort are commonly seen with corticosteroid use in dogs with appendicular osteosarcoma prior to amputation. The combination of NSAIDs and corticosteroids should be used with caution. In the authors' experience the risk of significant gastrointestinal side effects increases dramatically.

The agonist-antagonist and agonist opioids are the most effective agents for the management of moderate to severe pain. Morphine (0.1 to 0.4 mg/kg, IM in the dog) and oxymorphone (0.025 to 0.05 mg/kg, IM or IV in the dog) provide pain relief for 4 to 6 hours and 2 to 4 hours, respectively.[98] The mixed agonist-antagonist butorphanol (0.2 to 0.6 mg/kg, IM or IV in the dog, 2 to 4 hours' duration) is commonly used in veterinary medicine for the management of postoperative pain. It has the advantage of not being a controlled substance and has a reduced potential to cause respiratory or central nervous system depression. Transdermal administration of fentanyl using a patch delivery system appears to be effective for the management of acute pain in dogs and may be useful in the management of chronic cancer pain when the animal cannot be treated orally. Epidural administration of narcotics has been a useful technique for the management of perioperative and immediate postoperative pain in dogs receiving pelvic limb amputation for osteosarcoma.[99]

Palliative radiotherapy, as discussed above, can be used very effectively in the management of bone pain associated with primary or metastatic tumors. It is a viable alternative to oral analgesics for patients with painful, localized disease.

## REFERENCES

1. Jain, NC: Schalm's Veterinary Hematology. Philadelphia: Lea & Febiger, 1986.
2. Kaelin, WG Jr, Mayer, RH: Hematologic complications of cancer and cancer therapy. *In* Moossa, AR, Schimpff, SC, Robson, MC (eds): Comprehensive Textbook of Oncology. Baltimore: Williams & Wilkins, 1991, pp. 1754–1760.
3. Ogilvie, GK, Krawiec, DR, Gelberg, HB, et al: Evaluation of a short-term diuresis protocol for the administration of cisplatin. Am J Vet Res 49:1076–1078, 1988.
4. Couto, CG: Management of complications of chemotherapy. Vet Clin North Am, Small Anim Pract 20:1037–1053, 1990.
5. Plorde, JJ, Tenover, FC, Carlson, LG: Specimen volume versus yield in the blood culture system. J Clin Microbiol 22:292–295, 1985.
6. Dow, SW, Jones, RL: Bacteremia: Pathogenesis and diagnosis. Compend Contin Educ Pract Vet 11:432–443, 1989.
7. Dow, SW, Curtis, CR, Jones, RL, Wingfield, WE: Bacterial culture of blood from critically ill dogs and cats: 100 cases (1985–1987). J Am Vet Med Assoc 195:113–117, 1989.
8. Aucoin, DP: Rational use of antimicrobial drugs. *In* Kirk, RW, Bonagura, JD (eds): Current Veterinary Therapy XI. Philadelphia, WB Saunders, 1992, pp. 207–211.
9. Kirby, R: Sepsis/multiple organ systems failure. Proc Eleventh Annu Vet Med Forum, Am Coll Vet Intern Med 1993, 59–63 (Abstract).
10. MacVittie, TJ, Monroy, RL, Patchen, ML, et al: Therapeutic use of recombinant human G-CSF (rhG-CSF) in a canine model of sublethal and lethal whole-body irradiation. Int J Radiat Biol 57:723–736, 1990.
11. Ogilvie, GK, Obradovich, JE, Cooper, MF, et al: Use of recombinant canine granulocyte colony-stimulating factor to decrease myelosuppression associated with the administration of mitoxantrone in the dog. J Vet Intern Med 6:44–47, 1992.
12. Lothrop, CD Jr, Warren, DJ, Souza, LM, et al: Correction of canine cyclic hematopoiesis with recombinant human granulocyte colony-stimulating factor. Blood 72:1324–1328, 1988.
13. Ogilvie, GK, Obradovich, JE: Hematopoietic growth factors: Clinical use and implications. *In* Kirk, RW, Bonagura, JD eds: Current Veterinary Therapy XI. Philadelphia, WB Saunders, 1992, pp. 466–470.
14. Obradovich, JE, Ogilvie, GK, Powers, BE, Boone, T: Evaluation of recombinant canine granulocyte colony stimulating factor as an inducer of granulopoiesis. J Vet Intern Med 5:75–79, 1991.

15. Obradovich, JE, Ogilvie, GK, Stadler-Morris, S, et al: Effect of recombinant canine granulocyte colony-stimulating factor on peripheral blood neutrophil counts in normal cats. J Vet Intern Med 7:65–67, 1993.

16. Searcy, GP: Bone marrow failure in the dog and cat. *In* Kirk, RW (ed): Current Veterinary Therapy VII. Philadelphia, WB Saunders, 1980, pp. 413–416.

17. Couto, CG, Kallet, AJ: Preleukemic syndrome in a dog. J Am Vet Med Assoc 184:1389–1392, 1984.

18. Young, KM: Myeloproliferative disorders. Vet Clin North Am, Small Anim Pract 15:769–781, 1985.

19. Sherding, RG, Wilson, GPI, Kociba, GJ: Bone marrow hypoplasia in eight dogs with sertoli cell tumors. J Am Vet Med Assoc 178:497–501, 1981.

20. O'Donnell, MR, Slichter, SJ, Weiden, PL: Platelet and fibrinogen kinetics in canine tumors. Cancer Res 41:1379–1383, 1981.

21. Jain, NC, Switzer, JW: Autoimmune thrombocytopenia in dogs and cats. Vet Clin North Am, Small Anim Pract 11:421–434, 1981.

22. Helfand, SC, Couto, CG, Madewell, BR: Immune-mediated thrombocytopenia associated with solid tumors in the dog. J Am Anim Hosp Assoc 21:787–794, 1985.

23. Madewell, BR, Feldman, BF, O'Neill S: Coagulation abnormalities in dogs with neoplastic disease. Thromb Haemost 44:35–38, 1980.

24. MacEwen, EG, Drazner, FH, McClelland, AJ, Wilkins, RJ: Treatment of basophilic leukemia in a dog. J Am Vet Med Assoc 166:376–380, 1975.

25. Harvey, JW: Myeloproliferative disorders in dogs and cats. Vet Clin North Am, Small Anim Pract 11:349–381, 1981.

26. Cain, GR, Feldman, BF, Kawakami, TG, et al: Platelet dysplasia associated with megakaryoblastic leukemia in a dog. J Am Vet Med Assoc 188:529–530, 1986.

27. Harvey, JW, French, TW, Meyer, DJ: Chronic iron deficiency anemia in dogs. J Am Anim Hosp Assoc 18:946–960, 1982.

28. Madewell, BR, Feldman, BF: Characterization of anemias associated with neoplasia in small animals. J Am Vet Med Assoc 176:419–425, 1980.

29. Means, RT, Krantz, SB: Progress in the understanding of the pathogenesis of the anemia of chronic disease. Blood 80:1639–1647, 1992.

30. Giger, U, Gorman, NT: Acute complications of cancer and cancer therapy. *In* Gorman, NT (ed): Oncology. New York, Churchill-Livingstone, 1986, pp. 147–168.

31. Drazner, FH: Polycythemia. *In* Ettinger, SJ (ed): Textbook of Internal Medicine. Philadelphia, WB Saunders, 1989, pp. 101–104.

32. Helfand, SC: Principles and applications of chemotherapy. Vet Clin North Am, Small Anim Pract 20:987–1013, 1990.

33. Simonson, ER, Madewell, BR: A 5-hydroxytryptamine receptor antagonist for control of cisplatin-induced emesis: A pilot study. Proc Vet Cancer Soc 13th Annu Conf 1993, pp. 136–137 (Abstract).

34. LaRue, SM: Radiation therapy. *In* Kirk, RW (ed): Current Veterinary Therapy X. Philadelphia, WB Saunders, 1989, pp. 502–507.

35. Hahn, KA, Richardson, RC: Use of cisplatin for control of metastatic malignant mesenchymoma and hypertrophic osteopathy in a dog. J Am Vet Med Assoc 195:351–353, 1989.

36. Hansen, JF, Carpenter, RH: Fatal acute systemic anaphylaxis and hemorrhagic pancreatitis following asparaginase treatment in the dog. J Am Anim Hosp Assoc 19:977–980, 1983.

37. Moriello, KA, Bowen, D, Meyer, DJ: Acute pancreatitis in two dogs given azathioprine and prednisone. J Am Vet Med Assoc 191:695–696, 1987.

38. Morrison, WB: Pancreatitis associated with cytotoxic drug administration. Proc 10th Annu Vet Med Forum, Am Coll Vet Intern Med, 1992, pp. 632–633 (Abstract).

39. Cotter, SM: Renal disease in five tumor-bearing cats treated with adriamycin. J Am Anim Hosp Assoc 21:405–409, 1985.

40. O'Keefe, DA, Sisson, D, Gelberg, HB, et al: Systemic toxicity associated with doxorubicin administration in cats. J Vet Intern Med 7:309–317, 1993.

41. Page, R, Matus, RE, Leifer, CE: Cisplatin, a new antineoplastic drug in veterinary medicine. J Am Vet Med Assoc 186:288–290, 1985.

42. Ogilvie, GK: Approaches to ameliorate cisplatin-induced nephrotoxicity in the dog. Proc 10th Annu Vet Med Forum, Am Coll Vet Intern Med, 1992, pp. 637–639.

43. Forrester, SD, Saunders, GK, Kenny, JE: Prevention of cisplatin-induced nephrotoxicity using hypertonic saline as the vehicle of administration. Proc Vet Cancer Soc 13th Annu Conf, 1993, pp. 80–81 (Abstract).

44. Vail, DM, Elfarra, AA, Cooley, AJ, et al: Methimazole as a protectant against cisplatin induced nephrotoxicity using the dog as a model. Cancer Chemother Pharmacol 33:25–30, 1993.

45. Peterson, JL, Couto, CG, Hammer, AS, Ayl, RD: Acute sterile hemorrhagic cystitis after a single intravenous administration of cyclophosphamide in three dogs. Am Vet Med Assoc 201:1572–1574, 1992.

46. Crow, SE, Theilen, GH, Madewell, BR, et al: Cyclophosphamide-induced cystitis in the dog and cat. J Am Vet Med Assoc 171:259–262, 1977.

47. Henness, JF: Treatment of cyclophosphamide-induced cystitis [Letter]. J Am Vet Med Assoc 187:984, 1985.

48. Weller, RE: Intravesical instillation of dilute formalin for treatment of cyclophosphamide-induced cystitis in two dogs. J Am Vet Med Assoc 172:1206–1209, 1978.

49. Laing, EJ, Miller, CW, Cochrane, SM: Treatment of cyclophosphamide-induced hemorrhagic cystitis in five dogs. J Am Vet Med Assoc 193:233–236, 1988.

50. Weller, RE, Wolf, AM, Oyejide, A: Transitional cell tumor of the bladder associated with cyclophosphamide therapy in the dog. J Am Anim Hosp Assoc 15:733–736, 1979.

51. Doroshow, JH: Doxorubicin-induced cardiac toxicity. New Engl J Med 324:843–845, 1991.

52. Loar, AS, Susaneck, SJ: Doxorubicin-induced cardiotoxicity in five dogs. Semi Vet Med Surg (Small Animal) 1:68–71, 1986.

53. Mauldin, GE, Fox, PR, Patnaik, AK, et al: Doxorubicin-induced cardiotoxicosis—clinical features in 32 dogs. J Vet Intern Med 6:82–88, 1992.

54. Ogilvie, GK, Richardson, RC, Curtis, CR, Withrow, SJ, et al: Acute and short-term toxicoses associated with the administration of doxorubicin to dogs with malignant tumors. J Am Vet Med Assoc 195:1584–1587, 1989.

55. Kehoe, R, Singer, DH, Trapani, A, et al: Adriamycin-induced cardiac dysrhythmias in an experimental dog model. Cancer Treat Rep 62:963–978, 1978.

56. Page, RL, Keene, BW: Doxorubicin cardiomyopathy. In Kirk, RW, Bonagura, JD (eds): Current Veterinary Therapy XI. Philadelphia, WB Saunders, 1992, pp. 783–785.

57. Kanter, PM, Bullard, GA, Ginsberg, RA, et al: Comparison of the cardiotoxic effects of liposomal doxorubicin (TLC D-99) versus free doxorubicin in beagle dogs. In Vivo 7:17–26, 1993.

58. Couto, CG: Toxicity of anticancer chemotherapy. In Couto, CG (ed): Oncology: Kal Kan 10th Annu Symp. Vernon, CA, Kal Kan Foods, 1987, pp. 37–46.

59. MacEwen, EG, Rosenthal, RC, Fox, LE, et al: Evaluation of L-asparaginase: Polyethylene glycol conjugate versus native L-asparaginase combined with chemotherapy. J Vet Inter Med 6:230–234, 1992.

60. Ogilvie, GK, Atwater, SW, Ciekot, PA, et al: Prevalence of anaphylaxis associated with the intramuscular administration of L-asparaginase. J Am Anim Hosp Assoc 30:62–65, 1994.

61. Ogilvie, GK, Cockburn, CA, Tranquilli, WJ, et al: Hypotension and cutaneous reactions associated with intravenous administration of etoposide in the dog. Am J Vet Res 49:1367–1370, 1988.

62. Ogilvie, GK: Personal communication, 1994.

63. Bristow, MR, Sageman, WS, Scott, RH, et al: Acute and chronic cardiovascular effects of doxorubicin in the dog: The cardiovascular pharmacology of drug-induced histamine release. J Cardiovasc Pharmacol 2:487, 1980.

64. MacEwen, EG, Rosenthal R, Matus R, et al: A preliminary study on the evaluation of asparaginase polyethylene glycol conjugate against canine malignant lymphoma. Cancer 59:2011–2015, 1987.

65. Hamilton, TA, Cook, JA, Braund, KG, et al: Vincristine induced peripheral neuropathy in a dog. J Am Vet Med Assoc 198:635–638, 1991.

66. Harvey, HJ, MacEwen, EG, Hayes AA: Neurotoxicosis associated with use of 5-fluorouracil in five dogs and one cat. J Am Vet Med Assoc 171:277–278, 1977.

67. Hammer, AS, Carothers, MA, O'Keefe, DA, et al: Unexpected neurotoxicity in dogs receiving a cyclophosphamide, dactinomycin, and 5-fluorouracil chemotherapy protocol. J Vet Intern Med 8:240–243, 1994.

68. Dorman, DC, Coddington, KA, Richardson, RC: 5-fluorouracil toxicosis in the dog. J Vet Intern Med 4:254–257, 1990.

69. Steyn, PF, Wittum, TE: Radiographic, epidemiologic, and clinical aspects of simultaneous pleural and peritoneal effusions in dogs and cats: 48 cases (1982–1991). J Am Vet Med Assoc 202:307–312, 1993.

70. Gallagher, LA, Birchard, SJ, Weisbrode, SE: Effects of tetracycline hydrochloride on pleurae in dogs with induced pleural effusion. Am J Vet Res 51:1682–1687, 1990.

71. Laing, EJ, Norris, AM: Pleurodesis as a treatment for pleural effusion in the dog. J Am Anim Hosp Assoc 22:193–196, 1986.

72. Bartal, AH, Gazitt, Y, Zidan, G, et al: Clinical and flow cytometry characteristics of malignant pleural effusions in patients after intracavitary administration of methylprednisolone acetate. Cancer 67:3136–3140, 1991.

73. Viallat, JR, Boutin, C, Rey, F, et al: Intrapleural immunotherapy with escalating doses of interleukin-2 in metastatic pleural effusions. Cancer 71:4067–4071, 1993.

74. Ichinose, Y, Hara, N, Ohta, M, et al: Hypotonic cisplatin treatment for carcinomatous pleuritis found at thoracotomy in patients with lung cancer. J Thoracic Cardiovasc Surg 105:1041–1046, 1993.

75. Cascinu, S, Isidori, PP, Fedeli, A, et al: A phase 1 study of carboplatin and alpha-2 interferon in patients with malignant pleural effusions. Cancer 6:330–333, 1993.

76. Delgado, G, Potkul, RK, Treat, JA, et al: A phase I/II study of intraperitoneally administered doxorubicin entrapped in cardiolipin liposomes in patients with ovarian cancer. Am Obstet Gynecol 160:812–819, 1989.

77. Moore, AS, Kirk, C, Cardona, A: Intracavitary cisplatin chemotherapy experience with six dogs. J Vet Intern Med 5:227–231, 1991.

78. Berg, RJ, Wingfield, WE, Hoopes, PJ: Idiopathic hemorrhagic pericardial effusion in eight dogs. J Am Vet Med Assoc 185:988–992, 1984.

79. Sisson, D, Thomas, WP, Ruel, W.W, Zinkl, JG: Diagnostic value of pericardial fluid analysis in the dog. J Am Vet Med Assoc 184:51–55, 1984.

80. Belani, CP: Oncologic emergencies. In Moossa, AR, Schimpff, SC, Robson, MC (eds): Comprehensive Textbook of Oncology. Baltimore, Williams & Wilkins, 1991, pp. 1859–1863.

81. MacEwen, EG, Keller, ET: Current strategies for

management of metastatic disease. *In* Kirk, RW, Bonagura, JD (eds): Current Veterinary Therapy XI. Small Animal Practice. Philadelphia, WB, Saunders 1992, pp. 427–432.

82. Thrall, DE, Withrow, SJ, Powers, BE, et al: Radiotherapy prior to allograft limb sparing in dogs with osteosarcoma: A dose response assay. International J Radiat Oncol Biol Biophys *18*:1351–1357, 1990.

83. McEntee, MC, Page, RL, Novotney, CA, Thrall, DE: Palliative radiotherapy for canine appendicular osteosarcoma. Vet Radiol Ultrasound *34*:367–370, 1993.

84. Jeglum, KA, deGuzman, E, Young, K: Chemotherapy of advanced mammary adenocarcinoma in 14 cats. J Am Vet Med Assoc *187*:157–160, 1985.

85. Ogilvie, GK, Straw, RC, Jameson, VJ, et al: Evaluation of single-agent chemotherapy for treatment of clinically evident osteosarcoma metastases in dogs: 45 cases (1987–1991). J Am Vet Med Assoc *202*:304–306, 1993.

86. O'Brien, MG, Straw, RC, Withrow, SJ, et al: Resection of pulmonary metastases in canine osteosarcoma: 36 cases (1983–1992). Vet Surg *22*:105–109, 1993.

87. Bindal, RK, Sawaya, R, Leavens, ME, Lee, JJ: Surgical treatment of multiple brain metastases. J Neurosurg *79*:210–216, 1993.

88. Barr, LC, Skene, AI, Thomas, JM: Metastasectomy. Br J Surg *79*:1268–1274, 1992.

89. LeCouteur, RA, Turrel, JM: Brain tumors in dogs and cats. *In* Kirk, RW (ed): Current Veterinary Therapy IX. Philadelphia, WB Saunders, 1986, pp. 820–825.

90. Stewart, DJ, Molepo, JM, Eapen, L, et al: Cisplatin and radiation in the treatment of tumors of the central nervous system: Pharmacological considerations and results of early studies. Int J Radiat Oncol Biol Phys *28*:531–542, 1994.

91. Scott-Moncrieff, JCR, Chan, TCK, Samuels, ML, et al: Plasma and cerebrospinal fluid pharmacokinetics of cytosine arabinoside in dogs. Cancer Chemother Pharmacol *29*:13–18, 1991.

92. Dimski, DS, Cook, JR: Carmustine-induced partial remission of an astrocytoma in a dog. J Am Anim Hosp Assoc *26*:179–182, 1990.

93. Ingram, M, Jacques, DB, Freshwater, DB, et al: Adoptive immunotherapy of brain tumors in dogs. Vet Med Rep *2*:398–402, 1990.

94. Payne, R: Anatomy, physiology, and neuropharmacology of cancer pain. Med Clin North Am *71*:153–167, 1987.

95. Haskins, SC: Postoperative analgesia. Vet Clin North Am, Small Anim Pract *22*:353–356, 1992.

96. Swerdlow, M, Stjernsward, J: Cancer pain relief—an urgent problem. World Health Forum *3*:325–330, 1982.

97. Foley, KM, Inturrisi, CE: Analgesic drug therapy in cancer pain: Principles and practice. Med Clin North Am *71*:207–232, 1987.

98. Haskins, SC: Use of analgesics postoperatively and in a small animal intensive care setting. J Am Vet Med Assoc *191*:1266–1268, 1987.

99. Pascoe, PJ: Epidural morphine. *In* Short, CE, Van Poznak, A (eds): Animal Pain. New York: Churchill-Livingstone, 1992, pp. 269–274.

# 14

# New Developments in Cancer Therapy

Ilene D. Kurzman, Evan T. Keller, and E. Gregory MacEwen

Advances in veterinary oncology have been limited in part because most of the available therapeutic agents are associated with significant toxicity at therapeutic doses. Improvement in therapy requires agents that more specifically kill tumor cells while sparing normal cells. In the last decade, new developments have allowed (1) drugs to be targeted directly to the site of a tumor or metastasis, (2) preferential interference with the proliferation of tumor cells by agents that are not toxic to normal cells, (3) extension of the half-life of drugs in the body, (4) in vivo genetic alteration of cells to elicit an antitumor response, and (5) safer and more effective use of modes of treatment such as photodynamic therapy and bone marrow transplantation.

Many of the new developments in cancer therapy will be discussed in this chapter. Knowledge in veterinary oncology and in the treatment of cancer in all species is increasing at a rapid pace. One must stay aware of upcoming developments in the continuing war against cancer.

## SIGNAL TRANSDUCTION INHIBITION

An important mechanism in promoting the invasive and metastatic properties of tumor cells is altered transmembrane signaling, which leads to uncontrolled cell proliferation. Ortho-signaling therapy is the use of agents that block transmembrane signaling resulting in inhibition of tumor growth and metastasis. This section will discuss recent developments in the search for agents that inhibit signal transduction either by affecting isoprenylation or inhibiting protein kinases.

## Inhibition of Isoprenylation

*Ras* genes have a central role in the signaling pathways that cells use in response to growth factors. *Ras* genes are highly conserved across species and have been detected in dogs.[1] Mutations in the *ras* genes result in *ras* proteins that constantly promote cell growth in the absence of growth factor stimulation. This is of importance in cancer research because *ras* proteins are associated with the development of a variety of tumors. Normal or mutated *ras* proteins undergo post-translational modifications that enable them to adhere to the cell membrane, from which they relay growth signals to the interior of the cell. Investigators have been focusing on determining ways to interfere with the modifications of mutated *ras* proteins that would keep the protein from adhering to the cell membrane, and thus unable to relay growth signals.

Association of *ras* with the cell membrane is mediated by an isoprenyl group, farnesyl, that is covalently linked to *ras* and required for transformation of the cell. Farnesylation is the isoprenylation of *ras* proteins involving transfer of a farnesyl group from farnesyl diphosphate, a nonsterol metabolite of mevalonate, to the *ras* protein by farnesyltransferase (Fig. 14–1). Agents have recently been identified that interfere with farnesylation of the *ras* protein. Inhibition of farnesylation prevents adherence of the *ras* protein

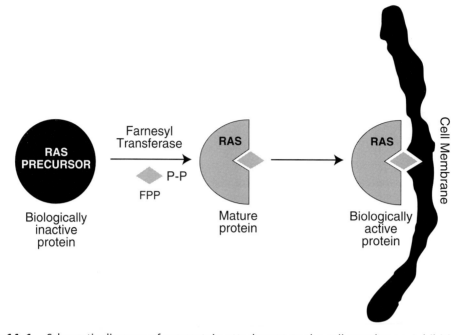

**Figure 14–1.** Schematic diagram of *ras* protein attachment to the cell membrane. Inhibition of farnesylation would block *ras* protein attachment FPP, farnesyl diphosphate. This figure was reproduced by permission from: Travis J: Novel anticancer agents move closer to reality. Science *260:*1877, 1993.

to the cell surface, resulting in inhibition of cell growth. In recent in vitro studies, two inhibitors of farnesyltransferase, L-731,734[2] and benzodiazepine,[3] were found to selectively inhibit the growth of cells transformed by mutated *ras* oncogenes in vitro. Cells transformed by other oncogenes and normal cells were not affected by these inhibitors. Other agents have also been identified that inhibit farnesylation. Farnesylamine, an analog of farnesyl, has been found to inhibit growth of *ras*-transformed NIH 3T3 cells, most likely accomplished by inhibiting farnesyltransferase.[4]

Monoterpenes inhibit isoprenylation of *ras* proteins and subsequent tumor cell growth both in vitro and in vivo. Their mechanism of action is not yet fully understood. In a recent study, limonene, the predominant monoterpene in the oil of orange peel, was found to be effective in inhibiting isoprenylation of the p21[ras] protein and growth of NIH 3T3 cells.[5] In this same study, it was shown that in rats limonene is metabolized, and these metabolites, perillic acid and dihydroperillic acid, were more potent than limonene in their ability to inhibit isoprenylation. Limonene is the first reported agent that specifically inhibits protein isoprenylation in cells in vitro and has antitumor activity in vivo.[6]

Oral administration of limonene resulted in complete regression of both DMBA- and NMU-induced rat mammary carcinomas with little or no observed toxicity. When limonene was discontinued, there were a significant number of tumor recurrences.

Research on the anticancer activity of inhibitors of isoprenylation is still in the very early phase. Studies suggest that these agents would be cytostatic rather than cytotoxic, and it is likely they would need to be chronically administered to sustain their anticancer activity. More work is necessary to determine long-term toxicity and anticancer activity in rodent models before these agents can be available for evaluation in larger species.

## Inhibition of Tyrosine Kinase

Control of cell growth is predominantly mediated by extracellular proteins that bind to specific receptors on the cell surface. Many of these receptors, such as those for epidermal growth factor (EGF), platelet-derived growth factor (PDGF), and insulinlike growth factors (IGFs) have intrinsic tyrosine kinase activity. Tyrosine kinase receptors have an extracellular ligand-binding domain connected to an intracellular tyrosine kinase domain that is responsible for transducing the mitogenic signal. Tyrosine protein kinases play a significant role in tumorigenesis, and many oncogenes activated by a variety of mechanisms have been shown to encode receptor and nonreceptor protein tyrosine kinases. Activation of receptor-associated tyrosine kinase or uncontrolled synthesis of tyrosine kinase oncoproteins results in uncontrolled cell proliferation. Inhibition of tyrosine kinase may represent a new approach to cancer therapy.[7,8]

Tyrosine kinases show distinct substrate specificities that should permit the design of selective inhibitors of each tyrosine kinase. Soybeans are the dietary source of Genistein, a natural isoflavonoid phytoestrogen, which is a strong inhibitor of protein tyrosine kinases and DNA topoisomerases. Genistein has been found to suppress a number of tumor cell lines in vitro. In vitro, genistein inhibited growth of Jurkat cells (a T-cell leukemia line) by arresting the cells in either G2/M- or S-phase (depending on dose) followed by apoptotic death.[7] In humans, the Philadelphia chromosome is associated with more than 90% of chronic myeloid leukemia and 20% of acute lymphoid leukemia patients. The Philadelphia chromosome contains a structurally altered gene (c-abl) that encodes an abnormally large protein with protein tyrosine kinase activity. In a recent in vitro study, Herbimycin A, a known inhibitor of tyrosine kinase, was found to preferentially inhibit the growth of Philadelphia-positive acute lymphoid leukemia and chronic myeloid leukemia cell lines.[9]

Ligand binding to the EGF receptor results in activation of tyrosine kinase activity. Overexpression of the EGF receptor or its ligands, EGF and the transforming growth factor-α, has been associated with a neoplastic phenotype in cells and transgenic mice. In human patients with breast cancer, squamous cell carcinoma of the lung and oral cavity, bladder carcinoma, and esophageal cancer, there is a correlation between the amount of EGF receptor and poor prognosis. In fibroblasts, and in human epidermoid carcinoma cells, the synthetic, very potent tyrosine kinase inhibitor PD 153035 has been found to rapidly suppress activation of the EGF receptor, resulting in selectively blocking EGF-mediated cellular processes such as mitogenesis and oncogenic transformation.[10]

Some investigators have taken a different approach to inhibition of tyrosine kinase. The *neu* oncogene (also called *erb*B-2), originally isolated from rat neuroblastomas, encodes a 185 Kd glycoprotein called p185neu, which is a tyrosine kinase receptor similar to the EGF receptor. Coexpression of EGF receptors and high levels of normal p185neu leads to transformation of rodent fibroblasts. It has also been found that the human homologue of c-*neu*, called c-*erb*B-2, is overexpressed in adenocarcinoma of the breast, pancreas, and ovary, suggesting that p185neu plays a role in neoplastic transformation of certain human tissues. Monoclonal antibodies to EGF receptor and p185neu have been found to inhibit in vivo tumorigenic growth of cells that had been transfected with cellular rat-*neu* and human EGF receptor c-DNA and then implanted into nude mice.[11]

## Inhibition of Protein Kinase C

In mammalian cells, protein kinase C is the major target for tumor-promoting phorbol esters. Aberrant or overexpression of protein kinase C has been associated with abnormal cell growth and metastatic potential of tumor cells. A mutated form of protein kinase C has been shown to induce highly malignant tumor cells with increased metastatic potential. The sphingosine derivatives, N,N-dimethylsphingosine (DMS) and (4E)-N,N,N-trimethyl-D-*erythro*-sphingenine (TMS), inhibitors of protein kinase C activity, have been found to inhibit in vitro growth of various human carcinoma cell lines and in vivo growth in mice. DMS and TMS inhibited tumor size in mice inoculated with human gastric carcinoma cells. After administration of DMS or TMS was stopped, increased tumor growth was observed.[12]

In comparison to DMS, TMS is a more potent inhibitor of protein kinase C, has greater antitumor and antimetastatic effects, and is more stable in solution. However, the dose of TMS that produced the antitumor effects was associated with toxicity, including hemolysis, hemoglobinuria, and an inflammatory response at the injection site. When TMS was encapsulated in egg phosphatidylcholine/cholesterol liposomes, it was found that the inhibitory effect on B16 melanoma cell growth and lung metastasis was the same or even greater than that of free TMS, without the observed toxicity of free TMS. In addition, multiple injections of the liposome-TMS did not result in an inflammatory response at the injection site, as observed with free TMS.[13]

Dexniguldipine hydrochloride has also been shown to be a potent inhibitor of mitogenic signal transduction dependent on protein kinase C activation. Dexniguldipine has strong antitumor activity against neuroendocrine lung tumors induced in hamsters, and an antiproliferative effect against mammary cancer and human lung carcinoid cell lines. Dexniguldipine is also a potent inhibitor of protein kinase C-stimulated cell proliferation in human small-cell and non-small-cell lung cancer lines that are responsive to autocrine or exogenous protein kinase C activation. Phase II trials are currently under way to evaluate dexniguldipine as a single agent for the treatment of human small-cell lung cancer.[14] There is currently an ongoing randomized trial comparing cisplatin (n=9) versus deniguldipine hydrochloride (n=10) as adjuvant treatment for dogs with osteosarcoma.[15] Although preliminary analysis shows no difference between the treatment groups with regard to survival, it is important to note that in this trial there were no adverse effects associated with administration of dexniguldipine hydrochloride (10 mg/kg/day given orally for up to 1 year).

## Inhibition of Calcium Influx

Another novel compound, known as carboxyamidoimidazole, has been shown to inhibit growth of primary ovarian cancer and melanoma cells in vitro and in vivo in nude mouse systems, as well as inhibiting in vitro growth of cells derived from ovarian and breast cancer metastases.[16] Carboxyamidoimidazole exerts its effect by blocking signal transduction pathways through inhibition of calcium influx into the cell via calcium channel blockade. The compound can be given orally and has low toxicity in animal models.

## ANTI-ANGIOGENESIS

Angiogenesis is a central mechanism for tumor cell survival and metastasis. The process entails an active, growth factor-triggered biochemical cascade resulting in the proliferation of endothelial cells to form new capillaries. This process is driven by proto-oncogenes and growth factors such as fibroblast growth factors (FGFs) and other cytokines produced by tumor cells and/or the surrounding supportive network of stromal cells and extracellular matrix.[17] The FGFs promote regeneration of several epithelial and endothelial tissues. The original members of this family, basic-FGF (b-FGF) and acidic-FGF (a-FGF), cause striking blood vessel proliferation.[18] Other cytokines such as interleukin-8, an inflammatory

molecule produced by monocytes that binds heparin, also have potent angiogenesis activity.[19]

Inhibition of angiogenesis is an important investigational approach in current cancer therapy. The heparin-binding agent suramin is a unique cytotoxic agent with remarkable in vitro activity against breast cancer cells and in vivo activity against aggressive prostate cancer, lymphomas, and other tumors. This drug is currently under study in a number of human cancers. This drug may inhibit the activity of FGFs by blocking the binding of FGFs to their appropriate transmembrane receptors.[20-22] The angiogenesis inhibitor O-(chloroacetyl-carbamoyl) fumagillin (TNP-470, AGM-1470), an analog of the "angioinhibin" fumagillin (a byproduct of the fungus *Aspergillus fumigatus*) inhibits b-FGF-induced endothelial cell proliferation.[23,24] Another mechanism of TNP-470 is to inhibit cell cycle of normal endothelial cells.[25] Phase I clinical trials are in progress evaluating TNP-470 in human malignancies.

Recent studies in in vitro models of both rat and human prostate suggest that retinoids (fenretinide-4HPR) may exhibit anti-angiogenesis activity, perhaps in part by augmenting the production of antithrombotic protein thrombomodulin and blocking the induction of coagulation-promoting tissue factor in endothelial cells exposed to TNF-$\alpha$.[26,27] Furthermore, $\alpha$-interferon possesses two potential mechanisms that confer anti-angiogenesis activity: inhibition of endothelial cell mobility; and down regulation of b-FGF gene expression (and thus b-FGF production) in tumor cells.[28,29]

Additional evidence for the role of b-FGF in angiogenesis and tumor metastasis is based on the fact that tumors that secrete high levels of b-FGF have a poor prognosis. This has been demonstrated in pancreatic cancer in humans.[30] Therapeutic approaches to down regulate b-FGF have strong potential benefit in controlling angiogenesis and tumor metastasis.

## ANTISENSE

Many cancers progress because of the overexpression of growth-enhancing factors such as oncogenes and cytokines. As mentioned elsewhere in this chapter, there are a variety of methods to inhibit these substances' actions biochemically. However, the drugs used to achieve inhibition are nonspecific in their actions and therefore are accompanied by significant toxicity.

The ability to target specifically the offending growth factor or oncogene should result in an increased therapeutic index. It is with this philosophy in mind that antisense technology has been developed.

Antisense molecules are nucleic acids that contain a nucleotide sequence complementary to the messenger RNA (mRNA) sequence of the target gene. Antisense molecules have a high degree of specificity for their target gene because of the complexity of the genome. Once bound to the mRNA, antisense may inhibit gene expression by a variety of mechanisms.

Antisense can be composed of either RNA or DNA. RNA antisense forms a stable duplex with the target mRNA, thus blocking translation. RNA antisense can also be designed to function in a catalytic fashion. These enzymatic RNA structures, called ribozymes, have RNA that is complementary to the target site at either end, but in the center of the molecule is an RNA structure that cleaves the target mRNA.[31]

The mechanism of DNA antisense action on the target mRNA is not well documented, but certain features are known. When DNA antisense binds the mRNA, it forms an RNA/DNA strand (heteroduplex), which is recognized by the enzyme RNase.[32] This enzyme degrades RNA that is bound to DNA and thus will destroy the mRNA in a heteroduplex. DNA antisense can also bind with the genomic DNA, resulting in the formation of a triple helix. This structure is very stable and will prevent transcription and thus gene expression.

An important parameter for the use of antisense is selection of the target site on the mRNA. In the case of many RNA antisense constructs, the entire region of the gene that encodes the protein is used, therefore the entire mRNA is targeted. Selection of an antisense binding site on the target mRNA is fairly empirical when using DNA antisense.

In the realm of cancer therapy, antisense will be most applicable for targeting oncogenes, growth factors, and their receptors. A variety of studies have demonstrated the efficacy of antisense for inhibiting tumor proliferation.[33,34] We have shown that oligonucleotide antisense to the interleukin-6 receptor can inhibit myeloma proliferation in vitro.[35] In addition to these growth-enhancing factors, antisense can be used to inhibit oncogenic viral replication.[36] This may develop into an important application for inhibiting FeLV replication. Though in its infancy, antisense technology has great potential to develop into an important contribution to veterinary cancer therapy.

## GENE THERAPY

Gene therapy refers to the introduction of genetic material into an organism to effect a therapeutic response. A variety of strategies are used to achieve gene therapy of cancer. Gene transfer to stimulate anticancer immunity is the most common use of gene therapy. Cytokine genes can be used to enhance immune effector cell activity directly or can stimulate tumor-specific antigen expression. Transfer of gene constructs encoding antisense to oncogenes may be able to inhibit cancer cell growth. Additionally, transfer of tumor suppressor genes can inhibit tumor cell growth.

Genes can be introduced into patients either by ex vivo or in vivo methods. Ex vivo transfection of cells followed by infusion into patients suffers from several drawbacks, including labor-intensive preparation of transfected cells, great time delays until treatment, and poor targeting of transfected cells to the tumor (only 1–2% of infused cells).[37] In vivo transfection of tumors can minimize treatment delay associated with ex vivo transfection protocols. Many mechanisms exist for in vivo introduction of genes,[38,39] including recombinant retroviruses or adenoviruses, lipofection, and direct injection of naked DNA. Retroviral vectors can efficiently target a variety of cells. Drawbacks to retroviral methods include the need for a viral receptor on the target cells and the production of infectious wild-type virus.[40,41] Drawbacks to adenoviral methods include the inhibition of host protein synthesis and the production of viral oncogenic proteins. Many nonviral methods of gene transfer depend on receptor-mediated endocytosis, which is limited by lysosomal degradation of DNA.[42] Direct injection of naked DNA works best in muscle; however, it is inefficient, requiring large amounts of nucleic acid.[43] In order to improve on these methods, alternative gene transfer strategies have been developed. Particle-mediated gene transfer is an effective method for in vivo gene transfection.[44–46] Particle-mediated gene transfer is based on the bombardment and penetration of target tissue with DNA-coated microscopic gold particles. The small nature of the particles (1–3 μM) results in minimal damage to the tissue surface and targets 10 to 20% of the cells for gene expression. As this method is not dependent on receptor-mediated endocytosis, any cell type can be targeted and DNA may be less subject to lysosomal action. Long-term reporter transgene expression occurs in tumor tissue in vivo.[46] Particle bombardment is up to 100-fold more efficient than currently used liposome-mediated gene-transfer methods.[47] Particle-mediated gene transfer was also shown to be much more efficient than direct injection of naked DNA into tissue.[48] We have demonstrated in dogs that particle-mediated gene transfer mediates cytokine gene expression (G-CSF, IL-6, IL-2) with acceptable toxicity, and cytokine proteins produced by particle-mediated gene transfer are biologically active.[49] Figure 14–2 shows a dog undergoing particle-mediated gene transfer.

Ex vivo retroviral-mediated gene transfer of various reporter and antibiotic resistance genes has been successful in the dog and cat.[50–54] In vivo transfer of retroviral vectors encoding either β-gal or factor IX cDNA into canine liver has also been performed.[55,56] Injection of liposome-encapsulated reporter genes into canine tumors in vivo results in measurable protein expression.[57] In a recent pilot study, dogs with oral melanoma were treated every 2 weeks for 12 weeks with intratumoral injections of canine GM-CSF cDNA by three methods: group 1, received allogeneic melanoma cells that were retrovirally transfected in vitro with GM-CSF and then radiated, group 2 received autologous melanoma cells that were retrovirally transfected in vitro with GM-CSF and then radiated, and group 3 received direct injection of plasmid DNA containing GM-CSF cDNA.[58] No response was seen in dogs in group 1, and in group 2, one of two dogs had a complete remission. In group 3, two of three dogs had a complete remission. While this was a small pilot study, the results indicate that in some dogs with oral melanoma, this gene therapy is effective at inducing complete remissions. Though in its infancy, continued exploration of gene transfer methods into canine tumor tissue will aid in the development of effective anticancer gene therapeutics.

## RETINOIDS

Retinoids are the group of molecules that consists of vitamin A and its natural and synthetic derivatives. Retinoids are known for their effects on various biologic functions, including cell proliferation, differentiation, and morphogenesis.[59] Interest in the retinoids as potential anticancer agents originated from findings of early studies on vitamin A deficiency. Animals deficient in vitamin A had a high incidence of epithelial cancers, which were prevented or reversed by supplementation with vitamin A.[60] In humans, epidemiologic studies have identified an inverse relationship between vitamin A and the risk of cancer development.[61] Cancer results from an arrest in normal cellular differentiation without loss of a cell's ability to proliferate. Given the role that vitamin A plays in growth and differentiation of normal cells, and the results of studies showing its ability to prevent carcinogenesis in experimentally induced tumors, retinoids have long been considered potential agents in the treatment of cancer.

Retinoids have been shown to prevent experimentally induced cancer of the bladder, breast, and skin, and there is evidence suggesting their potential for the prevention of cancers of the pancreas, prostate, lung, esophagus, and colon.[62] In vitro, retinoids are known to induce differentiation of some tumor cell lines, and growth inhibition of others.[63] Suggested mechanisms of

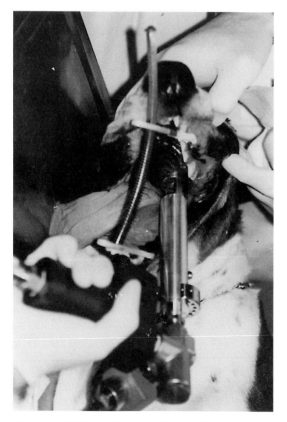

**Figure 14–2.**   A dog with oral melanoma undergoing particle-mediated gene transfer.

action are induction of transforming growth factor-β (TGFβ) and induction of apoptosis.[63] All-trans retinoic acid (RA), the natural metabolite of vitamin A, has received the most recent attention for its potential role in cancer therapy.

## Retinoic Acid

The most striking evidence of the anticancer effects of RA come from the recent studies in humans with acute promyelocytic leukemia (APL). APL is not a common malignancy in humans and is rarely seen in dogs and cats; however, it does represent a model for studying the differentiating ability of retinoids as a mechanism of their anticancer activity. In humans with APL treated with RA, tumor cells have been observed to undergo maturation as the patient enters remission, supporting the rationale for the use of differentiating agents in cancer therapy. As of 1993, approximately 1,500 patients with APL in various studies throughout the world have been treated with RA as a single agent. The studies included newly diagnosed patients and those that had relapsed after or were resistant to chemotherapy. When the studies were combined, there was an overall mean incidence of complete remission of 84%.[64] Induction of remission was associated with differentiation of immature neoplastic cells into mature granulocytes, followed by an emergence of normal hematopoietic cells.[64] In addition, it is suggested that after induction of an irreversible commitment to differentiation, RA may initiate apoptosis in the maturing cells. This is supported by the observation of a transient decrease in the peripheral blood leukocyte count below what is expected that may represent the final elimination of neoplastic cells followed by the delayed regrowth of normal hematopoietic cells.[64] It is important to note that the complete remissions observed were short-term (the median of one study was 3.5 months) and no further benefit was seen with continued treatment with RA.

RA is also receiving attention because of the recent identification of its multiple receptors. Its biologic activity is mediated by activation of nuclear retinoic acid receptors. The presence of multiple receptors may explain the varied biologic roles of RA. The identified receptors belong to a superfamily of nuclear receptors that include receptors for all steroid hormones, thyroid hormones, vitamin $D_3$, and others yet unknown.[65] Of particular interest is the observation in the majority of APL patients of a mutation leading to the expression of a defective RA nuclear receptor. In spite of this defect, RA is a very effective agent in this disease and it is postulated that at higher intranuclear concentrations of RA (as expected with administration of RA), the normal retinoid receptors would outcompete the defective ones.[64]

The use of retinoids for the treatment of solid tumors has been limited. Most clinical studies in humans have evaluated the use of 13-cis-retinoic acid. As a single agent, it has shown effectiveness in locally advanced or metastatic head and neck squamous cell carcinoma (SCC), basal and SCCs of the skin, and melanoma. No effect has been seen in the treatment of breast carcinoma or germ-cell tumors.[63] Topical RA has been shown to be effective (43% complete histologic response) in the treatment of moderate cervical epithelial dysplasia.[66]

It is unlikely that retinoids would be used as single agents for the treatment of cancer. In vitro studies have shown that the differentiating activity of retinoids can be enhanced by interferon-α (IFNα), tumor necrosis factor-α, granulocyte colony-stimulating factor (G-CSF), tamoxifen, and TGFβ.[59,67,68] In a recently completed study combining 13-cis-retinoic acid with IFN-α in the treatment of cutaneous SCC, there was an overall 68% response rate.[67] This same combination used in the treatment of locally advanced SCC of the cervix resulted in a greater than 50% response rate.[67] In patients with previously treated mycosis fungoides, a 44% response rate was observed.[59] Currently, there are ongoing and proposed phase I and II studies in humans of RA alone or combined with INFα, G-CSF, granulocyte-macrophage-CSF, florouracil, etoposide, cisplatin, or cytarabine, or some combination of these agents.[59,63]

The use of retinoids in veterinary oncology has been very limited. There is one recent report of dogs with epitheliotropic cutaneous lymphoma treated with the synthetic retinoids isotretinoin (11 dogs) or etretinate (1 dog). Remission was observed in 4 dogs treated with isotretinoin (5 to 13 months) and the 1 dog treated with etretinate (15 months).[69]

## LIPOSOME-ENCAPSULATED CHEMOTHERAPY

Liposomes are microscopic phospholipid vesicles composed of one or more lipid bilayers surrounding aqueous compartments (Fig. 14–3). As phospholipids have both hydrophilic and hydrophobic

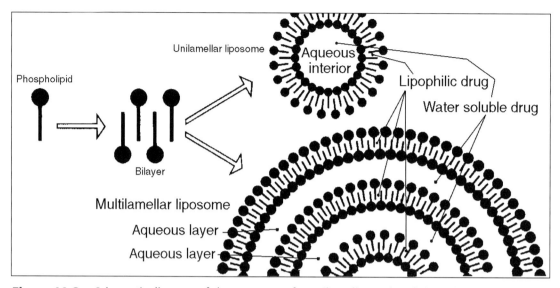

**Figure 14–3.** Schematic diagram of the structure of a unilamellar and multilamellar liposome.

moieties, they will naturally form structures that will facilitate both. The most studied lipsome formations include the small unilamellar vesicle (SUV), large unilamellar vesicle (LUV), and multilamellar vesicle (MLV). The LUVs and MLVs are commonly used for drug delivery.[70] Liposomes have been investigated extensively as carriers for anticancer drugs in an attempt to direct active agents to tumors in vivo or to protect sensitive tissue from toxicity. Both hydrophilic drugs and lipophilic drugs can be encapsulated within a liposome. Lipophilic drugs often have a better encapsulation efficiency due in part to the fact that they have an affinity for the lipid bilayers.[71]

Following intravenous injection, liposomes interact with cells in four ways.[71,72] The first method and most common is direct endocytosis into cells. This is performed primarily by circulating monocytes and tissue macrophages. The second method is adsorption onto cell surfaces. When this occurs, liposome contents may be released into the area of the cells and subsequently taken up by those cells. The third method is fusion of the liposome with the cell membrane. This event is very rare but does occur in a small percentage of adsorbed liposomes. The result is a release of liposome contents directly in the cytosol of the fused cell. The final method for liposomes to interact with the cell membrane is lipid exchange. In this method, lipids from the liposome bilayer are exchanged with lipids of the cell membrane without concurrent exchange of liposome contents.

Cellular interactions with liposomes is influ-enced by many factors.[72,73] Those factors that have been studied include size of the liposome, surface charge, and phospholipid composition. It is known that negatively charged liposomes are cleared more rapidly than positive or neutral liposomes. The composition of the phospholipids will determine the net charge of the vesicle.[74]

Natural targeting of liposome-encapsulated drugs is the form most commonly used in cancer therapy. Liposome-encapsulated drugs can be engulfed by monocytes and macrophages and these cells may "deliver" chemotherapy to the tumor vicinity.[72] Liposomes can also escape through fenestration in the capillaries of tumors and thus are able to concentrate drugs in the area. Liposomes have been shown to accumulate in areas of inflammation[75] and neoplasia.[76,77]

Liposome-encapsulation has been reported to alter the toxicity of several anticancer drugs. Significantly increased toxicity has been documented for liposomal methotrexate.[78] However, decreased toxicity has been noted for entrapped actinomycin D[79] and for several preparations of encapsulated anthracyclines.[80–82] Liposome-mediated decrease in anthracycline toxicity has generally been achieved without reduction in antineoplastic activity.[83–86] Liposome-encapsulation of doxorubicin has been shown to decrease cardiac toxicity in mice[87,88] and dogs.[89,90] Currently the most commonly evaluated liposome-delivered cancer chemotherapy drugs include liposome-encapsulated doxorubicin, daunorubicin, and a lipophilic cisplatin analog.[76,77,80–94]

Two formulations of liposome-encapsulated doxorubicin are currently being evaluated in human phase I and phase II clinical trials. One preparation is under development by the Liposome Company, Princeton, NJ (TLC D-99) that consists of liposomes composed of phosphatidylcholine/cholesterol (molar ratio 55/45). This preparation has been shown to be well tolerated in dogs, and studies have shown that this preparation does not induce doxorubicin cardiomyopathy.[90] We have administered this drug to more than 20 dogs without significant toxicity. We have also noted a particularly dramatic complete response using liposome-encapsulated doxorubicin (TLC D-99) in a dog with IgA multiple myeloma that was resistant to all conventional chemotherapy agents (including free doxorubicin). This dog received over 500 mg of liposome-encapsulated doxorubicin without any cardiac toxicity.[91] Another liposome preparation currently under study in humans and in dogs is the polyethylene glycol (PEG)-sterically stabilized liposome known as the "STEALTH" liposome.[77] The coating of the liposome with PEG increases surface hydrophilicity, decreases opsonization and reticuloendothelial system uptakes, and prolongs circulation time. Elimination half-life is approximately 30 hours in dogs[92] and 45 hours in humans.[76] Doxorubicin in this PEG-stabilized liposome*is currently under evaluation in our clinic in dogs with sarcomas, cutaneous lymphoma, and mast cell tumor.

Another liposome-encapsulated chemotherapeutic agent under study in veterinary oncology is a liposome-encapsulated cisplatin analog, cis-bis-neodecanoate-R-R-1,2-diaminocyclohexars platinum (II) (L-NDDP). NDDP is a lipophilic platinum analog specifically designed for liposome-encapsulation.[93] We have conducted studies in collaboration with Dr. L.E. Fox (University of Florida), to show that L-NDDP can be administered to cats safely at doses anywhere from 85 to 95 mg/m$^2$ every 3 weeks.[94] The major dose limiting toxicity is bone marrow suppression. We have not seen any pulmonary toxicity in cats.[95] Free cisplatin has been shown to be very toxic to cats as evidenced by the development of a lethal pulmonary edema.[96] Studies in dogs have shown that the maximum tolerated dose is 150 mg/m$^2$ and hemorrhagic enteritis was the limiting toxicity.[97] This drug is now in phase I and II studies in humans with various neoplastic diseases.[98]

*Dox-SL, Liposome Technology, Inc., Menlo Park, California 94025

Recent studies have also shown that liposome-encapsulated chemotherapy may be one way to circumvent multidrug resistance (MDR).[99–102] The exact mechanism is unknown, but it is thought that liposomes may fuse with membranes and allow a release of drugs into the cytosol of cells without having to enter cells through conventional mechanisms, thus bypassing the MDR efflux pumps. More studies will be needed to determine if this is truly a significant advantage with liposome-delivered chemotherapeutic agents.

In addition, liposomes are now being used to deliver cytokines.[103,104] The future for liposome-delivered drugs is very positive. By far, the most important advantage of liposome-encapsulated agents appears to be reduced toxicity and prolonged circulation times, without an apparent reduction in therapeutic activity.

## PHOTODYNAMIC THERAPY

Photodynamic therapy (PDT) has been found to be an effective anticancer treatment in a number of human and animal tumors. PDT induces cell death by the simultaneous action of a photosensitizer, light, and oxygen. When the sensitizer is exposed to light, cytotoxic singlet oxygen and other free radicals are generated as the excited sensitizer accepts or loses an electron. The sensitizer is preferentially retained in tumor tissue; however, the mechanism for this selectivity is unclear. Preferential targeting can be enhanced by delivering the sensitizer within liposomes or with tumor-associated monoclonal antibodies. PDT is accomplished with a laser light source. The depth of treatment is dependent on the wavelength required to activate the sensitizer used, and in most cases is only a few millimeters, limiting the use of PDT to superficial tumors or as an intraoperative adjuvant to marginal (incomplete) surgical resections. Most studies evaluating the effect and mechanism of action of PDT have used first-generation sensitizers, which are porphyrin-derived and activated at a wavelength of about 630 nm. Second-generation sensitizers, which are activated at longer wavelengths, allowing for an increase in the treatment depth, are now being evaluated. The main advantages of PDT are limited toxicity to normal tissue; it is usually given only once (although it can be repeated), treatment time is short, and it has been shown to be effective against tumors that are resistant to or have failed conventional therapy.

## Mechanism of Action

In vitro, most cell types are able to be destroyed by PDT, regardless of their inherent differences. Porphyrin studies have shown that these sensitizers initially bind with the plasma membrane, then migrate into intracellular regions. Within hours after PDT, there is evidence of severe membrane damage (blebbing of the cell membrane and leakage of cellular constituents). After cell blebbing, cell division stops, followed by cell lysis. Intracellular membranes (e.g., nuclear, mitochondrial) are also at risk. In vivo, the response to PDT, marked necrosis, is seen within 24 to 48 hours. Necrosis is due primarily to vascular injury. Stasis of blood flow in the immediate area occurs early following PDT. It is postulated that PDT induces release of clotting factors and blood cell agglutination, resulting in thrombus and subsequent collapse of the vessel. In addition, immunologic reactions to PDT have been noted. Macrophages release tumor necrosis factor in response to PDT, which may also be responsible for the vascular damage observed.[105]

The requirement of oxygen for PDT-induced cytotoxicity suggests that hypoxic cells would be resistant to PDT. This is of specific clinical interest since many tumors have significant populations of hypoxic cells. Using a murine radiation-induced fibrosarcoma model, it has been found that very high fractions of hypoxic cells have a poor prognosis to PDT but that low numbers do not necessarily limit tumor response to or cure by PDT.[106] Other mechanisms of action of PDT have been explored. In a recent study, PDT was found to be a highly efficient inducer of apoptosis in a mouse lymphoma cell line, resulting in extensive DNA fragmentation within 1 hour of treatment.[107]

## Photosensitizers

There are several families of photosensitizers of which the most commonly used are porphyrins. The hematoporphyrin derivative (Photofrin I, or the more pure and phototoxic Porphyrin II) have been the most widely used sensitizers in clinical studies. Factors restricting the use of porphyrins are that they absorb light in the 620–630 nm range, a process that limits the depth of the treatment, and there is significant skin photosensitization. New families of photosensitizers that cause less skin photosensitization and absorb at higher wavelengths, allowing deeper penetration, continue to emerge. Chlorins are cholorphyll derivatives that do not cause skin photosensitiza-

tion and absorb in the 640 to 700 nm range. Phthalocyanines are of particular interest because they are easily synthesized and absorb in the 675 to 700 nm range.[105,108]

The majority of studies utilizing PDT in veterinary medicine involve dogs and cats with SCC. In an early study of PDT using porphyrin in dogs and cats with a variety of tumors, complete remission was obtained in 7 of 11 dogs and 2 of 2 cats evaluated. Partial remission was observed in 4 dogs.[109] In a more recent study, 10 of 11 dogs with recurrent SCC of the head and neck region treated with PDT using Photofrin achieved complete remission and, of these, 2 relapsed at 4 and 5 months, 2 died at 2 months with no evidence of local disease, and 6 maintained local tumor control beyond 13 months.[110] In a study of dogs with oral SCC, 11 of 13 maintained long-term local tumor control following PDT using Photofrin. Six of 6 dogs with Stage I or II tumors of the rostral mandible were free of disease with a 20 month median follow-up. Two of 2 dogs with tumors of the rostral maxilla were free of disease at 8 and 10 months. Three other dogs that died of unrelated causes or metastatic disease had no evidence of local recurrence at 2, 18, and 33 months.[111] In the first reported study of PDT using a phthalocyanine (chloro-aluminum sulfonated phthalocyanine, CASPc) in 10 cats, 2 dogs, and 3 snakes with a variety of tumor types there was a 67% complete response, 22% partial response, and 11% no-response rate.[112] PDT with CASPc was also used to treat 30 cats with SCC of the nasal planum or pinna, and 18 cats achieved a complete remission (2 required a second treatment).[113] Eighteen cats with nasal or aural SCC have been treated with PDT using a different phthalocyanine, aluminum phthalocyanine tetrasulfhonate (ALPcS). There was a complete response in 9 of 14 nasal and 3 of 3 aural tumors.[114]

PDT has shown promise as an effective therapeutic approach to the treatment of cancer. Its use in veterinary medicine is currently inhibited by the availability of the equipment and the limitation as to the extent of the depth of treatment. New photosensitizers continue to emerge that can absorb at higher wavelengths or that may be delivered more efficiently to the tumor (e.g., via liposomes or monoclonal antibodies). Laser technology continues to improve, which may increase the benefit of this therapy while, hopefully, lowering the cost. The advantages of PDT, such as low toxicity, usually requiring a single treatment although multiple treatments are not associated with increased toxicity, and its potential use in combination with other treatment modalities, warrant further exploration of the use of PDT in clinical oncology.

## HYPERTHERMIA

Hyperthermia is defined as raising tissue temperature (as high as 42 to 50° C) for a specified time period in order to produce an antitumor effect. The rationale for using hyperthermia for the treatment of cancer is based on the knowledge that in general, temperatures above 42 to 43° C are cytotoxic if maintained for sufficient time periods. The inability of tumor tissue to maintain normal hemostatic conditions makes it more susceptible to heat effects than normal tissue. The microcirculation within a tumor is often vasodilated and poorly responsive to hyperthermia, whereas normal tissues in response to heat can vasodilate, causing increase in blood flow and subsequent cooling of the tissue. Heat-induced cytotoxicity is enhanced in cells that have a low pH or are nutritionally deprived, as is often the case in tumor tissues and uncommon in normal tissue. In addition, hyperthermia has been observed to act synergistically with radiation therapy and a number of chemotherapeutic agents.

There are various methods of induction of hyperthermia. Local hyperthermia can be induced using various sources of energy, including microwave, ultrasound, and ferromagnetic. Depending on the depth and location of the tumor, these techniques can be applied superficially or interstitially. Interstitial methods usually involve implanting into the tumor antennae or electrodes that need to be connected to an energy source. Thermoseeds, composed of metal alloys, can be implanted within a tumor and will absorb energy from an externally applied electromagnetic field. The advantage of this method is that deep tumors can be treated without the need for direct contact with the energy source. Depending on their composition, thermoseeds will reach a predetermined temperature and then lose their magnetic properties, allowing regulation of the hyperthermic conditions. This technique has been successfully used to heat spontaneous and transplanted tumors in dogs, with the major problem encountered being the migration of the implanted thermoseeds into local and distant tissues.[115] Various methods of localizing the thermoseeds (e.g., placing them in catheters, suturing them in place) are being evaluated. A limitation of local hyperthermia is the difficulty in heating the tumor uniformly. As the distance from the antennae, electrode, or thermoseed increases, the temperature begins to decline.

Larger and deeper tumors, and those that have metastasized, require whole-body or regional hyperthermia, which is usually accomplished with radiant heating devices or waterbaths. This method has the advantage of more uniformly heating the tumor, but because there is greater potential for damaging the normal tissues, the maximum temperature achieved must be lower than for local hyperthermia. To induce maximal temperatures with the optimal distribution of heat, a combination of local and whole-body hyperthermia may be indicated. In a recent study in tumor-bearing dogs, this approach was evaluated and it was found that the combination resulted in significantly higher and more uniform intratumor temperatures than local hyperthermia alone, and the treatment was well tolerated.[116] In addition, the power requirements of the local hyperthermia to meet the desired tumor temperature were reduced by 50%.

In the past few years, hyperthermia research has focused on improving the efficacy of hyperthermia by developing a better understanding of the effects of heat on tumor tissue, refining techniques for the delivery of hyperthermia, and combining hyperthermia with other treatment modalities. This section will discuss some of the recent studies evaluating the effects of hyperthermia in combination with heat-sensitizing agents, radiation and chemotherapy.

### Heat-Sensitizing Agents

Methods of manipulating the microenvironment of a tumor have been considered as a method of increasing the efficacy of hyperthermia. Acute reduction of extracellular pH increases tissue sensitivity to heat. Induction of hyperglycemia has been evaluated as an approach to decrease tumor pH. In rodents with transplanted tumors, administration of glucose induced a significant decrease in blood flow and tumor pH. Attempts to lower pH in humans by administration of glucose have had varying results. In one recent study in dogs with spontaneous soft tissue sarcomas, intravenous glucose administration was ineffective in lowering tumor pH.[117]

The efficacy of hyperthermia is directly related to the temperature produced in the tumor tissue. Methods of increasing tumor temperature above the normal tissue have been investigated.

One approach is preferentially to lower blood flow in the tumor, a procedure that would decrease heat loss and result in an increase in temperature within the tumor. Vasodilating agents act on smooth muscle of normal blood vessel walls but are ineffective in tumor blood vessels because of their lack of smooth muscle. It has been suggested that vasodilating agents could manipulate the distribution of blood flow between the normal and tumor tissues by selectively dilating the blood vessels in the normal tissue, resulting in a draining of blood from the tumor. In addition, tumors have a higher resistance to blood flow than normal tissue, which may add to the effect seen by dilating the normal tissue blood vessels. The use of the antihypertensive drug hydralazine has been evaluated in a small number of dogs as a method of increasing tumor temperature during hyperthermia.[118] It was found that the greater the decrease in blood pressure, the greater the increase in tumor temperature. Monitoring blood pressure and tumor tissue temperature, the maximum increase in tumor temperature that could be achieved without lowering the blood pressure below 60 mm Hg was 1° C. The effects of hydralazine lasted 40 to 45 minutes postadministration.

In a more recent study in normal and tumor-bearing dogs, nitroprusside was used to induce hypotension during local hyperthermia.[119] Blood pressure quickly returned to normal after cessation of nitroprusside. Nitroprusside resulted in a drop in blood pressure of approximately 40%. The results of this study showed a significant increase in tissue temperature (without changing the hyperthermia administration) once the nitroprusside was administered; however, there was no difference between normal and tumor tissue. Nitroprusside was more effective in increasing temperature than was increasing the power from the hyperthermia source.

## Radiation Therapy and Hyperthermia

Hyperthermia is known to produce radiosensitization. The combination of hyperthermia-induced cytotoxicity and radiosensitization results in a synergistic relationship when hyperthermia is combined with radiation therapy. This synergism may be due in part to the ability of hyperthermia to kill radio-resistant tumor cells that are in S-phase growth or are in a hypoxic environment. Numerous studies have been performed combining radiation with hyperthermia. This section will highlight a few of the more recent studies.

In one study, 51 dogs with varying inoperable tumors (45 with tumors in the head and neck region, 35 of which were oral tumors) were treated with once weekly radiation for a total of 36 to 40 Gy in 4 weeks. All dogs also received one or two treatments of local hyperthermia (44° C for 30 minutes, using a microwave system) given immediately postirradiation. The combination of hyperthermia and radiation resulted in an 88% response rate (61% complete, 27% partial response). Of the responders, 22 tumors recurred locally at a mean interval of 27 weeks (range: 11 to 76 weeks). Dogs that received two hyperthermia treatments did significantly better than those receiving one treatment, suggesting that the hyperthermia treatments were beneficial. Toxicity from this combined treatment was consistent with that seen in other studies. Within 1 week of hyperthermia 51% of dogs had gross tumor necrosis, which resolved as the tumor regressed.[120]

A randomized phase III study of 79 dogs with various solid tumors showed that dogs receiving a combination of radiation and local hyperthermia had a significantly higher complete response rate than dogs receiving radiation alone (65% and 37%, respectively). Radiation therapy consisted of 3.5 Gy fractions, 3 times per week for 14 treatments. There was no difference with regard to response between the dogs receiving hyperthermia immediately after radiation compared to the dogs treated several hours after radiation. Hyperthermia significantly enhanced the acute response of skin and oral mucosa, which required twice the healing time of the radiation-alone dogs.[121]

A randomized phase II study of 64 dogs with soft tissue sarcomas showed improvement in the duration of local tumor control when hyperthermia was combined with radiation compared to radiation alone. In this study, dogs were stratified by tumor volume and received 35 to 55 Gy in 10 fractions (3/week) with or without local ultrasound-induced hyperthermia (30 minutes at 42° C) twice weekly, given 3 hours after irradiation. No difference was observed between the treatment groups with regard to the complete response rate or frequency of distant metastases at 1 or 2 years post-treatment. The frequency of late normal tissue complications was the same for both treatment groups.[122]

The results of studies evaluating the combination of hyperthermia and radiation for the treatment of spontaneous tumors in dogs indicate a benefit from this combined therapy with regard to prolongation of tumor control; however, the effect on overall survival has been disappointing. Efforts to refine and optimize this combined therapy continue. Further studies will be focusing on the manipulation of factors such as radiation dose and frequency, duration, and temperature achieved by the hyperthermia method employed, and timing of the hyperthermia treatments in relationship to the radiation treatment.

## Chemotherapy and Hyperthermia

Hyperthermia has been shown to potentiate the in vitro antitumor effect of several chemotherapeutic agents, including cisplatin and doxorubicin. In human and rodent studies, however, the toxicity of these drugs is increased when administered with hyperthermia. Studies in dogs have focused on examining the distribution and pharmacokinetics of chemotherapy drugs when given concurrently with hyperthermia.

A normal dog study evaluated the effects of cisplatin given in combination with whole-body hyperthermia. This study found that hyperthermia altered tissue deposition of cisplatin in a nonuniform manner and that pharmacokinetic data collected at one temperature was not directly applicable to predict tissue concentrations at a different temperature. Drug distribution was significantly greater in many gastrointestinal tissues (esophagus, duodenum, ileum, colon, pyloric stomach region) and in the liver and lung of the hyperthermic dogs compared to control euthermic dogs. In addition, when uptake of cisplatin in lung tissue was compared to kidney or bone marrow, there was a suggestion that hyperthermia induced a potentially therapeutically favorable distribution to lung versus kidney and bone marrow. This finding supports further investigation into the combination of heat and cisplatin (altering the doses for optimal effect) for the treatment of tumors in the lung while potentially reducing the toxicity to the kidney and bone marrow.[123]

The increased toxicity observed when cisplatin is given concurrently with whole-body hyperthermia necessitates that the dose of cisplatin be reduced. In a recent study the maximum tolerated dose of cisplatin when combined with whole-body hyperthermia was determined in tumor-bearing dogs. Cisplatin was administered to 54 dogs, every 3 weeks for a minimum of two treatments. In 33 dogs, whole-body hyperthermia (41.9 to 42.1° C for 60 minutes) was induced at the time of cisplatin administration, using a radiant heating device. The starting dose of cisplatin was 60 and 20 mg/m² for normothermic and hyperthermic conditions, respectively. Dose escalation was done if three dogs at any dose level did not experience greater than mild toxic-

ity. Hematologic, acute renal, and chronic toxicity were evaluated for each dog. The maximum tolerated dose for acute and chronic (cumulative) toxicity for the hyperthermic dogs was 54.6 and 46.4 mg/m², respectively, and for the normothermic dogs, 73.6 and 70 mg/m², respectively. No difference in response was seen in a limited follow-up of these dogs. Further studies are now needed to determine the ability of whole-body hyperthermia to enhance the antitumor activity of cisplatin.[124]

One approach to avoid the increased systemic toxicity of combined cisplatin and hyperthermia therapy is to administer the cisplatin intralesionally. This approach has been evaluated in a small study of nine tumor-bearing dogs and one cat with fibrosarcoma. Cisplatin (mixed with collagen to restrict diffusion from the tumor) was administered intralesionally, once a week for 4 weeks. Local hyperthermia (42° C for 30 minutes using interstitial radio frequency or hot water bath technique) was induced immediately after cisplatin administration. The dose of cisplatin was dependent on the amount that could be placed within the tumor without leaking. There was an overall 50% response rate (including a complete response in the cat with fibrosarcoma) and no systemic toxicity was observed in these animals. The results of this study indicate that this approach is safe and may be effective for local tumor control.[125]

Tumor necrosis factor-α (TNFα) has been shown to act synergistically with hyperthermia.[126] TNF alters tumor vascular supply and causes hypoxia and a decreased pH within the tumor. These alterations in the tumor environment have been associated with increased sensitivity to heat. TNFα has been added to the cisplatin/hyperthermia approach in a recent study in rats. This combination may have potential as an anticancer therapy and needs to be further explored.[127]

Hyperthermia has also been evaluated for its effect when combined with doxorubicin. In a phase I study of increasing doses of doxorubicin combined with whole-body hyperthermia (using a radiant heating device), it was found that 30 mg/m² doxorubicin can be administered with hyperthermia to dogs with lymphoma without serious toxicity.[128] Results of a phase III study evaluating doxorubicin (30 mg/m²) combined with whole-body hyperthermia (using a radiant heating device) in 61 dogs with lymphoma showed a trend toward a longer disease-free survival for dogs receiving combined therapy compared to dogs receiving doxorubicin alone. There was no difference between the treatment groups with regard to clinical evidence of cardiac toxicity; however, on postmortem examination, dogs receiving the combined treatment had significantly greater cardiac myocyte degeneration and a trend toward increased cardiac fibrosis. The authors concluded that further refinement of this protocol may ultimately result in a significant prolongation of disease-free survival.[129]

In mice, the antitumor activity of the alkylating agent, melphalan, has been shown to be enhanced by hyperthermia. It has been proposed that repair of melphalan-induced DNA damage is inhibited by heat. In a phase I study in dogs with malignant melanoma, it was found that the maximum tolerated dose of melphalan was 1.9 times lower for dogs receiving whole-body hyperthermia (using a radiant heating device) than for dogs receiving melphalan alone.[130]

It is clear from the studies combining chemotherapeutic agents with hyperthermia, that dose reductions are necessary to avoid increased toxicity induced by heat. From the studies to date, there have been suggestions of increased benefit of this combination treatment, and as with the radiation therapy studies, larger clinical trials comparing the various combinations of drugs and whole-body or local hyperthermia are warranted.

## BONE MARROW TRANSPLANTATION

Bone marrow transplantation allows for high-dosage cancer therapy that would be lethal without bone marrow replacement. In humans, this procedure has been used to treat leukemia patients, as well as some selected solid tumors. Although much experimental work has been done in animals, particularly in the dog, there have been few reports on the use of bone marrow transplantation in clinical veterinary oncology.

### Autologous Bone Marrow Transplantation

Autologous bone marrow transplantation (ABMT) has been used in conjunction with total body irradiation (TBI) in the treatment of dogs with malignant lymphoma. In one study, 34 of 57 dogs (60%) treated with combination chemotherapy (nitrogen mustard, vincristine, prednisone, L-asparaginase, and 6-mercaptopurine) achieved complete remission. Twelve of the dogs in remission received no further therapy and had a median disease-free survival of 73.5 days. Sev-

enteen of the dogs in remission received 1100 rads TBI, followed by infusion of autologous bone marrow that had been aspirated immediately prior to the TBI. These dogs had a median disease-free survival of 205 days, which was significantly longer than the 73.5 days for the dogs receiving chemotherapy alone. These findings show that while dogs with malignant lymphoma are responsive to chemotherapy, the addition of TBI and rescue by infusion of the dog's own bone marrow markedly prolongs disease-free survival time.[131] More recent studies in the treatment of malignant lymphoma with TBI and ABMT have given similar results. These studies investigated the effects of varying the dose of radiation, and it was found that increasing the dose led to greater toxicity and no measurable decrease in the relapse rate after transplantation.[132]

One of the major concerns regarding the use of ABMT in dogs receiving TBI for lymphoma is the presence of tumor cells in the bone marrow. Relapse after ABMT may be due to the reinfusion of these tumor cells. In humans, numerous ways of purging the bone marrow of tumor cells in vitro, prior to reinfusion, have been investigated. Purging can be accomplished by cytotoxic drugs, physical manipulations, and immunologic methods. The limiting factors with regard to the use of cytotoxic agents are the sensitivity of normal bone marrow cells to the cytotoxic agent, and adverse effects related to infusion of the cytotoxic agent along with the bone marrow. Immunologic methods of bone marrow purging involve the use of monoclonal antibodies, either to the progenitor cells or to the tumor cells. In a recent study, anti-CD71 immunotoxin was found to be useful for bone marrow purging.[133] All proliferating committed progenitor cells express the transferrin receptor CD71. This receptor is not expressed on noncycling immature progenitors. In addition, CD71 is highly expressed on leukemic cells. Anti-CD71 immunotoxin kills the progenitor cells and is expected to kill the leukemic cells, allowing the immature progenitors to restore normal bone marrow.

### Allogeneic Bone Marrow Transplantation

The use of allogeneic bone marrow transplantation for restoration of hematopoiesis following bone marrow ablative chemotherapy or TBI has been extensively explored. Engraftment is reported to be generally successful (>90%) for dogs receiving TBI followed by infusion of bone marrow from genetically DLA-identical litter-mates;[134] however, such littermates are not often available in the clinical setting. In addition, a recent study has shown that if three blood transfusions from a DLA-identical donor precede transplantation, the graft will be rejected because of exposure to minor non-DLA histocompatibility antigens that are expressed on the surface of blood mononuclear cells, resulting in 100% rejection of the marrow from these same donors.[135] Irradiation (2000 CGy) of the blood prior to transfusion significantly reduced the risk of graft rejection (9 of 10 dogs engrafted). In a more recent study reported by these investigators, it was found that dogs receiving six blood transfusions from non-DLA-identical donors became sensitized to minor histocompatibility antigens, resulting in subsequent bone marrow rejection following TBI in 9 of 16 dogs transplanted with marrow from DLA-identical littermates.[136] As in their first study, these investigators found that irradiation of the unrelated blood prior to transfusion significantly reduced the incidence of marrow graft rejection (15 of 16 dogs engrafted).

Failure of engraftment is common (80–90%) for dogs receiving bone marrow from unrelated, DLA-nonidentical donors.[134] Graft resistance is mediated by immune cells of the host that survive TBI. Even with successful engraftment, development of graft versus host disease (GVHD) is a limiting factor for the clinical use of this approach. Immunosuppressive therapy following allogeneic transplants is used to prevent GVHD and to facilitate in the development of graft-host tolerance that is necessary once the immunosuppressive therapy is discontinued. Various immunosuppressive drugs are effective for this purpose in rodent models; however, these agents are not effective in inducing graft-host tolerance in dogs. Delay of GVHD and prolongation of survival have been seen with the use of methotrexate in combination with cyclosporin A.[137] In a recent investigation of FK-506, a macrolide lactone isolated from streptomyces and known to be highly immunosuppressive, it was found that FK-506 delayed the onset of acute GVHD and prolonged survival in dogs receiving DLA-nonidentical bone marrow following TBI. In combination with methotrexate, graft-host tolerance and long- term survival was induced in 50% of treated dogs, even though treatment was stopped after 90 days.[137] The limiting toxicities of FK-506 in dogs are gastrointestinal.

The clinical use of bone marrow transplantation for rescue following marrow ablative therapy has been slow to develop because of many of the encountered difficulties discussed above. However, advances are being made that will allow us to circumvent some of these difficulties. It is fortunate for the veterinary community that the majority of the research in bone marrow transplantation for humans is carried out in the dog, providing the development of refined techniques and protocols for successful transplantation and long-term survival that are directly applicable to the clinical canine patient. Bone marrow transplantation in cats has not been extensively studied, and a review of the literature revealed no reports of the use of transplantation in the treatment of cancer. In a small study in normal cats, it was found that following TBI, 5 of 5 cats receiving bone marrow transplants from siblings successfully engrafted (1 cat died of hepatic lipidosis following a prolonged period of anorexia).[138] In this study, an additional 2 cats received bone marrow from unrelated donors. One of the 2 cats rejected the marrow, the second cat also received immunosuppressive therapy and did successfully engraft. In a report of 78 cats (28 controls and 50 cats with varying disorders) treated with bone marrow transplant, the engraftment rate was 70.6%. Complications associated with the bone marrow transplantation were radiation-induced complications, failure to engraft with or without autologous recovery, graft-versus-host disease, anemia, thrombocytopenia, and infections secondary to transplant-related immunosuppression.[139]

# REFERENCES

1. Madewell BR, Gumerlock PH, Saunders KA, et al: Canine and bovine *ras* family expression detected and discriminated by use of polymerase chain reaction. Anticancer Res 9:1743–1749, 1989.
2. Kohl NE, Mosser SD, deSolms SJ, et al: Selective inhibition of *ras*-dependent transformation by a farnesyltransferase inhibitor. Science 260:1934–1937, 1993.
3. James GL, Goldstein JL, Brown MS, et al: Benzodiaszepine peptidomimetics: Potent inhibitors of Ras farnesylation in animal cells. Science 260:1937–1942, 1993.
4. Kothapalli R, Guthrie N, Chambers AF, et al: Farnesylamine: An inhibitor of farnesylation and growth of *ras*-transformed cells. Lipids 28:969–973, 1993.
5. Crowell PL, Chang RR, Ren Z, et al: Selective inhibition of isoprenylation of 21-26kDa proteins by the anticarcinogen d-limonene and its metabolites. J Biol Chem 266:7679–7685, 1991.

6. Haag JD, Lindstrom MJ, Gould MN: Limonene-induced regression of mammary carcionmas. Cancer Res 52:4021–4026, 1992.

7. Spinozzi F, Pagliacci MC, Migliorati G, et al: The natural tyrosine kinase inhibitor genistein produces cell cycle arrest and apoptosis in Jurkat T-leukemia cells. Leukemia Res 18:431–439, 1994.

8. Aaronson SA: Growth factors and cancer. Science 254:1146–1153, 1991.

9. Sato S, Honma Y, Hozumi M, et al: Effects of Herbamycin A and its derivatives on growth and differentiation of Ph1-positive acute lymphoid leukemia cell lines. Leukemia Res 18:221–228, 1994.

10. Fry DW, Kraker AJ, McMichael A, et al: A specific inhibitor of the epidermal growth factor receptor tyrosine kinase. Science 265:1093–1095, 1994.

11. Wade T, Myers JN, Kokai Y, et al: Anti-receptor antibodies reverse the phenotype of cells transformed by two interacting proto-oncogene encoded receptor proteins. Oncogene 5:489–495, 1990.

12. Endo K, Igarashi Y, Nisar M, et al: Cell membrane signaling as target in cancer therapy: Inhibitory effect of N,N-dimethyl and N,N,N-trimethyl sphingosine derivatives on in vitro and in vivo growth of human tumor cells in nude mice. Cancer Res 51:1613–1618, 1991.

13. Park YS, Hakomori S-I, Kawa S, et al: Liposomal N,N,N-trimethylsphingosine (TMS) as an inhibitor of B16 melanoma cell growth and metastasis with reduced toxicity and enhanced drug efficacy compared to free TMS: Cell membraned signaling as a target in cancer therapy III. Cancer Res 54:2213–2217, 1994.

14. Schuller HM, Orloff M, Reznik GK: Inhibition of protein-kinase-C-dependent cell proliferation of human lung cancer cell lines by the dihydropyridine dexniguildipine. J Cancer Res Clin Oncol 120:354–358, 1994.

15. Hahn KA, Schuller HM, Avenell JS, et al: Dexniguldipine as adjuvant treatment in canine osteosarcoma. Proc 14th Annu Vet Cancer Soc Conf, 1994, pp. 113–114.

16. Kohn EC, Sandeen MA, Liotta LA: In vivo efficacy of a novel inhibitor of selected signal transduction pathways including calcium, arachidonate and inosital phosphates. Cancer Res 52:3208–3212, 1992.

17. Scott PAE, Harris AL: Current approaches to targeting cancer using antiangiogenesis therapies. Cancer Treatment Rev 20:393–412, 1994.

18. Vlodavsky I, Fuks Z, Ishai-Michaeli R, et al: Extracellular matrix-residue basic fibroblast growth factor: Implication for the control of angiogenesis. J Cell Biochem 45:167–176, 1991.

19. Koch AE, Polverini PJ, Kunkel S, et al: Interleukin-8 as a macrophage-derived mediator of angiogenesis. Science 258:1798–1801, 1992.

20. Pesenti E, Sola F, Mongelli W, et al: Suramin prevents neovascularization and tumour growth though blocking of basic fibroblast growth factor activity. Br J Cancer 66:367–372, 1992.

21. Braddock P, Hu DE, Fan TP, et al: A structural-activity analysis of antagonism of the growth factor and angiogenic activity of basic fibroblast growth factor by suramin and related polyanions. Br J Cancer 69:890–898, 1994.

22. Takano S, Gately S, Neville ME, et al: Suramin, an anticancer and angiosuppressive agent, inhibits endothelial cell binding of basic fibroblast growth factor, migration, proliferation, and induction of urokinase-type plasminogen activator. Cancer Res 54:2654–2660, 1994.

23. Takamiya Y, Friedlander R, Brem H, et al: Inhibition of angiogenesis and growth of human nerve-sheath tumors by AGM 1470. J Neurosurg 78:470–476, 1993.

24. Yamaoka M, Yamamoto T, Masaki T, et al: Inhibition of tumor growth and metastasis of rodent tumors by the angiogenesis inhibitor O-(chloroacetyl-carbamoyl) fumagillin (TNP-470, AGM-1470). Cancer Res 53:4262–4267, 1993.

25. Antoine W, Greimers R, DeRoanne C, et al: AGM-1470, a potent angiogenesis inhibitor, prevents the entry of normal but not transformed endothelial cells into the $G_1$ phase of the cell cycle. Cancer Res 54:2073–2076, 1994.

26. Pienta KJ, Nguyen NM, Lehr JE: Treatment of prostate cancer in the rat with the synthetic retinoid fenretinide. Cancer Res 53:224–226, 1993.

27. Ischii H, Horie S, Kizak K, et al: Retinoic acid counteracts both the down-regulation of thrombomudulin and the induction of tissue factor in cultured human endothelial cells exposed to tumor necrosis factor. Blood 80:2556–2562, 1992.

28. Ezekowitz R, Mulliken J, Folkman J: Interferon alpha 2α therapy for life-threatening hemangiomas of infancy. N Engl J Med 326:1456–1463, 1992.

29. Guyer D, Adamis A, Gragoudes E, et al: Systemic antiangiogenesis therapy for choroidal neovascularization. Arch Ophthalmol 110:1383–1384, 1992.

30. Yamanaka Y, Friess H, Buchler M, et al: Overexpression of acidic and basic fibroblast growth factor in human pancreatic cancer correlates with advanced tumor stage. Cancer Res 53:5289–5296, 1993.

31. Torrence PF, Maitra RK, Lesiak K, et al: Targeting RNA for degradation with a (2'-5') oligoadenylate-antisense chimera. Proc Natl Acad Sci USA 90:1300–1304, 1993.

32. Giles RV, Tidd DM: Increased specificity for antisense oligodeoxynucleotide targeting of RNA cleavage by RNase H using chimeric methylphosphonodiester/phosphodiester structures. Nucl Acid Res 20:763–770, 1992.

33. Cho-Chung YS: Suppression of malignancy targeting cyclic AMP signal transducing proteins. Biochem Soc Trans 20:425–430, 1992.

34. Lu C, Kerbel RS: Interleukin-6 undergoes transition from paracrine growth inhibitor to autocrine stimulator during human melanoma progression. J Cell Biol 120:1281–1288, 1993.

35. Keller ET, Erschler WD: Antisense to interleukin-6 inhibits myeloma cell growth in vitro. J Immunol (in press).

36. Agrawal S, Goodchild J, Civeira MP, et al: Oligodeoxynucleoside phosphoramidates and phophrothioates as inhibitors of human immunodeficiency virus. Proc Natl Acad Sci USA 85:7079– 7083, 1988.

37. Rosenberg SA, Aebersold P, Cornetta K, et al: Gene transfer into humans—Immunotherapy of patients with advanced melanoma, using tumor-infiltrating lymphocytes modified by gene transduction. N Engl J Med 323:570–578, 1990.

38. Yang N-S: Gene transfer into mammalian somatic cells in vivo. Crit Rev Biotechnol 12:335–336, 1992.

39. Mulligan RC: The basic science of gene therapy. Science 260:926–932, 1993.

40. Miller AD, Buttimore C: Redesign of retrovirus packaging cell line to avoid recombination leading to helper virus production. Mol Cell Biol 6:2895–2902, 1986.

41. Miller AD, Rosman GJ: Improved retroviral vectors for gene transfer and expression. BioTechniques 7:980–990, 1989.

42. Wagner E, Zatloukal K, Cotten M, et al: Coupling of adenovirus to transferrin-polylysine/DNA complexes greatly enhances receptor-mediated gene delivery and expression of transfected genes. Proc Natl Acad Sci USA 89:6099–6103, 1992.

43. Barr E, Lin H, Parmacek MS, et al: Direct gene transfer into cardiac myocytes in vivo. Methods: Compar Methods Enzymol 4:169–176, 1992.

44. Yang N-S, Burkholder J, Roberts B, et al: In vivo and in vitro gene transfer to mammalian somatic cells by particle bombardment. Proc Natl Acad Sci USA 87:9568–9572, 1990.

45. Williams RS, Johnston SA, Riedy M, et al: Introduction of foreign genes into tissues of living mice by DNA-coated microprojectiles. Proc Natl Acad Sci USA 88:2726–2730, 1991.

46. Cheng L, Ziegelhoffer PR, Yang N-S: In vivo promoter activity and transgene expression in mammalian somatic tissues evaluated by using particle bombardment. Proc Natl Acad Sci USA 90:4455–4459, 1993.

47. Jiao S, Cheng L, Wolff JA, et al: Particle bombardment-mediated gene transfer and expression in rat brain tissues. Bio/Technol 11:497–502, 1993.

48. Fynan EF, Webster RG, Fuller DH, et al: DNA vaccines: Protective immunizations by parenteral, mucosal, and gene-gun inoculations. Proc Natl Acad Sci USA 90:11478–11482, 1993.

49. Keller ET, Burkholder JK, Shi F, et al: Particle-mediated cytokine gene transfer into canine oral mucosa and epidermis in vivo. Clin. Cancer Res (submitted), 1994.

50. Stead RB, Kwok WW, Storb R, et al: Canine model for gene therapy: Inefficient gene expression in dogs reconstituted with autologous marrow infected with retroviral vectors. Blood 71:742–747, 1988.

51. Flowers MED, Stockshlaeder MAR, Schuening FG, et al: Long-term transplantation of canine keratinocytes made resistant to G418 through retrovirus-mediated transfer. Proc Natl Acad Sci USA 87:2349–2353, 1990.

52. Lothrop, C Jr, al-Lebban ZS, Niemeyer GP, et al: Expression of a foreign gene in cats reconstituted with retroviral vector infected autologous bone marrow. Blood 78(1):237–245, 1991.

53. Deeg HJ, Huss R, de Oliveira JS, et al: Transduction and expression of canine MHC class II gene in murine cell lines and marrow-derived stromal cells. Exp Hematol 21, 1993 (Abstract no. 70).

54. O'Malley BW Jr, Adams RM, Sikes ML, et al: Retrovirus-mediated gene transfer into canine thyroid using an ex vivo strategy. Human Gene Therapy 4:171–178, 1993.

55. Cardoso JE, Branchereau S, Jeyaraj PR, et al: In situ retrovirus-mediated gene transfer in dog liver. Human Gene Therapy 4:411–418, 1993.

56. Kay MA, Rothenberg S, Landen CN, et al: In vivo gene therapy of hemophilia B: Sustained partial correction in factor IX-deficient dogs. Science 262:117–119, 1993.

57. Hickman MA, Malone RW, Madewell BR: Reporter gene expression in spontaneous canine and feline neoplasms following direct intratumoral injection of liposome/DNA complexes or DNA alone. J Vet Intern Med 8:147, 1994 (Abstract).

58. Elmslie RE, Dow SW, Potter TA: Genetic immunotherapy of canine oral melanoma. Proc 14th Annu Vet Cancer Soc Conf, 1994, pp. 111– 112.

59. Smith MA, Parkinson DR, Cheson BD, et al: Retinoids in cancer therapy. J Clin Oncol 10:839–864, 1992.

60. Ho RCS: Keynote Address: The past, the present, the future. Cancer 71(Suppl):1396–1399, 1993.

61. Tallman MS, Wiernik PH: Retinoids in cancer treatment. J Clin Pharmacol 32:868–888, 1992.

62. Goodman DS: Vitamin A and retinoids in health and disease. N. Engl J Med 310:1023–1031, 1984.

63. Parkinson DR, Smith MA, Cheson BD, et al: Trans-retinoic acid and related differentiating agents. Sem Oncol 19:734–741, 1992.

64. Warrell RP Jr, de The H, Wang ZY, et al: Acute promyelocytic leukemia. New Engl J Med 329:177– 189, 1993.

65. Wan YJY: Retinoic acid and its receptors. Am J Surg 166:50–53, 1993.

66. Meyskens FL, Surwit E, Moon TE, et al: Enhancement of regression of cervical intraepithelial neoplasia II (moderate dysplasia) with topically applied all-trans-retinoic acid: A randomized trial. J Natl Cancer Inst 86:539–543, 1994.

67. Lippman SM, Glisson BS, Kavanagh JJ, et al:

Retinoic acid and interferon combination studies in human cancer. Eur J Cancer 29A(Suppl 5):S9–S13, 1993.

68. Sparano JA, O'Boyle K: The potential role for biological therapy in the treatment of breast cancer. Sem Oncol 19:333–341, 1992.

69. White SD, Rosychuk RA, Scott KV, et al: Use of isotretinoin and etretinate for the treatment of benign cutaneous neoplasia and cutaneous lymphoma in dogs. J Am Vet Med Assoc 202:387–391, 1993.

70. Liliemark J: Liposomes for drug targeting in cancer chemotherapy. Eur J Cancer 5561:49–52, 1991.

71. Weinstein JN: Liposomes in the diagnosis and treatment of cancer. In Ostro MJ (ed): Liposomes: From Biophysics to Therapeutics. New York, Marcel Dekker, 1987, pp. 277–238.

72. Ostro MJ, Cullis PR: Use of liposome as injectable drug delivery systems. Am J Hosp Pharm 46:1576–1587, 1989.

73. Culis PR, Hope MJ, Bally MB, et al: Liposomes as pharmaceuticals. In Ostro MJ (ed): Liposomes: From Biophysics to Therapeutics. New York, Marcel Dekker, 1987, pp. 39–72.

74. New RRC, Black CDV, Parker RJ, et al: Liposomes in biological systems. In New RRC (ed): Liposomes: A Practical Approach. Oxford, IRL Press, 1990, pp. 221–252.

75. Morgan JR, Williams KA, Howard CB: Technetium-labelled liposome imaging for deep-seated infections. Br J Radiol 54:35–39, 1985.

76. Gabizon A, Papahadjopoulous D: Liposome formulation with prolonged circulation times in blood and enhanced uptake by tumors. Proc Natl Acad Sci USA 85:6949–6953, 1988.

77. Gabizon A, Catane R, Uziely B, et al: Prolonged circulation time and enhanced accumulation in malignant exudatesof doxorubicin encapsulated polyethylene-glycol coated liposomes. Cancer Res 54:987–992, 1994.

78. Kaye SB, Boden JA, Ryman BE: The effect of liposome (phospholipid vesicle) entrapment of actinomycin-D and metotrexate on the in vivo treatment of sensitive and resistant solid murine tumours. Eur J Cancer 17:279–289, 1981.

79. Rahmay YE, Hanson WR, Bharucha J, et al: Mechanisms of reduction of antitumor drug toxicity of liposome encapsulation. Ann NY Acad Sci 308:325–341, 1978.

80. Forssen EA, Tokes ZA: Use of anionic liposomes for reduction of chronic doxorubicin-induced cardiotoxicity. Proc Natl Acad Sci USA 78:1873–1877, 1981.

81. Rahman A, Kessler A, More N, et al: Liposomal protection of Adriamycin-induced cardiotoxicity in mice. Cancer Res 40:1532–1537, 1980.

82. Storm G, Roerdink FH, Steerenberg PA, et al: Influence of lipid composition on the antitumor activity exerted by doxorubicin-containing liposomes in a rat solid tumor model. Cancer Res 47:3366–3372, 1987.

83. Forssen EA, Tokes ZA: In vitro and in vivo studies with Adriamycin liposomes. Biochem Biophys Res Commun 91:1295–1301, 1979.

84. van Hoesel QGCM, Steerenberg PA, Crommelin DJA, et al: Reduced cardiotoxicity and nephrotoxicity with preservation of antitumor activity of doxorubicin entrapped in stable liposomes in the LOU/M Wsi rat. Cancer Res 44:3698–3705, 1984.

85. Forssen EA, Tokes ZA: Improved therapeutic benefits of doxorubicin by entrapment in anionic liposomes. Cancer Res 43:546–550, 1983.

86. Storm C, van Bloois L, Steerenberg PA, et al: Liposome encapsulation of doxorubicin: Pharmaceutical and therapeutic aspects. J Contr Release 9:215– 229, 1989.

87. Gabizon A, Meshorer A, Barenholz Y: Comparative long-term study of the toxicities of free and liposome-associated doxorubicin in mice after intravenous administration. J Natl Cancer Inst 77:459–469, 1986.

88. Gabizon A, Dagan A, Goren D, et al: Liposomes as in vivo carriers of Adriamycin: Reduced cardiac uptake and preserved antitumor activity in mice. Cancer Res 42:4734–4739, 1982.

89. Herman EH, Rahman A, Ferrans VJ, et al: Prevention of chronic doxorubicin cardiotoxicity in Beagles by liposomal encapsulation. Cancer Res 43:5427–5432, 1983.

90. Kanter PW, Bullard GA, Ginsberg RA: Comparison of the cardiotoxic effects of liposomal doxorubicin (TLC D-99) versus free doxorubicin in Beagle dogs. In Vivo 7:17–26, 1993.

91. Kisseberth WC, MacEwen EG, Helfand SC, et al: Complete response of drug-resistant plasma cell myeloma to treatment with liposome-encapsulated doxorubicin (TLC D-99) in a dog. J Vet Med (in press).

92. Gabizon A, Barenholz Y, Barber M: Prolongation of the circulation time of doxorubicin encapsulated in liposomes containing a polyethylene glycol-derivatized phospholipid: Pharmacokinetic studies in rodents and dogs. Pharm Res (NY) 10:703–708, 1993.

93. Al-Baker S, Perez-Soler R, Khokhar AR: Synthesis and biological studies of new lipid-soluble cisplatin analogues entrapped in liposomes. J Inorganic Biochem 47:99–108, 1992.

94. Toshach K, Fox LE, MacEwen EG, Perez-Soler R: An evaluation of liposome-encapsulated cisplatin analogue in normal cats. Proc 11th Annu Vet Cancer Soc Conf 1991, pp. 57–58.

95. Fox LE: Unpublished data.

96. Knapp DW, Richardson RL, DeNicola, et al: Cisplatin toxicity in cats. J Vet Intern Med 1:29–35, 1987.

97. Perez-Soler R, Lauterzstain J, Stephens LC, et al: Pre-clinical toxicity and pharmacology of liposome-entrapped cis-bis-neodecanoat-trans-R,R-

1,2-diaminocyclohexanep latinum(II). Can Chemo Pharmacol 24:1–8, 1989.

98. Perez-Soler R, Lopez-Berestein G, Lautersztain J, et al: Phase I clinical and pharmacological study of liposome-entrapped cis-bis-neodecanoate-trans-R-R-1,2-diaminocyclohexane platinum (II). Cancer Res 50:4254–4259, 1990.

99. Mickisch GH, Rahman A, Pastan I, et al: Increased effectiveness of liposome-encapsulated doxorubicin in multidrug-resistant transgenic mice compared with free doxorubicin. J Natl Cancer Inst 84:804–805, 1992.

100. Thierry AR, Vige D, Coughlin SS, et al: Modulation of doxorubicin resistance in multidrug-resistant cells by liposomes. FASEB J 7:572–579, 1993.

101. Oudard S, Thierry A, Jorgensen TJ, et al: Sensitization of multidrug-resistant colon cancer cells to doxorubicin encapsulated in liposomes. Cancer Chemother Pharmacol 28:259–265, 1991.

102. Fan D, Bucana CD, O'Brian CA, et al: Enhancement of murine tumor cell sensitivity to adriamycin by presentation of the drug in phosphatidylcholine-phosphatidylserine liposomes. Cancer Res 50:3619–3626, 1990.

103. Kedar E, Rutkowski Y, Braun E, et al: Delivery of cytokines by liposomes. I. Preparation and characterization of interleukin-2 encapsulated in long circulating sterically stabilized liposomes. J Immunother 16:47–59, 1994.

104. Kedar E, Braun E, Rutkowski Y, et al: Delivery of cytokines by liposomes. II. Interleukin-2 encapsulated in long circulating sterically stabilized liposomes: Immunomodulatory and antitumor activity. J. Immunother 16:115–124, 1994.

105. Pass HI: Photodynamic therapy in oncology: Mechanisms and clinical use. J Natl Cancer Inst 85:443–456, 1993.

106. Fingar VH, Wieman TJ, Park YJ, et al: Implications of a pre-existing tumor hypoxic fration on photodynamic therapy. J Surg Res 53:524–528, 1992.

107. Agarwal ML, Larkin HE, Zaidi SIA, et al: Phospholipase activation triggers apoptosis in photosensitized mouse lymphoma cells. Cancer Res 53:5897–5902, 1993.

108. Klein MK, Roberts WG; Recent advances in photodynamic therapy. Compendium 15:809–817, 1993.

109. Cheli R, Addis F, Mortellaro CM, et al: Photodynamic therapy of spontaneous animal tumors using the active component of hematoporphyrin derivative (DHE) as photosensitizing drug: Clinical results. Cancer Let 38:101–105, 1987.

110. Beck ER, Dunstan RW, Hetzel FW: Control of canine squamous cell carcinomas by photodynamic therapy. Proc 11th Annu Vet Cancer Soc Conf 1991, pp. 1–2.

111. Cyman JA, Young C, Beck ER: Phase II/III trial of PDT for canine oral squamous cell carcinomas. Proc 13th Annu Vet Cancer Soc Conf 1993, pp. 116–117.

112. Roberts WG, Klein MK, Loomis M, et al: Photodynamic therapy of spontaneous cancers in felines, canines, and snakes with chloro-aluminum sulfonated phthalocyanine. J Natl Cancer Inst 83:18–23, 1991.

113. Peaston AE, Leach MW, Higgins RJ, et al: Photodynamic therapy of squamous cell carcinoma using chloraluminum sulphonated phthalocyanine as photosensitizer: A pilot study in 30 cats. Proc 13th Annu Vet Cancer Soc Conf 1993, pp. 51–52.

114. Peaston AE, Leach MW, Higgins RJ: Photodynamic therapy for nasal and aural squamous cell carcinoma in cats. J Am Vet Med Assoc 202:1261–1265, 1993.

115. Brezovich IA, Lilly MB, Meredith RF, et al: Hyperthermia of pet animal tumours with self-regulating ferromagnetic thermoseeds. Int J Hyperthermia 6:117–130, 1990.

116. Thrall DE, Dewhirst MW, Page RL, et al: A comparison of temperatures in canine solid tumors during local and whole-body hyperthermia administered alone and simultaneously. Int J Hyperthermia 6:305–317, 1990.

117. Prescott DM, Charles HC, Sostman HD, et al: Manipulation of intra- and extracellular pH in spontaneous canine tumours by use of hyperglycaemia. Int J Hyperthermia 9:745–754, 1993.

118. Dewhirst MW, Prescott DM, Clegg S, et al: The use of hydralazine to manipulate tumour temperatures during hyperthermia. Int J Hyperthermia 6:971–983, 1990.

119. Prescott DM, Samulski TV, Dewhirst MW, et al: Use of nitroprusside to increase tissue temperature during local hyperthermia in normal and tumor-bearing dogs. Int J Radiation Oncol Biol Phys 23:377–385, 1992.

120. Thompson JM, Dhoodhat YA, Bleehan NM, et al: Microwave hyperthermia in the treatment of spontaneous canine tumours: An analysis of treatment parameters and tumour response. Int J Hyperthermia 4:383–399, 1988.

121. Denman DL, Legorreta RA, Kier AB, et al: Therapeutic responses of spontaneous canine malignancies to combinations of radiotherapy and hyperthermia. Int J Radiation Oncol Biol Phys 21:415–422, 1991.

122. Gillette SM, Dewhirst MW, Gillette EL, et al: Response of canine soft tissue sarcomas to radiation or radiation plus hyperthermia: A randomized phase II study. Int J Hyperthermia 8:309–320, 1992.

123. Riviere JE, Page RL, Rogers RA, et al: Nonuniform alteration of cis-diamminedichloroplatinum(II) tissue distribution in dogs with whole body hyperthermia. Cancer Res 50:2075–2080, 1990.

124. Page RL, Thrall DE, George SL, et al: Quantitative estimation of the thermal dose-modifying factor for cis-diamminedichloroplatinum (CDDP) in tumour-bearing dogs. Int J Hyperthermia 8:761–769, 1992.

125. Theon AP, Madewell BR, Moore AS, et al: Localized thermo-cisplatin therapy: A pilot study in spontaneous canine and feline tumours. Int J Hyperthermia 7:881–892, 1991.

126. Watanabe N, Niitsu Y, Umeno H, et al: Synergistic cytotoxic and antitumor effects of recombinant human tumor necrosis factor and hyperthermia. Cancer Res 48:650–653, 1989.

127. Ohno S, Strebel FR, Stephens LC, et al: Increased therapeutic efficacy induced by tumor necrosis factor α combined with platinum complexes and whole-body hyperthermia in rats. Cancer Res 52:4096–4101, 1992.

128. Novotney CA, Page RL, Macy DW, et al: Phase I evaluation of doxorubicin and whole-body hyperthermia in dogs with lymphoma. J Vet Intern Med 6:245–249, 1992.

129. Page RL, Macy DW, Ogilvie GK, et al: Phase III evaluation of doxorubicin and whole-body hyperthermia in dogs with lymphoma. Int J Hyperthermia 8:187–197, 1992.

130. Page RL, Thrall DE, Dewhirst MW, et al: Phase I study of melphalan alone and melphalan plus whole body hyperthermia in dogs with malignant melanoma. Int J Hyperthermia 7:559–566, 1991.

131. Weiden PL, Storb R, Deeg HJ, et al: Prolonged disease-free survival in dogs with lymphoma after total-body irradiation and autologous marrow transplantation consolidation of combination-chemotherapy-induced remissions. Blood 54:1039–1049, 1979.

132. Applebaum FR, Deeg HJ, Storb R, et al: Marrow transplant studies in dogs with malignant lymphoma. Transplantation 39:499–504, 1985.

133. Benedetti G, Bondesan P, Caracciolo D, et al: Selection and characterization of early hematopoietic progenitors using an anti-CD71/SO6 immunotoxin. Exp Hematol 22:166–173, 1994.

134. Raff RF, Storb R, Graham T, et al: What role for 15-deoxyspergualin in enhancing engraftment of unrelated histoincompatible canine marrow grafts and preventing graft-versus-host disease? Transplantation 55:684–688, 1993.

135. Bean MA, Storb R, Graham T, et al: Prevention of transfusion-induced sensitization to minor histocompatibility antigens on DLA-identical canine marrow grafts by gamma irradiation of marrow donor blood. Transplantation 52:956–960, 1991.

136. Bean MA, Graham T, Appelbaum FR, et al: γ-Irradiation of pretransplant blood transfusions from unrelated donors prevents sensitization to minor histocompatibility antigens on dog leukocyte antigen-identical canine marrow grafts. Transplantation 57:423-426, 1994.

137. Storb R, Raff RF, Appelbaum FR, et al: FK-506 and methotrexate prevent graft-versus-host disease in dogs given 9.2 Gy total body irradiation and marrow grafts from unrelated dog leukocyte antigen-nonidentical donors. Transplantation 56:800–807, 1993.

138. Cain JL, Cain GR, Turrel JM, et al: Clinical and lymphohematologic responses after bone marrow transplantation in sibling and unrelated donor-recipient pairs of cats. Am J Vet Res 51:839–844, 1990.

139. Fulton R, Gasper PW, Thrall MA, et al: Complications associated with bone marrow transplantation in the cat. Vet Clin Pathol 19:5, 1990 (Abstract).

# 15

# TUMORS OF THE SKIN AND SUBCUTANEOUS TISSUES

David M. Vail and Stephen J. Withrow

## INCIDENCE AND RISK FACTORS

Tumors of the skin and subcutaneous tissue are the most common tumors affecting dogs, accounting for approximately one third of all tumors encountered in the species.[1-4] In the cat, skin and subcutaneous tumors are second in frequency only to tumors of the lymphoid system and account for approximately one quarter of all tumors in the species.[1,3,5,6] Estimates of incidence rates for skin and subcutaneous tumors have been reported to be approximately 450 per 100,000 dogs and 120 per 100,000 cats.[1,7] Many tumor types occur in the skin, and a listing of the 10 most frequent tumors in the dog and the 5 most frequent in the cat based on larger North American (U.S.), Australian, and United Kingdom (U.K.) surveys are presented in Tables 15–1 and 15–2, respectively. Approximately 80% of the cutaneous tumors encountered in the dog and cat are represented in these two tables. Mast cell tumors represent the most commonly encountered cutaneous tumor in the dog and second most common in the cat will be discussed in Chapter 16. The only major discrepancy noted between the surveys is the predominance of fibrosarcomas in cats in the United Kingdom. Approximately 20 to 30% of primary tumors of the skin and subcutaneous tissues are histologically malignant in the dog, compared to 50 to 65% in the cat.[1,3,5-8] Occasionally, cutaneous tumors in dogs and cats may be secondary

**Table 15–1** Frequency (Percentage) of Top Ten Cutaneous Neoplasms in the Dog

| Neoplasm | U.S.A.[3] | U.K.[1] | Australia[4] | Australia[2] |
|---|---|---|---|---|
| Mast cell tumor | 21.3 | 19.2 | 17.6 | 16.1 |
| Hepatoid (perianal) adenoma | 18.3 | 9.8 | 8.3 | 5.0 |
| Lipoma | 8.6 | 8.5 | 6.0 | 5.0 |
| Sebaceous hyperplasia/adenoma | NR[a] | 8.2 | 6.8 | 7.7 |
| Fibrosarcoma | 5.9 | 7.4 | 3.6 | 6.6 |
| Melanoma | 5.0 | 6.3 | 6.8 | 5.3 |
| Histiocytoma | 2.5 | 6.0 | 7.8 | 14.0 |
| Squamous cell carcinoma | 3.9 | 5.4 | 5.2 | 6.9 |
| Hemangiopericytoma | 3.2 | 4.2 | 4.1 | 7.3 |
| Basal cell tumor | NR[a] | 4.1 | 12.0 | 5.5 |
| Total cases/study | 984 | 2616 | 1,000 | 1,000 |

[a]NR = not reported.

**Table 15–2**   Frequency (Percentage) of Top Five Cutaneous Neoplasms in the Cat

| Neoplasm | U.S.A.[6] | U.S.A.[5] | U.S.A.[3] | U.K.[1] |
|---|---|---|---|---|
| Basal cell tumor | 26.1 | 21.8 | NR[b] | 14.8 |
| Mast cell tumor | 21.1 | 20.0 | 21.3 | 7.69 |
| Squamous cell carcinoma | 15.2 | 4.5[a] | 12.1 | 17.4 |
| Fibrosarcoma | 14.7 | 15.3 | 12.0 | 25.4 |
| Sebaceous hyperplasia/adenoma | 4.4 | 3.2 | NR[b] | 2.3 |
| Total cases/study | 340 | 444 | 83 | 288 |

[a]Misleading, because ear tumors were dealt with separately in this survey and were not included.

[b]NR = not reported.

metastatic lesions, and clinicians should include this possibility in their list of differentials.

In general, cutaneous tumors occur in older animals and no significant difference in the incidence by sex is noted when all types are considered together. Such differences, where they exist, along with breed predilections, will be discussed under specific tumor types.

Specific etiologies have been proven for only a few tumors in the dog and cat. Several contributing factors in the development of skin tumors include viruses, solar and ionizing radiation, hormones, genetic influences, vaccines, thermal injuries, and immunologic influences.[5,9–21]

Long-term exposure to the ionizing effects of sunlight result in solar dermatosis, leading to documented increases in cutaneous hemangioma, hemangiosarcoma, and squamous cell carcinoma in beagles as well as squamous cell carcinoma in the cat.[13–15] Squamous papillomatosis (warts) in the young dog are of viral origin[22] as are rare instances of papillomatosis of aged animals.[10–12] Feline leukemia virus (FeLV) is associated with the development of cutaneous lymphoma, and the feline sarcoma virus has, under experimental conditions, produced malignant melanoma in cats.[5] Recently, a vaccine-associated sarcoma of cats (Chap. 17) has been described,[20] and injection-site epithelial tumors have been associated with vaccines produced from active canine oral papillomavirus.[19]

## PATHOLOGIC CLASSIFICATION

The heterogeneity of cutaneous structures that can be involved in a neoplastic process complicates the issue of classification. Generally, skin tumors are classified histologically according to the tissue of origin (epithelial, mesenchymal, melanotic, or round cell) and individual cell of origin if sufficient differentiation is present. Tumors are further classified as to the degree of malignancy based on several histologic characteristics. In some cases, there is not a clear differentiation between malignant and benign skin tumors.

Clinically, skin tumors are further classified, utilizing the TNM (tumor-node-metastasis) system devised by the World Health Organization and presented in Table 15–3.[23] This system allows the tumor to be described in exacting detail with regard to its clinical presentation. Finally, one must consider the tumor location when classifying a skin tumor. Some tumors behave differently when located in different areas of the body. An example of the difference in behavior because of location is canine oral melanoma (usually malignant) versus canine cutaneous melanoma arising from haired skin (usually benign). In addition, biologic behavior often varies for the same type of tumor in the dog versus the cat.

## HISTORY AND CLINICAL SIGNS

The history for an animal with a cutaneous tumor is variable. Commonly, owners will discover a growth while examining or grooming their pets. Benign tumors are more likely to have a history of slow growth from weeks to years. It is not unusual for benign epithelial tumors to be presented for ulceration due to self-trauma or secondary inflammation. Most benign tumors are well circumscribed, nonpainful, and freely movable and incite a minimal inflammatory response. Malignant tumors are often rapidly growing, fixed to underlying structures and ulcerated and will often have ill-defined margins. Invasion into vessels and regional lymphatics is often observed.

## DIAGNOSTIC TECHNIQUES AND WORKUP

One of the most important techniques used in the diagnosis and management of skin tumors is

**Table 15–3** Clinical Stages (TNM) of Canine or Feline Tumors of Epidermal or Dermal Origin (Excluding Lymphoma and Mastocytoma)

$T:$ *Primary Tumor*

| | |
|---|---|
| Tis | Preinvasive carcinoma (carcinoma in situ) |
| $T_0$ | No evidence of tumor |
| $T_1$ | Tumor < 2 cm maximum diameter, superficial, or exophytic |
| $T_2$ | Tumor 2–5 cm maximum diameter, or with minimal invasion irrespective of size |
| $T_3$ | Tumor > 5 cm maximum diameter, or with invasion of the subcutis, irrespective of size |
| $T_4$ | Tumor invading other structures such as fascia muscle, bone, or cartilage |

Tumors occurring simultaneously should have the actual number recorded. The tumor with the highest T category is selected and the number of tumors indicated in parentheses, e.g., $T_2(5)$. Successive tumors should be classified independently.

$N:$ *Regional Lymph Nodes (RLN)*

| | |
|---|---|
| $N_0$ | No evidence of RLN involvement |
| $N_1$ | Movable ipsilateral nodes |
| | $N_{1a}$ Nodes not considered to contain growth |
| | $N_{1b}$ Nodes considered to contain growth |
| $N_2$ | Movable contralateral or bilateral nodes |
| | $N_{2a}$ Nodes not considered to contain growth |
| | $N_{2b}$ Nodes considered to contain growth |
| $N_3$ | Fixed nodes |

$M:$ *Distant Metastasis*

| | |
|---|---|
| $M_0$ | No evidence of distant metastasis |
| $M_1$ | Distant metastasis detected—specify site(s) |

a thorough history and physical examination. The history should include queries about the duration of the lesion, rapidity of growth, change in appearance over time, travel history, presence of pruritus, response to previous therapy, and related medical history. Every tumor should be examined with respect to size, location, consistency, presence or absence of fixation to underlying tissue, and whether the overlying skin is ulcerated. Three-dimensional caliper measurements of the tumor and its location should become a permanent part of the medical record. In addition, a thorough examination of draining lymph nodes is important. Although the physical appearance, location, and growth pattern of a tumor may give the examiner a high degree of suspicion as to the type of tumor involved, it is imperative that some type of cytologic or histopathologic diagnosis be attained to plan therapy and prognosticate to the client properly. The two most common diagnostic procedures for skin tumors are cytology and tissue biopsy.

Aspiration cytology is an important screening tool to differentiate neoplastic from inflammatory lesions (Chap. 5). All cutaneous tumors should be evaluated by fine-needle aspiration cytology to aid in the planning of therapy. Romanowsky-type dip stains are quick and inexpensive and should be a part of every practice. Several tumors, such as mast cell tumors and melanocytic tumors, lend themselves well to cytologic diagnosis. Cytology often allows one to

differentiate between epithelial and connective tissue tumors; however, special training is necessary to further subclassify many of these tumors. Cytologic examination of enlarged regional lymph nodes should be performed prior to definitive therapy. It is important to bear in mind that ulcerated or inflamed tumors may cause reactive lymphadenopathy without metastasis.

Histologic examination of a suspected or known tumor is extremely important in planning therapy and determining prognosis. Histologic examination of an excised specimen will allow the pathologist to determine the degree of malignancy and invasion and whether surgical excision was adequate. The type of biopsy procedure is determined by size and location of the tumor. A small tumor in an easily accessible location amenable to adequate surgical margins is usually treated by excisional biopsy. It is important to submit the entire specimen for histologic examination and margin analysis (see Chap. 2). When dealing with large tumors, or tumors in locations that do not allow easy excision with wide margins (e.g., an extremity), an incisional biopsy should be performed to allow optimal therapeutic planning. Small, flat, or plaquelike skin lesions should not be prepped or scrubbed prior to incisional biopsy to ensure adequate assessment of undisturbed surface pathology.

With some neoplastic processes, in particular, the cutaneous round cell tumors, the degree of differentiation may not lend itself well to routine light-microscopic classification. Recently in the veterinary literature, immunohistochemical techniques have been developed and explored for their utility in differentiating such tumor types.[24–32] Monoclonal antibodies directed at specific tissue components including intermediate filament proteins (e.g., cytokeratin, vimentin) can be useful in identifying poorly differentiated tumors into epithelial or mesenchymal categories and in some cases specific histologic groupings. Examples will be discussed, when applicable, under specific tumor types.

Depending on the tumor type in question or the clinician's index of suspicion, an expanded diagnostic workup may be indicated to determine the presence of systemic spread as well as the patient's readiness for therapeutic intervention. If the lesion is likely a malignancy, such diagnostics are performed prior to definitive therapy. Occasionally, with skin tumors amenable to adequate surgical excision in otherwise healthy individuals, such diagnostics are performed after excisional biopsy and only if the histologic assessment warrants. The choice of expanded diagnostics is often driven by the known or suspected tumor type. For example, thoracic radiographs and abdominal ultrasound may be warranted for subungual melanoma, whereas a bone marrow aspirate would be appropriate when a poorly differentiated mast cell tumor is suspected.

Knowledge of the extent of cutaneous tumor margins prior to surgery, usually accomplished by digital palpation and occasionally local radiographs, may be enhanced with the use of diagnostic ultrasound (US), computed tomography (CT), or magnetic resonance imaging (MRI). In a study of dogs bearing cutaneous mast cell tumors or soft tissue sarcomas, the extent of local tumor margins was upgraded in 19 and 65% of cases using US and CT, respectively.[33] Such information allows more appropriate planning of definitive surgery or radiotherapy.

## TREATMENT AND PROGNOSIS OF SPECIFIC TUMOR TYPES

Many times the treatment of skin tumors is performed before the specific tumor type is known; therefore, the general principles of treatment of skin tumors will be discussed collectively. The specific form of therapy is determined by the nature of the primary disease, local and distant metastasis, the anticipated behavior of the tumor, and the patient's overall condition. When dealing with only local disease, the size and location will be important in determining the appropriate therapy.

Standard blade excision remains the treatment of choice for the majority of skin tumors. Standard surgical technique is employed, with emphasis on adequate surgical margins (Chap. 7). When attempting to excise a tumor completely, it is better to leave an open wound if necessary, rather than to leave tumor. A major advantage of surgical excision of skin tumors is that completeness of surgery can be determined histologically. In the case of very large tumors, cytoreduction surgery may be employed for palliation or to facilitate other forms of therapy. The leading cause of failure for surgical excision is inadequate surgical margins. When dealing with large malignant tumors on extremities, amputation should be considered.

Cryosurgery may be helpful in the treatment of select skin tumors (Chap. 8). The main advantages are speed, avoidance of general anesthesia in some cases, and low cost. Indications for cryosurgery are small or multiple tumors in older animals, for which anesthesia is a concern. Cryosurgery is also used for small, relatively noninvasive tumors of the nasal planum, pinnae, eyelid, lip, and perianal area. The major disadvantage of cryotherapy is the lack of histologic assessment of "surgical" margins.

Radiotherapy is now available in most areas of practice in the United States and Canada, primarily on a referral basis. It can be used as either the primary therapy, as an adjunctive form of therapy for residual tumor control, or on occasion to achieve preoperative cytoreduction. Radiotherapy, in some instances, is more cosmetic than surgery and may allow the retention of anatomical function; however, the cost and repetitive treatment protocols remain relative disadvantages.

Chemotherapy, both systemic and topical, has also been used in the treatment of skin tumors. It is usually reserved for those cases in which surgical or radiotherapeutic alternatives do not exist, or in the adjuvant setting in tumors with high metastatic potential. To date, with the exception of cutaneous lymphoma, little is known about the efficacy of this modality in the treatment of cutaneous tumors.

Other, less established forms of therapy, including hyperthermia, photodynamic therapy, intralesional chemotherapeutic implants, immunotherapy, and the use of vitamin A-related synthetic retinoids are showing promise for select groups of tumors and will be discussed along with those specific tumor types for which efficacy of therapy has been investigated.

## TUMORLIKE LESIONS

Several types of tumorlike cutaneous and subcutaneous masses are encountered in veterinary practice. These lesions are non-neoplastic but in some instances may mimic neoplastic lesions. The most common non-neoplastic lesions involving the skin of dogs and cats are cutaneous cysts. The most common of these are epidermoid cysts, dermoid cysts, and follicular cysts.

Epidermoid cysts (epidermal inclusion cyst, "sebaceous" cyst) are round to oval, firm to fluctuant, smooth, well-circumscribed lesions common in dogs but rare in cats. They may be solitary or multiple, and while found anywhere in the body, are more common on the extremities. These masses may contain gray to white-brown, cheesy material with bits of hair shafts and are usually covered by intact epithelium (Figs. 15–1A and 15–1B). These cysts may become ulcerated or inflamed if the cystic contents are extruded into the adjacent tissue. The treatment of choice is surgery or cryosurgery. An alternative therapy is to lance and drain the cyst, peel out the lining, and cauterize with silver nitrate. One dog with multiple epidermoid cysts was successfully

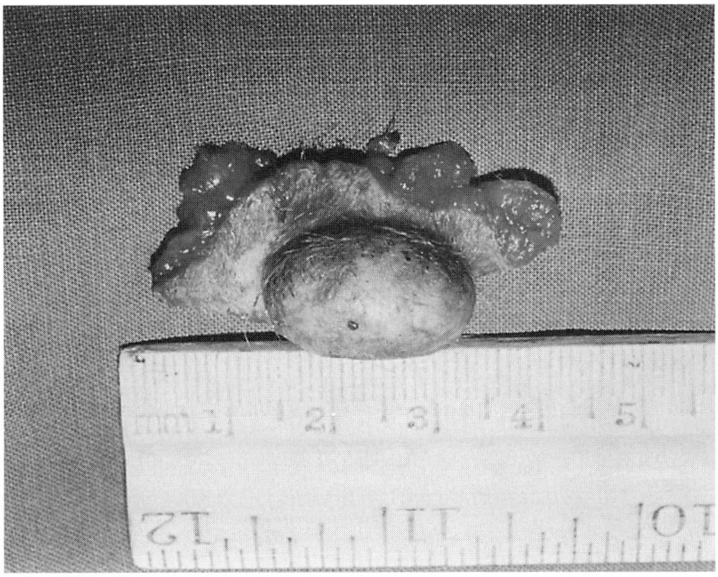

**Figure 15–1A.** Excised epidermoid cyst. Note hairless, circumscribed, dome-shaped appearance.

*A*

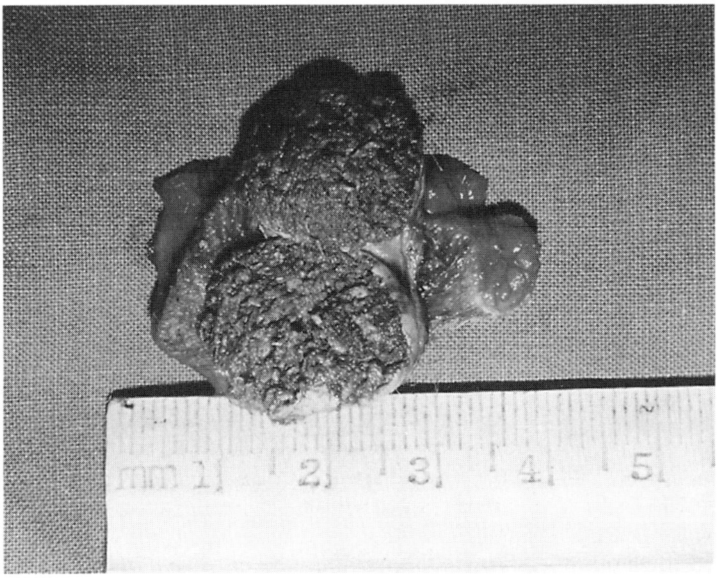

*B*

**Figure 15–1B.** Typical appearance of brown, greasy, and granular material inside the cyst pictured in Figure 15–1A.

treated with oral isotretinoin, a member of the vitamin A-related synthetic retinoids.[34]

Dermoid cysts are similar to epidermoid cysts but are more complex in structure. They appear to be congenital or hereditary lesions. Breeds that appear to be predisposed are boxers, Kerry blue terriers, and Rhodesian Ridgebacks.[35,36] The dermoid cysts of Rhodesian Ridgebacks and their crosses appear to be inherited. They are found on the dorsal midline, neck, and scrotum. In some cases, the lesion may extend deep into the dog's back to the level of the meninges and should be evaluated radiographically (including a fistulogram and/or myelogram) to ensure they do not communicate with the subarachnoid space. The treatment of choice is surgical excision and the prognosis is generally excellent.

Follicular cysts, which are keratinous cysts derived from epithelium of the outer root sheath, result from the retention of follicular or glandular products because of obliteration of follicular orifices. These cysts may be congenital or acquired. Therapy is again surgical excision with an excellent prognosis.

Other lesions that may be confused with cutaneous tumors include various forms of keratosis, xanthomas, calcinosis cutis/circumscripta, and cutaneous mucinosis. Actinic keratosis (solar keratosis) secondary to exposure to sunlight may be a precancerous lesion.[13–15] All of these are readily distinguished by histopathologic examination.

## Nodular Dermatofibrosis (Collagenous Nevi)

Numerous reports detail this unusual tumorlike syndrome confined to middle-aged German shepherd dogs.[37–41] Affected dogs typically present with numerous cutaneous nodules, which increase in number and location (limbs, head, and trunk) (Fig. 15–2). The nodules may become ulcerated and result in lameness. Histologically, these lesions represent hyperplastic dermal collagen (collagenous nevi). Strong evidence exists for inheritance in an autosomal-dominant fashion. Interestingly, in almost all cases, the benign skin lesions are associated with multiple bilateral renal cysts that progress to become cystadenocarcinoma with metastatic potential. Intact bitches with the condition usually develop multiple uterine leiomyomas. There is often a long history (months to years) associated with this condition, and dogs eventually succumb to either renal failure or widespread metastasis from renal carcinoma. No effective treatment exists, and skin masses are removed only for cosmesis or if they interfere with function.

## EPITHELIAL TUMORS

### Papillomas

Papillomas (cutaneous papillomatosis, warts, verrucae, squamous cell papilloma) are common skin tumors in the dog but relatively rare in the cat.[5,42] They appear as cauliflowerlike growths with a finely fissured surface. They may be sessile or pedunculated and when traumatized will often bleed. Two types of papillomas are recognized in the dog. In the young dog, papillomas are often multiple in nature and are most common on the head, eyelids, feet, and mouth (Fig. 15–3). These tumors are associated with a DNA virus that is species specific. It is contagious from dog to dog with an incubation period of 30 days. No treatment is usually necessary because lesions resolve within 3 months. If the severity of lesions is affecting mastication, surgery or cryotherapy may become necessary. That puppies

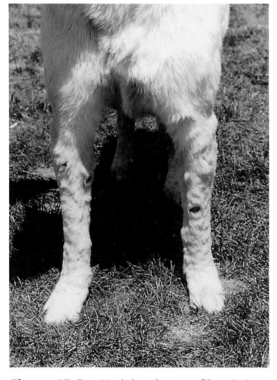

**Figure 15–2.** Nodular dermatofibrosis in a middle-aged German shepherd. Note multiple nodular growths, some ulcerated, on the limbs.

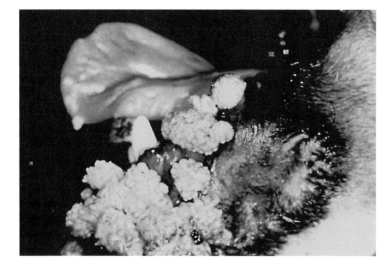

**Figure 15–3.** Multiple papillomas on the lip and gum of a young dog. These papillomas spontaneously regressed within 6 weeks.

treated with cyclosporin develop a generalized nonregressing form of the disease suggests the importance of an intact immune system in the regression of this disease.[43] Biologic response modification with levamisole, thiabendazole, and wart vaccines are for the most part ineffective. Autogenous vaccines have been implicated in the development of injection-site squamous cell carcinoma.[19] Viral papillomatosis has been reported in the bovine, equine, and human species as well as in the dog.[13,22]

The second type of papilloma is often seen in the older dog. These tumors are usually solitary but may be multiple and most commonly are located on the head, feet, eyelids, and genitalia. Papillomas of the older dog are generally not felt to be associated with a viral etiology; however, three recent reports of dogs with virus-associated multiple cutaneous inverted papillomas have been described.[10–12] Inverted papilloma is the endophytic variant of viral papilloma in dogs that present as cup-shaped lesions with a central core of keratin leading to an umbilicated surface similar in structure to intracutaneous cornifying epithelioma.[44] A papillomavirus distinct from that infecting young dogs is felt to be involved. The treatment for solitary papillomas is surgery or cryosurgery and the prognosis is excellent.

## Squamous Cell Carcinoma (Epidermoid Carcinomas)

Squamous cell carcinoma (SCC) is a common tumor involving the skin and accounts for approximately 15% of cutaneous tumors in the cat[1,3,5,6] and 5% of those in the dog.[1–4] SCCs are usually found in unpigmented or lightly pigmented skin. In many instances there is a recognized solar exposure relationship and these tumors are often referred to as "actinic" SCC.[1,13,14] The most common cutaneous locations for SCC in the dog are the nail bed (see the Subungual Tumors section of this chapter), scrotum, nose, legs, and anus. Tumors have also been reported to affect nonpigmented or lightly pigmented skin of the flank and abdomen in the dalmatian, beagle, whippet, and white English bull terrier dogs (Fig. 15–4).[21,45] The most common cutaneous locations for SCC in the cat are the sparsely haired areas of the nasal planum, eyelids, and pinnae (Figs. 15–5A and 15–5B). Multiple facial lesions are present in nearly 30% of affected cats. Squamous cell carcinoma usually afflicts older animals (mean age of 12 years in the cat, 8 years in the dog). Siamese cats are under-represented, as would be expected because of pigmented skin color.

SCC may present as either a proliferative or erosive lesion. Proliferative lesions may vary from a red firm plaque to a cauliflowerlike lesion that often ulcerates. The erosive lesion, which is most common in the cat, initially starts as a shallow crusting lesion that may develop into a deep ulcer. Histologically, the initial crusting lesions often represent carcinoma in situ or preinvasive carcinoma (i.e., Tis clinical stage, see Table 15–3).

Generally, SCCs involving the facial skin of cats are locally invasive but late to metastasize. The degree of local invasion can be quite severe and response to therapy is much more successful for Tis to $T_1$ lesions than for those with significant invasion. The behavior of subungual (nail-

**Figure 15–4.** Typical appearance of a red, raised, and ulcerated squamous cell carcinoma on the prepuce of a 5–year-old Dalmatian. The arrow denotes area of incisional biopsy. Surgical removal resulted in control for over 2 years, at which time a second lesion developed on the opposite flank.

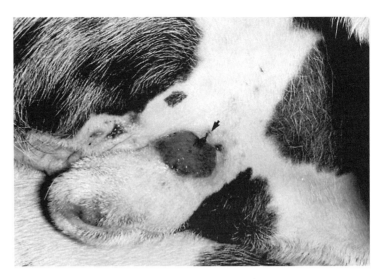

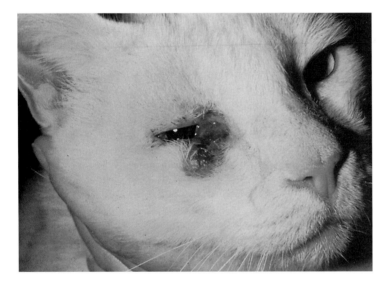

**Figure 15–5A.** Squamous cell carcinoma of the lower eyelid of a white cat. This represents a fairly advanced lesion, characterized by local invasion and ulceration.

*A*

*B*

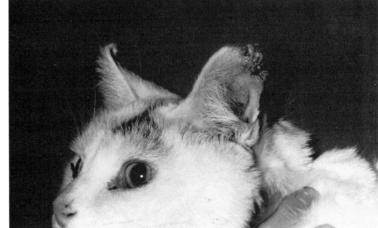

**Figure 15–5B.** Squamous cell carcinoma of the scarcely haired pinna of a cat.

bed) SCC is discussed at length in a later section. Tumors involving the skin of the flank and ventral abdomen in the dog are locally invasive with a low metastatic potential; however, multiple lesions are often present throughout the skin of the ventral abdomen, ranging from carcinoma in situ to more infiltrative and nodular SCC.

Many therapeutic modalities have been applied to SCC involving the facial skin in cats. Surgery or cryosurgery are most commonly used and remain the mainstay for treating these lesions, although numerous reports now exist detailing the use of radiotherapy and photodynamic therapy. Outcomes are generally good for most modalities if the tumors are treated early (i.e., Tis to $T_1$) in their course. In general, lesions of the pinna are more manageable than those of the nasal planum because the location allows a more aggressive surgical (Figs. 15–6A and 15–6B) or cryosurgical dose. Surgical excision of lesions of the pinnae result in long-term control (> 1.5 years) in the majority of cases.[46] The surgical procedure for infiltrative nasal planum SCC is discussed in Chapter 19. In a report of 102 cats with 163 lesions, aggressive cryotherapy was nearly 100% effective for managing pinnae and eyelid tumors; however, only 70% of nasal planum tumors responded.[47] Orthovoltage radiotherapy using 40 Gray total dosage in 10 fractions was applied in 90 cats with nasal planum SCC.[48] Tumor stage was found to be highly prognostic, as Tis and $T_1$ lesions enjoyed 5-year progression-free survivals of 56%, while tumors of higher stages responded poorly. Survival in this report could also be predicted by determining the proliferation fraction of the tumor using an immunohistochemical stain for PCNA (proliferating cell nuclear antigen). Similarly, the use of [90]strontium plesiotherapy, a form of superficial radiotherapy, has provided long-term control (1- and 3-year control rates of 89 and 82%, respectively) in 25 cats with early superficial lesions.[49] Plesiotherapy is limited to very early, shallow lesions because the radiation dose drops off significantly below depths of 2 mm. Photodynamic therapy has also been studied extensively for the treatment of superficial SCC in both the dog and cat.[50–55] Once again, if applied to early lesions, results are generally positive. Complete response rates of approximately 75% are reported for Tis to $T_2$ staged tumors and drop off quickly to 30% for tumors of higher stages. The bottom line with respect to treating local SCC lesions is to treat small lesions aggressively. Presently, combinations of surgery and radiation therapy for infiltrative nasal planum SCC are being evaluated and show early promise.

Chemotherapy for cutaneous SCC has shown little consistent efficacy in the veterinary literature. Agents that have been investigated on a limited basis for SCC in the dog and cat include mitoxantrone,[56,57] actinomycin D,[58] doxorubicin/cyclophosphamide combinations,[59] bleomycin,[60] and cisplatin (not used in cats).[61–63] Response rates are generally low and short-lived in duration. Chemotherapy in an adjuvant setting for microscopic disease following surgery or in conjunction with radiotherapy should be investi-

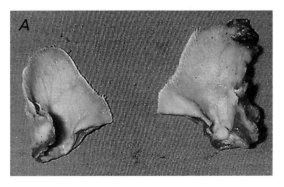

**Figure 15–6A.** Aggressive surgical resection of squamous cell carcinoma of the pinna from the cat pictured in Figure 15–5B. Early carcinoma in situ was present histologically throughout the peripheral edges of the pinna bilaterally.

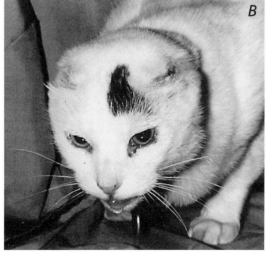

**Figure 15–6B.** The same cat 6 months following excision of pinnae for squamous cell carcinoma.

gated for high-grade lesions. Intralesional sustained release cisplatin and 5-FU have also been investigated in dogs, along with local hyperthermia and alone in cats with superficial SCC.[64,65] Long-term results are lacking; however, nearly half of the cats and dogs with actinic-related SCC have achieved a complete response.

The vitamin A-related synthetic retinoids have also been evaluated in dogs and cats with solar-induced cutaneous SCC. Only preneoplastic lesions were responsive to etretinate and early superficial lesions to a combination of isotretinoin and local hyperthermia in the dog.[66,67] No significant response was noted in 10 cats treated with isotretinoin.[68]

The nonsteroidal anti-inflammatory drug piroxicam, also known for its immunomodulating effects, has also been evaluated for efficacy in dogs with nonresectable SCC.[69] Partial responses were noted in half of the 10 patients treated, with a resulting median survival of 150 days.

A relatively new variation of SCC reported in cats is best referred to as multicentric SCC in situ (MSCCIS, also called Bowen's disease, or Bowenoid carcinoma in situ).[70-72] Unlike actinic or solar-induced SCC in situ, MSCCIS is found in haired, pigmented areas of the skin and is unrelated to sunlight exposure. It has not been associated with either FeLV or FIV viral infections. Multiple lesions are usually present in older cats, and lesions are confined to the epithelium, with no breachment of the basement membrane. The lesions are generally crusty, easily epilated, painful, and hemorrhagic when manipulated (Fig. 15–7). They are felt to be preneoplastic, because three cats had true SCC adjacent to sites of MSCCIS. When excision is possible, recurrence has not been reported; however, similar lesions often develop at other sites. They are unresponsive to antibiotics and corticosteroids, and variably responsive to [90]strontium plesiotherapy.

## Basal Cell Tumors

The basal cell tumors (BCTs) include basal cell epithelioma, basal cell carcinoma, and basiloid tumor. Since the tumor in domestic animals is almost always benign, the preferred nomenclature is basal cell tumor. BCT is the most common skin tumor affecting the cat, representing 15 to 26% of all feline skin tumors.[1,5,6] It is less common in the dog, representing 4 to 12% of canine skin tumors.[1,2,4] These tumors are generally found in middle-aged dogs (6–9 years) and slightly older cats with a mean age of 10 to 11

years.[5,6] In the dog, cocker spaniels and poodles have an increased incidence, and in cats, the Siamese were over-represented in one large study, while others have not documented a breed predilection.[5,6] BCTs are usually solitary, well circumscribed, firm, hairless, dome-shaped elevated masses from 0.5 to 10 cm in diameter (Figs. 15–8A and 15–8B). Most BCTs are freely movable and firmly fixed to the overlying skin but rarely invade underlying fascia. These tumors are most commonly located on the head, neck, and shoulders (Figs. 15–9A and 15–9B) in both the dog and cat. Feline BCTs can be pigmented, cystic, or solid, and are occasionally ulcerated and have a surprisingly high mitotic rate for tumors that are benign.[6] Most BCTs are benign, grow slowly, and may be present for months prior to diagnosis. The treatment of choice for BCTs is surgical excision, which carries a good prognosis. In 124 cases of BCTs in cats treated by surgical excision, none recurred nor metastasized.[73] In another report of 97 BCTs in cats, approximately 10% were classified as histologically malignant; however, only one developed metastasis to regional lymph nodes.[6] Rare recurrences and no metastasis have been reported in the dog. Cryosurgery is an alternative to surgery for smaller (< 1 cm) lesions.

## Sebaceous Gland Tumors

Sebaceous gland tumors represent a complex array of growths that can be divided into four groups based on histologic appearance. These are, in decreasing frequency, sebaceous hyperplasia, sebaceous epithelioma, sebaceous adenoma, and sebaceous adenocarcinoma. Sebaceous gland tumors are among the most common skin tumors in the dog, accounting for 6.8 to 7.9% of all skin tumors.[1,2,4,74] Sebaceous gland tumors are less common in the cat, accounting for 2.3 to 4.4 of all skin tumors.[1,5,6,75] Modified sebaceous glands are found in a variety of locations and may give rise to neoplastic growths, including eyelid meibomian gland tumors (Chap. 27) and perianal gland tumors (Chap. 18).

Sebaceous hyperplasia accounts for the majority of sebaceous gland tumors in the dog. They are characterized histologically by an accumulation of nearly mature sebaceous glands. Most are solitary; however, multiple lesions can occur. They are found on older animals (mean 9.1 years), and miniature schnauzers, beagles, poodles, and cocker spaniels appear to be over-represented.[74] They can occur anywhere on the body

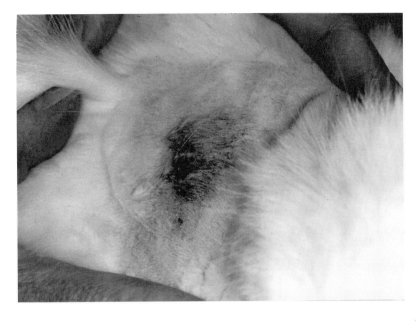

**Figure 15–7.** Lesion anterior to the tail head from a cat with multicentric squamous cell carcinoma in situ (Bowen's disease). The area has been shaved for illustration. The lesion is crusty, easily epilated, and hemorrhagic when manipulated.

*A*

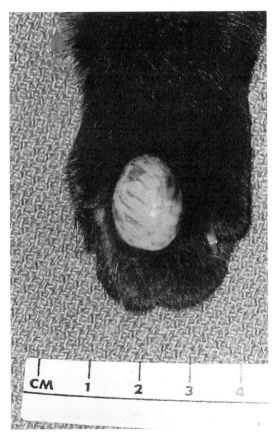

*B*

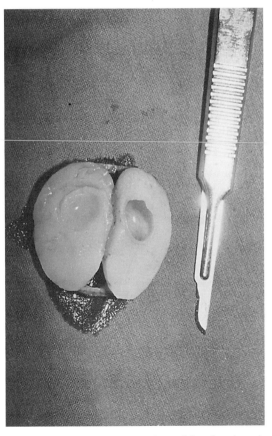

**Figure 15–8A.** Firm, circumscribed hairless basal cell tumor in the foot of a cat.

**Figure 15–8B.** Cross section of benign basal cell tumor seen in Figure 15–8A. Note cystic center and well-defined margins.

*A*

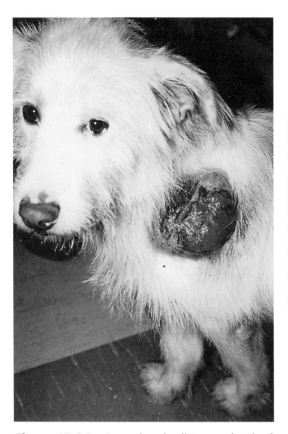

**Figure 15–9*A*.**    Large basal cell tumor that had been slowly growing for 2 years. In spite of its large size, fixation to underlying tissue, and ulceration, surgery was curative.

*B*

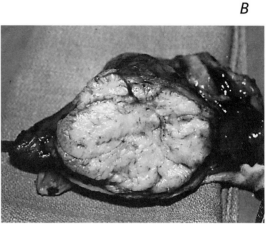

**Figure 15–9*B*.**    Cross section of basal cell tumor seen in Figure 15–9*A*.

*A*

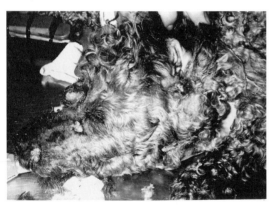

**Figure 15–10*A*.**    Multiple sebaceous gland adenomas on the head of an aged poodle.

*B*

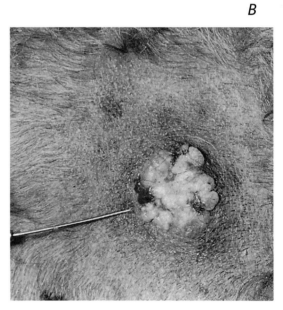

**Figure 15–10*B*.**    Close-up view of a sebaceous adenoma prior to cryosurgery (thermocouple in place). Note roughened surface that is often greasy to the touch.

but most are found on the limbs, trunk, and eyelids. Most are less than 1 cm in diameter, wartlike or cauliflowerlike, and can become ulcerated because of trauma (Figs. 15–10A and 15–10B). In a compilation of 92 cases in the dog, only one recurred following excision; however, nearly 10% of cases developed new lesions at other body sites.[74] Sebaceous hyperplasia is often found peripheral to and phasing into sebaceous adenomas or adenocarcinomas and is likely a precursor to their development. In the cat, sebaceous hyperplasia is typically a solitary lesion more common on the head, with a male predisposition.[5,75] Lesions may be present for many years. Recurrence has not been reported following excision.

Sebaceous epithelioma occurs primarily on the head (especially the eyelid) as a solitary lesion; however, generalized cases have been reported. Shih Tzus, Lhasa apsos, malamutes, Siberian huskies, and Irish setters appear to be over-represented. These lesions are nearly identical in appearance to sebaceous hyperplasia and the treatment of choice is excision. They are more likely to recur than sebaceous hyperplasia or adenoma, though the recurrence rate is still low, at approximately 6%.[74]

Sebaceous adenomas are relatively uncommon sebaceous gland tumors, similar in appearance and behavior to hyperplastic lesions. Sebaceous adenocarcinomas are rare in the cat and dog and appear to have a low potential for metastasis and recurrence.[5,74,75] They are characterized by ulceration and inflammation of surrounding tissues

(Fig. 15–11).[76] More aggressive surgical excision is indicated for these tumors.

## Sweat Gland Tumors

Sweat gland tumors can be of either apocrine gland derivation or eccrine gland derivation. Eccrine-derived tumors are rare in the dog, only occur on the foot pad, and have not been reported in the cat.

Cysts of the apocrine sweat glands, a benign tumorlike lesion is more common in the dog and appear as elevated, round, fluctuant intradermal nodules containing watery clear liquid. They are usually found on the head and are easily managed by surgical excision.

Tumors of the apocrine sweat glands (adenomas and adenocarcinomas) are rare in the dog, accounting for approximately 2% of all canine skin tumors.[77] They are more common than sebaceous gland tumors in the cat, accounting for 3.6 to 9.0% of all skin tumors in this species.[5,6,77] Adenocarcinomas appear to predominate, making up from 50 to 90% of cases in both the dog and cat. While most can be differentiated by routine light microscopy, immunohistochemistry has been utilized to discriminate between the adenoma and adenocarcinoma.[78] Sweat gland tumors usually occur in dogs greater than 8 years of age, and golden retrievers appear to be over-represented for this tumor type. In the dog, lesions can occur anywhere on the body and are usually solitary, raised, well circumscribed, and solid. Nearly half

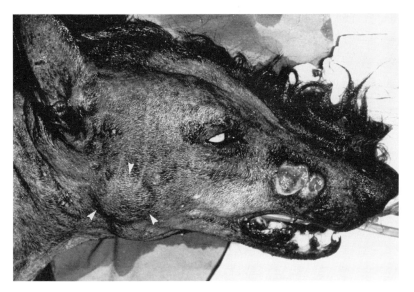

**Figure 15–11.** Scottish terrier with a sebaceous gland adenocarcinoma of the upper lip with metastasis to regional lymph nodes (arrows).

are ulcerated. While a quarter of cases have histopathologic evidence of lymphatic infiltrations, distant metastasis is uncommon. In one report, only 2 of 24 cases of malignant tumors treated with surgical excision recurred locally, and the remaining 22 were tumor free from 6 months to 3 years postexcision. While no case metastasized in this report, the authors' experience, along with sporadic reports of metastatic apocrine sweat gland tumors in the veterinary literature, suggests a guarded prognosis. The efficacy of radiotherapy for unresectable tumors and chemotherapy for metastatic lesions has not been established.

In the cat, benign apocrine sweat gland adenomas rarely ulcerate, are associated with little local inflammation, and have a cystic feel on palpation. Adenocarcinomas are more likely to be ulcerative, firm, and locally inflamed. Adenomas occur more commonly on the head, while adenocarcinomas can occur anywhere on the body. Both occur primarily in older cats averaging 12 years of age. Wide surgical excision is the therapy of choice and carries a good prognosis for adenomas and a guarded prognosis for adenocarcinomas. Local recurrence and widespread metastasis, while not common, have been reported to local lymph nodes, digits of the feet, liver, and lung.

Two modified apocrine gland tumors, those of the ceruminous glands of the ears (see Ear Canal Tumors in this chapter) and the anal sac (Chap. 18) will be discussed at length elsewhere.

## Intracutaneous Cornifying Epithelioma (Keratoacanthoma)

Intracutaneous cornifying epithelioma (ICE) is a benign epithelial proliferation arising from superficial epithelium between hair follicles, although they may appear to originate from adnexa. Only one case in the cat exists in the veterinary literature. Canine ICE may present as two distinct forms: (1) a solitary lesion, which may occur in any breed of dog, and (2) a multicentric form that usually occurs in Arctic Circle breeds (Norwegian elkhound and keeshond) (Fig. 15–12). Young male dogs appear to be at increased risk. The cause of ICE is unknown; however, some evidence suggests genetic factors in the multicentric forms.

Most tumors are between 0.5 and 4.0 cm in diameter with a pore opening to the surface. The pore usually contains a mass of keratin, which sometimes contains hair shafts. The tumors often contain a cheesy material that can be manually

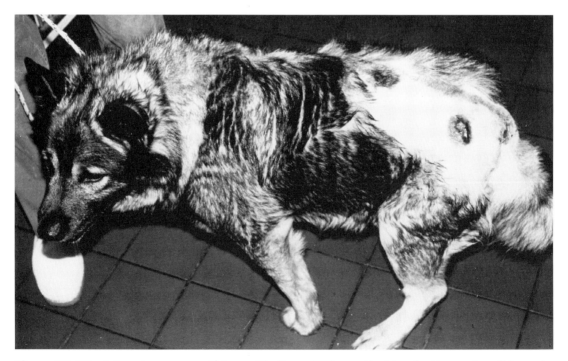

**Figure 15–12.**   Intercutaneous cornifying epithelioma (ICE) over the hip of a Norwegian elkhound. Surgical removal of this lesion was followed by the development of two new lesions, in different sites, within 2 years.

expressed, resulting in the "toothpaste tumor" acronym. Rupture of the cyst and extrusion of cystic contents into adjacent tissue may lead to a secondary inflammatory response. In some cases ICE may be located in the dermis and subcutaneous tissue without communication to the surface. Cytologically, these tumors are characterized by keratinous debris, clusters of squamous cells, and occasional cholesterol crystals. The treatment for solitary tumors is surgical excision and the prognosis is generally excellent. Multiple small tumors may be treated with cryosurgery. Recently, some success treating the multiple form of the disease with vitamin A-related synthetic retinoids has been reported.[34,79] Both isotretinoin and etretinate have been used successfully; however, the latter appears to be more effective. Long-term retinoid therapy is required and lesions may recur upon discontinuation. In one report of seven cases of multiple, generalized ICE, five complete responses and two partial responses occurred.[34]

## Tumors of the Hair Follicles (Hair Matrix Tumor)

Tumors of the hair follicles account for approximately 5% of all skin tumors in the dog.[80] They are extremely rare in the cat, accounting for less than 1% of all skin tumors.[5,6,81] Two histologically distinct types, trichoepitheliomas and pilomatrixomas, constitute the majority of cases, while two rare forms, tricholemmoma and trichofolliculomas, also exist.

Trichoepitheliomas are derived from the follicular sheath and account for nearly 80% of hair follicle tumors. These tumors are almost always solitary, round to oval, well-circumscribed intradermal masses 1 to 20 cm in diameter. The overlying skin may be atrophic, hairless, and often ulcerated from trauma. On cut section, small gray-white multiple foci are found separated by a thin connective tissue stroma. These tumors occur in older (mean age of 9.3 years) animals, and golden retrievers, basset hounds, and German shepherds are at increased relative risk. A histologically unique form with mucinous degeneration is reported to occur primarily in the golden retriever.[80] Most trichoepitheliomas occur over the dorsal lumbar and lateral thoracic region.

Pilomatrixomas are derived from hair matrix and account for approximately 20% of the hair follicle tumors in the dog. Miniature poodles and kerry blue terriers are at increased relative risk. They are solitary, solid tumors from 1 to 10 cm in diameter. The skin overlying them is hairless,

often ulcerated, and on a cut surface may be gritty because of mineral deposition. Approximately one quarter of tumors may be cystic and one third hyperpigmented.

In general, the tumors of hair follicles are benign and carry an excellent prognosis following surgical excision. No local recurrences nor metastasis was recorded in a compilation of 80 cases even though many had histologic evidence of malignancy. One report of metastatic pilomatrixoma exists in the dog.[82]

## MESENCHYMAL TUMORS

Mesenchymal tumors are derived from connective tissues. The most common mesenchymal tumors of the skin and subcutis in the dog are mast cell tumors (Chap. 16), lipomas (Chap. 17), the soft tissue sarcomas (Chap. 17), hemangiosarcomas (Chap. 29), melanomas, and histiocytomas.[1–4] The most common mesenchymal tumors in the cat are mast cell tumors (Chap. 16) and fibrosarcoma (Chap. 17).[1,3,5,6]

## ROUND CELL TUMORS

All round cell tumors can involve the skin and subcutis. Cytologically, these tumors are characterized by discrete round cells. There are primarily six different round cell tumors encountered in the skin and subcutis: histiocytoma, mast cell tumors, plasma cell tumors, lymphoma, transmissible venereal tumor (TVT), and neuroendocrine (Merkel cell) tumors. Many, especially in their poorly differentiated form, can be difficult to characterize by routine light microscopy, so occasionally specific histochemical stains are utilized.[25–30] For a discussion of mast cell tumors, cutaneous lymphoma, and TVT, the reader is referred to detailed discussions in Chapters 16, 28, and 29, respectively.

### Histiocytoma

Cutaneous histiocytomas are common in the dog and extremely rare in other species. These tumors arise from the monocyte-macrophage cells in the skin. Histiocytomas account for 3 to 14% of all skin tumors in the dog.[1–4] There is a predilection for young dogs but they may be seen in dogs of any age. Boxers, dachshunds, cocker spaniels, Great Danes, Shetland sheepdogs, and bull terriers may be at increased risk for their development. There is no reported sex predisposition. Only a few cases have been reported in the cat.[83]

Histiocytomas usually occur as solitary, fast-growing, nonpainful, dome-shaped intradermal lesions with a shiny, hairless, or ulcerated surface (Fig. 15–13). Tumors range from 0.5 to 4.0 cm in diameter, with the majority being 1 to 2 cm.

Histiocytoma can usually be diagnosed by fine-needle aspiration cytology. The tumor con-

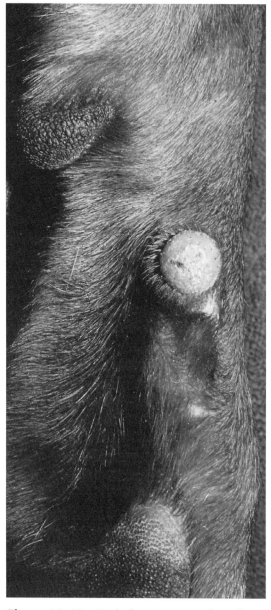

**Figure 15–13.** Typical appearance of a solitary histiocytoma on the foreleg of a young dog. Note hairless, circular, "buttonlike" appearance.

sists of pleomorphic cells resembling monocytes. The nuclei of histiocytoma cells are variable in size and shape, the mitotic index may be quite high, and the cytoplasm is variable in size and stains pale blue. Histiocytomas may have a large lymphocytic, plasmacytic, or neutrophilic infiltrate, depending on when the lesion is aspirated relative to its progression or regression. Although rapid growth and high mitotic index are suggestive of a malignancy, these are benign tumors that may regress spontaneously in approximately 3 months.

A variation of the disease involving multiple cutaneous lesions is referred to as cutaneous histiocytosis (histiocytic proliferative dermatitis). This is a benign proliferation of multiple erythematous dermal or subcutaneous plaques or nodules that may wax or wane with time. In the authors' experience this disease commonly afflicts young golden retrievers. Systemic involvement or lymphadenopathy is not present and should not be confused with malignant histiocytosis of primarily Bernese mountain dogs (Chap. 28).

The prognosis for canine cutaneous histiocytoma is excellent. The treatment of choice is conservative surgery or cryosurgery. Multiple cutaneous histiocytosis may also regress spontaneously; however, corticosteroids and rarely azathioprine have been effective in achieving regression of lesions.[84,85] Polyethylene glycosylated L-asparaginase (PEG-L-asparaginase) has also been used to achieve regression of multiple lesions.[86]

## Cutaneous Plasmacytoma

Within the last 5 years, a number of large case compilations of cutaneous plasmacytoma in the dog have been reported.[87–93] Technically, these are members of a group of plasmacytic tumors referred to as extramedullary plasmacytoma (i.e., they arise outside of bone). It is proposed that they have been previously diagnosed as *reticulum cell sarcomas*, a term that has lost favor in recent years. Only a handful of cases have been reported to occur in the cat.[5,93–95]

Cutaneous plasmacytoma is a tumor of older dogs (mean of 9–10 years). Large-breed dogs, in particular, German shepherds, may be overrepresented and no consistent sex predilection is reported. This tumor can occur on the trunk, limbs, head (especially the ear pinnae), and oral cavity, including the gingiva and tongue. Most lesions are solitary, smooth, raised pink nodules from 1 to 2 cm in diameter, although tumors as large as 10 cm have been reported.

Histologically, they are composed of circumscribed sheets of pleomorphic round cells consistent with plasma cells. Immunoreactivity has been demonstrated for canine IgG F(ab)2 and vimentin.[90] A variant characterized by an IgG reactive amyloid interspersed with the neoplastic cells has been described.[91] Systemic involvement is rarely evident and, unlike multiple myeloma, only one case has been associated with hypercalcemia and hypergammaglobulinemia, which resolved after surgical excision.[87]

Cutaneous plasma cell tumors in the dog are almost always benign and carry an excellent prognosis following conservative surgical excision. Combining recent reports in the literature, only 2 of 266 cases were accompanied by systemic multiple myeloma, only 11 recurred after surgery (most of these had incomplete surgical margins), and only 4 went on to develop distant disease consisting solely of cutaneous sites. Successful therapy with alkeran and prednisone has been reported for a local recurrence. Radiation therapy has been used infrequently for cases that are nonsurgical. DNA ploidy and p62[c-myc] oncoprotein content of biopsy samples were determined to be predictive for extramedullary plasmacytomas;[89] however, those that were malignant were all from noncutaneous sites (i.e., lymph node, colon, spleen); therefore location appears to be as predictive. The author has encountered one case of aggressive multiple cutaneous plasmacytoma that eventually resulted in the death of the animal. The prognosis for cutaneous plasmacytoma in the cat is unknown because of the paucity of reports. In the few cases that stated clinical outcomes, one cat presented with skin lesions as part of a systemic process, one metastasized to regional lymph nodes, and one was apparently cured by excision.[5,93,95]

## Melanocytic Tumors (Melanocytic Nevus, Melanocytoma, Melanosarcoma, Malignant Melanoma)

Tumors of melanocytes and melanoblasts are relatively common skin tumors in the dog, accounting for between 5 and 7% of all canine skin tumors.[1-4] They are a rare tumor in the cat, accounting for between 0.8 and 2.7% of all feline skin tumors.[1,5,6] Melanocytic tumors are most common in older dogs (average age 9 years) with darkly pigmented skin, although the literature varies in terms of which breeds are at risk. Early reports mention a male preponderance for tumor development; however, more recent reports do not support this. Melanocytic tumors are also more common in older cats (average age of 10–12 years), and no sex or breed predilection is known.

Cutaneous melanoma in the dog can be behaviorally benign or malignant and can occur anywhere on the body. Benign forms are often referred to as *melanocytic nevus*, a term that in its purest sense implies any congenital, melanin-pigmented lesion. Benign melanomas are typically well defined, deeply pigmented, less than 2 cm in diameter, dome shaped, firm, broad based, but mobile over underlying tissue (Fig. 15–14). These tumors can usually be diagnosed by simple fine-needle aspiration cytology. Behaviorally malignant melanomas tend to grow rapidly, can be greater than 2 cm, and are often ulcerated (Fig. 15–15). A summary of factors known to be prognostic for cutaneous melanoma in dogs is presented in Table 15–4. Over 85% of melanomas in dogs arising from haired skin are associated with benign behavior. The majority of oral and mucocutaneous junction melanomas (except eyelid), and approximately one third of melanomas arising in the nail bed (see Subungual Tumors in this chapter) are behaviorally malignant.[32,96,97] The histologic criteria of mitotic rate is highly predictive (approximately 90% accurate) of degree of malignancy. A mitotic rate of less than 3 per 10 high power field is strongly associated with benign behavior.[1,32,96,97] Breed has been reported to be of prognostic significance; more than 75% of melanoma in Doberman pinschers and miniature schnauzers are behaviorally benign, while

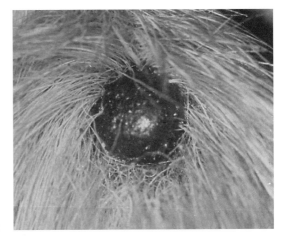

**Figure 15–14.** Typical appearance of a raised cutaneous melanoma. The vast majority of melanomas occurring on haired skin are benign in the dog. This mass was biopsied and treated with cryosurgery.

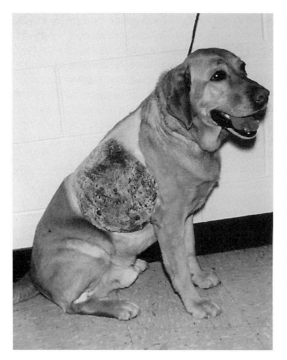

**Figure 15–15.** Behaviorally malignant cutaneous melanoma on the side of a Labrador retriever. Typically, the malignant variety of cutaneous melanomas are larger, poorly circumscribed, ulcerated and grow rapidly.

85% of melanomas in miniature poodles are behaviorally malignant.[96] Analysis of DNA ploidy with flow-cytometric analysis strongly correlates with degree of malignancy for melanoma in the dog.[96] However, it was no more predictive than routine light microscopy and therefore is not cost effective. Reactivity of tumor cells with a monoclonal antibody (MAB IBF9)

generated against a canine melanoma cell line has also been shown to be predictive.[32] Again, this time-consuming technique is not clinically useful as a prognostic index; however, it may have utility in differentiating amelanotic melanomas from other poorly differentiated tumors.

In the cat, melanogenic tumors can also be benign or malignant. While they can be induced experimentally with the feline sarcoma virus, it is unlikely to be associated with clinically observed cases.[5] The majority involve the head, and very rarely do they involve the extremities.[5,98] Most are ocular or on the eyelid (Chap. 27). Nonocular melanomas in the cat are similar in appearance to those in the dog; however, histologic assessment of malignancy does not appear to predict clinical outcome as in the dog. In general, ocular melanoma is behaviorally more malignant than oral melanoma, and dermal melanomas are more likely to have a benign clinical course in the cat.

The treatment of choice for local cutaneous melanoma in both the cat and dog is surgical excision. Those tumors in dogs with benign prognostic criteria (see Table 15–4) carry an excellent prognosis following complete excision. The prognosis for those with malignant criteria is guarded, as metastatic rates between 30 and 75% have been reported.[96,97] In the cat, prognosis is fair for nonocular dermal melanomas, as metastatic rates of 5 to 25% have been reported.[5,98] Alternatives to blade excision for local disease include radiotherapy, local hyperthermia, intralesional cisplatin,[65] and photodynamic therapy.[51,52] Radiotherapy has been used with success for local control of oral melanomas, and it is likely to be beneficial for dermal melanomas for which surgery is not an option. However, most dogs with malignant disease will succumb to systemic spread. Response to hyper-

**Table 15–4**   Prognostic Factors for Cutaneous Melanoma in the Dog

| Factor | Comment |
| --- | --- |
| Location | Tumors arising from haired skin are generally benign. Tumors arising from mucocutaneous junctions (except eyelid), nail bed, and oral lesions are generally malignant.[32, 96, 97] |
| Histology | Histologic determination of malignant versus benign is very predictive of biologic behavior. Determination based primarily on mitotic index.[1, 32, 96, 97] |
| Breed | More likely benign in Doberman pinscher and miniature schnauzer, likely malignant in miniature poodle.[96] |
| DNA ploidy | Prominent G2/M peaks predictive for malignant behavior. No more predictive than simple light microscopy, therefore not cost effective.[96] |
| MAB IBF9 reactivity[a] | Antigen expression by tumor reactive to MAB IBF9 is predictive of malignant behavior. Probably useful for identifying amelanotic tumors.[32] |

[a]MAB = monoclonal antibody.

thermia/intralesional cisplatin and photodynamic therapy appear to be short-lived.[51,52,65]

Chemotherapy for malignant melanoma in the dog has shown little promise in the veterinary literature. Agents that have been investigated on a limited bases include mitoxantrone,[56] doxorubicin,[61] intravenous melphelan,[99] cisplatin,[100] and decarbazine.[101] In general, response rates are very low and durations of response have been short-lived.

Limited investigations of immunotherapy have been undertaken for cutaneous malignant melanoma in the dog. No convincing evidence exists as yet for clinical efficacy.[31,102] More specific targeted approaches are currently being evaluated.

Two distinct histologic forms of melanoma, pilar neurocristic melanoma (discretely perifollicular) and "clear cell melanomas" have been reported in the dog.[103,104] No clinical information exists on pilar neurocristic melanoma. No recurrence or metastasis was reported in four cases of clear cell melanoma in dogs following excision.

## Cutaneous Neuroendocrine Tumors

Rare in dogs, the cutaneous neuroendocrine (Merkel cell) tumor is typically solitary and can occur on the lips, ears, digits, and in the oral cavity. Merkel cells are part of the diffuse neuroendocrine cell system and are believed to function as mechanoreceptors. In the few reports in the veterinary literature they appear to be behaviorally benign and are successfully managed by surgical excision.[105,106]

## EAR CANAL TUMORS IN DOGS AND CATS

Tumors of the ear canal will be discussed as a group for convenience and clarity. Both benign and malignant neoplasms occur with some frequency in the ear canal of both species, and large compilations of cases have been reported.[5,107] While inflammation may be secondary to tumor development in the area, the presence of longstanding otitis externa is believed to be a factor in tumor development, and observed increased glandular dysplasia suggests that chronic inflammation does indeed play a role.[107,108] Ear tumors occur in older cats (mean age of 7 and 11 years for benign and malignant tumors, respectively) and dogs (9 and 10 years of age). No sex predilection exists in either species. The cocker spaniel appears to be over-represented for both benign and malig-

nant tumor development and may be related to this breed's propensity to develop otitis externa.

The most frequently observed clinical presentations include the presence of a mass, aural discharge, odor, pruritus, and local pain. These signs are often present for months to years prior to presentation. Neurologic signs (e.g., Horner's syndrome, vestibular signs) are observed in approximately 10% of dogs with malignant tumors and 25% of cats with either benign polyps or malignant tumors. Benign tumors appear raised, pedunculated, and rarely ulcerated, while malignant tumors are more likely to be ulcerated, hemorrhagic, and have a broad base of attachment. Approximately 25% of malignant forms will have evidence of bulla involvement and skull radiographs are recommended as part of the diagnostic workup.

The most common benign tumors encountered in both species include inflammatory polyps, papillomas, basal cell tumors, and ceruminous gland adenomas. Inflammatory polyps in cats are discussed in detail in Chapter 18. Ceruminous gland cysts are a tumorlike lesions that occur in cats. They are sessile masses, usually blue or black in color, contain an oily black fluid, and can be mistaken clinically for melanomas or basal cell tumors.

The most common malignant tumor encountered in the dog is ceruminous gland adenocarcinoma (CGA), followed by squamous cell carcinoma (SCC), and carcinoma of unknown origin.[107,109] A report of 53 malignant ear canal tumors in cats indicated CGA (Fig. 15–16) and SCC are equally represented as the most common malignancy, while another report indicates CGA are four times more likely to occur than SCC.[5,107] Almost every other type of cutaneous tumor has been reported from time to time at lower frequencies in the ear canals of cats and dogs.

Malignant ear canal tumors in dogs are less aggressive than in cats. Survival data have recently been generated from 38 dogs and 39 cats with malignant ear canal tumors treated almost exclusively by surgical excision.[107] The majority of dogs live more than 2 years after surgery, compared to a median survival of 1 year in the cat. In general, ear canal tumors are locally invasive, with relatively low metastatic potential. Approximately 10% of dogs and 5 to 15% of cats have evidence of local lymph node or thoracic metastasis at initial diagnosis. Cats with SCC of the ear canal (as opposed to the pinna) are more likely to present with neurologic signs than other tumor types, reflecting a more invasive behavior.

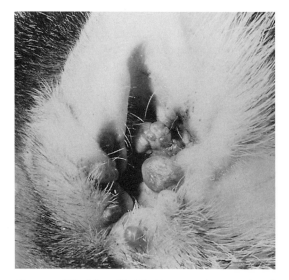

**Figure 15–16.** Multiple ceruminous gland tumors in the ear canal of a cat. Complete ear canal ablation was necessary to attain local control. The cat was free of disease 18 months postoperatively.

In the dog, bulla involvement and conservative surgery have both been identified as negative prognostic indices.[107,110] Aggressive ear canal ablation with lateral bulla osteotomy results in median survival times of 36 months compared to 9 months for dogs treated by more conservative lateral ear canal resection. In the cat, the presence of neurologic signs, histopathologic typing of SCC, or carcinoma of undetermined origin; histopathologic evidence of lymphatic or vascular invasion; and conservative surgery have been identified as negative prognostic indices. In cats with CGA a median disease-free interval (DFI) of 42 months, a 25% recurrence rate, and a 75% 1-year survival rate can be expected following aggressive ear ablation and bulla osteotomy. This compares favorably with a 10-month DFI, a 66% recurrence rate, and a 33% 1-year survival following conservative lateral ear resection.[111]

Most benign ear canal tumors in dogs and cats can be readily managed with conservative surgical resection. It appears that aggressive excision, including ear canal ablation and lateral bulla osteotomy, should be the treatment of choice for malignant ear canal tumors in both species. A good prognosis with a high likelihood of long-term survival results from such a procedure in the dog. A fair prognosis in the cat is warranted for CGC, and a guarded prognosis for SCC or carcinoma of undetermined origin.[107,111] Radiation therapy is a possible alternative to surgery and can be used as an adjuvant to incomplete resection. A median progression-free interval of 44 months and a 63% 1-year survival was achieved in one report of 5 dogs and 5 cats with CGA treated with 48 Gray external beam radiotherapy.[112] At present, no information exists on the efficacy of chemotherapy for ear canal tumors in the dog and cat.

## SUBUNGUAL TUMORS

Subungual (nail-bed) tumors are common in the dog and rare in the cat. A number of large case compilations exist on tumors of this location.[97,113–115] Approximately one third of subungual tumors in the dog are squamous cell carcinoma (SCC), followed in frequency by malignant melanoma, various soft tissue sarcomas (fibrosarcoma, neurofibrosarcoma), and mast cell tumors. Many other cutaneous tumor types have been reported at this site in lesser frequencies. Tumors comprise approximately 12% of all the disorders of the nail and nail bed and should be included in any differential list for disease in this area. Radiographs of the affected digit should be a routine part of the workup for nail-bed disease, because many tumors result in local bone lysis (Fig. 15–17). Subungual tumors are often secondarily infected and initially misdiagnosed as chronic paronychia or osteomyelitis. Prolonged histories prior to diagnosis result.

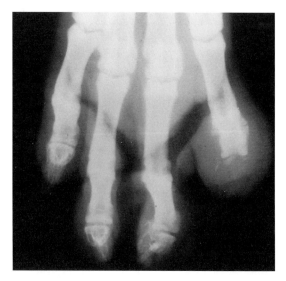

**Figure 15–17.** Radiograph from a dog with subungual squamous cell carcinoma of the second digit. Note almost complete osteolysis of $P_3$ with periosteal reaction of $P_2$ and the presence of a soft tissue mass in the surrounding tissues.

Subungual squamous cell carcinoma in the dog arises from the subungual epithelium and is locally invasive, almost always resulting in bony lysis of the third phalanx. It occurs in older dogs (mean age of 9 years) and no sex predilection is known. Approximately 75% of cases involve large-breed dogs and more than two thirds occur in dogs with primarily black coats (black Labradors and standard poodles), as opposed to the more common development of SCCs in other sites in lightly pigmented cats and dogs. They are usually solitary, ulcerative, occasionally hemorrhagic, and expansile (Fig. 15–18). The associated nail may be fractured or absent altogether. Subungual SCC is locally invasive, with a low metastatic potential contrary to previous reports. In 54 recently reported cases, none presented with radiographic evidence of distant metastasis, and only 5 (9%) went on to develop regional node or distant metastasis following complete excision (most involving wide digital amputation to the level of $P_1$).[113,114] In 21 cases managed by digital amputation, no recurrences were reported, resulting in 1- and 2-year survival rates of 76 and 43%, respectively. The rate of local recurrence increases if local excision is more conservative. It is therefore recommended that treatment for subungual SCC include a disarticulation amputation at the metacarpophalangeal, metatarsophalangeal, or proximal interphalangeal level. It does not appear that adjuvant therapy is required for the majority of cases.

A syndrome of multiple-digital SCC in dogs has been reported.[116,117] One report involved a standard poodle and a giant schnauzer, the other involved three related giant schnauzers that developed SCC in multiple digits over a period of several months to years.

Subungual melanomas are potentially malignant in the dog. Approximately one third to one half of melanomas originating in the nail bed will develop distant metastasis to lymph node, lung, and other systemic sites.[97,113] Digital amputation will usually control local disease (local recurrence rates of 30% can be expected); however, approximately half of dogs will die because of distant metastasis. It would appear that effective adjuvant systemic therapy is necessary for the majority of cases; however, as previously discussed, no consistent adjuvants exist for malignant melanoma, and a fair to guarded prognosis is warranted.

Soft tissue sarcomas involving the nail bed appear to behave similarly to their counterparts at other cutaneous sites (Chap. 17); that is, they are locally aggressive but uncommonly metastatic. Recently, four cases of "mesenchymal tumor of undetermined histogenesis" were described, two of which originated in the nail bed.[118] Long-term survival with local control was achieved following surgical excision. Mast cell tumors (Chap. 16) of the nail bed (not digital skin) are typically high-grade poorly differentiated tumors that carry a poor prognosis similar to mast cell tumors at other mucocutaneous sites.

In the cat, nail-bed tumors are rare. When they do occur they are usually metastatic lesions of carcinomas from other sites. In particular, several reports of pulmonary bronchiolar adenocarcinoma, pulmonary SCC, and cutaneous SCC metastasizing to multiple digits in the cat exist.[5,119–122]

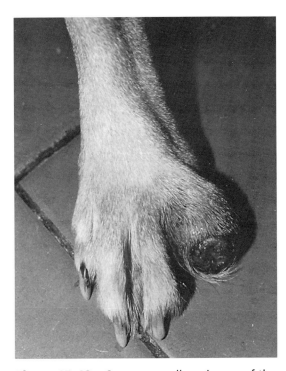

**Figure 15–18.** Squamous cell carcinoma of the digit. Extensive bone destruction was evident radiographically. A complete digital amputation was curative.

## REFERENCES

1. Bostock DE: Neoplasms of the skin and subcutaneous tissues in dogs and cats. Br Vet J *142*:1–19, 1986.
2. Rothwell TLW, Howlett CR, Middleton DJ, et al: Skin neoplasms of dogs in Sydney. Aust Vet J *64*:161–164, 1987.
3. Brodey RS: Canine and feline neoplasia. Adv Vet Sci Comp Med *14*:309–354, 1970.

4. Finnie JW, Bostock DE: Skin neoplasia in dogs. Aust Vet J 55:602–604, 1979.

5. Carpenter JL, Andrews LK, Holzworth J: Tumors and tumor like lesions. In Holzworth J (ed): Diseases of the Cat: Medicine and Surgery. Philadelphia, WB Saunders, 1987, pp. 406–596.

6. Miller MA, Nelson SL, Turk JR, et al: Cutaneous neoplasia in 340 cats. Vet Pathol 28:389–395, 1991.

7. Priester WA: Skin tumors in domestic animals: Data from 12 United States and Canadian colleges for veterinary medicine. J Natl Cancer Inst 50:457–466, 1973.

8. Priester WA, Mantel N: Occurrence of tumors in domestic animals. Data from 12 United States and Canadian colleges of veterinary medicine. J Natl Cancer Inst 47:1333–1344, 1971.

9. Allison AC: Viruses inducing skin tumors in animals. In Rook AJ, Walton CS (eds): Comparative Physiology and Pathology of the Skin. Oxford, Blackwell, 1965, pp. 665–684.

10. Shimada A, Shinya K, Awakura T, et al: Cutaneous papillomatosis associated with papillomavirus infection in a dog. J Comp Pathol 108:103–107, 1993.

11. Narama I, Ozaki K, Maeda H, Ohta A: Cutaneous papilloma with viral replication in an old dog. J Vet Med Sci 54:387–389, 1992.

12. Campbell KL, Sunberg JP, Goldschmidt MH, et al: Cutaneous inverted papillomas in dogs. Vet Pathol 25:67–71, 1988.

13. Dorn CR, Taylor D, Schneider R: Sunlight exposure and the risk of developing cutaneous and oral squamous cell carcinoma in white cats. J Natl Cancer Inst 46:1073–1078, 1971.

14. Madewell BR, Conroy JD, Hodgkins EM: Sunlight skin cancer association in the dog: A report of 3 cases. J Cutan Pathol 8:434–443, 1981.

15. Nikula KJ, Benjamin SA, Angleton GM, et al: Ultraviolet radiation, solar dermatosis, and cutaneous neoplasia in beagle dogs. Radiat Res 129:11–18, 1992.

16. Knowles DP, Hargis AM: Solar elastosis associated with neoplasia in two dalmatians. Vet Pathol 23:512–514, 1986.

17. Hayes JM, Wilson GP: Hormone-dependent neoplasms of the canine perianal gland. Cancer Res 37:2068–2071, 1977.

18. Moriello KA, Rosenthal RC: Clinical approach to tumors of the skin and subcutaneous tissues. Vet Clin North Am [Small Animal Pract] 20:1163–1190, 1990.

19. Bregman CL, Hirth RS, Sundberg JP, Christensen EF: Cutaneous neoplasms in dogs associated with canine oral papillomavirus vaccine. Vet Pathol 24:477–487, 1987.

20. Hendrick MJ, Goldschmidt MH, Shofer FS, et al: Postvaccinal sarcoma in the cat: Epidemiology and electron probe microanalytical identification of aluminum. Cancer Res 52:5391–5394, 1992.

21. Madewell BR, Theilen GH: Tumors and tumor-like conditions of epithelial origin. In Thielen GH, Madewell BR (eds): Veterinary Cancer Medicine. Philadelphia, Lea & Febiger, 1987, pp. 240–325.

22. Watach AM, Hanson LE, Meyer RC: Canine papilloma. The structural characterization of oral papilloma virus. J Natl Cancer Inst 43:453–458, 1969.

23. Owen LN (ed): TNM classification of tumors in domestic animals. Geneva, World Health Organization, 1980.

24. Castagnaro M, Canese MG: Lectin histochemistry on squamous metaplasia in different epithelial tumors of dogs. Vet Pathol 28:8–15, 1991.

25. Thoonen H, Broekaert D, Coucke P, et al: Expression of cytokeratines in epithelial tumours of the dog investigated with monoclonal antibodies. Schweiz Arch Tierheilk 132:409–484, 1990.

26. Rabanal RH, Fondevila CM, Montane V, et al: Immunocytochemical diagnosis of skin tumours of the dog with special reference to undifferentiated types. Res Vet Sci 47:129–133, 1989.

27. Cardona A, Madewell BR, Naydan DK, Lund JK: A comparison of six monoclonal antibodies for detection of cytokeratins in normal and neoplastic canine tissues. J Vet Diagn Invest 1:316–323, 1989.

28. Moore AS, Madewell BR, Lund JK: Immunohistochemical evaluation of intermediate filament expression in canine and feline neoplasms. Am J Vet Res 50:88–92, 1989.

29. Andreasen CB, Mahaffey EA, Duncan JR: Intermediate filament staining in the cytologic and histologic diagnosis of canine skin and soft tissue tumors. Vet Pathol 25:343–349, 1988.

30. Sandusky GE, Carlton WW, Wightman KA: Diagnostic immunohistochemistry of canine round cell tumors. Vet Pathol 24:495–499, 1987.

31. Helfand SC, Soergel SA, Gan J, et al: Expression of disialogangliosides on canine melanoma and effect of monoclonal anti-ganglioside antibody plus interleukin-2 on cell mediated lysis of canine melanoma. Proc Annu Conf Vet Cancer Soc 13:101–102, 1993.

32. Oliver JL, Wolfe LG: Antigen expression in canine tissues, recognized by a monoclonal antibody generated against canine melanoma cells. Am J Vet Res 53:123–128, 1992.

33. Hahn KA, Lantz GC, Salisbury SK: Comparison of survey radiography with ultrasonography and x-ray computed tomography for clinical staging of subcutaneous neoplasms in dogs. J Am Vet Med Assoc 196:1795–1798, 1990.

34. White SD, Rosychuk RAW, Scott KV, et al: Use of isotretinoin and etretinate for the treatment of benign cutaneous neoplasia and cutaneous lymphoma in dogs. J Am Vet Med Assoc 202:387–391, 1993.

35. Hofmeyer CFB: Dermoid sinus and the ridgeback dog. J Small Anim Pract 4:5–8, 1963.

36. Kral F, Schwartzman RM: Veterinary and comparative dermatology. Philadelphia, JB Lippincott, 1964.

37. Atlee BA, DeBoar DJ, Ihrke PJ, et al: Nodular dermatofibrosis in German shepherd dogs as a marker for renal cystadenocarcinoma. J Am Anim Hosp Assoc 27:481–487, 1991.

38. Gilbert PA, Griffin CE, Walder EJ: Nodular dermatofibrosis and renal cystadenoma in a German shepherd dog. J Am Anim Hosp Assoc 26:253–256, 1990.

39. Lium B, Moe L: Hereditary multifocal renal cystadenocarcinomas and nodular dermatofibrosis in the German shepherd dog: Macroscopic and histopatholgic changes. Vet Pathol 22:447–455, 1985.

40. Cosenza SF, Seely JC: Generalized nodular dermatofibrosis and renal cystadenocarcinomas in a German shepherd dog. J Am Vet Med Assoc 189:1587–1590, 1986.

41. Suter M, Lott-Stolz G, Wild P: Generalized nodular dermatofibrosis in six Alsatians. Vet Pathol 20:632–634.

42. Sundberg JP, O'Banion MK, Schmidt-Didier E, Teichmann ME: Cloning and characterization of a canine oral papillomavirus. Am J Vet Res 47:1142–1144, 1986.

43. Ruehl WW, Nizet V, Blum JR, et al: Generalized papillomatosis in narcoleptic dogs treated with cyclosporin A. Lab Anim Sci 37:518–519, 1987.

44. Walder EJ, Gross TL. Neoplastic diseases of the skin. In Gross TL, Ihrke PJ, Walder EJ (eds): Veterinary Dermatopathology. St. Louis, Mosby Yearbook, 1992, pp. 327–350.

45. Hargis AM, Thomassen RW, Phemister RD: Chronic dermatosis and cutaneous squamous cell carcinoma in the beagle dog. Vet Pathol 14:218–228, 1977.

46. Atwater SW, Powers BE, Straw RC, Withrow SJ: Squamous cell carcinoma of the pinna and nasal planum. Fifty-four cats (1980–1991). Proc Annu Conf Vet Cancer Soc 11:35–36, 1991.

47. Clarke RE: Cryosurgical treatment of feline cutaneous squamous cell carcinoma. Aust Vet Pract 21:148–153, 1991.

48. Theon AP, Madewell BR, Shearn V, Moulton JE: Irradiation of squamous cell carcinomas of the nasal planum in 90 cats. Proc Annu Conf Vet Cancer Soc 13:147–148, 1993.

49. Van Vechten MK, Theon AP: Strontium-90 plesiotherapy for treatment of early squamous cell carcinomas of the nasal planum in 25 cats. Proc Annu Conf Vet Cancer Soc 13:107–108, 1993.

50. Roberts WG, Klein MK, Weldy LS, Berns MW: Photodynamic therapy of spontaneous cancers in felines, canines, and snakes with chloroaluminum sulfonated phthalocyanine. J Natl Cancer Inst 83:18–23, 1991.

51. Cheli R, Addis F, Mortellaro CM, et al: Photodynamic therapy of spontaneous animal tumors using the active component of hematoporthyrin derivative (DHE) as photosensitizing drug: Clinic results. Cancer Lett 38:101–105, 1987.

52. Dougherty TJ, Thoma RE, Boyle DG, Weishaupt KR: Interstitial photoradiation therapy for primary solid tumors in pet cats and dogs. Cancer Res 41:401–404, 1981.

53. Magne ML, Rodriquez CO, Autry S, et al: Preliminary results of photodynamic therapy in cats with naturally occurring facial squamous cell carcinoma using the photosensitizer pyropheophorbide-hexyl-alpha-ether. Proc Annu Conf Vet Cancer Soc 13:114–115, 1993.

54. Peaston AE, Leach MW, Higgins RJ: Photodynamic therapy for nasal and aural squamous cell carcinoma in cats. J Am Vet Med Assoc 202:1261–1265, 1993.

55. Beck ER, Dunstan RW, Hetzel FW: Control of canine squamous cell carcinomas by photodynamic therapy. Proc Annu Conf Vet Cancer Soc 11:1–2, 1991.

56. Ogilvie GK, Obradovich JE, Elmslie RE, et al: Efficacy of mitoxantrone against various neoplasms in dogs. J Am Vet Med Assoc 198:1618–1621, 1991.

57. Ogilvie GK, Moore AS, Obradovich JE, et al: Toxicoses and efficacy associated with administration of mitoxantrone to cats with malignant tumors. J Am Vet Med Assoc 202:1839–1844, 1993.

58. Hammer AS, Couto CG, Ayl RD, Shank KA: Treatment of tumor-bearing dogs and cats with actinomycin D. J Vet Intern Med 8(3):236–239, 1994.

59. Mauldin GN, Matus RE, Patnaik AK, et al: Efficacy and toxicity of doxorubicin and cyclophosphamide used in the treatment of selected malignant tumors in 23 cats. J Vet Intern Med 2:60–65, 1988.

60. Buhles WC, Theilen GH: Preliminary evaluation of bleomycin in feline and canine squamous cell carcinoma. Am J Vet Res 34:289–291, 1973.

61. Moore AS: Recent advances in chemotherapy for nonlymphoid malignant neoplasms. Compend Contin Educ Pract Vet 15:1039–1050, 1993.

62. Himsel CA, Richardson RC, Craig JA: Cisplatin chemotherapy for metastatic squamous cell carcinoma in two dogs. J Am Vet Med Assoc 189:1575–1578, 1986.

63. Knapp DW, Richardson RC, Bonney PL, et al: Cisplatin therapy in 41 dogs with malignant tumors. J Vet Intern Med 2:41–46, 1988.

64. Kitchell BE, McCabe M, Luck EE, et al: Intralesional sustained-release chemotherapy with cisplatin and 5-fluorouracil therapeutic implants for treatment of feline squamous cell carcinoma. Proc Annu Conf Vet Cancer Soc 12:55, 1992.

65. Theon AP, Madewell BR, Moore AS, et al: Localized thermo-cisplatin therapy: A pilot study in spontaneous canine and feline tumours. J Hyperthermia 7:881–892, 1991.

66. Marks SL, Song MD, Stannard AA, Power HT:

Clinical evaluation of etretinate for the treatment of canine solar-induced squamous cell carcinoma and preneoplastic lesions. J Am Acad Dermato 27:11–16, 1992.

67. Levene N, Earle M, Wilson S: Controlled localized heating and isotretinoin effects in canine squamous cell carcinoma. J Am Acad Dermatol 23:68–72, 1990.

68. Evans AG, Madewell BR, Stannard AA: A trial of 13-cis-retinoic acid for treatment of squamous cell carcinoma and preneoplastic lesions of the head in cats. Am J Vet Res 46:2553–2557, 1985.

69. Jones SE, Knapp DW, HogenEsch H, DeNicola DB: Pilot study of piroxicam therapy of nonresectable squamous cell carcinoma in dogs. Proc Annu Conf Vet Cancer Soc 13:53–54, 1993.

70. Baer KE, Helton K: Multicentric squamous cell carcinoma in situ resembling Bowen's disease in cats. Vet Pathol 30:535–543, 1993.

71. Miller WH, Affolter V, Scott DW, Suter MM: Multicentric squamous cell carcinomas in situ resembling Bowen's disease in five cats. Vet Dermatol 3:177–182, 1992.

72. Turrel JM, Gross TL: Multicentric squamous cell carcinoma in situ (Bowen's disease) of cats. Proc Annu Conf Vet Cancer Soc 11:84, 1991.

73. Diters RW, Walsh KM: Feline basal cell tumors: A review of 124 cases. Vet Pathol 21:51–56, 1984.

74. Scott DW, Anderson WI: Canine sebaceous gland tumors: A retrospective analysis of 172 cases. Canine Pract 15:19–27, 1990.

75. Scott DW, Anderson WI: Feline sebaceous gland tumors: A retrospective analysis of nine cases. Feline Pract 19:16–21, 1991.

76. Strafuss AC: Sebaceous gland carcinoma in dogs. J Am Vet Med Assoc 169:325–326, 1976.

77. Kalaher KM, Anderson DWS: Neoplasms of the apocrine sweat glands in 44 dogs and 10 cats. Vet Rec 127:400–403, 1990.

78. Ferrer L, Rabanal RM, Fondevila D, Prats N: Immunocytochemical demonstration of intermediate filament proteins, S-100 protein and CEA in apocrine sweat glands and apocrine gland derived lesions of the dog. J Vet Med Series [A] 37:569–576, 1990.

79. Henfrey JI: Treatment of multiple intracutaneous cornifying epitheliomata using isotretinoin. J Small Anim Pract 32:363–365, 1991.

80. Scott DW, Anderson WI: Canine hair follicle neoplasms: A retrospective analysis of 80 cases (1986–1987). Vet Dermatol 2:143–150, 1991.

81. Scott DW, Anderson WI: Hair follicle neoplasms in three cats. Feline Pract 19:14–16, 1991.

82. Van Ham L, van Bree H, Maenhout T, et al: Metastatic pilomatrixoma presenting as paraplegia in a dog. J Small Anim Pract 32:27–30, 1990.

83. Macy DW, Reynolds HA: The incidence, characteristics and clinical management of skin tumors in cats. J Am Anim Hosp Assoc 17:1026–1034, 1981.

84. Bender WM, Muller GH: Multiple, resolving, cutaneous histiocytoma in a dog. J Am Vet Med Assoc 184:535–537, 1989.

85. Panich R. Scott DW, Miller WH. Canine cutaneous sterile pyogranuloma/granuloma syndrome: A retrospective analysis of 29 cases (1976–1986). J Am Anim Hosp Assoc 27:519–528, 1991.

86. Moriello KA, MacEwen EG, Schultz KT: PEG-L-asparaginase in the treatment of canine epitheliotrophic lymphoma and histiocytic proliferative dermatitis. In Ihrke PJ, Mason IS, White SR (eds): Advances in Veterinary Dermatology. New York, Pergamon Press, 1993, pp. 293–300.

87. Clark GN, Berg J, Engler SJ, Bronson RT: Extramedullary plasmacytomas in dogs: results of surgical excision in 131 cases. J Am Anim Hosp Assoc 28:105–111, 1992.

88. Rakich PM, Latimer KS, Weiss R, Steffens WL: Mucocutaneous plasmacytomas in dogs: 75 cases (1980–1987). J Am Vet Med Assoc 194:803–810, 1989.

89. Frazier KS, Hines ME, Hurvitz Al et al: Analysis of DNA aneuploidy and c-myc oncoprotein content of canine plasma cell tumors using flow cytometry. Vet Pathol 30:505–511, 1993.

90. Baer KE, Patnaik AK, Gilbertson SR, Hurvitz Al: Cutaneous plasmacytomas in dogs: A morphologic and immunohistochemical study. Vet Pathol 26:216–221, 1989.

91. Rowland PH, Valentine BA, Stebbins KE, Smith CA: Cutaneous plasmacytomas with amyloid in six dogs. Vet Pathol 28:125–130, 1991.

92. Kyriazidou A, Brown PJ, Lucke VM: An immunohistochemical study of canine extramedully plasma cell tumors. J Comp Pathol 100:259–266, 1989.

93. Lucke VM: Primary cutaneous plasmacytomas in the dog and cat. J Small Anim Pract 28:49–55, 1987.

94. Kryriazidou A, Brown PJ, Lucke VM: Immunohistochemical staining of neoplastic and inflammatory plasma cell lesions in feline tissues. J Comp Pathol 100:337–341, 1989.

95. Carothers MA, Johnson GC, DiBartola SP, et al: Extramedullary plasmacytoma and immunoglobulin-associated amyloidosis in a cat. J Am Vet Med Assoc 195:1593–1597, 1989.

96. Bolon B, Calderwood Mays MB, Hall BJ: Characteristics of canine melanomas amd comparison of histology and DNA ploidy to their biologic effect. Vet Pathol 27:96–102, 1990.

97. Aronsohn MG, Carpenter JL: Distal extremity melanocytic nevi and malignant melanomas in dogs. J Am Anim Hosp Assoc 26:605–612, 1990.

98. Patnaik Ak, Mooney S: Feline melanoma: A comparative study of ocular, oral, and dermal neoplasms. Vet Pathol 25:105–112, 1988.

99. Ruslander RM, Price GS, McEntree MC, et al: Intravenous melphalan: Phase II evaluation in dogs with malignant melanoma. Proc Annu Conf Vet Cancer Soc 13:82, 1993.

100. Guptill L, Knapp DW, Hahn K, et al: Retrospective study of cisdiaminedichloroplatinum (cisplatin) treatment for canine malignant melanoma. Proc Annu Conf Vet Cancer Soc 13:65–66, 1993.

101. Gillick A, Spiegle M: Decarbazine treatment of malignant melanoma in a dog. Can Vet J 28:204, 1987.

102. Moore AS, Theilen GH, Newell AD, et al: Preclinical study of sequential tumor necrosis factor and interleukin 2 in the treatment of spontaneous canine neoplasms. Cancer Res 51:233–238, 1991.

103. Anderson WI, Luther PB, Scott DW: Pilar neurocristic melanoma in four dogs. Vet Rec 123:517–518, 1988.

104. Diters RW, Walsh KM: Canine cutaneous clear cell melanomas: A report of three cases. Vet Pathol 21:355–356, 1984.

105. Whiteley LO, Leininger JR: Neuroendocrine (Merkel cell) tumors of the canine oral cavity. Vet Pathol 24:570–572, 1987.

106. Nickoloff BJ, Hill J, Weiss LM: Canine neuroendocrine carcinoma: A tumor resembling histiocytoma. Am J Dermatopathol 7:579–586, 1985.

107. London CA, Dubilzeig RR, Vail DM: Ear canal tumors of dogs and cats: A VCOG retrospective study (1978–1992). J Am Vet Med Assoc, in press.

108. Rogers KS: Tumors of the ear canal. Vet Clin North Am [Small Anim Pract] 18:859–867, 1988.

109. Little CJL, Pearson GR, Lane JG: Neoplasia involving the middle ear cavity in dogs. Vet Rec 124:54–57, 1989.

110. Marino DJ, MacDonald JM, Matthiesen DT, et al: Results of surgery and long-term follow-up in dogs with ceruminous gland adenocarcinoma. J Am Anim Hosp Assoc 29:560–563, 1993.

111. Marino DJ, MacDonald JM, Matthiesen DT, Patnaik AK: Results of surgery in cats with ceruminous gland adenocarcinoma. J Am Anim Hosp Assoc 30:54–58, 1994.

112. Barthez PY, Theon AP, Madewell BR: Radiation therapy in the treatment of ceruminous gland adenocarcinomas in dogs and cats: 10 cases. Proc Annu Conf Vet Cancer Soc 13:56–57, 1993.

113. Brewer WG: Personal communication, VCOG study coordinator for subungual neoplasms project, Auburn University, Auburn, AL, March 18, 1994.

114. O'Brien MG, Berg J, Engler SJ: Treatment by digital amputation of subungual squamous cell carcinoma in dogs: 21 cases (1987–1988). J Am Vet Med Assoc 201:759–761, 1992.

115. Scott DW, Miller WH: Disorders of the claw and clawbed in dogs. Compend Contin Educ Pract Vet 14:1448–1458, 1992.

116. Paradis M, Scott DW, Breton L: Squamous cell carcinoma of the nail bed in three related giant schnauzers. Vet Rec 125:322–324, 1989.

117. O'Rourke M: Multiple digital squamous cell carcinomas in 2 dogs. Mod Vet Pract 66:644–645, 1985.

118. Carpenter JL, Dayal Y, King NW, Moore FM: Distinctive unclassified mesenchymal tumor of the digit of dogs. Vet Pathol 28:396–402, 1991.

119. Pollack M, Martin RA, Diters RW: Metastatic squamous cell carcinoma in multiple digits of a cat: Case report. J Am Anim Hosp Assoc 20:835–839, 1984.

120. May C, Newsholme SJ: Metastasis of feline pulmonary carcinoma presenting as multiple digital swelling. J Small Anim Pract 30:302–310, 1989.

121. Scott-Moncrieff JC, Elliott GS, Radovsky A, Blevins WE: Pulmonary squamous cell carcinoma with multiple digital metastases in a cat. J Small Anim Pract 30:696–699, 1989.

122. Brown PJ, Hoare CM, Rochlitz I: Multiple squamous cell carcinoma of the digits in two cats. J Small Anim Pract 26:323–328, 1985.

# 16

# Mast Cell Tumors

## David M. Vail

The neoplastic proliferation of mast cells referred to as mast cell tumors (histiocytic mastocytoma, mast cell sarcoma) represents the most commonly encountered cutaneous tumor in the dog and the second most common cutaneous tumor in the cat.[1-6] Systemic forms of the disease are often referred to as mastocytosis. Canine and feline forms of the disease will be considered separately in this chapter, as many differences exist with regard to histologic type, biologic behavior, therapy, and prognosis.

## CANINE MAST CELL TUMORS

### Incidence and Risk Factors

Mast cell tumors (MCTs) represent the most common cutaneous tumor in the dog, accounting for somewhere between 16 and 21% of all cutaneous tumors in this species.[1-4] MCTs are primarily a disease of older dogs with a mean age of approximately 9 years, but have been reported in dogs from 3 weeks to 19 years of age.[1-4,7,8] Most occur in mixed breeds; however, boxers, Boston terriers, Labradors, terriers, beagles, and schnauzers have all been reported to be predisposed.[1,2,7,9] While boxers are at increased risk for development, accounting for nearly half of the dogs in one large series, they more commonly develop the histologically well-differentiated form of the disease, which carries a more favorable prognosis.[1] No sex predilection has been reported.

Multiple spontaneously regressing cutaneous MCTs in a 3-week-old Jack Russell terrier have

been described.[8] All the tumors regressed spontaneously within 27 weeks. Spontaneously regressing MCTs in young animals have been described in cats, pigs, foals, and humans. This syndrome of spontaneous regression in young animals implies a hyperplastic or dysplastic syndrome rather than a true neoplastic lesion.

The etiology of MCTs in the dog is for the most part unknown. On rare occasions MCTs have been associated with chronic inflammation or the application of skin irritants.[10-12] Unequivocal evidence is lacking for a viral etiology, although MCTs have been transplanted to susceptible laboratory dogs using tumor cell tissues and rarely by cell-free extracts.[13-15] Transplantation is only successful in very young or immunocompromized puppies. No C-type or identifiable virus particles have been observed, and no epidemiologic evidence exists to suggest horizontal transmission. Chromasomal fragile site expression, a phenomenon thought to predispose humans genetically to develop certain tumors, have been shown to be increased in boxer dogs with MCTs.[16] However, the control population for this study was young, non-tumor-bearing boxers, and the increased expression of chromasomal fragile sites is likely due to this age difference.

### Pathology and Natural History

Cutaneous MCTs are thought to arise from tissue mast cells in the dermis.[5] Well-differentiated mast cells contain cytoplasmic granules that become larger as the cell matures. These granules contain a number of bioactive constituents,

**Table 16–1** Histologic Classification of Mast Cell Tumors in Dogs

| Grade | Bostock[20] Grading | Patnaik[7] Grading | Microscopic Description |
|---|---|---|---|
| Anaplastic, undifferentiated | 1 | 3 | Highly cellular, undifferentiated cytoplasmic boundaries, irregular size and shape of nuclei; frequent mitotic figures; low number of cytoplasmic granules. |
| Intermediate differentiation | 2 | 2 | Cells closely packed with indistinct cytoplasmic boundaries; nucleus-to-cytoplasmic ratio lower than anaplastic; mitotic figures infrequent; more granules than anaplastic. |
| Well differentiated | 3 | 1 | Clearly defined cytoplasmic boundaries with regular spherical, or ovoid nuclei; mitotic figures rare or absent; cytoplasmic granules large, deep-staining, and plentiful. |

including histamine and heparin, which stain metachromatically with toluidine blue.

There is a wide variation in the histologic pattern seen in canine MCTs, and histologic grade has been clearly established as a strong prognostic factor highly predictive of biologic behavior and clinical outcome. Several investigators have applied histologic grading systems to canine mast cell tumors based on the degree of differentiation (Table 16–1). Because the number grades used in these studies are at odds, for the sake of clarity, the three differentiation groups should be simply referred to as undifferentiated grade, intermediate grade, and well-differentiated grade. Table 16–2 lists the relative distribution of MCT grades encountered in larger series. Highly anaplastic agranular MCTs may be difficult to diagnose by routine light microscopy. Immunohistochemical techniques have been applied in hopes they would be helpful in differentiating these from other anaplastic round cell tumors.[17,18] Mast cell tumors are vimentin positive and the majority are $\alpha$1-antitrypsin positive. In cases of high anaplasia, electron microscopic ultrastructural appearance is ultimately required for definitive conformation.

The true metastatic potential of canine MCTs is not entirely known. Histologic grade appears to be very predictive of such behavior. Early necropsy reports state the metastatic potential of MCTs is as high as 96% of all cases.[19] It must be stressed that these numbers are artificially overestimated, because the necropsy population in this generally untreated series either died or were euthanized as a direct result of their tumor. It is therefore likely the majority of dogs in the series suffered from anaplastic, undifferentiated tumors, which carry a poor prognosis. The clinical experience of the author and others suggests that the metastatic potential of well-differentiated tumors is low (i.e., less than 10%) and that of intermediate grades to be low to moderate.[7,20–22] Metastatic rates for undifferentiated tumors range from 55 to 96%. The majority disseminate first to local lymph nodes then to spleen and liver. Other visceral organs may be involved, though the lungs are infrequently involved. Neoplastic mast cells may be observed in the bone marrow and peripheral blood in cases of widespread systemic dissemination. Bone marrow involvement occurs in as many as half of the cases of anaplastic visceral MCTs.

Complications related to bioactive constituents of mast cell granules can occur with MCTs. Gas-

**Table 16–2** Relative Frequency of Mast Cell Tumors by Histologic Grade

| Investigator | Number of Dogs | Undiffer-entiated (%) | Intermediate Grade (%) | Well Differentiated (%) |
|---|---|---|---|---|
| Hottendorf[11] | 300 | 19 | 27 | 54 |
| Bostock[20] | 114 | 39 | 26 | 34 |
| Patnaik[7] | 83 | 20 | 43 | 36 |

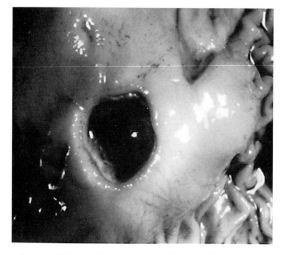

**Figure 16–1.** Perforated ulcer in the pylorus of a dog with an extensive cutaneous mast cell tumor.

trointestinal ulceration is common, reported to occur in 35 to 83% of necropsy specimens (Fig. 16–1).[23,24] A small percentage of these may go on to perforate. Histamine, released from MCT granules, is thought to act on parietal cells via $H_2$ receptors, resulting in increased hydrochloric acid secretion. Plasma histamine concentrations are increased in dogs with MCTs.[23] These dogs also have lowered concentrations of plasma gastrin normally released by antral G-cells in response to increased gastric hydrochloric acid concentrations, acting as a negative feedback loop. Increased gastric acid secretion in combination with vascular damage is likely the cause of gastric ulceration. Perioperative degranulation of MCTs and the subsequent release of histamine and other less characterized vasoative amines may also result in potentially life-threatening hypotensive events during surgery. Coagulation abnormalities, also reported in dogs with MCTs, are likely due to heparin release from mast cell granules.[25,26] While clinical evidence of hemorrhage is not typically associated with this phenomenon, at the time of surgery localized hemorrhage due to degranulation following tumor manipulation can become a serious event, even in the presence of normal presurgical coagulation parameters.

Delayed wound healing at the site of removal of MCTs has been attributed to local effects of proteolytic enzymes and vasoactive amines released by the tumor. Studies in mice suggest that histamine released from the tumor binds to $H_1$ and $H_2$ receptors of macrophages, resulting in the release of a fibroblastic suppressor factor that decreases normal fibroplasia and delays wound healing.[27]

## History and Clinical Signs

Cutaneous MCTS have an extremely varied range of clinical appearance. The majority of tumors are solitary; however, 11 to 14% of animals present with multiple lesions.[11,28,29] Their appearance has been correlated with the degree of histologic differentiation.[20] Well-differentiated MCTs tend to be solitary, slow-growing, rubbery tumors 1 to 4 cm in diameter, often present for at least 6 months. They are not typically ulcerated, but overlying hair may be lost (Fig. 16–2). Undifferentiated MCTs tend to be rapidly growing ulcerated lesions that cause considerable irritation and attain a large size (Fig. 16–3). Surrounding tissues may become inflamed and edematous. Small satellite nodules may develop in surrounding tissues. Tumors of intermediate-grade differentiation fill the spectrum between these two extremes. A subcutaneous form of MCT that is soft and fleshy on palpation is often misdiagnosed clinically as a lipoma (Fig. 16–4).

The history and clinical signs of dogs with MCTs may be complicated by signs attributable to release of histamine, heparin, and other vasoactive amines. Occasionally, mechanical manipulation during examination of the tumor results in degranulation and subsequent erythema and wheal formation in surrounding tis-

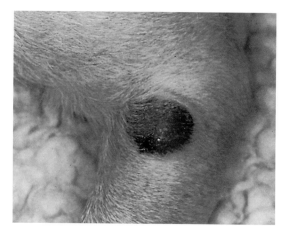

**Figure 16–2.** Well-differentiated mast cell tumor on the lateral aspect of the antebrachium. The overlying hair has been lost. This tumor had been present for 3 months prior to presentation.

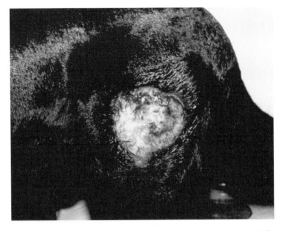

**Figure 16–3.** A large, rapidly growing undifferentiated mast cell tumor on the upper hindlimb of a black Labrador. Note significant ulceration. The subcutaneous tissues surrounding the mass were edematous and inflamed.

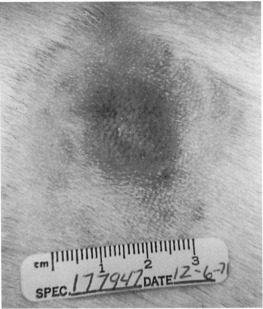

**Figure 16–5.** Erythema and wheal formation occurred in surrounding skin following manipulation of this cutaneous mast cell tumor. This phenomenon, resulting from release of vasoactive amines from mast cell granules, is known as Darier's sign.

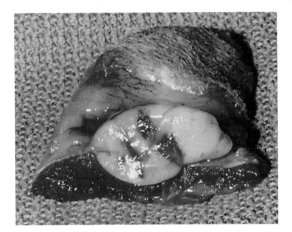

**Figure 16–4.** Subcutaneous mast cell tumor from the shoulder of a dog. This mass was originally misdiagnosed as a lipoma, based on palpation alone. Note tumor extension through fascia and muscle. Wide surgical excision to include the deep muscle layer is necessary to achieve complete ("clean") surgical margins.

sues. This phenomenon has been referred to as Darier's sign (Fig. 16–5).[29] As previously discussed, gastrointestinal ulceration can occur, and related signs of vomiting (possibly with blood), anorexia, melena, and abdominal pain may result.

Normal mast cells are found in abundance in the lung and gastrointestinal tract; however, these sites exhibit low prevalence rates for the development of MCTs. In the dog, cutaneous MCTs most frequently arise from the dermis and

subcutaneous tissues. They are most commonly found on the trunk, accounting for approximately 50 to 60% of all sites.[2,20] Tumors on the limbs account for approximately one quarter of all sites, and lesions are least common on the head and neck. Mast cell tumors have been reported to occur infrequently in other sites, including the conjunctiva, salivary gland, nasopharynx, larynx, and oral cavity.[30–33]

A visceral form of MCT, often referred to as disseminated mastocytosis, can also occur.[26,34] In the dog, visceral MCT is almost always preceded by the presence of an undifferentiated primary cutaneous lesion. Consistent abnormalities include lymphadenopathy, splenomegaly, and hepatomegaly, representing disseminated MCTs. Bone marrow and peripheral blood involvement with neoplastic mast cells are common. Pleural and peritoneal effusions containing abundant numbers of neoplastic mast cells have been observed in a number of dogs with visceral MCTs.

## Prognostic Factors

A discussion of the prognostic factors associated with canine MCTs will precede the sections on

**Table 16–3**   Prognostic Factor for Mast Cell Tumors in Dogs

| Factor | Comment |
| --- | --- |
| Histologic grade | Strongly predictive of outcome. Dogs with undifferentiated tumors typically die of their disease following local therapy, whereas those with well-differentiated tumors are usually cured with appropriate local therapy.[7, 20–22] |
| Clinical stage | Stage 0 and 1, confined to the skin without local lymph node or distant metastasis have a better prognosis than higher-stage disease.[20, 21, 38] |
| Location | Periprepucial, subungual, perianal, oral, and other mucocutaneous sites are associated with more undifferentiated tumors and poorer prognosis. Visceral or bone marrow disease carries a grave prognosis.[21, 35–37] |
| AgNOR count | Relative frequency of AgNOR's (agrophillic nucleolar orianizer regions) is predictive of postsurgical outcome. The higher the AgNOR count, the poorer the prognosis.[22] |
| Growth rate | MCT that remain localized and are present for prolonged periods of time (months or even years) are usually benign.[20] |
| Breed | MCT in boxers tend to be more well differentiated and carry a better prognosis.[1] |
| DNA ploidy | Trend toward shorter survivals and higher-stage disease in dogs with aneuploid tumors.[38] |
| Recurrence | Recurrence following surgical excision is felt by some to carry a more guarded prognosis.[36, 37] |
| Systemic signs | The presence of systemic illness (i.e., anorexia, vomiting, GI ulceration, melena) is associated with more aggressive forms of MCT.[26, 34] |

diagnosis and treatment because the steps followed in these sections are predicated on the presence or absence of these factors. Table 16–3 lists the factors known to be predictive of biologic behavior and clinical outcome in dogs with MCTs.

Histologic grade is the most consistent prognostic factor available for dogs with MCTs.[7,20–22] Survival following surgical excision based on grade is presented in Table 16–4. The vast majority of dogs with well-differentiated tumors (80–90%) and approximately 50 to 75% of dogs with intermediate-grade differentiation go on to enjoy long-term survival following complete surgical excision. Dogs with undifferentiated tumors typically die of their disease within 6 months of surgical excision, primarily because of local recurrence or metastasis to regional nodes and beyond. Recently, silver colloid staining of paraffin-embedded sections to determine the relative presence of so-called agrophillic nucleolar organizer regions (AgNORs) has been correlated with histologic grade and postsurgical outcome.[22]

**Table 16–4**   Survival of Dogs with Mast Cell Tumors Based on Histologic Grade

| Investigator | Number of Dogs | Percentage Alive | Months Postsurgery | Median Survival (Weeks) |
| --- | --- | --- | --- | --- |
| Bostock[20] | | | | |
| Well differentiated | 39 | 79 | 7 | |
| Intermediate differentiation | 30 | 37 | 7 | N/R |
| Undifferentiated | 45 | 15 | 7 | |
| Patnaik et al.[7] | | | | |
| Well differentiated | 30 | 83 | 48 | |
| Intermediate differentiation | 36 | 44 | 48 | N/R |
| Undifferentiated | 17 | 6 | 48 | |
| Bostock[22] | | | | |
| Well differentiated | 19 | 90 | | 40+ |
| Intermediate differentiation | 16 | 75 | N/R | 35+ |
| Undifferentiated | 15 | 27 | | 13 |

N/R = not reported; + = median dog still alive at time of writing.

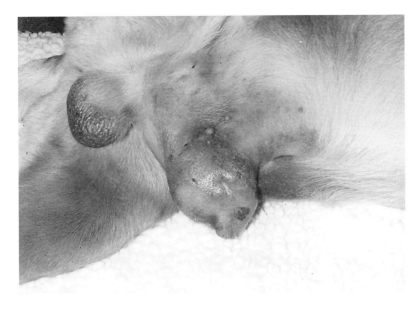

**Figure 16–6.** Mast cell tumors occurring in the prepucial area are nearly always anaplastic tumors, as was the case in this retriever. Tumors in this area have high metastatic potential, spreading to inguinal lymph nodes and beyond. Note edema and Darier's sign in the surrounding tissues.

AgNORs are thought to be an indirect measure of cell proliferation. In a study of 50 dogs with cutaneous MCTs, the AgNOR count was as reliable or even more predictive of biologic behavior than histologic grade. This relatively easy procedure can be performed on cytologic as well as histologic specimens and so may in the future provide simple, readily attainable prognostic information.

Several investigators feel that tumor location can be used to predict outcome.[21,35–37] Tumors in the prepucial/-inguinal area (Fig. 16–6), subungual (nail-bed) region (Fig. 16–7), and other mucocutaneous sites, including the oral cavity and perineum, are often associated with undifferentiated tumors that metastasize early in the course of their disease. One series of MCTs treated with radiotherapy following incomplete surgical excision reported a significant survival advantage for tumors present on extremities versus tumors occurring on the trunk.[21] This is felt to reflect the poor prognosis associated with inguinal and perineal sites.

Clinical stage, represented in Table 16–5, is also predictive of outcome.[20,21,38] Bostock[20] reported that growth rate, determined by dividing tumor volume by the time in weeks that the tumor is present, was significantly prognostic. More simply stated, recent rapid growth is a negative prognostic sign. A study of DNA ploidy determined by flow-cytometric analysis revealed a trend toward shorter survival and higher clinical stage of disease in aneuploid tumors when compared to diploid tumors.[38] Simple light microscopic criteria are of greater predictive value, however; therefore ploidy assessment is not a cost-effective procedure for MCTs.

Systemic signs of anorexia, vomiting, melena, widespread erythema, and edema associated with vasoactive substances from mast cell degranula-

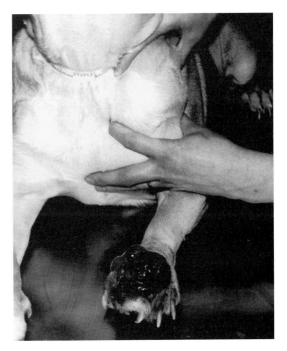

**Figure 16–7.** Subungual undifferentiated mast cell tumor in an English bulldog. As with most mast cell tumors in this location, early lymph node metastasis has occurred.

**Table 16–5**   World Health Organization Clinical Staging System for Mast Cell Tumors

| Stage | Description |
|---|---|
| 0 | One tumor incompletely excised from the dermis, identified histologically, without regional lymph node involvement.<br>    a. Without systemic signs<br>    b. With systemic signs |
| I | One tumor confined to the dermis, without regional lymph node involvement.<br>    a. Without systemic signs<br>    b. With systemic signs |
| II | One tumor confined to the dermis, with regional lymph node involvement.<br>    a. Without systemic signs<br>    b. With systemic signs |
| III | Multiple dermal tumors; large infiltrating tumors with or without regional lymph node involvement.<br>    a. Without systemic signs<br>    b. With systemic signs |
| IV | Any tumor with distant metastasis or recurrence with metastasis[a] |

[a]Including blood or bone marrow involvement.

tion are more commonly associated with visceral forms of MCTs and as such carry a more guarded prognosis.[26,34] In 16 cases of visceral MCTs a median survival of 90 days was reported and all

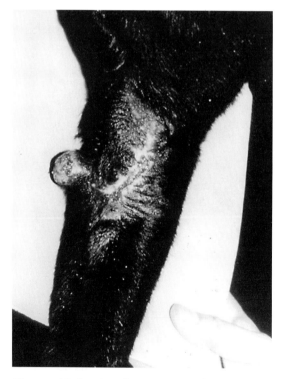

**Figure 16–8.** Local recurrence of a mast cell tumor within 1 month of attempted excision. Recurrence is often associated with more aggressive tumors.

dogs with follow-up died of their disease.[26] The recurrence of MCTs following surgical excision is felt by some to be associated with a more guarded prognosis (Fig. 16–8). This probably relates to the degree of differentiation because local recurrence rates increase as the degree of differentiation decreases.

## Diagnostic Technique and Workup

Mast cell tumors are initially diagnosed on the basis of fine-needle aspirate cytology. Rowmanovsky's or rapid hematologic-type stains present in most practices will suffice. Mast cells appear as small to medium-sized, round cells with abundant, small, uniform cytoplasmic granules that stain purplish red (metachromatic) (Fig. 16–9).[1,39] A small percentage of MCTs have granules that do not stain readily, giving them an epithelial-like or macrophage-like appearance. In these cases histologic assessment is necessary for diagnosis.

The extent of ancillary diagnostic workup following fine-needle aspirate cytologic diagnosis is predicated on the presence or absence of negative prognostic indices discussed previously. Figure 16–10 illustrates the diagnostic steps and the order in which they are pursued in the author's practice. If the MCT is in a location amenable to wide surgical excision and no negative prognostic indices are present (see Table 16–3), no further diagnostic staging is performed at that point and wide surgical excision is undertaken. The excised tumor is submitted for histopathologic assessment of grade and completeness of surgical removal (margins).

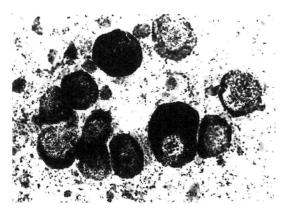

**Figure 16–9.** Fine-needle aspiration of a mast cell tumor in a dog. Note the presence of individual round cells with round to oval nuclei that are obscured by an abundance of fine basophilic cytoplasmic granules. Numerous mast cell granules are present in the background. (Wright stain, 1000X.)

both peripheral blood and buffy coat smears in determining systemic involvement. When performing ancillary tests for staging, it is important to realize that mast cells are also found in normal tissues. In 56 healthy non-tumor-bearing beagle dogs, approximately 24% of lymph node aspirates contained mast cells (range of 1–16 mast cells/slide, mean of 6.4/slide).[40] Of 51 bone marrow samples examined, 2 slides contained a single mast cell. No mast cells were observed in any of the 53 buffy coat smears examined from these normal beagles. This study was of normal beagles, and mast cell numbers could potentially be increased in dogs without MCTs who have inflammatory or allergic disease manifestations. Indeed, peripheral mastocytemia (1–90 mast cells/µl) is reported in dogs with acute inflammatory disease, in particular, parvoviral infections.[41]

Knowledge of the extent of the MCT margins

Fine-needle aspirate cytology is not sufficient to grade MCTs; therefore, histological assessment is strongly recommended. Further diagnostics and therapeutics may be performed if the excised specimen is determined to be an undifferentiated tumor or if surgical margins are incomplete.

If, however, the tumor presents at a site that is not amenable to wide surgical excision (e.g., distal extremity), or if negative prognostic factors exist in the history or physical exam, ancillary diagnostics to stage the disease thoroughly are undertaken prior to definitive therapy. These include cytologic assessment of regional lymph nodes, a complete blood count (CBC), and buffy coat smear to document peripheral mastocytosis, abdominal ultrasound with cytological assessment of spleen or liver if warranted, thoracic radiographs (usually negative), and a bone marrow aspirate. An incisional biopsy is often performed at this point to determine histologic grade. The results of the more thorough workup allow the clinician to prognosticate better the likelihood of response to further treatment and to help plan the type and extent of definitive therapy.

Careful examination of peripheral blood and bone marrow cytology is of particular importance to help rule out systemic or visceral dissemination of disease. Peripheral eosinophilia are observed in approximately 13% of visceral MCT cases, peripheral basophilia in 31%.[26] Buffy coat smears are positive for mast cells in 37% of cases, and 56% of bone marrow aspirates reveal mast cell dissemination in the visceral form. Bone marrow cytology appears to be superior to

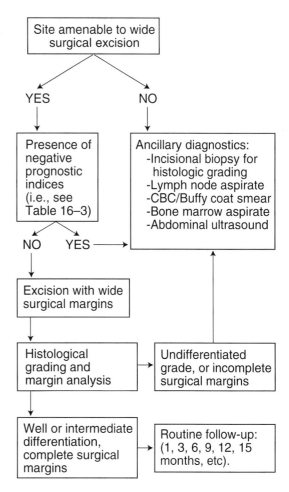

**Figure 16–10.** Suggested diagnostic steps for canine cutaneous mast cell tumors.

prior to surgery, usually accomplished by digital palpation and occasionally local radiographs, can be enhanced with the use of diagnostic ultrasound (US) or computed tomography (CT). Dogs bearing cutaneous mast cell tumors or soft tissue sarcomas have had the extent of local tumor margins upgraded in 19 and 65% of cases using US and CT, respectively.[42] Such information allows more appropriate planning of definitive surgery or radiotherapy. The cost effectiveness of such a study depends on the location of the tumor and whether wide excision is technically easy or difficult.

## Treatment

Treatment decisions are predicated on the presence or absence of negative prognostic indices and on the clinical stage of disease. Surgical excision and radiation therapy are the most successful treatment options available to date. In tumors staged just to the skin in areas amenable to wide excision, surgery is the treatment of choice. Surgical excision to include a 3 cm margin of surrounding normal tissue should be planned (Fig. 16–11). Extensive deep margins are as important as lateral margins, and if necessary fascial and muscle layers are removed in continuity with the tumor (e.g., see Fig. 16–4). As previously stated, all surgical margins should be evaluated histologically for completeness of excision. The tumors in areas not amenable to such wide surgical margins, such as distal extremities, should be evalu-

ated by incisional biopsy for histologic grade prior to definitive therapy. If the tumor is of well or intermediate-grade differentiation, three primary therapy options exist. The most aggressive option is amputation. Amputation generally guarantees wide margins but results in the least functional outcome of the three options. The second option is external beam radiotherapy alone, which produces varying control rates in the literature when used as a primary therapy.[21,43–47] Radiotherapy alone at dosages between 40 and 45 Gray result in 1-year control rates of approximately 50%. It is possible that more aggressive total doses of 48 to 57 Gray now employed by many veterinary radiotherapy facilities may improve on these results. The third, and in the author's opinion, the ideal option for well or intermediate-grade MCTs in areas where wide surgical excision is not possible is a combination of surgery and radiotherapy. The veterinary literature has established that the complementary use of surgery to achieve clinical stage 0 disease (i.e., microscopically incomplete margins) and external beam radiotherapy is associated with long-term control. Two-year control rates of 85 to 95% can be expected for stage 0 tumors of well or intermediate-grade differentiation.[21,48] Unfortunately, dogs with undifferentiated tumors do not fare nearly as well, with the majority developing distant metastasis within a few months of therapy. Regardless of the local therapy chosen, dogs with well and intermediate-grade tumors should be re-evaluated regularly for local recur-

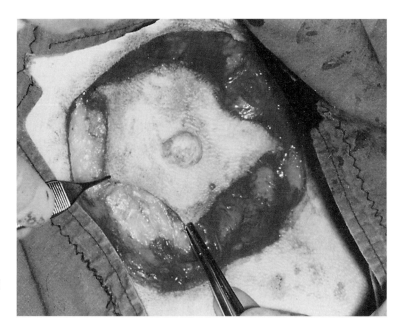

**Figure 16–11.**   Surgical excision of a cutaneous mast cell tumor from a dog. Note the wide, 3 cm surgical margins recommended to achieve complete excision.

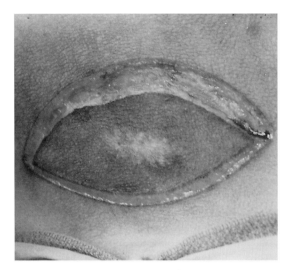

**Figure 16–12.** Re-excision of a mast cell tumor from the skin of a golden retriever whose first surgery resulted in incomplete surgical margins. The surgeon takes 3 cm margins around and wide of the previous incision and again submits the entire sample for margin analysis.

oughly investigated, clinically effective, or practical as surgery, radiation therapy, or combinations of the two. Despite its widespread use, there is no clinical data available to suggest that additional adjuvant corticosteroid therapy is of any benefit in cases of intermediate-grade MCTs that have been either excised completely or have been treated with local radiotherapy. Local immunostimulation of MCT excision sites has been studied using the biologic response modifier *C. parvum* and found to have no significant impact on recurrence rates.[49]

The treatment of anaplastic or undifferentiated MCTs remains a frustrating undertaking for both the client and the practicing clinician. This includes dogs with intermediate-grade tumors with regional or distant spread; in the author's opinion, such tumors behave similarly to undifferentiated tumors. Client education with respect to prognosis is essential in the decision-making process. Undifferentiated tumors should be treated with local surgery or radiotherapy only if thorough staging

rence and possible systemic spread. It is recommended patients be re-evaluated 1 month after definitive therapy, then every 3 months for 1.5 years, then every 6 months thereafter. Local site evaluation, complete physical exam, and buffy coat smears are performed at these intervals. More complete staging, including abdominal ultrasound and bone marrow aspirate, is pursued if warranted based on these findings.

For cases in which planned curative excisional surgery is unsuccessful and histologic margins are reported as incomplete, further local therapy is warranted. A second excision with additional wide margins of the surgical scar if possible (Fig. 16–12) or adjuvant radiotherapy is recommended. Not all MCTs with surgically incomplete margins will recur; in one report only 30% of MCTs with histologically confirmed incomplete margins did so.[49] This figure seems extremely low based on the personal experience of the author and may reflect confusion with normal cutaneous mast cells at the surgical margin. Figure 16–13 summarizes the treatment recommendations for clinical stage 1, histologically well-differentiated, or intermediate-grade MCTs. Alternative local therapies for confined MCTs have been reported and include hyperthermia in combination with radiotherapy,[50] intralesional brachytherapy,[51] photodynamic therapy,[52,53] intralesional corticosteroids,[54] cryotherapy, and intralesional deionized water.[55] None is as thor-

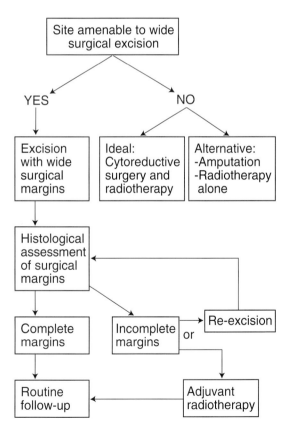

**Figure 16–13.** Suggested treatment of stage 1, histologically well or intermediately differentiated mast cell tumors in the dog.

fails to reveal dissemination and if the clients are fully informed as to the likelihood of future dissemination. The long-term prognosis for such dogs is poor because regional and distant metastasis is likely, especially in prognostically negative sites such as prepucial and perianal areas.

Poorly differentiated and metastatic MCTs will almost invariably kill the host in the absence of effective postsurgical intervention. Unfortunately, to date, no adjuvant therapy modalities (i.e., chemotherapy and immunotherapy) have been established that offer consistent, meaningful, or durable control of metastatic MCTs. Corticosteroids such as prednisone have been reported for many years in primarily preclinical or anecdotal settings to be of some benefit.[56-58] Recently the Veterinary Cooperative Oncology Group (VCOG) studied the efficacy of single-agent systemic prednisone therapy for intermediate-grade and undifferentiated canine MCTs.[59] Of 21 dogs receiving 1 mg/kg daily PO, only 1 complete response and 4 partial responses were noted. Responses were short-lived, lasting only a few weeks in the majority of cases. Corticosteroids may decrease peripheral tumor edema and give false impressions of partial response; however, no evidence exists that steroids are directly cytotoxic to neoplastic mast cells. Other chemotherapeutics have been used in attempts to control disseminated canine MCTs. These include COP (cyclophosphamide, vincristine, prednisone) combinations,[1,36] doxorubicin,[36] mitoxantrone,[60] and L-asparginase.[61] In general, the responses have been infrequent and short-lived. The vinca alkaloids vincristine and vinblastine have produced anecdotal responses in some dogs with MCTs, including a number of cases treated by the author. In the author's experience, both vinca alkaloids result in objective responses in approximately one third of cases, but they are not durable, and disease progression begins again within a few weeks.

The frequency to which we as clinicians must deal with MCTs, combined with our nearly complete lack of available adjuvant therapies, should make this a vital area of investigation in veterinary oncology. Another essential question that continues to be a source of controversy is what to do with MCTs of intermediate grade following complete (i.e., clean) surgical excision. We now know that incompletely excised intermediate-grade tumors can be effectively managed with follow-up radiotherapy, as previously stated. However, the management of those excised with complete margins remains controversial. From

Bostock's[20,22] and Patnaik's[7] work, one half to three quarters of the MCTs in this category are essentially cured; however, at present we have no way of predicting which of these cases are likely to disseminate. Some clinicians recommend adjuvant therapy with long-term corticosteroids, others with a number of cycles of vinca alkaloids, and still others recommend radiotherapy in the face of complete surgical margins. There is no clinical data to suggest any of these strategies has benefit in this setting. Other investigators feel, because of the lack of proven efficacy for adjuvant therapies in completely excised intermediate-grade MCTs, no further therapy be recommended and these animals be placed on a rigorous re-evaluation schedule. The suggested strategy in Figure 16–13 reflects that view.

Ancillary therapy for the systemic effects of MCTs related to degranulation is sometimes recommended. Blocking all or some of the effects of histamine release can be accomplished by administering the $H_1$ blocker diphenhydramine (2–4 mg/kg PO BID) and the $H_2$ blockers cimetidine (4 mg/kg PO TID) or ranitidine (2 mg/kg BID). The author generally reserves the use of these agents to those cases in which (1) systemic signs are present, (2) the tumor is likely to be entered or manipulated at surgery (i.e., cytoreductive surgery), and (3) treatment is undertaken when gross disease will remain and degranulation is likely to occur in situ (e.g., radiotherapy, corticosteroid, or chemotherapy for tumors that are not cytoreduced). These agents are not routinely used for cases in which surgical excision is to occur without excessive manipulation of the tumor proper. For cases with active evidence of gastric or duodenal ulceration, the addition of succralfate (0.5 to 1.0 gm PO TID) and occasionally misoprostol (3 mg/kg PO TID) to histamine blockers is prudent. The use of protamine sulfate, a heparin antagonist, has been mentioned by some for use in cases of intraoperative hemorrhage.[37]

## FELINE MAST CELL TUMORS

### Incidence and Risk Factors

MCTs represent the second most commonly encountered cutaneous tumor in the cat, accounting for approximately 20% of cutaneous tumors in this species in the United States.[3,5,6] The incidence of MCTs in cats appears to have increased dramaticaly since 1950.[5] MCTs in the United Kingdom appear to occur much less frequently, accounting for only 8% of all cutaneous tumors.[1] Two distinct forms of cutaneous MCTs in the cat have been reported: (1) the more typical mastocytic MCTs, histologically similar to MCTs in dogs, and (2) the less common histiocytic MCTs, with morphologic features characteristic of histiocytic mast cells. An overall mean age of 8 to 9 years is reported for cats with MCTs; however, the mastocytic and histiocytic forms occur at mean ages of 10 and 2.4 years, respectively.[5,6,62] Siamese cats appear to be predisposed to development of MCTs of both histologic types.[5,6,63,64] The distinct histiocytic form of MCTs in cats has been reported to occur primarily in young (< 4 years of age) Siamese cats, including two related litters. In contrast to these reports, Siamese cats have not been found any more likely to develop the histiocytic form of MCTs than the mastocytic form, as reported in another series of cases.[6] This report found only two of seven cases of histiocytic MCTs were from Siamese in their hospital population. Earlier studies reported a male predilection for development of MCTs;[62,65] however, larger more recent series have failed to confirm such a predilection.[5,6]

Visceral MCTs appear to be more common in the cat than in the dog, with up to 50% of MCT cases occurring in visceral sites in some series.[5,66] A splenic form (sometimes referred to as lymphoreticular MCT) represents the most common differential for "splenic disease" in cats, accounting for 15% of submissions in a series of 455 pathologic specimens.[67] The mean age of affected cats is approximately 10 years and no breed or sex predilection is known.[5] Intestinal MCT is the third most common primary intestinal tumor in cats after lymphoma and adenocarcinoma.[5] No breed or sex predilection is known. Older cats appear to be at risk, with a mean age of 13 years; however, cats as young as 3 years have been reported.[68]

The etiology for cats with MCTs is unknown. Viruslike particles have been reported in tissue samples from feline MCTs but failed to grow in tissue culture and were not transmissible to other cats, mice, or hamsters.[69] No association with feline leukemia virus (FeLV), feline immunodeficiency virus (FIV), or feline infectious peritonitis (FIP) has been reported. A genetic predisposition has been proposed because of the high incidence of MCTs in the Siamese breed.

## Pathology and Natural History

The granules present in feline MCTs stain blue with giemsa, and purple with toluidine blue.[1,5,6] They tend to appear more eosinophilic than their canine counterparts, with hematoxylin and eosin stains. As in the canine, granules present in feline mast cells contain vasoactive substances such as heparin and histamine.[5,70] In culture, feline mast cells contain surface-bound immunoglobulins and are capable of secreting histamine, heparin, and probably other vasoactive compounds when appropriately stimulated.[70] Complications associated with the degranulation of MCTs can also occur in the cat, including coagulation disorders, gastrointestinal ulceration, and anaphylaxis-type reactions.[5,71,72] Feline mast cells also have phagocytic capability and can endocytize erythrocytes in both experimental models and in clinical samples.[73]

As previously mentioned, feline cutaneous MCTs occur in two primary histologically distinct forms, referred to as the mastocytic and histiocytic variaties.[6,63,64] Table 16–6 lists a brief description of the histologic appearance of each.

**Table 16–6**  Histologic Classification of Mast Cell Tumors in Cats[1, 5, 6, 63, 64, 73]

| Type | Subtype | Microscopic Description |
|---|---|---|
| Mastocytic | Compact (well differentiated) | Homogenous cords and nests of slightly atypical mast cells with basophylic round nuclei, ample eosinophylic cytoplasm, and distinct cell borders. Eosinophils conspicuous only half the time. |
| | Diffuse (anaplastic) | Less discrete, infiltrate into subcutis, larger nuclei (> 50% of cell size). 2–3 mitosis/high-power field. Marked anisocytosis, including mononuclear and multinucleated giant cells. Eosinophils more commonly observed. |
| Histiocytic | | Sheets of histiocytelike cells with equivocal cytoplasmic granularity. Accompanied by randomly scattered lymphoid aggregates and eosinophils. Granules lacking in some reports; others readily demonstrate granules. |

The mastocytic form can be further subdivided on histological appearance into two categories, often referred to as compact and diffuse, which may be of prognostic significance.[5,64,74] The compact form, reportedly comprising 50 to 90% of cases in several series, are associated with a more benign behavior. The diffuse form are histologically more anaplastic and behaviorally more malignant. The histologic grading system described for canine mast cells provided no prognostic information for the cat in one series.[62] Immunohistochemical studies have also been performed on feline MCTs; all were vimentin positive, and the majority were positive for α-1 antitrypsin.[17] Metastatic rates for cutaneous MCTs in cats vary considerably, with reported rates of 0%,[62] 14%,[63] and 22%.[5] In two studies in which behavior was separated by compact and diffuse histologies, the relative majority of cases going on to recur or metastasize were of the diffuse type.[63,74] From this information, in general, it can be stated that the majority of feline cutaneous MCTs are behaviorally benign.

The uncommon histiocytic form of feline MCTs is more challenging to diagnose histologically.[63,64] Mast cells appear to comprise only 20% of the cells present, with the majority being sheets of histiocytes that lack distinct cytoplasmic granules and are accompanied by randomly scattered lymphoid aggregates and eosinophils. One report, in contrast, readily demonstrated metachromatic granules in seven cases of the histiocytic subtype. They can be initially misdiagnosed as granulomatous nodular panniculitis or deep dermatitis. For those cases in the literature with follow-up information, spontaneous regression of histiocytic MCTs occurred over a period of 4 to 24 months.[63,64]

With regard to visceral forms of MCTs in the cat (i.e., splenic and intestinal), widespread dissemination and metastasis are much more common. Necropsy data on 30 cats with splenic MCTs revealed dissemination in the following organs in decreasing order of frequency: liver (90%), visceral lymph nodes (73%), bone marrow (40%), lung (20%), and intestine (17%).[5] Up to a third of cases have peritoneal and pleural effusions rich in eosinophils and mast cells. Peripheral blood mastocytosis is present in as many as 40% of cases.[5] In one clinical report of 43 cases, 23% had bone marrow involvement.[72] Two gross forms of splenic involvement are possible, a diffuse and smooth splenomegalic form and a less common nodular form (Figs. 16–14A and 16–14B). In one report, 18% of cats with cutaneous MCTs went on to develop splenic dis-

ease.[5] Interestingly, in the face of widespread metastasis long-term survival following splenectomy is common with splenic MCTs (see Treatment and Prognosis section later). Intestinal MCT in cats is also associated with widespread dissemination and carries a poor prognosis.[5,68] It more commonly involves the small intestine (equally divided in the duodenum, jejunum, and ileum), with colonic involvement reported in less than 15% of cases. Lesions can be solitary or multiple. Peritoneal effusion, rich in mast cells, can occur. Unlike splenic MCTs, peripheral mastocytosis is not associated with intestinal MCTs, and only two reports exist in the literature of eosinophilia.[68] Metastasis is common to mesenteric lymph nodes and the liver, followed less commonly by the spleen, lung, and bone marrow. Most animals either die or are euthanized soon after diagnosis. Histologically, the mast cells from intestinal lesions appear less well differentiated than those of skin tumors, and cytoplasmic granules are harder to find. A cranial mediastinal form of MCT in cats has also been described.[5]

## History and Clinical Signs

The typical feline cutaneous MCT is a solitary, raised, firm, well-circumscribed, hairless, dermal nodule between 0.5 and 3 cm in diameter (Fig. 16–15).[5,6,62,63] It is often white in appearance, although a pink erythematous form is occasionally encountered. Approximately 20% are multiple, although one report from the United Kingdom found the majority to present as multiple lesions.[1] Ulceration is present in approximately one fourth of cases. Two other clinical forms have been described: one a flat pruritic plaquelike lesion similar in appearance to eosinophilic plaques and the other a discrete subcutaneous nodule.

Unlike the dog, the head and neck are the most common site for MCTs in the cat, followed by the trunk, limbs, and miscellaneous sites (Fig. 16–16A and 16–16B).[5,6,62] Those on the head often involve the pinnae near the base of the ear. They rarely occur in the oral cavity. Intermittent itching and redness are common, and self-trauma or vascular compromise may result in ulceration. Darier's sign, the erythema and wheal formation following mechanical manipulation of the tumor, has been reported in the cat.[71] Affected cats are usually otherwise healthy.

The spontaneously regressing histiocytic form of cutaneous MCTs are usually multiple, nonpruritic, firm, hairless, pink, and sometimes ulcerated subcutaneous nodules (Fig. 16–17).[6,64] Affected animals are otherwise healthy.

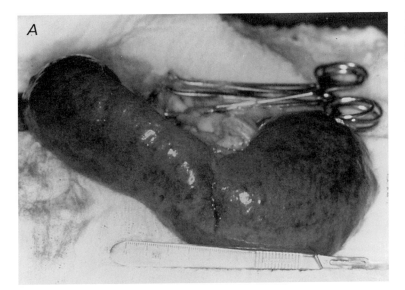

**Figure 16–14A.** Diffuse massive splenomegaly in a cat with splenic mast cell disease.

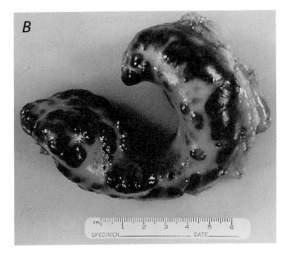

**Figure 16–14B.** The less common nodular form of splenic mast cell tumor in a cat.

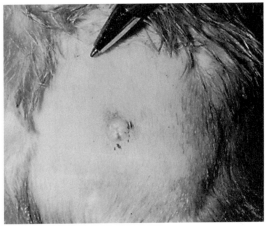

**Figure 16–15.** Typical solitary, raised, well-circumscribed, hairless dermal cutaneous mast cell tumor in a cat. Excision was curative in this case.

Cats with disseminated forms of MCTs may present with signs of systemic illness. Depression, anorexia, weight loss, and intermittent vomiting are most commonly associated with splenic and intestinal MCTs.[5,68,72,75] Abdominal palpation reveals massive splenomegaly in the majority of cases, and occasionally the presence of peritoneal effusion is suggested with splenic MCTs. Intestinal MCTs can often be palpated as well. Diarrhea with or without bloody stools is commonly seen with the intestinal form, and fever may be present. Affected cats usually have been ill for a number of months. The signs related to the release of vasoactive components of mast cell granules, including gastrointestinal ulceration, uncontrollable hemorrhage, altered smooth muscle tone, hypotensive shock, and labored breathing, are more likely to be observed with systemic forms. The signs related to vasoactive amines are often episodic in nature. Labored breathing may also occur secondary to pleural effusion or anemia, which is present in approximately one third of disseminated MCTs in cats.[5,72]

## Diagnostic Techniques and Workup

The diagnosis and staging of MCTs in cats is similar to those in the dog. Fine-needle aspiration (FNA) cytology is usually diagnostic. This includes FNA of cutaneous lesions as well as

**Figure 16–16A.** Multiple mast cell tumors on the head of a cat. The head and neck are the most commonly encountered location for these tumors in the cat. They often involve the area near the base of the ear. (Photograph courtesy of Dr. S. Helfand.)

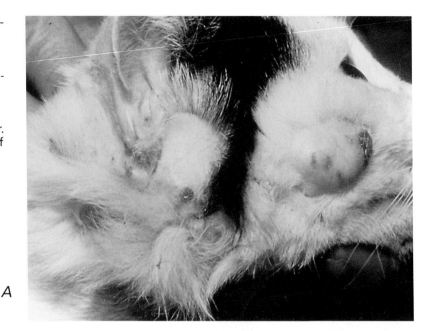

*A*

*B*

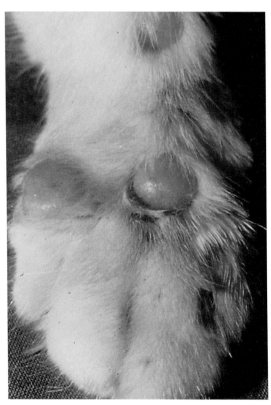

**Figure 16–16B.** Mast cell tumors in the cat are less common on the limbs. (Photograph courtesy of Dr. S. Helfand.)

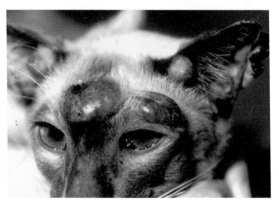

**Figure 16–17.** Histiocytic mast cell tumors on the head of a young Siamese cat. This form of mast cell tumors in cats typically regress spontaneously, as was the case in the cat pictured here. (Photo courtesy of Dr. K. Moriello.)

splenic aspirates and thoraco- and abdominocentesis in the case of pleural and peritoneal effusions. Less frequently, intestinal mass aspirates are diagnostic. Tissue biopsy and histologic assessment is typically required for the histiocytic form of MCTs, because FNA is only rarely diagnostic.

In cases in which disseminated (e.g., splenic or intestinal) disease is suspected, CBC, buffy coat smear, bone marrow aspirate, coagulation profile, and serum biochemistry profile will be helpful. One third of cats with visceral disease will be anemic, and up to 50% of cats with splenic MCTs will have evidence of bone marrow and buffy coat involvement.[5,72] Peripheral mastocytosis can be striking; peripheral mast cell counts up to 32,000 cell/μ have been reported.[5] Unlike the splenic form, intestinal MCT is not associated with peripheral mastocytosis, though eosinophilia has been reported on two occasions.[68] In one report of 43 cats with splenic MCTs, 90% had abnormalities on coagulation assessment, and while this was rarely of clinical significance, knowledge of its presence should allow preoperative precautions to be taken if surgery is contemplated.[72] Hyperglobulinemia has also been reported in cats with splenic MCTs, the cause of which remains unknown. Other common differential diagnoses for splenomegaly in the cat include lymphoma, myeloproliferative disease, accessory spleen, hemangiosarcoma, hyperplastic nodules, and splenitis.[67] The two most common differential diagnoses for intestinal masses in aged cats are lymphoma and adenocarcinoma.[5]

Thoracic and abdominal radiographs will confirm the presence of pleural and peritoneal effusions, present in up to one third of cats with splenic MCT.[5] Abdominal ultrasound may be required to determine the extent of intestinal involvement and indicate the presence of visceral dissemination. While most intestinal MCTs are either palpable or visible on abdominal radiographs or ultrasound, exploratory celeotomy may ultimately be required for definitive diagnosis.

## Treatment and Prognosis

Surgery is the treatment of choice for the mastocytic form of cutaneous MCTs in the cat. As previously discussed, most are behaviorally benign, and wide surgical margins may not be as critical as in the dog. This is fortunate, as most occur on the head, where such margins would be difficult to achieve. Frequency of local recurrence and systemic spread vary widely in the literature. Local recurrence rates of 0%,[62] 19%,[63] and 24%[5] have been reported following surgical excision. The frequency of systemic spread following surgical excision also varies, from 0%,[62] 14%,[63] and 22%.[5] Recurrence, should it take place, is usually noted within 6 months. For histologically anaplastic (i.e., diffuse) mastocytic tumors, a more aggressive approach similar to that for the dog may be prudent, because higher rates of recurrence and metastasis are associated with this type. Following biopsy confirmation, conserva-

tive resection or a wait-and-see approach may be taken with the histiocytic form in young cats with multiple masses, because the majority are reported to regress spontaneously.[5,6,64]

Little is known about the effectiveness of adjunctive therapy for cutaneous MCTs in the cat. Efficacy trials for corticosteroids, chemotherapeutics, and radiotherapy do not exist in the veterinary literature. Response to steroids in cats with the histiocytic form is equivocal.[64]

Cats with splenic MCTs will usually benefit from splenectomy. Surprisingly, even in the face of significant bone marrow and peripheral blood involvement, long-term survival with good quality of life is the norm following splenectomy, with median survivals from 12 to 19 months reported.[5,72,75-77] Anorexia, significant weight loss, and the male sex have been associated with a worsening prognosis. Frequent re-evaluation and buffy coat smears are used to follow response in such cases. Rarely does the peripheral mastocytosis resolve, but it will significantly decline, and its subsequent rise can serve as a marker of progression. Adjunctive therapy with various chemotherapy protocols, including prednisone, vincristine, cyclophosphamide, and methotrexate, have been attempted in a limited number of cases but do not appear to increase survival times.[5] Ancillary drugs to combat the effect of vasoactive amines (see discussion under canine MCTs) may transiently abate clinical signs.

The intestinal form of feline MCTs carries a poor prognosis. Metastasis at the time of diagnosis is common, and most cats either die or are euthanized soon after. If surgery is possible, wide surgical margins, including 5 to 10 cm of normal bowel on either side of the lesion are recommended, because tumor often extends histologically well beyond visible gross disease.[5]

## COMPARATIVE ASPECTS OF MAST CELL TUMORS

Mast cell cancer is rare in humans.[78] As is the case in dogs and cats, a wide range of syndromes exist from hyperplastic syndromes to malignant visceral forms and mast cell leukemia. The most common human mast cell neoplasm is a multiple cutaneous form occurring in infancy, known as urticaria pigmentosa. It is similar to mast cell disease described in kittens[5,63,64,] and an immature puppy[8] in that it arises during infancy and regresses spontaneously at the onset of puberty.

It is not, however, associated with a histiocytic histology as in the kitten. Other forms of MCTs in humans include benign systemic mastocytosis, malignant mastocytosis, and mast cell leukemia. Approximately one third of patients with urticaria pigmentosa will go on to develop malignant mastocytosis, a uniformly fatal disease. Many human patients are, like our veterinary patients, susceptible to systemic symptoms resulting from vasoactive substances released during degranulation of neoplastic mast cells. They will often benefic symptomatically from $H_1$ and $H_2$ blocking therapy. Because of the rarity of this condition, no standard treatment protocols are available for malignant mast cell disease in humans. The response to various chemotherapeutics has been disappointing.

# REFERENCES

1. Bostock DE: Neoplasms of the skin and subcutaneous tissues in dogs and cats. Br Vet J *142*:1–19, 1986.
2. Rothwell TLW, Howlett CR, Middleton DJ, et al: Skin neoplasms of dogs in Sydney. Aust Vet J *64*:161–164, 1987.
3. Brodey RS: Canine and feline neoplasia. Adv Vet Sci Comp Med *14*:309–354, 1970.
4. Finnie JW, Bostock DE: Skin neoplasia in dogs. Aust Vet J *55*:602–604, 1979.
5. Carpenter JL, Andrews LK, Holzworth J: Tumors and tumor like lesions. *In* Holzworth J (ed): Diseases of the Cat: Medicine and Surgery. Philadelphia, WB Saunders, 1987, pp. 406–596.
6. Miller MA, Nelson SL, Turk JR, et al: Cutaneous neoplasia in 340 cats. Vet Pathol *28*:389–395, 1991.
7. Patnaik AK, Ehler WJ, MacEwen EG: Canine cutaneous mast cell tumor: Morphological grading and survival time in 83 dogs. Vet Pathol *21*:469–474, 1984.
8. Davis BJ, Page R, Sannes PL, Meuten DJ: Cutaneous mastocytosis in a dog. Vet Pathol *29*:363–365, 1992.
9. Peters JA: Canine mastocytoma excess risk as related to ancestry. J Natl Cancer Inst *42*:435–443, 1969.
10. Peterson SL: Scar-associated canine mast cell tumor. Canine Pract *12*:23–29, 1985.
11. Hottendorf GH, Neilson SW: Survey of 300 extirpated canine mastocytomas. Zentralbl Veterinarmed [A] *14*:272–281, 1967.
12. Dunn TB, Patter H: A transplantable mast cell neoplasm in the mouse. J Natl Cancer Inst *18*:587–601, 1957.
13. Bowles CA, Kerber WT, Tangan SRS, et al: Characterization of a transplantable, canine, immature mast cell tumor. Cancer Res *32*:1434–1441, 1972.
14. Lombard LS, Moloney JB: Experimental transmission of mast cell sarcoma in dogs. Fed Proc *18*:490–495, 1959.
15. Nielson SW, Cole CR: Homologous transplantation of canine neoplasms. Am J Vet Res *27*:663–672, 1961.
16. Stone DM, Jacky PB, Prieur DJ: Chromasomal fragile site expression in dogs: Expression in boxer dogs with mast cell tumors. Am J Med Genetics *40*:223–229, 1991.
17. Fondevila D, Rabanal R, Ferrer L: Immunoreactivity of canine and feline mast cell tumors. Schweiz Arch Tierheilk *132*:409–484, 1990.
18. Bolon B, Calderwood Mays MB: Conjugated amidin-peroxidase as a stain for mast cell tumors. Vet Pathol *25*:523–525, 1988.
19. Hottendorf GH, Nielsen SW: Pathologic report of 29 necropsies on dogs with mastocytoma. Vet Pathol *5*:102–121, 1968.
20. Bostock DE: The prognosis following surgical removal of mastocytomas in dogs. J Small Anim Pract *14*:27–40, 1973.
21. Turrel JM, Kitchell BE, Miller LM, Theon A: Prognostic factors for radiation treatment of mast cell tumor in 85 dogs. J Am Vet Med Assoc *193*:936–940, 1988.
22. Bostock DE, Crocker J, Harris K, Smith P: Nuclear organiser regions as indicators of postsurgical prognosis in canine spontaneous mast cell tumors. Br J Cancer *59*:915–918, 1989.
23. Fox LE, Rosenthal RC, Twedt DC, et al: Plasma histamine and gastrin concentrations in 17 dogs with mast cell tumors. J Vet Intern Med *4*:242–246, 1990.
24. Howard EB, Sawa TR, Nielson SW, et al: Mastocytoma and gastroduodenal ulceration. Vet Pathol *6*:146–158, 1969.
25. Hottendorf GH, Nielson SW, Kenyon AJ: Canine mastocytoma. I. Blood coagulation in dogs with mastocytoma. Pathologica Veterinaria *2*:129–141, 1965.
26. O'Keefe DA, Couto CG, Burke-Schwartz C, Jacobs RM: Systemic mastocytosis in 16 dogs. J Vet Intern Med *1*:75–80, 1987.
27. Kenyon AJ, Ramos L, Michaels EB: Histamine-induced suppressor macrophage inhibits fibroblast growth and wound healing. Am J Vet Res *44*:2164–2166, 1983.
28. Van Pelt DR, Fowler JD, Leighton FA: Multiple cutaneous mast cell tumors in a dog: A case report and brief review. Can Vet J *27*:259–263, 1986.
29. Tams TR, Macy DW: Canine mast cell tumors. Compend Contin Educ Pract Vet *3*:869–877, 1981.
30. Johnson BW, Brightman AH, Whiteley HE: Conjunctival mast cell tumor in two dogs. J Am Anim Hosp Assoc *24*:439–442, 1988.
31. Carberry CA, Flanders JA, Anderson WI, Harvey HJ: Mast cell tumor in the mandibular salivary gland in a dog. Cornell Vet *77*:362–366, 1987.
32. Crowe DT, Goodwin MA, Greene CE: Total laryngectomy for laryngeal mast cell tumor in a dog. J Am Anim Hosp Assoc *22*:809–816, 1986.

33. Patnaik AK, MacEwen EG, Black AP, Luckow S: Extracutaneous mast-cell tumor in the dog. Vet Pathol 19:608–615, 1982.

34. Pollack MJ, Flanders JA, Johnson RC: Disseminated malignant mastocytoma in a dog. J Am Anim Hosp Assoc 27:435–440, 1991.

35. Moriello KA, Rosenthal RC: Clinical approach to tumors of the skin and subcutaneous tissues. Vet Clin North Am [Small Animal Pract] 20:1163–1190, 1990.

36. Richardson RC, Rebar AH, Elliott GS: Common skin tumors of the dog: A clinical approach to diagnosis and treatment. Compend Contin Educ Pract Vet 6:1080–1086, 1984.

37. O'Keefe DA: Canine mast cell tumors. Vet Clin North Am [Small Anim Pract] 20:1105–1115, 1990.

38. Ayl RD, Couto CG, Hammer AS, et al: Correlation of DNA ploidy to tumor histologic grade, clinical variables, and survival in dogs with mast cell tumors. Vet Pathol 29:386–390, 1992.

39. Clinkenbeard KD: Diagnostic cytology: Mast cell tumors. Compend Contin Educ Pract Vet 13:1697–1704, 1991.

40. Bookbinder PF, Butt MT, Harvey HJ: Determination of the number of mast cells in lymph node, bone marrow, and buffy coat cytologic specimens from dogs. J Am Vet Met Assoc 200:1648–1650, 1992.

41. Stockham SL, Basel DL, Schmidt DA: Mastocytemia in dogs with acute imflammatory diseases. Vet Clin Pathol 15:16–21, 1986.

42. Hahn KA, Lantz GC, Salisbury SK: Comparison of survey radiography with ultrasonography and x-ray computed tomography for clinical staging of subcutaneous neoplasms in dogs. J Am Vet Med Assoc 196:1795–1798, 1990.

43. Gillette EL: Indications and selection of patients for radiation therapy. Vet Clin North Am [Small Anim Pract] 4:889–896, 1974.

44. Gillette EL: Veterinary radiotherapy. J Am Vet Med Assoc 157:1707–1712, 1976.

45. Gillette EL: Radiation therapy of canine and feline tumors. J Am Anim Hosp Assoc 12:359–362, 1976.

46. Allan GS, Billette EL: Response of canine mast cell tumors to radiation. J Natl Cancer Inst 63:691–694, 1979.

47. McClelland RB: The treatment of mastocytomas in dogs. Cornell Vet 54:517–519, 1964.

48. Al-Sarraf R, Mauldin GN, Meleo KA, Patnaik A: A prospective study of radiation therapy for the treatment of incompletely resected grade 2 mast cell tumors in 32 dogs. Proc Annu Conf Vet Cancer Soc 13:64, 1993.

49. Misdorp W: Incomplete surgery, local immunostimulation, and recurrence of some tumour types in dogs and cats. Vet Q 9:279–286, 1987.

50. Legorreta RA, Denman DL, Kelley MC, Lewis GC: Use of hyperthermia and radiotherapy in treatment of a large mast cell sarcoma in a dog. J Am Vet Med Assoc 193:1545–1548, 1988.

51. Theon AP, Madewell BR, Castro J: High dose-rate remote afterloading brachytherapy: Preliminary results in canine and feline cutaneous and subcutaneous tumors. Proc Annu Conf Vet Cancer Soc 13:109–110, 1993.

52. Roberts WG, Klein MK, Weldy LS, Berns MW: Photodynamic therapy of spontaneous cancers in felines, canines, and snakes with chloro-aluminum sulfonated phthalocyanine. J. Natl Cancer Inst 83:18–23, 1991.

53. Dougherty TJ, Thoma RE, Boyle DG, Weishaupt KR: Interstitial photoradiation therapy for primary solid tumors in pet cats and dogs. Cancer Res 41:401–404, 1981.

54. Rogers KS: Common questions about diagnosing and treating canine mast cell tumors. Vet Med 88:246–250, 1993.

55. Grier RL, Guardo GD, Schaffer CB, et al: Mast cell tumor destruction by deionized water. Am J Vet Res 51:1116–1120, 1990.

56. Bloom F: Effect of cortisone on mast cell tumors (mastocytoma) of the dog. Proc Soc Exp Biol Med 88:79:651–654, 1952.
in a cat with multiple neoplasms. J Small Anim Pract 29:597–602, 1988.

57. Asboe-Hanson G. The mast cell: Cortisone action on connective tissue. Proc Soc Exp Biol Med 80:677–679, 1952.

58. Brodey RS, McGrath JT, Martin JE: Preliminary observations on the use of cortisone in canine mast cell sarcoma. J Am Vet Med Assoc 155:391–394, 1953.

59. McCaw DL, Miller MA, Ogilvie GK, et al: Response of canine mast cell tumors to treatment with oral prednisone. Proc Annu Conf Vet Cancer Soc 11:28, 1991.

60. Ogilvie GK, Obradovich JE, Elmslie RE, et al: Efficacy of mitoxantrone against various neoplasms in dogs. J Am Vet Med Assoc 198:1618–1621, 1991.

61. Hardy W, Old LJ: L-asparginase in the treatment of neoplastic disease of the dog, cat and cow. In Grundman E, Oettgen HF (eds): Experimental and Clinical Effects of L-asparginase. New York, Springer Verlag, 1970,. pp. 131–136.

62. Buerger RG, Scott DW: Cutaneous mast cell neoplasia in cats: 14 cases (1975–1985). J Am Vet Med Assoc 190:1440–1444, 1987.

63. Wilcock BP, Yager JA, Zink MC: The morphology and behavior of feline cutaneous mastocytomas. Vet Pathol 23:320–324, 1986.

64. Chastain CB, Turk MAM, O'Brien D: Benign cutaneous mastocytomas in two litters of Siamese kittens. J Am Vet Med Assoc 193:959–960, 1988.

65. Macy DW, Reynolds HA: The incidence, characteristics, and clinical management of skin tumors of cats. J Am Anim Hosp Assoc 17:1026–1034, 1981.

66. Neilson SW, Howard EB, Wolke RF: Feline mastocytosis. In Clark WJ, Howard EB, Hackett PL (eds): Myeloproliferative Disorders of Animals and Man. Oak Ridge, TN, U.S. Atomic Energy Commission, 1970, pp. 359–370.

67. Spangler WL, Culbertson MR: Prevalence and type of splenic diseases in cats: 455 cases (1985–1991). J Am Vet Med Assoc 201:773–776, 1992.

68. Bortnowski HB, Rosenthal RC: Gastrointestinal mast cell tumors and eosinophilia in two cats. J Am Anim Hosp Assoc 28:271–275, 1992.

69. Saar C, Opitz M, Lange W, et al: Mastzellenretikulose bei katzen. Berl Munch Tierarztl Wochenschr 82:438–444, 1969.

70. Mohr FC, Dunston SK: Culture and initial characterization of the secretory response of neoplastic cat mast cells. Am J Vet Res 53:820–828, 1992.

71. Macy DW: Darier's sign associated with a cutaneous mast cell tumour

72. Feinmehl R, Matus R, Maulden GN, Patnaik A: Splenic mast cell tumors in 43 cats (1975–1992). Proc Annu Conf Vet Cancer Soc 12:50, 1992.

73. Madewell BR, Munn RJ, Phillips LP: Endocytosis of erythrocytes in vivo and particulate substances in vitro by feline neoplastic mast cells. Can J Vet Res 51:517–520, 1987.

74. Holzinger EA: Feline cutaneous mastocytomas. Cornell Vet 63:87–93, 1973.

75. Schulman A: Splenic mastocytosis in a cat. California Vet 17:17–18, 1987.

76. Guerre R, Millet P, Groulade P: Systemic mastocytosis in a cat: Remission after splenectomy. J Small Anim Pract 20:769–772, 1979.

77. Liska WD, MacEwen EG, Zaki FA, et al: Feline systemic mastocytosis: A review and results of splenectomy in seven cases. J Am Anim Hosp Assoc 15:589–597, 1979.

78. Stone RM, Bernstein SH: Mast cell leukemia. In Holland JF, Frei E, Bast RC, Kufe DW, Morton DL, Weichselbaum RR (eds): Cancer Medicine, 3rd ed. Philadelphia, Lea & Febiger, 1993, pp. 2092–2096.

# 17

# Soft Tissue Sarcomas

E. Gregory MacEwen and Stephen J. Withrow

## INCIDENCE AND RISK FACTORS

Soft tissue sarcomas are a diverse group of cancers that collectively comprise 15% of all "skin" and subcutaneous cancers in the dog and 7% in the cat.[1] The annual incidence of soft tissue sarcomas in the dog is about 35 per 100,000 dogs at risk and 17 per 100,000 cats at risk.[2] With the exception of the feline very rare sarcoma virus-induced neoplasms of the young cat and vaccine-induced sarcomas in cats, the cause of these tumors is unknown. In dogs, sarcomas have been associated with radiation, trauma, and parasites (*Spirocerca lupi*).[3,4] Most sarcomas are solitary in the older dog or cat and no definite sex or breed predilection is known except for synovial sarcomas, in which the ratio of males to females is 3:2.[5] Rhabdomyosarcoma may occur in animals as young as 4 months. In the dog, soft tissue sarcomas tend to be reported in the larger breeds.

## PATHOLOGY AND NATURAL HISTORY

Soft tissue sarcomas develop from a variety of mesenchymal tissues (Table 17–1), although they are frequently classified inappropriately as skin or subcutaneous tumors. Both malignant and benign counterparts exist for each cell type, although this chapter will only emphasize the malignant varieties. The term *soft tissue sarcoma* generally excludes those tumors of hematopoietic or lymphoid origin. They are often considered collectively because of their similarity in clinical behavior. Hemangiosarcoma, lymphoma, mast cell sarcoma, oral sarcoma, osteosarcoma and chondrosarcoma, and feline virus-induced sarcoma are covered separately in other chapters.

Soft tissue sarcomas tend to have several important common features with regard to their biologic behavior.

- They may arise from any anatomic site in the body.
- They tend to appear as pseudoencapsulated fleshy tumors but have poorly defined histologic margins or infiltrate through facial planes.
- Local recurrence after conservative surgical excision is common.
- Sarcomas tend to metastasize through hematogenous methods in up to 25% of cases. Regional lymph node metastasis is unusual (except for synovial cell sarcoma).
- They generally have a poor response to chemotherapy and radiation therapy for measurable disease.

No other group of tumors present more of a diagnostic challenge than those originating in soft tissues. Many of these tumors present histologic patterns with overlapping features not only among themselves but also with a variety of other neoplasms with different histogenesis.[6] The development of immunocytochemical procedures and the availability of monoclonal antibodies and polyclonal antibodies to various tissue markers have significantly improved the diagnosis of soft tissue sarcomas in human pathology and to a limited degree in veterinary pathology.[7] Some of the markers used include intermediate filaments such as acidic and basic features, vimentin,

**Table 17–1**   Histiogenic Classification and Metastatic Potential of Common Soft Tissue Neoplasms

| Tissue of Origin[a] | Benign | Malignant | Metastatic Potential[b] | Other Chapters to See |
|---|---|---|---|---|
| Fibrous tissue and histiocyte | | Fibrous histiocytoma | + | |
| Fibrous tissue | Fibroma | Fibrosarcoma | +/++ | 18A |
| Myxomatous tissue | Myxoma | Myxosarcoma | +/++ | |
| Pericyte of blood vessel (unproven) | Hemangiopericytoma | Hemangiopericytoma | + | |
| Vessels | Lymphangioma | Lymphangiosarcoma | ++ | |
| | Hemangioma | Hemangiosarcoma | +++ | 29A |
| Adipose tissue | Lipoma | Liposarcoma | ++ | |
| Nerve | | Neurofibrosarcoma | + | |
| | | Malignant schwannoma | | 26 |
| Smooth muscle[c] | Leiomyoma | Leiomyosarcoma | + | 18, 22 |
| Synovial cell | Synovial cyst/ Synovioma | Synovial cell sarcoma | ++ | |
| Skeletal muscle | Rhabdomyoma | Rhabdomyosarcoma | ++ | |
| Miscellaneous | _____ | Granular cell tumor | + | 18A |
| | | Mesenchymoma | + | |

[a]Some neoplasms are so primitive and anaplastic that they can only be classified as undifferentiated sarcoma or undifferentiated spindle cell sarcomas.

[b]+ = Low, ++ = moderate, +++ = high.

[c]Probably of blood-vessel smooth muscle, as opposed to the more common gastrointestinal or reproductive tract neoplasms.

desmin, and neurofilament proteins. Actins are a major constituent of the microfilamentous cytoskeleton of virtually all eukaryotic cells. These markers are useful for both differentiation of smooth and striated muscle tissue. S-100 represents a group of small $Ca^{++}$ binding modulator proteins involved in cell-cycle progression, cell differentiation, and cytoskeletal-membrane interactions. The S-100 protein is found in glial, Schwann, and satellite cells in the nervous system. S-100 is expressed on both benign and malignant melanoma. The use of immunocytochemistry and ultrastructural features are increasing in veterinary pathology and will enhance the accuracy of diagnosis and prognosis.

**Table 17–2**   Histologic Grade of Sarcomas

| Low Grade | High Grade |
|---|---|
| Hypocellular | Hypercellular |
| Good maturation (well differentiated) | Poor maturation (poorly differentiated) |
| Much stroma | Minimal stroma |
| Hypovascular | Hypervascular |
| Minimal necrosis | Much necrosis |
| < 5 mitoses per 10 high-power fields | > 5 mitoses per 10 high-power fields |

The histologic nomenclature for some sarcomas may vary from pathologist to pathologist. Before the initiation of the best appropriate therapy for the treatment of soft tissue sarcomas, it is necessary to know the histologic type of sarcoma, the size, the site, the histologic grade, and the stage of disease. The majority of soft tissue sarcomas can occur in both low-grade and high-grade histologic forms. In general, histologic grading (low, intermediate, high) is assigned after histologic characterization (see Table 17–2).

## Fibrosarcoma

Most fibrosarcomas arise from the skin, subcutaneous tissue, or palate, and represent malignant or transformed fibrocytes. The tumor tissue is very cellular, with closely packed spindle-shaped fibroblasts showing many mitotic figures. Fibrosarcomas are malignant tumors with a tendency to grow to quite a large size, invade deeper structures such as tendons, fascia, and muscles, and ulcerate the epidermis.

## Hemangiopericytoma

Hemangiopericytomas are one of the most common tumors seen in dogs, with a mean age of onset of 10 years and no sex predilection. This is a malignant tumor of the subcutis that is considered to originate in adventitial pericytes of small vessels. They occur as nodular, lobulated, and poorly defined tumors, without histologic encapsulation; however, clinically they may appear encapsulated and discrete, mimicking a lipoma. Most of the tumors are adherent to deeper tissues and infiltrate underlying fascia, muscle, and skin. Although these tumors are considered malignant, they tend to have a relatively benign behavior; that is, they are locally invasive and rarely metastatic. Local recurrence is common following conservative surgery. They tend to grow slowly and can range in size from 0.5 cm to over 10 to 12 cm in diameter. In some cases, they can easily be confused with lipomas on initial clinical examination.

The tumor occurs most commonly on the extremities. The histologic criteria for making a diagnosis of hemangiopericytoma include typical whorling and the arrangement of plump spindle cells, which frequently form a circular pattern around open or collapsed vessels.

## Neurofibrosarcoma

The neurofibrosarcomas are malignant tumors of nerve sheath origin and have been referred to as neurogenic sarcomas, malignant schwannomas, and malignant neurolemmomas. These tumors can occur anywhere in the body. Close association with the nerve may be necessary in order to differentiate a neurofibrosarcoma from a fibrosarcoma.

Neurofibrosarcomas may cause nodular enlargement of nerves that results in the compression of nerves. They often involve the brachial or lumbosacral plexus, resulting in paralysis and pain. They can invade the spinal cord and metastasis can occur but is considered uncommon. (See Chap. 26.)

## Liposarcomas

Liposarcomas are rare malignant lesions of adipose tissue found in older animals. No breed or sex predilection is known.[8] Liposarcomas tend to be aggressive and locally invasive, and they may metastasize to the lungs, liver, and bone. They tend to occur in the subcutaneous ventral aspects of the body as well as the abdominal cavity.[9] Mitoses are frequent, as are infiltrations into the veins, lymphatics, and underlying muscle and fascia. On palpation these tumors tend to have a very firm texture and are poorly defined. Liposarcomas will not be confused with lipomas either clinically or cytologically.

## Infiltrative Lipoma

Infiltrative lipomas are rare tumors composed of well-differentiated adipose cells without evidence of anaplasia. They are considered benign and do not metastasize. Infiltrative lipomas commonly invade adjacent muscle, fascia, nerve, myocardium, joint capsule, and even bone.[10–12]

## Lipoma

Lipomas are benign neoplasms of well-differentiated lipocytes or adipocytes. These tumors occur in adult animals and are most frequently seen in females. Lipomas may occur as individual tumors or may be multiple. The most common sites are the ventral abdomen and the thorax. On rare occasions lipomas may be noted within body cavities.[13]

## Lymphangiosarcoma

Lymphangiosarcomas arise from lymphatic endothelial cells and are extremely rare in both dogs and cats.[14,15] They are usually soft and cystlike and may appear invasive. In most cases the clinical signs are associated with drainage of lymph through the skin or a cystic mass. Aspiration may reveal a fluid-filled mass. Lymphangiosarcomas usually arise from the subcutaneous tissues but can occur in such sites as the liver, pericardium, and nasopharynx. They tend to have a moderate metastatic potential.

## Rhabdomyosarcoma

Rhabdomyosarcomas are malignant tumors derived from striated muscle cells.[16] Rhabdomyosarcomas consist of large, pleomorphic, elongated tumor cells, so-called strap cells, which may show cross striation in their eosinophilic cytoplasm. These tumors tend to be locally invasive and can metastasize to the lungs, liver, spleen, kidneys, and adrenal glands. They tend to be diffuse, infiltrative, and poorly circumscribed. Rhabdomyosarcomas can also be termed "botryoid" because of their grapelike appearance. Botryoid rhabdomyosarcomas have usually been reported in the bladder of large young dogs.[17] (See Chap. 25.)

## Synovial Cell Sarcoma

Synovial sarcomas are malignant neoplasms thought to arise from tenosynovial tissue in either the joints, bursa, or tendon sheaths and are considered rare in dogs and cats. The tumor may occur at any age but is more common in middle age (6–8 years). The stifle joint is most often affected, and the elbow is the second most common site. Histopathologically, there is one of two cell populations: epithelioid or synovioblastic and spindle or fibrosarcomatous cell types.[18] Histologic grading has been shown to provide important prognostic information.[19] The synovial sarcoma tends to be invasive into tendons, muscles, and bone. The tumor tends to originate from periarticular tissue rather than the synovium of the joints, tendons, or bursa, and it commonly recurs following local surgical excision. Extensive bone destruction has been reported and metastasis is grade dependent.

## Leiomyoma and Leiomyosarcoma

Leiomyosarcomas are tumors that arise from smooth muscle and are found as firm, white, lobulated masses in any part of the gastrointestinal tract from the esophagus to the rectum.[16] They also are found to originate in the spleen and genitourinary tract. Benign lesions are usually small, localized, and encapsulated, with cells resembling normal intestinal smooth muscle. Many leiomyomas can occur within the gastrointestinal tract and have been associated with chronic blood loss

(see Chap. 18). Tumors affecting the vagina or vulva are usually pedunculated and will often protrude from the vulva (see Chap. 22).

Leiomyosarcomas commonly arise in the retroperitoneal space, the spleen, or the gastrointestinal tract. They tend to be highly aggressive and can metastasize widely.[20] Splenic leiomyosarcomas may commonly show leukocytosis (> 17,000 WBC/mm$^3$), anemia, and a large splenic mass.

## Malignant Fibrous Histiocytoma

Malignant fibrous histiocytomas (MFHs) are uncommon tumors and are characterized as primitive, pleomorphic sarcoma with partial fibroblastic and histiocytic differentiation.[21-23] This group of sarcomas have also been labeled as giant cell fascial sarcoma, epithelioid sarcoma, malignant histiocytoma, reticulum cell sarcoma, and giant cell tumor. They may be confused with fibrosarcoma or extraskeletal osteosarcoma. This neoplasm should not be confused with malignant histiocytosis or systemic histiocytosis, most commonly seen in Bernese Mountain dogs. MFHs are usually firm and invasive tumors arising in the subcutis and rarely metastasize. They are most commonly seen in middle-aged animals, with an average age of 9 years. These tumors seem to have the same biologic behavior in the cat as the dog, that is, invasive, high recurrence and low metastatic potential. The dorsal thoracic and scapular areas are the most common sites for MFH.[13]

*A*

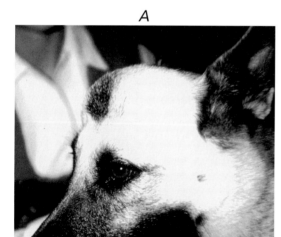

*B*

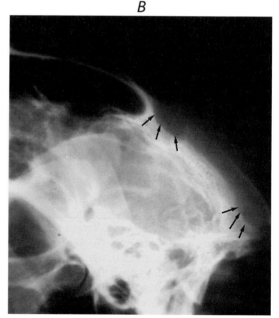

**Figure 17–1.** *A,* Dog with fibromatosis: 6-year-old dog with a large fibromatosis on the dorsum of the skull. *B,* Lateral radiograph of the skull of the same dog showing evidence of lysis in the skull (arrows).

## Malignant Mesenchymoma

Malignant mesenchymomas are rare tumors that have a fibrous tissue component plus two or more different varieties of sarcoma. These have been reported in the thigh muscles of the dog. They have a slow course of growth and tend to get very large, and metastasis has been reported.[24]

## Granular Cell Myoblastoma

Granular cell myoblastoma is a tumor of muscle origin, although it may not arise from myoblasts. These tumors are most commonly seen as bulging masses on the surface of the tongue.[25,26] (See Chap. 18.)

## Nodular Fasciitis (Fibromatosis, Pseudosarcomatous Fibromatosis)

Although considered a non-neoplastic condition, nodular fasciitis can be very invasive, nodular, and poorly circumscribed (Fig. 17–1). Nodular fasciitis is composed of large plump or spindle-shaped fibroblasts in a stromal network of variable amounts of collagen and reticulum fibers.[13] Scattered foci of inflammatory cells consisting of lymphocytes, plasma cells, and macrophages are characteristic. Complete excision, when possible, is usually curative.[13]

## HISTORY AND CLINICAL SIGNS

Most patients present with a slowly growing mass (weeks to months) anywhere in the body, although rapid cellular proliferation or intratumor hemorrhage or necrosis may result in a rapid increase in size. The symptoms are directly related to the site of involvement and the invasiveness of the lesion. There is marked variability in the physical features of soft tissue sarcoma, but the tumors are generally firm and adherent (fixed) to skin, muscle, or bone. Soft and lobulated sarcomas (especially hemangiopericytoma) are not uncommon.

Intra-abdominal tumors may present with vomiting, diarrhea, and melena. A mass may be palpable, and weight loss and anorexia can be seen. Leiomyosarcomas are seen most commonly in the gastrointestinal tract, spleen, and urogenital tracts. In the gastrointestinal tract the clinical signs are usually obstructive in nature and perforations may occur, leading to peritonitis. Rhabdomyosarcomas of the bladder present with signs of hematuria, dysuria, and hypertropic osteoarthropathy.[17] Nerve sheath tumors in the brachial or lumbar plexus can result in pain, lameness, and paralysis.

## DIAGNOSTIC TECHNIQUES AND WORKUP

Fine-needle aspiration cytology is a useful tool in helping rule out common differential diagnoses such as lipoma, seroma, inflammation, or abscess. Cytology has only a limited role in the diagnosis of soft tissue sarcoma because of limited sampling and the marked cytologic resemblance of reactive and benign neoplastic tumors. Many sarcomas have variable degrees of necrosis, and fine-needle aspirates may sample only those sites (false negatives). Additionally, sarcomas do not exfoliate cells for cytologic evaluation, as do epithelial tissues. Biopsy, either by incision or excision, is absolutely necessary for a definitive diagnosis. The biopsy should be positioned in such a location that it may be readily excised at surgery or included in a radiation field. Knowledge of the tumor type *before* curative intervention is vital for soft tissue sarcomas so that the

---

**Table 17–3** Modified Staging System for Soft Tissue Sarcomas

| | | |
|---|---|---|
| T Primary tumor | | |
| $T_1$ < 2 cm diameter | | |
| $T_2$ 2–5 cm diameter | | |
| $T_3$ > 5 cm diameter | | |
| $T_4$ Tumor invading muscle, bone, or cartilage | | |
| | | |
| N Regional lymph nodes | | |
| $N_0$ No histologically verified metastasis | | |
| $N_1$ Histologically verified metastasis | | |
| | | |
| M Distant metastasis | | |
| $M_0$ No distant metastasis | | |
| $M_1$ Distant metastasis | | |
| | | |
| Stage I | | |
| $I_A$ | | $= T_1 N_0 M_0$ |
| $I_B$ | | $= T_2 N_0 M_0$ |
| | | |
| Stage II | | |
| $II_A$ | | $= T_3 N_0 M_0$ |
| $II_B$ | | $= T_4 N_0 M_0$ |
| | | |
| Stage III | | |
| $III_A$ | | Any T $N_1 M_0$ |
| $III_B$ | | Any T Any N $M_1$ |

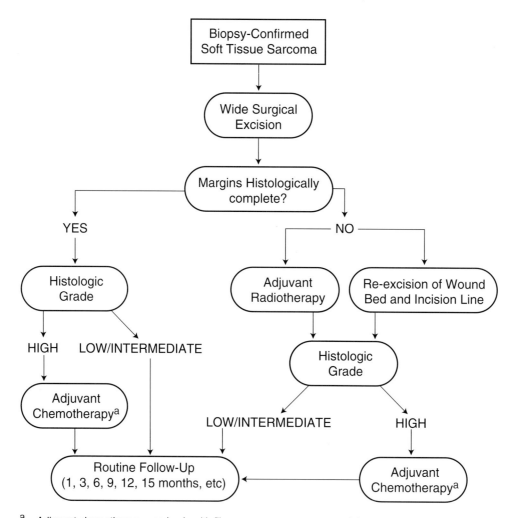

$^a$ = Adjuvant chemotherapy used only with fibrosarcoma, myxosarcoma, leiomyosarcoma, synovial sarcoma, rhabdomyosarcoma, and poorly differentiated sarcomas.

**Figure 17–2.**   Suggested treatment of stages I, II soft tissue sarcomas.

first therapy (usually surgery) can be properly planned and aggressively performed.

If the mass is fixed to bony structures, regional radiographs should be performed, depending on the location. Other imaging studies, such as ultrasound, computed tomography, magnetic resonance imaging, or angiographic studies, may be helpful for exact staging. Thoracic radiographs may be taken before or after biopsy but always before definitive treatment is undertaken.

Routine hematologic and serum biochemical evaluations are generally normal except for hemangiosarcoma. Hypoglycemia has been reported in dogs with intra-abdominal leiomyosarcoma.[20]

## Staging

The most important clinical information to obtain for staging is the size (< 2 cm, 2–5 cm, and > 5 cm diameter), fixation, site, status of regional lymph nodes, and clinically diagnosed distant metastasis. Table 17–3 summarizes a modified World Health Organization staging system useful for soft tissue sarcomas.

## THERAPY

Treatment decisions will be based on the location, clinical stage, histologic subtype, degree of differ-

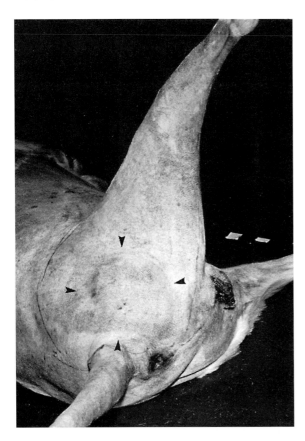

A

**Figure 17–3.** *A,* 15-year-old dog with a large fibrosarcoma (arrows) over the tuber ischii, with fixation to the ischium and tail and extended to the area of the greater trochanter. *B,* Tumor fixation and location mandated removal of the tail, ischium, acetabulum, and leg to achieve tumor-free margins. Function and cosmetics were excellent and patient remains free of disease 2 years later.

B

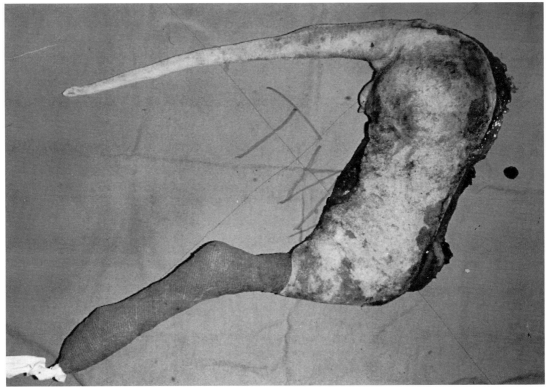

entiation (tumor grade), and completeness of surgery. Surgical excision and radiation therapy are the most successful treatment options reported to date. A suggested strategy to treat soft tissue sarcomas amenable to surgery is presented in Figure 17–2.

## Surgery

A multitude of treatments have been attempted for soft tissue sarcoma, but whenever possible surgery is the mainstay. Soft tissue sarcomas grow in the path of least resistance and push and invade surrounding tissue before them, forming a pseudocapsule of compressed tumor cells. Soft tissue sarcomas require aggressive removal (including amputation when necessary) in spite of what may appear to be an encapsulated lesion. This "capsule" is generally composed of compressed and viable tumor cells. A minimum of 3 cm margins should be strived for, and surgical planes of dissection should be through normal tissue only. Biopsy tracts should be excised in continuity with the main mass. Any areas of fixation (including bone and fascia) should be excised en bloc with the mass (Fig. 17–3). Any marginal area of concern to the surgeon should be tagged with fine suture, inked, or submitted as

a separate specimen for histologic analysis of margins (see Chap. 2). If incomplete (dirty) margins are reported, then one should consider reoperation of the entire previous surgery site or adjuvant radiation therapy. Soft tissue sarcomas cannot be "shelled out" or "peeled off" with the expectation of permanent control.

## Radiation

Measurable and palpable soft tissue sarcomas are generally felt to be resistant to conventional doses of irradiation (40–48 Gy).[27,28] Although higher doses of irradiation will have higher control rates, the chance of normal tissue complications also increases. These tumors do not rapidly regress after radiation, and "control" may be defined as a slowly regressing or stable-sized mass. In one study, radiation alone resulted in a 30% complete response rate.[29] In some studies, hyperthermia combined with irradiation showed promise for improved control versus irradiation alone.[30,31] In one recent study, the addition of hyperthermia with radiation increased the time to recurrence[29] (Fig. 17–4). Difficulty in the homogeneous heating of large tumors limits the routine use of hyperthermia for treating soft tissue sarcoma in conjunction with radiation.

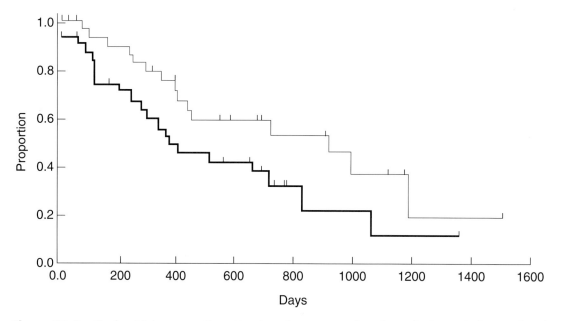

**Figure 17–4.**   Kaplan-Meier curves for estimates of recurrence time for radiation only (————) and radiation plus hyperthermia (——). Median time to recurrence was significantly increased with hyperthermia. (From McChesney G, Gillette S, Dewhirst MW, Gillette EL, et al: Response of canine soft-tissue sarcomas to radiation or radiation plus hyperthermia: A randomized phase II study. Int J Hyperthermia 8:309–320, 1992.)

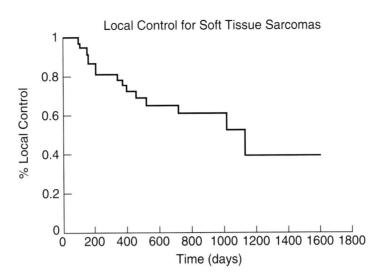

**Figure 17–5.** Local control for 39 dogs receiving radiation therapy after incomplete resection of soft tissue sarcomas.

Postoperative irradiation may be utilized if surgical removal is incomplete and further surgery is not feasible[32] (Fig. 17–5). Radiation for microscopic tumor, following excision, is generally superior to radiation of measurable tumors. The control rates for adjuvant radiation after histologically incomplete resection are 80% at 1 year and 60% at 2 years in histologically well-differentiated sarcomas, such as fibrosarcoma, hemangiopericytoma, and nerve sheath tumors (Fig. 17–5).[33]

Preoperative radiation therapy is rarely used in veterinary oncology, although it is used in human medicine. The principle reasons are that surgery alone will control more than 50% of cases and therefore do not need radiation; another reason is the cost of treatment.

## Chemotherapy

The evaluation of chemotherapy for soft tissue sarcomas has increased in the past 10 years.[34-41] At best, chemotherapy can be considered palliative for treating measurable soft tissue sarcomas.

Doxorubicin-based protocols and mitoxantrone have been shown to be the most active agents for treating soft tissue sarcomas.[35-37] Based on the author's experience, the histologic types most likely to show response to chemotherapy are fibrosarcoma, myxosarcoma, synovial sarcoma, and rhabdomyosarcoma.

Canine soft tissue sarcomas have shown complete or partial responses to vincristine, doxorubicin, and cyclophosphamide (VAC). Details of single chemotherapy agents that have shown antitumor activity in soft tissue sarcomas are presented in Table 17–4. The most effective combination chemotherapy protocols are presented in Table 17–5. Chemotherapy can be considered in the following clinical conditions:

1. Patients presenting for treatment following surgical removal of a high-grade sarcoma. Chemotherapy is used in the adjuvant setting, and response will be determined by the prevention or delay of local recurrence or distant metastasis. Increase in disease-free survival or overall survival analysis will be necessary to

**Table 17–4**  Chemotherapy Agents Shown to Have Antitumor Activity in Soft Tissue Sarcomas

| Single Agents | Usual Dosage | Comment | Reference |
|---|---|---|---|
| Doxorubicin | 30 mg/m² IV q 3 weeks × 6 | Best single agent | 35 |
| Mitoxantrone | 2.5 to 5.0 IV mg/m² q 3 weeks | Good substitute for doxorubicin in cats | 36, 39 |
| Vincristine | 0.7 mg/m² IV weekly | | 40 |

**Table 17–5**   Chemotherapy Protocols Used in Soft Tissue Sarcomas

| Combination Chemotherapy | Usual Dosage | Comment |
|---|---|---|
| VAC | | |
|    Vincristine | 0.7 mg/m² IV day 8, 15 | Prophylactic antibiotics may be needed |
|    Doxorubicin[a] | 30 mg/m² IV day 1 | |
|    Cyclophosphamide | 100–150 mg/m² IV day 1 | Repeat day 21 |
| Doxorubicin/Cyclophosphamide | | |
|    Doxorubicin[a] | 30 mg/m² IV day 1 | Repeat day 21 |
|    Cyclophosphamide | 50 mg/m² PO days 3, 4, 5, 6 or 150 mg/m² IV day 1 | |

[a]Cats dose at 20 mg/m² or 1 mg/kg doxorubicin.

determine the effectiveness of the chemotherapy; current proof of efficacy is lacking.

2. Patients presenting with a primary tumor, nonresectable, following a biopsy. If there is no response to VAC or single-agent therapy, then a different chemotherapy regimen should be considered. Response is determined by measurable reduction in tumor size.

3. Patients presenting with distant metastasis. If no response is seen to VAC or single-agent therapy, then a different chemotherapy regimen should be considered. Response is determined by measurable reduction in size and the extent of metastatic disease.

## Immunotherapy

Nonspecific immunomodulation using common microbial agents such as BCG, BCG cell walls, *Corynebacterium parvum*, and mixed bacterial vaccines have all been tested for antitumor effectiveness on soft tissue sarcomas and have demonstrated minimal therapeutic activity. Recently, a nonspecific immunomodulator has been reported to have some antitumor effect on fibrosarcomas[42]. Acemannan, a long-chain, polydispersed β-(1,4)-linked mannan, enhances macrophage release of IL-1, IL-6, TNFα and IFNγ.[43–45] Acemannan has shown antitumor activity in a murine sarcoma model.[46] In a recently published study in 43 dogs and cats with a variety of spontaneous tumors, 5 of 7 diagnosed with fibrosarcoma showed some tumor regression (6 animals) and tumor necrosis (7 animals).[42] In a more recent study, 14 fibrosarcomas treated with intralesional and intraperitoneal acemannan, 4 of 14 [31%] showed regression (29–85% reduction in size). All tumors were subsequently treated with surgery followed by radiation therapy. Survival and disease-free survival were compared to a historical control group treated by surgery and radiation; the median survival time for the acemannan-treated group was 303 days versus 161 days for the historical control group.[47] Unfortunately, randomized clinical trials have not been performed to prove that acemannan effectively improves disease-free survival and overall survival time in treated animals.

## PROGNOSIS

The metastatic potential of the various sarcomas is summarized in Table 17–1. Generally speaking, the prognosis is predicated more on local disease control than metastasis. The factors influencing the prognosis of sarcomas are summarized in Table 17–6. The overall metastatic rate for soft tissue sarcomas is less than 25%. Histologic grade has been correlated with response to radiation in soft tissue sarcomas[29] and survival of synovial sarcomas.[19]

**Table 17–6**   Factors Influencing Prognosis of Sarcomas

| Sarcoma | Favorable Factors | Unfavorable Factors |
|---|---|---|
| Size | Small | Large |
| Site | Superficial/extremities | Deep, trunk, invasive |
| Histologic grade | Low | High |
| Fixation | "Mobile" | Fixed and invasive |

## Hemangiopericytoma

A review of canine hemangiopericytoma cases treated principally by aggressive surgery revealed that local control can be achieved in 79% of cases at 2 years postoperatively (Fig. 17–6).[48] Another report indicated a 31% recurrence rate with surgery alone.[49] Size, site, histologic grade, and mitotic index were not prognostic.[49] Recurrent tumor was more difficult to control than primary cases, reinforcing the need to perform the first surgery aggressively and early in the course of the disease. Multiple surgeries are sometimes necessary, with the mean time to recurrence being 16 months.[48] Recurrence times tend to get shorter and shorter with multiple surgeries, and the metastatic potential may increase. Chemotherapy has not been shown to have any antitumor activity with hemangiopericytoma.

Adjuvant radiation therapy after incomplete surgical removal has yielded an approximate 40 to 90% control rate at 2 years.[48,50,51,53] Control rates (no increase in size) for radiation alone, without surgical debulking, is approximately 50% at 1 year and 20% at 2 years.[50] The tumor control dose for 50% of patients at 1 year ($TCD_{50}$) was 45.3 Gy in 10 fractions in 3 weeks (Fig. 17–7).

Normal tissue complications at higher doses can be significant, and the optimal dose, dose per fraction, and number of fractions to control soft tissue sarcomas are yet to be determined.[51,52] In one series of 29 dogs with soft tissue sarcoma, treated with radiation (45–56 Gy) and local hyperthermia, 5 had a complete regression, 14 had a partial regression, 9 had stable disease, and

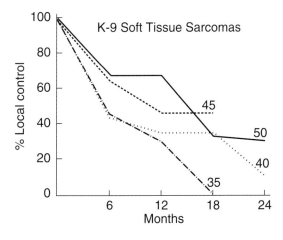

**Figure 17–7.** Probability of local control of various canine soft tissue sarcomas as a reflection of dosage. A clear-cut dosage response can be seen at 1 year. Patients were treated with radiation only for measurable disease. Radiation dose range 35 to 50 Gy.

1 had progressive disease. The median duration of response was 7 months and the overall median survival time was 15 months.[29,52]

## Synovial Sarcoma

Synovial sarcomas arise from primitive mesenchymal precursor cells outside the synovial membrane of the joints and bursa. The most common metastatic sites are the lungs and regional lymph nodes. In one published review, 20 of 37 cases showed evidence of metastasis at some time during the clinical course of the disease.[5] In a recent series of 36 cases, those dogs treated with amputation had a median survival time beyond 3 years.[19] Local excision failed in all cases and the median disease-free interval was 4.5 months. Negative prognostic factors included clinical stage (invasive into joints or bone), high-grade (Grade III) tumors, and a positive cytokeratin staining of the tumor (Figs. 17–8 and 17–9).[19] Long-term control of one dog with a synovial sarcoma has been reported using doxorubicin and cyclophosphamide chemotherapy.[37]

Synovial cysts have been reported in both dogs and cats.[54] These cysts appear clinically as a small, well-circumscribed tumor mass (< 2 cm), show no bony involvement, and are cured with complete surgical excision.[54]

## Infiltrative Lipoma

In a recently published study on dogs treated with surgery, 5 (30%) had recurrence, with a medium

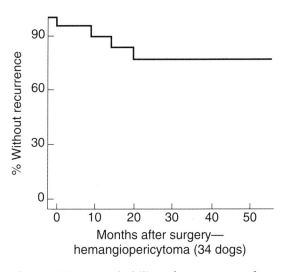

**Figure 17–6.** Probability of recurrence after aggressive surgical removal of hemangiopericytoma in 34 dogs.

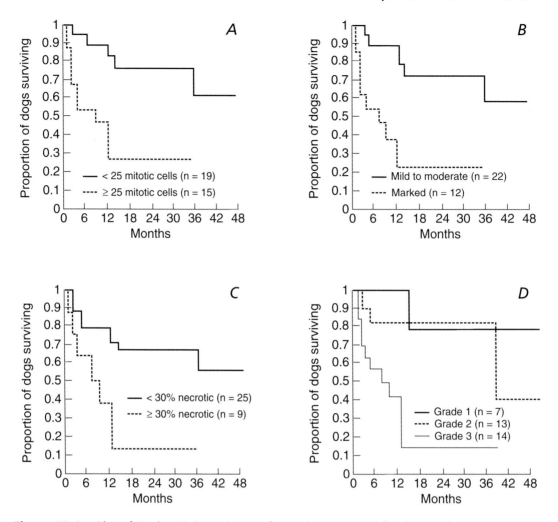

**Figure 17–8.** Plot of Kaplan-Meier estimate of cumulative survival for dogs with synovial sarcoma comparing, *A,* mitotic number; *B,* nuclear pleomorphism; *C,* percent tumor necrosis; and *D,* histologic grade. (Reprinted from Vail, DM, Powers BE, Getzy DM, et al: Evaluation of prognostic factors for dogs with synovial sarcoma: 36 cases (1986–1991). JAVMA 205:1300–1307, 1994.)

time to recurrence of 239 days, and 67% of the dogs were disease-free 1 year postsurgery.[55]

## Liposarcoma

Even with aggressive surgical resection, the prognosis of long-term control is poor. Chemotherapy and radiation therapy have not been shown to have any activity against liposarcoma.

## Malignant Fibrous Histiocytoma

The biologic behavior of malignant fibrous histiocytomas is similar to fibrosarcomas for which complete, radical, excision is usually curative.[22,23]

There are no reports of responsiveness to chemotherapy or radiation.

## Lymphangiosarcoma

Lymphangiosarcomas are tumors with a low metastatic potential; however, metastasis has been reported.[56] Treatment should include radical surgical excision (amputation if possible). No chemotherapy protocol has been shown to be effective, though radiation therapy has been used successfully in the treatment of lymphangioma in a dog.[57] Because of the rarity of these tumors, little has been reported on the prognosis following treatment.

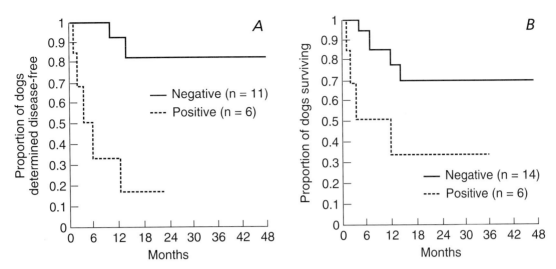

**Figure 17–9.** Plot of Kaplan-Meier estimate of, *A*, cumulative disease-free interval and, *B*, survival for dogs with synovial sarcoma comparing positive versus negative cytokeratin staining.(Reprinted from Vail, DM, Powers BE, Getzy DM, et al: Evaluation of prognostic factors for dogs with synovial sarcoma: 36 cases (1986–1991). JAVMA 205:1300–1307, 1994.)

### Splenic Leiomyosarcoma

Approximately one third of the dogs affected with splenic leiomyosarcoma will present with liver metastasis at the time of diagnosis.[20] In a series of 11 dogs undergoing splenectomy, the median survival time was reported to be 8 months, with 9 of the 11 dogs developing liver metastasis.[20]

### Fibrosarcoma

The prognosis for fibrosarcoma is based on location, degree of infiltrative growth, degree of anaplasia, and number of mitotic figures. The mitotic index is the most important criterion for predicting the behavior of fibrosarcomas.[58]

## FELINE SOFT TISSUE SARCOMAS

The cat is generally similar to the dog in terms of types and behavior of soft tissue sarcomas. Two exceptions are the rarity of feline hemangiopericytoma and synovial tumors and the presence of a virally induced multicentric fibrosarcoma in young cats.

Fibrosarcoma (nonvirally induced) accounts for more than 50% of soft tissue sarcomas in most published reports. Most patients are 8 to 12 years of age, and no sex or breed predilection is known. More than half of all fibrosarcomas occur on the limbs, making complete excision difficult, short of amputation.[59,60]

### Postvaccinal Sarcomas in Cats

In 1991, researchers published the first report of an increase in soft tissue fibrosarcomas, noted since 1987 at the University of Pennsylvania surgical biopsy service, an increase that coincided with the introduction of mandatory rabies vaccine and increased use of feline leukemia virus (FeLV) vaccine.[61] Since then, three additional papers have been published reporting on an increase in possible vaccine-associated sarcomas.[62-64] Most of these tumors are fibrosarcomas and are located in injection sites. The sites most commonly reported are the cervical/interscapular and femoral regions. The annual incidence is estimated to be 2 per 10,000 cats vaccinated.[65]

One study reported on a statistically significant association between FeLV vaccination within 1 year following vaccination.[64] Another study reported that the aluminum hydroxide or aluminum phosphate adjuvant may be associated with the pathogenesis.[62] In a recent review the authors make a comparison of postvaccinal sarcomas with feline ocular sarcomas caused by trauma.[65] It is believed that wounding of the eye sets up a chronic inflammatory reaction leading to neoplasia.[66]

The current recommendations specify that veterinarians keep accurate records of the vaccine type, manufacturer cited, and date administered and that they avoid simultaneously injecting multiple monovalent and/or multivalent vaccines at one site. In addition, it is advised to avoid vaccinating in the cervical/interscapular areas. The rear leg is preferable, because if a tumor develops, amputation can be considered.

Postvaccinal sarcomas need to be managed with aggressive surgical excision. Postoperative radiation therapy can be considered in cats with microscopic tumor left behind. Adjuvant chemotherapy has not been adequately tested. The use of chemotherapy to treat measurable tumors, using mitoxantrone or doxorubicin, has been disappointing.

As in the dog, wide resection is mandatory for the treatment of feline soft tissue sarcomas. Without always defining the aggressiveness of surgical removal, one report revealed a 2-year survival rate greater than 50%,[59] and another report revealed only a 40% 9-month survival rate.[60] The latter reported that histologic grade and tumor location were prognostic variables.[60] Tumors of the pinna and flank did not recur, while 70% of tumors located on the head, back, and leg recurred. Low-grade tumors (< 6 mitotic figures/high-power field) had a median survival of 128 weeks, while high-grade tumors had a median survival of 16 weeks. Most cats were euthanatized because of local recurrence and only 11% metastasized.[60]

The results of surgery and radiation therapy were recently reported in two separate studies. In one study, 24 cats with fibrosarcomas were treated with radiation therapy (48 Gy in 16 fractions) followed by surgical excision. Although follow-up continues, only 6 (25%) have had local recurrence, with a median progression-free interval of 280 days.[68] In another study, 9 cats were treated with radiation therapy (63 Gy in 21 fractions) following surgical excision. Four cats (44%) have died due to recurrence or metastasis, with an overall median survival time for all cats of 343 days.[69] These preliminary results indicate that cat fibrosarcomas are only moderately responsive to radiation when combined with surgery.

## COMPARATIVE ASPECTS[67]

In general, soft tissue sarcomas have a similar pathologic appearance, clinical presentation, and behavior in humans and animals. A specific difference is the higher incidence seen in young people as opposed to animals (rare rhabdomyosarcoma seen in young dogs). Most sarcomas seen in humans are recognized in animals, although the specific incidences may vary markedly. The more common histologic types in humans, in order, are fibrosarcoma, liposarcoma, rhabdomyosarcoma, malignant fibrous histiocytoma, synovial sarcoma, hemangiopericytoma, leiomyosarcoma, and neurofibrosarcoma.

As in animals, the most common site appears to be the limbs (61%), followed by the trunk (16%), retroperitonium (15%), breast (3.5%), and head and neck (3.5%). Metastasis would appear to be more common in human soft tissue sarcoma than in dogs, a phenomenon partially explained by the higher numbers of hemangiopericytomas (with their low metastatic rate) seen in the dog.

Well-defined prognostic variables in humans include clinical stage, histologic grade, necrosis, site, size, lymph node involvement, and aggressiveness of surgery or radiation.

Standard treatment is with aggressive surgical resection, but radiation and chemotherapy (often doxorubicin and DTIC combinations) used before or after resection may allow effective limb-sparing treatment in a significant number of patients. Ifosfamide is currently the most active salvage agent for patients who have failed doxorubicin-based protocols. Overall 5-year survival rates are 50 to 55% with surgery alone and 70 to 80% using adjuvant chemotherapy. Permanent local control with the first treatment is related to long-term survival.

## REFERENCES

1. Theilen GH, Madewell BR: Tumors of the skin and subcutaneous tissues. *In* Theilen GH, Madewell BR (eds): Veterinary Cancer Medicine. Philadelphia, Lea & Febiger, 1979, pp. 123–191.
2. Dorn ER: Epidemiology of canine and feline tumors. J Am Anim Hosp Assoc 12:307–312, 1976.
3. Hardy WD, Jr: The etiology of canine and feline tumor. J Am Anim Hosp Assoc 12:313–334, 1976.
4. Madewell BR, Theilen GH: Etiology of cancer in animals *In* Madewell BR, Theilen GH (eds): Veterinary Cancer Medicine, 2nd ed. Philadelphia, Lea & Febiger, 1987, pp. 13–25.
5. McGlennon NH, Houlton JEF, Gorman NT: Synovial sarcoma in the dog—A review. J Small Anim Pract 29:139–152, 1988.
6. Ordonez NG: Immunocytochemistry in the diagnosis of soft-tissue sarcomas. Cancer Bull 45:13–23, 1993.
7. Madewell BR, Munn RJ: The soft tissue sarcomas: Immunohistochemical and ultrastructural distinctions. Proc 9th ACVIM, 1991, pp. 717–720.
8. Doster AR, Tomlinson MJ, Mahaffey EA, et al: Canine liposarcoma. Vet Pathol 23:87–88, 1986.
9. Strafuss AC, Bozarth AJ: Liposarcoma in dogs. J Am Anim Hosp Assoc 9:183–187, 1973.
10. McChesney AE, Stephans LC, Lebel J, et al: Infil-

trative lipoma in dogs. Vet Pathol 17:316–322, 1980.

11. Kramek BA, Spackman CJA, Hayden DW: Infiltrative lipoma in three dogs. J Am Vet Med Assoc 186:81–82, 1982.

12. Frazier KS, Herron AJ, Dee JF, et al: Infiltrative lipoma in a stifle joint. J Am Anim Hosp 29:81–83, 1993.

13. Pulley LT, Stannard AA: Tumors of skin and soft tissue In Moulton JE (ed): Tumors in Domestic Animals, 3rd ed. Berkeley, University of California Press, 1990, pp. 23–87.

14. Kelly WR, Wilkinson GT, Allen PW: Canine angiosarcoma (lymphangiosarcoma): A case report. Vet Pathol 18:224–227, 1981.

15. Walsh K, Abbott DP: Lymphangiosarcoma in two cats. J Comp Pathol 94:611, 1984.

16. Hullard TJ: Tumors of the muscle. In JE Moulton (ed): Tumors of Domestic Animals, 3rd ed. Berkeley, University of California Press, 1990, pp. 88–101.

17. Pletcher JM, Dalton L: Botryoid rhabdomyosarcoma in the urinary bladder of a dog. Vet Pathol 18:695–697, 1981.

18. Pool RR: Tumors and tumor-like lesions of joints and adjacent soft tissues In JE Moulton (ed): Tumors of Domestic Animals, 3rd ed. Berkeley, University of California Press, 1990, pp. 102–156.

19. Vail DM, Powers BE, Getzy DM, et al: Evaluation of prognosis for dogs with synovial sarcoma: 36 cases (1986–1991). JAVMA, 205:1300–1307, 1994.

20. Kapatkin AS, Muller HS, Mathieson DT, et al: Leiomyosarcoma in dogs: 44 cases (1983–1988) J Am Vet Med Assoc 201:1077–1086, 1992.

21. Gibson KL, Blass CE, Simpson M, et al: Malignant fibrous histiocytoma in a cat. J Am Vet Med Assoc 194:1443–1445, 1989.

22. Gleiser CA, Raulston GL, Jardine JH, et al: Malignant fibrous histiocytoma in dogs and cats. Vet Pathol 16:199–208, 1979.

23. Allen SW, Duncan JR: Malignant fibrous histiocytoma in a cat. J Am Vet Med Assoc 192:90–91, 1988.

24. Moore RW, Snyder SP, Houchen JW, et al: Malignant mesenchymoma in a dog. J Am Vet Med Assoc 19:187–190, 1983.

25. Giles RC, Montgomery CA, Izen L: Canine lingual granular cell myoblastoma: A case report. Am J Vet Res 35:1357–1359, 1974.

26. Wyand DS, Wolke RE: Granular cell myoblastoma of the canine tongue: Case reports. Am J Vet Res 29:1309–1313, 1968.

27. Hilmas DE, Gillett EL: Radiotherapy of spontaneous fibrous connective-tissue sarcomas in animals. J Natl Cancer Inst 56:365–368, 1976.

28. Banks WC, Morris E: Results of radiation treatment of naturally occurring animal tumors. J Am Vet Med Assoc 166:1063–1064, 1975.

29. McChesney G, Gillette S, Dewhirst MW, et al: Response of canine soft-tissue sarcomas to radiation or radiation plus hyperthermia. A randomized phase II study. Int J Hyperthermia 8:309–320, 1992.

30. Brewer WG, Turrel JM: Radiotherapy and hyperthermia in the treatment of fibrosarcomas in the dog. J Am Vet Med Assoc 181:146–150, 1982.

31. Richardson RC, Anderson VL, Voorhees WD, et al: Irradiation-hyperthermia in canine hemangiopericytomas: Large-animal model for therapeutic response. J Natl Cancer Inst 73:1187–1194, 1984.

32. Atwater SW, LaRue SM, Powers BE, Withrow SJ: Adjuvant radiotherapy of soft-tissue sarcomas in dogs. Proc Vet Cancer Soc 1992, pp. 41–42.

33. Mauldin GN, Meleo KA, Burk RL: Radiation therapy for the treatment of incompletely resected soft tissue sarcomas in dogs: 21 cases. Proc Vet Cancer Soc 1993, p. 111.

34. Brown NO, Hayes AA, Mooney S, et al: Combined modality therapy in the treatment of solid tumors in cats. J Am Anim Hosp Assoc 16:719–722, 1980.

35. Ogilvie GK, Reynolds HA, Richardson RC, et al: Phase II evaluation of doxorubicin for treatment of various canine neoplasms. J Am Vet Med Assoc 195:1580–1583, 1989.

36. Ogilvie GK, Obradovich JE, Elmslie RE, et al: Efficacy of mitoxantrone against various neoplasms in dogs. J Am Vet Med Assoc 198:1618–1621, 1991.

37. Tilmant LL, Gorman WT, Ackerman N, et al: Chemotherapy of synovial cell sarcoma in a dog. J Am Vet Med Assoc 188:530–532, 1986.

38. Hammer AS, Couto CG, Filppi J, et al: Efficacy and toxicity of VAC chemotherapy (vincristine, doxorubicin and cyclophosphamide) in dogs with hemangiosarcoma. J Vet Intern Med 5:160–161, 1991.

39. Ogilvie GR, Moore AJ, Obradovich JE, et al: Toxicoses and efficacy associated with the administration of mitoxantrone to cats with malignant tumors. J Am Vet Med Assoc 202:1839–1844, 1993.

40. Hahn KA: Vincristine sulfate as single-agent chemotherapy in a dog and a cat with malignant neoplasms. J Am Vet Med Assoc 197:504–508, 1990.

41. Moore AS: Recent advances in chemotherapy for nonlymphoid malignant neoplasms. Compend Contin Educ Small Anim 15:1039–1052, 1993.

42. Harris C, Pierce K, King G, et al: Efficacy of acemannan in treatment of canine and feline spontaneous neoplasms. Mol Biother 3:207–213, 1991.

43. Marshall GD, Gibbons AS, Parnell LS: Human cytokines induced by acemannan. J Allergy Clin Immunol 91:295, 1993.

44. Tizard IR, Carpenter RH, McAnalley BH, et al: The biological activities of mannans and related complex carbohydrates. Mol Biother 1:290–296, 1989.

45. Kisseberth W, Shi F, MacEwen EG: Effect of acemannan on canine monocyte activation and peripheral neutrophil counts. Proc Vet Cancer Soc 1993, pp. 31–32.

46. Peng SY, Norman J, Curtin G, et al: Decreased

mortality of norman murine sarcoma in mice treated with the immunomodulator acemannan. Mol Biother 3:79–87, 1991.

47. King GK, Yates KM, Greenlee PG, et al: The effect of acemannan, surgery and radiation on spontaneous canine and feline fibrosarcoma. J Am Anim Hosp Assoc (in press) 1995.

48. Postorino NC, Berg RJ, Powers BE, et al: Prognostic variables for canine hemangiopericytoma: 50 cases (1979–1984). J Am Anim Hosp Assoc 24:501–509, 1988.

49. Graves GM, Bjorling DE, Mahaffey E: Canine hemangiopericytoma: 23 cases (1967–1984). J Am Vet Med Assoc 192:99–102, 1988.

50. Evans SM: Canine hemangiopericytoma. A retrospective analysis of response to surgery and orthovoltage radiation. Vet Radiol 28:13–16, 1987.

51. McChesney SL, Withrow SJ, Gillette EL, et al: Radiotherapy of canine soft tissue sarcomas. J Am Vet Med Assoc 194:60–63, 1989.

52. McChesney SL, Gillette EL, Dewhirst MW: Influence of WR 2721 on radiation response of canine soft tissue sarcomas. Int J Radiat Oncol Biol Phys 12:1957–1963, 1986.

53. Knapp DW, Richardson RC, Cantwell HD, et al: Radiation/hyperthermia therapy of hemangiopericytoma. Proc Vet Cancer Soc 1988, p. 5.

54. Pryma KC, Goldschmidt MH: Synovial cysts in five dogs and one cat. J Am Anim Hosp Assoc 27:151–154, 1991.

55. Bergman PJ, Withrow SJ, Straw RC, et al: Infiltrative lipoma in dogs: 16 cases (1981–1992). J Am Vet Med Assoc 205:322–324, 1994.

56. Rudd RG, Veatch JK, Whitehair JG, et al: Lymphangiosarcoma in dogs. J Am Anim Hosp Assoc 25:695–698, 1989.

57. Turrel JM, Lowenstine LJ, Cowgill LD: Response to radiation therapy of recurrent lymphangioma in a dog. J Am Vet Med Assoc 193:1432–1434, 1988.

58. Bostock DE, Dye MT. Prognosis after excision of canine fibrous connective tissue sarcomas. Vet Pathel 17:581–588, 1980.

59. Brown NO, Patnaik AK, Mooney S, et al: Soft tissue sarcomas in the cat. J Am Vet Med Assoc 173:744–749, 1978.

60. Bostock DE, Dye MT: Prognosis after surgical excision of fibrosarcomas in cats. J Am Vet Med Assoc 175:727–728, 1979.

61. Hendrick MJ, Goldschmidt MH: Do injection site reactions induce fibrosarcomas in cats? J Am Vet Med Assoc 199:968, 1991.

62. Hendrick MJ, Goldschmidt, MH, Shofer FS, et al: Postvaccinal sarcomas in the cat: Epidemiology and election probe microanalytical identification of aluminum. Cancer Res 52:5391–5394, 1992.

63. Esplin DG, McGill LD, Meininger A, et al: Postvaccinal sarcomas in cats. J Am Vet Med Assoc 202:1245–1247, 1993.

64. Kass PH, Barnes WG, Spangler WL, et al: Epidemiologic evidence for a causal relationship between vaccination and fibrosarcoma tumorigenesis in cats. J Am Vet Med Assoc 203:369–405, 1993.

65. Hendrick MJ, Kass PH, McGill LD, et al: Postvaccinal sarcomas in cats. J Natl Cancer Inst 86:341–343, 1994.

66. Dubielzig RR: Ocular sarcoma following trauma in three cats. J Am Vet Med Assoc 184:578–581, 1984.

67. Chang AE, Rosenberg SA, Glatstein EJ, et al. Sarcomas of soft tissues. In Devita VT, Hellman S, Rosenberg SA (ed): Cancer: Principles and Practice of Oncology, 3rd ed. Philadelphia, JB Lippincott, 1989, pp. 1345–1398.

68. Cronin KL, Page RL, Thrall DE. Radiation and surgery for treatment of feline fibrosarcomas. Proc 14th Ann Vet Cancer Soc, 1994, p. 22.

69. Meleok KA, Mauldin GN. Post-operative radiotherapy for the treatment of fibrosarcoma in 9 cats. Proc 14th Ann Vet Cancer Soc, 1994, pp. 127–128.

# 18

# Tumors of the Gastrointestinal System

## A. Cancer of the Oral Cavity

Stephen J. Withrow

## INCIDENCE AND RISK FACTORS

Collectively, oral cancer accounts for 6% of canine cancer and is the fourth most common cancer overall.[1] In the cat, it accounts for 3% of all cancers.[2] Tumors of unusual sites, types, and behavior will be covered at the end of this chapter (tonsillar squamous cell carcinoma, cancer of the tongue, viral papillomatosis, canine eosinophilic granuloma complex, epulis, inductive fibroameloblastoma, nasopharyngeal polyps, eosinophilic granuloma in cats, and malignancy of young dogs). A general summary of the common oral tumors is found in Table 18–1.

## PATHOLOGY AND NATURAL BEHAVIOR

The oral cavity is a very common site for a wide variety of malignant and benign cancers. Although most cancers are fairly straightforward histologically, some have confusing nomenclature or extenuating circumstances that warrant discussion.

Oral fibrosarcoma will often look surprisingly benign histologically, and even with large biopsy samples the pathologist is at pains to determine fibroma or low-grade fibrosarcoma. This syndrome, which is common on the maxilla and mandible of large-breed dogs (especially the golden retriever), has been termed "histologically low grade but biologically high grade" fibrosarcoma.[3] Even with a low-grade biopsy, if the can-

cer in question is rapidly growing, recurrent, or invading bone, the clinician should dictate treatment as for malignant cancer. Fibrosarcoma is very invasive locally but metastasizes in less than 20% of cases (usually to the lungs).

Malignant melanoma can present a confusing histopathologic picture if the tumor or the biopsy section does not contain melanin (one third of all cases). A histopathologic diagnosis of undifferentiated sarcoma should be looked upon with suspicion for possible underlying melanoma. Melanoma has a strong predilection to metastasize to regional lymph nodes and then lung. Metastasis to lung only or other sites is also common.

Squamous cell carcinoma is usually a straightforward histologic diagnosis. It is the most common feline oral malignancy. Severe and extensive involvement of bone is common in the cat. The metastatic rate in the cat is generally considered low but is somewhat unknown, since so few cats have their local disease controlled to observe the long-term metastatic potential. Metastasis in the canine is very site-dependent, with the rostral oral cavity having a low metastatic rate and the caudal tongue and tonsil having a high metastatic potential.

The terminology for the epulides and dental tumors has been revised by some authors.[4] The "traditional" epulides are similar to gingival hyperplasia in appearance and are usually confined to one or two sites at the gum margin. They are slow growing, firm, and generally covered by

**Table 18–1** Summary of Common Oral Cancers of the Dog and Cat

| | Canine | | | | Feline | |
|---|---|---|---|---|---|---|
| | Squamous Cell Carcinoma[a] (SCC) | Fibrosarcoma (FS) | Melanoma (MM) | Dental | Squamous Cell Carcinoma[a] (SCC) | Fibrosarcoma (FS) |
| Frequency (%) | 20–30 | 10–20 | 30–40 | 5 | 70 | 20 |
| Age (years) | 10 | 7 | 12 | 9 | 10 | 10 |
| Sex predilection | Equal | M > F | M > F | F > M | None | None |
| Patient size | Larger | Larger | Smaller | None | None | — |
| Site predilection | Rostral mandible | Palate | Buccal mucosa | Rostral mandible | Mandible or maxillary bone; tongue | Gingiva |
| Regional lymph node metastasis | Rare (except tonsil and tongue) | Rare | Common | Never | Rare | Rare |
| Distant metastasis | Rare (except tonsil and tongue) | Occasional | Common | Never | Rare | Occasional |
| Gross appearance | Red, cauliflower, raised, ulcerated | Flat, firm, ulcered | 2/3 pigmented, ulcerated | Like SCC | Proliferative in pharynx; minimal visible disease in oral cavity | Firm |
| %Bone involvement[b] | Variable | Common | Variable | Always | Common | Common |
| Radiation response[c] | Good | Poor–fair | Poor?[d] | Excellent | Poor | Poor |
| Surgery response | Good rostral; fair caudal | Fair–good (especially large lesions) | Fair–good | Excellent | Poor | Fair–good |
| Prognosis | Good rostral; poor caudal | Poor–fair | Poor–fair | Excellent | Very poor | Fair |
| Usual cause of death | Distant disease | Local disease | Distant disease | Rarely tumor related | Local disease | Local disease |
| Comments | Behavior varies dramatically from front (good) to back (poor) of oral cavity | Often looks low grade histologically but very invasive biologically | Presence or absence of pigment is not prognostic | May be confused with SCC histologically | Many tumors of mandible and maxilla have little or no visible oral disease but have severe deep invasion of bone | Local disease |

[a]Nontonsillar.

[b]Varies with site; if adherent to bone, the bone involved must be considered.

[c]Adjuvant microscopic postoperative residual disease is generally better than treating large-volume macroscopic disease.

[d]Coarsely fractionated radiation (large dose/fraction) may achieve transient clinical response but is rarely curative.

intact epithelium. Most are firmly attached, while some are pedunculated. These are classified as fibrous epulis or ossifying epulis, depending on the presence or absence of bone. A third class has been termed *acanthomatous epulis* instead of the previous term of *adamantinoma*. Some pathologists use the terms interchangeably. These are much more locally invasive and virtually always invade bone. They do not metastasize.

## HISTORY AND SIGNS

Most patients present with a mass in the mouth noticed by the owner. Cancer in the caudal pharynx, however, is rarely seen by the owner, and the patient will present for signs of increased salivation, weight loss, halitosis, bloody discharge, dysphagia, or occasionally cervical lymphadenopathy. Loose teeth, in a patient with generally good dentition, should alert the clinician to possible underlying neoplastic bone lysis (especially in the cat).[5]

## DIAGNOSTIC TECHNIQUES AND WORKUP

The diagnostic evaluation for oral cancers is critical because of the wide range of cancer behavior and available therapeutic options. If the cancer is suspected of being malignant, thoracic radiographs can be performed prior to biopsy. The most likely cancers to have positive thoracic radiographs at the time of diagnosis are melanoma and squamous cell carcinoma of the caudal oral and pharyngeal area. Most animals will require a short general anesthesia for careful palpation, regional radiographs, and a biopsy. Patients with exophytic or ulcerated masses will generally tolerate a wedge biopsy without anesthesia.

Cancers that are adherent to bone, other than simple epulis, should have regional radiographs taken under anesthesia (Figs. 18–1*A* and 18–1*B*). When 40% or more of the cortex is destroyed, lysis may be observed. However, apparently normal radiographs do not rule out bone invasion.

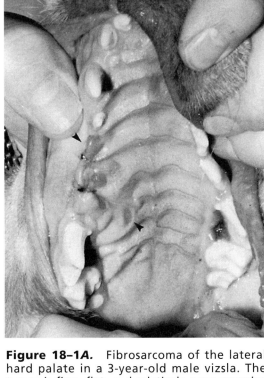

**Figure 18–1*A*.** Fibrosarcoma of the lateral hard palate in a 3-year-old male vizsla. The tumor is firm, flat, and relatively nonaggressive in appearance.

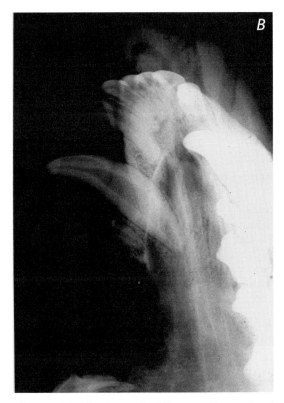

**Figure 18–1*B*.** Lateral oblique radiograph of the dog in Figure 18A–1*A*. Note the marked destruction of the maxilla and the loss of teeth. This dog was treated with a partial maxillectomy and remains free of cancer at 3 years postoperatively.

This evaluation will assist in determining the clinical stage of cancer and the extent of resection when surgery is indicated. Computed tomography can be a very valuable staging tool, especially for evaluation of possible tumor extension into the nasal cavity or in the caudal pharynx and orbit.

Regional lymph nodes (mandibular and retropharyngeal) should be carefully palpated for enlargement or asymmetry. When abnormal (or even just palpable), they should be aspirated via a fine needle. This is especially important for melanoma and caudally situated squamous cell carcinoma.

The last step, under the same anesthesia, is a large incisional biopsy. Oral cancers are commonly infected, inflamed, or necrotic and it is important to obtain a large specimen. Electrocautery may distort the specimen and should only be used for hemostasis after blade incision. Large samples of healthy tissue at the edge and center of the lesion will increase the diagnostic yield. The biopsy site should be located in such a position as to be easily included in a possible resection. For small lesions (epulides, papillomas, or small labial mucosa melanoma), curative-intent resection (excisional biopsy) may be undertaken at the time of initial evaluation. For more extensive disease, waiting for biopsy results to plan treatment accurately is encouraged.

Cytologic preparations of oral cancers may not be rewarding because of the necrosis and inflammation that commonly accompany these conditions.

## THERAPY

Surgery, cryosurgery, and irradiation are the principal therapies utilized in the mouth. When feasible, surgical excision is the most economical, fastest, and most curative treatment. Radical surgeries such as mandibulectomy and partial maxillectomy are well tolerated by the patient and indicated for lesions with extensive bone invasion that are not felt to be radiation responsive or are too large for cryosurgery (Table 18–2 and 18–3).[6–16] Margins of at least 2 cm are necessary for malignant cancers such as squamous cell carcinoma, malignant melanoma, and fibrosarcoma in the dog. Squamous cell carcinoma in the cat should have wider margins yet, because of their high local recurrence rates.

Cryosurgery may be indicated for lesions less than 2 cm in diameter that are fixed or minimally invasive into bone (see Chap. 8). Larger

lesions should generally be surgically resected. More extensive lesions in bone will often result in a fracture (mandible) or oronasal fistula (maxilla) if aggressively frozen. Cancer of soft tissue only should be surgically excised rather than frozen.

If it is used alone, hyperthermia offers no advantage over cryosurgery or surgery. In fact, bone penetration is less reproducible with heat versus cold treatment. Hyperthermia at moderate temperatures (42 to 43°C) may, however, be used as an adjunct to irradiation.[17–19]

Radiation therapy is utilized under three general settings:

1. Known responsiveness for such tumors as dental (acanthomatous epulis or adamantinoma),[20,21] squamous cell carcinoma,[17,22,23] and possibly malignant melanoma.[24]
2. An inoperable cancer of any histology (radiation will generally be only palliative).
3. Known postoperative residual disease to "clean up" the remaining cancer.

Local and regional disease control is the goal of treatment. No known effective adjuvant chemotherapeutic agents exist for cancers likely to metastasize (malignant melanoma, squamous cell carcinoma, or fibrosarcoma). Intralesional cisplatin was utilized in 20 dogs with oral melanoma with some success, but this treatment remains investigational.[25] Adjuvant immunotherapy with a BCG (Bacillus Calmette-Guérin) or levamisole has failed to improve survivals for malignant melanoma in the dog. A slight improvement in survival was demonstrated for patients with advanced local stage malignant melanoma when treated with surgery and *Corynebacterium parvum* versus surgery alone.[26]

## PROGNOSIS

The prognosis for acanthomatous epulis/ adamantinoma is excellent with surgery or irradition or a combination of the two. Recurrence rates for these tumors after aggressive resection is less than 5%.[6,8,27,28] Radiation therapy will control in excess of 90% of these tumors.[20,21] A peculiar syndrome of a malignant cancer developing in the irradiated site may occur in up to 20% of patients, especially if treated with orthovoltage radiation.[20,29] The tumors may be of epithelial or mesenchymal origin and usually take several years to develop.

**Table 18–2** Various Mandibulectomies

| Mandibulectomy Procedure | Area Removed | Indications | Comments | |
|---|---|---|---|---|
| Unilateral rostral | A | Lesions confined to rostral hemimandible; not crossing midline | The most common tumor types are squamous cell carcinoma and acanthomatous epuli that do not require removal of the entire affected bone; the tongue lags to resected side | A |
| Bilateral rostral | B | Bilateral rostral lesions crossing the symphysis | The tongue will be "too long" and some cheilitis of chin skin will occur; mandibulectomy has been performed as far back as PM4 but preferably at PM 2. | B |
| Vertical ramus | C | Low-grade bony or cartilaginous lesions confined to vertical ramus | These tumors are variously called chondroma rodens or multilobular osteoma; the temporomandibular joint (TMJ) may be removed; cosmetics and function are excellent | C |
| Complete unilateral | D | High-grade tumors with extensive involvement of horizontal ramus or invasion into medullary canal of ramus | Mandibulectomy usually reserved for aggressive tumors; function and cosmetics are good | D |
| Segmental | E | Low-grade midhorizontal ramus cancer, preferably not into medullary cavity | Segmental mandibulectomy is a poor choice for highly malignant cancer in medullary cavity, since growth along mandibular artery, vein, and nerve is common | E |

**Table 18–3** Various Maxillectomies

| Maxillectomy Procedure | Area Removed | Indications | Comments |
|---|---|---|---|
| Unilateral rostral | A | Lesions confined to hard palate on one side | One-layer direct lip to palate closure |
| Bilateral rostral | B | Bilateral lesions of rostral hard palate | Usually requires double-layer closure of overlapping or opposing lip but may be closed by direct single layer lip apposition. |
| Lateral | C | Laterally placed midmaxillary lesions | Single-layer closure if small defect, two layer if large |
| Bilateral | D | Bilateral palatine lesions | High rate of closure dehiscence, since lip flap rarely reaches side to side; may result in permanent oronasal fistula |

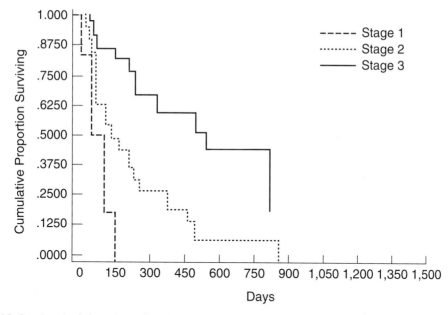

**Figure 18–2.** Survival duration of 89 dogs with oral melanoma treated with surgery or surgery and *Corynebacterium parvum*. Stage 1 is a tumor diameter less than 2 cm, and stage 2 is a tumor diameter between 2 and 4 cm. Both stages 1 and 2 have negative lymph nodes. Stage 3 is a tumor diameter greater than 4 cm or any size tumor with positive lymph nodes. Stage 1 was associated with a significant increase in survival time (*p* = 0.024).[26] (Reprinted by courtesy of Marcel Dekker Inc.)

The outlook for squamous cell carcinoma is very site-and species-dependent. Cancers of the canine in the rostral mouth are curable with surgery[6] or irradiation,[23] while those of the tonsil or base of tongue are highly metastatic and likely to recur locally or regionally.[22,30] Local control of feline squamous cell carcinoma is poor with either surgery, hyperthermia, chemotherapy, or radiation therapy.[9,31,32,33–37] One-year survivals rarely exceed 10% in the cat.

Overall, approximately 25% of canine oral malignant melanomas will survive 1 year or more.[26,38] The only known variables that have prognostic significance are size (< 2 cm diameter do better) and the ability of the first treatment to afford local control.[18,26,38] Dogs with tumors less than 2 cm in diameter have a median survival of 511 days as opposed to dogs with lymph node involvement or tumors greater than 2 cm in diameter whose median survival is 164 days (Fig. 18–2).[26] Recurrent malignant melanoma does worse than primarily treated disease that achieves local control.[38] Age, breed, sex, degree of pigmentation, and microscopic appearance are not prognostic.

Local control of fibrosarcoma is more of a problem than metastasis. The best 1-year survivals with almost any treatment are no better than 25 to 40%.[6–10] Fibrosarcomas are generally considered radiation resistant.[39,40] Mean survival after radiation of 17 dogs was only 7 months.[41] Radiation combined with regional hyperthermia improved local control rates to 50%, as measured at 1 year in a series of 10 cases.[19]

Several reports entailing more than 500 dogs with various oral malignancies, undergoing mandibulectomy or maxillectomy, recently have been described. Most cases were treated with surgery alone. Unfortunately the methods of reporting and end results vary with each paper, but an attempt to combine cases by tumor type and outcome is shown in Table 18–4. Local recurrence was lowest for acanthomatous epulis and squamous cell carcinoma. Fibrosarcoma locally recurred in almost half the cases, and melanoma and osteosarcoma locally recurred in 25%. Survivals were best for acanthomatous epulis and squamous cell carcinoma; melanoma, fibrosarcoma, and osteosarcoma had worse survival rates. Most of these reports suggest that histologically complete resection and a rostral location are favorable prognostic indicators. Rostral locations are generally detected at an earlier stage, are easier to operate, and may be more likely to have a complete resection. It is also clear that fibrosarcoma continues to have an unacceptable local

**Table 18–4**[6-16]   Summary of Various Papers on Mandibulectomy or Maxillectomy

|                         | Number | % Local Recurrence | Median Survival (Months) | % 1 Year |
|-------------------------|--------|--------------------|--------------------------|----------|
| Acanthomatous epulis    | 149    | 4                  | 36                       | 90       |
| Squamous cell carcinoma | 92     | 15                 | 18                       | 70       |
| Osteosarcoma            | 69     | 25                 | 8                        | 50       |
| Melanoma                | 126    | 25                 | 8                        | 35       |
| Fibrosarcoma            | 92     | 46                 | 11                       | 35       |

recurrence rate and needs to be addressed with wider resections or other adjuvant therapies, especially postoperative radiation after incomplete resection, which has shown benefit in dogs with other soft tissue sarcomas. On the other hand, melanoma is controlled locally in 75% of cases, but metastatic disease requires effective adjuvant therapy.

Osteosarcoma of the mandible was evaluated in a series of 51 dogs. Treatment was principally with mandibulectomy and the 1-year survival for dogs treated with surgery alone was 71%.[42] Mandibular osteosarcoma appears to carry a naturally better survival pattern than dogs with appendicular osteosarcoma, and there may not be as compelling a need for use of adjuvant chemotherapy.

## SELECTED SITES OR CANCER CONDITIONS IN THE ORAL CAVITY

### Tonsillar Squamous Cell Carcinoma

Tonsillar squamos cell carcinoma is 10 times more common in animals living in urban areas than in rural ones, implying an etiologic association with environmental pollutants.[43] Most primary tonsillar cancer is squamous cell carcinoma. Lymphoma can affect the tonsils but is usually accompanied by generalized lymphadenopathy. Other cancer, especially malignant melanoma, may metastasize to the tonsil as well. Cervical lymphadenopathy, ipsi- or contralateral, is a common presenting sign, even with very small primary cancers. Fine-needle aspirates of these lymph nodes or excisional biopsy of the tonsil will confirm the diagnosis. Thoracic radiographs will be positive for metastasis in 10 to 20% of cases at presentation. In spite of disease apparently confined to the tonsil, this disease is considered systemic at diagnosis in more than 90% of patients. Simple tonsillectomy is almost never

curative but probably should be done bilaterally because of the high percentage of bilateral disease.[44] Cervical lymphadenectomy, especially for large and fixed nodes, is rarely curative and should be considered diagnostic only. Regional radiation (pharynx and cervical lymph nodes) is capable of controlling local disease in more than 75% of the cases; however, survival still remains poor, with only 10% of affected animals alive after 1 year.[22,45] The cause of death is local disease early and systemic disease (usually lung metastasis) later. To date, no known effective chemotherapeutic agents exist for canine or feline squamous cell carcinoma, although cisplatin and bleomycin have been utilized with very limited success.[45,46]

### Tongue[30,47]

Cancer confined to the tongue is rare. White dogs appear to be at higher risk for squamous cell carcinoma, even though lack of protective pigment would not seem to be as much a problem as it is in other, more exposed areas of the body (nose, eyelids, and ears). The most common cancer of the canine tongue is squamous cell carcinoma (~50%), followed by granular cell myoblastoma, melanoma, mast cell, fibrosarcoma, and a wide variety of histologic types. Feline tongue tumors are usually squamous cell carcinoma and most are located on the ventral surface near the frenulum. The presenting signs are similar to other oral cancers and mass lesions.

Under general anesthesia, the tongue may be biopsied with a wedge incision and closed with horizontal mattress sutures. The regional lymph nodes should be aspirated for staging purposes, if palpable. The treatment is generally with surgery, and irradiation is reserved for inoperable cancer or cancer metastatic to the lymph nodes. Partial glossectomy can be performed for more than half of the mobile tongue. Eating and drinking may be slightly impaired, but good hydration and nutrition can be maintained postoperatively.[47] Grooming in cats will be compromised, with up to 50% removal and may result in poor hair-coat hygiene. Long-term control of feline tongue tumors is rarely reported.

The prognosis for tongue tumors will vary with the site, type, and grade of cancer.[47] Cancer in the rostral (mobile) tongue has a better pattern of behavior for any of the following reasons:

1. Earlier detection, since the owner can see the lesion.
2. The rostral tongue may have less abundant lymphatic and vascular channels as opposed to the caudal tongue, whose richer systems may allow metastasis.
3. Rostral lesions are easier to operate with wide margins.

In a series of 10 dogs, the 1-year survival with surgery or radiation for squamous cell carcinoma of the tongue is as high as 50% for histologically complete resection of as much as 60 to 80% of the tongue in dogs with low-grade histology.[47] Granular cell myoblastoma is a curable cancer.[48] These lesions may look large and invasive but are almost always removable with conservative and close margins (Fig. 18–3). Permanent local control rates exceed 80%. The tumors may recur late, but serial surgeries are usually possible. This cancer is rarely metastatic. Local control in four of five tongue melanomas was obtained by surgery and the metastatic rate was less than 50% in this small series.[30] The behavior of other tongue cancers is generally unknown because of the rarity of these conditions.

## Viral Papillomatosis[49]

Viral papillomatosis is horizontally transmitted by a viral agent (papovavirus) from dog to dog. Affected animals are generally young. The lesions appear wartlike and are generally multiple in the oral cavity, pharynx, tongue, or lips. A biopsy can be performed if necessary but visual examination is usually diagnostic. Most patients never suffer any significant side effects of this disease, while an occasional dog will have such marked involvement that surgical debulking will be required to permit swallowing. The majority of patients will undergo a spontaneous regression of disease within 4 to 8 weeks that resists a subsequent viral challenge. For resistant cases, a wide

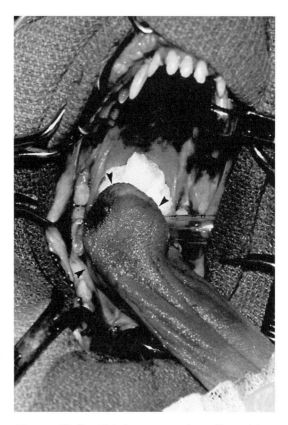

**Figure 18–3.** This large granular cell myoblastoma was easily removed surgically. The patient had a recurrence at 2 years postoperatively; the lesion was again removed and the dog is free of disease 3 years after the last surgery.

variety of treatments have been tried: crushing of lesions in situ to "release" antigen; autogenous vaccines; and chemotherapy.[50] These methods are seldom required or effective, and the prognosis is generally excellent.

## Canine Oral Eosinophilic Granulomas[51,52]

Oral eosinophilic granulomas affect young dogs (1 to 7 years) and may be heritable in the Siberian husky. The disease is histologically similar to the feline disease, with eosinophils and granulomatous inflammation predominating. The granulomas typically occur on the lateral and ventral aspects of the tongue. They are raised, are frequently ulcerated, and may mimic more malignant cancers in appearance. Treatment with corticosteroids or surgical excision is generally

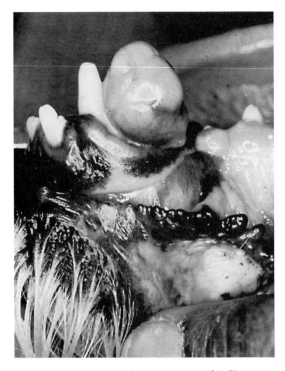

**Figure 18–4.** Typical appearance of a fibromatous epulis on the gum line of an 8-year-old dog. The mass is firmly adherent to underlying bone but noninvasive on radiographs. Conservative removal was curative.

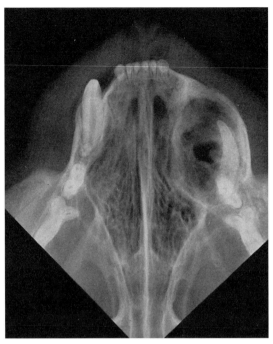

**Figure 18–5.** Radiograph of a 1-year-old cat with a large inductive fibroameloblastoma of the entire lateral maxilla. Note the displacement of the teeth and expansile nature of the bone distortion. This patient was treated with radiation therapy and is in clinical remission 3 years after treatment.

curative, although spontaneous regression may occur. Recurrences are uncommon.

## Epulis

Benign, gingivally located proliferations of tissue in the dog are termed *epulides* and may be fibromatous or ossifying.[4] Acanthomatous epulides are covered elsewhere in this chapter. Epulides are usually firm, 1 to 4 cm, and variably fixed to the bone at the gum line (Fig. 18–4). Mild ulceration may occur, but most epulides are covered by epithelium. Epulides do not significantly invade bone, and treatment is with conservative blade excision. The rare recurrent lesion may require more aggressive destruction of the base with electrocautery or cryosurgery. Epulides are rare in the cat.

## Inductive Fibroameloblastoma[53–55]

The rare odontogenic tumor known as inductive fibroameloblastoma affects primarily young cats (6 months to 2 years) and has a predilection for the

region of the upper canine teeth and maxilla. Radiographically the tumor site shows variable degrees of bone destruction, production, and expansion of the maxillary bones (Fig. 18–5). Teeth deformity is common. Smaller lesions are treated with surgical debulking and cryosurgery or premaxillectomy. Larger lesions will respond to radiation. Local treatment needs to be aggressive but control rates are good and metastasis has not been reported.

## Nasopharyngeal Polyps in Cats

Nasopharyngeal polyps tend to affect young cats, most less than 2 years old. No definitive breed or sex predilection is known.[56] Clinical signs include sneezing, change in voice, swallowing problems, rhinitis, and difficulty in breathing. Firm, fleshy masses can be seen or palpated in the caudal pharynx or above the soft palate (Fig. 18–6). Occasionally, masses can be visualized in the external ear canal.[57,58] Skull radiographs may reveal fluid or tissue in the tympanic bullae.[59] Most lesions originate in the bullae or eustachian

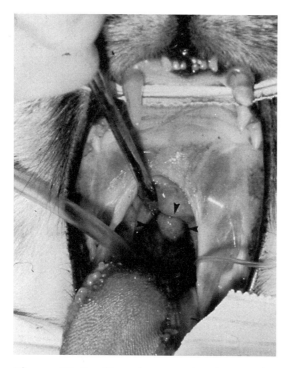

**Figure 18–6.** Nasopharyngeal polyp can be visualized as the soft palate is pulled forward. This lesion is attached to a stalk emanating from the eustachian tube.

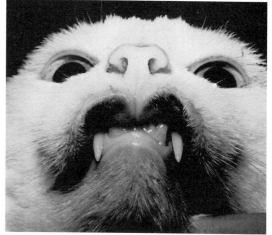

**Figure 18–7.** Typical erosive eosinophilic granuloma on the upper lip of a female cat.

tube and grow toward the pharynx to become a pedunculated mass. Treatment through the oral cavity or external ear canal is by traction and ligation of as much of the stalk as possible; however, recurrences are common if that is the sole treatment. If radiographs reveal tissue in the bullae, a combined oral removal and bullae osteotomy may be required to effect a cure.[58,60] The disease is probably not truly neoplastic but rather primarily or secondarily inflammatory.

## Eosinophilic Granuloma in the Cat[61–63]

Most commonly known as eosinophilic granuloma, this condition is also known as rodent ulcer or indolent ulcer. It occurs more commonly in female cats with an average age of 5 years. The etiology is unknown.

Any oral site is at risk, but the disease is most common on the upper lip near the midline (Fig. 18–7). The history is usually that of a slowly progressive (months to years) erosion of the lip. Biopsies are often necessary to differentiate the condition from true cancers.

Various treatments are proposed, including (in order of author preference): prednisone at 1 to 2 mg/kg BID × 30 days orally or IM methyl prednisolone acetate* at 20 mg/cat SQ every two weeks; megestrol acetate;** hypoallergenic diets; radiation; surgery; immunomodulation; or cryosurgery. The prognosis for complete and permanent recovery is only fair, although rare cases may undergo spontaneous regression.

## Malignancy of Young Dogs[64]

Undifferentiated malignancy is seen in dogs under 2 years of age (range 6 to 22 months). Most patients are large breeds and there is no sex predilection. The disease manifests as a rapidly growing mass in the area of the hard palate, upper molar teeth or maxilla or both, and orbit. Biopsies reveal an undifferentiated malignancy of undetermined histogenesis. Most patients present with lymph node metastasis, and at necropsy five of six had metastasis beyond the head and neck. No effective treatment has been proposed although, conceptually, chemotherapy would be necessary. Most patients are euthanatized within 30 days of diagnosis because of progressive and uncontrolled tumor growth.

Papillary squamous cell carcinoma has been reported to occur in the oral cavity of very young dogs (2 to 5 months). Treatment was with surgical debulking and curettage followed by radiation (40 Gy in 20 fractions). No dog had metastasis, and long-term control was achieved in all dogs for periods up to 4 years.[65]

*a Depo-Medrol, UpJohn.
**b Ovaban, Schering.

## COMPARATIVE ASPECTS[66]

The vast majority of oral cavity cancer in humans is squamous cell carcinoma. It is associated with alcohol and tobacco use and usually occurs in patients more than 45 years old.

Treatment is generally with surgery, radiation, or both. Chemotherapy has a limited role for local disease but has shown promise, often in combination with radiation, for advanced-stage cancer.

Prognosis is strongly correlated to histologic grade, stage, and site (the pharynx and caudal tongue fare worse than the rostral tongue and oral cavity).

## REFERENCES

1. Hoyt RF, Withrow SJ: Oral malignancy in the dog. J Am Anim Hosp Assoc 20:83–92, 1984.
2. Stebbins KE, Morse CC, Goldschmidt MH: Feline oral neoplasia: A ten-year survey. Vet Pathol 26:121–128, 1989.
3. Ciekot PA, Powers BE, Withrow SJ, et al: Histologically low grade yet biologically high grade fibrosarcomas of the mandible and maxilla of 25 dogs (1982 to 1991). J Am Vet Med Assoc 204:610–615, 1994.
4. Dubielzig RR: Proliferative dental and gingival diseases of dogs and cats. J Am Anim Hosp Assoc 18:577–584, 1982.
5. Madewell BR, Ackerman N, Sesline DH: Invasive carcinoma radiographically mimicking primary bone cancer in the mandibles of two cats. J Am Vet Radiol Soc 27:213–215, 1976.
6. Withrow SJ, Holmberg DL: Mandibulectomy in the treatment of oral cancer. J Am Anim Hosp Assoc 19:273–286, 1983.
7. Withrow SJ, Nelson AW, Manley PA, Biggs DR: Premaxillectomy in the dog. J Am Anim Hosp Assoc 21:49–55, 1985.
8. White RAS, Gorman NT, Watkins SB, Brearley MJ: The surgical management of bone-involved oral tumors in the dog. J Small Anim Pract 26:693–708, 1985.
9. Bradley RL, MacEwen EG, Loar AS: Mandibular resection for removal of oral tumors in 30 dogs and 6 cats. J Am Vet Med Assoc 184:460–463, 1984.
10. Salisbury SK, Richardson DC, Lantz GC: Partial maxillectomy and premaxillectomy in the treatment of oral neoplasia in the dog and cat. Vet Surg 15:16–26, 1986.
11. Salisbury SK, Lantz GC: Long-term results of partial mandibulectomy for treatment of oral tumors in 30 dogs. J Am Anim Hosp Assoc 24:285–294, 1988.
12. White RAS: Mandibulectomy and maxillectomy in the dog: long-term survival in 100 cases. J Small Anim Pract 32:69–74, 1991.
13. Kosovsky JK, Matthiesen DT, Marretta SM, Patnaik AK: Results of partial mandibulectomy for the treatment of oral tumors in 142 dogs. Vet Surg 20:397–401, 1991.
14. Wallace J, Matthiesen DT, Patnaik AK: Hemimaxillectomy for the treatment of oral tumors in 69 dogs. Vet Surg 21:337–341, 1992.
15. Schwarz PD, Withrow SJ, Curtis CR, et al: Mandibular resection as a treatment for oral cancer in 81 dogs. J Am Anim Hosp Assoc 27:601–610, 1991.
16. Schwarz PD, Withrow SJ, Curtis CR, et al: Partial maxillary resection as a treatment for oral cancer in 61 dogs. J Am Anim Hosp Assoc 27:617–624, 1991.
17. Gillette EL, McChesney SL, Dewhirst MW, Scott RJ: Response of canine oral carcinomas to heat and radiation. Int J Radiat Oncol Biol Phys 13:1861–1867, 1987.
18. Dewhirst MW, Sim DA, Forsyth K, et al: Local control and distant metastases in primary canine malignant melanomas treated with hyperthermia and/or radiotherapy. Int J Hyperthermia 1:219–234, 1985.
19. Brewer WG, Turrel JM: Radiotherapy and hyperthermia in the treatment of fibrosarcomas in the dog. J Am Vet Med Assoc 181:146–150, 1982.
20. Thrall DE: Orthovoltage radiotherapy of acanthomatous epulides in 39 dogs. J Am Vet Med Assoc 184:826–829, 1984.
21. Langham RF, Mostosky UV, Schirmer RG: X-ray therapy of selected odontogenic neoplasms in the dog. J Am Vet Med Assoc 170:820–822, 1977.
22. MacMillan R, Withrow SJ, Gillette EL: Surgery and regional irradiation for treatment of canine tonsillar squamous cell carcinoma: Retrospective review of eight cases. J Am Anim Hosp Assoc 18:311–314, 1982.
23. Gillette EL: Radiation therapy of canine and feline tumors. J Am Anim Hosp Assoc 12:359–362, 1976.
24. Bateman KE, Catton PA, Pennock PW, et al: Radiation therapy for the treatment of canine oral melanoma. J Vet Intern Med 8:267–272, 1994.
25. Kitchell BE, Brown DM, Luck EE, et al: Intralesional implant for treatment of primary oral malignant melanoma in dogs. J Am Vet Med Assoc 204:229–236, 1994.
26. MacEwen EG, Patnaik AK, Harvey HJ, et al: Canine oral melanoma: Comparison of surgery versus surgery plus Corynebacterium parvum. Cancer Invest 4:397–402. Marcel Dekker Inc, New York, 1986.
27. Bjorling DE, Chambers JN, Mahaffey EA: Surgical treatment of epulides in dogs: 25 cases (1974–1984). J Am Vet Med Assoc 190:1315–1318, 1987.
28. White RAS, Gorman NT: Wide local excision of acanthomatous epulides in the dog. Vet Surg 18:12–14, 1989.
29. Thrall DE, Goldschmidt MH, Biery DN: Malig-

nant tumor formation at the site of previously irradiated acanthomatous epulides in four dogs. J Am Vet Med Assoc 178:127–132, 1981.

30. Beck ER, Withrow SJ, McChesney AE, et al: Canine tongue tumors: A retrospective review of 57 cases. J Am Anim Hosp Assoc 22:525–532, 1986.

31. Bostock DE: The prognosis in cats bearing squamous cell carcinoma. J Small Anim Pract 13:119–125, 1972.

32. Cotter SM: Oral pharyngeal neoplasms in the cat. J Am Anim Hosp Assoc 17:917–920, 1981.

33. Evans SM, Shofer F: Canine oral nontonsillar squamous cell carcinoma. Vet Radiol 29:133–137, 1988.

34. Reeves NCP, Turrel JM, Withrow SJ: Oral squamous cell carcinoma in the cat. J Am Anim Hosp Assoc 29:438–441, 1993.

35. Hutson CA, Willauer CC, Walder EJ, et al: Treatment of mandibular squamous cell carcinoma in cats by use of mandibulectomy and radiotherapy: Seven cases (1987–1989). J Am Vet Med Assoc 201:777–781, 1992.

36. Evans SM, LaCreta F, Helfand S, et al: Technique, pharmacokinetics, toxicity, and efficacy of intratumoral etanidazole and radiotherapy for treatment of spontaneous feline oral squamous cell carcinoma. Int J Radiat Oncol Biol Phys 20:703–708, 1991.

37. Mauldin GN, Matus RE, Patnaik AK, et al: Efficacy and toxicity of doxorubicin and cyclophosphamide used in the treatment of selected malignant tumors in 23 cats. J Vet Intern Med 2:60–65, 1988.

38. Harvey HJ, MacEwen GE, Braun D, et al: Prognostic criteria for dogs with oral melanoma. J Am Vet Med Assoc 178:580–582, 1981.

39. Hilmas DE, Gillette EL: Radiotherapy of spontaneous fibrous connective-tissue sarcomas in animals. J Natl Cancer Inst 56:365–368, 1976.

40. Creasey WA, Phil D, Thrall DE: Pharmacokinetic and anti-tumor studies with the radiosensitizer misonidazole in dogs with spontaneous fibrosarcomas. Am J Vet Res 43:1015–1018, 1982.

41. Thrall DE: Orthovoltage radiotherapy of oral fibrosarcomas in dogs. J Am Vet Med Assoc 172(2):159–162, 1981.

42. Straw RC, Powers BE, Klausner J, et al: Canine mandibular osteosarcoma: 51 cases (1980–1992). J Am Anim Hosp Assoc, submitted.

43. Reif JS, Cohen D: The environmental distribution of canine respiratory tract neoplasms. Arch Environ Health 22:136–140, 1971.

44. Todoroff RJ, Brodey RS: Oral and pharyngeal neoplasia in the dog: A retrospective survey of 361 cases. J Am Vet Med Assoc 175:567–571, 1979.

45. Brooks MB, Matus RE, Leifer CE, et al: Chemotherapy versus chemotherapy plus radiotherapy in the treatment of tonsillar squamous cell carcinoma in the dog. J Vet Intern Med 2:206–211, 1988.

46. Buhles WC, Theilan GH: Preliminary evaluation of bleomycin in feline and canine squamous cell carcinomas. Am J Vet Res 34:289–291, 1973.

47. Carpenter LG, Withrow SJ, Powers BE, et al: Squamous cell carcinoma of the tongue in 10 dogs. J Am Anim Hosp Assoc 29:17–24, 1993.

48. Turk MAM, Johnson GC, Gallina AM: Canine granular cell tumour (myoblastoma): A report of four cases and review of the literature. J Small Anim Pract 24:637–645, 1983.

49. Norris AM, Withrow SJ, Dubielzig: Oropharyngeal neoplasms. In Harvey CE (ed): Oral Disease in the Dog and Cat: Veterinary Dentistry. Philadelphia, WB Saunders, 1985, pp. 123–139.

50. Calvert CA: Canine viral and transmissible neoplasias. In Greene CE (ed): Clinical Microbiology and Infectious Diseases of the Dog and Cat. Philadelphia, WB Saunders, 1984, pp. 461–478.

51. Potter KA, Tucker RD, Carpenter JL: Oral eosinophilic granuloma of Siberian huskies. J Am Anim Hosp Assoc 16:595–600, 1980.

52. Madewell BR, Stannard AA, Pulley LT, et al: Oral eosinophilic granuloma in Siberian husky dogs. J Am Vet Med Assoc 177:701–703, 1980.

53. Dubielzig RR, Adams WM, Brodey RS: Inductive fibroameloblastoma: An unusual dental tumor of young cats. J Am Vet Med Assoc 174:720–722, 1979.

54. Hawkins CD, Jones BR: Adamantinoma in a cat. Aust Vet J 59:54–55, 1982.

55. Poulet FM, Valentine BA, Summers BA: A survey of epithelial odontogenic tumors and cysts in dogs and cats. Vet Pathol 29:369–380, 1992.

56. Bradley RL, Noone KE, Saunders GK, et al: Nasopharyngeal and middle ear polypoid masses in five cats. Vet Surg 14:141–144, 1985.

57. Harvey CE, Goldschmidt MH: Inflammatory polypoid growths in the ear canal of cats. J Small Anim Pract 19:669–677, 1978.

58. Faulkner JE, Budsberg SC: Results of ventral bulla osteotomy for treatment of middle ear polyps in cats. J Am Anim Hosp Assoc 26:496–499, 1990.

59. Parker NR, Binnington AG: Nasopharyngeal polyps in cats: Three case reports and a review of the literature. J Am Anim Hosp Assoc 21:473–478, 1985.

60. Trevor PB, Martin RA: Tympanic bulla osteotomy for treatment of middle-ear disease in cats: 19 cases (1984–1991). J Am Vet Med Assoc 202:123–128:1993.

61. Scott DW: Disorders of unknown or multiple origin (Chap. 11). J Am Anim Hosp Assoc 16:406–411, 1980.

62. McClelland RB: X-ray therapy in labial and cutaneous granulomas in cats. J Am Vet Med Assoc 125:469–470, 1954.

63. MacEwen EG, Hess PW: Evaluation of effect of immunomodulation on the feline eosinophilic granuloma complex. J Am Anim Hosp Assoc 23:519–526, 1987.

64. Patnaik AK, Lieberman PH, Erlandson RA, et al: A clinicopathologic and ultrastructural study of undifferentiated malignant tumors of the oral cavity in dogs. Vet Pathol 23:170–175, 1986.

65. Ogilvie GK, Sundberg JP, O'Banion MK, et al: Papillary squamous cell carcinoma in three young dogs. J Am Vet Med Assoc 192:933–936, 1988.

66. Schantz SP, Harrison LB, Hong WK: Tumors of the nasal cavity and paranasal sinuses, nasopharynx, oral cavity and oropharynx. In DeVita VT et al (eds): Cancer: Principles and Practice of Oncology. Philadelphia, JB Lippincott, 1993, pp. 574–630.

# B. Cancer of the Salivary Glands

## Stephen J. Withrow

### INCIDENCE AND RISK FACTORS

Primary salivary gland cancer is rare in the dog and cat. Most cases are reported in older patients (10–12 years) and no breed or sex predilection has been determined.[1,2]

### PATHOLOGY

The vast majority of salivary cancers are adenocarcinomas, but a wide range of specific histologic variants have been reported.[1] They can arise from major (parotid, mandibular, sublingual, zygomatic) or minor glands. Benign salivary gland tumors are rare in animals compared to humans. The mandibular gland is most commonly affected.[3] Salivary cancers are variably locally invasive and metastasis to regional lymph nodes is common. Distant metastasis has been reported but may be slow to develop. Metastasis is more common in the cat than in the dog.[4]

### HISTORY AND CLINICAL SIGNS

The symptoms are nonspecific and generally include a unilateral, firm, painless swelling of the upper neck (mandibular and sublingual), base of the ear (parotid), upper lip or maxilla (zygomatic), or mucous membrane of the lip or tongue (accessory salivary tissue).

The major differential diagnoses are mucoceles, abscesses, salivary gland infarction, sialadenitis, lymphoma, or reactive lymphadenopathy.[3] Of 245 submissions of salivary tissue for histologic diagnosis, 30% were neoplastic.[3]

### DIAGNOSTIC TECHNIQUES AND WORKUP

Fine-needle aspiration cytology of masses in these locations should help differentiate noncancer diseases from cancer. Regional radiographs will usually be normal but may reveal periosteal reaction on adjacent bones or displacement of surrounding structures. Needle-core or wedge biopsies will usually be necessary to make a definitive diagnosis.

### THERAPY

When possible, aggressive surgical removal should be performed. Unfortunately, most lesions are extracapsular and widely extensive throughout the regional area, which contains numerous vital structures. Radiation therapy after surgery resulted in good local control and prolonged survival in three reported cases.[5] Chemotherapy for salivary gland adenocarcinoma has been largely unreported.

### PROGNOSIS

The prognosis for salivary gland cancer is generally unknown. Clinical experience on a limited number of cases seems to indicate that aggressive local resection (usually histologically incomplete) followed by adjuvant radiation can attain permanent local control and long-term survival.[5] Incomplete removal will invariably result in local recurrence.[2] The median survival rate for dogs and cats treated with surgical resection with or without adjuvant radiation was 12 months.[4]

## COMPARATIVE ASPECTS[6]

Salivary gland tumors are more common in older people than in animals and account for 4% of head and neck neoplasms. The parotid gland is most commonly affected. A wide array of benign and malignant neoplasms are recognized. Treatment is with surgical excision, and radiation is utilized for inoperable disease or after incomplete removal. Five-year survival usually exceeds 75% but is dependent on stage and histologic type.

## REFERENCES

1. Koestner A, Buerger L: Primary neoplasms of the salivary glands in animals compared to similar tumors in man. Vet Pathol 2:201–226, 1965.
2. Carberry CA, Glanders JA, Harvey HJ, Ryan AM: Salivary gland tumors in dogs and cats: A literature and case review. J Am Anim Hosp Assoc 24:561–567, 1988.
3. Spangler WL, Culbertson MR: Salivary gland disease in dogs and cats: 245 cases (1985–1988). J Am Vet Med Assoc 198:465–469, 1991.
4. Hammer AS: Interim analysis of 90 dogs and cats with salivary gland tumors. Vet Coop Oncol Group, 1994.
5. Evans SM, Thrall DE: Postoperative orthovoltage radiation therapy of parotid salivary gland adenocarcinoma in three dogs. J Am Vet Med Assoc 182:993–994, 1983.
6. Sessions RB, Harrison LB, Hong WK: Tumors of the salivary glands and paragangliomas. In DeVita VT et al (ed): Cancer: Principles and Practice of Oncology. Philadelphia, JB Lippincott. 1993, pp. 655–672.

# C. Esophageal Cancer

## Stephen J. Withrow

## INCIDENCE AND RISK FACTORS

Cancer of the esophagus is very rare and accounts for less than 0.5% of all cancer in the dog and cat.[1] Sarcomas, secondary to *Spirocerca lupi* infestation, have been reported in indigenous areas (Africa and southeastern United States).[2] No cause is known for the more common carcinomas. Most animals are older and no sex or breed predilection is evident.

## PATHOLOGY AND NATURAL BEHAVIOR

The more commonly reported histologic types include squamous cell carcinoma, leiomyosarcoma, fibrosarcoma, and osteosarcoma. Rarely, benign neoplasms such as leiomyoma and plasmacytoma may be encountered, especially in the area of the terminal esophagus and cardia.[3,4] Paraesophageal tumors such as thymic, heart base, or thyroid may also invade the esophagus.[1] In cats, squamous cell carcinomas are usually seen in females and are located in the middle third of the esophagus just caudal to the thoracic inlet.[5,6]

Most esophageal cancers are locally invasive and metastasis is to draining lymph nodes, or hematogenously.

## HISTORY AND SIGNS

The signs of disease, other than those of general debilitation and weight loss, include pain on swallowing, dysphagia, and regurgitation of undigested food. Pneumonia, secondary to aspiration, may also be noted. Hypertrophic osteopathy has been reported, especially with *Spirocerca lupi*-induced sarcomas.[2]

## DIAGNOSTIC TECHNIQUES AND WORKUP

It is generally evident from the history that the patient is suffering from a partial or complete upper gastrointestinal obstruction. Plain radiographs may reveal retention of gas within the esophageal lumen, a mass, or esophageal dilatation proximal to the cancer. A positive contrast esophagram with or without fluoroscopy will generally reveal a stricture or mass lesion in the lumen. Esophagoscopy allows visualization of the lesion, which is frequently ulcerated. Several biopsies should be taken, since necrosis and inflammation are often prominent. The risk of esophageal perforation during the biopsy is generally minimal.

Open surgical biopsy via thoracotomy or cervical exploration is another option to obtain tissue for a diagnosis. *Spirocerca lupi* ova may be detected in the feces.

## THERAPY

Therapy for malignant cancer of the esophagus is difficult at best because of the advanced stage of disease in most cases.[7] Intrathoracic resections are further complicated by poor exposure, lengthy resections, tension on the anastomosis, and the unique healing problems of the thoracic esophagus. For lesions in the caudal esophagus or cardia, gastric advancement through the diaphragm can be attempted.

Various procedures to partially replace the resected esophagus have been described, including microvascular transfer of the colon or small bowel, but clinical reports on their use in the cancer patient are lacking.[8–10] Chemotherapy has rarely been attempted. Radiation therapy for the cervical esophagus can be attempted but is of limited value for the intrathoracic esophagus because of the poor tolerance of normal tissues such as the lung and heart.

Benign leiomyomas of the esophagus or cardia can be approached via thoracotomy or celiotomy. Short-term palliation can be achieved via esophagotomy or gastrostomy tubes.

## PROGNOSIS

Except for the rare, benign lesion[3,4] or lymphoma, the prognosis is very poor for cure or palliation because of poor resection options and the high metastatic rate.

## COMPARATIVE ASPECTS[11]

Esophageal cancer (principally squamous cell carcinoma) is rare in humans but still accounts for 7,000 deaths per year in the United States. Marked geographic variance in worldwide incidence implies numerous environmental influences on development (including tobacco, alcohol, hot food, and nitrosamines).

Most esophageal cancers have extensive local tumor growth and lymph node involvement, which preclude curative treatment. Combinations or single use of surgery, radiation, and chemotherapy have resulted in 5-year survivals of less than 20% for the more common advanced-stage disease. A variety of palliative bypass procedures for inoperable disease are also performed (esophagogastrostomy, intraluminal intubation, dilatation, and feeding gastrostomies).

## REFERENCES

1. Ridgeway RL, Suter PF: Clinical and radiographic signs in primary and metastatic esophageal neoplasms of the dog. J Am Vet Med Assoc 174:700–704, 1979.
2. Bailey WS: *Spirocerca lupi:* A continuing inquiry. J Parasitol 58:3–22, 1972.
3. Culbertson R, Branam JE, Rosenblatt LS: Esophageal/gastric leiomyoma in the laboratory Beagle. J Am Vet Med Assoc 183:1168–1171, 1983.
4. Hamilton TA, Carpenter JL: Esophageal plasmacytoma in a dog. J Am Vet Med Assoc 204:1210–1211, 1994.
5. Carpenter JL, Andrews LN, Holzworth J: Tumor and tumor-like lesion. In, Holzworth J (ed): Diseases of the Cat. Philadelphia, WB Saunders, 1987, p.492.
6. Cotchin E: Neoplasms in cats. Proc R Soc Med 45:671, 1952.
7. McCaw D, Pratt M, Walshaw R: Squamous cell carcinoma of the esophagus in a dog. J Am Anim Hosp Assoc 16:561–563, 1980.
8. Gregory CR, Gourley IM, Bruyette DS, Schultz LJ: Free jejunal segment for treatment of cervical esophageal stricture in a dog. J Am Vet Med Assoc 193:230–232, 1988.
9. Kuzma AB, Holmberg DL, Miller CW, Barker I, Roth J: Esophageal replacement in the dog by microvascular colon transfer. Vet Surg 18:439–445, 1989.

10. Straw RC, Tomlinson JL, Constantinescu G, Turk MAM, Hogan PM: Use of a vascular skeletal muscle graft for canine esophageal reconstruction. Vet Surg 16:155–156, 1987.

11. Roth JA, Lichter AS, Putnam JB, Forastiere AA: Cancer of the esophagus. *In*, DeVita VT et al (eds): Cancer: Principles and Practice of Oncology. Philadelphia, JB Lippincott, 1993, pp. 776–817.

# D. Exocrine Pancreas

## Stephen J. Withrow

### INCIDENCE AND RISK FACTORS

Exocrine cancer of the pancreas is very rare (< 0.5%) in the dog and even more uncommon in the cat.[1] Older female dogs have been described as being at higher risk.[2,3] Experimentally, N-ethyl-N′-nitro-N-nitrosoquanidine has been shown to induce pancreatic duct adenocarcinoma when administered intraductally.[4]

### PATHOLOGY AND NATURAL BEHAVIOR

Almost all cancers of the pancreas are epithelial and most are adenocarcinoma of ductular or acinar origin. Nodular hyperplasia is a common asymptomatic finding in older dogs or cats. In the vast majority of cases, malignant cancer has metastasized to regional or distant sites before a diagnosis can be made.[1]

### HISTORY AND CLINICAL SIGNS

The history and clinical signs of pancreatic cancer are vague and nonspecific. Weight loss, anorexia, vomiting, abdominal distention, icterus (with common bile duct obstruction), and depression are common symptoms. Alternatively, patients may present for symptoms of metastatic disease. Abdominal effusions can develop because of tumor implants on the peritoneum or compression of the post cava.

### DIAGNOSTIC TECHNIQUES AND WORKUP

Most hematologic and biochemical evaluations are nonspecific but may include mild anemia, neutrophilia, and bilirubinemia (if occluding the common bile duct).[1] Elevations of serum amylase and lipase are inconsistent. In extreme cases, signs of pancreatic insufficiency may be exhibited.[5] Positive contrast upper gastrointestinal radiographs may reveal slowed gastric emptying and occasionally compression or invasion of the duodenum.

Ascites may be a clinical sign and, when present, may reveal malignant cells on cytologic examination. Most tumors are not palpable through the abdominal wall.

Ultrasonography should be a useful diagnostic tool but few reports exist to document its efficacy. Most diagnoses are made at exploratory laparotomy.

### THERAPY

Most nonislet cell carcinomas of the pancreas are metastatic (regional lymph nodes and liver) or very locally invasive at the time of diagnosis. If the liver, peritoneal cavity, or draining lymph nodes are positive for tumor, heroic surgery should generally not be performed. Complete pancreatectomy or pancreaticoduodenectomy (Whipple's procedure) has been described in man but carries a high operative morbidity and mortality without significant cure rates.[6,7] Palliative gastrointestinal bypass (gastrojejunostomy) is a short-term option if bowel obstruction is imminent. Radiation and chemotherapy have shown limited value in humans and animals.

### PROGNOSIS

The outlook for this disease in animals is very poor because of its critical location and advanced stage at diagnosis. One-year survival after diagnosis, regardless of treatment, has not been reported.[1]

## COMPARATIVE ASPECTS[7]

Pancreatic exocrine carcinoma affects over 20,000 humans per year in the United States. Most patients have disease progression beyond the pancreas at the time of initial diagnosis; 75% of tumors are located in the head of the pancreas and the remainder in the body and tail. Direct extension to the duodenum, bile duct, and stomach as well as common metastasis to the lymph node and liver make treatment difficult.

When possible, pancreaticoduodenectomy (Whipple's procedure) or complete pancreatectomy is the treatment of choice. However, operative mortality ranges from 5 to 30%. Palliative bypass of the biliary tree and duodenum is commonly performed for inoperable lesions.

Traditional external beam radiation therapy is generally palliative rather than curative. Intraoperative and interstitial radiation are being explored as means for high-dose delivery to the tumor while sparing normal radiosensitive structures.[8,9] Chemotherapy alone or in combination with radiation or surgery has demonstrated some improvement in survival. Overall, 5-year survival for all patients remains less than 5%.

## REFERENCES

1. Davenport D: Pancreatic carcinoma in twenty dogs and five cats. Proc Annu Conf Vet Cancer Soc, 1985 (Abstract).
2. Kircher CH, Nielsen SW: Tumors of the pancreas. Bull WHO 53:195–202, 1976.
3. Anderson NV, Johnson KH: Pancreatic carcinoma in the dog. J Am Vet Med Assoc 150:286–295, 1967.
4. Kamano T, Azuma N, Katami A, Tamura J, et al: Preliminary observation on pancreatic duct adenocarcinoma induced by intraductal administration of N1-ethyl-N′-nitro-N-nitrosoquanidine in dogs. Jpn J Cancer Res 79:1–4, 1988.
5. Bright JM: Pancreatic adenocarcinoma in a dog with a maldigestion syndrome. J Am Vet Med Assoc 187:420–421, 1985.
6. Cobb LF, Merrell RC: Total pancreatectomy in dogs. J Surg Res 37:235–240, 1984.
7. Brennan MF, Kinsella TJ, Casper ES: Cancer of the pancreas. In DeVita VT et al (eds): Cancer: Principles and Practice of Oncology. Philadelphia, JB Lippincott, 1993, pp. 849–882.
8. Ahmadu-Suka F, Gillette EL, Withrow SJ, et al: Pathologic response of the pancreas and duodenum to experimental intraoperative irradiation. Int J Radiat Oncol Biol Phys 14:1197–1204, 1988.
9. Dobelbower RR, Konski AA, Merrick HW, et al: Intraoperative electron beam radiation therapy (IOEBRT) for carcinoma of the exocrine pancreas. Int J Radiat Oncol Biol Phys 20:113–119, 1991.

# E. Gastric Cancer

## Stephen J. Withrow

## INCIDENCE AND RISK FACTORS

Gastric cancer is more common than esophageal cancer but still accounts for less than 1% of all malignancies. No definitive etiology is known, although long-term administration of nitrosamines may induce carcinomas in dogs.[1] One article has described a high incidence of gastric carcinoma in related Belgian shepherds, implying a genetic mechanism in the development of this disease.[2] The average age of affected carcinoma patients is 8 years, with a 2.5:1 male to female ratio. Males are also more commonly affected with gastric lymphoma than females.[3] No clear-cut breed predilection has been identified.[4,5] Leiomyomas tend to occur in very old dogs (average age 15 years).[6,7]

## PATHOLOGY AND NATURAL BEHAVIOR

Adenocarcinoma accounts for 60 to 70% of cancer of the canine stomach. The lesions are often scirrhous (firm and white serosally) and have been termed *linitis plastica* ("leather bottle") because of their firm and nondistensible texture. They can be diffusely infiltrative, expansile (often with a central crater and ulceration) or may look more polypoid.[8] Other reported canine malignancies include leiomyosarcoma,[9] lymphoma,[3] extramedullary plasmacytoma,[10] and fibrosarcoma. Adenocarcinoma will frequently spread to regional lymph nodes (70 to 80% at necropsy), followed by the liver and lung.[2,5,8,11] Adenocarcinomas have been described as diffuse or interstitial, but little clinical significance can be associated with these variants.[5] Benign lesions are generally leiomyomas, hypertrophic gastropathy, or adenomas.[7,12–17] Feline gastric adenocarcinoma is rare and the stomach is the least commonly affected gastrointestinal site in the cat.[17,18] Lymphoma is the most common gastric tumor in the cat and may be solitary or one component of systemic involvement. Most cats with gastric lymphoma are feline leukemia virus negative.

## HISTORY AND CLINICAL SIGNS

The most common history is one of progressive vomiting (often blood tinged or "coffee grounds" in nature), anorexia, and weight loss. The weight loss may be a result of poor digestion, loss of protein and blood from an ulcer, or generalized tumor cachexia. The duration of the symptoms is from weeks to many months.

## DIAGNOSTIC TECHNIQUES AND WORKUP

Routine laboratory tests and noncontrast radiographs are generally not diagnostic. A microcytic hypochromic anemia is common. Occult blood in the feces may be detected. Liver "enzymes" may be elevated because of hepatic metastasis or obstruction of the common bile duct. Thoracic radiographs are only rarely positive for metastasis at the time of initial presentation.

Positive or double contrast gastric radiographs may reveal a mass lesion extending into the lumen (Fig. 18–8). Ulceration is also a common sign. Delayed gastric emptying, poor motility, or delayed adherence of contrast material to an ulcerated tumor may also be detected. Fluoroscopy may aid in determining motility alterations. Malignancies tend to be sessile, and adenocarcinoma tends to occur most commonly on the lesser curvature and gastric antrum (Fig. 18-9).

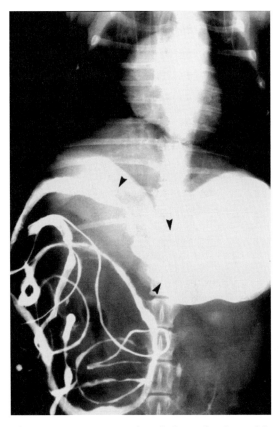

**Figure 18–8.** Ventrodorsal view of a dog with gastric cancer. Note the filling defect and partial outflow obstruction of the gastric antrum and pylorus (arrows).

Benign lesions may be pedunculated or well circumscribed. Leiomyomas often occur at the cardia and will grow into the lumen as a smooth circumscribed mass.[7]

Gastroscopy with a flexible endoscope will generally reveal larger lesions that can be biopsied. Several "large" samples should be taken, since most gastric tumors have superficial necrosis, inflammation, and ulceration. In some patients, the lesions are submucosal only, making endoscopic biopsy difficult. False-negative biopsies through the gastroscope are common. Open surgical biopsy is the most definitive method of diagnosis.

## THERAPY

Except for lymphoma, surgery is the most common form of treatment for gastric cancer. As with esophageal cancer, curative resection is compli-

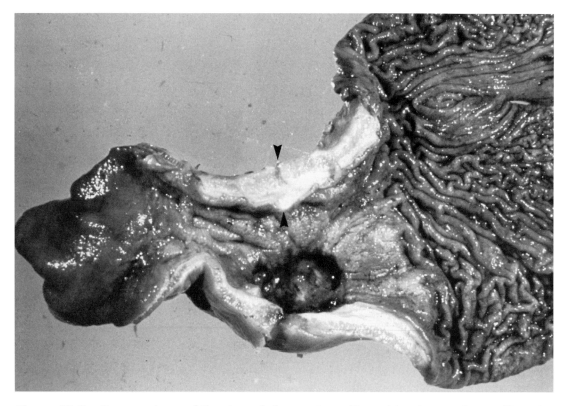

**Figure 18–9.**   Gross specimen of the stomach from a dog with gastric adenocarcinoma. Note the large ulcer and fibrous thickening of the stomach wall in the area of the gastric antrum (arrows). This patient had metastasis to the regional lymph nodes and liver.

cated by advanced-stage disease in a difficult operative area (lesser curvature, antrum, and pylorus) with a frequently debilitated patient. At the time of surgery, a careful evaluation of the liver and regional lymph nodes should be made to stage the cancer adequately. Lymph node metastasis can be quite varied, and all abdominal lymph nodes should be examined. If the cancer is felt to be localized to the stomach at laparotomy, a curative resection may be attempted. If possible, wide partial gastrectomy or antrectomy followed by a gastroduodenostomy (Billroth I) should be performed because of the increased morbidity associated with more extensive surgery, such as partial gastrectomy and gastrojejunostomy (Billroth II).[19] Lesions requiring biliary bypass and very extensive surgery (complete gastrectomy) are generally too advanced to make these procedures worthwhile in terms of survival. For obstructive lesions felt to be inoperable for cure, or metastatic, it is possible to perform a palliative gastrojejunostomy to allow passage of food into

the intestine, although this procedure is associated with significant postoperative morbidity.[19]

Leiomyomas are usually discrete, solitary lesions in the area of the cardia. They are not premalignant but can cause symptoms because of a mass effect. They can be easily "shelled out" via midline laparotomy, gastrotomy and submucosal removal or via intercostal thoracotomy if the side of the lesion can be clearly delineated.[7]

Radiation therapy is rarely utilized because of the poor radiation tolerance of surrounding normal tissue (liver and intestine). Nonresectable lymphoma may be dramatically reduced with lower doses of irradiation than those required for other tumors. No effective chemotherapy is known for adenocarcinoma.

Lymphoma may be excised if localized but does not generally respond well to conventional chemotherapy.[3,20] The need for postoperative chemotherapy after "complete" resection of lymphoma is unknown. If a careful search of other body sites fails to reveal cancer and if the margins of resection are free of tumor, chemotherapy may not be necessary.

## PROGNOSIS

The prognosis for most malignant gastric cancer is poor. Even if surgery can be performed, most patients are dead within 6 months as a result of recurrent or metastatic cancer.[21–24] Few adenocarcinoma patients are operable for cure and the short-term morbidity with radical resection can be high. Palliation via bypass can be achieved for 1 to 6 months. The median survival for seven dogs with gastric leiomyosarcoma that lived at least 2 weeks postoperatively was 1 year.[9] Patients with benign lesions can be cured with complete surgical excision.[7]

## COMPARATIVE ASPECTS[25]

Gastric cancer is the sixth most common cause of cancer death in humans. Adenocarcinoma comprises more than 90% of all malignant gastric cancer. Multiple socioeconomic, geographic, and environmental factors are associated with the risk of tumor development.

Most lesions will be firm, ulcerative, and located in the antrum or lower third of the stomach, as in the dog. Most lesions are detected late in the course of the disease and have direct tumor extension to surrounding organs, lymph node metastasis, or systemic metastasis, as with the dog.

Treatment is with surgical resection when possible or with less effective radiation and chemotherapy. Five-year survival for all patients is less than 10%, with a 30% survival for patients deemed operatively to have "localized" disease.

## REFERENCES

1. Sasajima K, Kawachi T, Sano T, et al: Esophageal and gastric cancers with metastasis induced in dogs by N-ethyl-N'-nitro-N nitrosoquanidine. J Natl Cancer Inst 58:1789–1794, 1977.
2. Scanziani E, Giusti AM, Gualtieri M, Fonda D: Gastric carcinoma in the Belgian shepherd dog. J Small Anim Pract 32:465–469, 1991.
3. Couto CG, Rutgers HC, Sherding RG, Rojko J: Gastrointestinal lymphoma in 20 dogs. J Vet Intern Med 3:73–78, 1989.
4. Sautter JH, Hanlon GF: Gastric neoplasms in the dog: A report of 20 cases. J Am Vet Med Assoc 166:691–696, 1975.
5. Patnaik AK, Hurvitz AI, Johnson GF: Canine gastric adenocarcinoma. Vet Pathol 15:600–607, 1978.
6. Patnaik AK, Hurvitz AI, Johnson GF: gastrointestinal neoplasms. Vet Pathol 14:547–555, 1977.
7. Kerpsack SJ, Birchard SJ: Removal of leiomyomas and other noninvasive masses from the cardiac region of the canine stomach. Proc Annu Conf Vet Cancer Soc, 1993, p. 61.
8. Murray M, Robinson PB, McKeating FJ, et al: Primary gastric neoplasia in the dog: A clinico-pathological study. Vet Rec 91:474–479, 1972.
9. Kapatkin AS, Mullen HS, Matthiesen DT, Patnaik AK: Leiomyosarcoma in dogs: 44 cases (1983–1988). J Am Vet Med Assoc 201:1077–1079, 1992.
10. Brunnert SR, Dee LA, Herron AJ, Altman NH: Gastric extramedullary plasmacytoma in a dog. J Am Vet Med Assoc 200:1501–1502, 1992.
11. Lingeman CH, Garner FM, Taylor DON: Spontaneous gastric adenocarcinomas of dogs: A review. J Natl Cancer Inst 47:137–149, 1971.
12. Walter MC, Goldschmidt MH, Stone EA, et al: Chronic hypertrophic pyloric gastropathy as a cause of pyloric obstruction in the dog. J Am Vet Med Assoc 186:157–161, 1985.
13. Kipnis RM: Focal cystic hypertrophic gastropathy in a dog. J Am Vet Med Assoc 173:182–184, 1978.
14. Happe RP, Van Der Gaag W, Wolvekamp THC, Van Toorenburg J: Multiple polyps of the gastric mucosa in two dogs. J Small Anim Pract 18:179–189, 1977.
15. Culbertson R, Branam JE, Rosenblatt LS: Esophageal/gastric leiomyoma in the laboratory beagle. J Am Vet Med Assoc 183:1168–1172, 1983.
16. Hayden DW, Nielsen SW: Canine alimentary neoplasia. Zbl Vet Med A20:1–22, 1973.
17. Brodey RS: Alimentary tract neoplasms in the cat: A clinicopathologic survey of 46 cases. Am J Vet Res 27:74–80, 1966.
18. Turk MAM, Gallina AM, Russell TS: Nonhematopoietic gastrointestinal neoplasia in cats: A retrospective study of 44 cases. Vet Pathol 18:614–620, 1981.
19. Beaumont PR: Anastomotic jejunal ulcer secondary to gastrojejunostomy in a dog. J Am Anim Hosp Assoc 17:133–237, 1981.
20. MacEwen EG, Mooney S, Brown NO, et al: Management of feline neoplasms. In Holzworth J (ed): Diseases of the Cat, Vol. 1. Philadelphia, WB Saunders, 1987, pp. 597–606.
21. Olivieri M, Gosselin Y, Sauvageau R: Gastric adenocarcinoma in a dog: Six-and-one-half month survival following partial gastrectomy and gastroduodenostomy. J Am Anim Hosp Assoc 20:78–82, 1984.
22. Elliott GS, Stoffregen DA, Richardson DC, et al: Surgical, medical, and nutritional management of gastric adenocarcinoma in a dog. J Am Vet Med Assoc 185:98–101, 1984.
23. Walter MC, Matthiesen DT, Stone EA: Pylorec-

tomy and gastroduodenostomy in the dog: Technique and clinical results in 28 cases. J Am Vet Med Assoc *187*:909–914, 1985.

24. McDonald AE: Primary gastric carcinoma of the dog: Review and case report. Vet Surg *3*:70–73, 1978.

25. Alexander HR, Kelsen DP, Tepper JE: Cancer of the stomach. *In* DeVita VT et al (eds): Cancer: Principles and Practice of Oncology. Philadelphia, JB Lippincott, 1993, pp. 818–848

# F. Hepatic Tumors

## Rodney C. Straw

## INCIDENCE AND RISK

Primary hepatic tumors are rare. They account for 0.6 to 1.3% of all canine neoplasms,[1,2] and 1.5 to 2.3% of all feline neoplasms.[3–10]

Most malignant hepatic tumors occur in older animals at an average age of 10 years.[1] No breeds appear to be at increased risk of developing primary liver tumors. The etiology is unknown, but experimental exposure to certain carcinogens, especially aflatoxins, pyrollizidine alkaloids, and diethylnitrosamine has been shown to induce primary hepatic tumors.[11,12] Metastatic tumors are more common than primary neoplasms in the liver because of the dual afferent blood supply of the hepatic artery and portal vein.[13]

## PATHOLOGY AND NATURAL BEHAVIOR

Five neoplasms of epithelial origin affect the hepatobiliary system of domestic animals. These include hepatocellular carcinoma, bile duct carcinoma, hepatocellular adenoma, bile duct adenoma, and hepatoblastoma.[1,14,15] Carcinoid tumors of neuroectodermal origin also arise from the hepatobiliary system.[1,14,15] In the dog, bile duct adenomas are not clinically significant and hepatoblastomas have not been documented. Therefore, hepatocellular carcinoma, bile duct carcinoma, hepatocellular adenoma, and carcinoid tumors are the clinically significant tumor types. Hepatocellular carcinomas are the most common malignant tumor of the canine and feline liver.[1,3–5] Males appear to be at increased risk for developing these tumors.[1,2] Grossly, hepatocellular carcinoma may be massive, nodular, or diffuse.[1] The massive form is the most common and

consists of a large mass affecting a single liver lobe with smaller metastatic masses often scattered throughout other lobes of the liver. The left liver lobes are more often affected by massive hepatocellular carcinomas.[1,15] The nodular form of the disease consists of multiple discrete nodules of variable size within several lobes. In the diffuse form of hepatocellular carcinoma, large areas of the liver are infiltrated by nonencapsulated neoplastic tissue. The metastatic rate of these tumors is high and somewhat dependent on subtype; 100% of the diffuse, 93% of the nodular, and 36.6% of the massive type demonstrate metastasis at the time of diagnosis.[1] The most common metastatic sites are the hepatic lymph nodes, lung, and peritoneum.[1,15]

Bile duct carcinomas are the second most common primary hepatobiliary tumor of dogs.[16] Bile duct carcinomas occur more frequently in female dogs.[1] Three sites give rise to these tumors: intrahepatic bile ducts, extrahepatic bile ducts, and the gallbladder.[1,2] In dogs, intrahepatic bile ducts are the most common site of origin.[16] As with hepatocellular carcinoma, the disease has three gross forms: massive, nodular, and diffuse.[16] Bile duct carcinomas are highly metastatic tumors; the reported rate of metastasis is 87.5%.[2,16] The most common sites of metastasis are the hepatic lymph nodes, lung, and peritoneum.[17] The nodular and diffuse forms can sometimes be difficult to differentiate from nodular hyperplasia, cirrhosis, or chronic active hepatitis. The highly metastatic nature of this tumor helps differentiate it clinically from these other diseases.[16]

Hepatocellular adenomas are benign tumors that are more common than their malignant counterpart. They are usually single masses but can occur as multiple tumors and often are pedunculated. They can be difficult to differentiate histologically from nodular hyperplasia. However, compression of the surrounding hepatic parenchyma is characteristic of adenomas.

Carcinoid tumors arise from neuroectodermal tissue or the amine precursor uptake and decarboxylation (APUD) cells of the biliary epithelium. They are rare, accounting for less than 15% of all hepatic tumors.[18,19] They require specific silver stains to identify their characteristic intracytoplasmic granules.[18] Grossly they are diffuse, micronodular, or nodular tumors that affect all lobes of the liver.[18] Hemorrhage, necrosis, and calcification occur throughout these tumors. Because of their APUD origin, they may be capable of secreting vasoactive peptides and amines. A metastatic rate of 90% is reported,[18] most commonly to the hepatic lymph nodes and peritoneum.

The cat may develop primary liver tumors as well.[3,4,5] Benign and malignant tumors of hepatocellular origin occur. Carcinomas may be nodular, massive, or diffuse. Tumors of the intrahepatic bile ducts are more common. Bile duct adenocarcinoma is the most frequently reported feline liver tumor. Females are more commonly affected; the incidence is reported to be 11 females to 3 males. Once again, the signs are nonspecific, and 78% of the tumors will have metastasized to the lungs, lymph nodes, and intestinal serosa by the time of diagnosis.[6] Intrahepatic bile duct adenocarcinomas have been associated with liver fluke infestations.[6,7] Bile duct adenomas are also seen, being the third most common primary tumor type affecting the feline liver.[6] Other tumor types are rare; they include tumors of the extrahepatic bile ducts, gallbladder, plasmacytoma, and cystadenomas.[3–6,20,21]

Myelolipomas are tumorlike nodules composed of mature adipose tissue and bone marrow elements, most commonly found in the adrenal glands, tissues of the paravertebral, intrathoracic, retroperitoneal, and presacral regions and the mesentery of man. They have been reported in both wild and domestic cats.[8–10,22]

Metastatic liver tumors are more common than primary ones in both the dog and the cat. Metastasis from any site may occur, but the most common primary tumors are gastrointestinal tumors, hemangiosarcomas, pancreatic tumors, and mammary adenocarcinomas. The history and clinical presentation will often mimic primary hepatic tumors.[2]

## HISTORY AND CLINICAL SIGNS

Animals with hepatic tumors usually present with variable histories of vague, nonspecific clinical signs, such as anorexia, weight loss, vomiting, and polydipsia.[2,12,15] Most gallbladder tumors do not show clinical signs until the common bile duct is occluded. Occasionally, an animal may show signs of central nervous system disease due to hepatoencephalopathy or hypoglycemia secondary to the tumor.

Physical examination may reveal a palpable cranial abdominal mass as well as abdominal distention from ascites or hemoperitoneum.[4,12,15] Pale mucous membranes are a common finding, but it is quite rare for the animal to be clinically icteric.[1,4,15,16]

## DIAGNOSIS AND WORKUP

The most consistent laboratory abnormalities are increased serum alkaline phosphatase (ALP) secondary to cholestasis and increased serum alanine aminotransferase (SALT) and serum aspartate aminotransferase (SAST) caused by hepato-cellular necrosis or increased enzyme production by neoplastic tissues.[2,23,24] In humans, the ratio of SAST to SALT is suggestive of histologic type. Hepatocellular carcinomas are associated with a ratio of greater than 1:1, and bile duct carcinomas usually give ratios of less than 1:1. In a series of canine patients, a ratio of less than 1:1 was associated with hepatocellular or bile duct carcinoma, and a ratio of greater than 1:1 was associated with sarcomas or carcinoid tumors.[1,23] Serum and $\propto$-fetoprotein has been shown to be elevated in approximately half of dogs with hepatic tumors.[24] It is rare for the serum bilirubin or sulfobromophthalein (BSP) retention to be elevated. Serum protein levels are usually within normal limits, although one study showed elevations in globulin levels along with decreases in albumin levels.[2] These changes may be explained by alterations in hepatic synthesis and degradation as well as possible increased antigenic stimulation resulting in increased globulin production. Serum bile acid levels will be elevated with hepatic neoplasia, but this is not definitive for tumors.[24,25] A nonregenerative anemia is a common finding due to anemia of chronic disease. However, regenerative anemia can occur if the tumor actively bleeds into the peritoneum.

Hypoglycemia is another reported abnormality that can be attributed to the tumor's increased use of glucose or production of hormones with insulinlike activity.[2] The liver's decreased production of clotting factors can cause coagulation abnormalities. The most consistent clotting abnormalities associated with hepatic neoplasia are shortened thrombin clotting time, decreased Factor VIII:C levels, and increased Factor VIII:Ag levels.[26] A coagulogram should be performed in all cases prior to biopsy or any surgical procedure.

Abdominocentesis should be performed in animals presented with ascites. In some cases, neoplastic cells can be identified in the fluid, especially when peritoneal metastases are present. Other diagnostic tests include abdominal radiography to help localize the abdominal mass to the liver. Abdominal ultrasound may be used to characterize the internal structure of the tumor, to confirm the organ of origin, to aid in defining the extent of the disease, and possibly to identify previously undetected metastases.[13,27] Thoracic radiographs should be performed on patients with suspect hepatic tumors to identify pulmonary metastases but will usually be negative.

Despite all these noninvasive techniques, neoplastic tissue must be obtained to arrive at a definitive diagnosis of hepatic tumor. Tissues may be obtained via percutaneous biopsy, laparoscopy, or laparotomy. Laparotomy is the most definitive method and has the advantage of being both diagnostic and in some cases therapeutic as well. Percutaneous liver biopsy or laparoscopic biopsy is considered when the disease is diffuse and surgical treatment is considered unlikely.

## TREATMENT

Surgical excision is the treatment of choice for hepatic tumors (Fig. 18–10).[4,15,21,28] Because they are insidious in onset, many tumors are nonresectable by the time of presentation. Up to 75% of the liver may be resected without significant clinical dysfunction.[12,15,28] Hepatic regeneration occurs rapidly and is usually complete within 6 to 8 weeks. There are no controlled studies in veterinary medicine to support the use of chemotherapy for nonresectable hepatic tumors or as an adjuvant treatment. Hepatic dearterialization has been described in the dog[29] and may be a palliative treatment for unresectable primary hepatic tumors.

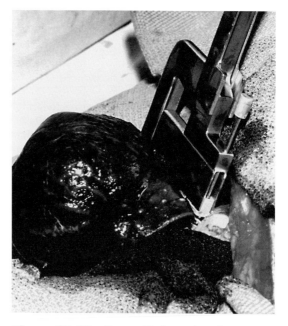

**Figure 18–10.**   Dog with hepatic adenoma at surgery. Mass was removed with staples, and dog is alive and free of disease at 18 months.

## PROGNOSIS

The prognosis for benign hepatic tumors following excision is good; survival times greater than 2 years have been reported.[4,12,21] Diffuse hepatic neoplasia carries a grave prognosis, but localized hepatic neoplasia can be resected with occasional good prognosis. The solitary nature and resectability of the tumor may be more prognostic than histologic type.[12, 15] The size of the tumor is not a reliable indicator of prognosis because many large, solitary, well-encapsulated tumors can be successfully removed.[12,15] It appears that the degree of invasiveness and resectability, as well as the presence of metastases, are the most reliable indicators of survival.[12,15]

The prognosis for cats with primary liver tumors is poor because most of the tumors have metastasized by the time of diagnosis.[6] The prognosis following surgical excision of myelolipomas and cystadenomas is good; most animals are free of the disease more than 1 year after treatment.[4,8,21]

## COMPARATIVE ASPECTS

Primary tumors of the hepatobiliary system are rare and highly lethal tumors in man. Gallbladder carcinoma is the most common tumor type, followed by hepatocellular carcinoma and cholangiocarcinoma. Two-thirds of hepatocellular carcinomas are the nodular form, 30% are massive, and 5% are diffuse. An encapsulated form also occurs in 4% of the cases and is less aggressive than other forms of the disease. Adenocarcinomas represent 85% of all the tumors that occur in the gallbladder and bile duct.[30]

The etiology of hepatobiliary tumors is unknown, but an increased frequency has been associated with preexisting liver disease, especially cirrhosis, hepatitis B infections, steroid and hormone therapy, cholelithiasis, liver fluke infestations, and ulcerative colitis.[30]

As in other animals, clinical signs are nonspecific; abdominal pain, jaundice, weight loss, and an acute onset of ascites are common. Unfortunately, the similarity of symptoms of benign and malignant disease often confuses the diagnosis. Surgery is the treatment of choice, but because the symptoms are vague, the disease is often advanced beyond the limits of excision at the time of diagnosis. Radiation therapy can be effective, though the liver tolerates only a limited dosage of radiation. Chemotherapy is used for advanced neoplasms. Mitomycin-C has shown the best results, and responses have been reported with combinations of doxorubicin, bleomycin, and 5-fluorouracil. Hepatic artery infusion is useful for delivering chemotherapy directly to the tumor.[30]

Prognosis is poor. Patients treated with resection have a 5-year survival rate of less than 20%, and in advanced, unresectable tumors, the 5-year survival rate is zero.[30]

## REFERENCES

1. Patnaik AK, Hurvitz AI, Lieberman PH: Canine hepatic neoplasms: A clinicopathologic study. Vet Pathol 17:553–564, 1980.
2. Strombeck DR: Clinicopathologic features of primary and metastatic neoplastic disease of the liver in dogs. J Am Vet Med Assoc 173:267–269, 1978.
3. Patnaik AK: A morphologic and immunocytochemical study of hepatic neoplasms in cats. Vet Pathol 29:405–415, 1992.
4. Lawrence HJ, Erb HN, Harvey HJ: Nonlymphomatous hepatobiliary masses in cats: 41 cases (1972 to 1991). Vet Surg 23:365–368, 1994.
5. Post G, Patnaik AK: Nonhematopoietic hepatic neoplasms in cats: 21 cases (1983–1988). J Am Vet Med Assoc 201:1080–1082, 1992.
6. Carpenter JL, Andrews LK, Holzworth J: Tumors and tumor-like lesions. In Holzworth J (ed): Diseases of the Cat. Philadelphia, WB Saunders, 1987, pp. 500–505.
7. Feldman BF, Strafuss AC, Gabbert N: Bile duct carcinoma in the cat: Three case reports. Fel Pract (January): 33–39, 1976.
8. Gourley IM, Popp JA, Park RD: Myelolipomas of the liver in a domestic cat. J Am Vet Med Assoc 158:2053–2057, 1974.
9. Ikede BO, Downey RS: Multiple hepatic myelolipomas in a cat. Can Vet J 13:160–163, 1972.
10. Lombard LS, Fortna HM, et al: Myelolipomas of the liver in captive wild felidae. Vet Pathol 5:127–134, 1968.
11. Hirao K et al: Primary neoplasms in dog liver induced by diethylnitrosamine. Cancer Res 34:1870–1882, 1974.
12. Liska W: Canine hepatomas and hepatocellular carcinomas. Resident seminar presented at the Animal Medical Center, New York, April 9, 1975.
13. Nyland TG, Park RD: Hepatic ultrasonography in the dog. Vet Radiol 24:74–84, 1983.
14. Strombeck DR: Hepatic neoplasms. In DR Strombeck (ed): Small Animal Gastroenterology. Santa Barbara, Stonegate Publishing, 1979.
15. Kosovsky JE, Manfra-Marretta S, et al: Results of partial hepatectomy in 18 dogs with hepatocellular carcinoma. J Am Anim Hosp Assoc 25:203–206, 1989.
16. Patnaik AK, Hurvitz AI, et al: Canine bile duct carcinoma. Vet Pathol 18:439–444, 1981.
17. Strafuss AC: Bile duct carcinoma in dogs. J Am Vet Med Assoc 169:429, 1976.
18. Patnaik AK, Lieberman PH, et al: Canine hepatic carcinoids. Vet Pathol 18:445–453, 1981.
19. Willard MD, Dunstan RW, Faulkner J: Neuroendocrine carcinoma of the gall-bladder in a dog. J Am Vet Med Assoc 192:926–928, 1988.
20. Larsen AE, Carpenter JL: Hepatic plasmacytoma and biclonal gammopathy in a cat. J Am Vet Med Assoc 205:708–710, 1994.
21. Trout NJ, Berg RJ, et al: Surgical treatment of hepatobiliary cystadenomas in cats: Five cases (1988–1993). J Am Vet Med Assoc 206:505–507, 1995.
22. McCaw DL, da Silva Curiel JMA, Shaw DP: Hepatic myelolipomas in a cat. J Am Vet Med Assoc 197:243–245, 1990.
23. Center SA, Slater MR, et al: Diagnostic efficacy of serum alkaline phosphatase and γ-glutamyltransferase in dogs with histologically confirmed hepatobiliary disease: 270 cases (1980–1990). J Am Vet Med Assoc 201:1258–1264, 1992.
24. Lowseth LA, Gillett NA, et al: Detection of serum α-fetoprotein in dogs with hepatic tumors. J Am Vet Med Assoc 199:735–741, 1991.
25. Center SA, Baldwin BH, et al: Bile acid concentrations in the diagnosis of hepatobiliary disease in the dog. J Am Vet Med Assoc 187:935–940, 1985.
26. Badylak SF, Dodds WJ, Van Vleet JF: Plasma coagulation factor abnormalities in dogs with naturally

occurring hepatic disease. Am J Vet Res 44:2336–2340, 1983.

27. Feeney DA, Johnston GR, Hardy RM: Two-dimensional gray-scale ultrasonography for assessment of hepatic and splenic neoplasia in the dog and cat. J Am Vet Med Assoc 184:68–81, 1984.

28. Bjorling DE, Prasse KW, Holmes RA: Partial hepatectomy in dogs. Comp. Cont. Ed. Pract. Vet. 7:257–265, 1985.

29. Gunn C, Gourley IM, Koblick PD: Hepatic dearterialization in the dog. Am J Vet Res 47:170–175, 1986

30. MacDonald JS, Gunderson LL, Adson MA: Cancer of the hepatobiliary system. In DeVita VT (ed): Cancer: Principles and Practice of Oncology, pp. 590–615. Philadelphia, JB Lippincott, 1982.

# G. Tumors of the Intestinal Tract

## Rodney C. Straw

### INCIDENCE AND RISK FACTORS

Tumors of the intestine are uncommon in domestic animals and represent less than 1% of all malignancies. They occur most commonly in the rectum or colon of dogs, and the small intestine of cats. No definitive etiologic factors for development of intestinal neoplasia are known for the dog or cat.

Adenocarcinoma is the most common intestinal tumor in the dog,[1] and leiomyosarcoma is the most common sarcoma.[2] Adenomatous polyps are reported to be the most common tumor in the canine rectum.[3] In the feline intestinal tract, lymphoma is reported most frequently,[4–7] followed by adenocarcinoma and mast cell tumor.[8] Other tumors affecting the intestinal tract include fibrosarcoma,[9,10] undifferentiated sarcoma,[1] carcinoids,[11–15] leiomyomas,[1,3] and plasmacytoma.[3,16]

Carcinoma of the intestine occurs in older animals. The mean age of affected dogs is 9 years (range, 1 to 14 years) and 10 years for cats (range, 2 to 17 years). One study of nonlymphoid intestinal neoplasia reported that male dogs outnumbered females (21:11) and that female cats were affected more often than male cats (9:5),[1] although others have reported no sex predisposition for feline nonlymphoid gastrointestinal neoplasia.[17,18]

Siamese cats are reported to have a higher frequency of small intestinal adenocarcinoma than other breeds.[1,17–19] In one report 70% of cats with small intestinal adenocarcinoma were Siamese; however cats with adenocarcinoma of the cecum, colon, and rectum were more commonly domestic cats.[8] Boxers,[20] collies,[8] and German shepherds[8] may be predisposed to development of intestinal cancer, although in one series none of the canine breeds were over-represented.[1]

Leiomyosarcomas of the intestines of dogs were diagnosed in less than 0.2% of 10,270 canine necropsies reviewed.[21] They occur most commonly in the cecum and jejunum, and the mean and median age of affected dogs is 11 and 10.5 years.[1,2,21] One report indicated that younger dogs may be affected with small intestinal leiomyosarcoma.[22] There is no apparent breed predilection and females may be more commonly affected than males.[21]

Lymphoma occurs predominantly in middle-aged dogs, and there are conflicting data in the literature regarding a possible sex predilection. In one study of 144 canine lymphoma cases, 6.9% were alimentary in origin.[23] Lymphosarcoma of the feline intestine is often part of a multicentric disease.[17] In a study of 76 cases of feline alimentary lymphoma that excluded cats with multicentric disease, there appeared to be no breed or sex predilection.[24] The mean age of affected cats was 10.6 years (range, 4 to 17 years) and the intestine was the most common site (41/76), with the jejunum and ileum most frequently affected.[24] These tumors are thought to arise from B-lymphocytes in the lamina propria.[8,25] In one study, 41 cats with intestinal lymphoma were tested for the presence of feline leukemia virus and 4.9% were positive.[24] (See Chap. 28A.)

Mast cell tumors are more common in the feline than in the canine intestine. The mean age for cats with mast cell tumors of the intestine is 13 years (range, 7 to 21 years). All reported cases, in a series of 28, occurred in domestic short- or long-hairs and there was no sex predilection.[8] A primary mast cell tumor in the ileocecal region has been described in a dog.[26]

Intestinal carcinoids occur rarely and affect older dogs. No sex or breed predisposition has been determined. In dogs, carcinoids are mainly located in the duodenum, colon, and rectum.[20] Six cases of intestinal carcinoids and one case of adenocarcinoid have been reported in dogs.[13–15] Intestinal carcinoid has been reported in the cat; most feline carcinoids develop in the stomach or small intestine.[11]

## PATHOLOGY AND NATURAL BEHAVIOR

Intestinal neoplasms in dogs and cats are usually malignant. Of nonlymphoid intestinal neoplasms in 32 dogs and 14 cats, 88% of the canine tumors and all of the feline tumors were malignant.[1] Half of the canine rectal tumors showed transition from benign polypoid lesions to adenocarcinomas in one study.[13] In a study of 12 dogs with colorectal adenomatous polyps and 22 dogs with carcinoma in situ, only 2 dogs with adenomatous polyps had recurrence, whereas 12 dogs with carcinoma in situ had recurrence after tumor removal.[27] Progression from adenomatous polyp to carcinoma in situ to invasive carcinoma was demonstrated in 6 dogs. Some polypoidlike lesions are malignant and those greater than 1.0 cm in diameter will generally have a more anaplastic appearance, may recur after excision, and may progress to invasive adenocarcinoma.[20] Care in histologic evaluation is necessary to identify the focal areas of dysplasia, which may herald a high probability of recurrence.[27]

Adenocarcinoma of the canine and feline intestine is usually in an advanced stage at the time of diagnosis. Extension of the neoplasm beyond the bowel wall was found in 86% of dogs at necropsy;[1] lymph nodes, liver, lungs, and adjoining sections of the gastrointestinal wall were the most common sites of metastasis.[13] Results of a study of small intestinal adenocarcinoma in 32 cats indicated that 71% had gross or histologic evidence of metastatic disease at the time of diagnosis.[18] In cats, the most common metastatic sites are abdominal serosa, followed by lymph nodes, lung, and liver.[17] Regional lymph node metastasis was identified in 5 of 11 cats with gastrointestinal carcinoma.[28]

Adenocarcinoma has been described as annular when the lumen is constricted 360 degrees by tumor (Fig. 18–11), or intraluminal when there is neoplastic growth into the lumen as well as infiltration into the wall.[13] One histologic classification divides canine adenocarcinoma into four groups that may overlap: acinar, solid, mucinous, and papillary.[29] Acinar adenocarcinoma may be either annular or intraluminal. Papillary forms are usually intraluminal, and mucinous adenocarcinomas are annular in the small intestine but intraluminal in the rectum.[13]

Tumors involving large segments of bowel may be slow-growing, with predominantly horizontal spread and few distant metastases; this is often the case with papillary adenocarcinoma.[13,29] Acinar, solid, and mucinous adenocarcinoma tend

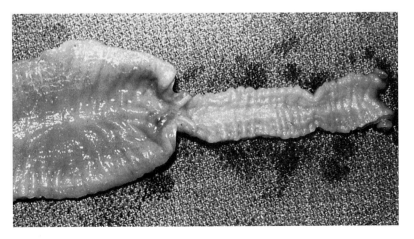

**Figure 18–11.** Gross specimen of annular intestinal adenocarcinoma removed from the cat in Figure 18–15. This patient survived 18 months and succumbed to lymph node and omental metastasis.

**Figure 18–12.** Gross specimen of a an intestinal leiomyosarcoma removed from the dog in Figure 18–14. This patient was alive and free of disease more than 2 years postoperatively, after which the dog was lost to follow-up.

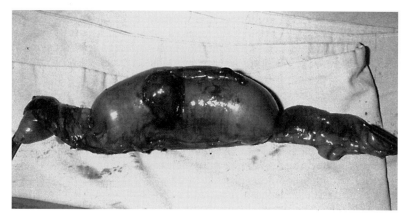

to show more vertical growth and extend into bowel wall, serosa, and other organs. There is one case report of a signet ring carcinoma of the colon with secondary meningeal carcinomatosis.[29]

The clinical and gross appearance of feline intestinal adenocarcinoma is similar to that in dogs.[20] In cats, the tumors have been reported to be located most frequently in the jejunum; the second most frequent location is the ileum and least frequent the ileocecal region.[28] Similar morphologic types are described and osteochondroid metaplasia is a frequent feature of adenocarcinoma in the cat.[17,20]

Leiomyosarcomas of the canine intestine are locally invasive malignant smooth muscle neoplasms that are slow to metastasize, although extension to regional lymph nodes has been reported.[2] Dogs with these tumors can be asymptomatic, and the diagnosis may be an incidental finding at necropsy or exploratory surgery (Fig. 18–12). Some animals are presented because of melena and may have anemia.

Animals with the alimentary form of lymphoma may have focal or diffuse neoplastic infil-

trates of the bowel wall (Fig. 18–13) that may also involve mesenteric lymph nodes, liver, and spleen.

Carcinoids can be expansile and infiltrative, and larger neoplasms are usually more malignant and likely to metastasize, especially to the liver.[13,20] Feline intestinal mast cell tumors metastasize to the mesenteric lymph nodes most commonly; other metastatic sites include liver, spleen, and, rarely, the lungs.[20]

## HISTORY AND SIGNS

The most common finding in animals with intestinal neoplasia is weight loss of several days to more than 6 months' duration.[1,17] The tumor may cause ulceration of the intestinal mucosa and resultant hemorrhage. Intestinal obstruction or abscessation may also occur. Septic peritonitis was associated with a duodenal leiomyosarcoma in a dog.[22] Dogs may present with pale mucous membranes and have microcytic anemia.[30] Vomiting, anorexia, and depression are also commonly found. Less common signs include constipation,

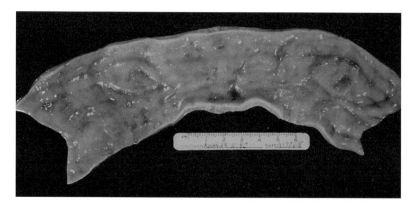

**Figure 18–13.** Gross specimen of bowel from a cat with diffuse alimentary form of lymphoma.

icterus, diarrhea, ascites, melena, and dehydration. Tenesmus, hematochezia, dyschezia, and occasionally intermittent anal eversion may be seen in dogs with colorectal neoplasia.[3,13,19,31,32] Signs of obstructive bowel disease may be present[33] or a malabsorption syndrome may occur, especially with diffuse lymphoma. Tumor infiltrates may occasionally obstruct lymphatics and lead to steatorrhea due to lymphangiectasia. Carcinoids of the small bowel are usually slow-growing. The clinical signs may be related to the primary tumor—that is, nonspecific pain, intermittent obstruction, with associated vomiting. Bleeding is unusual. Although not documented in dogs, carcinoid tumors may be associated with clinical features dependent on hormones or amines produced by the tumor. The most common clinical signs are chronic diarrhea and weight loss. Serotonin (5-HT) is commonly associated with carcinoids in humans.

## DIAGNOSTIC TECHNIQUES AND WORKUP

An abdominal mass, dilated intestinal loops, thickened bowel, or intra-abdominal lymphadenomegaly may be detected on careful abdominal palpation. Adenomatous polyps or carcinoids may evert through the anus. Most rectal cancer can be detected on digital palpation as firm annu-lar rings. In a study of canine colorectal adenocarcinoma, 63% (49/78) of the dogs had masses that were palpable on rectal exam.[32]

Hematologic and biochemical profiles are often normal, although anemia or hypoproteinemia may be present because of bleeding into the intestine.

Pulmonary metastases are rarely detected on thoracic radiography. Plain abdominal radiographs may reveal a mass, enlarged lymph nodes, or signs of intestinal obstruction. Positive-contrast upper gastrointestinal studies may delineate an intramural (Fig. 18-14) or annular (Fig. 18-15) lesion, and diffuse intestinal neoplasia may appear as ragged filling defects along the bowel wall. Barium enemas may help establish the extent of colorectal tumors (Fig. 18-16) and double-contrast studies may define small lesions.[34] Colonoscopy and proctoscopic examination can be a valuable diagnostic aid in the identification and biopsy of lesions of the colon and rectum, and because adenocarcinoma can be diffuse or have multiple lesions, endoscopy is recommended for staging and planning treatment.[32,35] However, biopsies retrieved by endoscopy may underestimate the severity of the lesion. In one study, 30% of canine rectal lesions were incorrectly diagnosed by endoscopic biopsies probably because the biopsies retrieved were small and only contained material from the surface of the lesions.[27] A definitive diagnosis of

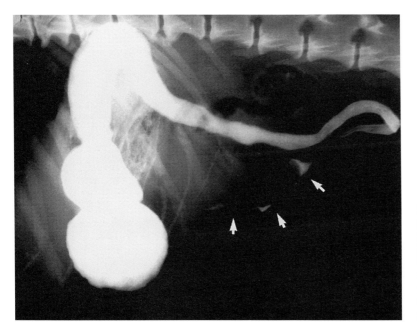

**Figure 18–14.** Lateral projection of an upper gastrointestinal contrast study of a dog with intestinal leiomyosarcoma. Note the intramural filling defect in the small intestine (arrows).

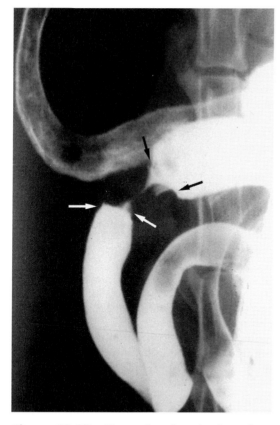

intestinal neoplasia can only be made on histologic examination of sufficiently representative biopsy material.

## THERAPY

The most common treatment for intestinal neoplasia is surgical resection. Margins of at least 4 to 8 cm should be strived for. Suspicious lesions (especially in the liver and regional lymph nodes) should be biopsied during intra-abdominal procedures. Careful attention to surgical technique in anastomosis is important, owing to the frequent debilitated state of the patient and potential for poor healing.

Tumors of the small intestine, cecum, and colon are treated via a midline abdominal approach. Tumors of the rectum (especially adenocarcinoma) pose special problems for the surgeon (Fig. 18-17). About one-half of dogs with midrectal adenocarcinoma (a site where > 50% of these tumors occur) have luminal obstruction requiring resection to alleviate signs.[32] Various techniques such as end-to-end anastomosis (usually requiring a pelvic osteotomy for access), rectal pull-through, or the dorsal rectal approach have been described.[36–38] A technique of sagital pubic osteotomy has been described as a surgical approach for the treatment of intrapelvic neoplasia.[39] However, the short length of mesorectum, the location of the affected segment within the bony pelvis, and the problems associated with surgery of the large intestine cause significant

**Figure 18–15.** Ventrodorsal projection of an upper gastrointestinal contrast study of a cat with annular intestinal adenocarcinoma. Note the typical "apple core"-like lesion. (arrows)

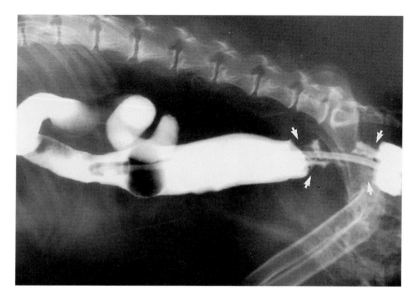

**Figure 18–16.** Positive-contrast barium enema in a dog showing a pre-pelvic and intrapelvic rectal adenocarcinoma (arrows).

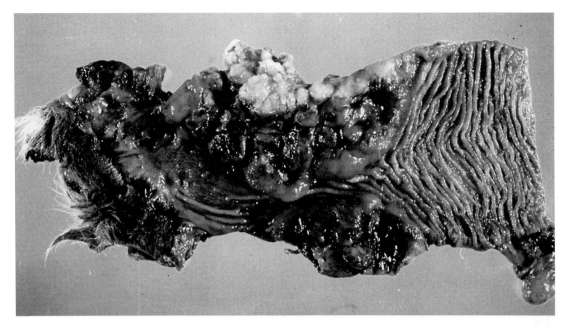

**Figure 18–17.** Gross specimen of rectal adenocarcinoma from a dog. This tumor usually occurs at the pelvic brim, making resection difficult.

morbidity (infection, incontinence, dehiscence, and stricture) and mortality when wide removals are undertaken. Considering the morbidity, mortality (3 out of 4 in one report[32]), it is questionable whether surgery should be undertaken in some cases. Local excision and cryosurgery for adenocarcinoma of the colon have significantly extended the life of dogs compared with other methods of surgical treatment; however, 82% (9/11) treated with cryosurgery suffered complications (rectal prolapse, stricture, perineal hernia, and recurrence).[32] Electrosurgery may be a viable treatment method when rectal adenocarcinoma is not annular and is in a distal location so it can be completely prolapsed.

Rectal adenomatous polyps may be pedunculated or have a sessile base (Figs. 18-18 and 18-19). Most polyps are within 2 cm of the anus. They may be multiple but usually appear singularly. They are treated by surgical excision, electrosurgery or cryosurgery.[32,35,40,41] Masses that are not accessible by digital exteriorization require rectal prolapse.[40] Epidural anesthesia provides excellent muscle relaxation, and gentle traction applied to four stay sutures placed equidistant around the rectum in the mucosal folds allows exposure of the lesion. Polyps with sessile bases are best managed with cryosurgery or electrosurgery.[40] Once the mass is exposed, its stalk is transfixed with a ligature and the mass is removed. The base is then frozen with a cryoprobe.

Surgery is indicated in obstructive intestinal lymphoma or when bowel perforation has occurred. Biopsies and cytologic evaluation of impression smears of adjacent intestine, lymph nodes, spleen, and liver should be performed to clinically stage the disease. Chemotherapy protocols for lymphoma can be employed as adjuvant therapy or as the major form of therapy in diffuse disease (see Chap. 28B and C). Diffuse canine alimentary lymphoma does not respond as well to chemotherapy as does multicentric disease, but solitary or nodular gastrointestinal lymphoma does respond better to chemotherapy. In a study of 23 cats with alimentary lymphoma treated with L-asparaginase, vincristine, cyclophosphamide, methotrexate, and prednisone, the mean survival time was 25.3 weeks.[24] The method of diagnosis (lesional biopsy versus resection of a solitary tumor) did not affect survival time. In this report, four cats received prednisone alone; their mean survival was 7.3 weeks.

High-dose radiotherapy has been reported as a treatment for adenocarcinomas of the distal half of the rectum and anal canal.[42] The rectum was prolapsed with stay sutures, and doses of between 15 and 25 Gy were delivered from an

**Figure 18–18.** Pedunculated rectal polyp in a dog. This mass was biopsied and then frozen and has not recurred in more than 2 years.

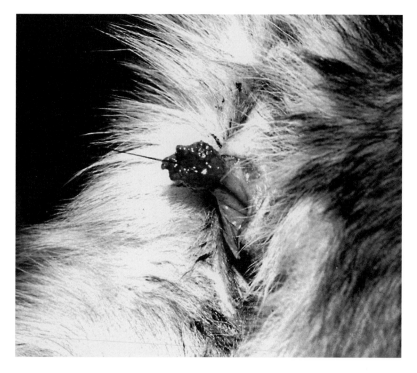

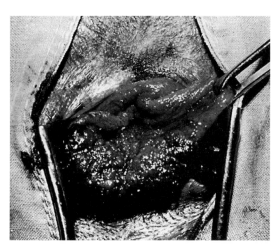

**Figure 18–19.** Canine adenomatous polyp with a sessile base.

orthovoltage X-ray teletherapy unit with the beam restricted by a cone. The cone diameter was 1 cm greater than the diameter of grossly visible tumor. In early or small recurrent lesions in six dogs ($T_1N_0M_0$ and $T_2N_0M_0$), the treatment was technically feasible and safe; toxicity was limited to occasional, transient tenesmus. Three dogs had no evidence of disease at 5, 6, and 31 months, and three others had local recurrence at 1, 6, and 7 months. High-dose radiotherapy may represent a suitable alternative to surgery for selected cases.

Adjuvant chemotherapy for intestinal adenocarcinoma and leiomyosarcoma has been recommended,[43] but the efficacy of such treatment has not been reported in the dog and cat.

## PROGNOSIS

Twenty-three dogs with large intestinal adenocarcinoma treated only with fecal softners had a mean survival time of 15 months.[32] Clinical signs of metastasis were not observed in any of the 78 dogs with colorectal adenocarcinoma in the same study. In another study, dogs with surgically managed malignant epithelial tumors had a mean survival time of 6.9 months; local recurrence was the reason for euthanasia in every case.[35] Dogs with single, pedunculated, polypoid adenocarcinoma lesions had a mean survival time of 32 months; those with nodular or cobblestone-like lesions had a mean survival time of 12 months, and dogs with annular masses causing strictures had a mean survival time of 1.6 months.[32]

Dogs with colonic or rectal adenocarcinoma are usually euthanatized because of failure to control dyschezia and hematochezia. The surgeon must consider control of these clinical signs as an important goal. A prognosis is based on the ability to achieve this goal. The form and severity of disease are also prognostic indicators. In one report, 23 cats with small intestinal adenocarcinoma were treated with intestinal resection and end-to-end anastomosis. Eleven cats either died or were euthanatized within 2 weeks of surgery. Twelve cats survived an average of 15 months following surgery (range 1.5 to 50 months). Five of these cats were staged with extension to mesenteric lymph nodes, 2 had disease confined to the bowel, and 5 were not staged. Five cats died with known or suspected recurrence, 5 died of unknown causes, 1 was euthanatized for an unrelated cause, and 1 was alive at 50 months after surgery. The 5 cats with known lymph node metastasis had a mean survival time of 12 months.[18] The median survival of 10 cats with gastrointestinal adenocarcinoma treated surgically was 2.5 months (range 0 to 24 months). However, in this report, those cases that died of nontumor or treatment causes were not censored from the survival statistics.[28]

An excellent prognosis can be expected with completely excised polyps; however, recurrence is possible, especially with large or sessile lesions. Malignant transformation is also possible. In one study of 12 dogs with adenomatous polyps and 22 dogs with carcinoma in situ treated by surgical resection with or without cryosurgery, only 2 dogs with adenomatous polyps developed recurrence at 270 and 365 days whereas 12 dogs with carcinoma in situ developed recurrence with a median disease-free interval of 80 days.[27] In the same study, 4 dogs developed invasive carcinoma at 8, 10, 19, and 37 months, and 2 dogs with adenomatous polyps developed carcinoma in situ 9 and 17 months after diagnosis.

Diffuse intestinal lymphoma carries a poor prognosis; solitary nodular lymphoma does better. Insufficient data are available to evaluate adequately the prognosis for patients with intestinal carcinoids; however, surgical resection is recommended where possible. One report suggested a favorable prognosis after complete surgical resection of canine intestinal leiomyosarcoma.[2] In this study, three of five dogs treated with surgical resection were alive a minimum of 12 months following resection, with no evidence of recurrence of metastasis. Two dogs developed metastasis, 3 months and 12 months postexcision, and one dog died one month postexcision with no evidence of metastasis or local recurrence. In one report of dogs with small intestinal carcinomas,

four were treated with surgical excision and three of these survived 6 months or longer.[34]

## COMPARATIVE ASPECTS[44,45]

Cancers of the duodenum and small intestine are uncommon in humans and account for about 1% of all gastrointestinal tract malignancies.[45] Adenocarcinoma of the large bowel, however, affects approximately 1 person in every 20 in the United States and in most westernized countries. This cancer constitutes a major health problem, with more than 140,000 new cases diagnosed annually in the United States. This represents 15% of all cancers. Worldwide, the incidence rates of colorectal cancer vary widely, from 3.4 cases per 100,000 population in Nigeria to 35.8 cases per 100,000 population in Connecticut. Although it is not possible to identify a specific cause of colon cancer, epidemiologic studies of nutritional habits and migration patterns point to a clear association with certain diets. People eating diets rich in animal fats and meat and poor in fiber appear to be at high risk. Increasing dietary fiber, particularly by ingesting cellulose and bran fiber, appears to be of value in prevention, as supported by numerous case-control and population studies. Limitation of total dietary fat has also been proposed to help reduce the risk of colon cancer. Antioxidants such as vitamin C, tocopherol, and selenium have been suggested as protective agents; however, simple dietary supplimentation with these agents has not proved to be of dramatic benefit. There are several clinical risk factors that can be identified for colorectal cancer. These factors are genetic (familial adenomatous polyposis syndrome, Gardner, Oldfield, or Turcot syndrome, Peutz-Jegher syndrome), familial (familial colorectal cancer syndrome, hereditary adenocarcinomatosis syn- drome, family history of colorectal cancer), pre-existing disease (inflammatory bowel disease, colorectal cancer, pelvic cancer post irradiation, neoplastic colorectal polyps), and age (all men and women over age 40). Early detection of colorectal cancer is potentially associated with a dramatic reduction in disease-related mortality. Aggressive screening with colonoscopy and air contrast barium enema is justified, particularly where clinical risk factors exist.

Surgery remains the mainstay in the treatment of colorectal cancer, but treatment strategies with multimodal therapies may depend on the classification of the patient into the following groups: (1) resectable colon cancer, (2) resectable rectal cancer, (3) potentially curable but primarily surgically unresectable colorectal cancers, and (4) recurrent or metastatic disease. Adjuvant radiation therapy has a role to play in the management of certain stages of colorectal cancer. Adjuvant chemotherapy includes 5-fluorouricil, floxuridine, methyl-CCNU, and vincrystine. Bacillus Calmette-Guérin (BCG) or BCG-MER (BCG with methanol extraction) or levamisole has also been used in treating colorectal cancer.

Many variables affect the curability of colorectal cancer. Multivariate analysis indicates that surgical-pathological stage is the most important. For node-negative patients the 5-year survival rate when the tumor involved the mucosa or submucosa is in excess of 90%. Muscle-wall invasion decreases the 5-year survival rate slightly, to 80%. Transmural penetration is still associated with a cure in the majority of patients, with survival in the 60 to 80% range. Patients with one to four nodes positive have a survival rate of 56%.

# REFERENCES

1. Birchard SJ, Couto CG, Johnson S: Nonlymphoid intestinal neoplasia in 32 dogs and 14 cats. J Am Anim Hosp Assoc 22:533–537, 1986.
2. Bruecker KA, Withrow SJ: Intestinal leiomyosarcoma in six dogs. J Am Anim Hosp Assoc 24:281–284, 1988.
3. Holt PE, Lucke VM: Rectal neoplasia in the dog: A clinicopathological review of 31 cases. Vet Rec 116:400–405, 1985.
4. Brodey RS: Alimentary tract neoplasms in the cat: A clinicopathologic study of 46 cases. Am J Vet Res 27:74–80, 1966.
5. Cotchin E: Some tumors of dogs and cats of comparative veterinary and human interest. Vet Rec 71:1040–1050, 1959.
6. Engle GG, Brodey RS: A retrospective study of 395 feline neoplasms. J Am Anim Hosp Assoc 5:21–31, 1969.
7. Head KW: Tumors of the lower alimentary tract. Bull WHO 53:167–186, 1976.
8. Carpenter JL, Andrews LK, Holzworth J: Tumors and tumor-like lesions. In Holzworth J (ed): Diseases of the Cat: Medicine and Surgery. Philadelphia; WB Saunders, 1987, pp. 406–596.
9. Howard DR, Schirmer RG, Ulrey VM, Michel RL; Adenocarcinoma in the ileum of a young dog. J Am Vet Med Assoc 162:956–8958, 1973.
10. Brodey RS, Cohen D: An epizootiological and clinicopathologic study of 95 cases of gastrointestinal neoplasms in the dog. Proc Am Vet Med Assoc 101:167–179, 1964 (Abstract).
11. Carakostas MC, Kennedy GA, Kittleson MD, Cook JE: Malignant foregut carcinoid in a domestic cat. Vet Pathol 16:607–609, 1979.
12. Sykes GP, Cooper BJ: Canine intestinal carcinoids. Vet Pathol 19:120–131, 1982.
13. Patnaik AK, Hurvitz AI, Johnson GF: Canine intestinal adenocarcinoma and carcinoid. Vet Pathol 17:149–163, 1980.
14. Patnaik AK, Leiberman PH: Canine goblet cell carcinoid. Vet Pathol 18:410–413, 1981.
15. Giles RC, Hildebrandt PK, Montgomery CA: Carcinoid tumor in the small intestine of the dog. Vet Pathol 11:340–349, 1974.
16. MacEwen EG, Patnaik AK, Johnson GF, Hurvitz AI, Erlandson SI, Lieberman PH: Extramedullary plasmacytoma of the gastrointestinal tract in two dogs. J Am Vet Med Assoc 184:1396–1398, 1984.
17. Turk MAM, Gallina AM, Russel TS: Non-hemopoietic gastrointestinal neoplasia in cats: A retrospective study of 44 cases. Vet Pathol 18:614–620, 1981.
18. Kosovsk JG, Matthiesen DI, Patnaik AK: Small intestinal adenocarcinoma in cats: 32 cases (1978–1985). J Am Vet Med Assoc 192:233–235, 1988.
19. Patnaik AK, Liu SK, Johnson GF: Feline intestinal adenocarcinoma: A clinicopathologic study of 22 cases. Vet Pathol 13:1–10, 1976.
20. Barker IK, VanDreumel AA: The alimentary system. In Jubb KVF (ed): Pathology of Domestic Animals. New York, Academic Press, 1985, pp. 1–237.
21. Patnaik AK, Hurvitz AI, Johnson GF: Canine gastrointestinal neoplasms. Vet Pathol 14:547–555, 1977.
22. Larahu LJ, Center SA, Flanders JA, Dietze AE, Laratta LJ, Castleman WL: Leiomyosarcoma in the duodenum of a dog. J Am Vet Med Assoc 183:1096–1097, 1983.
23. Theilen GH, Madewell BR: Tumors of the digestive tract. In Theilen GH, Madewell BR (eds): Veterinary Cancer Medicine. Philadelphia, Lea & Febiger, 1979, pp. 307–331.
24. Fulton LM, Mooney S, Matus RE, Hayes AA: Alimentary lymphosarcoma in 76 cats. The Animal Medical Center, personal communication, 1988.
25. Hardy WD, Jr: Hematopoetic tumors of cats. J Am Anim Hosp Assoc 17:921–940, 1981.
26. Patnaik AK, Twedt DC, Marretta SM: Intestinal mast cell tumor in a dog. J Small Anim Pract 21:207–212, 1980.
27. Valarius KD, Powers BE, McPherron MA, Mann FA, Withrow SJ: Adenomatous polyps and carcinoma in situ of the canine colon and rectum. J Am Anim Hosp Assoc (in press).
28. Cribb AE: Feline gastrointestinal adenocarcinoma: A review and retrospective study. Can Vet J 29:709–711, 1988.
29. Strampley AR, Swayne DE, Prasse KW: Meningeal carcinomatosis secondary to a colonic signet-ring carcinoma in a dog. J Am Anim Hosp Assoc 23:655–658, 1987.
30. Comer KM: Anemia as a feature of primary gas-

trointestinal neoplasia. Compend Contin Educ Pract Vet 12:13–19, 1990.

31. Seiler RJ: Colorectal polyps of the dog: A clinicopathologic study of 17 cases. J Am Vet Med Assoc 174:72–75, 1979.

32. Church EM, Hehlhaff CJ, Patnaik AK: Colorectal adenocarcinoma in dogs: 78 cases (1973–1984). J Am Vet Med Assoc 191:727–730, 1987.

33. Feeney DA, Klausner J, Johnston GR: Chronic bowel obstruction caused by primary intestinal neoplasia: A report of five cases. J Am Anim Hosp Assoc 18:67–77, 1982.

34. Gibbs C, Pearson H: Localized tumors of the canine small intestines: A report of 20 cases. J Small Anim Pract 27:507–519, 1986.

35. White RAS, Gorman NT: The clinical diagnosis and management of rectal and pararectal tumors in the dog. J Small Anim Pract 28:87–107, 1987.

36. McKeown DB, Cockshutt JR, Partlow GD, Dekleer VS: Over-the-top approach to the caudal pelvic canal and rectum in the dog and cat. Vet Surg 13:181–184, 1984.

37. Anderson GI, McKeown DB, Partlow GD, Percy DH: Rectal resection in the dog: A new surgical approach and the evaluation of its effect on fecal continence. Vet Surg 16:119–125, 1987.

38. Walshaw R: Removal of rectoanal neoplasms. In Bojrab MJ (ed): Current techniques in Small Animal Surgery. Philadelphia, Lea & Febiger, 1990, pp. 274–290.

39. Davies JV, Read HM: Sagital public osteotomy in the investigation and treatment of intrapelvic neoplasia in the dog. J Small Anim Pract 31:123–130, 1990.

40. Seim HB: Diseases of the anus and rectum. In Kirk RW (ed): Current Veterinary Therapy, IX. Philadelphia, WB Saunders, 1986, pp. 901–921.

41. Palmintieri A: The surgical management of polyps of the rectum and colon of the dog. J Am Vet Med Assoc 148:771–776, 1966.

42. Turrel JM, Theon AP: Single high-dose irradiation for selected canine rectal carcinomas. Vet Radiol 27:141–145, 1986.

43. Walshaw R: The small intestine. In Gourley IM, Vasseur PB (eds): General Small Animal Surgery. Philadelphia, JB Lipincott, 1985, pp. 343–384.

44. Cohen AM, Shank B, Friedman MA: Colorectal cancer. In DeVita VT, Hellman S, Rosenberg SA (eds): Cancer Principles and Practice of Oncology. Philadelphia, JB Lippincott, 1989, pp. 895–964.

45. Sindelar WF: Cancer of the small intestine. In DeVita VT, Hellman S, Rosenberg SA (eds): Cancer Principles and Practice of Oncology. Philadelphia, JB Lippincott, 1989, pp. 875–894.

# H. Perianal Tumors

## Stephen J. Withrow

### INCIDENCE AND RISK FACTORS

Perianal tumors (circumanal, hepatoid tumors) are very common in the male and rare in the female dog or the cat. Perianal adenomas comprise more than 80% of all perianal tumors and are the third most common tumor in the male dog.

Risk factors vary from male to female and from benign to malignant (Table 18-5). The older, intact male is at high risk for perianal adenomas, implying an androgen dependency, whereas perianal adenocarcinoma occurs in castrated or intact males, implying no hormonal dependency. Adenomas are more prevalent in the cocker spaniel, beagle, bulldog, and Samoyed.[1]

A high incidence of associated testicular interstitial cell tumors has been reported for males with adenomas, suggesting testosterone production as a cause.[1] However, a true cause-and-effect relationship has not been clarified, since interstitial cell tumors are such common incidental findings in nontumor-bearing, older, intact males. Perianal adenomas in the female occur almost exclusively in ovariohysterectomized animals in which estrogen does not suppress tumor growth. Rarely, testosterone secretion from the adrenal glands (with or without signs of Cushing's disease) may stimulate perianal adenoma formation.[2] Large-breed males appear to be overrepresented for development of sebaceous gland adenocarcinoma. Most older females with apocrine gland (anal sac) adenocarcinoma are ovariohysterectomized, but a true hormonal dependence has not been shown, since most older females have been ovariohysterectomized.

Perianal tumors are not commonly recognized in the cat, since the cat has no glands analogous to the perianal sebaceous glands in the dog.

**Table 18-5** Perianal Tumors

| | Male | | Female | |
|---|---|---|---|---|
| | Benign | Malignant | Benign | Malignant |
| Cell type | Sebaceous | Sebaceous (rarely apocrine) | Sebaceous | Apocrine (anal sac) |
| Tumor type | Perianal adenoma | Perianal adenocarcinoma | Perianal adenoma | Anal sac adenocarcinoma |
| Frequency | Common | Rare | Rare | Rare |
| Hormonal factors | Usually intact, testosterone dependent (?) | None | Ovariohysterectomized (i.e., lack of estrogen)[a] | Often ovariohysterectomized but no proven hormone regulation |
| Location and appearance | Superficial hairless perineum; single, multiple, or diffuse; may be on prepuce or tailhead | Usually single, invasive, often ulcerated | Superficial and single | Subcutaneous at 4 or 8 o'clock, firm and fixed (anal sacs) |
| Paraneoplastic syndromes | None | None (very rarely hypercalcemia) | None | 50 to 90% have hypercalcemia |
| Metastatic pattern | None | First to regional nodes, then further; up to 50% of time, especially with multiple recurrence | None | Very common to regional lymph nodes and then further |
| Special workup | None; cytology may have difficulty telling benign from malignant | Caudal abdominal X rays or ultrasound | None | Caudal abdominal X rays or ultrasound, possibly thoracic X rays; calcium levels and renal function |
| Treatment | Castration, surgical or cryosurgical removal of tumors[b] | Wide excision and lymphadenectomy if involved; radiation or chemotherapy if inoperable; castration of little benefit | Surgery or cryosurgery[b] | Wide excision of primary, lymphadenectomy; consider radiation postop to primary and metastatic lymph node sites |
| Prognosis | Excellent, less than 10% recurrence rate | Fair to good (tumors <5 cm do well); recurrence is common but many take many months and several surgeries can be done | Excellent | Poor to fair; less than 40% 1-year survival |

[a]If multiple or large (malelike), consider testosterone secretion from adrenal (with or without Cushing's signs).

[b]Estrogens will cause tumor regression but carry risk of bone marrow suppression. Adenomas will respond to radiation therapy, but surgery is cheaper, faster, and safer.

## PATHOLOGY AND NATURAL BEHAVIOR

Almost any tumor can occasionally affect the perianal region, including lymphoma, soft tissue sarcoma, squamous cell carcinoma, melanoma, and mast cell tumor: however, the most common are those of the sebaceous cells of the perineum. These have been called circumanal hepatoid cells because of their morphologic resemblance to liver cells. The histologic distinction between adenomas and adenocarcinomas may not always be clear and clinically there may be an intermediate condition called invasive perianal adenoma that may look benign under the microscope yet be invasive in the patient.

The malignant anal sac (apocrine gland) adenocarcinoma is most commonly seen in the female and is distinct from the male perianal sebaceous gland adenocarcinoma clinically and histologically. Both the male and female forms of adenocarcinoma are locally invasive. Metastasis to regional lymph nodes is detectable in approximately 50% of females at the time of presentation[3,4] and only 13% of the time in males.[5,6] Metastasis to other organs, especially lung, is rare but may occur.

## HISTORY AND CLINICAL SIGNS

The history for the benign lesions is that of a slow-growing (months to years) mass or masses, which are nonpainful and usually asymptomatic. These may be single, multiple, or diffuse (similar to generalized hyperplasia or hypertrophy of the perianal tissue) (Fig. 18-20A,B). Most occur on the hairless skin area around the anus, although they may extend to haired regions and can develop on the prepuce, scrotum, or tailhead (stud tail or "caudal tail gland") (Fig. 18-21). Benign lesions may ulcerate and become infected but are rarely adherent or fixed to deeper struc-

*A*

*B*

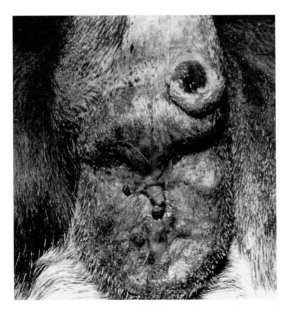
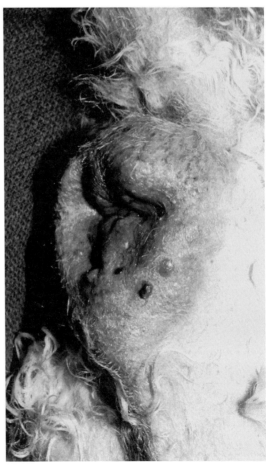

**Figure 18–20.** *A,* Typical small and ulcerated perianal adenoma can be seen at 1 o'clock. Treatment with castration and cryosurgery was curative. *B,* Diffuse 360-degree involvement of the perianal region with perianal adenoma. Aggressive resection or cryosurgery should not be performed, but rather castration, a waiting period of several months for partial regression, and then local treatment for residual disease.

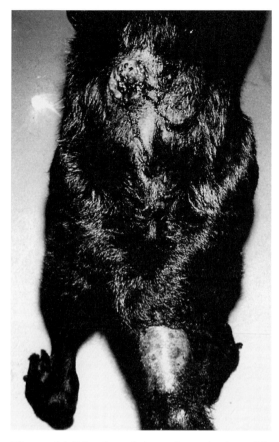

**Figure 18–21.** Dorsal view of a male dog with an ulcerated skin mass over the lumbar region and a thickened, hairless area over the tailhead. Both lesions were perianal adenoma.

tures. They are usually fairly well circumscribed, 0.5 to 3 cm in diameter, and elevated from the perineum.

The male perianal adenocarcinoma may look similar to adenomas but tends to grow faster, be firmer, become ulcerated, adhere to deeper tissues (or the anal and rectal tissues), recur following treatment, and will generally be larger than adenomas. Obstipation or dyschezia can be seen with larger masses. Castrated males with new or recurrent perianal tumors should raise the clinician's suspicion for malignant rather than benign disease, since adenocarcinomas are not hormonally dependent.

Females (and rarely males) with anal sac adenocarcinoma will generally present for systemic signs of hypercalcemia (see paraneoplastic syndromes) or occasionally obstruction of the anal canal.[7,8] Rarely, regional bone metastasis or direct extension of tumor from sublumbar (iliac) lymph nodes into the lumbar vertebrae with associated pain or fracture may be seen. An externally visible mass, as seen in the male, is not commonly observed by the owner or the clinician.

## DIAGNOSTIC TECHNIQUES AND WORKUP

In the male, a routine geriatric workup prior to anesthesia is desirable. Thoracic radiographs to evaluate for lung metastasis are probably not cost effective unless indicated for other cardiopulmonary evaluation. Caudal abdominal radiographs to evaluate regional lymph node size is indicated if one suspects adenocarcinoma (castrated dog, recurrent disease, or physical-examination characteristics of malignancy) (Fig. 18-22). A rectal exam may reveal palpable evidence of sublumbar lymphadenopathy. Fine-needle aspiration and cytology, to differentiate benign from malignant tumors in the male, has been unrewarding in the author's experience although it is very helpful in ruling out other forms of cancer or mass development.

The anal sac adenocarcinoma of the female requires careful evaluation for stage of disease and the systemic effects of hypercalcemia. Caudal abdominal radiographs are always indicated and, if positive, should be followed by thoracic radiographs. Ultrasonographic or computed tomographic evaluation of the sublumbar lymph nodes are probably better staging tools than plain radiographs, which can both under- and overestimate lymph node disease. It is uncommon to discover pulmonary metastasis without obvious regional lymph node metastasis. A fine-needle aspirate is helpful in differentiating cancer from infection and usually demonstrates pleomorphic malignant cells. Benign tumors of the anal sac are very rare. Most females with this cancer will have an elevated calcium level, although one paper demonstrated only 26% of dogs with hypercalcemia.[3,4,8] This may result in significant renal damage, which will modify the prognosis and anesthetic risk. Depending on the level of hypercalcemia and renal function, aggressive saline diuresis and diuretic administration may be in order prior to surgery (see paraneoplastic disorders, Chap. 4).

A careful rectal exam should be performed to detect possible lymphadenopathy and the clinical degree of fixation prior to surgery. The tumors in the female have characteristic clinical appear-

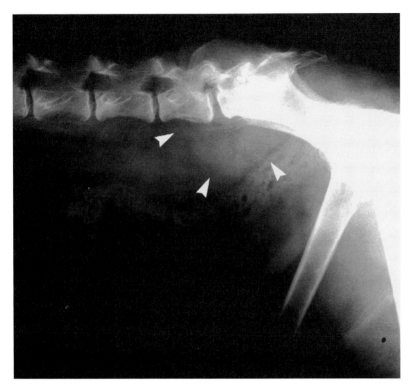

**Figure 18–22.** A lateral radiograph of the caudal abdomen in a male dog with perianal adenocarcinoma. Note metastatic involvement of sublumbar/iliac lymph nodes (arrows) and displacement of large bowel.

ances and rarely require a tissue biopsy before treatment. Males with clinical (fixed, large, ulcerated) or historical (previously castrated, recurrent) evidence of malignancy may require a wedge or punch biopsy to determine benign from malignant so that the desired extent of surgery can be determined.

## THERAPY

Castration and tumor removal with surgery or cryosurgery will be effective for the vast majority of adenomas.[9] Cryosurgery should only be used for focal lesions less than 1 to 2 cm in diameter (see Chap. 8). For diffuse or large lesions situated on or in the anal sphincter, castration followed by an observation period of several months to allow reduction in tumor volume may permit safer and easier mass removal. This will only be effective for the benign lesions that are hormone dependent. Estrogens have been used in the past to reduce tumor volume but carry a significant risk of bone marrow suppression. They should only be used when owners absolutely refuse castration or anesthesia for their dog. Rarely, estrogens are used to help reduce the size of a large tumor prior to surgery. In one study, 69% of irradiated adeno-

mas regressed for at least one year.[10] The cost and added morbidity of radiation makes this treatment a last alternative with most clinicians. Adenomas in the female are managed by simple excision or cryosurgery.

Perianal adenocarcinomas in the male are more locally invasive than their benign counterpart and generally do not respond to castration. Aggressive surgical removal with adequate margins is indicated. Removal of one-half or more of the anal sphincter is possible with only rare transient loss of continence. Recurrent disease becomes more difficult to resect. Regional lymph node metastasis can be excised in more than half the cases. Resectability cannot be reliably predicted preoperatively, and large volume is not a contraindication to caudal abdominal exploratory and lymphadenectomy. Some nodes "shell out" readily, while others are very invasive. For inoperable local or regionally confined (lymph node) disease, radiation therapy may be effective in slowing the disease progression but is only rarely curative. A subtotal lymphadenectomy (almost always the case) can also be followed with adjuvant radiation. On a limited number of cases, we have had success with lymphadenectomy, intraoperative radiation to the lymph node bed (15 Gy), and external beam radiation to the lymph node site. Doxorubicin (± cyclophosphamide) or cisplatin has resulted in some short-term partial remissions.

Anal sac adenocarcinoma in the female is generally locally invasive and has spread to regional lymph nodes in most cases regardless of radiographic findings. Treatment with surgery is similar to the malignant male disease, with the exception of routine abdominal exploratory and lymphadenectomy. Radiation and chemotherapy may be utilized as in the male. Total or near total removal of the tumor results in reversal of the hypercalcemia within 1 to 2 days. Return of hypercalcemia postoperatively usually signals recurrence or metastasis.

## PROGNOSIS

The prognosis for the various subsets of this disease location are widely divergent. For benign adenomas in the male or the female, more than 90% will be cured with castration (male) and mass removal. Occasional recurrences are usually treated successfully but should be rebiopsied to rule out carcinoma.

Adenocarcinoma in the male is difficult to cure because of common local recurrence and

may require numerous palliative resections over several years.[1,6] Unfortunately, most adenocarcinomas are not suspected or known until after a conservative resection, which contaminates further tissue planes, making the second resection problematic. If the clinician is more sensitized to preoperatively diagnosing malignancy, more aggressive initial resection should improve survivals. The emergence of regional or distant metastasis may take many years in the male.

In a series of 41 dogs with perianal adenocarcinoma, 15% had demonstrable metastasis at presentation. Stage of disease ($T_2N_0M_0$, or less) had an influence on survival, with tumors less than 5 cm in diameter ($T_2$) having survivals in excess of 70% at 2 years with surgical resection (Fig. 18–23).[6]

Anal sac adenocarcinoma in the female carries the worst prognosis, with mean survivals of 1 year. Local recurrence occurred in 50% of cases. Metastasis at diagnosis and hypercalcemia were poor prognostic signs.[4] Cause of death is either renal failure secondary to hypercalcemia or local and metastatic disease symptoms.[3,4,8,11] Most reports to date have concentrated on the pathophysiology of the disease rather than therapy. Aggressive resection with intraoperative and postoperative radiation has resulted in remissions

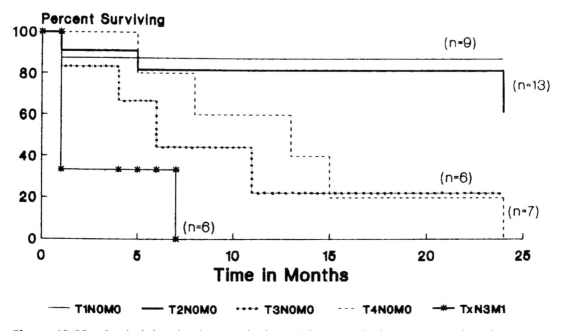

**Figure 18–23.**  Survival duration in 41 male dogs with perianal adenocarcinoma based on stage. Note that dogs with small tumors ($T_1$ or $T_2$) without lymph node involvement will do well after aggressive removal of the primary.

of longer than 1 year at CSU in a limited number of cases.

## COMPARATIVE ASPECTS[12]

No similar hormonally dependent disease state exists in humans. The most common cancer of the perianal skin is squamous cell carcinoma (epidermoid carcinoma). Chronic anal irritation (fissure, fistulas, etc.) may precede tumor development. Surgical resection is slowly being replaced with combination treatment with chemotherapy (5-FU and mitomycin) and radiation.

## REFERENCES

1. Wilson GP, Hayes HM: Castration for treatment of perianal gland neoplasms in the dog. J Am Vet Med Assoc *174*:1301–1303, 1979.
2. Dow SW, Olson PN, Rosychuk RAW, Withrow SJ: Perianal adenomas and hypertestosteronemia in a spayed bitch with pituitary-dependent hyperadrenocorticism. J Am Vet Med Assoc *192*:1439–1441, 1988.
3. Meuten DJ, Cooper BJ, Capen CC, Chew DJ, Kociba GJ: Hypercalcemia associated with an adenocarcinoma derived from the apocrine glands of the anal sac. Vet Pathol *18*:454–471, 1981.
4. Ross JT, Scavelli TD, Matthiesen DT, Patnaik AK: Adenocarcinoma of the apocrine glands of the anal sac in dogs: A review of 32 cases. J Am Anim Hosp Assoc *27*:349–355, 1991.
5. Nielsen SW, Aftosmis J: Canine perianal gland tumors. J Am Vet Med Assoc *144*:127–135, 1964.
6. Vail DM, Withrow SJ, Schwarz PD, Powers BE: Perianal adenocarcinoma in the canine male: A retrospective study of 41 cases. J Am Anim Hosp Assoc *26*:329–334, 1990.
7. Rubin S, Shivaprasad HL: Hypercalcemia associated with an anal sac adenocarcinoma in a castrated male dog. Compend Contin Educ Pract Vet *7*:348–352, 1985.
8. Hause WR, Stevenson S, Meuten DJ, Capen CC: Pseudohyperparathyroidism associated with adenocarcinomas of anal sac origin in four dogs. J Am Anim Hosp Assoc *17*:373–379, 1981.
9. Liska WD, Withrow SJ: Cryosurgical treatment of perianal gland adenomas in the dog. J Am Anim Hosp Assoc *14*:457–463, 1978.
10. Gillette EL: Veterinary radiotherapy. J Am Vet Med Assoc *157*:1707–1712, 1970.
11. Goldschmidt MH, Zoltowski C: Anal sac gland adenocarcinoma in the dog: 14 cases. J Small Anim Pract *22*:119–128, 1981.
12. Shank B, Cohen AM, Kelsen D: Cancer of the anal region. *In* DeVita VT (ed): Cancer, Principles and Practice of Oncology. Philadelphia, JB Lippincott, 1993, pp. 1006–1022.

# 19

# Tumors of the Respiratory System

Stephen J. Withrow

## A. Cancer of the Nasal Planum

### INCIDENCE AND RISK FACTORS

Cancer of the nasal planum is rare in the dog and fairly common in the cat. The development of squamous cell carcinoma (SCC) has been correlated with ultraviolet light exposure and lack of protective pigment.[1] It is classically seen in older, lightly pigmented cats.

### PATHOLOGY AND NATURAL BEHAVIOR

By far the most common cancer is SCC. Depending on the timing of biopsy, these tumors may be reported as carcinoma in situ, superficial SCC, or deeply infiltrative SCC. They may be very locally invasive but only rarely metastasize.

Other cancers reported in this site are lymphoma, fibrosarcoma, hemangiomas, melanoma, mast cell tumors, fibromas, and eosinophilic granulomas. Immune-mediated disease may present as erosive or crusty lesions on the nose but are rarely proliferative and usually have other sites on the body affected.

### HISTORY AND CLINICAL SIGNS

Invasive SCC is usually preceded by a protracted course of disease (months to years) that progresses through the following stages (Figs. 19–1A, 19–1B, 19–1C): crusting and erythema, superficial erosions and ulcers (carcinoma in situ

or early SCC), and finally deeply invasive and erosive lesions. Associated eyelid and ear pinna lesions may be seen if these sites lack pigment. Patients have often been treated with corticosteroids or topical ointments with little response.

### DIAGNOSTIC TECHNIQUES AND WORKUP

Erosive or proliferative lesions should have a deep wedge biopsy to determine the degree of invasion and histologic type of disease. These biopsies will require a brief general anesthetic because of sensitivity of the nasal planum. Hemorrhage can be profuse and will usually require one or two sutures to appose the edges. Rarely, dilute epinephrine (1 : 10,000) can be injected or topically applied to arrest capillary oozing. Cytologic scrapings or superficial biopsies are of little value, since they only reveal the inflammation that may accompany both cancer and noncancerous conditions. Lymph nodes are rarely involved except in very advanced disease, and thoracic radiographs are invariably negative for metastasis.

### THERAPY

It may be possible to prevent or arrest the course of the preneoplastic disease by limiting exposure to the sun or tattooing to add pigment protection. Topical sunscreens are readily licked off and

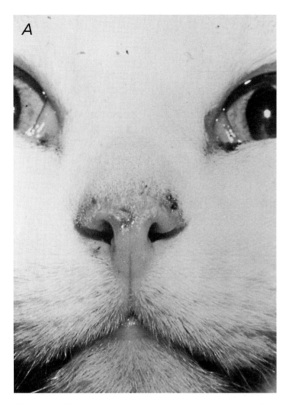

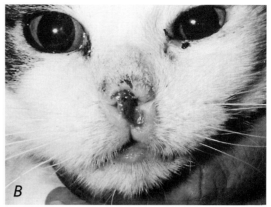

**Figure 19–1B.** This cat has an invasive squamous cell carcinoma that has caused some erosion of the nasal planum but is still confined to the nasal planum. Nosectomy was curative.

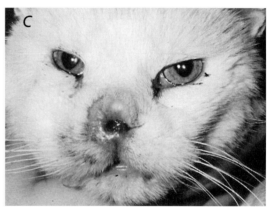

**Figure 19–1A.** Crusting and erythema of a white cat's nose that had been slowly progressive for 8 months. Six months later the lesion was biopsy confirmed as carcinoma in situ.

**Figure 19–1C.** This cat had a 2-year history of progressive nasal ulceration and deformity. The nasal planum is markedly deformed, and the surrounding skin up to the eyelids is swollen and infiltrated with squamous cell carcinoma. Even nosectomy would not be curative. Note concomitant eyelid lesions that were carcinoma in situ.

rarely help. When inflammation and ulceration are present, it is very difficult to maintain the tattoo, since it is rapidly removed by macrophages. Even under the best of circumstances, tattooing will have to be repeated at regular intervals. Attempts to increase epithelial differentiation with synthetic derivatives of vitamin A generally have been unsuccessful for advanced disease but may be of help in reversing or limiting the growth of preneoplastic lesions.[2,3]

SCC, and probably other neoplasms as well, fall into two general categories: (1) superficial minimally invasive disease and (2) deeply infiltrating disease. Superficial cancers can be managed effectively by almost any method, including cryosurgery, phototherapy,[4] hyperthermia, or irradiation.[5] A distinct disadvantage with these techniques is the inability to get a surgical margin to document the adequacy of the treatment. Deeply invasive cancer, on the other hand, is generally resistant to these treatments. In particular, radiation therapy, which would have the greatest

chance of preserving the cosmetic appearance of the nose, has had poor local control rates for bigger and more invasive SCC in the dog and the cat.[6,7] The expectations for radiation with other tumor types would have to be extrapolated from the radiation results achieved in more conventional sites.

Complete excision of invasive cancer of the nasal planum can be performed in the cat with an acceptable cosmetic result.[8] The nasal planum is completely removed with a 360-degree skin incision that also transects the underlying turbinates

(Fig. 19–2). A single cutaneous purse-string suture of 3-0 nylon is then placed to pull the skin into an open circle (1 cm diameter) around the airways. The purse string should not be pulled too tight because it may heal across the airway. The site will crust and scab over. This scab is removed at suture removal (often requiring sedation) and the healing of the skin with two patent "nostrils" is complete by 1 month. Functional and cosmetic results are good in the cat (Fig. 19–3) and fair in the dog. This probably is the treatment of choice for invasive lesions that have not extended extensively to the lip or surrounding skin. If the margins of removal are incomplete, adjuvant radiation therapy has been successfully used by the author. Combined removal

of the premaxilla and nasal planum has been reported in the dog.[9]

## PROGNOSIS

The outlook for SCC is good for early, noninvasive disease. Later development of new sites of neoplasia on other areas of the planum is common, however, since the underlying causes are not reversed. Later-stage disease can be cured with aggressive surgery but is poorly responsive to most other treatments. Fifteen of 20 cats with invasive SCC of the nasal planum treated at CSU with wide resection (nosectomy) were free of recurrent disease at 1 year.[8] Photodynamic ther-

**Figure 19–2.** Operative view of the resected nasal planum in a cat with invasive carcinoma that was confined to the nasal planum.

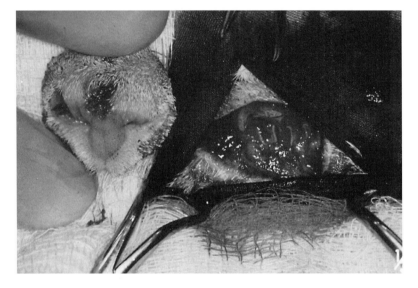

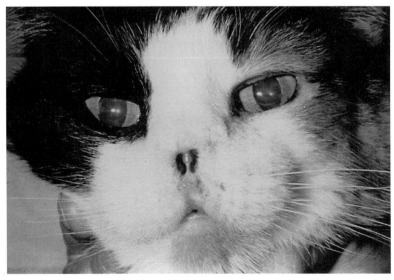

**Figure 19–3.** One-year postoperative view of a cat after nosectomy for squamous cell carcinoma. Note well-healed skin around patent airways. This cat remains free of disease 28 months postoperatively.

apy was effective in treating 9 of 16 cats with SCC of the nose, but the lesions had to be small and minimally invasive for a good result.[4] Since SCC rarely metastasizes from this site, even untreated animals with advanced cancer can live a long time, albeit with an ulcerated and deforming cancer.

## COMPARATIVE ASPECTS[10]

Cancer of the human nasal skin and nasal vestibule (anterior entrance to the nasal cavity) may be ultraviolet light induced, as in the cat. Lack of protective pigment is also a contributing factor. SCC of the vestibule is treated with radiation (interstitial or external beam) or surgery. Surgery generally entails resection of the nasal skin and cartilage, with reconstruction via composite ear skin and cartilage, nasolabial flaps, or a prosthesis. Local control is generally good.

## REFERENCES

1. Hargis AM: A review of solar-induced lesions in domestic animals. Compend Contin Educ Pract Vet 3:287–294, 1981.
2. Evans AG, Madewell BR, Stannard AA: A trial of 13-cis-retinoic acid for treatment of squamous cell carcinoma and preneoplastic lesions of the head in cats. Am J Vet Res 46:2553–2557, 1985.
3. Marks SL, Song MD, Stannard AA, Power HT: Clinical evaluation of etretinate for the treatment of canine solar-induced squamous cell carcinoma and preneoplastic lesions. J Am Acad Dermatol 27:11–16, 1992.
4. Peaston AE, Leach MW, Higgins RJ: Photodynamic therapy for nasal and aural squamous cell carcinoma in cats. J Am Vet Med Assoc 202:1261–1265, 1993.
5. Grier RL, Brewer WG, Theilen GH: Hyperthermic treatment of superficial tumors in cats and dogs. J Am Vet Med Assoc 177:227–233, 1980.
6. Carlisle CH, Gould S: Response of squamous cell carcinoma of the nose of the cat to treatment with x-rays. Vet Radiol 23:186–192, 1982.
7. Thrall DE, Adams WM: Radiotherapy of squamous cell carcinomas of the canine nasal plane. Vet Radiol 23:193–195, 1982.
8. Withrow SJ, Straw RC: Resection of the nasal planum in nine cats and five dogs. J Am Anim Hosp Assoc 26:219–222, 1990.
9. Kirpensteijn J, Withrow SJ, Straw RC: Combined resection of the nasal planum and premaxilla in three dogs. Vet Surg, 23:341–346, 1994.
10. Safai B: Cancers of the skin. In DeVita VT, et al: Cancer: Principles and Practice of Oncology Philadelphia, JB Lippincott 1993, pp. 1567–1611.

# B. Cancer of the Larynx and Trachea

## INCIDENCE AND RISK FACTORS

Cancer in either the larynx or trachea is rare. Young patients with active osteochondral ossification sites are at higher risk for benign tracheal osteocartilaginous tumors that grow in synchrony with the rest of the musculoskeletal system.[1] Laryngeal oncocytomas also appear to occur in younger mature dogs.[2,3] No breed or sex predilection is known for either site.

## PATHOLOGY AND NATURAL BEHAVIOR

Reported canine laryngeal tumors include rhabdomyoma (oncocytomas), osteosarcoma, chondrosarcoma, undifferentiated carcinoma, fibrosarcoma, mast cell, adenocarcinoma, and squamous cell carcinoma.[4–6] Rhabdomyomas in the dog may attain a large size, are minimally invasive, and do not appear to metastasize.[2,3,7,8] Most other laryngeal tumors are very locally invasive with a significant metastatic potential. Feline laryngeal neoplasms are most commonly lymphoma, although squamous cell carcinoma and adenocarcinoma have been reported.[5–7]

Reported tracheal cancer includes lymphoma, plasmacytoma, chondrosarcoma, adenocarcinoma, and squamous cell carcinoma. Tracheal leiomyomas and polyps have also been reported.[10–12] Several reports of benign tracheal osteochondral tumors exist in the literature.[1,13] These lesions grow from the cartilaginous rings and are composed of cancellous bone capped by cartilage. They may reflect a malfunction of osteogenesis rather than true cancer and are benign.[13]

The larynx and trachea may be secondarily invaded by neoplasms such as lymphoma and thyroid adenocarcinoma.

## HISTORY AND CLINICAL SIGNS

Patients with laryngeal tumors usually present with a progressive change in the voice or bark, exercise intolerance, or dysphagia. Tracheal

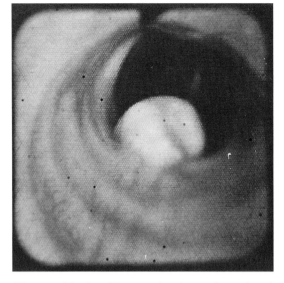

**Figure 19–4.** Fiberoptic view of tracheal osteochondroma in a 5-month-old dog.

tumor patients will usually present with coughing and exercise intolerance. Since osteochondral lesions of young dogs grow at the same rate as the rest of the skeleton, they will cause the greatest symptoms during or after the skeletal growth spurt.

Laryngeal and tracheal tumors are generally not palpable externally.

## DIAGNOSTIC TECHNIQUE AND WORKUP

Laryngeal tumors can usually be biopsied under direct visualization. Regional radiographs may reveal the lesion but are rarely necessary.[4]

Tracheal tumors offer more of a diagnostic challenge but can be biopsied with the use of fiberoptic instruments or a rigid bronchoscope (Fig. 19–4). Alternately, open surgical biopsy, often coupled with excision, can be performed. Plain radiographs or a tracheogram may reveal a mass narrowing the lumen (Fig. 19–5).

## THERAPY

Benign laryngeal cancers such as rhabdomyomas can be successfully removed with preservation of function.[2,7,8] Complete laryngectomy with a permanent tracheostomy is another option used in humans but has had limited utilization in veterinary medicine.[6,14–16] Depending on suspected radioresponsiveness, invasive cancers can be treated with irradiation to better preserve laryngeal function. Radiation should control lymphoma or plasmacytoma in the dog or cat larynx or trachea. Chemotherapy (with or without surgery) may also be effective.[17]

Tracheal tumors should be treated with resection, especially benign osteochondral tumors (Fig. 19–6).[1,18] Full-thickness removal with end-

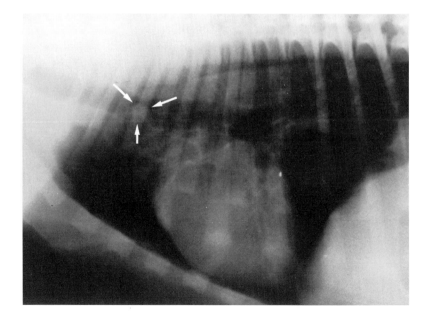

**Figure 19–5.** Lateral thoracic radiograph of the dog in Figure 19–4. Note the intraluminal mass on the floor of the trachea (arrows).

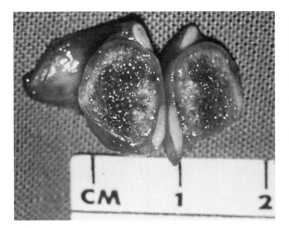

**Figure 19–6.** Resected tumor and associated tracheal cartilage rings of the dog in Figures 19–4 and 19–5. The tumor is bisected and has the typical appearance of cancellous bone with a cartilaginous cap. The patient recovered uneventfully from surgery and survived for more than 5 years, when it was lost to follow-up.

to-end anastomosis can be easily performed on up to three or four rings. Experimentally, up to 50% of tracheal length has been removed with successful closure.[19]

Phototherapy via bronchoscopy has been successfully utilized in humans for small lesions (carcinoma in situ or early carcinoma) but these lesions are only rarely recognized in the dog.

## PROGNOSIS

Benign lesions of the trachea or larynx carry a good prognosis if they can be surgically resected. Most dogs with resectable rhabdomyomas will live more than a year and may be presumed cured.[2,7,8] Very limited information is available for malignancies, since very few have been treated and reported.[6]

## COMPARATIVE ASPECTS[20]

Laryngeal cancer is common in man (2% of all cancers) and is related to smoking and alcohol consumption. Squamous cell carcinoma accounts for nearly all cancers. Earlier detection due to changes in voice make treatment more feasible.

The disease appears to progress through stages of development, from dysplasia, to carcinoma in situ, to minimally invasive carcinoma, to invasive carcinoma. Sixty percent of patients with carcinomas are presented with local disease only, 30% with regional nodal metastasis, and 10% with distant metastasis. Treatment is with surgery (partial or complete laryngectomy) or radiation. Local control and cure rates are good to excellent.

Tracheal cancer (independent of lung cancer) is very rare.

## REFERENCES

1. Withrow SJ, Holmberg DL, Doige CE, Rosychuk RAW: Treatment of a tracheal osteochondroma with an overlapping end-to-end tracheal anastomosis. J Am Anim Hosp Assoc 14(4):469–473, 1978.
2. Meuten DJ, Calderwood-Mays MB, Dillman RC, Cooper BJ, et al: Canine laryngeal rhabdomyoma. Vet Pathol 22:533–539, 1985.
3. Pass DA, Huxtable CR, Cooper BJ, Watson ADJ, Thompson R: Canine laryngeal oncocytomas. Vet Pathol 17:672–677, 1980.
4. Wheeldon EB, Suter PF, Jenkins T: Neoplasia of the larynx in the dog. J Am Vet Med Assoc 180:642–647, 1982.
5. Saik JE, Toll SL, Diters RW, Goldschmidt MH: Canine and feline laryngeal neoplasia: A 10-year survey. J Am Anim Hosp Assoc 22:359–365, 1986.
6. Carlisle CH, Biery DN, Thrall DE: Tracheal and laryngeal tumors in the dog and cat: Literature review and 13 additional patients. Vet Radiol 32:229–235, 1991.
7. Henderson RA, Powers RD, Perry L: Development of hypoparathyroidism after excision of laryngeal rhabdomyosarcoma in a dog. J Am Vet Med Assoc 198:639–643, 1991.
8. Calderwood Mays MB: Laryngeal oncocytoma in two dogs. J Am Vet Med Assoc 185:677–679, 1984.
9. Vasseur PB: Laryngeal adenocarcinoma in a cat. J Am Anim Hosp Assoc 17:639–641, 1981.
10. Bryan RD, Frame RW, Kier AB: Tracheal leiomyoma in a dog. J Am Vet Med Assoc 178:1069–1070, 1981.
11. Black AP, Liu S, Randolph JF: Primary tracheal leiomyoma in a dog. J Am Vet Med Assoc 179:905–907, 1981.
12. Hendricks JC, O'Brien JA: Tracheal collapse in two cats. J Am Vet Med Assoc 187(4):418–419, 1985.
13. Carb A, Halliwell WH: Osteochondral dysplasias of the canine trachea. J Am Anim Hosp Assoc 17:193–199, 1981.
14. Nelson AW, Wykes PM: Upper respiratory system. In Textbook of Small Animal Surgery. Philadelphia, WB Saunders, 1985, pp. 950–990.
15. Harvey CE: Speaking out. J Am Anim Hosp Assoc 22:568, 1986.
16. Crowe DT, Goodwin MA, Greene CE: Total laryn-

gectomy for laryngeal mast cell tumor in a dog. J Am Anim Hosp Assoc 22:809–816, 1986.

17. Schneider PR, Smith CW, Feller DL: Histiocytic lymphosarcoma of the trachea in a cat. J Am Anim Hosp Assoc 15:485–487, 1979.

18. Pearson GR, Lane JG, Holt PE, Gibbs C: Chondromatous hamartomas of the respiratory tract in the dog. J Small Anim Pract 28:705–712, 1987.

19. Nelson AW: Lower respiratory system. In Slatter DH (ed): Textbook of Small Animal Surgery. Philadelphia, WB Saunders, 1985, pp. 950–990.

20. Sessions RB, Harrison LB, Hong WK: Cancer in the head and neck. In DeVita VT, et al (eds): Cancer: Principles and Practice of Oncology. Philadelphia, JB Lippincott, 1993, pp. 631–654.

# C. Lung Cancer

## INCIDENCE AND RISK FACTORS

Compared to humans, primary canine lung cancer is very rare and accounts for only 1% of all cancers diagnosed. It is even more uncommon in the cat. The attempts to correlate urban living[1] and passive cigarette smoking have not as yet shown a convincing positive etiologic association.[2] However, dogs trained to smoke cigarettes (with or without concomitant asbestos instillation) through a tracheostomy will develop lung cancer at a dramatically increased rate.[3,4] Plutonium[239] and other forms of radiation have been shown to induce lung cancer in normal dogs when inhaled as an aerosol.[5] The average age at diagnosis is 10 years, and there is no apparent sex or breed predilection for dogs. Female cats are more commonly affected than male cats. Metastatic lung cancer is much more common than primary lung cancer in the dog and the cat.[6,7]

## PATHOLOGY AND NATURAL BEHAVIOR

Almost all primary cancers of the lung are carcinomas, the most common being adenocarcinoma.[6] Adenocarcinomas are further classified by location, such as bronchial, bronchoalveolar, or alveolar carcinoma. Carcinomas can be further graded as differentiated or undifferentiated, either grade being correlated to the incidence of metastasis.[6,8] Squamous cell carcinoma is less commonly reported. Benign tumors and primary sarcomas are rare.[6,9] A rare neoplasm of the lung is lymphomatoid granulomatosis.[10]

Metastasis can occur via lymphatics, through the airways, hematogenously, or transpleurally.[11] Lung cancer in humans and animals seems to have a propensity to spread to the central nervous system.[12–14] More than 50% of undifferentiated adenocarcinomas and more than 90% of squamous cell carcinomas will metastasize.[6]

## HISTORY AND CLINICAL SIGNS

Most symptomatic animals present with nonproductive coughing, exercise intolerance, or other respiratory signs that have been present for several weeks to months. An occasional animal may be presented peracutely, secondary to hemothorax, pneumothorax, or malignant pleural effusion.[15]

Paraneoplastic syndromes, common in humans, are rare (or unrecognized) in animals, with the most common being hypertrophic osteopathy.[11] When present, the animal may be seen for lameness or swollen legs.

## DIAGNOSTIC TECHNIQUES AND WORKUP

Many diagnostic techniques are theoretically available but only rarely are they indicated. Once a thoracic radiograph demonstrates a solitary lung mass, the next step is generally surgical removal. Deciding which lung lesions are likely to be primary lung cancer and treatable with surgery, versus those that should not be operated or treated in another fashion, is the clinical dilemma. However, a strong presumptive diagnosis can be made before surgery.

Radiographs will usually demonstrate a well-demarcated, spherical mass that is usually solitary. Occasionally, primary or metastic lung cancer can be cavitary on radiographs.[16] The caudal lung lobes are the most commonly affected (Fig. 19–7). Multiple or miliary lesions can be seen but are less common. Hilar lymphadenopathy is uncommonly seen on radiographs, even though

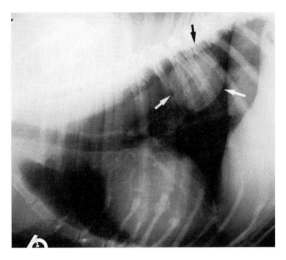

**Figure 19–7.** Lateral radiograph of 12-year-old dog with a well-circumscribed mass in the caudal lung lobe (arrows). This mass was surgically removed via lobectomy and diagnosed as adenocarcinoma. The patient died 26 months later of noncancer causes and the autopsy revealed no evidence of cancer.

positive lymph nodes may be removed at surgery. Pleural effusion may also be detected, but only rarely contains cancer cells.[17] Other imaging techniques such as MRI and CT scans may allow more accurate staging for resectability as well as detection of occult metastasis or lymph node enlargement.

Bronchoscopy can be performed and may be of diagnostic value for centrally located lesions that extend into the bronchus for tissue or brush biopsy.[18] Transtracheal lavage can also be performed but only rarely is diagnostic except in diffuse lymphoma, for which the clinician should have at their disposal other more simple and safe diagnostics, which negate the need for lavage.[19,20] Transthoracic fine-needle aspirates can be quite rewarding for larger lesions located in a peripheral site, but it is common for these tumors to have a necrotic center that may confuse interpretation.[21–23] However, bronchoscopy, tracheal lavage, and fine-needle aspirates are really not necessary before surgery for solitary lesions because the treatment (i.e., lobectomy) is the same for all etiologies. Unless the owner desires an accurate diagnosis or prognosis before surgery, the diagnosis and treatment should be combined. Unfortunately, an *accurate and precise* diagnosis before surgery is rarely attained.

Pleural effusions, on the other hand, should be carefully assessed because malignant pleural effusions carry very poor prognoses and may preclude the need for surgical intervention.

## THERAPY

Once a diagnosis of solitary lung mass is made in a patient who has disease apparently confined to the thorax and who can tolerate anesthesia, thoracotomy is generally the next step. Regardless of etiology, surgical removal is the treatment of choice. At the very least, an accurate diagnosis and stage can be attained.

A standard intercostal incision over the fourth to sixth interspace or a sternotomy midline will generally allow complete lung lobe removal and hilar lymph node biopsy. Partial lobectomy can be accomplished for very peripherally located tumors, but a complete lobectomy is the rule. Careful palpation of other lobes may reveal further nodules for removal. The use of stapling equipment (TA-55 or 90)* has allowed quick and secure lobectomy to be performed in most patients but is not required (Figs. 19–8A, 19–8B, 19–8C)[23,24]

Other methods of therapy such as radiation and chemotherapy have been largely untried. Normal lung tissue will generally not accept the doses of irradiation required to kill tumor cells without serious consequences to normal tissues such as fibrosis. In a very limited series of cases, multidrug chemotherapy with vindesine with or without cisplatin may have shown some benefit.[23] Isolated lung perfusion with chemotherapy for unresectable disease has been tested in dogs and humans but is technically demanding and associated with significant toxicity.[25]

Malignant pleural effusions can be treated with systemic chemotherapy or intrapleural chemotherapy with agents such as cisplatin.[26] Alternatively, sclerosing agents such as tetracycline or talc have been used.[27]

Metastatic lung cancer is treatable on rare occasions.[28–31] The criteria to operate a patient with metastasis are relative but include complete control of the primary cancer (the longer the better, but at least 300 days); no other metastatic sites known; prior exposure to "effective" chemotherapy that hopefully will have eradicated other disease sites; a "favorable histology" (this is not established in veterinary medicine but gener-

*U.S. Surgical, Autosuture, Norwalk, Connecticut.

*C*

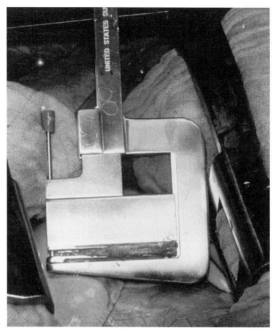

*A*

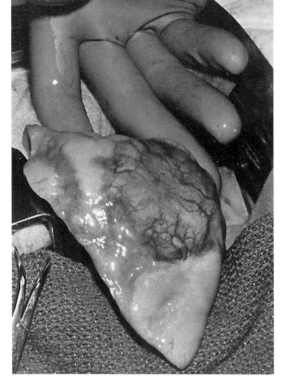

**Figure 19–8C.**   A stapler has been fired that releases a double row of capital B-shaped stainless steel staples. The lung mass is then removed and the instrument is released. The artery, vein, and bronchus are then inspected for possible small leaks, which are sutured.

**Figure 19–8A**.   Operative view of lung cancer from the paient in Figure 19–7. Note the typical raised lesion with superficial neovascularization.

*B*

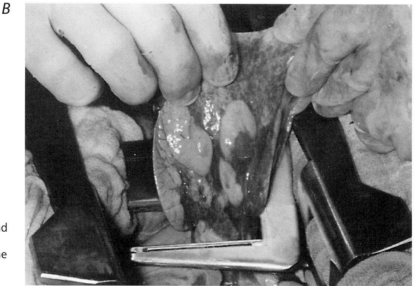

**Figure 19–8B**.   The lung lobe is lifted up and surgical staples are placed at the level of the proximal main-stem bronchus.

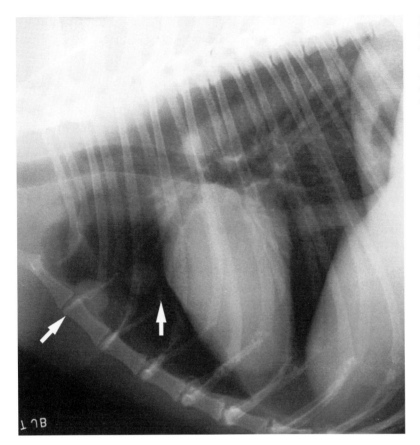

**Figure 19–9.** Lateral radiographs of a 10-year-old Irish setter who had undergone forelimb amputation for osteosarcoma 8 months previously. Note two spherical lesions in the apical lung lobes (arrows). The diameter of these lesions increased only 25% in 40 days and they were surgically removed with a partial lobectomy. This paient did well for 8 more months, when a rib metastasis was noted. No further metastatic lung cancer was noted.

ally includes sarcomas); a slow doubling time (greater than 40-day doubling of tumor diameter); and less than three radiographically visible lesions. Even for dogs that fit most of the above criteria, one fourth to one third can expect greater than 1-year survival after metastasectomy.[31] (See Figure 19–9.)

## PROGNOSIS

The best prognosis is seen in dogs with solitary lesions of small diameter (< 2 inches), negative lymph nodes, no malignant pleural effusion, and well-differentiated adenocarcinoma.[8,23] In this group of patients, more than 50% can be expected to live at least 1 year postoperatively. Of the malignant cancers, adenocarcinomas have a better prognosis than squamous cell carcinoma, which is often diffuse at diagnosis. One study reported a mean survival of 8 months for three squamous cell carcinomas and a mean of 19 months for eight adenocarcinomas in dogs.[23]

Canine patients with tumors located in the periphery had better survivals than those involving the entire lobe (mean of 16 months versus 8 months). Similarly, small tumors (< 100 cc$^3$, 5 cm diameter) had a mean survival of 20 months, while large tumors (> 100cc$^3$) had a mean survival of 8 months.[23] In another case series, patients with lymph node involvement had a median survival of 60 days, while dogs without lymph node involvement lived a median of 12 months.[8] Hypertrophic osteopathy, if present, can be expected to resolve after complete removal of the lung mass.

## COMPARATIVE ASPECTS[32]

Primary lung cancer develops in more than 100,000 people per year in the United States. It is the leading cause of cancer death in males and females over 35 years of age and it is strongly associated with smoking.

Bronchial or bronchoalveolar carcinomas and

bronchial mucinous gland carcinomas comprise more than 90% of lung cancers. The most common histologic types, in order, are adenocarcinoma, squamous cell carcinoma, small cell carcinoma (oat cell), and large cell carcinoma.

Paraneoplastic syndromes seen in more than 50% of cases are common and diverse.

Surgical resection is the treatment of choice for most lesions. If resection for cure can be performed, up to 30% of non-small-cell cancer patients may survive 5 years. Small cell carcinoma has historically carried the worst prognosis. Although small cell carcinoma may originally respond well to chemotherapy or radiation, long-term control is poor. Radiation is generally reserved for nonresectable tumors or for palliation.

## MISCELLANEOUS CONDITIONS OF THE LUNG

### Canine Pulmonary Lymphomatoid Granulomatosis[10,33]

In a series of seven cases, canine pulmonary lymphomatoid granulomatosis (PLG) affected young to middle-aged dogs with no breed or sex predilection. The most consistent laboratory abnormalities were circulating basophilia (6/7) and leukocytosis (4/7). Radiographic changes include lung lobe consolidation or large pulmonary granulomas (6/7) and tracheobronchial

lymph node enlargement (6/7) (Fig. 19–10A). Transthoracic fine-needle aspirates yielded eosinophilic and neutrophilic inflammation and were not diagnostic. All dogs were negative for heartworm. The major differential diagnosis is heartworm granulomas and either metastatic or primary lung cancer.[34] The definitive diagnosis was based on histologic examination of involved tissues (generally an open biopsy) and was characterized by angiocentric and angiodestructive infiltration of the pulmonary parenchyma by large lymphoreticular and plasmacytoid cells, along with normal lymphocytes, eosinophils, and plasma cells. This infiltrate was characteristically centered around the small- to medium-sized arteries and veins. A less than ideal but practical approach to diagnosis is diagnosis by response to therapy. Open lung biopsy via thoracotomy is not a low-risk procedure in dogs with diffuse lung disease. To our knowledge, PLG is the only diffuse neoplastic primary lung disease that will rapidly respond to chemotherapy. If the dog has a complete response in 1 or 2 weeks, one may be able to back into a diagnosis of PLG. However, another report on PLG reported only moderate response to therapy.[33] The full characterization of this unusual disease awaits further study.

The treatment consisted of immunosuppressive therapy and was attempted in five dogs. The drugs utilized included cyclophosphamide, vincristine, and prednisone. Three of the five treated dogs achieved a complete response, as evidenced by both clinical and radiographic resolution of

*A*

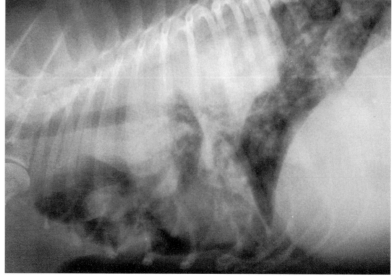

**Figure 19–10A.** Lateral radiograph of a 3-year-old dog, demonstrating a large perihilar mass with additional peripheral parenchymal lung pathology.

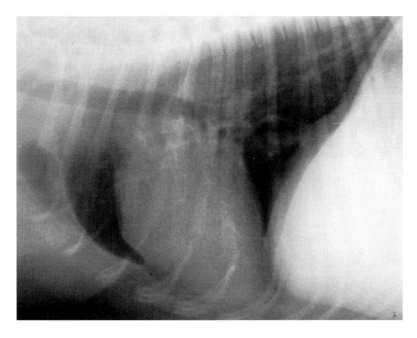

**Figure 19–10B.** Lateral radiograph of the dog in Figure 19–10A one year after chemotherapy with cyclophosphamide, vincristine, and prednisone. Chemotherapy was given for 6 months, and the dog remains in remission 4 years later.

*B*

the signs of disease (Fig. 19–10B). These three animals remained in complete remission at 7, 12, and 48 months from the time of diagnosis and initiation of therapy. One dog was euthanatized because of progression of signs after treatment with prednisone alone, and one dog who was treated with combination chemotherapy developed lymphoblastic leukemia 2 months after initiating therapy. Two dogs were euthanatized at the time of diagnosis.

The etiology of lymphomatoid granulomatosis remains unknown and may represent a preneoplastic, immune-mediated, or allergic disease. The disease responds to combination chemotherapy and carries a good prognosis with proper treatment. Lymphomatoid granulomatosis must be recognized as a distinct disease entity with a better prognosis than other more commonly diagnosed primary or metastatic diseases affecting the canine lung.[10,33]

## Malignant Histiocytosis

Malignant histiocytosis was reported originally in 10 male and 1 female Bernese Mountain dogs.[35] Nine dogs were closely related, suggesting a genetic predisposition. Other breeds are also at risk, however, including the rottweiler and golden retriever.[36,37] Most of the patients were middle-aged (range 4–10 years, mean 7 years). Respiratory signs were the most common complaint, although weight loss, lethargy, and

anorexia were also noted. Most patients had radiographic evidence of a large pulmonary nodule, with smaller nodules visible as well. Clinically or at necropsy, all patients had metastasis beyond the lung tissue. The most common sites of metastasis were the lymph node, liver, kidney, and central nervous system. The histologic diagnosis is not always straightforward and may require special stains for confirmation.[38] Treatment with various chemotherapies has been generally unrewarding.

## Lung Cancer in the Cat

The general principles of canine lung cancer apply to the cat as well. Cats have far less frequency of developing primary lung cancer than the dog, and metastatic disease to the lung is far more common than primary lung cancer. The general distribution of histologic types is similar between species, but very little has been written in terms of prognosis after treatment.[7,39]

An unusual syndrome in the cat is that of primary carcinoma of the lung (usually squamous cell carcinoma) with metastasis to multiple digits and other sites.[40–42] Most cats present with swelling of several toes and concomitant radiographic evidence of a lung mass. It is presumed that the lung mass (often solitary) has metastasized to the digits. Why the digit is a suitable "soil" for metastasis is unclear. Treatment has been unrewarding to date.

## REFERENCES

1. Reif JS, Cohen D: The environmental distribution of canine respiratory tract neoplasms. Arch Environ Health 22:136–140, 1971

2. Reif JS, Dunn K, Ogilvie GK, Harris CK: Passive smoking and canine lung cancer risk. Am J Epidemiol 135:234–239, 1992.

3. Auerbach O, Hammond EC, Kirman D, et al: Pulmonary neoplasms. Arch Environ Health 21:754–768, 1970.

4. Humphrey EW, Ewing SL, Wrigley JV, et al: The production of malignant tumors of the lung and pleura in dogs from intratracheal asbestos instillation and cigarette smoking. Cancer 47:1994–1999, 1981.

5. Gillett NA, Stegelmeier BL, Kelly G, et al: Expression of epidermal growth factor receptor in plutonium-239-induced lung neoplasms in dogs. Vet Pathol 29:46–52, 1992.

6. Moulton JE, von Tscharner C, Schneider R: Classification of lung carcinomas in the dog and cat. Vet Pathol 18:513–528, 1981.

7. Koblik PD: Radiographic appearance of primary lung tumors in cats. Vet Radiol 27:66–73, 1986.

8. Ogilvie GK, Weigel RM, Haschek WM, et al: Prognostic factors for tumor remission and survival in dogs after surgery for primary lung tumor: 76 cases (1975–1985). J Am Vet Med Assoc 195:109–112, 1989.

9. Ogilvie GK, Haschek WM, Withrow SJ: Classification of primary lung tumors in dogs: 210 cases (1975–1985). J Am Vet Med Assoc 195:106–108, 1989.

10. Postorino NC, Wheeler SL, Park RD, et al: A syndrome resembling lymphomatoid granulomatosis in the dog. J Vet Intern Med 3:15–19, 1989.

11. Brodey RS, Craig PH: Primary pulmonary neoplasms in the dog: A review of 29 cases. J Am Vet Med Assoc 147:1628–1643, 1965.

12. Sorjonen DC, Braund KG, Hoff EJ: Paraplegia and subclinical neuromyopathy associated with a primary lung tumor in a dog. J Am Vet Med Assoc 180:1209–1211, 1982.

13. Moore JA, Taylor HW: Primary pulmonary adenocarcinoma with brain stem metastasis in a dog. J Am Vet Med Assoc 192:219–221, 1988.

14. MacCoy DM, Trotter EJ, DeLahunta A, MacDonald JM: Pelvic limb paralysis in a young miniature pinscher due to metastatic bronchogenic adenocarcinoma. J Am Anim Hosp Assoc 12:774–777, 1976.

15. Dallman MJ, Martin RA, Roth L: Pneumothorax as the primary problem in two cases of bronchioloalveolar carcinoma in the dog. J Am Anim Hosp Assoc 24:710–714, 1988.

16. Silverman S, Poulos PW, Suter PF: Cavitary pulmonary lesions in animals. J Am Vet Radiol Soc 17:134–146, 1976.

17. Biery DN: Differentiation of lung diseases of inflammatory or neoplastic origin from lung diseases in heart failure. Vet Clin North Am 4:711–721, 1974.

18. Venker-van Haagen AJ, Vroom MW, Heijn A, et al: Bronchoscopy in small animal clinics: An analysis of the results of 228 bronchoscopies. J Am Anim Hosp Assoc 21:521–526, 1985.

19. Hawkins EC, DeNicola DB, Kuehn NF: Bronchoalveolar lavage in the evaluation of pulmonary disease in the dog and cat. J Vet Intern Med 4:267–274, 1990.

20. Hawkins EC, Morrison WB, DeNicola DB, Blevins WE: Cytologic analysis of bronchoalveolar lavage fluid from 47 dogs with multicentric malignant lymphoma. J Am Vet Med Assoc 203:1418–1425, 1993.

21. Berquist TH, Bailey PB, Cortese DA, et al: Transthoracic needle biopsy. Accuracy and complications in relation to location and type of lesion. Mayo Clin Proc 55:475–481, 1980.

22. Roudebush P, Green RA, Digilio KM: Percutaneous fine-needle aspiration biopsy of the lung in disseminated pulmonary disease. J Am Anim Hosp Assoc 17:109–116, 1981.

23. Mehlhaff CJ, Leifer CE, Patnaik AK, et al: Surgical treatment of primary pulmonary neoplasia in 15 dogs. J Am Anim Hosp Assoc 20:799–803, 1984.

24. LaRue SM, Withrow SJ, Wykes PM: Lung resection using surgical staples in dogs and cats. Vet Surg 16:238–240, 1987.

25. Minchin RF, Johnston MR, Schuller HM, et al: Pulmonary toxicity of doxorubicin administered by in situ isolated lung perfusion in dogs. Cancer 61:1320–1325, 1988.

26. Moore AS, Kirk C, Carcona A: Intracavitary cisplatin chemotherapy experience with six dogs. J Vet Intern Med 5:227–231, 1991.

27. Laing EJ, Norris AM: Pleurodesis as a treatment for pleural effusion in the dog. J Am Anim Hosp Assoc 2:193–196, 1986.

28. Spanos PK, Payne WS, Ivins JC, et al: Pulmonary resection for metastatic osteogenic sarcoma. J Bone Jt Surg 58A:624–628, 1976.

29. Huth JF, Holmes EC, Vernon SE: Pulmonary resection for metastatic sarcoma. Am J Surg 140:9–16, 1980.

30. Roth JA, Putnam JB, Wesley MN, et al: Differing determinants of prognosis following resection of pulmonary metastases from osteogenic and soft tissue sarcoma patients. Cancer 55:1361–1366, 1985.

31. O'Brien MG, Straw RC, Withrow SJ, et al: Resection of pulmonary metastases in canine osteosarcoma: 36 cases (1983–1992). Vet Surg 22:105–109, 1993.

32. Ginsberg RJ, Kris MG, Armstrong JG: Cancer of the lung. In DeVita VT, et al (eds): Cancer: Principles and Practice of Oncology. Philadelphia, JP Lippincott, 1993, pp. 673–758.

33. Berry CR, Moore PF, Thomas WP, et al: Pulmonary lymphomatoid granulomatosis in seven

dogs (1976–1987). J Vet Intern Med 4:157–166, 1990.

34. Calvert CA, Mahaffey MB, Lappin MR, Farrell RL: Pulmonary and disseminated eosinophilic granulomatosis in dogs. J Am Anim Hosp Assoc 24:311–320, 1988.

35. Rosin A, Moore P, Dubielzig R: Malignant histiocytosis in Bernese Mountain dogs. J Am Vet Med Assoc 188:1041–1045, 1986.

36. Shaiken LC, Evans SM, Goldschmidt MH: Radiographic findings in canine malignant histiocytosis. Vet Radio 32:237–242, 1991.

37. Hayden DW, Waters DJ, Burke BA, Manivel JC: Disseminated malignant histiocytosis in a golden retriever: Clinicopathologic, ultrastructural, and immunohistochemical findings. Vet Pathol 30:256–264, 1993.

38. Moore PF: Utilization of cytoplasmic lysozyme immunoreactivity as a histiocytic marker in canine histiocytic disorders. Vet Pathol 23:757–762, 1986.

39. Barr F, Gruffydd-Jones TJ, Brown PJ, Gibbs C: Primary lung tumours in the cat. J Small Anim Pract 28:1115–1125, 1987.

40. Pollack M, Martin RA, Diters RW: Metastatic squamous cell carcinoma in multiple digits of a cat: Case report. J Am Anim Hosp Assoc 20:835–839, 1984

41. May C, Newsholme SJ: Metastasis of feline pulmonary carcinoma presenting as multiple digital swelling. J Small Anim Pract 30:302–310, 1989.

42. Scott-Moncrieff JC, Elliott GS, Radovsky A, Blevins WE: Pulmonary squamous cell carcinoma with multiple digital metastases in a cat. J Small Anim Pract 30:696–699, 1989.

# D. Nasal Tumors

## INCIDENCE AND RISK

Intranasal cancer comprises approximately 1% of all neoplasms.[1] It has been speculated, but unproven, that dolichocephalic breeds (long-nose) or dogs living in urban environments with resultant nasal filtering of pollutants may be at higher risk.[2,3] The average age of patients is 10 years and medium to large breeds may be more commonly affected. Chondrosarcoma will occur in a younger age group than other cancers.[4] A slight male predilection has been reported.[2]

This cancer is less common in the cat.

## PATHOLOGY AND NATURAL BEHAVIOR

Carcinomas (mainly adenocarcinoma, squamous cell carcinoma, and undifferentiated carcinoma) comprise nearly two thirds of intranasal cancers.[5] Sarcomas (fibrosarcoma, chondrosarcoma, osteosarcoma, and undifferentiated sarcoma) comprise the bulk of the remaining cancer.[6] All of the above malignancies are characterized by progressive local invasion. The metastatic rate is generally considered low at the time of initial diagnosis but may be as high as 50% in dogs subjected to a full necropsy. Lymph node and lung are the most common metastatic sites.[4,7]

Rarely, transmissible venereal cell cancer and polyps/fibromas will be seen.[8] The cat will have a higher percentage of lymphoma (usually feline leukemia virus negative) than will the dog.[9,10]

## HISTORY AND CLINICAL SIGNS

Although many intranasal diseases will have overlapping clinical signs, a strong presumption of cancer can be made for older animals with an intermittent and progressive history of initially unilateral epistaxis. The average length of signs before diagnosis is 3 months.[1] If facial deformity, and to a lesser degree epiphora, are present, the diagnosis is almost always cancer. "Apparent" response to a variety of symptomatic treatments is commonly seen.

On rare occasions animals may present with only neurologic signs from direct invasion of the cranial vault.[11]

## DIAGNOSTIC TECHNIQUES AND WORKUP

A definitive diagnosis of intranasal cancer requires a tissue biopsy, even though radiographs and historical information can be highly suggestive. Before skull radiographs and biopsy are performed, it is important to rule out a systemic bleeding disorder as carefully as possible. Attention to platelet count, the clotting of venipuncture sites, the presence of hematuria, retinal changes (hemorrhage or hypervisocity), the presence of petechial hemorrhages, and possibly a clotting time should determine if serious bleeding will occur subsequent to the biopsy.

Nasal radiographs are generally required to help define the extent of disease, provide a presumptive diagnosis, and locate that area within the nasal cavity most likely to yield diagnostic material with a biopsy.[12] Standard radiographs include lateral, dorsal ventral (DV), frontal sinus, and open-mouth oblique views. Probably the most rewarding views are an open-mouth DV oblique (to show the caudal nasal cavity and cribriform plate) or the isolated nasal cavity exposure with the film placed in the mouth and exposed in the DV plane (Fig. 19–11). Asymmetrical destruction of turbinates and the superimposition of a soft tissue mass over the turbinates, especially in the caudal half of the nose, are both classic radiographic changes of cancer. Bone destruction or

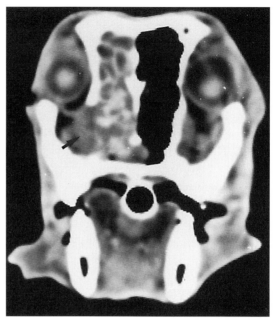

**Figure 19–12.** Computerized tomographic image of a dog with nasal cancer taken in the transverse plane at the level of the orbit. Note the involvement of the left side of the nasal cavity with invasion and destruction of the medial bony orbit (arrow).

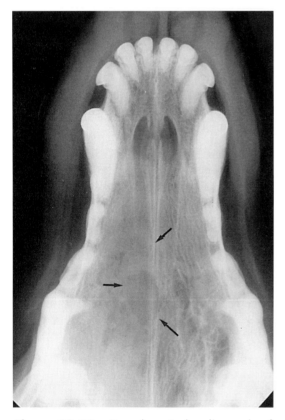

**Figure 19–11.** Dorsal ventral radiograph of the nasal cavity whereby the film is placed in the mouth. Note the asymmetry from side to side. Bone lysis (small arrows) and loss of turbinate detail imply tumor in the caudal half of the nasal cavity.

erosion is also common with cancer. Fluid in one or both frontal sinuses without bony erosion is usually secondary to outflow obstruction of the normal mucoid secretions and not neoplastic infiltration. Computerized tomography is an ideal diagnostic tool, especially as it relates to cribriform plate and orbital invasion (Fig. 19–12).[13–15]

Under the same anesthesia as the radiographs, a tissue biopsy should be obtained. This biopsy is usually easily procured via a transnostril core sample.[16] Based on the location of the lesion on radiographs, either a punch biopsy needle or a large bore (3–5 mm) plastic cannula is passed up the nostril and directed to the tumor.[16] With either technique, it is important to avoid penetrating the cribriform plate. The biopsy instruments should be marked with tape (punch) or cut off (plastic core) so as to never penetrate farther than the distance from the tip of the nares to the medial canthus of the eye (Fig. 19–13). Tumors are usually strongly suspected when white to yellow tissue is obtained rather than turbinate or mucous only. Mild to moderate hemorrhage is to be expected and will subside within a few minutes. If hemorrhage is severe, the unilateral carotid artery

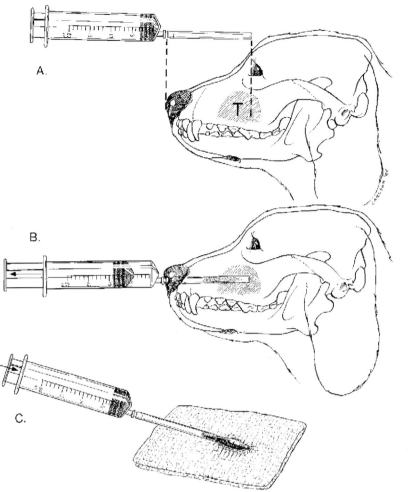

**Figure 19–13.** *A,* Illustration of a dog showing caudally situated tumor (T). The plastic cannula for the core aspirate has been shortened to extend no deeper than the medial canthus of the eye to avoid injury to the brain. *B,* The cannula is introduced into the nasal cavity through the nares. Slight resistance is usually felt as the tumor is entered. Negative pressure is applied as the cannula is redirected in various angles. *C,* Tissue and blood are expelled onto a gauze sponge, where blood is separated from tissue. The tissue is then submitted for histologic evaluation.[16]

can be permanently ligated in the neck. Cats or small dogs may also be biopsied with a curette passed up the nostril and into the tumor.

Attempts at nasal washing and fluid retrieval for cytological examination have been generally unrewarding and are not recommended as the sole means of diagnosis.[1] Rhinoscopy is only rarely needed to facilitate tissue procurement but is advocated by some authors.[17,18]

Lymph node aspirates are positive in as many as 10% of cases (especially carcinomas) and thoracic radiographs are usually normal at presentation.[1,4]

If any central nervous system signs exist, a cerebrospinal fluid (CSF) sample should be procured to help in determining the potential extension of disease to the dura or farther across the cribriform plate.[11] Increased CSF pressure, protein, and rarely cell count are suggestive of brain involvement.[19]

Culture and sensitivity testing for bacterial evaluation is seldom helpful in the therapy of primary bacterial rhinitis or rhinitis secondary to a tumor.

## THERAPY

Therapy is directed principally at local disease control. Unfortunately, this disease usually presents in a relatively advanced stage in a critical location near the brain and eyes (Fig. 19–14). Bone invasion occurs early and curative surgery is virtually impossible. Although surgical removal via rhinotomy has been recommended, its higher rate of acute and chronic morbidity, without significant extension of life,[1,5,20,21] makes it rarely indicated unless other therapies such as radiation are available.

Radiation therapy has the advantage of treat-

**Figure 19–14.** Cross section of a dog's skull with atypical intranasal carcinoma. Note the mid- to caudal position of the tumor, in the nasal cavity; the erosion of dorsal nasal bones; the dark mucous in frontal sinus secondary to obstruction; and the close proximity of the tumor to the cribriform plate. Complete surgical resection is impossible.

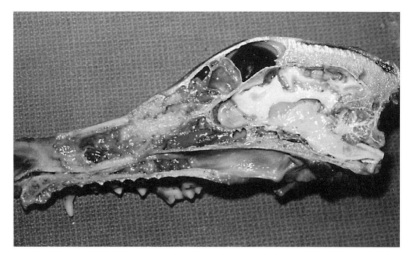

ing the entire nasal cavity, including bone extension, which surgery cannot remove. It is unclear whether surgical debulking before radiation is of benefit. It is probably necessary when using orthovoltage radiation but may not be for high-energy radiation such as cobalt or megavoltage.[22,23] Doses of 40 to 48 Gy are usually delivered in 10 to 12 fractions over 3 to 4 weeks to the caudal three fourths of the nasal cavity and frontal sinuses if indicated.[23] Either a single dorsal portal or bilateral opposed portals (preferred) are utilized. Although rhinitis as a result of surgery and radiation can be severe, it will usually subside within 1 or 2 months. Owners may be required to clean the nostrils several times a day, and rarely is the patient completely normal relative to its nasal cavity. Ocular changes can be expected if both eyes receive irradiation to 40 Gy in 3 weeks. Keratoconjunctivitis sicca is very common, and corneal ulcers and cataract formation will often occur at doses over 40 Gy.[24]

Cats are usually treated with radiation therapy only because of their poor tolerance to rhinotomy and the marked radiosensitivity of their tumors, especially if these are lymphoma.[9]

Unilateral or bilateral carotid artery ligation will palliate the symptoms of epistaxis for up to 3 months or longer without damage to the brain.[25]

Immunotherapy and cryosurgery have done nothing to improve survivals.[1,26] Cisplatin has shown slight benefit in dogs with nasal adenocarcinoma (27% response rate) but median survival was only 20 weeks.[27] A combination of cisplatin (a known radiation sensitizer) and radiation (with or without surgery) is potentially indicated in the dog.

## PROGNOSIS

Overall, the prognosis for canine nasal tumors is poor (Table 19–1). The mean survival for surgery, chemotherapy, immunotherapy, cryosurgery, or no treatment is 3 to 6 months, and most dogs will die or be euthanatized as a result of local disease progression.[1,20,21,26–28]

The only improvements in survival have been with radiation therapy, with or without surgical debulking. Mean and median survivals from various reports in dogs range from 8 to 25 months.[7,23,28–31] One-year survivals range from 20 to 59% and 2-year survivals range from 10 to 48%.[7,23,29–32] The prognosis for sarcomas is better than that for carcinomas, and adenocarcinomas respond better than squamous cell carcinoma or undifferentiated carcinoma.[7,29]

A problem exists in analyzing the end results after radiation with or without surgical debulking, since clinical symptoms as a result of treatment may be similar to those of the tumor before treatment.[23] Additionally, radiation therapy has been applied in such a varied manner (total dosage, number of fractions, duration of treatment, energy of radiation, portals of treatment, with or without surgery) that true comparisons between reports are impossible. Added to the above problems are those of a diverse group of tumor types, extent of surgery, and tumor stage, for which tumor response may vary. Few dogs are truly cured if followed to autopsy. In a series of autopsied patients treated with radiation, most had evidence of local recurrence, and almost 50% had lymph node metastasis and metastasis beyond the head and neck (usually lung).[7] As

**Table 19–1** Summary of Selected Articles on Treatment of Nasal Cancer in Dogs with Radiation Therapy

|  | Thrall[23] | Adams[29] | Evans[31] | Theon[30] | McChesney[b,7] |
|---|---|---|---|---|---|
| Number of dogs | 21 | 67 | 70 | 77 | 68 |
| Surgery | 18/21 | 41/67 | 64/70 | 217 | None |
| Survival |  |  |  |  |  |
|   Mean | 25 mo |  |  |  | 9.8 |
|   Median | 23 mo[a] | 8.5 mo | 16.5 mo | 21 mo,12 mo |  |
| % 1 year | 57 | 38 | 54 | 60 | 20 |
| % 2 years | 48 | 30 | 43 | 25 | 10 |
| Dose (rads) |  |  |  |  |  |
|   Mean |  | 4,300 |  |  |  |
|   Median | 4,500 |  | 4,500 | 4,800 | 44–6,800 |
| Number of fractions | 10 | 5–10 | 10 | 12 | 8–45 |
| Type radiation | Orthovoltage | Varied | Orthovoltage | Cobalt | Megavoltage |
| Prognostic indicators | None | adeno[c] > SCC[d] sarc[e] = adeno[c] Sx if low-energy energy radiation | None | Sarc[e] > car[cf] Chondro[g] > adeno | adeno[c] > SCC[d] |

[a]Not by life table analysis.
[b]Carcinoma only.
[c]adeno = adenocarcinoma.
[d]SCC = squamous cell carcinoma.
[e]sarc = sarcoma.
[f]carc = carcinoma.
[g]chondro = chondrosarcoma.

improvements in local control and survival continue to progress, the true metastatic potential of nasal malignancies in the dog will increase.

Far fewer cats have been treated, but survival, especially for lymphoid neoplasms, appears excellent.[9,10] The clinical improvement of patients with lymphoid tumors is very fast, complete, and possibly permanent.[9,10] Another study of non-lymphoid neoplasia in the cat had a 1-year survival of 44% and a 2-year survival of 17%, a rate very similar to that of the canine.[33]

## COMPARATIVE ASPECTS[34]

Cancer of the nasal cavity and paranasal sinuses is rare in humans. It generally affects persons more than 40 years of age and is twice as common in males as females. The most common cancer is squamous cell carcinoma. The etiologic factors for adenocarcinoma include occupations associated with wood dust, boot making, and the flooring industry.

The disease is variably locally invasive and reasonably late to metastasize. Surgery or irradiation or both are the standard treatment, depending on the stage, site, and type of cancer. Five-year control rates vary from 50 to 75%.

## REFERENCES

1. MacEwen EG, Withrow SJ, Patnaik AK: Nasal tumors in the dog: Retrospective evaluation of diagnosis, prognosis, and treatment. J Am Vet Med Assoc 170:45–48, 1977.
2. Stunzi H, Hauser B: XX. Tumours of the nasal cavity. Bull WHO 53:257–263, 1976.
3. Reif JS, Cohen D: The environmental distribution of canine respiratory tract neoplasms. Arch Environ Health 22:136–140, 1971.
4. Panaik AK: Canine sinonasal neoplasms: Clinicopathological study of 285 cases. J Am Anim Hosp Assoc 25:103–114, 1989.
5. Madewell BR, Priester WA, Gillette EL, et al: Neoplasms of the nasal passages and paranasal sinuses in domesticated animals as reported by 13 veterinary colleges. Am J Vet Res 851–856, 1976.
6. Patnaik AK, Lieberman PH, Erlandson RA, et al: Canine sinonasal skeletal neoplasms: Chondrosarcomas and osteosarcomas. Vet Pathol 21:475–482, 1984.

7. McChesney-Gillette S, Gillette EL, Thrall DE, et al: Response of canine nasal tumors and normal tissues to nonstandard fractionation. Radiat Res, in press.

8. Weir EC, Pond MJ, Duncan JR, et al: Extragenital occurrence of transmissible venereal tumor in the dog: Literature review and case reports. J Am Anim Hosp Assoc 14:532–536, 1978.

9. Straw RC, Withrow SJ, Gillette EL, et al: Use of radiotherapy for the treatment of intranasal tumors in cats: Six cases (1980–1985). J Am Vet Med Assoc 189:927–929, 1986.

10. Evans SM, Hendrick M: Radiotherapy of feline nasal tumors. Vet. Radiol. 30:128–132, 1989.

11. Smith MO, Turrel JM, Bailey CS, Cain GR: Neurologic abnormalities as the predominant signs of neoplasia of the nasal cavity in dogs and cats: Seven cases (1973–1986). J Am Vet Med Assoc 195:242–245, 1989.

12. Gibbs C, Lane JG, Denny HR: Radiological features of intra-nasal lesions in the dog: A review of 100 cases. J Small Anim Pract 20:515–535, 1979.

13. Thrall DE, Robertson ID, McLeod DA, et al: A comparison of radiographic and computed tomographic findings in 31 dogs with malignant nasal cavity tumors. Vet Radiol 30:59–66, 1989.

14. Park RD, Beck ER, LeCouteur RA: Comparison of computed tomography and radiography for detecting changes induced by malignant nasal neoplasia in dogs. J Am Vet Med Assoc 201:1720–1724, 1992.

15. Codner EC, Lurus AG, Miller JB, et al: Comparison of computed tomography with radiography as a noninvasive diagnostic technique for chronic nasal disease in dogs. J Am Vet Med Assoc 202:1106–1110, 1993.

16. Withrow SJ, Susaneck SJ, Macy DW, et al: Aspiration and punch biopsy techniques for nasal tumors. J Am Anim Hosp Assoc 21:551–554, 1985.

17. Rudd RG, Richardson DC: A diagnostic and therapeutic approach to nasal disease in dogs. Compend Contin Educ Pract Vet 7:103–112, 1985.

18. Lent SEF, Hawkins EC: Evaluation of rhinoscopy and rhinoscopy-assisted mucosal biopsy in diagnosis of nasal disease in dogs: 199 cases (1985–1989). J Am Vet Med Assoc 201:1425–1429, 1992.

19. Bailey CS, Higgins RJ: Characteristics of cisternal cerebrospinal fluid associated with primary brain tumors in the dog: A retrospective study. J Am Vet Med Assoc 188:414–417, 1986.

20. Laing EJ, Binnington AG: Surgical therapy of canine nasal tumors: A retrospective study (1982–1986). Canine Vet J 29:809–813, 1988.

21. Holmberg DL, Fries C, Cockshutt J, VanPelt D: Ventral rhinotomy in the dog and cat. Vet Surg 18:446–449, 1989.

22. Feeney DA, Johnston GR, Williamson JF, et al: Orthovoltage radiation of normal canine nasal passages: Assessment of depth dose. Am J Vet Res 44:1593–1596, 1983.

23. Thrall DE, Harvey CE: Radiotherapy of malignant nasal tumors in 21 dogs. J Am Vet Med Assoc 183:663–666, 1983.

24. Roberts SM, Lavach JD, Severin GA, et al: Ophthalmic complications following megavoltage irradiation of the nasal and paranasal cavities in dogs. J Am Vet Med Assoc 100:43–47, 1987.

25. Clendenin MA, Conrad MC: Collateral vessel development after chronic bilateral common carotid artery occlusion in the dog. Am J Vet Res 40:1244, 1979.

26. Withrow SJ: Cryosurgical therapy for nasal tumors in the dog. J Am Anim Hosp Assoc 18:585–589, 1982.

27. Hahn KA, Knapp DW, Richardson RC, Matlock CL: Clinical response of nasal adenocarcinoma to cisplatin chemotherapy in 11 dogs. J Am Vet Med Assoc 200:355–357, 1992.

28. Norris AM: Intranasal neoplasms in the dog. J Am Anim Hosp Assoc 15:231–236, 1979.

29. Adams WM, Withrow SJ, Walshaw R, et al: Radiotherapy of malignant nasal tumors in 67 dogs. J Am Vet Med Assoc 191:311–315, 1987.

30. Theon AP, Madewell BR, Harb MF, Dungworth DL: Megavoltage irradiation of neoplasms of the nasal and paranasal cavities in 77 dogs. J Am Vet Med Assoc 202:1469–1475, 1993.

31. Evans SM, Goldschmidt M, McKee LJ, Harvey CE: Prognostic factors and survival after radiotherapy for intranasal neoplasms in dogs: 70 cases (1974–1985). J Am Vet Med Assoc 194:1460–1463, 1989.

32. McEntee MC, Page RL, Heidner GL, et al: A retrospective study of 27 dogs with intranasal neoplasms treated with cobalt radiation. Vet Radiol 32:135–139, 1991.

33. Theon AP, Peaston AE, Madewell BR, Dungworth DL: Irradiation of nonlymphoproliferative neoplasms of the nasal cavity and paranasal sinuses in 16 cats. J Am Vet Med Assoc 204:78–83, 1994.

34. Schantz SP, Harrison LB, Hong WK: Cancer in the head and neck. In DeVita VT, et al (eds): Cancer: Principles and Practice of Oncology. Philadelphia, JB Lippincott, 1993, 574–672.

# 20

# Tumors of the Skeletal System

Rodney C. Straw

## OSTEOSARCOMA IN DOGS

### Incidence and Risk Factors

Osteosarcoma (OS) is the most common primary bone tumor in dogs, accounting for up to 85% of malignancies originating in the skeleton.[1–5] Osteosarcoma is estimated to occur in over 8,000 dogs each year in the United States; however, this is probably an underestimation, since not all cases are confirmed or recorded.[6,7] The demographics of canine OS have been well reported.[1–5,8–24] It is largely a disease of middle-aged to older dogs, with a median age of 7 years. There is a large range in age of onset, with a reported case in a 6-month-old pup,[25] and a small peak in age incidence at 18–24 months.[11] Primary rib OS tends to occur in younger adult dogs with a mean age of 4.5 to 5.4 years.[26,27] Osteosarcoma is classically a cancer of large and giant breeds. In a review of 1,462 cases of canine OS, dogs weighing more than 40 kg accounted for 29% of all cases, and only 5% of their tumors occurred in the axial skeleton. Only 5% of OS occur in dogs weighing less than 15 kg, but 59% of their tumors originated in the axial skeleton.[23] The breeds most at risk for OS are Saint Bernard, great Dane, Irish setter, Doberman pinscher, German shepherd, and golden retriever; however, size seems to be a more important predisposing factor than breed.[1,3,5,8,9,11,12,14,20,24,28] Males are reported to be slightly more frequently affected than females (1.1–1.5:1),[1,4,8,11,13,15,17–19,28] with the exception of the Saint Bernard, Rottweiler, and great Dane and of dogs with primary OS of the axial skeleton (except rib and spine), where affected females outnumber males.[1,17,18,26] However, in 544 cases of canine OS of all sites treated at Colorado State University between 1986 and 1994, the male to female ratio was 1:1.2 (unpublished data). Overall, approximately 75% of OS occurs in the appendicular skeleton, with the remainder occurring in the axial skeleton.[1,26] The metaphyseal region of long bones is the most common primary site, with the front limbs affected twice as often as rear limbs and the distal radius and proximal humerus being the two most common locations.[16] It is extremely rare for OS to be primarily located in bones adjacent to the elbow. In the rear limbs, tumors are fairly evenly distributed between the distal femur, distal tibia, and proximal tibia, with the proximal femur a slightly less common site.[1] Primary OS distal to the antebrachiocarpal and tarsocrural joints is relatively rare in dogs.[29] In a study of 116 cases of canine primary OS in the axial skeleton, it was reported that 27% were located in the mandible, 22% in the maxilla, 15% in the spine, 14% in the cranium, 10% in ribs, 9% in the nasal cavity or paranasal sinuses, and 6% in the pelvis.[26] Documentable multicentric OS at the time of initial diagnosis occurs in less than 10% of all cases.[30] Osteosarcoma of extraskeletal sites is rare, but primary OS has been reported in mammary tissue, spleen, bowel, liver, kidney, testicle, vagina, eye, gastric ligament, and adrenal gland.[31]

The etiology of canine OS is generally unknown. Some have speculated a viral cause because OS can occur in litter mates, and OS may be experimentally induced by injecting OS cells into canine fetii.[32,33] However, this is currently not a popularly held view, and an etiologic virus has not been isolated. A simplistic theory based on circumstantial evidence is that, since OS tends to occur in major weight-bearing bones adjacent to late-closing physes, and heavy dogs are predisposed, multiple minor trauma and subsequent injury to sensitive cells in the physeal region may occur. This may initiate the disease by inducing mitogenic signals, increasing the probability for the development of a mutant lineage. There are reports of OS associated with metallic implants used for fracture repair, with chronic osteomyelitis, and with fractures in which no internal repair was used.[34–38] Ionizing radiation can induce osteosarcoma. In one study, 43 of 403 beagles fed strontium-90 developed primary bone sarcomas.[39] Three of 87 spontaneous tumor-bearing dogs, or 3.4% of dogs treated for soft tissue sarcomas, developed OS within the field of radiation.[40] Secondary OS developed between 1.7 to 5 years after radiation in that study, and the authors speculated that a high dose of radiation per fraction may predispose to this serious late effect of irradiation. Osteosarcoma is a rare, late complication of radiation therapy in people and is even less common in dogs.[41,42] Postirradiation OS in people comprises approximately 2% to 4% of all osteosarcomas reviewed in two large series.[43,44] Osteosarcomas have been concurrently seen in dogs with bone infarcts.[45,46] Bone infarcts are uncommon, are of unknown etiology, and may be identified as incidental findings by radiography. Bone infarcts are probably not associated with tumor emboli. Osteosarcomas associated with bone infarcts appear to be more common in smaller breeds. It is not clear whether there is any causal relationship between bone infarcts and osteosarcoma. There has recently been a flurry of experimental work and clinical data to support molecular genetic models by which OS may develop.[47–54] Osteosarcoma tumorigenesis in humans results if both alleles at the retinoblastoma susceptibility locus (Rb gene) are altered. Some workers conclude that Rb gene alteration is pertinent to the genesis of most human OS cases and some other bone and soft tissue tumors.[53] Additional genetic evidence suggests that another event in the development of OS is the homozygous alteration of another gene, p53.[51] Both the Rb gene and p53 have been proposed to act as tumor-suppressor genes. Therefore, OS tumorigenesis may be a loss of function of these two, and perhaps other, genes.

## Pathology and Natural Behavior

Osteosarcoma (or osteogenic sarcoma) is a malignant mesenchymal tumor of primitive bone cells.

These cells produce an extracellular matrix of osteoid, and the presence of tumor osteoid is the basis for the histological diagnosis differentiating OS from other sarcomas of bone. There are many histological subclassifications of OS based on the type and amount of matrix and characteristics of the cells: osteoblastic, chondroblastic, fibroblastic, poorly differentiated, and telangiectatic osteosarcoma (a vascular subtype). In dogs, it has not been demonstrated that there is a difference in the biological behavior of the different histological subclassifications. The histological pattern may vary between tumors or even within the same tumor. Small biopsy samples of an OS may lead to misdiagnoses such as chondrosarcoma, fibrosarcoma, or hemangiosarcoma. These histological diagnoses from small biopsies must be interpreted with caution. It is important to obtain histologic analysis of the entire tumor following definitive excision to confirm the diagnosis.

Osteosarcoma has very aggressive local effects and causes lysis, production of bone, or both processes. The local disease is usually attended by soft tissue swelling. Pathological fracture of the affected bone can occur. Metastasis is very common and arises early in the course of the disease, although usually subclinically. Although less than 5% of dogs have radiographically detectable pulmonary metastasis at presentation, approximately 90% will die with metastatic disease, usually to the lungs, within 1 year when amputation is the only treatment.[1,13] Metastasis via the hematogenous route is most common; however, on rare occasions extension to regional lymph nodes may occur. Although the lung is the most commonly reported site for metastasis, tumor spread to bones or other soft tissue sites occurs with some frequency. The biological behavior of OS of the mandible is probably an exception. Dogs with OS of the mandible treated with mandibulectomy alone had a 1-year survival rate of 71% in one study.[55] Survival of dogs with OS distal to the antebrachiocarpal or tarsocrural joints was somewhat longer (median of 466 days) than survival of dogs with OS of more common appendicular sites; however, OS in these sites is aggressive, with a high potential for metastasis.[29]

## History and Clinical Signs

Dogs with OS of appendicular sites generally present with a lameness and swelling at the primary site. Sometimes there is a history of mild trauma just prior to the onset of lameness. This history can often lead to misdiagnosis as a strain, sprain, or other orthopedic injury such as cranial cruciate rupture. The pain is likely due to microfractures or disruption of the periosteum induced by osteolysis of cortical bone with tumor extension from the medullary canal. The lameness worsens, and a moderately firm to soft, variably painful swelling arises at the primary site. Dogs may present with acute, severe lameness associated with pathologic fractures. Large and giant breed dogs that present with lameness or localized swelling at metaphyseal sites should be evaluated with OS as the most likely diagnosis.

The signs associated with axial skeletal OS are site dependent. Signs vary from localized swelling with or without lameness to dysphagia (oral sites), exophthalmos and pain on opening the mouth (caudal mandibular or orbital sites), facial deformity and nasal discharge (sinus and nasal cavity sites), and hyperesthesia with or without neurological signs (spinal sites). Dogs with tumors arising from ribs usually present because of a palpable, variably painful mass, and respiratory signs are not common even where the lesions have large intrathroacic components. Dyspnea as a sign of malignant pleural effusion is quite rare.

Dogs rarely have respiratory signs as the first clinical evidence of pulmonary metastasis; rather, their first signs are usually vague. With radiographically detectable pulmonary metastasis dogs may remain asymptomatic for many months, but most dogs develop decreased appetites and nonspecific signs such as malaise within 1 month. Hypertrophic osteopathy may develop in dogs with pulmonary metastasis.

## Diagnostic Techniques and Workup

Initial evaluation of the primary site involves interpretation of good-quality radiographs taken in lateral and craniocaudal projections. Special views may be necessary for lesions occurring in sites other than in the appendicular skeleton. The overall radiographic abnormality of bone varies from mostly bone lysis to almost entirely osteoblastic or osteogenic changes. There is also an entire spectrum of changes between these two extremes, and the appearance of OS can be quite variable. There are some features, however, that are commonly seen. Cortical lysis is a common feature of OS and may be severe enough to leave obvious areas of discontinuity of the cortex leading to pathological fracture. There is often soft tissue extension with an obvious soft tissue swelling, and new bone (tumor bone) may form in these areas in a palisading pattern perpendicu-

lar or radiating from the axis of the cortex ("sunburst"). As tumor invades the cortex the periosteum is elevated, and new bone is laid down by the cambium layer, providing a triangular-appearing deposition of dense new bone on the cortex at the periphery of the lesion. This periosteal new bone has been called *Codman's triangle* but this is not pathognomonic for osteosarcoma. Osteosarcoma does not directly cross articular cartilage, and primary lesions usually remain monostotic. The tumors may extend into periarticular soft tissues, however, and adjacent bones are at risk because of extension through adjacent soft tissue structures. Other radiographic changes that can attend OS are loss of the fine trabecular pattern in the metaphysis, a vague transition zone at the periphery of the medullary extent of the lesion (rather than a sharp sclerotic margin), or areas of fine punctate lysis (Figure 20–1). Any one or combinations of these changes may be seen depending on the size, histological subtype, location, and duration of the lesion.

Based on signalment, history, physical exam findings, and radiographic findings a presumptive diagnosis of OS can be made. Differential diagnoses of lytic, proliferative, or mixed pattern aggressive bone lesions identified on radiographs include other primary bone tumors (chondrosarcoma, fibrosarcoma, hemangiosarcoma); metastatic bone cancer; multiple myeloma or lymphoma of bone; systemic mycosis with bony localization; and bacterial osteomyelitis.

Other primary bone tumors are far less common but may be suspected, especially in dogs with unusual signalment or tumor location. Metastatic cancer can spread to bone from almost any malignancy. A careful physical exam is important, including a rectal exam with special attention paid to the genitourinary system to help rule out the presence of a primary cancer. Dogs with a history of cancer should have their original biopsy reviewed and should be restaged for the original disease. Common sites for metastatic bone cancer are lumbar and sacral vertebrae, pelvis, and diaphyses of long bones. There are usually other clues for the diagnosis of multiple myeloma such as hyperproteinemia (Chapter 28E), and both multiple myeloma and lymphoma of bone are usually attended by radiographic lesions that are almost entirely lytic. The classic radiographic appearance of myeloma bone lesions is described as "punched-out" areas of lysis.

Systemic mycoses with tendency for bone localization are caused by either Coccidioides chronic or disseminated form, and the lung lesions do not usually resemble metastatic cancer nodules. The radiographic appearance of the osteomyelitis caused by these fungal organisms is predominantly of productive and blastic changes in the distal diaphyses, metaphyses, epiphyses, or, rarely, the axial skeleton (Figure 20–2). Serology may be helpful but is rarely definitive, and diagnosis depends on identification of the organisms from histological evaluation of biopsy tissue. An unusual fungal infection that may localize in bone is disseminated aspergillosis caused by *Aspergillus terreus* (Figure 20–3). This infection is thought to arise because of immunosuppression, but predisposing causes have not been identified in infected dogs. Most affected dogs are young to middle-aged German shepherds.[58–60]

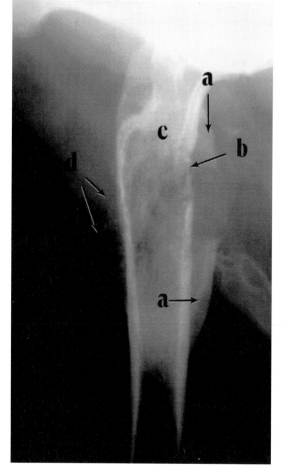

**Figure 20–1.** Lateral radiograph of the proximal end of the femur of a dog with stage IIB osteosarcoma: *a*, Codman's triangle, *b*, cortical lysis, *c*, loss of fine trabecular pattern in the metaphysis, *d*, "sunburst" tumor bone in the soft tissues.

immitis or Blastomyces dermatitidis.[56,57] These are soil-borne organisms found in certain locations in North America (the Southwest for coccidioidomycosis and the Mississippi, Missouri, and Ohio river valleys and Mid-Atlantic states for blastomycosis), Mexico, and Central and South America. Dogs are infected through the respiratory tract or, rarely, from contamination of open wounds. Dogs from endemic areas are at risk, and a travel history to such areas is cause for increased suspicion. There may be radiographic evidence of pulmonary disease, although this is more common in the acute phase of the infection. Hilar lymphadenopathy may persist in the

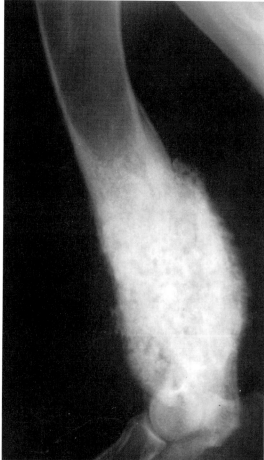

**Figure 20–2.** Radiograph of a humerus of a dog with fungal osteomyelitis due to systemic blastomycosis.

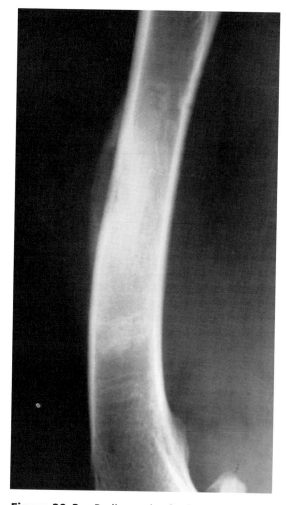

**Figure 20–3.** Radiograph of a femur of a German shepherd dog with osteomyelitis due to *Aspergillus terreus.*

Fever or changes in the leukogram consistent with infection do not always accompany this diagnosis, especially in chronic cases.

A diagnosis of primary malignant bone tumor may be suggested by signalment, history, and physical examination and radiographic findings. However, a definitive diagnosis lies in correct procurement and interpretation of tissue for histopathology. With new treatments such as limbsparing, knowledge of the specific tumor type may avoid overextensive or inappropriate treatment of bone tumors thought to be osteosarcoma (e.g., chondrosarcoma or lymphoma). It is crucial to the success of a limbsparing surgery that the biopsy procedure is planned and performed carefully with close attention to asepsis, hemostasis, and wound closure. The skin incision for the biopsy must be small and placed so that it can be completely excised with the tumor at limbsparing without compromising the procedure. Transverse incisions must be avoided. It has been recommended that the surgeon who is to perform the definitive surgical procedure (especially if this is limbsparing) should be the person to perform the preoperative bone biopsy.[61]

Bone biopsy may be performed as an open incisional or as a closed needle or trephine biopsy. The advantage of the open techniques is that a large sample of tissue is procured, which presumably improves the likelihood of establishing an accurate histologic diagnosis. Unfortunately, this advantage is outweighed by the disadvantages of (1) an involved operative procedure and (2) risk of postsurgical complications such as hematoma formation, wound breakdown, infection, local seeding of tumor, and pathological fracture.[62,63] Although closed biopsy with a Michelle trephine yields a diagnostic accuracy rate of 93.8%, there is greater risk of creating pathologic fracture than with a smaller-gauge needle.[64] This underscores some of the advantages of a closed biopsy using a Jamshidi bone marrow biopsy needle (Figure 20–4) or similar type of needle.* Jamshidi needle biopsy has an accuracy rate of 91.9% for detecting tumor versus other disorders and an 82.3% accuracy rate for diagnosis of specific tumor subtype.[65]

The biopsy site is selected carefully. Radiographs (two views) are reviewed and the center of the lesion chosen for biopsy. The skin incision is made so the biopsy tract and any potentially

One dog was reported to be infected with *Aspergillus fumigatum.*[60] These dogs may have lameness, spinal pain, weight loss, inflammatory ocular disease, diskospondylitis, pyrexia, weakness, or any combination. Fungal hyphae may be identified in the urine sediment, and the organism may be cultured from the urine.

The pathogenesis of bacterial osteomyelitis in adult dogs requires pathogenic bacteria to gain access directly to the bone and is usually not a sequel to bacteremia or septicemia. Common history is of recent surgery or other penetrating injury that carries bacteria directly to the bone. These lesions usually drain purulent material, and sequestra are often seen on radiographs.

---

*Jamshidi bone marrow needle, American Pharmaseal Company, Valencia, California. Bone marrow biopsy needle, Sherwood Medical Company, St. Louis, Missouri

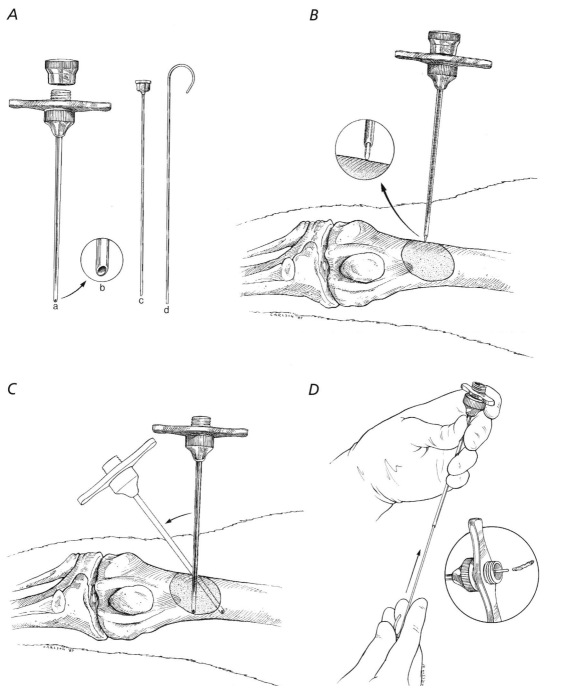

**Figure 20–4.** *A,* The Jamshidi needle: cannula and screw on cap (a), tapered point (inset b), pointed stylet to advance cannula through soft tissue (c), and probe to expel specimen from cannula (d). *B,* With the stylet locked in place, the cannula is advanced through soft tissue until bone is reached. Inset: close-up of portion of bone with stylet up to cortex. *C,* The stylet removed and the bone cortex penetrated with the cannula. The cannula is withdrawn and the procedure is repeated with redirection of the needle. *D,* The probe is then inserted into the tip of the cannula and the specimen expelled through the cannula base (inset). Reprinted with permission, J Am Vet Med Assoc *193*:(2), 205–210, 1988.[65]

seeded tumor cells can be completely removed at the time of definitive surgery. Care is used to avoid major nerves, vessels, and joint spaces. A 4-inch 8- or 11-gauge needle is used. With the dog anesthetized and prepared and draped for surgery, a small stab incision (2 to 3 mm) is made in the skin with a #11 scalpel blade. The bone needle cannula, with the stylet locked in place, is pushed through the soft tissue to the bone cortex (Figure 20–4). The stylet is removed and the cannula is advanced through the bone cortex into the medullary cavity using a gentle twisting motion and firm pressure. The opposite cortex is not penetrated. The needle is removed and the specimen is gently pushed out of the base of the cannula by inserting the probe into the cannula tip. One or two more samples can be obtained by redirecting the needle through the same skin incision so that samples of the transition zone may also be obtained. Ideal specimens should be 1 or 2 cm in length and not fragmented. Biopsy is repeated until solid tissue cores are obtained. Material for culture and cytology may be taken from the samples prior to fixation in 10% neutral buffered formalin. Diagnostic accuracy is clearly improved when samples are evaluated by a pathologist thoroughly familiar with bone cancer. After tumor removal (amputation or limbsparing) histology should be performed on a larger specimen to confirm the preoperative diagnosis.

Examination for evidence of apparent spread of the disease is important. Regional lymph nodes should be palpated and fine needle cytology performed on any enlarged node. Sites of bone metastasis may be detected by a careful orthopedic examination with palpation of long bones and the accessible axial skeleton. Organomegaly may be detected by abdominal palpation. Usually pulmonary metastases are undetectable by clinical exam, but careful thoracic auscultation is important to detect intercurrent cardiopulmonary disorders. High detail thoracic radiographs should be taken during inspiration with the patient awake and should include three views: a ventrodorsal view or a dorsoventral view and both right and left lateral views. Osteosarcoma pulmonary metastases are generally soft tissue dense and cannot be detected radiographically until the nodules are 6 to 8 mm in diameter. It is relatively rare to detect pulmonary metastatic disease at the time of diagnosis (less than 10% of dogs). Computerized tomography (CT) of the lungs may increase the number of dogs detected with lung lesions at presentation. Bone survey radiography has been useful in detecting dogs with second skeletal sites of osteosarcoma.[30] Bone surveys include lateral radiographs of all bones in the body and a ventrodorsal projection of the pelvis using standard radiographic technique appropriate for the region radiographed. One hundred and seventy-one dogs with primary bone tumors underwent radiographic bone surveys and thoracic radiography in one study.[66] The findings were that, at presentation, there was a higher yield in finding other sites of OS with radiographic bone survey (6.4%, 11 of 171 dogs) than with thoracic radiographs (4%, 7 of 171 dogs). There are conflicting reports on the usefulness of nuclear scintigraphy (bone scan) for clinical staging of dogs with osteosarcomas. Bone scintigraphy was used in one study to identify suspected second bone sites of OS in 14 of 25 dogs with appendicular primaries.[67] Seven of these lesions were biopsied and confirmed to be osteosarcoma. Another study of 70 dogs with appendicular primary bone tumors resulted in only one scintigraphically detectable occult bone lesion.[68] In a third report, of 23 dogs with suspected skeletal neoplasia that were evaluated with scintigraphy and radiography, 4 dogs had second skeletal sites suspected to be neoplastic.[69] The suspicious site in one of these dogs was found on histologic evaluation to be normal bone. A nuclear bone scan can be a useful tool for the detection and localization of bone metastasis in dogs presenting for vague lameness or signs such as back pain (Figure 20–5). Nuclear bone scans are very sensitive but not specific for identifying sites of skeletal tumor location. Any region of osteoblastic activity will be identified by this technique, including osteoarthritis and infection. Computerized tomography may be useful to plan surgery, especially for tumors located in the axial skeleton. Magnetic resonance imaging can also be used to stage local disease. This is a valuable tool to determine the extent of the soft tissue component of the tumor, especially within the medullary canal and in the soft tissue outside the cortex.

A surgical staging system for sarcomas of the skeleton has been devised for people.[70] This system is based on the histologic grade (G), the anatomic setting of the primary tumor (T), and regional or distant metastasis (M). There are three stages: stage I, the low-grade ($G_1$) lesions without metastasis; stage II, the high-grade ($G_2$) lesions without metastasis; and stage III, the lesion with regional or distant metastasis regardless of histologic grade. The stages are subdivided by the anatomic setting, A being intracompart-

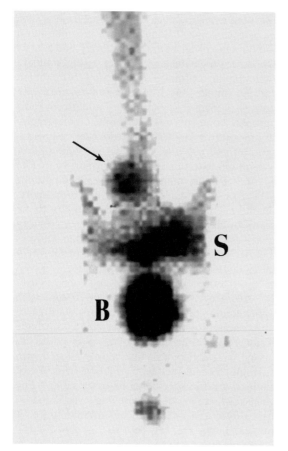

**Figure 20–5.** Scintigram using technetium M[99] from a 10-year-old Shetland sheep dog with back pain. No radiographic abnormalities were detectable. The sacrum is indicated by the letter "S" and the bladder by the letter "B". A "hot spot" is clearly identified in the body of L7 (arrow) and the sacrum. This was confirmed histologically as a metastatic lesion from a prostatic carcinoma. The treatment for the primary lesion had been external beam radiation therapy completed one year previously.

mental ($T_1$) and B extracompartmental ($T_2$). According to this system, most dogs with OS present with stage IIB disease.

The patient's overall health status requires careful assessment. Advancing years do not preclude treatment; however, prolonged anesthesia and chemotherapy may not be tolerated in dogs with organ compromise. Particular attention to the cardiovascular system is important. Coexisting cardiomyopathy or any degree of heart failure may lead to serious complications, particularly during fluid diuresis at surgery or during admin-

istration of cisplatin chemotherapy. An electrocardiogram and echocardiogram should be performed on dogs where the history or physical findings implicate a cardiac disorder. Renal function may be evaluated prior to administration of cisplatin.* A minimum database should include a complete blood count, platelet count, serum biochemical analysis, and urinalysis. For safe administration of cisplatin, dogs should have > 3,000 polymorphonuclear leukocytes per $\mu$l, > 150,000 platelets per $\mu$l, a normal BUN and creatinine, and urine specific gravity of 1,030, with no proteinuria or casts in the urine sediment.[71]

## Therapy and Prognosis

Occult metastatic disease is present in approximately 90% of dogs at presentation, and the median survival is only 3 to 4 months if amputation is the only treatment; therefore some form of systemic therapy is necessary if survival is to be improved. With no treatment at all, dogs experience pain because of extensive destruction of bone and surrounding tissue by their primary tumors, and most owners elect euthanasia for their pets soon after diagnosis if no treatment is given. In a multi-institutional study of 162 dogs with appendicular OS treated with amputation alone, dogs younger than 5 years of age had worse survival than older dogs.[13] There is no clear-cut evidence that any other easily measured variable, other than mandibular site, has prognostic significance. Some studies, however, have weakly related large tumor size[11] and humerus location[72] to poor outcome. Large tumor size has been reported to be a negative prognostic factor for people with osteosarcoma.[73–75] Dogs presented with stage III disease (measurable metastasis) have a very poor prognosis.

**Adjuvant Treatment**   Early work to identify treatments for micrometastatic disease with various adjuvant therapies was generally unsuccessful.[76–78] In a later study, the median survival was 222 days for dogs treated with amputation and intravenously administered liposome-encapsulated muramyl tripeptide-phosphatidylethanolamine (liposome/MTP-PE).[79] The agent MTP-PE is a lipophilic derivative of muramyl dipeptide, which is a synthetic analog of a fragment of Mycobacterium cell wall. There is evidence that liposome/MTP-PE can activate

*Platinol, Bristol-Meyers Company, Syracuse, New York

**Table 20–1**  Survival Data for Dogs with OS Treated with Amputation or Limbsparing with Varying Total Cumulative Doses of Cisplatin

| Number of Dogs Studied | Number of Doses of Cisplatin at 70/mg/m$^2$ | Median Disease-Free Interval (Days) | Median Survival (Days) | % 1-Year Survival |
|---|---|---|---|---|
| 117 | 2 | 229 | 280 | 41.3 |
| 40 | 4 | 244 | 414 | 51.8 |
| 12 | 6 | 392 | 392 | 55.6 |

macrophages to destroy malignant cells. Although this study showed that liposome/MTP-PE significantly delayed the time to metastasis and prolonged survival when compared to dogs that received empty liposomes, more than 50% of the dogs were dead by 8 months after surgery. In a follow-up study, dogs randomized to liposome/MTP-PE following 4 doses of cisplatin (70 mg/m$^2$q 4 weeks) had a median survival time of 432 days (14.5 months) versus 291 days (9.7 months) for the dogs receiving 4 doses of cisplatin.[79] The National Cancer Institute is coordinating a national U.S. trial with the Children's Cooperative Oncology Group (CCOG) and the Pediatric Oncology Group (POG) using liposome/MTP-PE in combination with chemotherapy in children following surgery.

Cisplatin used either alone or in combination with doxorubicin* on an alternating basis has been demonstrated to improve survival in dogs with OS after amputation.[80,81] In a report of 36 dogs with appendicular OS treated with cisplatin and amputation,[14] 17 dogs (group 1) were treated with two doses of IV cisplatin 21 days apart, beginning on average 18 days after amputation, and 19 dogs (group 2) were treated at diagnosis with IV cisplatin and received a second dose 21 days later immediately after amputation. The median survival for group 1 was 262 days, with 1- and 2-year survival rates of 38% and 18%. The median survival for group 2 was 282 days, with 1- and 2-year survival rates of 43% and 16%. The survival of dogs receiving two doses of cisplatin was significantly longer than 35 amputation-alone historic control dogs (median survival 119 days, 1- and 2-year survival rates of 11% and 4%). There was no significant difference between the survival of group 1 and group 2. There is a large body of evidence, however, reported in clinical studies of human OS[82–85] and laboratory studies with rodents[86,87] that supports

perioperative use of chemotherapy. It seems reasonable to recommend the earliest possible administration of chemotherapy, which is usually at the time of amputation. At Colorado State University (CSU), between 3 and 6 doses of cisplatin 21 days apart at 70 mg/m$^2$ body surface area has been safely administered to 191 dogs with OS after amputation or limbsparing. Some of these dogs also received cisplatin as implanted OPLA-Pt, which is a biodegradable polylactic acid polymer containing cisplatin (unpublished data). The median survival was 392 days, with a 1-year survival rate of 52% and a 2-year survival rate of 31%. An increasing cumulative dose of cisplatin appears to increase the probability for survival (see Table 20–1).[88,89]

The recommended dose for cisplatin is 70 mg/m$^2$ body surface area. In one study a single dose of 90 mg/m$^2$ was given to 12 dogs, and there was no apparent nephrotoxicity over the short term.[90] However, myelosuppression and renal toxicity become serious and life-threatening complications as the dose of cisplatin is increased. Saline diuresis helps prevent nephrotoxicity, which is the dose-limiting toxicity in dogs. The protocol recommended is that described by Ogilvie et al.[91] (see Chapter 9).

Carboplatin* is a second-generation platinum compound that is less nephrotoxic than cisplatin with apparently similar antitumor effects.[92–96] In a multi-institutional study of 48 dogs with appendicular OS treated with amputation and up to 4 doses of carboplatin, the median disease-free interval was 257 days, the median survival was 321 days, and 35.4% of dogs were alive at one year (see Table 20–2).[72] One of the advantages of carboplatin is that it can be given intravenously without the saline diuresis necessary for cisplatin administration. The drug can be given at amputation and every 21 days, provided there are no

*Adriamycin, Adria Laboratories, Columbus Ohio

**Paraplatin, Bristol-Meyers, Squibb Laboratories, Evansville, Indiana

**Table 20–2**   Commonly Used Adjuvant Chemotherapy Agents and the Survival Outcome for Dogs with Osteosarcoma Where Amputation Has Been Performed

| Drug | Dose Regime and Number of Dogs | Disease Free | Survival | Comments |
|---|---|---|---|---|
| Cisplatin[14] | 70 mg/m² IV on 2 occasions, every 21 days n = 26 | Median 177–226 days | 38–43% at 1 year, 16–18% at 2 years Median 262–282 days | No significant difference between survival data for dogs given cisplatin before amputation and those treated after amputation |
| Cisplatin[109] Some dogs treated with limbsparing | 60 mg/m² IV on 1 to 6 occasions, every 21 days n = 22 | Not reported | 45.5% at 1 year, 20.9% at 2 years Median 325 days Median 300 days | Apparent increase in treatment failures due to bone metastases |
| Cisplatin[81] | 40–50 mg/m² IV on 2 to 6 occasions, every 28 days n = 11 | | | |
| Cisplatin[184] | 50 mg/m² IV on 2 occasions, 2 and 7 weeks after amputation n = 15 | Not reported | 30% at 1 year Median 290 days | |
| Cisplatin[185] | 50 mg/m² IV on up to 9 occasions, every 28 days n = 16 | Not reported | 62% at 1 year Median 413 days | Trend for dogs receiving higher cumulative doses of cisplatin to have long survival times |
| Carboplatin[72] | 300 mg/m² on 4 occasions every 21 days n = 48 | Median 257 days | 35.4% at 1 year Median 321 days | Maximum tolerated cumulative dose has not been described for dogs. |
| Doxorubicin and cisplatin[80] | Doxorubicin at 30 mg/m² IV day 1 and cisplatin at 60 mg/m² IV on day 21. Cycle repeated once in 21 days n = 19 | Median 210 days | 37% at 1 year Median 300 days | No significant difference was found between survival data from this study and survival data from a single-agent cisplatin study.[14] |
| Doxorubicin[97] | 30 mg/m² on 5 occasions every 2 weeks | Not reported | 50.5% at 1 year, 9.7% at 2 years | Percentage of necrosis of tumor predicted survival |
| OPLA-Pt[105] | 80 mg/m² implanted at the time of amputation n = 37 | Median 256 days | 41.2% at 1 year Median 278 days | New trials ongoing with an injectable polymer containing cisplatin |

signs of severe bone marrow suppression. The dose recommended for use in dogs is 300 mg/m² administered every 3 weeks for 4 treatments; however, the maximum tolerated cumulative dose has not been described.

A poor response to adjuvant doxorubicin as a single agent was determined by one report of 16 dogs with osteosarcoma.[78] In that study, doxorubicin was given intravenously at a dosage of 30 mg/m² every 3 weeks, beginning 3 weeks after surgery. In a more recent study, doxorubicin was given at the same dosage but every 2 weeks for 5 treatments to 35 dogs with appendicular OS, and surgical excision was performed either 13 days after the second or third treatment, with the subsequent treatment given on the day after surgery.[97] The 1- and 2-year survival rates were 50.5% and 9.7% respectively. Why the 2-year survival rate is so poor is unclear.

There have been several reports of adjuvant chemotherapy protocols for dogs with osteosarcoma. The results of some of these studies appear in Table 20–2. It would seem reasonable that combinations of cisplatin, carboplatin, and doxorubicin, drugs shown to be efficacious alone, could further improve survival times.

A measure of the effectiveness of chemotherapy may be the percentage of tumor necrosis measured in the resected tumor specimen if the chemotherapy was given prior to surgery (neoadjuvant chemotherapy). Evaluation of the response of the primary tumor by determining the necrosis percentage is considered a valuable determinant of the effectiveness of preoperative treatment in people.[84,98–102] If the percentage of tumor necrosis is low, the response is considered inadequate, and the postoperative chemotherapy regimen is often modified.[84] Percentage of tumor necrosis was evaluated in resected specimens from dogs with OS treated with various preoperative regimes.[103] Mean percentage tumor necrosis was: untreated tumors (n = 94) 27%, radiation therapy alone (n = 23) 82%, 2 doses of intra-arterial (IA) cisplatin at 70 mg/m$^2$ dose (n = 14) 45%, 2 doses of IV cisplatin at 70 mg/m$^2$ dose (n = 6) 24%, 2 doses of IA cisplatin at 70 mg/m$^2$ dose and radiation therapy (n = 45) 82%, and 10 doses of IV cisplatin at 10 mg/m$^2$ dose and radiation therapy (n = 8) 78%. There was no significant difference between percentage of tumor necrosis in untreated osteosarcoma compared to those receiving IV cisplatin alone, but a significant increase in percentage of tumor necrosis was present in all other groups. Percentage of tumor necrosis was strongly correlated with local tumor control after limbsparing, as 91% of dogs with > 90% tumor necrosis had local control, whereas 78% of dogs with 80% to 89% tumor necrosis had local tumor control, and only 30% of dogs with > 79% tumor necrosis had local control. Since those dogs with radiation as part of their preoperative treatments had a higher mean percentage of tumor necrosis, radiation in combination with chemotherapy may still play a role in the local preoperative management of osteosarcoma. Percentage of tumor necrosis in resected primary tumors from dogs with OS treated with intravenous doxorubicin ranged from 0% to 87% (mean, 24.9%) in one report.[97] Interestingly, there was a significant direct correlation between survival time and percentage of necrosis in that study.

A drug delivery system has been developed that can release a very high dose of chemotherapy into a surgical wound and cause slow release of relatively low concentrations of chemotherapy systemically. The system is a biodegradable polymer called open cell polylactic acid containing cisplatin (OPLA-Pt). When OPLA-Pt was implanted in normal dogs no systemic toxicity and no impedance of cortical allograft healing was identified at doses of up to 80.6 mg/m$^2$.[104] Serum pharmacology data revealed approximately a 30-fold increase in area under the curve (AUC) for systemic platinum exposure compared to a similar dose of intravenous cisplatin. Local wound concentrations of platinum are up to 50 times that achievable from a single intravenous dose. This drug delivery system may potentially be important in controlling microscopic local cancer after limbsparing because very high doses of cisplatin can be delivered to the tumor bed after incomplete surgical removal. Also, control of the microscopic distant disease may be achieved because cisplatin escapes from the implanted device to the circulation for an extended period of time. Thirty-nine dogs with stage IIB appendicular OS were treated with amputation and 1 dose of OPLA-Pt implanted in the muscles of the amputation stump at the time of surgery.[105] The median survival was 256 days and the 1-year survival rate was 41.2% (see Table 20–2). This is at least equivalent to the improvement in survival probability when two intravenous doses of cisplatin are used with amputation. We are now investigating the effect of repeated doses of slow-release chemotherapy for control of micrometastatic cancer in the canine OS amputation model.

**Surgery**    Amputation of the affected limb is the standard treatment for canine appendicular osteosarcoma. Even large and giant breed dogs can function well after limb amputation, and most owners are pleased with their pets' mobility and quality of life after surgery.[106,107] *Severe* preexisting orthopedic or neurologic conditions may cause poor results in some cases, and careful preoperative examination is important. With no treatment dogs experience increasing pain from the primary tumor site. Surgery alone must be considered palliative for osteosarcoma. After surgery alone euthanasia is usually requested by owners when their dogs become symptomatic for metastatic disease.

Although most dogs function well with amputation, there are some dogs where limbsparing would be preferred over amputation, such as dogs with severe pre-existing orthopedic or neurologic disease, very large dogs, or dogs with owners who absolutely will not permit amputation. Until recently, only a few reports of limbsparing in dogs, with limited follow-up, have appeared in the literature.[108–112] More than 200 limbsparing procedures have been performed at CSU through September 1994. Limb function has been good to excellent in most dogs, and survival has not been adversely affected by removing the primary tumor with marginal resection as compared to radical margins, as with amputation.

Suitable candidates for limbsparing are dogs with osteosarcoma clinically and radiographically confined to the leg, where the primary tumor affects < 50% of the bone determined radiographically and dogs that are in otherwise good general health. Most dogs treated at CSU with limbsparing received either some form of preoperative treatment (IA cisplatin, IV cisplatin, radiotherapy to the tumor bone, or a combination of radiotherapy with IV or IA cisplatin) or OPLA-Pt implantation at surgery. Most dogs had cisplatin given intravenously after surgery. Results from 21 dogs treated with radiation therapy alone given in large doses per fraction prior to limbsparing were unsatisfactory for preservation of life and limb.[111] Many of the dogs treated with preoperative IA cisplatin on two occasions 21 days apart, with the last treatment 21 days prior to surgery, showed marked decrease in the degree of vascularization of the tumor. This usually represented a high degree of induced tumor necrosis in the resected specimen, especially when combined with radiation therapy, and facilitated limbsparing.[89,112]

The most suitable cases for limbsparing are dogs with tumors in the distal radius or ulna. Dogs with tumors in proximal humeral sites may also be potential limbsparing candidates. Dogs with tumors located in the distal tibia are not as suitable because the infection rate is high in these dogs due to minimal soft tissue coverage. Tumors located in the proximal tibia or distal femur present special problems, since it is usually impossi-

ble to save the knee joint. Dogs with limbsparing and stifle arthrodeses generally have poor function. Preservation of knee function using osteochondral allografts has been attempted in three dogs. In one dog with a small chondrosarcoma of the medial femoral condyle, a hemicondylectomy was performed, with reconstruction with an osteochondral allograft. This dog had excellent function for 8.5 months, at which time euthanasia was performed because of symptomatic pulmonary metastases. In one dog, a distal femoral OS was removed and the distal femur was replaced with an osteochondral allograft. This dog had only fair function and died due to metastatic disease 5 months after diagnosis. The lateral half of the proximal tibia with half of the tibial plateau was removed from a dog with chondrosarcoma. The tibia was reconstructed with an osteochondral allograft and OPLA-Pt was implanted. This dog is alive, free of measurable cancer, and has excellent function 3 years after surgery (Figure 20–6).

Limbsparing is a complicated process that requires a supply of allografts (bone bank) and, more important, a coordinated team effort among surgical and medical oncologists, radiologists, pathologists, and technical staff. A description of the surgery follows. Second-generation cephalosporin antibiotics are administered IV immediately preoperatively, intraoperatively, and for 24 hours postoperatively. Meticulous aseptic technique is used.

For a distal radial site, the dog is placed in lateral recumbency, with the affected limb uppermost. A skin incision is made on the dorsolateral aspect of the antebrachium from a point just distal to the elbow to just proximal to the metacarpophalangeal joint. Any biopsy tracts are excised en bloc. Soft tissue is dissected to the level of the tumor pseudocapsule. Care is taken not to enter the tumor. The bone is cut with an oscillating bone saw 3 to 5 cm proximal to the proximal radiographic margin of the tumor. The extensor carpi radialis muscle is transected, and the distal part of this muscle and its tendon are removed with the tumor. The common digital extensor

**Figure 20–6.** *(Facing page) A,* Radiograph of the stifle of a 5-year-old golden retriever with chondrosarcoma of the lateral aspect of the proximal end of the tibia. *B,* CT scan showing lesion confined to the lateral side of the tibial plateau. *C,* Radiograph after en bloc removal of the tumor and reconstruction with fresh frozen osteochondral allograft. There were tumor cells to the surgical margins, however, and OPLA-Pt was placed adjacent to the allograft at the time of surgery. *D,* Radiograph 3 years after surgery. The dog has excellent range of motion of the stifle joint, has excellent function, and remains disease free.

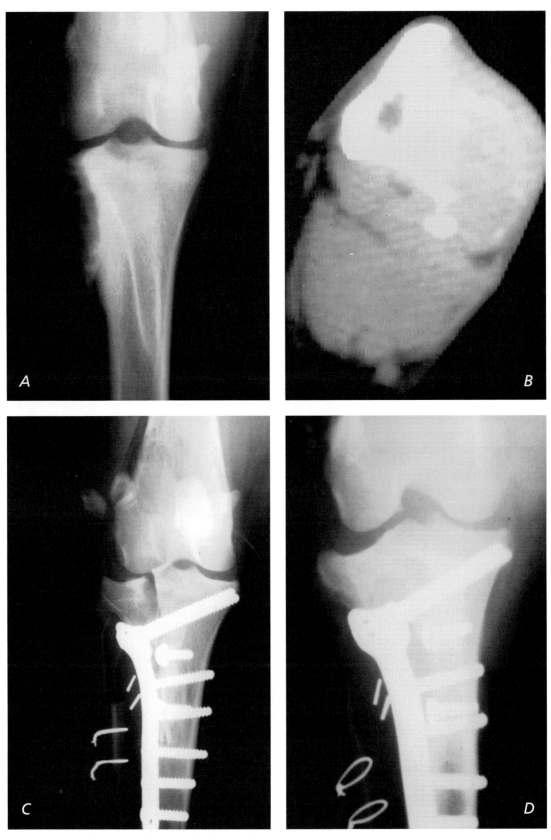

**Figure 20–6.** *(See opposite page for legend.)*

tendon usually is closely involved with the tumor pseudocapsule, and it is usually transected proximal and distal to the tumor and removed with the mass. The distal margin is usually at the level of the radiocarpal joint. The joint capsule is incised, keeping close to the proximal row of carpal bones. The ulna is sectioned sagitally with an osteotome, and the medial ulnar cortex adjacent to the tumor is removed en bloc with the radius. For tumors that have extension to the ulna, the ulna is also cut with a bone saw and the distal one third or more is removed with the radius. Care is taken to preserve as much vasculature as possible, especially on the palmar surface. Large vessels associated with the tumor are ligated and divided. Surgical hemostatis staples* are very useful. The specimen is radiographed and then submitted for histological evaluation, including assessment of completeness of surgical margins and percentage of tumor necrosis.

A fresh-frozen cortical allograft[113] is thawed in 1 liter of an antibiotic in saline solution,** the articular cartilage is removed, the graft is cut to fit, and the medullary cavity reamed to remove fat and cellular debris. The articular cartilage of the proximal carpal bones is removed, and the allograft is stabilized in compression using Association for the Study of Internal Fixation (ASIF/AO) principles. A dynamic compression plate with a minimum of three screws proximal and four screws distal to the graft is used; 3.5 mm broad plates of up to 22 holes size are appropriate in most cases, but for very large dogs 4.5 mm narrow or broad plates are selected. The plate is fastened in the patient to the allograft with two or three screws, removed from the surgery site, and the medullary canal of the allograft is filled with polymethyl methacrylate† bone cement containing amikacin (1 g amikacin to 40 g of polymer powder). This provides support for the screws during revascularization of the graft and acts as a reservoir for antibiotics. The healing of the allograft is not significantly impeded by the presence of the cement.[114] The plate extends proximally in the host radius for at least three screws and distally to a level just proximal to the metacarpophalangeal joint.

*Surgiclip, United States Surgical Corporation, New York, New York
**Neomycin 1 g, polymyxin B 500,000 U, potassium penicillin 5,000,000 U
†Palacos radiopaque bone cement, Smith and Nephew Richards Inc, Memphis, Tennessee

The wound is thoroughly lavaged with saline, and at this point OPLA-Pt may be implanted. A closed suction drain is inserted adjacent to the allograft and the wound is closed. The leg is supported in a padded bandage. The drain is removed the day after surgery in most cases. It is most important to prevent self-mutilation (licking) after surgery, and Elizabethan collars should be used as necessary. No external coaptation is used, and most dogs use the limb fairly well by 10 days after surgery. Postoperative swelling can be considerable but usually resolves by 2 weeks. Although decreased exercise is recommended for the first 3 to 4 weeks to allow soft tissues to heal, no exercise restriction need apply after this time. In fact, it is important to encourage limb use, even in early postoperative times so that flexure contracture of the digits does not occur.

The principles of resection are the same for other sites; however, because of abundant soft tissue in the area, wider margins are often attained with proximal humerus resections. Proximal humerus resections are, however, more difficult, and limb use immediately following surgery is usually poor but improves to good but rarely excellent over about 1 to 2 months. The allograft selected for reconstruction of proximal humeral defects can be a distal femur from the opposite side. The femoral allograft is placed so that the medial condyle sits in the glenoid and the femoral diaphysis contacts the distal humerus with the caudal part of the allograph facing cranially. That is, the femur is placed upside-down and back to front. The plate then extends from the dorsocranial side of almost the entire length of the scapular spine to cover the dorsal aspect of the humerus with the allograft in compression, and scapulohumeral arthrodesis is performed. Vigorous physiotherapy is important after surgery in these dogs.

There is no significant difference in survival rates for dogs treated with amputation and cisplatin compared to dogs treated with limbsparing and cisplatin. Overall, limb function has been satisfactory, with approximately 80% of dogs experiencing good to excellent limb function.

Limbsparing requires a dedicated owner and clinical team. Complications can arise in any or all phases of treatment (chemotherapy, radiation, or surgery). Serious complications as a result of chemotherapy (e.g., sepsis and renal failure) are extremely rare. High-dose radiation therapy may complicate wound and allograft healing and potentiate allograft infection.[111] Moderate-dose radiation in combination with chemotherapy may, however, be useful for control of local disease, as indicated by percentage of tumor necrosis data.[103,112] The major complications related mainly to surgery are recurrent local disease and allograft infection. In the first 200 dogs that have had limbsparing surgeries performed at CSU, the 1-year local recurrence-free rate determined by Kaplan-Meier life tables was 76.3%. Local disease control was improved with certain treatments such as pretreatment with moderate doses of radiation and intra-arterial cisplatin. When OPLA-Pt was implanted at the time of tumor removal, the 1-year local recurrence-free rate was 89.9%. Some dogs had their locally recurrent disease resected en bloc and remained disease free for an extended period. Eighty-eight dogs (40%) developed allograft infections. The majority had their infections adequately controlled with systemic antibiotics with or without local antibiotics (antibiotic-impregnated polymethyl methacrylate beads).[115] Many of these dogs continued to have evidence of infection; however, their function was not severely affected. In severe and uncontrolled infections, allografts had to be removed, and a small number of dogs required amputation. An unexpected finding was that dogs with allograft infections were twice as likely to survive compared to dogs with limbsparings without infected allografts. The reason for this result is unclear, but it could be related to activation of immune effector cells and a response to cytokines, such as interleukins or tumor necrosis factor, elaborated in the face of chronic bacterial infection.

Bone tumors originating in proximal sites of the scapula can be successfully removed by partial scapulectomy.[116] Dogs function well with partial scapulectomy; however, gait abnormalities may occur after scapulectomy by disarticulation at the scapulohumeral joint.[116] Mandibulectomy and maxillectomy are appropriate surgeries for bone tumor primaries of oral sites.[117–120] Tumors of periorbital sites can be removed in orbitectomy.[121] Rib tumors can be removed by thoracic wall resection and the defect reconstructed with polypropylene mesh* with plastic plates** for large defects, or by diaphragmatic advancement for caudally located defects.[122] Small primary tumors of the ulna can be removed by partial ulnectomy, and reconstruction with allografts or

bone substitutes may not be necessary. Certain primary bone tumors of the pelvis can be removed by techniques of hemipelvectomy[123] and, although these surgeries are difficult, function and cosmetic outcome have been excellent (Figure 20–7).

**Radiation**   The combination of external beam radiation therapy and limbsparing has been described.[111,112] It appears that radiation therapy can cause considerable necrosis of primary OS in dogs. Palliative radiation for metastatic bone disease is discussed in the next section; palliative radiation for primary OS has also been described.[124] This may be a treatment option for dogs with stage III disease at presentation (that is, distant metastasis to lung, for example) or where the owner does not want to pursue attempts at permanent local control. Another area in which radiation likely plays a role in treating OS in dogs is for OS of vertebrae. At CSU, 14 dogs with spinal OS and 6 dogs with spinal fibrosarcoma were treated from 1986 to 1994. Fourteen of these dogs had surgery to decompress the spinal cord, and 9 dogs were treated with OPLA-Pt implanted in a distant intramuscular site. Twelve were given intravenous cisplatin. Fourteen dogs were treated with fractionated external beam radiation therapy. All dogs had surgery, radiation therapy, or both, whereas no dog was treated with chemotherapy alone. Eight dogs improved neurologically after treatment and 7 remained the same. All 3 dogs presenting with nonambulatory paraparesis regained ambulatory status after treatment. The median survival after treatment was relatively short, however, at approximaely 4.5 months.[125]

## Metastatic Disease

The usual cause of death in humans and dogs following amputation as the sole treatment for osteosarcoma is diffuse pulmonary metastasis. Resection of pulmonary metastasis from osteosarcoma or other solid tumors has been reported in people.[126] There is a report of 36 dogs treated with pulmonary metastasectomy for osteosarcoma.[127] Lesions located subpleurally were gently lifted from the lung parenchyma by thumb forceps and a single pursestring of 2-0 or 3-0 polygalactan 910 suture† was tied around the base of normal tissue. Larger lesions located

---

*Marlex mesh, CR Bard Inc., Billerica, Maryland
**Lubra plates, Fort Collins, Colorado

†Vicryl, Ethicon, Sommerville, New Jersey

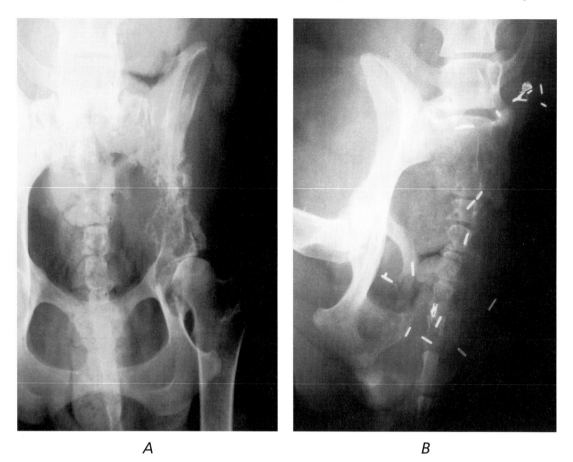

A                                          B

**Figure 20–7.** *A,* Radiograph of the pelvis of an 8-year-old chow-chow with osteosarcoma of the ilium. *B,* radiograph of the pelvis 3 years after hemipelvectomy and cisplatin chemotherapy. This dog continues to be disease free and has excellent function.

deeper in the lung parenchyma were removed by complete or partial lobectomy using surgical staples.* No chemotherapy was given after these surgeries. Although the initial treatments varied among dogs, the median survival time of the entire group was 487 days. The median survival after pulmonary metastasectomy was 176 days (range 20–1,495 days). The criteria established for case selection for pulmonary metastasectomy in order to maximize the probability of long survival periods are: (1) primary tumor in complete remission, preferably for a long relapse-free interval (> 300 days); (2) one or two nodules visible on plain thoracic radiographs; (3) cancer

found only in the lung (negative bone scan); and perhaps (4) long doubling time (> 30 days) with no new visible lesions within this time.

In another study, 45 dogs with measurable metastatic OS were treated with various chemotherapy regimes (cisplatin, doxorubicin, mitoxantrone**).[128] Only one dog had a partial remission, which lasted 21 days. All other dogs experienced progressive disease, and the median survival time from the time metastatic disease was diagnosed was 61 days (range, 14–192 days). Cisplatin, doxorubicin, and mitoxantrone chemotherapy appears to be ineffective for the treatment of *measurable* metastatic OS in the dog.

*TA30 or TA55, United States Surgical Corporation, New York, New York

**Novantrone, Lederle Laboratories, Pearl River, New York

A change over recent years in the pattern of metastatic disease in human osteosarcoma has been described.[129–132] This change is primarily an increase in bone metastases. Possible explanations for this change include a change in the behavior of this cancer independent of treatment; selective killing of metastatic cancer by chemotherapy in certain sites, such as lung, which allows metastasis in other sites to become clinically relevant; lung resection and chemotherapy have improved survival, and bone sites become clinically relevant; more sensitive detection methods, which allow previously undetectable metastases to be seen; and more complete and detailed necropsies compared to those performed previously, which identify asymptomatic metastatic sites. Since the advent of adjuvant chemotherapy with increasing survival times there has been an increase in the number of treated dogs presenting with signs referable to bone metastases. In one report of 35 dogs treated with doxorubicin, 32 dogs were euthanized because of distant metastasis. Approximately one third were euthanized because of bone metastases.[97]

Nuclear scintigraphy is a useful way of identifying sites of bone metastasis. For dogs with solitary bone metastases and no evidence of cancer elsewhere, metastasectomy may be indicated, although the subsequent disease-free interval is generally short. An alternative is to treat metastatic bone lesions with palliative radiation. A protocol of three 10 Gy fractions of high-energy photons delivered over a 3-week period on days 0, 7, and 21, for a total dose of 30 Gy, has been described for palliative treatment of OS in dogs.[124] A useful and safe protocol used at CSU is a coarse fractionation scheme delivered as high-energy photons at 4.5 Gy per fraction for 5 consecutive daily fractions to a total dose of 22.5 Gy. Dogs can remain pain free for over 6 months. Unfortunately, the metastatic lesions usually become symptomatic in about 2 to 3 months after radiation. A second course, using the same fractions, has been successful as further temporary pain relief in a few dogs. For short-term pain control, the nonsteroidal anti-inflammatory drug piroxicam* may be given at 0.1 to 0.4 mg/kg daily for 3 to 5 days, then every 48 hours. This appears to give temporary pain relief to most dogs with OS lesions. Dogs must be carefully monitored for signs of gastrointestinal toxicity and the drug withdrawn if these signs occur. Cor-

ticosteroids must not be administered at the same time because this combination can predispose to the development of gastric or duodenal ulceration. It is also not advisable to give corticosteroids or piroxicam concurrently with cisplatin or in dogs with decreased renal function. There has been some work that suggests piroxicam may have some antitumor effects.[133] Radiopharmaceuticals (such as strontium-90), bisphosphonates, diphosphonates, and other compounds have been used to palliate pain from metastatic bone cancer in people.[134–137] Samarium-153-ethylenediamine-tetramethylene-phosphonic acid ($^{153}$Sm-EDTMP) is a radiopharmaceutical that has been used to treat metastatic and primary bone tumors in dogs.[138] In both normal beagle dogs and in tumor-bearing dogs, $^{153}$Sm-EDTMP caused transient bone marrow depression (for approximately 4 weeks) of all cell lines.[138,139]

## Comparative Aspects

Animal models for the study of human diseases are important to our understanding of the mechanism and etiology of disease and for the development and refinement of therapeutic strategies. Spontaneously developing diseases in animal populations are particularly useful for study.[140] Canine osteosarcoma has many similarities to human osteosarcoma and can serve well as a valuable comparative model for study (see Table 20–3).[7,141] Osteosarcoma is more common in dogs than in humans; therefore, case accrual can be rapid in dogs.[142,143] Since disease progression is more rapid in dogs than in humans, results of treatment protocols can be reported earlier than would those of similar trials in humans. Research costs are less for clinical trials in dogs compared to those in human clinical trials and, from an animal welfare standpoint, no disease is induced and dogs with cancer can be helped through the course of the research.

Osteosarcoma is an uncommon cancer of humans affecting mainly children in their second decade of life and it remains a very serious, aggressive solid tumor. Fortunately, there has been a great improvement in survival rates with the use of established multidrug adjuvant protocols. Some centers boast 5-year survival rates of 80%–90%, which contrasts to the 20% expected 5-year survival rates of 15 years ago. Limbsparing programs are becoming more common, and many survivors of OS retain functional, pain-free limbs.

*Feldene, Pfizer, New York, New York

**Table 20–3**

| Variable | Dog | Human |
| --- | --- | --- |
| Incidence in U.S. | >8,000/year | 1,000/year |
| Mean age | 7 years | 14 years |
| Race/breed | Large or giant purebreds | None |
| Body weight | 90% > 20 kg | Heavy |
| Site | 77% long bones | 90% long bones |
| | Metaphyseal | Metaphyseal |
| | Distal radius > proximal humerus | Distal femur > proximal tibia |
| | Distal femur > tibia | Proximal humerus |
| Etiology | Generally unknown | Generally unknown |
| Percentage clinically confined to the limb at presentation | 80–90% | 80–90% |
| Percentage histologically high grade | 95% | 85–90% |
| DNA index | 75% aneuploid | 75% aneuploid |
| Metastatic rate without chemotherapy | 90% before 1 year | 80% before 2 years |
| Metastatic sites | Lung > bone > soft tissue | Lung > bone > soft tissue |
| Improved survival with chemotherapy | Yes | Yes |

Modified with permission from Withrow SJ, Powers BE, Straw RC, Wilkins RM: Comparative aspects of osteosarcoma: Dog versus man. Clin Orthop Rel Res. *270*:159–167, 1991.[7]

## BONE SURFACE OSTEOSARCOMA

Osteosarcoma usually originates from elements within the medullary canal of bones (intra-osseous-OS); however, some forms of this cancer originate from the outside surface of bones. Periosteal OS is a high-grade form of surface OS and seems to arise from the periosteal surface but has invasive characteristics seen radiographically. There is cortical lysis with extension of the tumor into the bone and surrounding soft tissues. These tumors are histologically similar to intraosseous OS and have similar aggressive biological behavior. Parosteal OS, or juxtacortical OS, arises from the periosteal surface of bones but appears less aggressive than periosteal OS both radiographically and in terms of biological behavior. Parosteal osteosarcomas are relatively uncommon and have a moderately well circumscribed radiographic appearance. The tumors grow out from the periosteal side of a cortex, and cortical lysis is usually very mild if apparent at all on radiographs. Histologically, these tumors look more benign compared to intraosseous or periosteal-osteosarcoma. These tumors contain well-differentiated cartilage, fibrous tissue, and bone with sparse regions of sarcoma cells adjacent to tumor osteoid. Histologic specimens must be evaluated carefully because it is often easy to miss the areas of tumor cells and misdiagnose the lesion as osteoma, chondroma, or reactive bone. These tumors generally do not invade the medullary canal and tend to grow out from the bone on broad pedicles. Diagnosis is based on typical histologic and radiographic findings.

Parosteal OS is usually slow growing but can induce pain at the local site. Metastases can occur, but the prognosis for survival is much better than for intra-osseous osteosarcoma.[144,145] Control of parosteal OS can be achieved by en bloc resection of the tumor with the adjacent cortical bone. This has been reported for tumors of the zygomatic arch.[145] If the full thickness cortex needs to be removed for tumors on long bones, reconstruction may be performed using autogenous corticocancellous bone such as a rib, ileal crest, or allogeneic cortical bone. The margins of resection must be carefully evaluated for signs of tumor infiltration. Extension of malignant cells up to the cut edge signifies the need for either further surgery (removal of more cortical bone with the entire previous surgical field or limb amputation) or perhaps adjuvant radiation or chemotherapy.

## MULTILOBULAR OSTEOCHONDROSARCOMA

Multilobular osteochondrosarcoma (MLO) is an uncommon tumor that generally arises from the skull of dogs. Many names have been used to describe this disease, including chondroma rodens and multilobular osteoma. These tumors have a characteristic radiographic appearance: Generally the borders of the tumor are sharply demarcated with limited lysis of adjacent bone, and there is a coarse granular mineral density throughout (Figure 20–8). Histologically, these tumors are composed of multiple lobules, each centered on a core of cartilaginous or bony matrix that is surrounded by a thin layer of spindle cells. A histologic grading system has been described.[146] These tumors have the potential to recur locally following incomplete resection, and metastasis can occur. In one report[146] the average

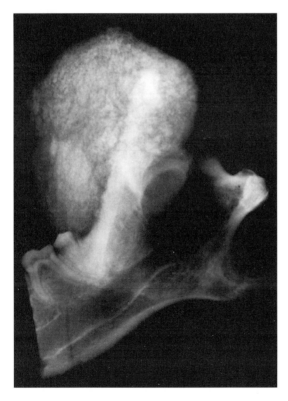

**Figure 20–8.** Radiograph of a specimen removed by caudal mandibulectomy. The margins are well defined, and the granular mineral density is a characteristic of multilobular osteochondrosarcoma.

age of affected dogs was 7.5 years, and there was no breed or sex predilection. A little over half the dogs developed metastases after treatment with a median time to metastasis of 14 months. The median survival time was 21 months. Local tumor recurrence and metastasis after treatment appear to be partially predicted by histologic grade. When metastatic lesions are identified by thoracic radiography, dogs may remain asymptomatic for their lung disease for up to one year or more. Local tumor excision with histologically complete surgical margins appears to offer good opportunity for long-term tumor control. The role of chemotherapy and radiation therapy in the management of MLO is not well defined.

## OTHER PRIMARY BONE TUMORS OF DOGS

It can be difficult to distinguish chondroblastic osteosarcoma from chondrosarcoma and fibroblastic osteosarcoma from fibrosarcoma and telangiectatic osteosarcoma from hemangiosarcoma when only small amounts of biopsy tissue are evaluated.[65] This makes interpretation of older reports difficult in terms of trying to establish the true incidence of the different types of primary bone tumors. This also underscores the importance of evaluating the entire excised specimen to validate the preoperative biopsy. All too often a bone malignancy thought to be relatively low grade from preoperative biopsy is upgraded to a true OS once the histology of the surgical specimen is reviewed. This changes both the prognosis and the postsurgical treatment plan. Primary bone tumors other than OS make up somewhere between 5% and 10% of bone malignancies in dogs. These tumors are chondrosarcomas, hemangiosarcomas, and fibrosarcomas.

### Chondrosarcoma

Chondrosarcoma (CS) is the second most common primary tumor of bone in humans and dogs and accounts for approximately 5% to 10% of all canine primary bone tumors.[2,3,5,147] Chondrosarcomas are characterized histologically by anaplastic cartilage cells that elaborate a cartilaginous matrix. There is a spectrum of degree of differentiation and maturation of the cells within and between each tumor. Histologic grading systems have been devised.[148,149] The etiology is generally unknown, although CS can arise in dogs with multiple cartilaginous exostosis.[150,151] In a recent clinicopathological study of 97 dogs with CS, the mean age was 8.7 years (range, 1–15 years) and golden retrievers were at a higher risk of developing CS than any other breed.[152] There was no sex predilection, and 61% of the tumors occurred on flat bones. Chondrosarcoma can originate in the nasal cavity, ribs, long bones, pelvis, extraskeletal sites (such as the mammary gland, heart valves, aorta, larynx, trachea, lung, and omentum), vertebrae, facial bones, digits and *os* penis.[31,148,149,152–159] The nasal cavity is the most common site for canine chondrosarcoma.[148,149,152]

Chondrosarcoma is generally considered to be slow to metastasize. Tumor location rather than histologic grade was prognostic in one study;[149] however, histologic grade was found to be important for predicting survival for tumors of the same anatomic site of origin.[148] The reported median survival of dogs with nasal CS ranges from 210 days to 510 days with various treatments (radiation therapy, rhinotomy and radiation therapy, and rhinotomy alone).[148,152] Clinical signs were present for a long time, up to one year, before treatment in one study.[148] Metastatic disease is not a feature of nasal CS in dogs.[148,149] The reported median survival for dogs with CS of ribs varies widely.[27,147–149,160,161] Reports prior to 1992 contained few cases that were treated with intent to cure, but 15 dogs with rib CS treated with en bloc resection in a recent study had a median survival of 1,080 days.[122] The median survival for dogs with CS of long bones was 201 days in one report of 7 dogs treated with amputation with or without adjuvant chemotherapy[148] and 540 days in another study of 5 dogs treated with amputation alone.[152] Death was usually associated with metastatic disease. A reliable adjuvant chemotherapeutic agent is not known for canine chondrosarcoma.

## Hemangiosarcoma

Primary hemangiosarcoma (HS) of bone is rare and probably accounts for less than 5% of all bone tumors. This disease generally affects middle-aged to older dogs and can occur in dogs of any size. This is a highly metastatic tumor, and virtually all dogs affected will develop measurable metastatic disease within six months of diagnosis. Metastases can be widely spread throughout various organs such as lungs, liver, spleen, heart, skeletal muscles, kidney, brain, and other bones. Dogs can present with multiple lesions, making it difficult to determine the site of pri-

mary disease. Histologically, HS is composed of highly anaplastic mesenchymal cells, which are precursors to vascular endothelium. The cells are arranged in chords separated by a collagenous background and may appear to be forming vascular channels or sinuses. Cellular pleomorphism and numerous mitotic figures are features of this highly malignant disease. There is profound bone lysis, and the malignant cells aggressively invade adjacent normal structures. The lesion, however, may be confused with telangiectatic osteosarcoma, especially if the diagnosis is based on small tissue samples. Often the dominant radiographic feature is lysis; however, HS does not have an unequivocally unique radiographic appearance, and diagnosis is based on histopathology.

If HS is diagnosed, the dog must be thoroughly staged with thoracic and abdominal films, bone survey radiography or bone scintigraphy, and ultrasonographic evaluation, particularly of the heart and abdominal organs. Right atrial HS may be present without clinical or radiographic signs of pericardial effusion. The prognosis is very poor, and even dogs with HS clinically confined to one bony site have less than a 10% probability of surviving one year if the tumor can be completely excised. Cyclophosphamide,* vincristine,** and doxorubicin have been used in combination as an adjuvant protocol, and the reported median survival of dogs with nonskeletal HS is 172 days.[162] Doxorubicin as a single agent adjuvant seems to be as effective as the combination of drugs, with some long-term survivors, although the overall survival prognosis is still poor[163] (see Chapter 29A).

## Fibrosarcoma

Primary fibrosarcoma (FS) is also a rare tumor of dogs and probably accounts for less than 5% of all primary bone tumors of dogs.[3] Unfortunately, the difficulty in distinguishing FS from fibroblastic OS histologically (especially from small tissue samples) renders study of this tumor difficult. In a recent study, 11 dogs thought to have FS were studied. On re-evaluation of complete resection specimens the histologic diagnosis was changed to OS in 6 dogs.[164] Histologic characteristics of FS have been described as interwoven bundles of fibroblasts within a collagen matrix permeating cancellous and cortical bone but not associated with osteoid produced by the tumor cells. Host

*Cytoxan
**Oncovin

bone–derived new bone can be seen, however, especially at the periphery of the tumor.[164]

Complete surgical resection of the primary lesion is recommended for dogs with FS clinically confined to the primary site. This treatment may be curative, although metastatic potential may be considerable. There is no good evidence that adjuvant chemotherapy is of any benefit in preventing metastatic disease. It has been postulated that primary FS of bone has a propensity to metastasize to such sites as heart, pericardium, skin, and other bones rather than lung.[164]

## METASTATIC TUMORS OF BONE

Almost any malignant tumor with the capacity to metastasize can spread to bone via the hematogenous route. The lumbar vertebrae and the pelvis are common sites for cancer spread, possibly because these are predilection sites for bone metastasis from the common urinogenital malignancies such as prostate, bladder, urethral, and mammary cancer.[165] Metastatic lesions in long bones frequently affect the diaphysis, probably because of the proximity to the nutrient foramen. Nuclear scintigraphy is a very sensitive technique to detect bone metastasis. A whole skeleton bone scan is recommended when metastatic bone cancer is suspected because it is common for there to be multiple sites of bone metastasis even if the patient is symptomatic for tumor in only one bone.

## BENIGN TUMORS OF BONE

### Osteomas

Osteomas are benign tumors of bone. Radiographically, these are well circumscribed, dense bony projections that are usually not painful to palpation. Histologically, they are composed of tissue almost indistinguishable from reactive bone. The diagnosis is made after considering physical exam and radiographic and histologic findings. The most important differential diagnosis is MLO when the lesion occurs on the skull. Treatment for osteoma is simple surgical excision, which is usually curative.

### Multiple Cartilaginous Exostoses

Multiple cartilaginous exostoses (MCE) is considered a developmental condition of growing dogs.[17] There is evidence that the etiology of this condition may have a heritable component.[166,167] The actual incidence of MCE is difficult to determine since affected dogs may show no signs, and the diagnosis is often incidental. Lesions occur by the process of endochondral ossification when new bone is formed from a cartilage cap analogous to a physis. Lesions are located on bones that form from endochondral ossification, and lesions stop growing at skeletal maturity. Malignant transformation of MCE lesions has been reported,[151] but generally they remain as unchanged, mature, bony projections from the surface of the bone from which they arose.

Dogs typically are presented because of a moderately painful palpable mass on the surface of a bone or bones. The pain and lameness are thought to be due to mechanical interference of the mass with the overlying soft tissue structures. Radiographically, there is a bony mass on the surface of the affected bone, which has quite a benign appearance, with fine trabecular pattern in the body of the mass. To obtain a histologic diagnosis, biopsy material must be collected so sections can include the cartilaginous cap and the underlying stalk of bone. Histologically, this cartilaginous cap gives rise to an orderly array of maturing bone according to the sequence of endochondral ossification. The cortical bone surfaces of the mass and the adjacent bone are confluent.[150] A strong presumptive diagnosis is made by evaluation of the physical findings, history, and radiographic findings.

Treatment involves conservative surgical excision but this is necessary only if signs do not abate after the dog is skeletally mature. Because of the likelihood of a heritable etiology, affected dogs should not be bred. Owners should also be advised of the possibility of late malignant transformation. Dogs with a previous history of MCE should be carefully evaluated for bone malignancy if signs return later in life.

### Bone Cysts

Cysts are rare, benign lesions of bone. Affected animals are often young and present because of mild or moderate lameness; however, pathologic fracture can occur through cystic areas of long bones, leading to severe lameness. There appears to be a familial tendency in Doberman pinschers and Old English sheepdogs. The majority of the veterinary literature pertaining to bone cysts centers on several small series of cases or single case reports.[168-172] The nomenclature in various reviews of canine bone cysts is confusing. By definition, a cyst is a fluid-filled sac lined by epithelium. The only true cyst of primary intraosseous origin is a simple bone cyst (SBC, or unicameral bone cyst). These lesions are usually in metaphyseal regions of long bones, and they can adjoin an open growth plate. Sometimes, however, unicameral bone cysts can be diaphyseal or epiphyseal. Neither the etiology nor the pathogenesis is known, but it is speculated that the lesions may be the result of trauma to the growth plate, interfering with proper endochondral ossification. Others have theorized that with the rapid resorption and deposition of bone occurring in the metaphysis of a young animal, a cyst might develop if resorption is so rapid that a focus of loose fibrous tissue forms. The focus of fibrous tissue may then obstruct the thin-walled sinusoids, causing interstitial fluid to build up and form a cyst. The theory that appears to be at least partially substantiated is the synovial "rest" thesis.[173] It is suggested that during fetal development a "rest" of synovial or presynovial tissue becomes misplaced or incorporated into the adjacent osseous tissue. If this tissue remains or becomes functional, then by the effect of synovial secretion a cyst would develop in the bone. Cysts have been described to occur in bone just below articular cartilage (subchondral bone cysts or juxtacortical bone cysts).[171,172] In these it has often been possible to demonstrate direct communication with the articular synovial membrane. Malignant transformation of SBC is not known to occur in small animals, although there has been one documented case in a human patient.[174] Radiographically, SBC are single or, more commonly, multilocular, sharply defined, centrally located, radiolucent defects in the medullary canal of long bones (Figure 20–9). Variable degrees of thinning of the cortex with symmetrical bone "expansion" is often a feature of the radiographs. The diagnosis cannot, however, be reliably made from interpretation of radiographs. Lytic OS can be misdiagnosed as SBC. Diagnosis of an SBC relies on the histologic finding of a thin fibrous wall lined by flat to slightly plump layers of mesothelial or endothelial cells. Treatment consists of meticulous curettage and packing the space with autogenous bone graft.

Aneurysmal bone "cysts" (ABC) are spongy, multiloculated masses filled with free-flowing blood. The walls of an ABC are rarely lined by epithelium, and the lesion is probably an arteriovenous malformation. A proposed pathogenesis

of ABCs is that a primary event such as trauma or a benign bone tumor occurs within the bone or periosteum. This event disrupts the vasculature, resulting in a rapidly enlarging lesion with

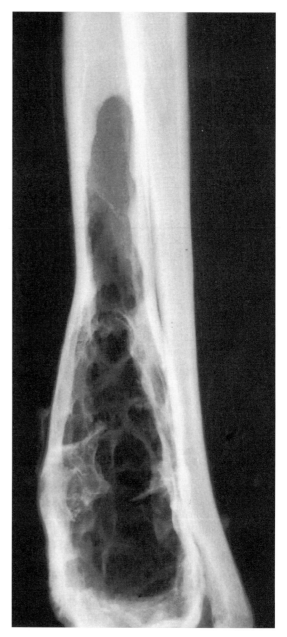

**Figure 20–9.** Radiograph of the distal antebrachium from a dog with a simple bone cyst. Note the multilocular, sharply defined, centrally located, radiolucent defect in the distal metaphysis of the radius.

anomalous blood flow that damages the bone mesenchyme. The bone reacts by proliferating. As the vascular anomaly becomes stabilized, the reactive bone becomes more consolidated and matures.[173] It is important to differentiate these lesions from OS or other malignant lesions of bone. The age of affected dogs ranges from 2 to 14 years.[175] Treatment can be achieved by en bloc resection and reconstruction, but extensive curettage with packing of the defect with autogenous bone graft can be effective. Cryosurgery has also been recommended.

## PRIMARY BONE TUMORS OF CATS

### Incidence and Risk

Cancer involving bones of cats is rare. An estimate of the incidence of all bone tumors in cats is 4.9 per 100,000.[176] Anywhere between 67% to 90% of bone tumors in cats are histologically malignant, and tumors occur in long bones approximately twice as often as in axial skeleton sites. The hind limbs are affected nearly twice as often as the front limbs. Osteosarcomas account for 70% to 80% of all primary malignant cancer of cats. The disease in cats differs from that in dogs in that the primary lesions occur more often in hind limbs in cats, and the disease is far less metastatic than in dogs. Osteosarcoma generally affects older cats (mean 10.2 years[177]), but the age range of reported cases is large (1–20 years). In one study, males outnumbered females, but the opposite was found in a second study.[177,178] Osteosarcoma was reported to arise after a limb fracture was repaired with an intramedullary pin in one cat.[35] A case of suspected radiation-induced osteosarcoma has been reported in a cat.[179]

Multiple cartilaginous exostosis (MCE) is a disease that occurs after skeletal maturity in cats. This is in contrast to the disease in dogs, where exostoses develop before closure of growth plates. Also in contrast to the disease in dogs, the lesions seldom affect long bones, are rarely symmetric, and are probably of viral rather than familial origin. There does not appear to be any breed or sex predisposition, although early reports of this condition were in the Siamese.[179–181] Affected cats range in age from 1.3 years to 8 years (mean 3.2 years).[178] Virtually all cats with multiple cartilaginous exostosis will test positive for the FeLV virus. This disease is included in the discussion of primary bone tumors because of its aggressive natural behavior.

### Pathology and Natural Behavior

Osteosarcoma of cats is composed of mesenchymal cells embedded in malignant osteoid. There may be a considerable amount of cartilage present, and osteoid may be scant. A feature of some feline OS cases is the presence of multinucleate giant cells, which may be numerous. Reactive host bone and remnants of host bone are often present in specimens. Tumors are seen to be invasive; however, some surrounding soft tissue may be compressed rather than infiltrated. There is often variation of the histologic appearance within the tumor, with some portions having more fibrosarcomatous appearance, others more cartilaginous, and so on. Some authors have described subtypes that resemble those seen in dogs: chondroblastic, fibroblastic, and telangiectatic, as well as the giant cell variant. These features, however, do not appear to confer any prognostic predictive balue. Osteosarcomas in cats can be of the juxtacortical type.

In cats with OS of a limb where there are no clinically detectable metastatic lesions, amputation alone may be curative. In one study of 15 cats, the median survival after amputation alone was 24 months.[177] The metastatic potential is much less than for the same disease in dogs or humans.

Osteochondroma may occur singly in cats, but there is a form that is multicentric (osteochondromatosis). The lesions are composed of hard, irregular exostoses having a fibrous and cartilaginous cap.[178] Endochondral ossification occurs from the cartilage cap, which extends to a variable thickness. This cap tends to blend with adjacent tissue, making its surgical removal difficult. Cats usually develop multiple sites of disease, and there is a potential for malignant transformation and metastasis. The presence of FeLV virus is also foreboding for these cats.

### History and Clinical Signs

The most common signs of OS are deformity and lameness depending on the location of the lesion. The lesions may appear radiographically similar to the OS in dogs; however, some cats have lesions arising from the periosteal surface (juxtacortical OS). It is very rare for cats to have metastatic osteosarcoma.

Cats with multiple cartilaginous exostosis

have rather rapidly progressing, conspicuous, hard swellings over affected sites, causing pain and loss of function. Common sites for lesion development are the scapula, vertebrae, and mandible; however, any bone can become affected. Radiographically, the lesions are either sessile or pedunculated protuberances from bone surfaces with indistinct borders with the normal bone. There may be a loss of smooth contour with evidence of lysis, particularly if there is malignant transformation.

## Diagnostic Workup

Both OS and MCE may be suspected by the radiographic appearance of the lesions and the FeLV status of the cat. Definitive diagnosis is made by histopathologic evaluation of properly collected biopsy tissue.

## Therapy and Prognosis

For OS of a limb, amputation is recommended. No adjuvant therapy is known to be efficacious, and without adjuvant treatment the median survival of cats with OS is 2 years.

Cats with MCE have a guarded prognosis. Lesions may be removed surgically for palliation; however, local recurrences are common, and new, painful, debilitating lesions may occur. No reliably effective treatment is known for this condition in cats.

## OTHER PRIMARY BONE TUMORS OF CATS

Fibrosarcoma is the second most common primary bone tumor of cats.[182] Chondrosarcoma is reported to be next in terms of frequency, and hemangiosarcomas rarely involve bones of cats. Little is known about the biologic behavior of these rare lesions; however, metastases have been seen in cats with chondrosarcoma and hemangiosarcoma.[177,179,183]

## REFERENCES

1. Brodey RS, Riser WH: Canine osteosarcoma: A clinicopathological study of 194 cases. Clin Orthop 62:54–64, 1969.
2. Ling GV, Morgan JP, Pool RR: Primary bone tumors in the dog: A combined clinical, radiologi-

cal, and histologic approach to early diagnosis. J Am Vet Med Assoc 165:55–67, 1974.
3. Lui SK, Dorfman HD, Hurvitz AI, Patnaik AI: Primary and secondary bone tumors in the dog. J AM Vet Med Assoc 18:313–326, 1977.
4. Brodey RS, Sauer RM, Medway W: Canine bone neoplasms. J AM Vet Med Assoc 143:471–495, 1963.
5. Brodey RS, McGrath JT, Reynolds H: A clinical and radiological study of canine bone neoplasms: Part I. J Am Vet Med Assoc 134:53–71, 1959.
6. Priester WA, ed: The occurrence of tumors in domestic animals. NCI Monograph No. 54. November 1980.
7. Withrow SJ, Powers BE, Straw RC, Wilkins RM: Comparative aspects of osteosarcoma: Dog vs. man. Clin Orthop 270:159–167, 1991.
8. Brodey RS, Abt DA: Results of surgical treatment in 65 dogs with osteosarcoma. J Am Vet Med Assoc 168:1032–1035, 1976.
9. Smith RL, Sutton RH: Osteosarcoma in dogs in the Brisbane area. Aust Vet Pract 18:97–100, 1988.
10. Tjalma RA: Canine bone sarcoma: Estimation of relative risk as a function of body size. J Natl Cancer Inst 36:1137–1150, 1966.
11. Misdorp W, Hart AA: Some prognostic and epidemiological factors in canine osteosarcoma. J Natl Cancer Inst 62:537–545, 1979.
12. Wolke RE, Nielsen SW: Site incidence of canine osteosarcoma. J Small Anim Pract 7:489–492, 1966.
13. Spodnick GJ, Berg RJ, Rand WM, Straw RC, et al: Prognosis for dogs with appendicular osteosarcoma treated by amputation alone: 162 cases (1978–1988). J Am Vet Med Assoc 200:995–999, 1992.
14. Straw RC, Withrow SJ, Richter SL, et al: Amputation and cisplatin for treatment of canine osteosarcoma. J Vet Int Med 5:205–210, 1991.
15. Misdorp W: Skeletal osteosarcoma. Am J of Path 98:285–288, 1980.
16. Knecht CD, Priester WA: Musculoskeletal tumors in dogs. J Am Vet Med Assoc 172:72–74, 1978.
17. LaRue SM, Withrow SJ: Tumors of the skeletal system. In Withrow SJ, MacEwen EG (eds): Clinical Veterinary Oncology. Philadelphia, JB Lippincott, 1989, pp. 234–252.
18. Goldschmidt MH, Thrall DE: Malignant bone tumors in the dog. In Newton CD, Nunamaker DM (eds): Textbook of Small Animal Orthopedics. Philadelphia, JB Lippincott, 1985, pp. 887–902.
19. Owen LN, Owen LN (eds): Bone tumors in man and animals. London: Butterworth and Co, 1969, pp. 29–52.
20. Alexander JW, Patton CS: Primary tumors of the skeletal system. Vet Clin North Am 13:181–195, 1983.
21. Jongeward SJ: Primary bone tumors. Vet Clin North Am 15:609–641, 1985.

22. Nielsen SW, Schroder JD, Smith DTL: The pathology of osteogenic sarcoma in dogs. J Am Vet Med Assoc 124:28–35, 1954.

23. Kistler KR: Canine osteosarcoma: 1462 cases reviewed to uncover patterns of height, weight, breed, sex, age and site involvement. Phi Zeta Awards, University of Pennsylvania, School of Veterinary Medicine, 1981.

24. Riser WH: Bone tumors in the dog. Vet Annual 16:147–150, 1976.

25. Phillips L, Hagar H, Parker R, Yanik D: Osteosarcoma with a pathological fracture in a six-month-old dog. Vet Radiol 27:18–19, 1986.

26. Heyman SJ, Diefenderfer DL, Goldschmidt MH, Newton CD: Canine axial skeletal osteosarcoma: A retrospective study of 116 cases (1986 to 1989). Vet Surg 21:304–310, 1992.

27. Feeney DA, Johnston GR, Grindem CB: Malignant neoplasia of canine ribs: Clinical, radiological, and pathological findings. J Am Vet Med Assoc 180:927–933, 1982.

28. Pool RR: Tumors of bone and cartilage. In Moulton JE (ed): Tumors of domestic animals. Berkeley, University of California Press, 1990, pp. 157–230.

29. Gamblin RM, Straw RC, Powers BE, Park RD, Bunge MM, Withrow SJ: Primary osteosarcoma distal to the antebrachiocarpal and tarsocrural joints in nine dogs (1980–1992). J Am Anim Hosp Assoc 31:86–91, 1995.

30. LaRue SM, Withrow SJ, Wrigley RH: Radiographic bone surveys in the evaluation of primary bone tumors in dogs. J Am Vet Med Assoc 188:514–516, 1986.

31. Patnaik AK: Canine extraskeletal osteosarcoma and chondrosarcoma: A clinicopathological study of 14 cases. Vet Pathol 27:46–55, 1990.

32. Bech-Nielsen S, Haskins ME, Reif JS, Brodey RS, Patterson DF, Spielman R: Frequency of osteosarcoma among first-degree relatives of St. Bernard dogs. J Natl Cancer Inst 60:349–353, 1978.

33. Owen LN: Transplantation of canine osteosarcoma. Eur J Cancer 5:615–620, 1969.

34. Rosin A, Rowland GN: Undifferentiated sarcoma in a dog following chronic irritation by a metallic foreign body and concurrent infection. J Am Anim Hosp Assoc 17:593–598, 1981.

35. Bennett D, Campbell JR, Brown P: Osteosarcoma associated with healed fractures. J Small Anim Pract 20:13–18, 1979.

36. Stevenson S, Holm RB, Pohler OEM, Fetter AW, Olmstead ML, Wind AP: Fracture-associated sarcoma in the dog. J Am Vet Med Assoc 180:1189, 1982.

37. Sinibaldi K, Rosen H, Liu S, DeAngelis M: Tumors associated with metallic implants in animals. Clin Orthop 118:257–266, 1976.

38. Knecht CD, Priester WA: Osteosarcoma in dogs: A study of previous trauma, fracture and fracture fixation. J Am Anim Hosp Assoc 14:82–84, 1978.

39. White RG, Raabe OG, Culbertson MR, Perks NJ, Samuels SJ, Rosenblatt LS: Bone sarcoma characteristics and distribution in beagles fed strontium-90. Radiat Res 136:178–189, 1993.

40. McChesney-Gillette S, Gillette EL, Powers BE, Withrow SJ: Radiation-induced osteosarcoma in dogs after external beam or intraoperative radiation therapy. Can Res 50:54–57, 1990.

41. Tillotson C, Rosenberg A, Gebhardt M, Rosenthal DI: Postradiation multicentric osteosarcoma. Cancer 62:67–71, 1988.

42. Robinson E, Neugut AI, Wylie P: Clinical aspects of postirradiation sarcomas. J Natl Cancer Inst 80:233–240, 1988.

43. McKenna RJ, Schwinn CP, Soong KY, Higinbotham NL: Sarcomata of the osteogenic series (osteosarcoma, fibrosarcoma, chondrosarcoma, parosteal osteogenic sarcoma, and sarcomata arising in abnormal bone): An analysis of 552 cases. J Bone and Jt Surg 48A:1–26, 1966.

44. Dahlin DC, Coventry MB: Osteogenic sarcoma: A study of 600 cases. J Bone and Jt Surg 49A:101–110, 1967.

45. Dubielzig TF, Biery DN, Brodey RS: Bone sarcomas associated with multifocal medullary bone infarction in dogs. J Am Vet Med Assoc 179:64–68, 1981.

46. Prior C, Watrous BJ, Penfold D: Radial diaphyseal osteosarcoma with associated bone infarction in a dog. J Am Anim Hosp Assoc 22:43–48, 1986.

47. Hansen WH: Molecular genetic considerations in osteosarcoma. Clin Orthop 270:237–246, 1991.

48. Meyer WH: Recent developments in genetic mechanisms, assessment, and treatment of osteosarcomas. Curr Opin Oncol 3:689–693, 1991.

49. Strauss PG, Mitreiter K, Zitzelsberger H, et al: Elevated p53 RNA expression correlates with incomplete osteogenic differentiation of radiation-induced murine osteosarcomas. Int J Cancer 50:252–258, 1992.

50. Toguchida T, Yamaguchi T, Dayton SH, et al: Prevalence and spectrum of germline mutations of the p53 gene among patients with sarcoma. N Engl J Med 326:1301–1308, 1992.

51. Chandar N, Billig B, McMaster J, Novak J: Inactivation of p53 gene in human and murine osteosarcoma cells. Br J Cancer 65:208–214, 1992.

52. Yamaguchi T, Toguchida J, Yamamuro T, et al: Allelotype analysis in osteosarcomas: Frequent allele loss on 3q, 13q, 17p, and 18q. Cancer Res 52:2419–2423, 1992.

53. Araki N, Uchida A, Kimura T, et al: Involvement of the retinoblastoma gene in primary osteosarcomas and other bone and soft tissue tumors. Clin Orthop 270:271–277, 1991.

54. McIntyre JF, Smith-Sorensen B, Friend SH, et al: Germline mutations of the p53 tumor suppressor gene in children with osteosarcoma. J Clin Oncol 12:925–930, 1994.

55. Straw RC, Powers BE, Klausner J, et al: Canine mandibular osteosarcoma: 51 cases, (1980–1992). J Am Anim Hosp Assoc (in press).

56. Legendre AM: Blastomycosis. *In* Greene CG (ed): Infectious diseases of the dog and cat. Philadelphia, W.B. Saunders Company, 1990, pp. 669–678.

57. Barsanti JA, Jeffrey KL: Coccidioidomycosis. *In* Greene CE (ed): Infectious diseases of the dog and cat. Philadelphia, W.B. Saunders Company, 1990, pp. 696–706.

58. Neer M: Disseminated aspergillosis. Comp Contin Educ Pract Vet 10:465–471, 1988.

59. Kabay MJ, Robinson WF, Huxtable CRR, McAleer R: The pathology of disseminated *Aspergillus terreus* infection in dogs. Vet Pathol 22:540N547, 1985.

60. Oxenford CJ, Middleton DJ: Osteomyelitis and arthritis associated with *Aspergillus fumigatus* in a dog. Aust Vet J 63:59–60, 1986.

61. Mankin HJ, Lange TA, Spanier SS: The hazards of biopsy in patients with malignant bone and soft-tissue tumors. J Bone and Jt Surg 64A:1121–1127, 1982.

62. DeSantos LA, Murray JA, Ayala AG: The value of percutaneous needle biopsy in the management of primary bone tumors. Cancer 43:735–744, 1979.

63. Simon MA: Current concepts review, biopsy of musculoskeletal tumors. J Bone and Jt Surg 64-A:1253–1257, 1982.

64. Wykes PM, Withrow SJ, Powers BE: Closed biopsy for diagnosis of long bone tumors: Accuracy and results. J Am Anim Hosp Assoc 21:489–494, 1985.

65. Powers BE, LaRue SM, Withrow SJ, Straw RC, Richter SL: Jamshidi needle biopsy for diagnosis of bone lesions in small animals. J Am Vet Med Assoc 193:205–210, 1988.

66. Straw RC, Cook NL, LaRue SM, Withrow SJ, Wrigley RH: Radiographic bone surveys. J Am Vet Med Assoc 195 (letters):1458, 1989.

67. Hurd C, Cantwell HD, Hahn KA: Nuclear scintigraphy as a diagnostic tool for canine osteogenic sarcoma. Proc Vet Cancer Soc 8th Ann Conf, Estes Park, CO, 1, 1988.

68. Berg J, Lamb CR, O'Callaghan MW: Bone scintigraphy in the initial evaluation of 70 dogs with primary bone tumors. J Am Vet Med Assoc 196:917–920, 1990.

69. Parchman MB, Flanders JA, Erb HN: Nuclear medical bone imaging and targeted radiography for evaluation of skeletal neoplasms in 23 dogs. Vet Surg 18:454–458, 1989.

70. Enneking WF: Staging of musculoskeletal neoplasms. *In* Enneking WF (ed.): Current concepts of diagnosis and treatment of bone and soft tissue tumors. New York: Springer-Verlag, 1984, pp. 1–21.

71. Ogilvie GK, Straw RC, Jameson VJ, Walters LM, et al: Prevalence of nephrotoxicosis associated with four hour saline solution diuresis protocol for the administration of cisplatin to dogs with malignant tumors: 64 cases (1989–1990). J Am Vet Med Assoc 1991.

72. Bergman PJ, MacEwen EG, Kurzman ID, et al: Amputation and carboplatin for treatment of dogs with osteosarcoma: 48 cases (1991–1993). J Vet Int Med (in press).

73. Brostrom LA, Strander H, Nilsonne U: Survival in osteosarcoma in relation to tumor size and location. Clin Orthop 167:250–254, 1982.

74. Spanier SS, Shuster JJ, Vander Griend RA: The effect of local extent of the tumor on prognosis with osteosarcoma. J Bone and Jt Surg 72A:643–653, 1990.

75. Taylor WF, Ivins JC, Unni KK, Beabout JW, Golenzer HJ, Black LE: Prognostic variables in osteosarcoma: A multi-institutional study. J Natl Cancer Inst 81:21–31, 1989.

76. Colter SM, Parker LM: High dose methotrexate and leucovoran rescue in dogs with osteogenic sarcoma. Am J Vet Res 39:1943–1945, 1978.

77. Hamilton HB, LaRue SM, Withrow SJ: Effect of RA233 on metastasis in dogs with osteosarcomas. Am J Vet Res 48:1380–1382, 1987.

78. Madewell BR, Leighton RC, Theilen GH: Amputation and doxorubicin for treatment of canine and feline osteogenic sarcoma. Eur J Cancer 4:287–293, 1978.

79. MacEwen EG, Kurzmann ID, Rosenthal RC: Therapy for osteosarcoma in dogs with intravenous injection of liposome-encapsulated muramyl tripeptide. J Natl Cancer Inst 81:935–938, 1989.

80. Mauldin GN, Matus RE, Withrow SJ: Canine osteosarcoma treatment by amputation versus amputation and adjuvant chemotherapy using doxorubicin and cisplatin. J Vet Int Med 2:177–180, 1988.

81. Shapiro W, Fossum TW, Kitchell BE: Use of cisplatin for the treatment of appendicular osteosarcoma in dogs. J Am Vet Med Assoc 4:507–511, 1988.

82. Kalifa C, Dubousset J, Contesso G: Osteosarcoma—An attempt to reproduce T-10 protocol in a single institution. Proc Am Soc Clin Oncol 4:236–248, 1985.

83. Rosen G: Neo-adjuvant chemotherapy for osteogenic sarcoma. A model for treatment of malignant neoplasms. Recent results. Cancer Res 103:148–157, 1986.

84. Rosen G, Capassas B, Huros AG: Preoperative chemotherapy for osteogenic sarcoma: Selection of postoperative adjuvant chemotherapy based on the response of the primary tumor to preoperative chemotherapy. Cancer 49:1221–1230, 1982.

85. Winkler K, Beron G, Kotz RS: Neoadjuvant chemotherapy for osteogenic sarcoma: Results of a cooperative German/Austrian study. J Clin Oncol 2:617–624, 1984.

86. Bell RS, Roth YF, Gebhardt MC: Timing of chemotherapy and surgery in a murine osteosarcoma model. Cancer Res 48:5533–5538, 1988.

87. Fisher B, Saffer E, Rudock C: Effect of local or systemic treatment prior to primary tumor

removal on the production and response to a serum growth-stimulating factor in mice. Cancer Res 49:2002–2004, 1989.

88. Dernell WS, Straw RC, Powers BE, Withrow SJ: The effect of increasing doses of cisplatin on disease free interval and survival outcome for dogs with appendicular osteosarcoma. J Am Vet Med Assoc (in press).

89. O'Brien MG, Withrow SJ, Straw RC: Recent advances in the treatment of canine appendicular osteosarcoma. Comp Contin Educ Pract Vet 15:613–616, 1993.

90. Fallin EA, Forrester SD: Comparison of two loading protocols for preventing nephrotoxicosis associated with high-dose cisplatin. Vet Cancer Soc News Let 18:1–5 (abstract), 1994.

91. Ogilvie GK, Krawiec DR, Gelberg HB: Evaluation of a short-term saline diuresis protocol for the administration of cisplatin. Am J Vet Res 49:1076–1078, 1988.

92. Curt AH, Grygiel JJ, Corden BJ, et al: A phase I pharmacokinetic study of diammine cyclobutanedicarboxylatoplatinum (NSC 241240). Cancer Res 43:4470–4473, 1983.

93. Calvert AH, Harland SJ, Newell DL, Siddak ZH, Harrap KR: Phase I studies with carboplatin at the Royal Marsden Hospital. Cancer Treat Rev 12 (suppl A): 51–57, 1985.

94. Koeller JM, Trump DL, Tutsch KD, Earhart RH, Davis TE, Tormey DC: Phase I clinical trial and pharmacokinetics of carboplatin (NSC 241240) by single monthly 30-minute infusion. Cancer 57:222–225, 1986.

95. Canetta R, Bragman K, Smaldone L, Rozencweig M: Carboplatin: Current status and future prospects. Cancer Treat Rev 15:17–32, 1988.

96. Canetta R, Franks C, Smaldone L, Bragman K, Rozencweig M: Clinical status of carboplatin. Oncology-Huntingt 1:61–69, 1987.

97. Berg J, Weinstein MJ, Springfield DS, Rand WM: Response of osteosarcoma in the dog to surgery and chemotherapy with doxorubicin. J Am Vet Med Assoc 206(10):1555–1560, 1995.

98. Ayala AG, Raymond AK, Jaffe N: The pathologist's role in the diagnosis and treatment of osteosarcoma in children. Hum Pathol 15:258–266, 1984.

99. Bacci G, Springfield D, Campanner R: Neoadjuvant chemotherapy for osteosarcoma of the extremity. Clin Orthop Rel Res 24:268–276, 1987.

100. Chuang VP, Wallace S, Benjamin RS: The therapy of osteosarcoma by intra-arterial cis-platinum and limb preservation. Cardiovasc Intervent Radiol 4:229–235, 1981.

101. Jaffe N, Knapp J, Chuang VP: Osteosarcoma: Intra-arterial treatment of the primary tumor with cis-diamine-dichloroplatinum-II (CDP): Angiographic, pathologic and pharmacologic studies. Cancer 51:402–407, 1983.

102. Winkler K, Beron G, Delling G: Neoadjuvant chemotherapy of osteosarcoma: Results of a randomized cooperative trial (COSS-82) with salvage chemotherapy based on histological tumor response. J Clin Oncol 6:329–337, 1988.

103. Powers BE, Withrow SJ, Thrall DE, Straw RC, et al: Percent tumor necrosis as a predictor of treatment response in canine osteosarcoma. Cancer 67:126–134, 1991.

104. Straw RC, Withrow SJ, Douple EB, et al: The effects of cis-diamminedichloroplatinum II released from D,L,-polylactic acid implanted adjacent to cortical allografts in dogs. J Orthop Res 12:871–877, 1994.

105. Withrow SJ, Straw RC, Brekke JH, et al: Slow release adjuvant cisplatin for the treatment of metastatic canine osteosarcoma. European J. Musculoskeletal Research, submitted.

106. Carberry CA, Harvey HJ: Owner satisfaction with limb amputation in dogs and cats. J Am Anim Hosp Assoc 23:227–232, 1987.

107. Withrow SJ, Hirsch VM: Owner's response to amputation of a pet's leg. Vet Med Small Anim Clin 10:332–334, 1979.

108. Vasseur P: Limb preservation in dogs with primary bone tumors. Vet Clin North Am 17:889–993, 1987.

109. Berg J, Weinstein MJ, Schelling SH, Rand WM: Treatment of dogs with osteosarcoma by administration of cisplatin after amputation or limb-sparing surgery: 22 cases (1987–1990). J Am Vet Med Assoc 200:2005–2008, 1992.

110. LaRue SM, Withrow SJ, Powers BE, et al: Limb sparing treatment for osteosarcoma in dogs. J Am Vet Med Assoc 195:1734–1744, 1989.

111. Thrall DE, Withrow SJ, Powers BE, et al: Radiotherapy prior to cortical allograft limb sparing in dogs with osteosarcoma: A dose response assay. Int J Rad Onc Biol Phys 18:1354–1357, 1990.

112. Withrow SJ, Thrall DE, Straw RC, et al: Intraarterial cisplatin with or without radiation in limbsparing for canine osteosarcoma. Cancer 71:2484–2490, 1993.

113. Tomford WW, Doppelt SH, Mankin HJ: 1983 bone banking procedures. Clin Orthop Rel Res 174:15–21, 1983.

114. Straw RC, Powers BE, Withrow SJ, Cooper MF, Turner AS: The effect of intramedullary polymethylmethacrylate on healing of intercalary cortical allografts in a canine model. J Orthop Res 10:434–439, 1992.

115. Calhoun JH, Mader JT: Antibiotic beads in the management of surgical infection. Am J Surg 157:443–449, 1989.

116. Kirpensteijn J, Straw RC, Pardo AD, Adams WH, Withrow SJ, Calhoon CS: Partial and total scapulectomy in the dog. J Am Anim Hosp Assoc 30:313–319, 1994.

117. Schwarz PD, Withrow SJ, Curtis CR, Straw RC, Powers BE: Partial maxillary resection as a treatment of oral cancer in 61 dogs. J Am Anim Hosp Assoc 27:617–624, 1991.

118. Schwarz PD, Withrow SJ, Curtis CR, Straw RC, Powers BE: Mandibular resection as a treatment of oral cancer in 81 dogs. J Am Anim Hosp Assoc 27:601–610, 1991.

119. Schwarz PD, Withrow SJ: Mandibulectomy. *In* Bojrab MJ (ed): Current techniques in small animal surgery. Philadelphia, Lea & Febiger, 1994, pp. 850–861.

120. Schwarz PD, Withrow SJ: Maxillectomy and premaxillectomy. *In* Bojrab MJ (ed): Current techniques in small animal surgery. Philadelphia, Lea & Febiger, 1990, pp. 861–870.

121. O'Brien MG, Withrow SJ, Straw RC, Powers BE, Kirpensteijn T: Total and partial orbitectomy for the treatment of periorbital tumors in 23 dogs and 6 cats. Vet Surg (in press).

122. Pirkey-Ehrhart N, Withrow SJ, Straw RC, et al: Primary rib tumors in 54 dogs. J Am Anim Hosp Assoc 31:65–69, 1995.

123. Straw RC, Withrow SJ, Powers BE: Partial or total hemipelvectomy in the management of sarcomas in seven dogs and two cats. Vet Surg 21:183–188, 1992.

124. McEntee MC, Page RL, Novotney CA, Thrall DE: Palliative radiotherapy for canine appendicular osteosarcoma. Vet Radiol and Ultrasound 34:367–370, 1993.

125. Van Vechten BJ, Withrow SJ, Straw RC, LaRue SM: Vertebral tumors in 20 dogs. Proc Vet Cancer Soc 14th Ann Conf (Abstract), 1994.

126. Kern KA, Pass HI, Roth JA: Surgical treatment of pulmonary metastasis. *In* Rosenburg SA (ed): Surgical Treatment of Metastatic Cancer. Philadelphia, JB Lippincott, 1987, pp. 69–100.

127. O'Brien MG, Straw RC, Withrow SJ, et al: Resection of pulmonary metastases in canine osteosarcoma: 36 cases (1983–1992). Vet Surg 22:105–109, 1993.

128. Ogilvie GK, Straw RC, Jameson VJ, et al: Evaluation of single agent chemotherapy for the treatment of clinically evident osteosarcoma metastasis in dogs (1987–1991). J Am Vet Med Assoc 202:304–306, 1993.

129. Bacci G, Avella M, Picci P: Metastatic patterns in osteosarcoma. Tumori 74:421–427, 1988.

130. Campanacci M, Bacci G, Bertoni F: Treatment of osteosarcoma of the extremities. Cancer 48:1569–1581, 1981.

131. Giuliano AE, Feig S, Eilber FR: Changing metastatic patterns of osteosarcoma. Cancer 54:2160–2164, 1984.

132. Huth JF, Eilber FR: Patterns of recurrence after resection of osteosarcoma of the extremity: Strategies for treatment of metastasis. Arch Surg 124:122–126, 1989.

133. Knapp DW, Richardson RC, Chan TCK, et al: Piroxicam therapy in 34 dogs with transitional cell carcinoma of the urinary bladder. J Vet Int Med 8:273–278, 1994.

134. Goeckeler WF, Stoneburner LK, Kasi LP, Fossella FV: Analysis of urine samples from metastatic bone cancer patients administered 153Sm-EDTMP. Nucl Med Biol 20:657–661, 1993.

135. Pecherstorfer M, Schilling T, Janisch S, Woloszczuk W, Baumgartner G: Effect of clodronate treatment on bone scintigraphy in metastatic breast cancer. J Nucl Med 34:1039–1044, 1993.

136. Holmes RA: Radiopharmaceuticals in clinical trials. Semin Oncol 20(3 Suppl 2):22–26, 1993.

137. Clarke NW, Holbrook IB, McClure J, George NJ: Osteoclast inhibition by pamidronate in metastatic prostate cancer: A preliminary study. Br J Cancer 63:420–423, 1991.

138. Lattimer JC, Corwin LA, Stapleton J, et al: Clinical and clinicopathologic response of canine bone tumor patients to treatment with samarium-153-EDTMP. J Nucl Med 31:1316–1324, 1990.

139. Lattimer JC, Corwin LA, Stapleton J, et al: Clinical and clinicopathologic effects of samarium-153-EDTMP administered intravenously to normal beagle dogs. J Nucl Med 31:586–593, 1990.

140. MacEwen EG: Spontaneous tumors in dogs and cats: Models for the study of cancer biology and treatment. Cancer Met Rev 125:125–136, 1990.

141. Brodey RS: The use of naturally occurring cancer in domestic animals for research into human cancer: General considerations and a review of canine skeletal osteosarcoma. Yale J Biol Med 52:345–361, 1979.

142. Goorin AM, Abelson HT, Frei EI: Osteosarcoma: Fifteen years later. N Engl J Med 313:1637–1643, 1985.

143. Lane JM, Hurson B, Boland PJ: Osteogenic sarcoma. Clin Orthop Rel Res 204:93–110, 1986.

144. Banks WC: Parosteal osteosarcoma in a dog and cat. J Am Vet Med Assoc 158:1412–1415, 1971.

145. Withrow SJ, Doige CE: En bloc resection of a juxtacortical and three intra-osseous osteosarcomas of the zygomatic arch in dogs. J Am Anim Hosp Assoc 867:872, 1980.

146. Straw RC, LeCouteur RA, Powers BE, Withrow SI: Multilobular osteochondrosarcoma of the canine skull: Sixteen cases. J Am Vet Med Assoc 195:1764–1769, 1989.

147. Brodey RS, Riser WH, van der Heul RO: Canine skeletal chondrosarcoma: A clinicopathological study of 35 cases. J Am Vet Med Assoc 165:68–78, 1974.

148. Obradovich JE, Straw RC, Powers BE, Withrow SJ: Canine chondrosarcoma: A review of 55 cases (1983–1990). J Am Vet Med Assoc (in press).

149. Sylvestre AM, Brash ML, Atilola MAO, Cockshutt JR: A case series of 25 dogs with chondrosarcoma. Vet Comp Orthop Traum 5:13–17, 1992.

150. Doige CE: Multiple cartilagenous exostosis in dogs. Vet Pathol 24:276–278, 1987.

151. Doige CE, Pharr JW, Withrow SJ: Chondrosarcoma arising in multiple cartilagenous exostosis in a dog. J Am Anim Hosp Assoc 14:605–611, 1978.

152. Popovitch CA, Weinstein MJ, Goldschmidt MH, Shofer FS: Chondrosarcoma: A retrospective study of 97 dogs (1987–1990). J Am Anim Hosp Assoc 30:81–85, 1994.

153. Southerland EM, Miller RT, Jones CI: Primary right atrial chondrosarcoma in a dog. J Am Vet Med Assoc 203:1697–1701, 1993.

154. Anderson WI, Carberry CA, King JM, Trotter EJ, De-Lahunta A: Primary aortic chondrosarcoma in a dog. Vet Pathol 25:180–181, 1988.

155. Patnaik AK, Mattiesen DT, Zawie DA: Two cases of canine penile neoplasm: Squamous cell carcinoma and mesenchymal chondrosarcoma. J Am Anim Hosp Assoc 24:403–406, 1988.

156. Flanders JA, Castleman W, Carberry CA, Tseng FS: Laryngeal chondrosarcoma in a dog. J Am Vet Med Assoc 190:68–70, 1987.

157. Aron DN, DeVries R, Short CE: Primary tracheal chondrosarcoma in a dog: A case report with description of surgical and anesthetic techniques. J Am Anim Hosp Assoc 16:31–37, 1980.

158. Weller RE, Dagle GE, Perry RL, Park JF: Primary pulmonary chondrosarcoma in a dog. Cornell Vet 82:447–452, 1992.

159. Greenlee PG, Lui SK: Chondrosarcoma of the mitral leaflet in a dog. Vet Pathol 21:540–542, 1984.

160. Matthiesen DT, Clark GN, Orsher, Pardo AO, Glennon J, Patnaik AK: En bloc resection of primary rib tumors in 40 dogs. Vet Surg 21:201–204, 1992.

161. Montgomery RD, Henderson RA, Powers BE, et al: Retrospective study of 26 primary thoracic wall tumors in dogs. J Am Anim Hosp Assoc 29:68–72, 1993.

162. Hammer AS, Couto CG, Filippi J, Getzy D, Shank K: Efficacy and toxicity of VAC chemotherapy (vincristine, doxorubicin, and cyclophosphamide) in dogs with hemangiosarcoma. J Vet Int Med 5:160–166, 1991.

163. Ogilvie GK, Powers BE, Mallinckrodt CH, Withrow SJ: Doxorubicin chemotherapy and surgery for hemangiosarcoma in the dog. Proc Vet Cancer Soc (Abstract), 1994.

164. Wesselhoeft Ablin L, Berg J, Schelling SH: Fibrosarcoma in the canine appendicular skeleton. J Am Anim Hosp Assoc 27:303–309, 1991.

165. Brodey RS, Reid CF, Sauer RM: Metastatic bone neoplasms in the dog. J Am Vet Med Assoc 148:29–43, 1966.

166. Chester DK: Multiple cartilaginous exostoses in two generations of dogs. J Am Vet Med Assoc 159:895–897, 1971.

167. Gee BR, Doige CE: Multiple cartilaginous exostoses in a litter of dogs. J Am Vet Med Assoc 156:53–59, 1970.

168. Hunt GB, Johnson KA: What is your diagnosis? J Am Vet Med Assoc 199:1071–1072, 1991.

169. Pernell RT, Dunstan RW, DeCamp CE: Aneurysmal bone cyst in a six-month-old dog. J Am Vet Med Assoc 201:1897–1899, 1992.

170. Biery DN, Goldschmidt M, Riser WH, Rhodes WH: Bone cysts in the dog. J Am Vet Radiol 17:202–212, 1976.

171. Basher AWP, Doige CE, Presnell KR: Subchondral bone cysts in a dog with osteochondrosis. J Am Anim Hosp Assoc 24:321–326, 1988.

172. Schrader SC, Burk, Lui S: Bone cysts in two dogs and a review of similar cystic bone lesions in the dog. J Am Vet Med Assoc 182:490–495, 1983.

173. Mirra JM: Cysts and cyst-like lesions of bone. In Mirra JM, Picci P, Gold RH (eds): Bone Tumors: Clinical, Radiographic and Pathologic Correlations. Philadelphia, Lea & Febiger, 1989, pp. 1233–1234.

174. Grabias S, Mankin H: Chondrosarcoma arising in histologically proved unicameral bone cyst. J Bone and Jt Surg 56A:1501–1503, 1973.

175. Halliwell WH: Tumorlike lesions of bone. In Bojrab MJ (ed): Disease mechanisms in small animal surgery. Philadelphia, Lea & Febiger, 1993, pp. 932–943.

176. Dorn CR, Taylor DON, Schneider R: Survey of animal neoplasms in Alameda and Contra Costa Counties, California. II. Cancer morbidity in dogs and cats from Alameda County. J Natl Cancer Inst 40:307–318, 1968.

177. Turrel JM, Pool RR: Primary bone tumors in the cat: A retrospective study of 15 cats and a literature review. Vet Radiol 23:152–166, 1982.

178. Carpenter JL, Andrews LK, Holzworth J: Tumors and tumor-like lesions. In Holzworth J (ed): Diseases of the cat: Medicine and surgery. Philadelphia, W. B. Saunders Company, 1987, pp. 406–596.

179. Berman E, Wright JF. What is your diagnosis? (osteosarcoma of tibia and hemangiosarcoma of femur metastatic to lungs in an irradiated cat). J Am Vet Med Assoc 162:1065–1066, 1973.

180. Riddle WEJ, Leighton RI: Osteochondromatosis in a cat. J Am Vet Med Assoc 156:1428–1430, 1970.

181. Pool RR, Carrig CB: Multiple cartilagenous exostoses in a cat. Vet Pathol 9:350–359, 1972.

182. Lui S, Dorfman HD, Patnaik AK: Primary and secondary bone tumors in the cat. J Small Anim Pract 15:141–156, 1974.

183. Quigley PJ, Leedale AH: Tumors involving bone in the domestic cat: A review of fifty-eight cases. Vet Pathol 20:670–686, 1983.

184. Thompson JP, Fugent MJ: Evaluation of survival times after limb amputation, with and without subsequent administration of cisplatin, for treatment of osteosarcoma in dogs: 30 cases (1979–1990). J Am Vet Med Assoc, 200:531–533, 1992.

185. Kraegel SA, Madewell BR, Simonsen E: Osteogenic sarcoma and cisplatin chemotherapy in dogs: 16 cases (1986–1989). J Am Vet Med Assoc 199:1057–1059, 1991.

# 21

# Tumors of the Endocrine System

Gregory K. Ogilvie

There are many tumors of the endocrine system that can cause a wide variety of diseases with either subtle or dramatic manifestations. The diagnosis of endocrine system malignancies can be quite simple or it can be complex and convoluted. Few areas in the disciplines of internal medicine and surgery are more challenging. This chapter reviews the most common tumors of the endocrine system and the pathophysiology, diagnosis, management, and prognosis of each tumor.

## TUMORS OF THE THYROID GLAND

### Background

The thyroid gland of dogs and cats has two distinct lobes that adjoin the first five to eight rings of the trachea. There are two parathyroid glands associated with each of the two thyroid lobes. The external parathyroid gland is located outside the thyroid gland capsule and is usually found in the cranial pole of the thyroid gland. The internal parathyroid glands are within the thyroid gland capsule in the caudal and medial aspect of each respective lobe and are rarely identified by gross examination. The parathyroid is white to gray in color and may have its own vascular supply. The thyroid gland is quite vascular. In both the dog and the cat, ectopic thyroid tissue is present, located primarily within the cervical region, but it may be located anywhere from the thorax to the base of the tongue. Thus, malignancies of the thyroid gland may be located in ectopic sites in either species. When a thyroid malignancy is suspected but is not identified in the normal loca-

tion, one should evaluate those areas where ectopic thyroid glands have been identified. This is especially true in the cat, which frequently presents with hyperthyroidism.

### Canine Thyroid Neoplasia

Thyroid tumors are uncommon in the dog and account for approximately 10 to 15% of all head and neck tumors.[1-9] The average age of dogs with thyroid adenomas and adenocarcinomas is approximately 9 to 10 years, with a range of 7 to 18 years.[1-4,7] There is no sex predilection. Boxers have been reported to be predisposed to the development of thyroid adenomas.[1-4,9] Beagles, boxers, and golden retrievers may have a higher prevalence of carcinomas. Although it has been suggested that these tumors are more prevalent in iodine-deficient geographic locations, this has not been confirmed in subsequent reports.[9]

### Pathobiology

Thyroid carcinomas are identified clinically far more than thyroid adenomas.[1-9] Approximately 90 to 95% of thyroid tumors identified clinically are carcinomas, and tumor volumes usually exceed 100 cm³ at the time of diagnosis.[5] Two thirds of thyroid carcinomas are unilateral at initial presentation.[7] Bilateral tumors are generally more extensive and fixed to underlying tissue, which can be a poor prognostic sign. As stated earlier, thyroid carcinomas and adenomas may arise from ectopic mediastinal thyroid tissue and occasionally occur from the base of the tongue.[10]

Carcinomas may be encapsulated but often invade surrounding structures, including the esophagus, trachea, larynx, cervical musculature, nerves, and blood vessels (Fig. 21–1). The common sites of metastases are the lung and cervical lymph nodes, cervical vertebrae, followed by the adrenal glands, kidneys, myocardium, liver, and brain.[2,3,7] Most carcinomas are follicular but histopathologically they can be identified as compact or papillary carcinomas. Determining the specific histopathologic classification is not of prognostic value. From a clinical perspective, very small thyroid tumors are rarely identified. From a pragmatic point of view, thyroid tumors fixed to underlying structures are a poor prognostic sign, whereas those freely movable are more amenable to subsequent surgical resection.

## History and Clinical Signs

Adenomas of the thyroid gland, although rarely detected clinically, are seen when dogs are presented without associated clinical signs due to their thyroid neoplasia.[2,7] Owners are prompted to present their dogs with thyroid carcinomas primarily because of a palpable cervical mass. Dysphagia, dyspnea, and a change in vocalization may be described.[1–7] In addition, regurgitation, precaval syndrome (Fig. 21–2), weight loss, or extensive hemorrhage secondary to disseminated intravascular coagulation may be present. The duration of clinical signs prior to presentation is generally less than 3 months. One investigator in the Netherlands noted that approximately 20% of all thyroid tumors were hyperfunctional and resulted in a thyrotoxic state.[11] This appears to be rare in the United States (< 5%). The clinical signs commonly seen in hyperthyroid dogs are very similar to those of the cat (polydipsia, polyuria, increased appetite despite the presence

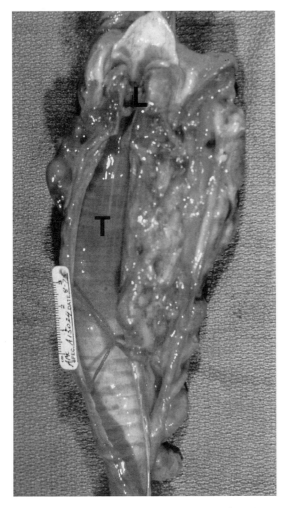

**Figure 21–1.** Thyroid carcinoma invading into larynx (L), trachea (T), and cervical blood vessels.

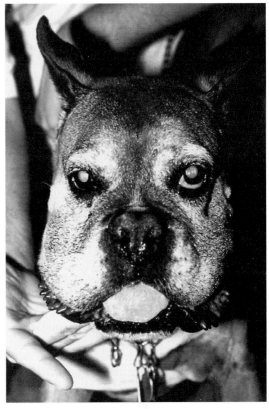

**Figure 21–2.** Precaval syndrome, resulting in pronounced facial edema, secondary to an invasive thyroid carcinoma in a boxer.

of weight loss, panting, restlessness, heat intolerance, occasionally weakness). The dog may appear cachectic on physical examination, with muscle atrophy and rapid heart rate with bounding pulses. Although hyperthyroidism is reported less commonly in other studies,[3] it has occurred in dogs with either bilateral or unilateral tumors. Hypothyroidism secondary to a unilateral tumor may result from the production of biologically inactive thyroid hormone, which feeds back on the brain to inhibit pituitary thyrotropin (thyroid-stimulating hormone, or TSH) secretion, which subsequently results in the atrophy of normal thyroid tissue.

## Diagnosis

A nonpainful large cervical swelling must stimulate thoughts of several differential diagnoses, including abscess, granuloma, salivary mucocele, metastatic neoplasia, lymphoma, carotid body tumor, and regional soft tissue sarcoma.[1-3,9] When a cervical mass is present, fine-needle cytology may aid diagnosis. Because thyroid tumors are frequently very vascular, cells from the thyroid tumor may be obtained by repeatedly advancing a 22-gauge, three-fourths-inch needle into the suspected thyroid gland through a single puncture site in the skin. Aspiration usually is not recommended because of subsequent hemodilution, which may obscure the presence of tumor cells. Carcinoma cells consistent with thyroid carcinoma are usually found at the feathered edge of the slide and often are rare in number and may not look malignant. Histopathology is necessary to confirm the diagnosis. When surgery or biopsy is contemplated, thoracic radiographs and coagulogram (platelet count, one-step prothrombin time, activated partial thromboplastin time) should be performed to ensure there is no metastatic disease and to identify coagulopathies that would be a risk to the dog. A cervical radiograph, ultrasound, and computerized tomography, although optional, may help identify the location of the mass and other vital structures in the area. If biopsy is required, a percutaneous needle biopsy or open surgical biopsy can be performed. Because significant hemorrhage can result in large hematoma formation within the cervical area, many experienced surgeons proceed with a definitive excisional procedure if thoracic radiographs fail to identify any metastatic disease; a complete blood count (CBC), biochemical profile, urinalysis, coagulogram, and

thyroid hormone assessment fail to identify any metabolic disease that would preclude performing anesthesia and surgery; and if the mass is "mobile" and compatible with a thyroid carcinoma based on fine-needle aspiration cytology.[1-9] Nuclear scans using radioactive iodine or sodium pertechnetate can be helpful in identifying the location and extent of primary and metastatic neoplasia. Unlike the cat, in dogs not all thyroid tumors take up $I^{123}$ or pertechnetate uniformly.[3,4,9] When thyroid assessment is made, a resting $T_4$ should be performed. If it is clearly within normal limits, the dog is probably euthyroid. If there is any question, then a TSH test should be performed. In one study that evaluated the tumors by flow cytometry, abnormal numbers of chromosomes (aneuploid) were more frequent in carcinomas from dogs with distant metastases (78%) than from dogs with less advanced stages of disease.[14]

## Treatment

Complete surgical excision is the best treatment for canine thyroid carcinomas or adenomas. Because freely movable carcinomas and adenomas are usually amenable to complete surgical excision, it is the treatment of choice[9,15] (Figs. 21-3 to 21-6). At the time of surgery the surgeon will face three general possibilities:

1. Freely mobile (unilateral or bilateral). These are mobile masses that have a well-defined capsule without invasion into the surrounding tissue. Surgery is straightforward and often curative.
2. Partially adherent to adjacent tissue and unilateral. The mass is excised in continuity with fixed tissue with the only nonexpendable tissue (on one side) being the esophagus and trachea.
3. Totally fixed and often bilaterally by direct extension of one side to the other. Complete removal is impossible and a cautious incisional biopsy is in order.

Distinguishing category 2 from 3 is not easy and may occasionally be determined only at the time of neck exploration.

Surgery is performed by making an incision on the ventral midline.[9,15] When possible, vital structures such as the carotid artery (and associated vagosympathetic trunk), jugular vein, recurrent laryngeal nerve, and esophagus should be

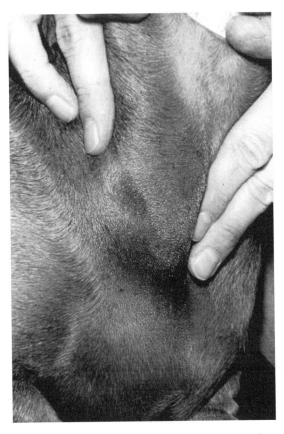

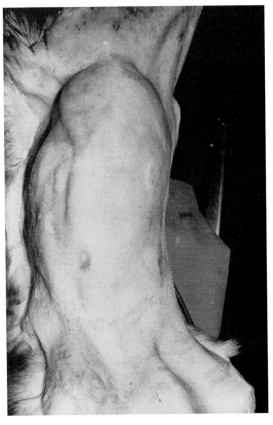

**Figure 21–3.** Freely movable noninvasive thyroid carcinoma in a dog. Surgical removal alone resulted in local and systemic control for more than 4 years.

**Figure 21–4.** Large fixed invasive thyroid carcinoma in a dog. (Head is toward the top.)

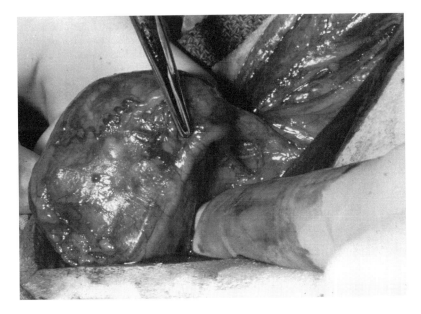

**Figure 21–5.** Encapsulated noninvasive thyroid carcinoma at surgery. (Same patient as in Figure 21–3.)

**Figure 21–6.** Flow diagram outlining treatment for thyroid carcinoma in the dog.* Currently being investigated as promising therapeutic modalities.

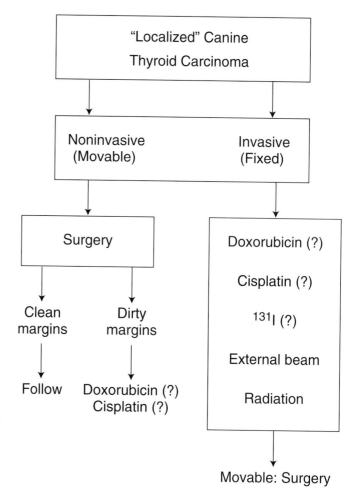

identified and preserved. If necessary, however, the jugular, carotid, vagosympathetic, recurrent laryngeal nerve on one side may be resected. Strict attention should be made to ensure ligation of all blood supply to the tumor. The cervical lymph nodes should be examined and biopsied when possible. If only one thyroid gland and adjoining parathyroid tissue is involved, hypoparathyroidism and hypothyroidism are rarely postoperative complications. Because approximately one third of carcinomas are bilateral,[7] a bilateral thyroidectomy should be performed when indicated as one mass or two distinct lesions. Parathyroid tissue usually cannot be preserved; thus it is necessary to supply calcium and vitamin D postoperatively, and probably vitamin D for the rest of the animal's life.[16] If untreated, hypoparathyroidism often results in a hypocalcemic crisis with neurologic signs that range from nervousness, irritability, panting, increased body temperature, muscle tremors,

tetany, convulsions, and death. Hypocalcemia should be treated with 10% calcium gluconate administered slowly intravenously at a dose of 1.0 to 1.5 ml/kg over 10 to 20 minutes. Bradycardia or shortening of the QT interval may indicate that the infusion is resulting in toxicosis from hypercalcemia. When this occurs, the infusion should be discontinued temporarily. After the emergency situation has resolved, then 2.5 ml/kg 10% calcium gluconate should be added to intravenous fluids and administered every 6 to 8 hours. In these cases, vitamin D and calcium therapy should be initiated for long-term maintenance. Dihydrotachysterol (Hytakerol) is administered initially at 0.05 mg/kg/day, followed by 0.02 mg/kg/day for 2 days, followed by 0.01 mg/kg/day. During the initial 4-day loading period, oral calcium gluconate should be administered at 0.05 to 1 gm/kg given in three to four divided doses per day. For those animals that seizure from hypocalcemia, parenteral calcium can be discontinued, usually within 2 to 3 days after oral vitamin D and calcium loading. For maintenance therapy, the dosage of oral vitamin D and calcium should be adjusted according to the calcium and phosphorus determinations. Hypercalcemia should be avoided because hypercalcemic nephropathy can be just as fatal as hypocalcemia. Hypothyroidism should be treated with L-thyroxine at a dosage of 20 to 30 $\mu$g/kg given in two divided doses and adjusted according to $T_4$ values that are determined 4 to 6 hours after pill administration. If a bilateral thyroidectomy is performed, one should monitor for laryngeal paralysis in the postoperative course.

For thyroid carcinomas that are diffusely fixed to underlying structures in which complete surgical removal is unlikely, surgery should be avoided because of the high morbidity, mortality, and cost associated with the procedure. Using a midline approach, these tumors should be biopsied and the owner advised of the impending prognosis.

Some authors suggest that doxorubicin (30 mg/m$^2$) every 3 weeks for five total treatments can result in partial remission in about one half of all cases.[5,6] It is theoretically possible that surgical removal can be performed after partial remission occurs in dogs with tumors that respond well. Experience at Colorado State University suggests that dogs with measurable malignant thyroid tumors do not respond substantially to chemotherapy.[15] However, in those with microscopic disease or with a minimal amount of tumor present at the time doxorubicin chemotherapy is administered, a favorable response (improved disease-free interval) may be noted.

Another form of treatment is external beam radiation therapy and I[131] therapy.[17] External beam radiation is a local treatment that should be employed only when there is no metastatic disease. Unfortunately, the large-volume nonresectable tumor is unlikely to respond to external beam radiation. I[131] will be effective if the malignant thyroid tumor or any metastatic disease will uniformly take up the radionuclide. Controlled trials of radiation treatment of thyroid carcinomas have not been reported. (See Fig. 21–6.)

## Prognosis

Tumor volume was directly related to metastatic behavior in one study. Fourteen percent of dogs with tumor volumes less than 20 cm$^3$ had metastases, versus 74 to 100% of dogs that had metastases with tumor volumes from 21 to greater than 100 cm$^3$, respectively.[7]

Adenomas that are completely excised surgically have an excellent prognosis. Small, noninvasive, freely movable encapsulated carcinomas also have an excellent survival time of from 1 to 4 years with surgery alone.[2,3,15] Large tumors that are fixed to underlying structures warrant a poor prognosis. DNA ploidy was recently measured by flow cytometry in 36 primary malignant thyroid tumors in the dog, including six bilateral tumors.[14] Ploidy status (diploid versus aneuploid) was identical in the primary and metastatic sites in 10 of 14 dogs. Aneuploidy occurred more frequently in the carcinomas from dogs with distant metastases (78%) than from dogs with less advanced stages of disease (53%). In another study, circulating thyroglobulin was measured in 20 dogs with thyroid cancer, using a homologous polyclonal radial immunoassay. Plasma thyroglobulin levels exceeded the normal range in 70% of the dogs. Plasma thyroglobulin levels were higher in scintigraphically hot tumors (functional) than in cold ones (nonfunctional), a finding that may help indicate whether I[131] therapy would be beneficial in certain cases. It was concluded in the study that the measurement of plasma thyroglobulin levels might be useful for monitoring the postoperative course of the disease in certain dogs with thyroid cancer because the thyroglobulin levels decreased to within normal limits after the thyroid tumors had been successfully removed.[18] Cisplatin chemotherapy has been used to treat at least one dog with thyroid adenocarcinoma, which resulted in partial remission. The results of studies evaluating a large number of cases that have been treated with chemotherapy, external beam radiation therapy, or I[131] do not exist.

## Comparative Aspects[19]

Papillary carcinomas are the most common thyroid tumor type in people but are rare in the dog. Previous radiation therapy to the cervical area has been associated with the development of thyroid neoplasia in people. Medullary carcinomas are also common in people. Although high concentrations of calcitonin exist, these individuals usually are not hypocalcemic or hypophosphatemic. Medullary carcinomas are uncommon in dogs; however, when they occur they also tend to have normal serum calcium and phosphorus levels. People and dogs with medullary carcinomas have been reported to experience diarrhea from excess secretion of serotonin or prostaglandins or both.[19]

# FELINE HYPERTHYROIDISM

Hyperthyroidism was first described in the literature in 1979. Since then, thyrotoxicosis has emerged as the most common endocrine disorder of the domestic cat.[20,21] The most common cause of the condition is a functional adenomatous hyperplasia (or adenoma), a benign change involving thyroid tissue. Functional thyroid carcinomas occur in only 1 to 2% of cases.[20,21] There appears to be no breed or sex predilection; however, there appears to be a higher incidence on the East and West coasts; the reason for this is unknown. The average age of cats with hyperthyroidism is 13 years, with a range of 6 to 20 years.[20,21] In approximately 70% of cats with functional thyroid adenomas or adenomatous hyperplasia, both lobes are involved and only one lobe is involved in the remaining 30% (Fig. 21–7). Adenomas that arise from accessory thyroid tissue located within the mediastinum are rare.

## History and Clinical Signs

Because of secretion of large amounts of thyroid hormone, a variety of clinical signs may be due to the hormone's effect on different systems. In some cases, alterations in one organ system will predominate. There is evidence to suggest that the most common clinical signs may have changed to more vague or nondescript problems due to earlier diagnosis and greater awareness of this clinical condition. In one early study of 131 cases of hyperthyroidism, the most common clinical signs were weight loss, polyphagia, increased activity, polydipsia, polyuria, and vomiting.[20] Diarrhea, anorexia, panting, heat intolerance, muscle weakness, muscle tremors, increased nail growth, dyspnea, alopecia, and behavioral changes along with ventral neck flexion, were less commonly seen. Many cats with thyrotoxicosis are hyperexcitable and polyphagic; however, 10% are depressed and anorectic. These cats are described as having the apathetic form of hypothyroidism and they frequently have concurrent cardiac abnormalities.[9,20–22] Practitioners are more commonly identifying cats that have an elevated $T_4$ and only subtle clinical signs because of early detection.

On physical examination, a thyroid mass or masses may be noted peritracheally in about 90% of affected cats.[9,20] The enlarged lobes may actually descend toward and into the thoracic inlet. Shaving the neck may facilitate palpation and visualization of very small tumors, which may be several millimeters to several centimeters in diameter. In some cases, the clinical signs secondary to the hormone's effect on the cardiovascular system predominate.[22] They include tachycardia, gallop rhythm, systolic murmur, and bounding pulses. Ten percent of cats with thyro-

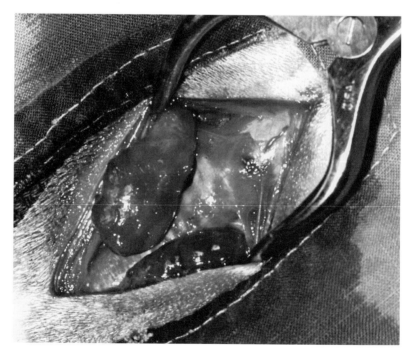

**Figure 21–7.**  Bilaterally enlarged thyroids in a cat at surgery. Bilateral thyroidectomy is indicated in this case. Generally this will entail extracapsular removal on one side and intracapsular removal on the side with the most delineated parathyroid.

toxicosis are presented in congestive heart failure. These cases may develop pleural effusion and secondary respiratory compromise.

## Diagnosis

When thyrotoxicosis is suspected, a CBC, biochemical profile, urinalysis, basal $T_4$ echocardiogram, and electrocardiogram should be performed.[9,20–22] The most common hematologic abnormalities are a stress leukogram, mild to moderate erythrocytosis, and macrocytosis. The macrocytosis may be a result of the premature release of red blood cells from the bone marrow.[20] Elevated liver enzymes are seen in many cases, with increases in serum alkaline phosphatase, lactate dehydrogenase, alanine aminotransferase (ALT), and aspartate aminotransferase (AST). An elevated total bilirubin may also be seen. Histopathologic evaluation of the liver usually reveals nonspecific changes.[20] Interestingly, an increased phosphorus is seen in 20% of the cases, sometimes secondary to renal insufficiency or from increased bone reabsorption mediated by the elevated thyroid hormone. Most, if not all, of these hematologic and biochemical abnormalities return to normal after the cat has reverted to a euthyroid state.[9,20] Thoracic radiographs rarely identify any evidence of thyroid tissue within the thoracic cavity, but frequently they are valuable for determining the extent of changes to the cardiovascular system. Early data suggest that approximately 50% of cats with hyperthyroidism have evidence of cardiomegaly on thoracic radiographs.[20,22,23] Early detection has resulted in the identification of a large group of cats with normal cardiac structure and function. Less commonly, pulmonary edema or pleural effusion is identified. Eighty percent of cats with hypothyroidism have abnormalities on the electrocardiogram because of a cardiomyopathic-like state.[22] Sinus tachycardia, increased QRS complex amplitude, and atrial and ventricular arrhythmias are sometimes identified. Therefore, any middle-aged to older cats with cardiovascular disease should always be evaluated for hyperthyroidism. Echocardiography helps in the identification of the common asymmetrical hypertrophy of the myocardial walls and septum and frequently identifies a hyperdynamic state associated with the cardiomyopathic-like state of thyrotoxicosis. When cats are reverted to a euthyroid state, most if not all of these cardiovascular changes return to within normal limits.

The definitive diagnosis for hyperthyroidism in cats is made by a demonstration of an elevated serum $T_4$ and $T_3$.[20] TSH stimulation tests are generally not recommended in most cats because they may induce a thyroid storm and result in life-threatening cardiac arrhythmias. Nuclear scintigraphy using $I^{125}$ or sodium pertechnetate often helps identify whether the condition is bilateral or unilateral and whether there is ectopic thyroid tissue present and affected by the condition.[20] Therefore, scintigraphy is especially valuable in those cases in which hyperthyroidism is strongly suspected, yet no cervical masses are identified. In rare cases of thyroid carcinomas, scintigraphy also can identify distant metastatic disease. The appearance of mild clinical signs of hyperthyroidism when normal or equivocally high basal serum thyroid hormone concentrations are present is termed *occult hyperthyroidism*.[9,20,24] Frequently there are very subtle clinical signs that over time progress to overt hyperthyroidism. Serum concentrations of $T_4$ and $T_3$ fluctuate in and out of normal range for a period of days in some cats with mild or moderate hyperthyroidism. These fluctuations explain why some cats have "normal" thyroid hormone levels despite clinical evidence of thyrotoxicosis. A diagnosis can be made simply by repeating thyroid levels at a later date.[25] If repeat thyroid hormone levels do not confirm a diagnosis of hyperthyroidism, a $T_3$ suppression test or thyrotropin-releasing-hormone (TRH) stimulation is recommended.[24,25] To perform a $T_3$ suppression test, a blood sample is drawn to determine the basal thyroid concentrations of total $T_4$ and $T_3$. The owners are instructed to administer $T_3$ orally (liothyronine cytomel*) at a dosage of 25 μg given three times daily for 2 days beginning the morning after blood is drawn. The morning of the third day a seventh 25 μg dose of liothyronine is given and the cat is returned for subsequent sampling for serum $T_4$ and $T_3$ levels. When the $T_3$ suppression test is performed in normal cats, there is a marked fall in $T_4$ concentrations after excess $T_3$ administration. In hyperthyroid cats, minimal if any suppression of serum $T_4$ concentrations are noted. In normal cats the intravenous administration of TRH at a dosage of 0.1 mg/kg intravenously causes a twofold or greater increase in serum $T_4$ concentrations over basal values in four hours. In cats with mild hyperthyroidism, there is little if any increase in the $T_4$ levels after the TRH administration. The TRH response test can be

---

*Pfizer/Smith Kline and French Laboratories

performed in less time than the $T_3$ suppression test. The major disadvantage of the TRH suppression test is the potential for transient side effects from hormone administration (salivation, vomiting, tachypnea, defecation). As noted above, a thyroid storm may result in cardiovascular problems.

## Therapy

There are three options for the treatment of hyperthyroidism in cats: chronic antithyroid drug administration, surgical removal of the affected thyroid gland(s), or $I^{131}$ treatment.[25-33] Other treatments such as stable iodine solutions, beta-adrenergic blocking drugs, and sedatives can also be used in the management of these cases. Essentially the average cat with thyrotoxicosis is evaluated by a baseline $T_4$, CBC, biochemical profile, urinalysis, electrocardiogram, echocardiogram, and when possible nuclear scintigraphy to determine the gland(s) involved. The owners should then be given the option of surgery, $I^{131}$, or medical management alone. If there is evidence of cardiomyopathy or metabolic disease that would preclude the safe use of anesthetics or if these problems are at great risk for the cat's short-term survival, antithyroid medication (e.g., methimazole) and appropriate cardiac therapy (e.g., diltiazem, atenolol, enalapril, propranolol, furosemide) is prescribed. If surgery is anticipated, the patient is anesthetized when stable (generally 2 to 3 weeks). An intracapsular surgery (30% relapse by 3 years) is not as effective as an extracapsular thyroid resection (5% relapse in 3 years). $I^{131}$ is approximately as effective as surgery. More specific details of therapy follow.

**Thioureylenes**[26,27]    Thioamides are a category of drugs that share antithyroid activity. The drugs currently recommended are methimazole (Tapazole*) and carbimazole (Neo-Mercazole**). Methimazole is available in the United States; carbimazole is available only in Europe currently but is expected to be marketed in the United States soon.[26] Propylthiouracil was the first thioureylene used in cats; however, it caused severe hematologic complications and is not recommended.

Methimazole safety has been evaluated in 262 cats. Carbimazole was evaluated in a series of 47 thyrotoxic cats (preoperative evaluation in 39 cats, long-term therapy in 8 cats).[25,33] The results of these two studies indicate that both drugs are the antithyroid drugs of choice for preoperative

*Eli Lilly
**Nicholas

and long-term medical management of feline hyperthyroidism.

When methimazole is used preoperatively or exclusively, it should be administered at a dosage of 10 to 15 mg/kg/day in divided doses every 8 to 12 hours. $T_4$ concentrations decrease to at or below the high normal values in 2 to 3 weeks. Complete blood and platelet counts should be determined to ensure there are no adverse reactions associated with the administration of this drug (e.g., immune-mediated neutropenia and thrombocytopenia). The dosage should be increased or decreased based on $T_4$ values obtained after the initial 2- to 3-week period.

Carbimazole, when administered at 5 mg every 8 hours, induces euthyroidism in 91% of cats in approximately 6 days.[25,26] Some cats are resistant to this dosage and may require higher ones. For maximum efficacy, carbimazole must be administered on a regular 8-hour schedule. To confirm euthyroidism, serum $T_4$ and $T_3$ concentrations should be evaluated approximately 2 weeks after the initiation of carbimazole therapy. The use of methimazole for long-term medical management is most effective when the dosages are split and given every 8 to 12 hours. Serum $T_4$ and $T_3$ evaluations should be repeated when the lowest possible effective dose is determined. In cases in which the owners cannot administer the drug two or three times a day, it may be possible to administer the drug once daily and still maintain the cat euthyroid most of the time. Carbimazole therapy usually requires a dose of 5 mg administered twice daily to maintain euthyroidism during long-term medical management of this condition; once-a-day therapy is inadequate; therefore owner compliance may be a problem.

Adverse reactions associated with methimazole therapy are more common than those noted with carbimazole treatment.[25,33] Twenty-two percent of hyperthyroid cats treated with methimazole developed antinuclear antibodies in approximately 46 days.[33] Approximately 10% of the cats developed clinical signs (anorexia, vomiting, lethargy, eosinophilia, lymphocytosis) 2 to 3 weeks after therapy began. Other less common abnormalities (noted in fewer than 5% of the patients) include excoriation of skin, bleeding, hepatopathy, thrombocytopenia, agranulocytosis, leukopenia, and a positive Coomb's test. Mild side effects associated with carbimazole can include vomiting with or without associated anorexia, depression, and hematologic evidence of lymphocytosis and leukopenia. These occur in approximately 15% of the cases, but the abnormalities are easily reversed with discontinuation of therapy. The adverse effects are noted 2 weeks after therapy. Serious adverse effects are very rare but should be watched for. Therefore, carbimazole may be a better tolerated drug than methimazole in cats. However, to identify any hematologic abnormalities, a complete blood count and platelet count should be repeated every 2 weeks for the first 3 months when either drug is used.

**Stable Iodine**    Iodine[127] was the first agent used to treat human thyrotoxicosis.[9,25] This treatment can result in the reduction of thyroid hormone synthesis and the rate of thyroid hormone release. The effects of stable iodine are inconsistent and short-lived; therefore the drug should not be used as the sole method for treatment of feline thyrotoxicosis.

**Beta-Adrenergic Blocking Drugs[7,25]**    Propranolol, a nonselective beta-1 adrenoceptor blocking drug, will frequently reverse many signs of feline hyperthyroidism. Its mechanism of action is not clearly understood. Propranolol corrects the elevated metabolic rate, heat intolerance, fever, diarrhea, and steatorrhea. It is frequently prescribed to control cardiovascular abnormalities such as tachycardia, prominent precordial impulse, and bounding pulse, as well as neurologic abnormalities such as increased activity and restlessness. Generally, propranolol should be used in conjunction with other more definitive therapy. Propranolol should be administered at an initial oral dosage of 2.5 mg every 8 hours for 3 days. If the resting heart rate does not decrease below 200 bpm, then the dose can be increased to 5 mg every 8 hours. Diltiazem (Cardizem), a drug with similar effects, can also be used to treat many of the cardiovascular abnormalities at a dosage of 1.75 to 2.4 mg/kg every 8 to 12 hours orally. Atenolol, a newer beta-blocking agent, is currently being evaluated; one major advantage of this drug is its longer half-life and resulting longer dosing interval.

## Surgery[20,30,34]

Frequently surgery is the quickest and the most economical way to resolve thyrotoxicosis in the cat. Before surgery is performed, each patient should be evaluated to determine the extent of thyrotoxicosis, and often the cat should be treated preoperatively to return it to a euthyroid state prior to surgical thyroidectomy. This is usually accomplished with methimazole, carbimazole, propranolol, atenolol, or diltiazem, as noted previously. In certain cases oral potassium iodide can be given at 50 to 100 mg/day for 7 to 14 days to decrease thyroid hormone concentrations. As noted previously, oral iodine should always be used in conjunction with other treatments such as propranolol.[25] Scintigraphy performed prior to surgery will give the surgeon an excellent idea of whether one or both thyroid glands should be removed but is not mandatory. Regardless, at surgery both lobes of the thyroid gland should be evaluated. Bilateral thyroidectomy is performed in more than 70% of cats. Bilateral enlargement of the thyroid glands is easily identified at surgery and bilateral thyroidectomy can be performed without removal of the cranial parathyroid glands on at least one side (see Fig. 21–9). When unilateral tumors are present, there should be almost complete atrophy of the contralateral lobe; in these cases, only the affected lobe should be removed by extracapsular resection. When a unilateral parathyroidectomy is performed, it is not necessary to save the cranial parathyroid gland on the affected lobe (Fig. 21–8). When there is question regarding the involvement of the contralateral thyroid gland, both lobes should be removed. If one thyroid gland is removed and hypothyroidism ensues, it usually occurs within 12 and 24 months after surgery (Fig. 21–9).[30] However, recurrence as late as 44 months has been reported. Possible complications after thyroidectomy include Horner's syndrome, laryngeal paralysis, and hypocalcemia resulting from extirpation of all functional parathyroid tissue.[30] Postoperatively a catheter should be in place and the animal should be closely watched for hypocalcemia after bilateral removal. The clinical signs of hypocalcemia include restlessness, panting, irritability, facial twitching, elevated body temperature, tremors, tetany, and seizures. Hypoparathyroidism can occur within hours to up to 3 days after surgery. Treatment for hypoparathyroidism is discussed on page 320 of this chapter. Maintenance therapy is often required and includes vitamin D therapy, which may be discontinued in 2 to 3 months. Although rare, hypocalcemia may persist for the life of the cat. One author reported that when both thyroids and parathyroid glands were surgically removed from a group of normal cats, hypocalcemia was identified shortly after thyroid and parathyroidectomy. However, with no supportive care normal calcium levels were maintained despite low normal parathormone levels for the duration of the study. Despite the results of the report, the owner should be warned of the potential clinical problems associated with hypoparathyroidism after surgery. After unilateral thyroidectomy, thyroid supplementation is not necessary. After bilateral thyroidectomy, cats

**Figure 21–8.** Unilateral thyroid tumor after extracapsular surgical removal from a cat. The arrow indicates the cranial parathyroid gland. Because the contralateral thyroid lobe and associated parathyroid tissue were not removed, it was not necessary to dissect the cranial parathyroid gland on the affected lobe.

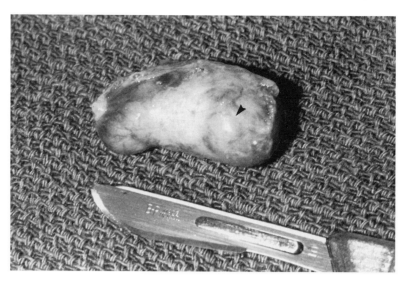

should receive 0.1 mg/day thyroxine daily to treat hypothyroidism. Thyroid hormone should be evaluated shortly after completion of therapy and then every 6 months to monitor for recurrence after thyroidectomy.

## Surgical Techniques[9,30]

Surgical treatment of feline hyperthyroidism is accomplished by either extracapsular or intracapsular thyroidectomy (see Fig. 21–9). In the extracapsular technique, without the capsule being opened, the entire thyroid gland, parathyroid gland, and capsule are removed. In the intracapsular technique, the capsule is opened and the thyroid gland is teased away from the capsule, leaving the cranial parathyroid gland, using Q-tips or other surgical tools to bluntly dissect the capsule from the gland. In the modified intracapsular technique, the thyroid capsule is

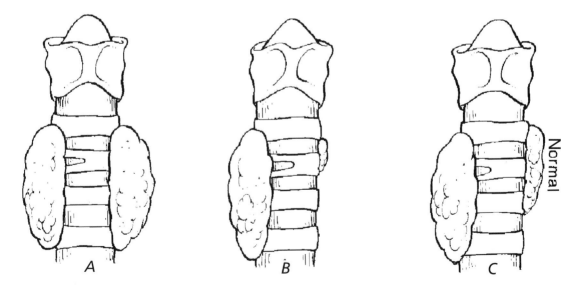

**Figure 21–9.** The surgeon is faced with 3 possibilities: *A,* Obvious bilateral thyroid enlargement. Bilateral thyroidectomy is indicated. *B,* Unilateral enlargement with atrophy of the contralateral lobe. Unilateral extracapsular thyroidectomy of the enlarged lobe is indicated. *C,* Unilateral thyroid enlargement with a "normally sized" contralateral lobe. Unilateral thyroidectomy is indicated, but serum T4 assay should be performed every 3 months to check for the recurrence of hyperthyroidism.

removed after the gland has been removed, while preserving the parathyroid gland. In either case, a ventral midline surgical approach with the neck in slight hyperextension is used. The incision should extend from the larynx to a point just cranial to the manubrium. The sternohyoid and sernothyroid muscles are bluntly separated and retracted with a Gelpi retractor. The thyroid glands are exposed and removed, but care is taken to leave at least one of the parathyroid glands intact using intracapsular resection technique.

**Radioactive Iodine Therapy[28,29,31,32]** Radioactive iodine therapy involves a single intravenous or oral administration of radioactive iodine.[131] The I[131] is taken up by the hyperfunctional tissue very rapidly; therefore normal tissue is generally preserved. A persistent hyperthyroidism has been reported in up to 18% of the cases treated intravenously and this may require additional therapy. Hypothyroidism is identified in approximately the same percentage of cases after treatment. Recently 40 cats with hyperthyroidism were evaluated. Each was treated using 200 to 300 mEq of orally administered I[131]. Thirty-six cases (90%) were successfully treated, as assessed by the resolution of clinical signs and reduction of plasma thyroxine concentrations to normal or reduced values after treatment. Higher doses of I[131] are required when the radioisotope is administered orally than when administered intravenously. Oral administration is less stressful and offers possible advantages for treating thyrotoxic cats. Hypoparathyroidism is generally not a risk in this procedure. Although radioactive iodine therapy appears to be a safe form of treatment, it has disadvantages because the animals must be contained within a special room and handled with specific guidelines for 2 to 3 weeks after treatment because of the highly radioactive excrement. Few institutions are licensed to apply this therapy. I[131] may be most valuable for treating small functional nodules of metastatic disease that are hard to find or treat surgically.

## Prognosis

With appropriate therapy, the prognosis for cure is excellent (Fig. 21–10). Operative mortality has been documented to be as high as 9%, but in the cats that died, thyroid function frequently was not normalized prior to surgery. Therefore, to minimize the anesthetic risk for thyrotoxic cats, appropriate preoperative management should be employed. Cats with cardiomyopathy should be appropriately treated and stabilized prior to surgery. Medical management of hyperthyroidism is directly related to the owner's ability to treat their cats appropriately.[25] The probability for adverse effects of medical management is low but still a concern. Radioactive iodine[131] is generally safe and effective despite the time required to employ this treatment. A few cats must be retreated because of underdosing or inability of the active thyroid tissue to take up the I[131].

## Comparative Aspects[19]

The biologic behavior of canine and feline thyroid tumors is markedly different (Table 21–1). Grave's disease in people (a type of hyperthyroidism) is an immune-mediated disorder whereby circulating autoantibodies release excess thyroid hormone and is most common in young women. Exophthalmos is seen in people with this disorder. The Grave's disease syndrome that occurs in people is rarely identified in cats. Histologic changes seen in cats with hyperthyroidism closely resemble toxic nodular goiter, which is characterized by one or more hyperfunctioning adenomas and is seen in elderly people.[19]

## HYPERADRENOCORTICISM

Hyperadrenocorticism is a common systemic disease in dogs and a less common condition in cats. It results from an excessive amount of circulating cortisol. The disorder occurs most commonly secondary to pituitary-dependent hyperadrenocorticism (PDH) and less commonly is caused by an adrenocortical tumor (AT). The two disorders (PDH and AT) have very similar clinical signs.

## Incidence and Risk Factors

Hyperadrenocorticism is the most common endocrinopathy in the dog.[9] Eighty to 90% of dogs with hyperadrenocorticism have the pituitary-dependent form of the disease, whereas the remainder have adrenocortical tumors. The condition is rare in the cat, with pituitary-dependent adrenal adenomas and bilateral adrenocortical hyperplasia being reported.[35–37] Middle-aged to older (> 6 years of age) dogs are affected, with poodles, dachshunds, and boxers at increased risk. There is no sex predilection for dogs with pituitary-dependent hyperadrenocorticism. Dogs with adrenal-dependent tumors are generally

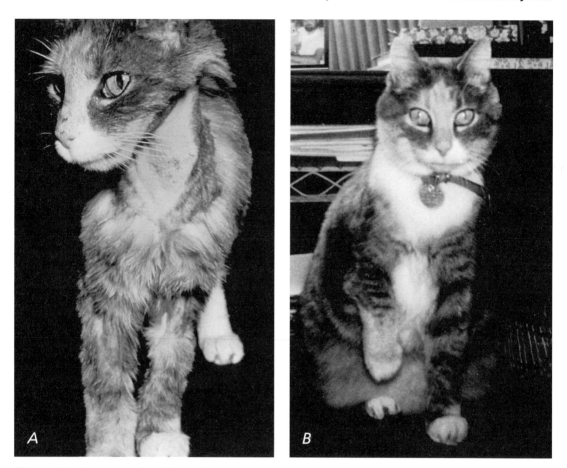

**Figure 21–10.** Hyperthyroid cat shown A, at presentation, and B, 2 years after bilateral thyroidectomy. This cat demonstrates that with appropriate therapy all clinical signs are reversible and the prognosis is good.

older (mean 10.5 years, range 5 to 15 years) and of larger body size.[39] Seventy to 75% of dogs with adrenal tumors are females. Cats with hyperadrenocorticism are middle-aged to older (mean 10.4 years, range 7 to 15 years) and it occurs more frequently in females (70%).[35–37]

## Pathology and Natural Behavior

PDM in dogs and cats is most often caused by adenomas that arise from the pars distalis, but pars intermedia tumors have also been described. The pituitary tumors secrete variable amounts of adrenocorticotropic hormone (ACTH), which subsequently results in bilateral adrenocortical hyperplasia and subsequently elevated cortisol levels. Adrenal tumors occur very infrequently in the dog (10–15%), and they are seen in the cat (approximately 19%).[35,51] In dogs and cats with adrenal tumors, there is excessive production of cortisol by the adrenocortical tumors that feed back on the hypothalamic pituitary-adrenal axis and cause decreased pituitary ACTH production. Adrenal adenomas and carcinomas occur with equal frequency and the right and left adrenal glands are equally affected. About 50% of adrenal carcinomas have gross evidence of liver metastases, and invasion of the caudal vena cava, renal vein, and phrenicoabdominal vein has been reported.

## History and Clinical Signs

Dogs with pituitary-dependent and adrenal-dependent hyperadrenocorticism have clinical signs that result from excessive circulating cortisol.[38] The most common clinical sign is polyuria/polydipsia, which occurs in about 85% of the cases. Other clinical signs seen are pendulous abdomen, hepatomegaly, skin atrophy, hair

**Table 21–1** Comparison of Canine and Feline Thyroid Tumors

|  | Canine | Feline |
|---|---|---|
| Incidence rate | Low | Moderate |
| Geographic incidence | None | Possibly higher on East and West coasts |
| % Malignant | 80–90% | < 1% |
| Local invasion | Common | Rare |
| Metastatic behavior | Common with larger primary tumors | Rare |
| Association with hyperthyroidism | < 5% | > 90% |
| Association with cardiac disease | None | 50–70% |
| Appropriate therapeutic modalities | Surgery, doxorubicin, cisplatin, radiation | Antithyroid drugs, surgery, $I^{131}$ |

loss, lethargy, polyphagia, muscle weakness, anestrus, and obesity. Muscle atrophy, comedones, increased panting, testicular atrophy, hyperpigmentation, calcinosis cutis, facial dermatosis, and facial nerve palsy may also occur. If a large pituitary mass is present, then central nervous system (CNS) signs may be present (e.g., seizures, blindness, dementia). It should be noted that pituitary tumors are generally quite small but occasionally can be large and result in CNS problems. Other less common signs in the dog include secondary bacterial infections of the skin, lungs, and urinary tract caused by cortisol-induced immunosuppression. Thromboembolism has also been described.[39–42] Diabetes mellitus occurs in about 20% of affected dogs from the antagonistic effect of cortisol and insulin.[43] Dogs with adrenal carcinomas display a rapid onset of progressive signs, often without the severe dermatologic signs seen with pituitary-dependent hyperadrenocorticism. Cats with hyperadrenocorticism frequently have polyuria, polydipsia, a pendulous abdomen, and polyphagia.[35–37] Truncal and abdominal alopecia, unkempt haircoat, thin skin, bruising, and abscesses are also seen, along with muscle wasting, weight gain, hepatomegaly, infection, or depression. In dogs, polyuria and polydipsia occur early in the syndrome, whereas in cats the polyuria and polydipsia occur later because of a glucocorticoid-induced hyperglycemia. Indeed 81% of cats with hyperadrenocorticism have concurrent diabetes mellitus, whereas only 10 to 15% of dogs with hyperadrenocorticism develop diabetes mellitus.[35–37,38] Therefore any cat with diabetes mellitus should be evaluated for hyperadrenocorticism, especially when other clinical signs associated with this disease occur.

## Diagnosis

The diagnosis of hyperadrenocorticism in the dog and cat can be complex and at times frustrating. The following general points should be kept in mind during the diagnostic workup.[35–38,43–56]

1. The diagnosis of hyperadrenocorticism is made in part by having a supportive history and the results of a physical examination.
2. The results of routine laboratory tests will support a diagnosis of hyperadrenocorticism.
3. The low-dose dexamethasone suppression test and the ACTH stimulation test (corticotropin) are the most reliable screening tests for hyperadrenocorticism.
4. The diagnosis of hyperadrenocorticism is made by evaluating all of the parameters: history, physical examination, supporting laboratory tests, and screening tests.
5. More definitive diagnostic tests should be employed after strong supportive evidence has been obtained for hyperadrenocorticism.

Endogenous ACTH (corticotropin) concentrations and a high-dose dexamethasone suppression test can be definitive; however, these tests sometimes need to be combined with computerized tomography, magnetic resonance imaging, ultrasonography, or plain radiography. The diagnosis of hyperadrenocorticism in the dog and cat should begin with a CBC, a biochemical profile, a urinalysis, radiographs, and other miscellaneous tests. In the dog, the most common abnormality on the hemogram is a stress leukogram.[38] Occasionally the packed cell volume is slightly above normal.

## Diagnosis in the Dog

The following biochemical abnormalities are seen commonly in dogs with hyperadrenocorticism:[38,56] increased alkaline phosphatase (45–85%), increased alanine transaminase (50 to 60%), elevation in serum cholesterol (80 to 90%), mild elevations in plasma glucose (50 to 60%), and overt diabetes mellitus (5 to 10% of cases). Other abnormalities seen on the biochemical profile include decreased blood urea nitrogen, lipemia, and an increased bromsulphalein (BSP) retention. A urinalysis is essential for the workup of these patients. Eight-five percent of the dogs have a specific gravity below 1.015, caused by the polyuria and polydipsia. In addition, glucosuria is seen in most cases that have diabetes mellitus. Because urinary tract infections are common in dogs with hyperadrenocorticism, a sediment should be evaluated and, if indicated, appropriate cultures should be submitted. Mild proteinuria may result from steroid-induced systemic hypertension and subsequent glomerulonephritis. Radiographs frequently demonstrate hepatomegaly; excellent abdominal contrast due to the increased fat within the abdomen; a potbellied appearance; distended bladder; osteoporosis; calcinosis cutis or dystrophic calcification; adrenal calcification in animals with adrenal tumors; and, rarely, evidence of congestive heart failure, pulmonary thromboembolism, calcification of the trachea and main-stem bronchi, and pulmonary metastases of adrenal carcinomas.[28,38] Other tests that may be supportive but not diagnostic for hyperadrenocorticism include low basal concentrations of an adequate $T_4$ and $T_3$ response to TSH, and systemic hypertension.

## ACTH Stimulation Test[37,44]

An ACTH stimulation test is a valuable screening test for diagnosing hyperadrenocorticism in the dog.[37,42–49] It is performed by sampling before and 2 hours after giving 2.2 units/kg, up to a maximum dose of 20 units, of ACTH gel intramuscularly for sampling before and 1 hour after giving 0.5 units/kg of the aqueous ACTH intravenously. Hyperadrenocorticism is strongly suspected when there is an excessive increase in serum cortisol concentrations. Each laboratory should be queried to obtain their normal values for these tests. About 85% of PDH cases and only about 50% of AT cases will show a diagnostic hyperresponse with the ACTH stimulation test.

## Low-Dose Dexamethasone Suppression Test[38,44,46]

The low-dose dexamethasone suppression test is an accurate screening test for hyperadrenocorticism in the dog. The test is performed by sampling before, and 3 and 8 hours after giving 0.01 to 0.015 mg/kg dexamethasone intravenously or intramuscularly. The serum cortisol concentration after the administration of dexamethasone is less than 1 µg/dl in normal dogs 3 and 8 hours after the test dose of dexamethasone has been administered. Dogs with hyperadrenocorticism generally will not suppress less than 1 µg/dl. The test is diagnostic for 100% of dogs with adrenal tumors and 96% of dogs with PDH.

## High-Dose Dexamethasone Suppression Test[38,44]

To differentiate PDH from AT, the high-dose dexamethasone suppression test should be performed or an endogenous ACTH level obtained. The high-dose dexamethasone suppression test is performed by taking serum samples before and 3 and 8 hours after the IV administration of 1 to 2 mg/kg dexamethasone. The suppression of serum cortisol concentrations below 1.5 µg/dl is diagnostic for PDH and rules out ATs.

## ACTH Test

Plasma ACTH levels are elevated (> 40 pg/ml) in dogs with PDH and are low to low normal (< 20 pg/ml) in dogs with adrenal tumors.[50] Because ACTH is a highly labile peptide, blood samples should be taken as specifically directed by the laboratory performing the assay. This frequently involves obtaining samples in plastic containers and placing them on ice, centrifuging them in a cold centrifuge, and freezing the plasma immediately after the red cells have been removed. Only the ACTH assays validated for the dog should be used.

## Miscellaneous Tests[44,47]

Unfortunately, 15% of dogs with PDH will not show suppression with the high-dose dexamethasone suppression test. If calcification in the area of the adrenal gland is seen on abdominal radiographs, a diagnosis of adrenocortical tumor can be made and no additional testing is needed. If calcification of the adrenal gland is not seen, or if a single adrenal mass is not identified by other diagnostic methods, performing an endogenous plasma ACTH level may be helpful. In addition, exploratory laparotomy, adrenal gland scintigraphy, computerized tomography, or magnetic resonance imaging can be done to establish an etiology for the disease.

### Urine Cortisol Test[47]

The measurement of urine cortisol metabolites is a viable screening test for hyperadrenocorticism in dogs. The measurement of urine cortisol concentrations from a randomly obtained single urine sample has been evaluated recently. In addition, urine cortisol-creatinine ratios have also been evaluated. The advantage over other screening tests of measuring the urine cortisol-creatinine ratio is that the test can be performed with only one free-catch urine sample. A recent study demonstrated that the urine cortisol-creatinine ratio is highly sensitive in separating normal dogs from those with hyperadrenocorticism.[47] This procedure, however, did not adequately separate dogs with hyperadrenocorticism from dogs with polyuria/polydipsia related to other causes. Therefore, the test is highly sensitive but not specific.

### Diagnosis in the Cat[34–36]

As in the dog, there are many laboratory abnormalities associated with hyperadrenocorticism in the cat. Ninety-three percent of cats have hyperglycemia, 87% have glucosuria, 77% have hypercholesterolemia, and more than half have evidence of a corticosteroid leukogram. Approximately 40 to 50% have increased serum alkaline phosphatase and alanine aminotransferase. A decreased blood urea nitrogen is seen in approximately 20% of the cats with this condition. Hepatomegaly is observed on radiographs in more than half of the cats. Calcification of the adrenal gland occurs in some normal cats; therefore it should be evaluated with caution when diagnosing an adrenal tumor.

### ACTH Stimulation Test

An ACTH stimulation test is an effective screening test for hyperadrenocorticism in the cat. The test is performed by collecting blood for plasma cortisol concentrations before, and 1 and 2 hours after the intramuscular injection of ACTH gel given at a dose of 2.2 units/kg. Synthetic ACTH (Cosyntropin 0.125 mg/cat) can be administered intramuscularly and samples can be taken at 30 and 60 minutes. Most cats show an exaggerated response to the administration of ACTH, which is similar to that seen in dogs.

### Dexamethasone Suppression Tests

When the ACTH stimulation test is not supportive of a diagnosis or if it is equivocal, then a low- or high-dose dexamethasone suppression test can be performed. In a low-dose dexamethasone suppression test, serum cortisol concentrations are determined prior to and 8 hours after the administration of 0.01 to 0.015 mg/kg dexamethasone IV. Failure to suppress below 50% of the basal levels may suggest the presence of hyperadrenocorticism. It should be noted that low-dose dexamethasone suppression is not as useful for diagnosing hyperadrenocorticism in cats as it is in dogs. Therefore, a high-dose dexamethasone suppression test is often used to diagnose hyperadrenocorticism more accurately. In the high-dose suppression test, the dexamethasone is administered intravenously at a dose of 1.0 mg/kg IV. In a normal cat this dose causes a consistent and reliable suppression of cortisol values, whereas cats with hyperadrenocorticism do not suppress 2 hours after the administration of dexamethasone. In summary, it is currently suggested that a dexamethasone suppression test using 0.1 mg/kg may be a reliable screening test for feline hyperadrenocorticism. A dexamethasone suppression test using 1 mg/kg is appropriate for distinguishing pituitary-dependent from adrenal tumors in cats.

### Therapy

Canine PDH can be treated with surgical hypophysectomy (rarely performed), bilateral adrenalectomy, and more commonly medical therapy. Cyproheptadine and bromocriptine have been reported to lower pituitary ACTH secretion. The treatment of choice for PDH is o,p'-DDD (mitotane, lysodren).[38,41,51,54] o,p'-DDD causes necrosis and atrophy of the adrenal cortex, which secretes glucocorticoids but spares the zona glomerulosa that produces mineralocorticoids. Many dosing regimens are recommended, including administering lysodren at a dosage of 50 mg/kg divided twice daily for 10 to 14 days. This loading dose of lysodren results in a rapid decline in serum cortisol concentrations. Because adverse effects (e.g., anorexia, weakness, vomiting, diarrhea) can occur even without an excessive reduction in cortisol concentrations, frequently either prednisone or prednisolone is administered concurrently at a dosage of 0.2 mg/kg daily during the loading period. If clinical signs of glucocorticoid deficiency occur, the o,p'-DDD therapy should be discontinued and higher dosages of prednisone should be administered.

Dogs with concurrent diabetes mellitus and hyperadrenocorticism should be treated with a less aggressive protocol using 25 mg/kg for a loading dose because reduction in cortisol concentrations may cause a substantial decrease in the insulin requirements of some dogs. After the loading dose, an ACTH stimulation test should be performed to assess treatment efficacy. Forty-eight hours prior to the administration of the test, the glucocorticoids that are being administered should be discontinued to prevent interference with the test. The goal of loading therapy is to suppress adrenocortical functions so that both the pre- and post-ACTH serum cortisol concentrations are in the normal resting range (i.e., both pre- and postvalues are in the range normally expected prior to the administration of ACTH). If the ACTH stimulation test reveals pre- and postcortisol concentrations that are in the range of normal dogs, additional (e.g., 3 to 5 days) loading is required.[38,41,51,54] After supplemental loading, an ACTH test should again be performed. In rare cases, 30 to 60 days of loading are required. In animals that have an excessive decrease in their ACTH cortisol concentrations, glucocorticoids should be administered for 2 to 6 weeks while further o,p'-DDD therapy is withheld. These animals should be reassessed with an ACTH stimulation test in approximately 4 to 6 weeks. Once adequate loading has been achieved, then o,p'-DDD is given in maintenance dosages of 50 mg/kg/week divided into 2 to 3 weekly doses. Exogenous glucocorticoids generally are not administered unless stress or illness occurs. If the animal exhibits signs of glucocorticoid deficiency, then o,p'-DDD should be discontinued and glucocorticoids again should be administered. Irreversible glucocorticoid and mineralocorticoid deficiency (Addison's disease) may occur but is uncommon. In these cases, a mineralocorticoid should be administered along with glucocorticoids. In all cases, ACTH stimulation tests should be repeated at 4, 8, and 12 months, and every 6 months thereafter when the dogs are well controlled. If it is obvious that a patient is coming out of remission, then another 5-day standard loading dose should be performed.

Other treatments for PDH include ketoconazole therapy, deprenyl, and radiation treatment.[55] Ketoconazole is an expensive antifungal drug that is effective for treating both pituitary-dependent and adrenal tumors. Ketoconazole given at 15 mg/kg twice daily orally results in rapid normalization of serum cortisol concentrations. The drug may cause vomiting and occa-

sionally hepatic damage. Halting ketoconazole therapy results in the immediate increase of serum cortisol concentrations. In cases of a large and symptomatic pituitary macroadenoma, radiation therapy is the treatment of choice. In addition, radiation therapy should be used for patients that are unresponsive to medical management, even if neurologic signs are not present. Deprenyl is currently being evaluated for use in dogs with PDH.

## Therapy—Cats with PDH

In cats with PDH, the therapeutic options are bilateral adrenalectomy, o,p'-DDD therapy, and megavoltage irradiation. The use of o,p'-DDD in cats is generally discouraged because the species is dramatically sensitive to hydrocarbons. Bilateral adrenalectomy followed by mineralocorticoid and glucocorticoid replacement is perhaps the most successful treatment for pituitary-dependent hyperadrenocorticism in the cat. Radiation therapy may be effective, especially for cats with macroadenomas.[9]

## Therapy—Dogs and Cats: ADH

Surgical removal is the treatment of choice for dogs and cats with adrenal tumors. A ventral midline approach is used to evaluate both adrenal glands and to examine all internal organs for metastatic disease, including regional lymph nodes and liver. Atrophy of the contralateral adrenal gland is a consistent finding with ATs. Histology is confusing (i.e., malignant tumors look like benign, and vice versa), so malignant or benign tumors are best determined clinically. Because removal of the affected adrenal tumor can result in glucocorticoid deficiency because of the atrophied contralateral gland, large doses of IV steroids should be administered the morning prior to surgery (5 mg/kg soluble hydrocortisone; 2 mg/kg prednisone sodium succinate; or 0.1 to 0.2 mg/kg dexamethasone). The steroids should be repeated after surgery. The day after surgery, 0.5 mg/kg prednisolone should be administered twice daily, subsequent doses tapered every 7 to 10 days, and then discontinued in 2 months. If both adrenal glands are enlarged, nonsuppressible PDH should be suspected. Biopsy should be performed; however, in the cat bilateral adrenalectomy and subsequent supplementation of glucocorticoids and mineralocorticoids may be beneficial. In dogs with ATs that undergo surgery, complication rates are minimal to as great as 50%.[39,53] Complications include cardiac arrest, pneumonia, pulmonary artery thromboembolism, pancreatitis, and acute renal failure. If metastatic disease is identified, then ketoconazole or a high dose (50 to 150 mg/kg/day) of o,p'-DDD can be used, but this treatment is rarely successful. Indeed, 32 dogs with cortisol-secreting adrenocortical neoplasms were treated with mitotane (o,p'-DDD) with a mean survival time of 16.4 months.[56]

## Prognosis[34–38]

Untreated dogs and cats with hyperadrenocorticism usually die from their disease. The causes of death include hypertension, cardiovascular disease, thromboembolism, diabetes mellitus, or serious bacterial infections. With surgical removal, the prognosis for adrenal adenomas is excellent. The prognosis for dogs with adrenal carcinomas, even after surgical excision, is often poor. Medical treatment for PDH generally prolongs and improves the quality of life in the dog and cat. As noted previously, about 10% of dogs with PDH can be successfully managed for more than 4 years.[38]

## Comparative Aspects[19]

Hyperadrenocorticism is not as common in people as it is in dogs. In people, as in dogs and cats, PDH is much more common than adrenal tumors. The incidence of adrenal adenomas and carcinomas is approximately equal in people, dogs, and cats.

## PANCREATIC HORMONE-SECRETING NEOPLASMS

Normally, pancreatic islets contain four specific cell types. A-cells secrete glucagon, B-cells secrete insulin, D-cells secrete somatostatin, and F- or P-cells secrete pancreatic polypeptide. In addition, tumors of islet cells may produce gastrin and ACTH, which normally are not produced by the pancreas. The most common functional islet cell tumors of small animals are insulin-secreting beta cell tumors known as insulinomas, and the less common gastrin-secreting tumor known as a gastrinoma.[51–75] A pancreatic polypeptide-secreting tumor has been documented in one dog.[70] Glucagon-secreting tumors in dogs are not clearly defined.

## Insulinoma

Pancreatic insulin-secreting tumors are also known as insulinomas, insulin-producing islet cell tumors, beta cell tumors, islet cell tumors, and insulin-producing pancreatic tumors. These pancreatic insulin-secreting tumors are uncommon in the dog but extremely rare in the cat (Fig. 21–11). It is a condition common in ferrets, and males predominate.[59] The tumor occurs in middle-aged to older dogs (mean age 9 years, range 2.5 to 15

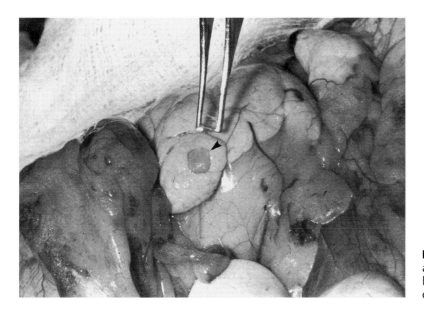

**Figure 21–11.** The arrow indicates a nodular insulin-secreting pancreatic mass in a dog.

years), with no sex predilection.[58] The most common breeds affected include boxers, German shepherds, Irish setters, standard poodles, collies, Labrador retrievers, and fox terriers.[58]

## Pathobiology

In the dog, both lobes of the pancreas are affected equally by insulin-producing tumors.[63] Almost all insulinomas are malignant, with metastases occurring via lymphatics to the regional lymph nodes and liver in about 50% of the cases.[9] Metastases have been documented in the mesentery, omentum, portal vessels, lungs, spleen, myocardium, and spinal meninges. It is frequently difficult to predict the metastatic behavior of insulinomas based on their histologic characteristics. Therefore, many pathologists prefer to classify them simply as islet cell tumors.

## History and Clinical Signs

The clinical signs associated with insulinomas in almost all affected species are a result of hypoglycemia that results from the release of insulin by the tumor.[57-71] In most cases, the initial historical and physical exam findings are subtle and often dismissed because of their obscure nature. As the disease progresses, the history and clinical signs include seizures, hind limb weakness, collapse, generalized weakness, ataxia, and muscle tremors.[60-64] Occasionally, owners describe exercise intolerance, depression, bizarre behavior or hysteria, irritability, polyphagia, and polydipsia/polyuria; the tumor may cause a relatively rapid decline and serum glucose levels that are not significantly below normal values. However, when blood glucose levels drop more slowly, the patient is able to adapt to extremely low levels of blood glucose before clinical signs are noted. The stimuli reported to induce hypoglycemia include fasting; exercise, excitement, or stress; and feeding that can induce insulin production by the tumor and result in hypoglycemia. The duration of clinical signs prior to diagnosis varies from 1 day to 3 years but in most studies averages approximately 3 months.[60-62] In one study, 29% of the cases were initially misdiagnosed and placed on anticonvulsant therapy.[68] Physical examination is usually unremarkable.

## Diagnosis

The diagnosis of an insulin-producing tumor in the dog, cat, or ferret is confirmed by noting a low blood glucose in association with the development of clinical signs and a concurrent, inappropriately high insulin level. In many studies, 95% of dogs have been hypoglycemic upon initial presentation.[60-63] The remaining dogs developed hypoglycemia after 8 to 12 hour periods of fasting. In rare cases, fasting for 72 hours may be necessary to induce the hypoglycemia. Dogs with insulinomas almost always display Whipple's triad, which includes clinical signs associated with hypoglycemia, fasting blood glucose $\leq$ 40 mg/dl, and the disappearance of clinical signs with dextrose administration.[64] Although insulinoma is most likely associated with Whipple's triad, other differentials must be considered, including improper blood sample handling; hypoadrenocorticism; sepsis; end-stage liver disease; hunting-dog hypoglycemia; starvation; extrapancreatic tumors (especially carcinomas of the liver); hepatoma of the liver; renal failure; heart failure; congenital hepatic enzyme deficiencies of glycogen storage diseases; exogenous insulin administration; oral hypoglycemic agents (e.g., sulfonylurea agents); ethanol, salicylate, and propranolol toxicity; and laboratory error.[64] Other routine laboratory tests such as a CBC, serum biochemical profile, and urinalysis are usually normal with the exception of hypoglycemia on the biochemical profile and the presence of elevated transaminases that do not necessarily correlate with hepatic metastases. Thoracic and abdominal radiographs may be taken but are usually normal. Hepatic, pancreatic, and regional lymph node ultrasonography may aid in identifying the extent of the disease. Serum insulin concentrations are elevated in 67 to 76% of dogs with insulinomas.[62,63] Insulin-glucose ratios of greater than 0.3 $\mu$U/mg and glucose-insulin ratios of < 2.5 suggest that an insulinoma is present. False negatives can occur in either case. The insulin-glucose ratio is defined by the following formula: serum insulin $\mu$U/ml $\times$ 100 divided by plasma glucose [mg/dl] – 30. When plasma glucose is $\leq$ 30, a value of 1 should be used for the denominator.[60,63] Ratios above 30 are indicative of insulin-secreting tumors. It should be noted that an elevated insulin-glucose ratio has also been identified in dogs with hypoglycemia secondary to sepsis or nonpancreatic tumors.[65,66] Provocative testing with a high-dose IV glucose tolerance test, a glucagon tolerance test, a L-leucine tolerance test, and tolbutamide has been described, but the risk for inducing symptomatic hypoglycemia is significant; therefore these provocative tests generally are not recommended. In all cases of hypoglycemia when an insulinoma is suspected, exploratory laparotomy is often the simplest, cheapest way to identify and potentially treat the problem.

## Treatment

The goals of treatment for an insulinoma include specific treatment for the tumor, reduction of insulin secretion, and correction of hypoglycemia. Surgery is the treatment of choice to obtain a biopsy and histologically confirm the etiology of the hypoglycemia, to reduce tumor burden and hopefully the severity of clinical signs, and to stage extent of the disease.[59–64,66] Surgery is rarely curative but in many patients it may prolong survival and improve the quality of life. Surgery results in longer survival than medical management, including chemotherapy.[60,63,67] To avoid hypoglycemic seizures, several small feedings are administered every 4 hours until 4 hours prior to surgery. If this is not feasible, the animal can be fasted overnight and maintained on dextrose-containing intravenous fluids. Blood glucose should be monitored frequently and the animal observed for any occurrence of seizures. In addition, during anesthesia the animal should be continuously monitored and glucose-containing fluids should be administered to maintain glucose levels within normal or near normal limits. A ventral midline incision is made from the xiphoid to the pubis and a routine abdominal exploratory performed.[9] The entire pancreas should be inspected and gently palpated. Intrapancreatic tumor masses are generally firm and often white or gray in color. They frequently are discrete nodules approximately 0.5 to 2 cm in diameter, although multiple nodular masses and diffuse infiltration of the pancreas have been rarely reported.[63] As noted previously, tumors equally involve both the right and left lobes of the pancreas. Therefore, if no discrete tumor is identified, partial pancreatectomy and subsequent histopathologic evaluation should be performed if possible. If at least one pancreatic duct cannot be preserved, a total pancreatectomy can be performed, although careful preservation of the common bile duct and the blood vessels to the duodenum is imperative. Discrete tumors of the head of the pancreas may be "shelled out" with a small cuff of normal surrounding tissue, whereas tumors of the right or left limbs are usually treated with resection of the limb and preservation of necessary blood vessels supplying the bowel (especially the pancreaticoduodenal artery on the right limb of the pancreas. The liver and regional lymph nodes should be examined carefully for any metastatic disease. The duodenal,

splenic, hepatic, and greater mesenteric lymph nodes should all be inspected. Suspicious nodes should be excised and examined histopathologically. It should be noted that dogs with diffuse metastatic disease have been medically managed for more than 1 year; therefore euthanasia at the time of surgery is not mandatory unless that is the owner's desire. In the ferret, multiple nodules are usually identified at surgery.[59]

Pancreatitis is a potential postoperative complication in the dog and ferret. This can result in tender abdomen and vomiting; therefore patients should be maintained on dextrose-containing fluids postoperatively and nothing per os.[59,67] If hypoglycemia persists for 2 days after surgery, then residual tumor should be suspected even when residual neoplastic tissue is not identified at surgery. Insulin-producing tumors can cause atrophy of normal islet tissue, and therefore persistent hyperglycemia, which may require insulin therapy for variable periods of time, can occur postoperatively. Medical management for hypoglycemia can be divided into short-term and chronic therapy.[64] Short-term therapy for acute episodes of hypoglycemia can involve placing corn syrup or other sources of high concentrations of glucose on the animal's gums and mouth if mild symptoms occur at home. If neurologic signs are significant, then 0.1 to 0.5 gm/kg dextrose is administered slowly intravenously in a 25% dextrose solution. Occasionally animals do not respond to this therapy if the hypoglycemic seizures are prolonged as a result of cerebral laminar necrosis, and anticonvulsive therapy may be required. Once the animal can swallow safely and when the risk of pancreatitis is past, small meals of a high-protein and high-fat diet should be fed frequently. When carbohydrates are provided, they should be complex rather than simple sugars. Therefore, semimoist diets that are very high in simple sugar should be avoided. When frequent feedings are ineffective for controlling clinical signs, prednisone is often a useful agent to prevent hypoglycemia. Prednisone acts by increasing hepatic gluconeogenesis and by inhibiting the effect of insulin on peripheral tissues.[64] Dosages starting at 0.25 mg/kg twice daily orally can be increased to 2 to 4 mg/kg twice a day as needed. Iatrogenic Cushing's disease frequently results from high dosages of prednisone. To manage hypoglycemia, diazoxide can also be utilized either alone or in combination with prednisone or hydrochlorothiazide diuretic.[64] Hydrochlorothiazide potentiates the effect of diazoxide. Diazoxide should be started at 5 mg/kg twice daily, but if necessary the dosage can be increased to 40 mg/kg twice daily.[64] Diazoxide increases serum glucose by inhibiting insulin secretion, decreasing peripheral uptake of glucose and increasing hepatic glycogenolysis and gluconeogenesis by adrenergic stimulation. Anorexia, vomiting, and diarrhea are sometimes seen as side effects. Other less common side effects of diazoxide therapy are diabetes mellitus, cataracts, sodium and fluid retention, bone marrow suppression, and tachycardia. Phenytoin, propranolol, and L-asparaginase have been suggested as other therapies for insulinomas, but their efficacy is unconfirmed. Streptozotocin and alloxan have been used to treat insulinomas in people, but these drugs are severely nephrotoxic and they should be used with caution in the dog.[69] Recently 50 dogs with metastatic insulinomas were treated with alloxan at a dosage of 65 mg/kg given once intravenously.[70] Other research is necessary to confirm the efficacy of this treatment.

Sandostatin (Octreotide, Sandoz) is a somatostatin analog that has been effective treatment in about 50% of people and two of five dogs with insulinomas.[68] This drug inhibits insulin synthesis and secretion. The initial dosage in dogs is 10 to 20 μg two to three times daily. Dogs become refractory after 1 to 2 weeks of therapy; therefore the value of sandostatin is unknown at this time.

## Prognosis

The average survival of dogs after surgery is approximately 10 to 14 months.[60–63] Survival is not correlated with breed, body weight, type of clinical signs, severity or frequency of clinical signs, preoperative serum glucose concentrations, or tumor location within the pancreas as long as it is resectable. Younger dogs tend to have shorter survival than older dogs.[63] Dogs with metastases to organs beyond the regional lymph nodes have a significantly shorter survival time (Figs. 21–12 and 21–13).[62] Dogs that present with clinical stage 1 (tumor confined to the pancreas) have a significantly longer disease-free interval after surgery than dogs with stage 2 (tumor located within the pancreas and regional lymph node) or 3 (tumor metastasizing beyond regional lymph

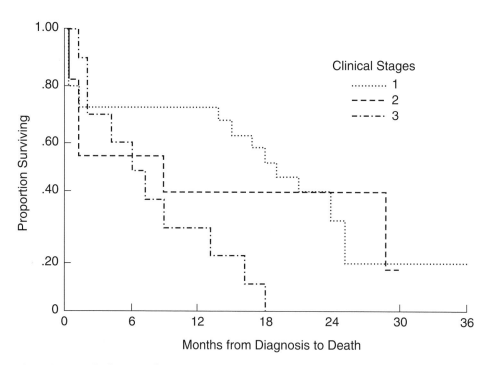

**Figure 21–12.** Survival curve after surgery in dogs with insulin-secreting islet cell tumors based on clinical stage. Dogs with metastasis of the tumor beyond the regional lymph nodes (clinical stage 3; $T_1$, $N_0$, $M_1$, or $N_1$, $M_1$) have significantly shorter survival times. However, dogs with metastasis to regional lymph nodes only (clinical stage 2: $T_1$, $N_1$, $M_0$) appear to show survival similar to dogs with tumor that appears to be confined to the pancreas (clinical stage 1: $T_1$, $N_0$, $M_0$) at the time of surgery. (Reprinted with permission.)[63]

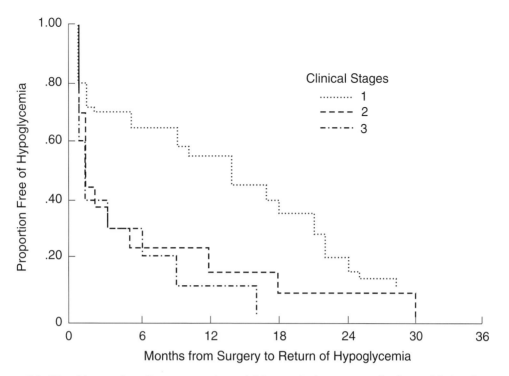

**Figure 21–13.** Disease-free (i.e., normoglycemia) interval after surgery in dogs with insulin-secreting islet cell tumors based on clinical stage. Dogs with tumor that appears to be confined to the pancreas (clinical stage 1; $T_1$, $N_0$, $M_0$) have a significantly longer disease-free interval after surgery than dogs with more advanced disease (clinical stages 2 and 3). Clinical stage 2 denotes the spread of tumor to local lymph nodes but not distant metastasis ($T_1$, $N_1$, $M_0$), while clinical stage 3 denotes distant metastasis with or without spread to local lymph nodes ($T_1$, $N_1$, $M_1$, or $N_0$, $M_1$). (Reprinted with permission.[63])

node). Fifty percent of the dogs with stage 1 disease have normal glucose levels for 14 months after surgery, whereas only 20% of the dogs with stages 2 and 3 have normal glucose levels for the same length of time. Reoperations may be considered in dogs with recurrence of clinical signs in hopes that further resection of the pancreas or regional nodes may be possible. Unfortunately, however, most will have unresectable liver metastasis. In ferrets, the median disease-free interval is 240 days and the median survival is 483 days.[59] Medical management with prednisone, diazoxide, alloxan, etc, is very effective for minimizing clinical signs in this species.

## Comparative Aspects[19]

Ninety percent of all insulin-secreting tumors in people are benign. Like the dog, the distribution of the tumor is throughout the pancreas. Surgery and medical management are similar in all species.

## GASTRIN-SECRETING ISLET CELL TUMORS

Islet cell tumors that secrete excessive amounts of gastrin are known as gastrinomas or Zollinger-Ellison syndrome.[71–75] Gastrin stimulates hydrochloric acid secretion from the gastric parietal cells of the stomach. It also exerts a trophic effect on the mucosa of the gastrointestinal tract. Gastric acid output is stimulated by gastrin, histamine, and acetylcholine. Therefore gastric acid secretion is controlled therapeutically by use of specific receptor antagonist for these three secretagogues.

## History and Clinical Signs

Gastrinomas usually occur in middle-age, dogs, with females more commonly affected than males.[70] Older cats are usually affected; however, the condition is extremely uncommon in cats.[70–75] The most common clinical signs are vomiting and weight loss, followed by depression, lethargy, anorexia, and intermittent diarrhea.[70–75] The duration of clinical signs ranges from 2 weeks to 2 years prior to presentation. The average time clinical signs have persisted in cats prior to presentation is about 8 weeks.[70,74]

## Diagnosis

CBC documents a regenerative anemia in approx- imately 44% of the cases, leukocytosis in 44%, neutrophilia in 30%, and increased band cells in 11%.[70] Hyperglycemia, hypoalbuminemia, hypocalcemia, hypokalemia, and increased alkaline phosphatase levels are infrequent but are the most common biochemical abnormalities.[70] A barium series may reveal plaquelike lesions within the stomach or duodenum, consistent with ulceration. These may also be identified on gastroscopy. In addition, gastroscopic examination may reveal thickened gastric rugae, gastric ulceration and hemorrhage, excessive liquid in the stomach, duodenal ulceration, and a hypertrophic pyloric antrum. A definitive diagnosis is made by the identification of elevated fasting gastrin concentrations and basal gastric acid secretion, or by use of provocative tests such as secretin and calcium challenge. These findings, in combination with the clinical signs and confirmation of ulceration and proliferation of the stomach and duodenum, are often diagnostic. At surgery dogs and cats with gastrinoma have an islet cell tumor of the pancreas.[70–75] The tumor appears more commonly in the right lobe and body of the pancreas. Frequently there is a solitary nodule, but multiple masses are found in approximately 30 to 40% of cases.[70] Seventy-two percent of the cases have metastases with the liver and regional lymph nodes as the most common site.[70–75]

## Treatment

Treatment includes removal of the specific tumor.[70–75] The same surgical procedure as for insulinoma should be used. Medical management involves direct medical manipulation of gastrin production from the tumor and by management of gastric acid hypersecretion. Management of gastrin production from the tumor may be successfully accomplished by using sandostatin, a somatostatin analog noted previously. Somatostatin inhibits serum gastrin levels and parietal cell hydrogen secretion. Management of gastric

acid production includes anticholinergics, histamine blockers, proton pump inhibitors, and somatostatin analogs. $H_2$ receptor antagonists are effective in modulating gastric acid production and include cimetidine at a dosage of 5 to 10 mg/kg every 4 to 6 hours.[70–75] It should be noted that because of the ulcerogenic potential of the gastrin-secreting tumors, this dosage is somewhat higher than that routinely used for the treatment of gastric ulcers from other causes. Ranitidine is another $H_2$ receptor antagonist that is administered at 2 mg/kg orally or intravenously every 8 hours. Omeprazole* is a proton pump inhibitor and a potent inhibitor of gastric acid secretion. Although it is very effective, it is also expensive. The dosage most commonly used is 2 $\mu$Mol/kg orally daily. Other treatments for gastric ulceration include sucralfate given at a dosage of 1 gm every 8 hours for large dogs and half a gram every 8 hours for small dogs. Cats can be dosed with sucralfate at 0.5 to 0.25 gm every 8 to 12 hours. Caution should be used when other drugs are combined with sucralfate because sucralfate may inhibit the absorption of these drugs.

## Prognosis

As mentioned previously, gastrinomas are highly malignant, with approximately 75% of cases having metastatic disease at the time of diagnosis.[70–75] Surgery and medical management have resulted in survival times ranging from 1 week to 18 months, with an average of 4.8 months.

## PANCREATIC PEPTIDOMA

Pancreatic peptidoma is rare in the pancreas of dogs and cats.[70] Clinical signs resemble those of gastrinoma and include chronic vomiting, hypertrophic gastritis, duodenal ulceration, and fasting hypergastrinemia.[70] No studies have been performed in dogs or cats to confirm the efficacy of various diagnostic and therapeutic modalities.

## NON-ENDOCRINE-PRODUCING PITUITARY TUMORS

A variety of nonfunctional tumors of the pituitary gland in the dog and cat are described.[76–78]

*Losec, Merck, Sharpe and Dohme

They include adenomas of the pars distalis, aci-dophil adenoma of the pars distalis, basal cell ade-noma of the pars distalis, pituitary chromophobe carcinoma, and craniopharyngiomas. Many of these tumors cause hypopituitarism. Because the diaphragm sella is incomplete in dogs, these tumors can invade dorsally and cause brain dam-age that results in cranial nerve abnormalities and thalamic functional abnormalities. When there is decreased growth hormone secretion prior to clo-sure of the epiphyseal plates, there can be decreased long-bone growth. Diabetes insipidus can occur as a result of structural impedance, with the release of antidiuretic hormone, which can result in polyuria and subsequent polydipsia. In addition, there can be reduction in the secretion of ACTH and TSH, which result in hypoadrenocor-ticism and hypothyroidism.

## GROWTH HORMONE EXCESS

In cats, people, and rarely dogs, a growth hor-mone-secreting tumor of the pituitary gland may cause excess secretion, which results in acromegaly.[79-81] This problem occurs primarily in the cat but is quite rare in any species.

### Clinical Features

Acromegaly in any species, especially a cat, results from excess secretion of growth hormone in mature animals. Dogs and cats with this condition are middle-aged or older.[80,81] Mixed-breed cats are most commonly affected, with soft tissue swelling and hypertrophy of the face and extremities. Increased proliferation of connective tissue causes increased body size, weight gain, and enlargement of the abdomen and face. In addition, the skin becomes thickened and develops excessive folds, especially around the head and neck. Growth hypertrophy of all the organs of the body occurs, including the heart, liver, kidneys, and tongue. Clinicians frequently become aware of this partic-ular problem because the animals, especially cats, are presented for polyuria/ polydipsia, which sub-sequently is found to be associated with diabetes mellitus.[79-81] Growth hormone excess has a pow-erful diabetogenic activity, which can result in hyperglycemia from peripheral insulin resistance. Any cat that has refractory diabetes mellitus and any of the systemic or morphologic changes asso-ciated with acromegaly should be investigated for growth hormone excess.[81]

## Diagnosis

The most common clinicopathologic features of feline growth hormone excess and resultant acromegaly include hyperglycemia, glycosuria without ketonuria, increased liver enzyme con-centrations, hyperphosphatemia, hyperproteine-mia, hypercholesterolemia, and an increase in red blood cell mass and numbers.[81] Similar findings are noted in the dog. A definitive diagnosis of acromegaly from growth hormone excess is made by documenting the marked elevation in circulating growth hormone concentrations. Because many conditions, such as renal failure, result in growth hormone concentration eleva-tions, this elevated growth excess should be con-firmed by identifying the presence of a pituitary mass or by evaluation of pituitary growth hor-mone responsiveness to a glucose suppression test. To perform the glucose suppression test, glucose is administered at 1 gm/kg either orally or intravenously.[79-81] An animal will have sup-pression in the circulating growth hormone con-centrations to less than 5 µg/ml within 60 min-utes, whereas growth hormone concentrations remain elevated in acromegaly. Computerized tomography or magnetic resonance imaging enhances the identification of a mass in the area of the pituitary gland or hypothalamus.

## Treatment

Treatment involves either surgery, radiation ther-apy, or medical management. Surgery to remove the pituitary tumor requires substantial expertise and is not a viable option in clinical practice. Radi-ation therapy delivered to the tumor may reduce growth hormone excess.[79-81] To date no large studies exist that document the efficacy of radia-tion therapy for pituitary tumors that induce growth hormone excess. Medical therapy for growth hormone excess includes estrogen ther-apy, dopaminergic agents, and long-acting somatostatin analogs.[79-81] Cats with growth hor-mone excess are frequently diagnosed with refractory diabetes mellitus; therefore persistent therapy for the diabetes mellitus is essential.

## Prognosis

Survival times for cats with acromegaly range from 8 to 30 months.[79-81] All cats eventually die or are euthanatized because of severe congestive heart failure, renal failure, or expanding pituitary tumor.

# PARATHYROID TUMORS

Parathyroid tumors can cause altered calcium homeostasis but are very rare clinical disorders in the dog and cat. Older dogs (7 to 13 years) of either sex are most commonly affected.[82] Keeshonds may be over-represented. Cats with hyperparathyroidism are usually older and, like the dog, are presented for nonspecific mild clinical signs. The dog is more likely to be presented with signs such as polyuria/polydipsia, normal phosphatemia, and urinary tract bacteria and calculi, whereas the cat is less likely to have polydipsia, bacteremia, and calculi. Dogs and cats are more likely to have adenomas than carcinomas of the parathyroid gland.[81–86] Because the most common clinical manifestation of parathyroid tumors is hypercalcemia, other etiologies must be considered, including lymphoma, adenocarcinoma of the apocrine glands of the anal sac, multiple myeloma, vitamin D toxicity, hypoadrenocorticism, renal failure, and skeletal disorders. Treatment of hypercalcemia is discussed elsewhere in this text (Chap. 4).

## Diagnosis

A good history, a physical examination, a serum biochemical profile, thoracic and abdominal radiographs, a biopsy of any palpable lymph nodes, a rectal examination for any perirectal masses, and thorough questioning regarding the possible exposure of the dog or cat to vitamin D supplementation or a rodenticide are all essential. Because it is very important to rule out lymphoma, an evaluation of the lymph nodes must be made. Bone marrow biopsy is recommended to rule out occult sources of malignant lymphocytes. Cervical palpation in affected dogs and cats rarely identifies parathyroid masses,[81–86] because usually they are quite small in size. The most common complication associated with hypercalcemia is hypercalcemic nephropathy, which can result in the typical changes associated with compromised renal function. Measurement of serum parathormone- or parathormone-related peptide (PTH-rp) may help differentiate the presence of primary hyperparathyroidism or hyperparathyroidism caused by a malignant condition. Ideally, these are performed prior to surgical exploration of the neck. The diagnosis of primary hyperparathyroidism is frequently a diagnosis for exclusion because parathyroid adenomas are so uncommon. When all other etiologies have been ruled out, then surgical exploration of the thyroid/parathyroid area should be performed.

## Treatment

Parathyroid tumors are usually visible as distinct nodules separate from the associated thyroid and are larger than normal parathyroid glands. Surgical removal can be performed by blunt dissection. Other parathyroid glands, if visible, frequently are substantially diminished in size because of atrophy. Ectopic parathyroid tumors are rare. If the normal parathyroids are small bilaterally, more extensive exploration of the lower cervical area should be employed.

## Prognosis

After surgery, serum calcium concentrations must be monitored for at least 48 to 72 hours. Postoperative complications are very rare in the cat and more common in the dog. Complications include hypocalcemia, transient Horner's syndrome (damage to the vagus nerve), and persistent harsh vocalization (due to damage to the recurrent laryngeal nerve). Hypocalcemia is managed by vitamin D and calcium therapy, which is discussed elsewhere. Recurrence of parathyroid carcinomas and metastasis is possible.

# PHEOCHROMOCYTOMA

Pheochromocytomas are functional tumors that arise from the adrenal medulla and secrete catecholamines that cause vague and unusual clinical signs.[87–90] These tumors are rare in the dog and even rarer in the cat. Affected dogs and cats are generally older, with no sex or breed predisposition. The tumors usually do not metastasize and are locally invasive into the vena cava, liver, and kidneys. Increased release of catecholamines from these tumors can result in hypertension, panting, alterations in behavior, dyspnea, tremors, polydipsia/polyuria, anorexia, and reluctance to sleep. Severe hypertension can result in epistaxis, seizures, and cerebrovascular accidents. Occasionally the hypertension can result in ruptured vascular structures within the tumor or elsewhere, and a shock state from hypovolemia may ensue. These findings are usually episodic and frequently have a vague and prolonged history. Physical examination is usually nonspecific. Because of the episodic nature of the catecholamine release, hypertension may not be identified on a random blood pressure evaluation.[89] Occasionally partial obstruction of the vena cava by the tumor has resulted in ascites, edema of the rear legs, and distention of the caudal superficial

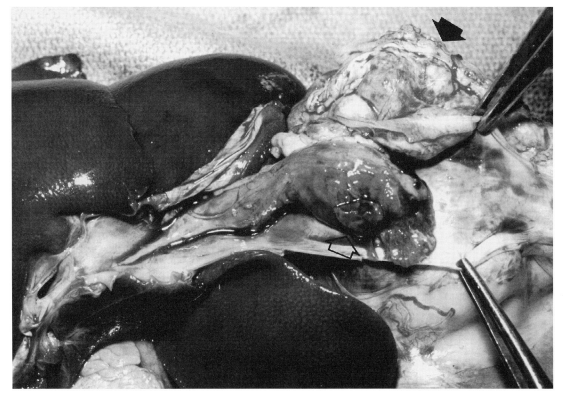

**Figure 21–14.** Pheochromocytoma (indicated by closed arrow) with local invasion into the caudal vena cava by tumor thrombus (indicated by open arrow).

epigastric veins (Fig. 21–14). Cardiac auscultation may reveal periods of tachycardia, arrhythmias, and cardiac murmurs. Dilated pupils are seen in some cases. Routine laboratory tests are usually nonspecific; however, occasionally hemoconcentration, anemia, neutrophilia, and proteinuria are noted. Abdominal radiographs and ultrasonography may reveal an adrenal mass. Venography is an essential study with or without ultrasonography of the vena cava and the adrenal gland to determine the extent of the tumor and its invasion into the caudal vena cava. When a venogram is performed, contrast media is rapidly injected into the lateral saphenous vein, followed by a series of abdominal radiographs. Constant measurement of blood pressures may aid in the identification of hypertension, which is usually episodic. Provocative testing using phentolamine, an alpha-adrenergic blocking agent, may cause significant and sustained falling blood pressure in hypertensive dogs with pheochromocytomas but have little effect on normal dogs.[89] Demonstration of circulating concentrations of catecholamines and increased urinary excretion of catecholamine metabolites is also very effective in the definitive diagnosis of this problem. Several excellent references review this procedure.[9,87–89]

## Therapy

Surgery is the treatment of choice.[9,87–89] The major role of medical therapy is to minimize the adverse effects associated with catecholamine release and to minimize the risk of surgery. Phenoxybenzamine hydrochloride, an alpha-adrenergic blocking agent, can be administered at 0.2 to 1.5 mg/kg orally twice daily for 10 to 14 days prior to surgery.[89] It may be advisable to start at the low end of the dose and slowly progress to the most effective dosage. Propranolol can also be used at 0.15 to 0.5 mg/kg three times a day to control cardiac arrhythmias and hypertension that is not controlled with phenoxybenzamine therapy.[89] Propranolol is a beta-adrenergic blocking agent and should not be administered without concurrent phenoxybenzamine therapy, or severe hypertension may be precipitated. Phenothiazines such as acepromazine should be avoided because they possess alpha blocking effect that may stimulate a hypotensive crisis.[87,89]

Narcotics are frequently considered for preanesthetics. Atropine is generally contraindicated because these animals frequently have tachycardia. In these cases, insoflurane is the agent of choice for maintenance. Arterial line monitoring of blood pressure and an electrocardiogram are essential to identify hypertensive or tachycardic crises. When they occur, they are treated with repeated intravenous boluses of phentolamine (0.02 to 0.1 mg/kg).[87,89] Hypotension is treated with fluid administration. Propranolol is frequently helpful for the treatment of intraoperative arrhythmias. Dissection of the tumor can be difficult because the vasculature may be abundant. Invasive tumors, especially those that involve thrombi growing into the vena cava, require sophisticated surgical techniques for removal. The preoperative venogram will hopefully have determined the presence or absence of a tumor thrombus in the vena cava and how far cranially it extends. The ventral thorax should be prepared for surgery (sternal split) in case the thrombus extends through the diaphragm. Even thrombi extending to the right atrium can occasionally be removed, because they are only minimally adherent to the wall of the vena cava.[89] In one study,[89] local tumor invasion was seen at surgery in 52% of the dogs, lymph node metastases were seen in 12%, and distant metastases were identified in 24%. The cause of death was tumor-related in 38% of dogs and non-tumor-related in 54%. For proper histopathologic evaluation, the tumor should be placed in Zenker's fixative without acetic acid rather than in formalin.[90] After surgery the patient should be monitored carefully for hypertension for several days. If hypertension is identified, then an incompletely resected tumor should be suspected.

## MULTIPLE ENDOCRINE NEOPLASIAS

Multiple endocrine neoplasia is a syndrome in which two or more neoplastic endocrine tumors simultaneously induce clinical signs.[19,91] There are three types of multiple endocrine neoplasia (MEN) in people. MEN-1 is parathyroid hyperplasia associated with pancreatic islet cell adenoma or carcinoma or hyperplasia of the anterior pituitary gland. MEN-2 or -2a is a medullary carcinoma of the thyroid associated with pheochromocytoma or parathyroid hyperplasia. MEN-3 or -2b is a medullary carcinoma of the thyroid gland associated with a pheochromocytoma or multiple mucosal neuromas. MEN-2a has been identified in dogs.

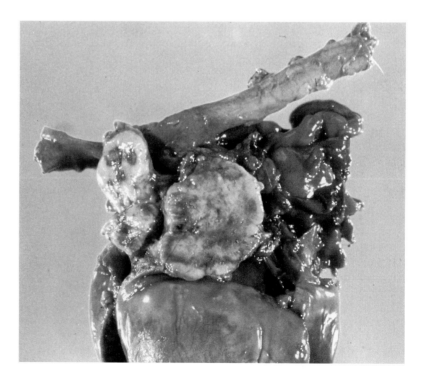

**Figure 21–15.** Invasive aortic body tumor at the heart base of a dog.

## CHEMODECTOMA

Chemodectoma or nonchromaffin paraganglioma occurs as an aortic body tumor or a carotid body tumor (Fig. 21–15).[9,19,92–97] These tumors are more common in the dog than the cat, but are uncommon in both species. Aortic body tumors account for 80 to 90% of chemodectomas; carotid body tumors account for the remainder.[94,95] Affected dogs are usually 10 to 15 years of age, with boxers and Boston terriers most commonly affected. There is no sex predilection in dogs with carotid body tumors, but male dogs may be more predisposed to aortic body tumors. The tumors range in size from 1 to 13 cm and are sometimes difficult to differentiate clinically from a thyroid carcinoma of that location. Larger tumors may cause congestive heart failure. The most common presenting clinical complaint for dogs with carotid body tumors is a neck mass with dysphagia, dyspnea, and regurgitation. At least 20% of these cases metastasize to the lungs, liver, myocardium, kidneys, lymph nodes, adrenal gland, brain, and bone. Local invasion, especially into the blood vessels, occurs in about 50% of the cases. Arteriovenous fistula has been documented in carotid body tumors in the dog. Mobile masses in the neck or on the heart are surgically excised and have good outcomes. However, most are fixed to underlying tissue and are quite difficult to excise completely. Most carotid body tumors are unilateral and may invade adjacent tissue, requiring rmoval of the carotid artery, vagosympathetic trunk, jugular vein, and associated neck muscles. Except for a unilateral Horner's syndrome, no permanent disability results from this surgery. Aortic body tumors are usually quite invasive and rarely completely resectable. Establishing a definitive diagnosis preoperatively is difficult and other neoplastic conditions such as ectopic thyroid carcinoma and hemangiosarcoma must be considered. The role of primary or adjuvant chemotherapy for these tumors is unknown.

## REFERENCES

1. Birchard SJ, Roesel OF: Neoplasia of the thyroid gland in the dog: A retrospective study of 16 cases. J Am Anim Hosp Assoc 17:369–372, 1981.
2. Brodey RS, Kelly DF: Thyroid neoplasms in the dog. Cancer 22:406–416, 1968.
3. Harari JR, Patterson JS, Rosenthal RC: Clinical and pathologic features of thyroid tumors in 26 dogs. J Am Vet Med Assoc 188:1160–1164, 1994.
4. Mitchell M, Hurov LI, Troy GC: Canine thyroid carcinomas: Clinical occurrence, staging by means of scintiscans, and therapy of 15 cases. Vet Surg 8:112–118, 1979.
5. Loar AS: Canine thyroid tumors. In Kirk RW (ed): Current Veterinary Therapy IX. Philadelphia, WB Saunders, 1986, pp. 1033–1039.
6. Jeglum KA, Whereat A: Chemotherapy of canine thyroid carcinoma. Compend Contin Educ Pract Vet 5:96–98, 1983.
7. Leav I, Schiller AL, Rijnberk A, et al: Adenomas and carcinomas of the canine and feline thyroid. Am J Pathol 83:61–93, 1976.
8. Harmelin A, Nyska A, Aroch I, et al: Canine thyroid carcinoma with unusual distant metastases. 5(2):284–288, 1983.
9. Wheeler S: Tumors of the endocrine system. In Withrow SJ, MacEwen EG (eds): Clinical Veterinary Oncology. Philadelphia, JB Lippincott, 1989, pp. 72–105.
10. Walsh KM, Diters RW: Carcinoma of ectopic thyroid in a dog. J Am Anim Hosp Assoc 20:665–668, 1982.
11. Rijnberk A: Iodine metabolism and thyroid diseases in the dog. PhD dissertation. Utrecht, Drukkerj Elinkwijk, 1971.
12. Haley PJ, Hahn FF, Muggonbury BA, Griffith WC: Thyroid neoplasms in a colony of beagle dogs. Vet Pathol 26(5):438–441, 1989.
13. Branum JE, Leighton RL, Hornoff WJ: Radioisotope imaging for the evaluation of thyroid neoplasia and hypothyroidism in the dog. J Am Vet Med Assoc 180:1077–1079, 1982.
14. Verschaeren CP, Rutteman GR, Kuiper-Dijkschoorn NJ, et al: Flow-cytometric DNA ploidy in primary and metastatic canine thyroid carcinomas. Anticancer Res 11(5):1755–1761, 1991.
15. Klein MK, Powers BE, Withrow SJ, et al: Treatment of carcinoma in dogs by surgical resection alone: 20 cases (1981–1989). JAVMA 206(7):1007–1009, 1995.
16. Peterson ME: Hypoparathyroidism. In Kirk RW (ed): Current Veterinary Therapy IX. Philadelphia, WB Saunders, 1986, pp. 1039–1045.
17. Mauldin GN: Radiation therapy for endocrine neoplasia. In Kirk RW, Bonagura D (eds): Current Veterinary Therapy XI. Philadelphia, WB Saunders, 1992, pp. 319–321.
18. Verschnaren CP, Selman PI, Mol JA, et al: Circulating thyroglobulin measurements by homologous radioimmunoassay in dogs with thyroid carcinoma. ACTA Endocrinol 125(3):291–298, 1991.
19. Norton JA, Doppman JL, Jensen RU: Cancer of the endocrine system. In DeVita VT et al (eds): Cancer: Principles and Practice of Oncology, 2nd ed. Philadelphia, JB Lippincott, 1985, pp. 1179–1241.
20. Peterson ME, Kintzer PP, Cavanagh PG, et al: Feline hyperthyroidism: Pretreatment clinical and laboratory evaluations of 131 cases. J Am Vet Med Assoc 183:103–110, 1983.

21. Peterson ME, Turrel JM: Feline hyperthyroidism. *In* Kirk RW (ed): Current Veterinary Therapy IX. Philadelphia, WB Saunders, 1986, pp. 1026–1033.

22. Peterson ME, Keene B, Ferguson DC, et al: Electrocardiographic findings in 45 cats with hyperthyroidism. J Am Vet Med Assoc *180*:934–938, 1982.

23. Lui SK, Peterson ME, Fox PR: Hypertrophic cardiomyopathy and hyperthyroidism in the cat. J Am Vet Med Assoc *185*:52–57, 1984.

24. Peterson ME, Graves TK, Gamble DA: Triiodothyronine (T$_3$) suppression test: An aid in the diagnosis of mild hyperthyroidism in cats. J Vet Intern Med *4*:233–240, 1990.

25. Peterson ME: Thyroid function testing. *In* August JR (ed): Consultations in Feline Internal Medicine II. Philadelphia, WB Saunders, 1994, pp. 143–155.

26. Thoday KL, Mooney CT: Medical management of feline hyperthyroidism. *In* Kirk RW, Bonagura JD (eds): Current Veterinary Therapy IX. Philadelphia, WB Saunders, 1992, pp. 338–345.

27. Peterson ME, Hurvitz AI, and Leib MS, et al: Propylthiouracil-associated hemolytic anemia, thrombocytopenia, and antinuclear antibodies in cats with hyperthyroidism. J Am Vet Med Assoc *184*:806–808, 1984.

28. Meric SM, Hawkins EC, Washabau RJ, et al: Serum thyroxine concentrations after radioactive iodine therapy in cats with hyperthyroidism. J Am Vet Med Assoc *188*:1038–1040, 1986.

29. Turrel JM, Feldman ED, Hays M, et al: Radioactive iodine therapy in cats with hyperthyroidism. J Am Vet Med Assoc *184*:554–559, 1984.

30. Birchard SJ, Peterson ME, Jacobson A: Surgical treatment of feline hyperthyroidism: Results of 85 cases. J Am Anim Hosp Assoc *20*:705–709, 1984.

31. Maln CR, Lamb WA, Church DB: Treatment of feline hyperthyroidism using orally administered radioiodine: A study of 40 consecutive cases. Austr Vet J *70*(6):218–219, 1993.

32. Meric SM, Rubin SI: Serum thyroxine concentrations following fixed dosese of radioactive iodine treatment in hyperthyroid cats: 62 cases (1986–1989). *197*(5):621–623, 1990.

33. Peterson ME, Kintzer PP, K/Hurvitz AL: Methimazole treatment of 262 cats with hyperthyroidism. J Vet Intern Med *2*:150–157, 1988.

34. Birchard SI: Thyroidectomy and parathyroidectomy in the dog and cat. Problems in Vet Med *3*(2):277–289, 1991.

35. Zerbe CA: Feline hyperadrenocorticism. *In* Kirk RW (ed): Current Veterinary Therapy X. Philadelphia, WB Saunders, 1989, 1038–1042.

36. Peterson ME, Steele P: Pituitary-dependent hyperadrenocorticism in a cat. J Am Vet Med Assoc *189*:680–683, 1986.

37. Bruyette DS: Adrenal function testing. *In* August JR (ed): Feline Internal Medicine 2. Philadelphia, WB Saunders, 1994, pp. 129–132.

38. Peterson ME: Canine hyperadrenocorticism. *In* Kirk RW (ed): Current Veterinary Therapy IX. Philadelphia, WB Saunders, 1986, pp. 963–972.

39. Scavelli TD, Peterson ME, Mattheisen DT: Results of surgical treatment for hyperadrenocorticism caused by adrenocortical neoplasia in the dog: 25 cases (1980–1984). J Am Vet Med Assoc *189*:1360–1364, 1986.

40. Peterson ME, Drieger DT, Drucker WD, et al: Immunocytochemical study of the hypophysis in 25 dogs with pituitary-dependent hyperadrenocorticism. Acta Endocrinol *101*:15–24, 1982.

41. Rijnberk AD, Relshaw BE: o,p ′-DDD treatment of canine hyperadrenocorticism: An alternative protocol. *In* Kirk RW, Bonagura JD (eds): Current Veterinary Therapy XI. Philadelphia, WB Saunders, 1992, pp. 345–364.

42. Burns MG, Kelly AB, Hornoff WJ, et al: Pulmonary artery thrombosis in 3 dogs with hyperadrenocorticism. J Am Vet Med Assoc *178*:388–393, 1981.

43. Peterson ME, Nesbitt GH, Schaer M: Diagnosis and management of concurrent diabetes mellitus and hyperadrenocorticism in thirty dogs. J Am Vet Med Assoc *179*:66–69, 1981.

44. Peterson ME, Drucker WD: Advances in the diagnosis and treatment of canine Cushing's syndrome. Proc Gaines Vet Symp, 1981, pp. 17–24.

45. Peterson ME, Gilbertson DR, Drucker WD: Plasma cortisol response to exogenous ACTH in 22 dogs with hyperadrenocorticism caused by adrenocortical neoplasia. J Am Vet Med Assoc *180*:542–544, 1982.

46. Feldman EC: Comparison of ACTH response and dexamethasone suppression as screening tests in canine hyperadrenocorticism. J Am Vet Med Assoc *182*:506–510, 1983.

47. Stolp R, Rijnberk A, Meijer JC, et al: Urinary corticoids in the diagnosis of canine hyperadrenocorticism: Res Vet Sci *34*:141–144, 1983.

48. Kaufman J, Macy DW: The glucagon tolerance test as a screening method for canine hyperadrenocorticism. *In* American College of Veterinary Internal Medicine Proceedings, 1984, p. 30.

49. Roberts SM, Lavach JD, Macy DW, et al: Effect of ophthalmic prednisolone acetate on the canine adrenal gland and hepatic function. Am J Vet Res *45*:1711–1714, 1984.

50. Feldman EC: Effect of functional adrenocortical tumors on plasma cortisol and corticotropin concentrations in dogs. J Am Vet Med Assoc *178*:823–826, 1981.

51. Kintzer PP, Peterson ME: Use of o,p′-DDD in treatment of 200 dogs with pituitary-dependent hyperadrenocorticism. J Vet Intern Med *3*:182–195, 1991.

52. Enns SG, Johnston DE, Eigenmann JE, et al: Adrenalectomy in the management of canine hyperadrenocorticism. J Am Anim Hosp Assoc *23*:557–564, 1987.

53. Stolp R, Croughs RJM, Rijnberk A: Results of cyproheptadine treatment in dogs with pituitary-

dependent hyperadrenocorticism in a dog. J Am Vet Med Assoc 187:276–278, 1985.

54. Willard MD, Schall WD, Nachreiner RF, et al: Hypoadrenocorticism following therapy with o.p'-DDD for hyperadrenocorticism in four dogs. J Am Vet Med Assoc 180:638–641, 1982.

55. Bruyette DS, Feldman EC: Efficacy of ketoconazole in the management of spontaneous canine hyperadrenocorticism. In American College of Veterinary Internal Medicine Proceedings, 1987, p. 885.

56. Kintzer PP, Peterson ME: Mitotane treatment of 32 dogs with cortisol secreting adrenocortical neoplasms. J Am Vet Med Assoc 205:54–59, 1994.

57. McMillan FD, Barr B, Feldman EC: Functional pancreatic islet cell tumor in a cat. J Am Anim Hosp Assoc 21:741–746, 1985.

58. Priester WA: Pancreatic islet cell tumors in domestic animals. Data from 11 colleges of veterinary medicine in the United States and Canada. J Natl Cancer Inst 53:227–229, 1974.

59. Ehrhart N, Withrow SJ, Wimsatt J, et al: Insulin secreting tumors in the ferret: A retrospective study. J Am Vet Med Assoc 1994, submitted.

60. Kruth SA, Feldman EC, Kennedy PC: Insulin-secreting islet cell tumors: Establishing a diagnosis and the clinical course for 25 dogs. J Am Vet Med Assoc 181:54–58, 1982.

61. Mehlhaff CJ, Peterson ME, Patnaik AK, et al: Insulin-producing islet cell neoplasms: Surgical considerations and general management in 35 dogs. J Am Anim Hosp Assoc 21:607–612, 1985.

62. Leifer CE, Peterson ME, Matus RE: Insulin-secreting tumor: Diagnosis and medical and surgical management in 55 dogs. J Am Vet Med Assoc 188:60–64, 1986.

63. Caywood DD, Klausner JK, O'Leary TP, et al: Pancreatic insulin-secreting neoplasms: Clinical, diagnostic, and prognostic features in 73 dogs. J Am Anim Hosp Assoc 31(4), 1995.

64. Leifer CE: Hypoglycemia. In Kirk RW (ed.): Current Veterinary Therapy IX. Philadelphia, WB Saunders, 1986, pp. 982–987.

65. Leifer CE, Peterson ME, Matus RE, et al: Hypoglycemia associated with nonislet cell tumor in 13 dogs. J Am Vet Med Assoc 186:53–55, 1985.

66. Breitschwerdt EB, Loar AS, Hribernik TN, et al: Hypoglycemia in four dogs with sepsis. J Am Vet Med Assoc 178:1072–1076, 1981.

67. Chrisman CL: Postoperative results and complication of insulinomas in dogs. J Am Anim Hosp Assoc 16:677–684, 1980.

68. Shahar R, Rousseaux C, Steiss J: Peripheral polyneuropathy in a dog with functional islet B-cell tumor and widespread metastasis. J Am Vet Med Assoc 187:175–176, 1985.

69. Meyer DJ: Pancreatic islet cell tumor in a dog treated with streptozotocin. Am J Vet Res 37:1221–1223, 1976.

70. Zerbe CA: Islet cell tumors secreting insulin, pancreatic polypeptide, gastrin or glucagon. In Kirk RW, Bonagura JD (eds): Current Veterinary Therapy XI. Philadelphia, WB Saunders, 1992, pp. 368–375.

71. Feldman EC, Nelson RW: Canine and Feline Endocrinology and Reproduction. Philadelphia, WB Saunders, 1987, p. 325.

72. Happe HP, Van Der Gaag I, Lamers CRHW, et al: Zollinger-Ellison syndrome in three dogs. Vet Pathol 17:177–186, 1980.

73. Jones BR, Nicholls MR, Badman R: Peptic ulceration in a dog associated with an islet cell carcinoma of the pancreas and an elevated plasma gastrin level. J Small Anim Pract 17:593–598, 1976.

74. Middleton DJ, Watson ADJ: Duodenal ulceration associated with gastrin-secreting pancreatic tumor in a cat. J Am Vet Med Assoc 183:461–462, 1983.

75. Straus E, Johnson GF, Yalow RS: Canine Zollinger-Ellison syndrome. Gastroenterology 72:380–381, 1977.

76. Zaki FA, Harris JM, Budzilovich G: Cystic pituicytoma of the neurohypophysis in a Siamese cat. J Comp Pathol 85:467–471, 1975.

77. Zaki FA, Lui SK: Pituitary chromophobe adenoma in a cat. Vet Pathol 11:232–237, 1973.

78. Capen CC, Martin SC, Koestner A: Neoplasms in the adenohypophysis of dogs. Pathol Vet 4:301–325, 1967.

79. Eigenmann JE, Wortman JA, Haskins ME: Elevated growth hormone levels and diabetes mellitus in a cat with acromegalic features. J Am Anim Hosp Assoc 20:747–752, 1984.

80. Randolph JF, Peterson ME: Acromegaly (Growth Hormone Excess) Syndromes in Dogs and Cats. In Kirk RW, Bonagura JD (eds): Current Veterinary Therapy XI. Philadelphia, WB Saunders, 1992, pp. 322–327.

81. Greco DS: Acromegaly. In August JR (ed): Consultations in Feline Internal Medicine 2. Philadelphia, WB Saunders, 1994, pp. 169–176.

82. Berger B, Feldman EC: Primary hyperparathyroidism in dogs: 21 cases (1976–1986). J Am Vet Med Assoc 191:350–356, 1987.

83. Thompson KG, Jones LP, Smylie WA, et al: Primary hyperparathyroidism in German shepherd dogs: A disorder of probable genetic origin. Vet Pathol 21:370–376, 1984.

84. Kallet AJ, Richler KP, Feldman EC, et al: Primary hyperparathyroidism in seven cats. J Am Vet Med Assoc 197:1767–1771, 1991.

85. Meuten DJ: Hypercalcemia. Vet Clin North Am 14:891–910, 1984.

86. Meuten DJ, Cew DJ, Kociba GJ, et al: Relationship of calcium to albumin and total proteins in dogs. J Am Vet Med Assoc 180:63–67, 1982.

87. Twedt DC, Tilley LP, Ryan WW, et al: Grand rounds conference: Pheochromocytoma in a canine. J Am Anim Hosp Assoc 11:491–496, 1975.

88. Schaer M: Pheochromocytoma in a dog: A case report. J Am Anim Hosp Assoc 16:583–587, 1980.

89. Gilson SD, Withrow SJ, Wheeler SL, Twedt DC:

Pheochromocytoma in 50 dogs. J Vet Intern Med 8:228–232, 1994.

90. Wheeler SL: Canine pheochromocytoma. *In* Kirk RW (ed.): Current Veterinary Therapy IX. Philadelphia, WB Saunders, 1986, pp. 977–981.

91. Peterson ME, Randolph JF, Zaki FA, et al: Multiple endocrine neoplasia in a dog. J Am Vet Med Assoc 180:1476, 1982.

92. Buergelt CD, Das KM: Aortic body tumor in a cat: A case report. Pathol Vet 5:84–90, 1968.

93. Collins DR: Thoracic tumor in a cat. Vet Med/ Small Anim Clin 59:459, 1964.

94. Hayes HM: An hypothesis for the aetiology of canine chemoreceptor system neoplasms, based upon an epidemiological study of 73 cases among hospital patients. J Small Anim Pract 16:337–343, 1975.

95. Patnaik AK, Liu SK, Hurvitz AI, et al: Canine chemodectoma (extra-adrenal paragangliomas)— A comparative study, J Small Anim Pract 16:785– 801, 1975.

96. Blackmore J, Gorman NT, Kagan K, et al: Neurologic complications of a chemodectoma in a dog. J Am Vet Med Assoc 184:475–478, 1984.

97. Hopper PE, Jongeward SJ, Lammerding JJ, et al: Carotid body tumor associated with an arteriovenous fistula in a dog. Compend Contin Educ Pract Vet 5:68–72, 1983.

# 22

# Tumors of the Female Reproductive System

## Mary Kay Klein

## OVARIAN TUMORS

### Incidence

Ovarian tumors are uncommon in dogs and cats. The reported incidence in the intact female dog is 6.25%,[1] comprising 0.5% to 1.2% of all canine tumors.[2,3] Incidence rates in the cat range from 0.7% to 3.6%.[4] The low incidence rate in both species is undoubtedly biased by the large segment of the population that is surgically neutered at an early age.

Epithelial tumors have been reported in dogs ranging in age from 4 to 15 years, with medians near 10 years.[3,5] Granulosa cell tumors have been reported in dogs ranging in age from 14 months to 16 years.[3,5–7] In one study 10 of 13 bitches with this tumor were nulliparous.[1] Teratomas have been reported in animals ranging in age from 20 months to 9 years, with the majority of animals 6 years old or younger.[5,8,9] Pointers were found to be at increased risk for epithelial tumors and English bulldogs at increased risk for granulosa-theca cell tumors in one series.[10] Ovarian tumors have been reported in cats ranging from 2 months to 20 years of age, with a mean of 6.7 years.[11]

### Pathology and Natural Behavior

**Canine Ovarian Tumors** Three general categories of canine ovarian tumors are described according to the cell of origin: epithelial cell, germ cell, and sex-cord stromal cell (Table 22–1). Epithe-lial and sex-cord stromal tumors account for the majority of recorded cases (80–90%).[3,8–10,12–14]

*Epithelial Cell Tumors.* Epithelial tumors include the papillary adenoma, papillary adenocarcinoma, cystadenoma, and undifferentiated carcinoma. They account for 40 to 50% of reported canine ovarian neoplasms.[3,5,13,14]

Papillary adenomas and adenocarcinomas can be bilateral.[5,6,13] Differentiation between the two forms can be difficult and is usually based on size, mitotic index, invasion into ovarian stoma, and extension into the ovarian bursa and adjacent peritoneum.[6,14] Classically the papillary adenocarcinoma is associated with widespread peritoneal implantation and the formation of malignant effusion. Malignant effusions may develop by several mechanisms:[2,15]

1. Edema within the ovarian tumor may cause leakage of fluid throughout the tumor capsule.
2. The tumor may exfoliate cells, resulting in transcoelomic metastasis, and these tumor implants can exert pressure and obstruct peritoneal and diaphragmatic lymphatics.
3. Secretions from metastatic peritoneal implants can also occur.

Papillary adenocarcinomas have been noted to metastasize to the renal and para-aortic lymph nodes, omentum, liver, and lungs.[3]

The cystadenoma appears to originate from the rete ovarii, is generally unilateral, and consists of multiple thin-walled cysts containing clear, watery fluid.[6,13]

**Table 22–1**  Classification of Canine Ovarian Tumors

|  | Epithelial Cell Tumors | Germ Cell Tumors | Sex-Cord Stromal Tumors |
|---|---|---|---|
| Histologic classifications | Papillary adenoma<br>Papillary adenocarcinoma<br>Cystadenoma<br>Undifferentiated carcinoma | Dysgerminoma<br>Teratocarcinoma<br>Teratoma | Thecoma<br>Luteoma<br>Granulosa cell tumor |
| % of cases | 40–50 | 6–12 | 35–50 |
| Bilateral incidence | occasional | rare | rare |
| Functional incidence | rare | rare | ~50% |
| Metastatic rate in malignant classification | ~50% | ~30% | <20% |

*Undifferentiated carcinoma* is the term used to denote tumors whose embryonic morphology and absence of hormonal secretion does not allow the identification of a specific epithelial cell of origin.

*Germ Cell Tumors.* The primordial germ cells of the ovary are thought to be the origin of dysgerminomas, teratomas, and teratocarcinomas. Germ cell tumors comprise 6% to 12% of canine ovarian tumors.[3,5] Dysgerminomas arise from undifferentiated germ cells and so closely resemble their testicular counterparts that they have been referred to as "ovarian seminomas."[3,6,13,15,16] Bilateral dysgerminomas have been reported; however, most are unilateral.[17,18] Dysgerminomas grow by expansion,[6,15] and have a reported metastatic rate of 10% to 30%.[3,9,13–15,17,18] The most common metastatic site is the abdominal lymph nodes; however, involvement of the liver, kidney, omentum, pancreas, and adrenal glands has been reported.[3,6,9,17,18]

Teratomas are composed of cells arising from more than one germ cell layer. Any combination of ectodermal, mesodermal, and endodermal tissues can be seen. These tissues are generally well differentiated histologically. Teratocarcinomas have both mature elements and undifferentiated elements resembling those of the embryo. A cumulative review[9] of the literature revealed a 32% metastatic rate in canine teratomas and teratocarcinomas. Metastases were noted in multiple abdominal sites as well as the lungs, anterior mediastinum, and bone. The metastatic lesions were noted to be composed predominantly of undifferentiated elements.

*Sex-Cord Stromal Tumors.* The most common sex-cord stromal tumor is the granulosa cell tumor, which accounts for approximately 50% of ovarian tumors in several reviews.[1,3,5,6,13] Because the sex-cord stromal tumor arises from the specialized gonadal stroma of the ovary, which is responsible for estrogen and progesterone production, all of these tumors have the potential to elaborate hormones that may manifest clinical signs.

Granulosa cell tumors are usually unilateral and tend to be firm and lobulated, although cysts are commonly apparent on cross section. These tumors can be quite large.[3,5] Sertoli-Leydig cell tumors can occur bilaterally.[5] Up to 20% of granulosa cell tumors demonstrate malignant behavior in the dog,[3,5–7,13,14,16] with metastasis to the sublumbar lymph nodes, liver, pancreas, and lung[3] as well as peritoneal carcinomatosis.[7]

Thecomas are generally benign in their behavior, growing by expansion without metastasis.[13,14] Luteomas are rarely seen but have been reported in the dog[13,14] and are considered benign.

*Tumorlike Conditions and Metastatic Involvement.* Numerous tumorlike conditions can exist and often must be differentiated histologically. Ovarian cysts are common in the dog and can be very large and easily confused with a neoplastic process.[1] Paraovarian cysts, arising from mesonephric tubules, can be single or multiple. Less common conditions include cystic rete tubules, vascular hematomas, and adenomatous hyperplasia of the rete ovarii.[13,14]

The ovary is rarely a site for metastatic disease; however, metastasis to the ovary has been recorded in cases of mammary, intestinal, and pancreatic carcinomas and lymphomas.[1,13]

**Feline Ovarian Tumors**  Feline ovarian tumors are also defined as epithelial, germ cell, or sex-cord stromal tumors. The latter category is by far the most common, accounting for at least 50% of reported cases.[19,20] More than half of the granulosa cell tumors in cats are malignant.[11,16,19–21] As is true in the dog, they often show evidence of hormonally induced changes and are most commonly unilateral.[11,19,20] Reported metastatic sites include the peritoneum, lumbar lymph nodes, omentum, diaphragm, kidney, spleen, liver, and lungs.[11,20,21]

In one series of 14 sex-cord stromal tumors, the author classified 5 as interstitial gland tumors (luteomas). All were benign in behavior.[11] A similarly described tumor appeared to have virilizing effects in a 9-year-old cat.[20]

Approximately 15% of feline ovarian neoplasms are dysgerminomas.[11,16,19] In one study, two of six tumors were noted to be bilateral.[11] Dysgerminomas are generally considered to be hormonally inactive and slow to metastasize; yet metastasis has been reported in 20%[16] to 33%[11] of cases. These tumors tend to be encapsulated, smooth, dense tissue masses that can attain a large size within the ovary.[16,20] Teratomas are reported only rarely[11,19,20] and in at least one case demonstrated malignant behavior.[20]

Epithelial tumors are extremely rare in the cat.[11,19,20] Cystadenomas and ovarian adenocarcinomas have been reported.[11,20] Metastasis to the lungs, liver, and abdominal peritoneum was seen in one case of ovarian adenocarcinoma.[20]

Lymphomas and endometrial carcinomas have been noted to involve the ovaries in the cat secondarily.[19]

## History and Clinical Signs

**Canine Ovarian Tumors** The history and clinical signs of canine ovarian tumors can be quite variable, depending on their tissue of origin. With the exception of teratomas, which can be seen in young dogs,[8–10,12] the tumors occur most commonly in middle-aged to older animals.

Most epithelial cell tumors are asymptomatic until signs referable to a space-occupying mass occur.[6,15,16] Epithelial tumors may present with malignant ascites.[6,15] Pleural effusions have also been noted secondary to thoracic metastasis.[15] Cytologic analysis of fluid may reveal signet ring and rosette cellular patterns suggestive of adenocarcinoma.[6,15]

Germ cell tumors have been associated with evidence of hormonal dysfunction, but more commonly are associated with the clinical signs of a space-occupying mass. Teratomas in particular can attain large size,[6,8] and areas of calcification are often seen on routine abdominal radiographs.[6,8,9]

Sex-cord stromal tumors are well documented to have the ability to produce steroid hormones (estrogen and progesterone).[3,5–7,13,16] Excessive estrogen production leads to vulvar enlargement, sanguineous vulvar discharge, persistent estrus, alopecia, or aplastic pancytopenia. Excessive progesterone production leads to cystic endometrial hyperplasia/pyometra complex. Sex-cord stromal tumors may produce one or both hormones, or none at all.[2,3,5,13,22] Rarely, thecomas may produce estrogens, and luteomas can have secondary masculinizing effects. If functional neoplasia is suspected, evaluation of vaginal cytology for evidence of estrogen-induced cornification and serum progesterone measurement for values exceeding 2 ng/ml are indicated.[23] Regardless of whether or not they are functional, most sex-cord stromal tumors are unilateral and large enough to be palpable by the time of presentation.[5–7]

**Feline Ovarian Tumors** The granulosa cell tumor is most often recognized.[11,14,19,20] The clinical signs of hyperestrogenism are commonly reported, including persistent estrus, alopecia, and cystic or adenomatous hyperplasia of the endometrium.[11,19–21] Granulosa cell tumors are generally unilateral and large enough to be detected on palpation at presentation.[14,19–21] In at least one case, a functional androgenic interstitial gland tumor resulted in virilizing clinical signs.[20]

Dysgerminomas can be found bilaterally and may attain large size.[11,19,20] Signs of depression, vomiting, abdominal distention, and ascites are usually referable to the mass lesion.[19] The reported mean age of occurrence is 7 years.[20] Teratomas have also been reported on rare occasions, and the clinical signs noted were referable to their large size.[11,20]

Epithelial tumors are reported only rarely and can be found bilaterally.[11,20]

## Diagnostic Techniques and Workup

There are no consistently abnormal laboratory findings with ovarian tumors. The presence of an abdominal mass in an intact female animal with or without signs referable to the reproductive tract should place an ovarian tumor on the list of differentials. Small tumors are in proximity to the caudal pole of the kidney, while larger tumors are pendulous and mimic any midabdominal mass in location. Intravenous pyelography can be of benefit in differentiating ovarian from renal masses. Ultrasonography may aid in defining the size and location of the tumor. Cytologic evaluation of abdominal or pleural fluid may be suggestive of malignant effusions. Radiographic evidence of calcification within the mass is suggestive of teratomas; however, definitive diagnosis rests with histopathologic evaluation of resected tissue. Transabdominal needle biopsies are not recommended because of the propensity for many of these tumors to implant readily and grow on peritoneal surfaces. Thoracic radiographs should be evaluated for any evidence of metastatic disease, but they only rarely are positive at the time of diagnosis.

## Therapy

Surgery remains the mainstay of treatment for ovarian tumors. A complete ovariohysterectomy is recommended, although oophorectomy alone is possible. Gentle handling of tissues to minimize transcoelomic tumor spread is warranted. Careful examination of all serosal surfaces and removal or biopsy of any lesions suspected of metastatic disease are recommended for staging purposes.

One case of metastatic granulosa cell tumor was successfully treated with serial and combination use of cyclophosphamide, chlorambucil, 1-2 chloroethyl-3-cyclohexyl-1-nitrosourea, and bleomycin for longer than 10 months.[15] While cisplatin-based combination chemotherapy regimens are of benefit in human cases, they are largely unevaluated in veterinary patients. Intracavitary instillation of cisplatin has been of benefit in controlling malignant effusions.[24,25] Radiation therapy is rarely indicated or used because animals with disease confined to the ovary (amenable to radiation) are usually successfully treated with surgery.

## Prognosis

Very little survival data are available for canine ovarian tumors. Survival times up to 4 years following the removal of ovarian dysgerminomas, and 6 years following the removal of teratomas, are reported.[9] The prognosis for all ovarian tumors would appear to be the same, regardless of histology. The prognosis is good when single tumors are completely excised at surgery. If there is any evidence of metastatic disease, the prognosis must be considered poor.

Chemotherapy would appear to have the potential to lengthen survival times in patients with evidence of metastatic disease. A dog with metastatic ovarian papillary cystadenocarcinoma survived longer than 10 months with adjuvant chemotherapy.[15] Survival for longer than 2 years following treatment with an immunotherapeutic regimen was reported in a dog with metastatic

granulosa cell tumor.[2] Intracavitary instillation of cisplatin was effective in controlling a malignant effusion of 8 months in a canine ovarian carcinoma case.[25]

Treated survival times are unavailable for feline ovarian tumor cases.

## Comparative Aspects

Ovarian cancer is the fourth most common cause of cancer death in women.[26] Most human patients present with advanced, disseminated disease. Ovarian tumors are localized to the reproductive system in less than 25% of patients at the time of diagnosis.[26–28] Human and canine tumors share many characteristics:

1. A similar incidence rate: 4% of human female tumors,[27] 6.25% of intact female canine tumors.[1]
2. An increasing incidence with age in the epithelial tumor classification and a younger set of patients with teratomas.[27]
3. A tendency for transcoelomic metastasis in epithelial tumor cases.[13,27]

Eighty percent of human ovarian tumor cases are epithelial in origin.[26] Several prognostic factors have been elucidated in human clinical studies, including histologic grade, the extent of residual disease postoperatively, the stage of the disease at presentation, and the age of the patient.[26,28–30]

Human ovarian epithelial tumors are well documented to be chemoresponsive; however, long-term patient survival is still low.[26–29] Single-agent chemotherapeutic agents that have demonstrated efficacy against human ovarian tumors include doxorubicin, cisplatinum, carboplatin, taxol, and melphalan.[26] Combination regimens have demonstrated significantly improved response over melphalan and cyclophosphamide singly.[29,30] Platinum-based combination chemotherapy regimens appear to have the best chance for effecting a complete response in advanced ovarian carcinoma.[26] A steep dose-response curve exists for cisplatin and full therapeutic doses should be implemented.[26] Progestational agents have demonstrated a 5% to 15% response rate.[26] Whether or not intraperitoneal therapies will play an important role is as yet undetermined.[26] Radiation therapy is also of benefit in some cases.[30]

Teratomas and dysgerminomas are most commonly reported in women less than 35 years of age.[27] Teratomas are most commonly reported in young dogs, and show evidence of being more malignant than their human counterparts.[5,9,31]

## UTERINE TUMORS

### Incidence

Uterine tumors are rare in both the dog and the cat; the reported incidence rates are 0.3% to 0.4% of all canine tumors,[6,16,32,33] 0.2% to 1.5% in the cat.[34-36] Middle-aged to older animals are most commonly affected, and no breed predilections have been reported in either species.[16,19,33]

### Pathology and Natural Behavior

The majority of canine uterine tumors are mesenchymal in origin; leiomyomas account for 85% to 90% and leiomyosarcomas for 10% of mesenchymal tumors.[16,32] On rare occasions adenomas, adenocarcinomas, fibromas, fibrosarcomas, and lipomas have been reported.[6,32,37,38]

Leiomyomas are generally noninvasive, nonmetastatic, and slow growing.[6] Grossly, it is difficult to distinguish them from their malignant counterparts.[32,38] A syndrome characterized by multiple uterine leiomyomas, bilateral renal cystadenocarcinomas, and nodular dermatofibrosis has been characterized in German shepherd dogs and noted to have a hereditary component.[39] (See Chap. 25.)

In the cat, uterine adenocarcinomas account for the majority of cases and arise from the endometrium.[19,40] Metastases to the cerebrum, eyes, ovaries, adrenal glands, lungs, liver, kidneys, bladder, colon, diaphragm, and regional lymph nodes have been reported.[40] Other uterine neoplasms reported less commonly in the cat include leiomyoma, leiomyosarcoma, fibrosarcoma, lymphosarcoma, fibroma, and lipoma.[19]

### History and Clinical Signs

Canine leiomyomas and leiomyosarcomas are rarely associated with clinical signs, and, in fact, many are incidental findings at the time of necropsy or ovariohysterectomy.[6,32,33] They can gain sufficient size to compress adjacent viscera.[6,32] Vaginal discharge and pyometra may accompany malignant or benign uterine tumors.[6,32,33] Clinical signs secondary to metastatic disease may be the presenting complaint in cases of uterine and cervical carcinoma.[38,41]

Clinical signs may not be associated with feline uterine adenocarcinomas until the tumor gains large proportions. A vaginal discharge is common and can vary from purulent to mucoid to darkly hemorrhagic. Other reported clinical signs include abnormal estrous cycles, polydipsia, polyuria, vomiting, and abdominal distention.[19,40] Clinical signs may occur as a result of metastatic disease prior to any clinical indication of the primary tumor.[40-42]

### Diagnostic Techniques and Workup

No consistent laboratory abnormalities are noted, and abdominal radiographs only confirm the presence of an abdominal or uterine mass. A definitive diagnosis is usually attained upon histologic examination of surgically excised specimens. Ultrasonography may further delineate the origin of the mass; however, the uterus of cats and dogs generally cannot be visualized by this technique unless it contains fluid, a fetus, or a mass.

### Therapy

A complete ovariohysterectomy is recommended, and attempts should be made to remove all tumors and metastatic foci. Chemotherapy and radiation therapy are largely untried in veterinary cases.

### Prognosis

The prognosis associated with leiomyomas and other benign tumors is excellent, as surgery is nearly always curative. In the case of leiomyosarcomas and other malignant tumors, the prognosis remains good if there is no evidence of metastatic disease at the time of surgery and complete excision is possible. Because clinical signs are rarely evident until late in the course of disease, the prognosis should always be considered guarded until histopathology and staging are complete. Nonresectable or metastatic disease warrants a grave prognosis.

Feline uterine adenocarcinomas have well-documented metastatic potential and their prognosis must be considered guarded.[19,37] Again, the presence of metastatic disease indicates a grave prognosis.

### Comparative Aspects

In women, carcinoma of the endometrium is the most common malignant tumor in the genital tract, comprising approximately 13% of all malignant tumors. Most cases are diagnosed in the 55- to 60-year-old age group.[26] The pathology and natural behavior of the disease in humans most closely resembles the disease in the cat.

Approximately 85% to 90% of cases of carcinoma of the endometrium are diagnosed while disease is still confined to the uterus. Prognostic factors include age, stage at diagnosis, histologic grade, depth of myometrial penetration, and lymph node status.[26]

Postoperative radiotherapy is used extensively in human cases. Chemotherapy has not been studied in any detail; however, doxorubicin has been well evaluated in adequate numbers of patients, and results in one study indicate a 37% response rate.[43]

## VAGINAL AND VULVAR TUMORS

### Incidence

Vulvar and vaginal tumors account for 2.4% to 3% of canine neoplasms.[33,44] They are the second most common canine female reproductive tumor after those of the mammary gland. The vast majority are benign, arise from smooth muscle, are found in intact female dogs, and affect dogs from 2 to 18 years of age, with an average of 10.8 years.[16,33,44,45] One study found the boxer to be at an increased risk over other breeds.[44] Vaginal and vulvar leiomyomas can be characterized as a disease of older, sexually intact dogs. The incidence rate of these tumors is significantly higher in nulliparous bitches.[33] Lipomas tend to occur in younger dogs with an age range of 1 to 8 years and a mean of 6.3 years.[33]

Incidence rates are not available for the cat. Leiomyomas and a fibroma have been reported.[19,46] The vaginal leiomyomas were noted in older intact queens.[46]

### Pathology and Natural Behavior

As many as 86% of vulvar and vaginal tumors are reported to be benign smooth muscle tumors.[44,45] These are variably referred to as leiomyomas, fibroleiomyomas, fibromas, and polyps, and vary only in the amount of connective tissue present. Because the clinical course of the tumor does not appear to be affected by histologic variations,[33,44] it is justified to consider these tumors collectively. In endemic areas, transmissible venereal tumors (TVTs) are common (see Chap. 29C).

Most leiomyomas arise from the vestibule of the vulva rather than from the vagina.[33,44] Extra- and intraluminal forms are described. Extraluminal forms present as a slow-growing perineal mass. On cut section these tumors are gray to white to tan in color, well encapsulated, and poorly vascularized.[6,32,33]

Intraluminal tumors are attached to the vestibular or vaginal wall by a thin pedicle. They are often firm and ovoid, and although their mucosa is generally intact, ulceration may occur with exposure or irritation.[32,44] Intraluminal tumors can be multiple.[44,45] All pedunculated or polypoid tumors were found to be benign in one study.[44]

Subjective data indicate that leiomyomas may be hormone dependent. In two studies, none of the dogs diagnosed with the leiomyoma, fibroma, or polypoid tumors had prior ovariohysterectomies.[44,45] There was a 15% recurrence rate in dogs left intact after treatment and no recurrences in dogs ovariohysterectomized at that time.[44] In another study, leiomyomas were not seen in bitches ovariectomized prior to 2 years of age.[33] Concurrent uterine, ovarian, and mammary gland changes, including cystic endometrial glandular hyperplasia, ovarian cysts, and mammary gland tumors, were present in approximately one third of the cases.[33,45]

Other benign vaginal and vulvar tumors that have been reported include lipomas, sebaceous adenomas, fibrous histiocytomas, benign melanomas, myxomas, and myxofibromas.[6,16,33,44]

The most common malignant tumor seen is the leiomyosarcoma.[6,32,33,44] Distant metastases have been reported.[33] Other tumors with malignant potential that have been reported include TVT, adenocarcinoma, squamous cell carcinoma, hemangiosarcoma, osteosarcoma, mast cell tumor, and epidermoid carcinoma.[6,16,32,33,44] The labia of the vulva may be the site for any tumor associated with cutaneous tissues. Carcinomas arising from the bladder or urethra may also present with palpable vaginal masses near the urethral papilla.[45,47]

### History and Clinical Signs

The duration of clinical signs tends to be longer in cases of extraluminal tumors.[33] The presenting clinical sign is generally a slow-growing perineal mass (Fig. 22–1). Intraluminal tumors, by virtue of their tendency toward pedunculation, often appear externally when straining causes the mass to extrude through the vulvar lips, especially at the times of estrus (Fig. 22–2). The most common owner complaint recorded is that of a mass "popping out" of the vulva. Clinical signs seen less frequently include vulvar bleeding or discharge, an enlarging vulvar mass, dysuria, hematuria, tenesmus, excessive vulvar licking, and dystocia.[33,44,45] A greater proportion of malig-

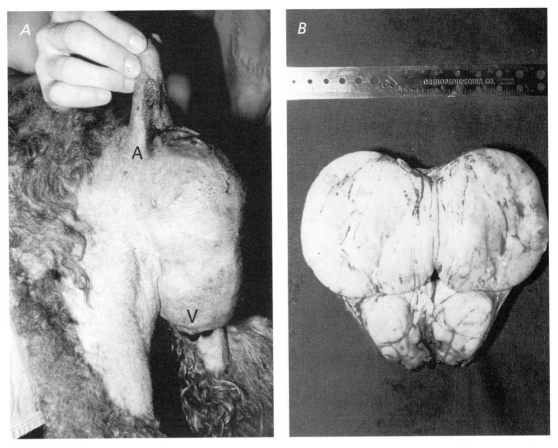

**Figure 22–1.** *A,* Slow-growing perineal mass typical of an extraluminal leiomyoma (anus = A, vulva = V). *B,* A midline perineal incision allowed the removal of this well-encapsulated mass. Histology confirmed a benign leiomyoma.

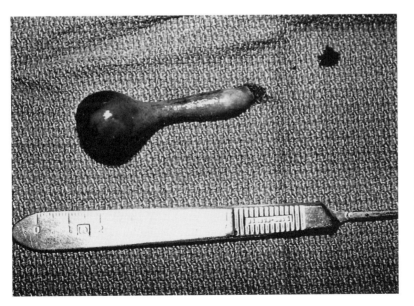

**Figure 22–2.** Pedunculated intraluminal vaginal leiomyoma. This tumor often prolapses during estrus, and the exposed surface may ulcerate when traumatized. Treatment included removal by simple ligation of the pedicle and concomitant ovariohysterectomy.

nancy is noted in vaginal and vulvar tumors, demonstrating frequent recurrence and a lack of pedunculation.[33]

The only clinical sign reported with lipomas is a slow-growing mass and subsequent impingement on adjacent structures. The tumors can arise from the perivascular and perivaginal fat and lie within the pelvic canal. They may attach to the tuber ischium. All are reported to be well circumscribed and relatively avascular.[32,33]

The tumor masses in feline cases of leiomyoma were quite firm, and the presenting clinical sign, constipation, was secondary to the dorsal compression of the rectum and dilation of the colon anterior to the tumor.[46] One cat also had cystic ovaries and a mammary adenocarcinoma.[46]

## Diagnostic Techniques and Workup

Although the older, intact female signalment of the animal combined with the location and gross appearance are suggestive, a definitive diagnosis rests upon histopathologic examination of excised tissue. Vaginoscopic examination, retrograde vaginography, or urethrocystography may help delineate a suspect mass. Caudal abdominal radiographs may be indicated for an extraluminal mass with extension cranially.

## Therapy

In light of the evidence of hormonal dependence and high incidence of disease associated with an intact reproductive system in an aging bitch, it would appear prudent to perform an ovariohysterectomy at the time of treatment. This also permits examination of abdominal organs for evidence of metastatic disease. Conservative surgical excision combined with ovariohysterectomy is usually curative for benign tumors. Intraluminal tumors can be easily removed by placing one or more sutures in the pedicle. Wide removal is not necessary if ovariohysterectomy is performed, even though these tumors probably arise in the smooth muscle of the vaginal wall. If the pedicle or urethral papilla cannot be adequately visualized, a dorsal episiotomy ensures complete resection and avoids any damage to the urethra.

Surgical removal of extraluminal tumors can also be readily accomplished through a dorsal episiotomy. Because they tend to be well encapsulated and poorly vascularized, blunt dissection generally removes them entirely. On rare occasions, a perineal approach or pelvic split may be required. Catheterization of the urethra aids in preventing accidental damage to that structure. If complete excision of the primary tumor and metastatic foci cannot be accomplished, local radiation therapy may be of benefit.[32] Malignant, infiltrative vaginal neoplasms can be addressed with complete vulvovaginectomy and perineal urethostomy.[48]

## Prognosis

Surgery for benign lesions is nearly always curative, and vulvovaginal tumors are rarely identified as a cause of death. Many are incidental findings at necropsy. The prognosis associated with adenocarcinomas and squamous cell carcinomas is generally poor because of high local recurrence and metastatic rates.[32,44] Surgery with ovariohysterectomy was curative in the feline leiomyoma cases reported.

## Comparative Aspects

Vaginal fibroids are rare in women but common in the dog.[43] Conversely, uterine fibroids affect 20% of all women over 30 years of age but are very uncommon in the canine uterus.[43] Human genital leiomyomas typically cease growth after menopause and resume growth if estrogens are administered. However, the majority of women with these tumors have normal ovarian function, and there is no objective data to indicate that an endocrine imbalance precedes their formation.[43]

## REFERENCES

1. Dow C: Ovarian abnormalities in the bitch. J Comp Pathol 70:59–69, 1960.
2. Hayes A, Harvey HJ: Treatment of metastatic granulosa cell tumor in a dog. J Am Vet Med Assoc 174:1304–1306, 1979.
3. Cotchin E: Canine ovarian neoplasms. Res Vet Sci 2:133–142, 1961.
4. Cotchin E: Some tumours of dogs and cats of comparative veterinary and human interest. Vet Rec 71:1040–1054, 1959.
5. Patnaik AK, Greenlee PG: Canine ovarian neoplasms: A clinicopathologic study of 71 cases, including histology of 12 granulosa cell tumors. Vet Pathol 24:509–514, 1987.
6. Herron MA: Tumors of the canine genital system. J Am Anim Hosp Asoc 19:981–994, 1983.
7. Anderson GL: Granulosa cell tumor in a dog. Compend Contin Educ 8:158–168, 1986.
8. Wilson RB, Cave JS, Copeland JS, Onks J: Ovarian teratoma in 2 dogs. J Am Anim Hosp Assoc 21:249–253, 1985.

9. Greenlee PG, Patnaik AK: Canine ovarian tumors of germ cell origin. Vet Pathol 22:117–122, 1985.

10. Hayes HM, Young JL: Epidemiologic features of canine ovarian neoplasms. Gynecol Oncol 6:348–353, 1978.

11. Gelberg HB, McEntee K: Feline ovarian neoplasms. Vet Pathol 22:572–576, 1985.

12. Jergens AE, Knapp DW: Ovarian teratoma in a bitch. J Am Vet Med Assoc 191:81–83, 1987.

13. Nielsen SW, Misdorp W, McEntee K: Tumours of the ovary. Bull WHO 53:203–215, 1976.

14. Nielsen SW: Classification of tumors in dogs and cats. J Am Anim Hosp Assoc 19:13–52, 1983.

15. Greene JA, Richardson RC, Thornhill JA, Boon GD: Ovarian papillary cystadenocarcinoma in a bitch. Case report and literature review. J Am Anim Hosp Assoc 15:351–356, 1979.

16. Theilen GH, Madewell BR: Tumors of the urogenital tract. In Veterinary Cancer Medicine. Philadelphia, Lea & Febiger, 1979, pp. 367–373.

17. Andrews EJ, et al: A histopathological study of canine and feline ovarian dysgerminomas. Can J Comp Med 38:85–89, 1974.

18. Dehner LP, et al: Comparative pathology of ovarian neoplasms. 3. Germ cell tumors of canine, bovine, feline, rodent and human species. J Comp Pathol 80:299–306, 1970.

19. Stein BS: Tumors of the feline genital tract. J Am Anim Hosp Assoc 17:1022–1025, 1981.

20. Norris HJ, Garner FM, Taylor HB: Pathology of feline ovarian neoplasms. J Pathol 97:138–143, 1969.

21. Arnberg J: Extra-ovarian granulosa cell tumor in a cat. Fel Pract 10:26–32, 1980.

22. McCandlish IAP, et al: Hormone producing ovarian tumors in the dog. Vet Rec 105:9–11, 1979.

23. Johnston SD: Reproductive systems. In Slatter D (ed): Textbook of Small Animal Surgery. Philadelphia, WB Saunders, 1993, pp. 2177–2192.

24. Moore AS, Kirk C, Cardona A: Intracavitary cisplatin chemotherapy: Experience with six dogs. J Vet Intern Med 5:227–231, 1991.

25. Olsen J, Komtebedde J, Lackner A, Madewell BR: Cytoreductive treatment of ovarian carcinoma in a dog. J Vet Intern Med 8:133–134, 1994.

26. Young RC, Perez CA, Hoskins WJ: Cancer of the Ovary. In DeVita VT, Hellman S, Rosenberg SA (eds): Cancer: Principles and Practice of Oncology, 4th ed. Philadelphia, JB Lippincott, 1993, pp. 1226–1263.

27. Barber HRK: Ovarian cancer. CA-A Cancer Journal for Clinicians 36:149–184, 1986.

28. Kerstin S, Silfversward C, Einhorn M: Ovarian cancer: The challenge of local tumor control: Its impact on survival. Int J Radiat Oncol Phys 12:567–571, 1986.

29. Ozols RF, Young RC: Chemotherapy of ovarian cancer. Semin Oncol 11:251–263, 1984.

30. Dembo AJ: Radiotherapeutic management of ovarian cancer. Semin Oncol 11:238–250, 1984.

31. Patnaik AK, Schaer M, Parks J, Liu SK: Metastasizing ovarian teratocarcinoma in dogs. J Small Anim Pract 17:235–246, 1976.

32. Withrow SJ, Susaneck SJ: Tumors of the canine female reproductive tract. In Morrow DA (ed): Current Therapy in Theriogenology 2. Philadelphia, WB Saunders, 1986.

33. Brodey RS, Roszel JF: Neoplasms of the canine uterus, vagina, vulva: A clinicopathologic survey of 90 cases. J Am Vet Med Assoc 151:1294–1307, 1967.

34. Cotchin E: Neoplasia in the cat. Vet Rec 69:425–434, 1957.

35. Engle CG, Brodey RS. A retrospective study of 395 feline neoplasms. J Am Anim Hosp Assoc 5:21–25, 1969.

36. Schmidt RE, Langham RF: A survey of feline neoplasms. J Am Vet Med Assoc 151:1325–1328, 1967.

37. Wardrip SJ, Esplin DG: Uterine carcinoma with metastasis to the myocardium. J Am Anim Hosp Assoc 20:261–264, 1984.

38. Vos JH: Uterine and cervical carcinomas in five dogs. J Vet Med A 35:385–390, 1988.

39. Lium B, Moe L: Hereditary multifocal renal cystadenocarcinomas and nodular dermatofibrosis in the German shepherd: Macroscopic and histopathologic changes. Vet Pathol 22:447–455, 1985.

40. O'Rourke MD, Geib L: Endometrial adenocarcinoma in a cat. Cornell Vet 60:598–604, 1970.

41. Bellhorn R: Secondary ocular adenocarcinoma in three dogs and a cat. J Am Vet Med Assoc 160:302–307, 1972.

42. Prieser H: Endometrial adenocarcinoma in a cat. Vet Pathol 1:485–487, 1964.

43. Perez CA, Knapp RC, Young RC: Gynecologic tumors. In DeVita VT, Hellman S, Rosenberg SA (eds): Cancer: Principles and Practice of Oncology. Philadelphia, JB Lippincott, 1982, pp. 849–860.

44. Thacher C, Bradley RL: Vulvar and vaginal tumors in the dog: A retrospective study. J Am Vet Med Assoc 183:690–692, 1983.

45. Kydd DM, Burnie AG: Vaginal neoplasia in the bitch: A review of 40 clinical cases. J Small Anim Pract 27:255–263, 1986.

46. Wolke RE: Vaginal leiomyoma as a cause of chronic constipation in the cat. J Am Vet Med Assoc 143:1103–1105, 1963.

47. Magne ML, Hoopes PJ, Kainer RA, Olson P, Husted PW, Allen RA, Wykes PM, Withrow SJ: Urinary tract carcinomas involving the canine vagina and vestibule. J Am Anim Hosp Assoc 21:767–772, 1985.

48. Bilbrey SA, Withrow SJ, Klein MK, et al: Vulvovaginectomy and perineal urethrostomy for neoplasms of the vulva and vagina. Vet Surg 18:450–453, 1989.

# 23

# Tumors of the Mammary Gland

E. Gregory MacEwen and Stephen J. Withrow

## CANINE MAMMARY TUMORS

Mammary neoplasms are the most common tumors of the female dog and are estimated to occur in 2 per 1,000 female dogs at risk.[1] Mammary gland tumors have been historically reported to comprise 52% of all neoplasms in the bitch, although the incidence is declining because of the common practice of ovariohysterectomy in young dogs. The median age is between 10 and 11 years of age, and mammary gland tumors are very rare in dogs less than 5 years of age. The breeds with the highest incidence are the poodle, English spaniel, Brittany spaniel, English setter, pointer, fox terrier, Boston terrier, and cocker spaniel.[2] Boxers, greyhounds, beagles, and chihuahuas are considered to have a decreased risk of developing malignant mammary tumors.[2,3]

Canine mammary tumors are clearly a hormonally dependent tumor. The risk of developing mammary tumors in dogs spayed prior to the first estrus is 0.05%, 8% after the first estrus, and after the second estrus the risk will increase to 26%.[4] Additional evidence for a hormonal component with this disease is based on the fact that increased levels of both estrogen and progesterone receptors, have been identified in mammary gland tumors. Most studies indicate that 40 to 60% of all malignant tumors will contain either estrogen or, to a lesser degree, progesterone receptors,[5-10] and receptors are present in about 70% of the benign tumors.[5,7,10] The more malignant tumors (less differentiated) tend to be receptor negative. In addition, some malignant tumors have been positive for prolactin receptors, but the level of receptor expression has been lower in malignant tissue than nonmalignant tissue.[11]

It is well known that, in the female dog, progesterone or synthetic progestin such as chlormadinone acetate (CMA) or medroxyprogesterone acetate (MPA) induces full lobuloalveolar development of the mammary gland, with hyperplasia of secretory and myoepithelial elements, while estradiol stimulates ductal growth. However, prolonged administration of estrogens has not been shown to increase the incidence of mammary tumors in dogs. Conversely, progesterone administered to young female beagles will produce a higher percentage of benign nodules.[12] In a recently published study, long-term, high-dose, (125× human dose) 19-Nortestosterone produced mammary carcinoma in 40% of the intact dogs treated.[13] Injectable progestins used to prevent estrus in dogs have been shown to increase the incidence of benign tumors, but not malignant tumors.[14] Moderate-to-high doses of progestins have been shown to increase growth hormone (GH) secretion, but it has not been proven that increased secretion of GH results in mammary tumor development.[12] Recently, a study has shown that GH gene expression is present in the normal and neoplastic mammary tissue of the dog. The expression in normal tissue is strongly stimulated by progestins and may act as an intermediate in the progestin-stimulated development in canine mammary tumors. It is hypothesized that after malignant transformation the mammary GH messenger RNA (mRNA) expression may become progesterone independent.[15]

Experiments in rodents and epidemiologic studies in humans have shown that a high-fat diet and obesity increase the risk of mammary cancer. In a recent study in pet dogs diagnosed with mammary cancer, it was found that among spayed dogs, the incidence was reduced if the dogs were thin at 9 to 12 months of age.[16] Thus, nutritional factors may play a role in canine mammary tumor development.

## Pathology and Natural Behavior

Between 41 and 53% of the mammary tumors that occur in the bitch are considered malignant (Table 23–1).[17–18] Histologic evidence of malignancy does not invariably imply a malignant clinical course. In some studies, histologic malignancy may be under-reported and in others it may be over-reported. A major problem with canine mammary tumors is that a number of histologic criteria are used to define malignancy, and the criteria will differ from one institution to another and often within individuals from the same institution. Additionally, histologic appearance may vary markedly within the same mass. Most malignant mammary tumors will be classified as epithelial tumors or carcinomas. Depending on the classification system used, the carcinomas may be further subdivided into simple

carcinoma, complex carcinoma, adenocarcinoma, and solid carcinoma (see Table 23–1). A malignant tumor composed of cells morphologically resembling the epithelial and connective tissue components, both of which are malignant, is termed a *malignant mixed tumor* or *carcinosarcoma*. Most histologic classification systems are based on recognition of histologic tissue patterns, with little, if any, reference to disease behavior. Using a classification system adopted from a significantly prognostic human pathologic staging system, 232 dogs with mammary gland tumors were evaluated. This system was found to be of significant prognostic value for the dog.[18] In this study, dogs were characterized into one of four histologic grades as follows:

1. Histologic Grade 0—Malignant proliferation limited to the anatomic borders of the mammary duct system, i.e., in situ carcinoma.
2. Histologic Grade I—Malignant proliferation extending beyond the anatomic borders of the mammary duct system into the surrounding stroma, i.e., invasive carcinoma, but without identifiable vascular or lymphatic invasion.
3. Histologic Grade II—Invasive carcinoma with vascular or lymphatic invasion or metastasis to regional lymph nodes, or both.
4. Histologic Grade III—Pathologic evidence of distant metastasis.

**Table 23–1** Distribution of Canine Mammary Neoplasms Based on Histologic Examination

| Tumor Type | Relative Frequency |
|---|---|
| *Benign* (50%) | |
| Fibroadenomas (benign mixed tumor) | 45.5 |
| Simple adenomas | 5.0 |
| Benign mesenchymal tumors | 0.5 |
| *Malignant* (49%) | |
| Solid carcinomas | 16.9 |
| Tubular adenocarcinomas | 15.4 |
| Papillary adenocarcinomas | 8.6 |
| Anaplastic carcinomas | 4.0 |
| Sarcomas | 3.1 |
| Carcinosarcoma (malignant mixed tumors) | 1.0 |

*Sources:* Figures were obtained from an unselected series of 1,625 canine mammary tumors submitted by general practioners to the Department of Clinical Veterinary Medicine, Cambridge, England, for diagnosis. Reproduced with the permission of WB Saunders, Philadelphia, from Bostock R: Neoplasia of the skin and mammary glands in dogs and cats. *In* Kirk RW (ed): Current Veterinary Therapy: VI. Small Animal Practice, 1977, pp. 493–496.

Furthermore, these tumors can be histologically evaluated on the basis of their degree of nuclear differentiation. The nuclear differentiation can be categorized into poorly differentiated, moderately differentiated, and well differentiated. The degree of differentiation is usually inversely related to tumor aggressiveness.

Sarcomas comprise less than 5% of all mammary tumors and are much less common than carcinomas. It is uncertain whether these arise from myoepithelial tissue that has undergone neoplastic change or from the intralobular connective tissue. There is no evidence that sarcomas arise from pre-existing mixed cell tumors. Sarcomas can be subdivided into various groups, including osteosarcoma, fibrosarcoma, and chondrosarcoma.

Another histologic form of malignant mammary tumors is termed *inflammatory carcinoma*.[19] These neoplasms grow with extreme rapidity and invade lymphatics in the skin, resulting in marked edema and inflammation (Fig. 23–1). Histologically, there is evidence of a poorly differentiated carcinoma with extensive

**Figure 23–1.** Bilateral inflammatory carcinoma with vaginal edema and edema of the leg in a dog. Vaginal cytology and fine-needle cytology of the popliteal lymph node were positive for cancer.

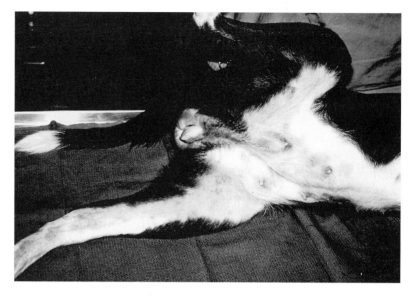

evidence of both mononuclear and polymorphonuclear cellular infiltrates.

## History and Signs

Mammary tumors are characterized clinically as single (~75%) or multiple (~25%) nodules located within the mammary gland. They may be associated with the nipple or they may be associated with the glandular tissue itself. In many animals with benign mammary tumors such as the adenomas, the tumor will be small, well circumscribed, and firm on palpation. The dog has five pairs of glands, all of which can develop one or more benign or malignant tumors. Roughly 65 to 70% of canine tumors occur in glands 4 and 5, probably because of the greater volume of breast tissue in these glands. In some animals, the tumor may have undergone ulceration and may present with inflammation (Fig. 23–2).

As previously mentioned, the inflammatory carcinomas tend to be diffusely swollen, and there is poor demarcation between normal and abnormal tissue. All or part of one mammary

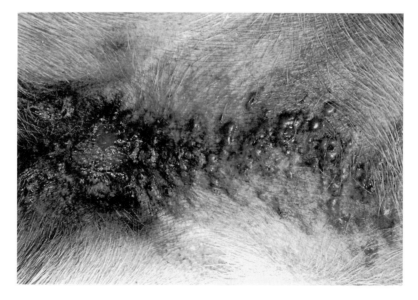

**Figure 23–2.** Cutaneous involvement in a dog of a recurrent mammary carcinoma with ulceration and nodular plaque formation. This is a poor prognostic sign.

chain may be involved or bilateral involvement may also be observed. Extensive lymph edema of a limb or limbs adjacent to this type of mammary cancer may also occur (see Fig. 23–1). Such edema is due to occlusion of the affected lymphatics, with accompanying retrograde growth down the limb. Inflammatory carcinomas are often initially misdiagnosed as an acute mastitis and are treated as such with antibiotics and corticosteroids. It is important to differentiate this type of malignancy with that of inflammatory mastitis. The inflammatory carcinomas tend to be quite firm and have a diffuse type of swelling, whereas mastitis tends to be more localized and is usually seen after estrus or false pregnancy.

Carcinoma that metastasizes to the inguinal lymph nodes may enter the pudendal lymphatics and spread to the internal iliac nodes. Metastasis from the internal iliac nodes may be palpable and cause compression of the colon.

## Diagnostic Techniques and Workup

Diagnostic workup should include a thorough physical examination, and a routine hematologic and serum chemistry profile prior to anesthesia is desirable. A coagulogram may be indicated in dogs with inflammatory carcinoma because of the concurrent association with disseminated intravascular coagulation. Thoracic radiographs in both the right and left lateral and ventrodorsal planes should be taken prior to surgery to evaluate the lungs and sternal lymph node for possible metastasis. In some cases, if the mammary tumors are involving the caudal two glands, it is desirable to evaluate the sublumbar region for metastic lymphadenopathy with caudal abdominal radiographs or ultrasound. Also, a rectal exam may reveal palpable evidence of internal iliac lymphadenopathy. Fine-needle aspiration and cytology to differentiate benign from malignant tumors has been reported to be an insensitive method, and the distinction between benign and malignant does not change the operative procedure.[20]

The most definitive way to obtain a diagnosis is through an excisional biopsy. If lymph node metastasis is suspected, cytology can be used to assess these nodes for metastasis. We have found that fine-needle aspiration for cytological evaluation has also been very beneficial in the diagnosis of inflammatory carcinomas.

**Clinical Staging**   Accurate and precise staging is important prior to undertaking treatment. The most important features of staging are to evalu-

ate (1) the primary tumor and regional lymph nodes and (2) attempt to identify any distant metastatic sites. The most important features to note with the primary tumor are size, clinical evidence of invasiveness (fixation to skin or fascia), evidence of inflammatory carcinoma, ulceration, and recent rapid growth. The sites most common for distant metastasis will be the lung, sublumbar lymph nodes, liver, and rarely bone. Table 23–2 summarizes a modified World Health Organization (WHO) clinical staging system for dogs.

## Therapy

Surgery remains the treatment of choice for all dogs with mammary gland tumors, with the exception of those with inflammatory carcinomas or distant metastasis. The type of surgery will depend on the extent of disease.

**Surgical Technique**   No prospective clinical trial has shown an improved survival for canine patients undergoing "radical" mastectomy versus local mass removal. The theoretical and practical pros and cons of radical versus local excision have been extensively debated.[21] In a published prospective clinical trial of 144 dogs to compare simple to radical mastectomy, there was no dif-

---

**Table 23–2**   Canine Mammary Tumor Staging Modified*

T: Primary Tumor
   $T_1$   < 3 cm maximum diameter
   $T_2$   3–5 cm maximum diameter
   $T_3$   > 5 cm maximum diameter

N: Regional lymph node status
   $N_0$   Histologic— No metastasis
   $N_1$   Histologic— Metastasis

M: Distant metastasis
   $M_0$   No distant metastasis detected
   $M_1$   Distant metastasis detected

*Excluding inflammatory carcinoma.

*Stage Grouping*

| Stage | | | |
|-------|-------|-------|-------|
| I | $T_1$ | $N_0$ | $M_0$ |
| II | $T_2$ | $N_0$ | $M_0$ |
| III | $T_3$ | $N_0$ | $M_0$ |
| IV | Any T | $N_1$ | $M_0$ |
| V | Any T | Any N | $M_1$ |

ference in recurrence rate and survival time.[22] The proponents in favor of radical removal argue that it is the most likely procedure to remove all tumor (known or occult) and that it reduces future risk by reducing the volume of breast tissue at risk. The proponents opposed to routine radical resection argue that it is too much surgery, when more than 50% of canine breast masses are benign and no published data exist to prove benign lesions transform to malignant; a radical procedure can always be performed later on the 40 to 50% of patients with a malignant histology; radical surgery increases the morbidity, time, and expense of the treatment; and, most compellingly, radical mastectomy does *not* improve survival over lesser procedures. The goal of surgery in canine breast cancer is to remove all tumor by the simplest procedure. More surgery is not better surgery for the dog.

A variety of procedures exist for removing canine breast tumors, and the choice of procedure is determined by size, fixation to surrounding tissue, and the number of lesions rather than any expected change in survival. Definitions of the various procedures and their indications are described below:

**Lumpectomy, or Nodulectomy**   Lumpectomy, or nodulectomy, is indicated for small (< 0.5 cm), firm, superficial, nonfixed nodules that are usually benign. The skin is incised and the nodule bluntly dissected from the breast tissue with a small rim of normal tissue surrounding the tumor nodule.

After resection, the tumor is classified as benign or malignant and the completeness of the removal is evaluated. For benign lesions, even close and incomplete removal is probably adequate. If the lesion is malignant, close but clean margins is acceptable. Clearly, incomplete resection warrants more aggressive removal of the entire gland or previous biopsy site..

**Mammectomy**   Removal of one gland is indicated for lesions centrally located within the gland, bigger than 1 cm, and exhibiting any degree of fixation to skin or fascia. Skin and abdominal wall fascia should be removed with the mass, if involved.

Based on individual patient gland confluency, it may be easier to remove glands 4 and 5 as a unit or glands 1, 2, and 3 as a unit rather than extensively divide mammary tissue. In other words, if the individual gland is a distinct anatomic unit, single-gland removal is acceptable.

**Regional Mastectomy**   Regional mastectomy was originally proposed based on the known venous and lymphatic drainage of the mammary tissue.[23,24] In the dog, mammary glands have been identified, depending on their position, as the cranial thoracic (gland 1), caudal thoracic (gland 2), cranial abdomen (gland 3), caudal abdominal (gland 4), and inguinal (gland 5). Lymphatic drainage from the mammary glands has been documented to the axillary, superficial inguinal, sublumbar, and cranial sternal nodes, depending on the gland involved.

The lymphatic drainage of canine mammary tumors is complex. Although there can be lymphatic drainage between all the glands, it has recently been reported that major connections occur between glands 1 and 2, and between glands 4 and 5.[24] Mammary glands 1, 2, and 3 drain to axillary and cranial sternal lymph nodes. The superficial inguinal lymph nodes, usually numbering two, provide lymphatic drainage to mammary glands 3, 4, 5, and occasionally 2. The superficial inguinal lymph nodes have efferent drainage to the medial iliac lymph nodes, which then continue to the lumbar trunks and finally to the cisterna chyli. Based on the premise of lymphatic drainage, the tumors involving glands 1, 2, or 3 should be removed en bloc. Conversely, the tumors involving 4 or 5 should be removed en bloc, and adjoining lymph nodes should always be removed whenever possible. The axillary lymph node is removed only if enlarged or cytologically positive for malignant cells.

In patients with several mammary masses, it is presumed that the tumor spreads from one gland to another, rather than started as synchronous primaries. Although either presumption is hard to prove, the latter is likely, making regional mastectomy more of a theoretical consideration than a necessity.

**Unilateral or Bilateral Mastectomy**   Glands 1 through 5 can be removed as a unit if multiple tumors or several large tumors preclude rapid and wide removal by lesser procedures. Simultaneous bilateral mastectomy has also been proposed and can be accomplished in dogs and cats with pendulous mammae.[21] These procedures are done because they may be faster than multiple lumpectomies or mammectomies, not because they improve survival in the dog.

**Lymph Nodes**   The axillary lymph nodes are rarely involved with mammary cancer in the dog and should not be removed prophylactically.

Fixed, adherent, and large axillary nodes can only rarely be removed completely. When enlarged and cytologically positive for cancer or whenever gland 5 is removed, the inguinal lymph node should be removed, since it is intimately associated with this gland.

In summary, mammary cancer in the dog should be removed by the simplest procedure that will remove known cancer in the mammary gland. This does not mean that incomplete resection or debulking surgery is acceptable.

**Chemotherapy**   No therapeutic or adjuvant chemotherapy protocol has been reported to be effective in the dog. We have evaluated two chemotherapeutic combinations and have found minimal antitumor activity. We have seen some antitumor activity in dogs with mammary adenocarcinoma using doxorubicin and cyclophosphamide or cisplatin as a single agent. Using established canine mammary tumor cell lines, doxorubicin has been shown to have antitumor activity using in vitro clonogenic assays.[25] Additional studies are needed to determine the optimal chemotherapeutic agent(s) for the treatment of canine malignant mammary tumors. Future clinical trials should concentrate on adjuvant chemotherapy of dogs with poor prognostic factors, such as large, invasive, high-grade tumors, following complete surgical removal.

**Radiation Therapy**   As with chemotherapy, no reliable information on the value of radiation is yet available. Radiation therapy, like surgery, is mainly limited by the extent of the tumor and may only be considered useful in dogs that have tumors that are too extensive for surgery. Radiation therapy has been tried in a few inoperable patients and in inflammatory carcinoma cases, but the short-term morbidity is high, and accentuation of already present inflammatory disease is a complication. More carefully designed studies are needed before any efficacy can be placed on the value of radiation for canine mammary tumors.

**Biologic Response Modifiers**   Studies with nonspecific immunomodulation using levamisole[22] and *Corynebacterium parvum* with the bacillus Calmette-Guérin (BCG) show little effectiveness over surgery alone.[26] In a double-blind prospective WHO comparative oncology group study of 130 bitches with confirmed mammary cancer treated by chain resection, dogs were treated with IV BCG (live Pasteur strain) or *C. parvum* vaccine (Burrough Wellcome) or IV

saline. No statistical differences were reported in 1-, 2-, and 3-year survival rates for the three treatment groups.[27] Another study reported that IV BCG (Glaxo-live) following mastectomy increased median survival time from 24 weeks (control) to 100 weeks (BCG).[28] In another study, mammary tumor cells treated with neuraminidase and used as a vaccine showed temporary regression in 4 of 23 dogs treated.[29] These approaches, though, are still considered experimental and have questionable therapeutic effectiveness.

**Hormonal Therapy**   The issue of ovariohysterectomy for potential therapeutic benefit for mammary tumors remains unresolved. In one study of 154 dogs treated with mastectomy and ovariohysterectomy (OHE), the mean survival time was reported to be 8.4 months,[30] and this compares to mean survival times of 10 and 8 months in other studies treated by mastectomy alone.[17] There have been no well-designed prospective studies to clearly address the issue of ovariohysterectomy as an adjunctive treatment for dogs with malignant mammary tumors. Routine OHE at the time of mastectomy is not recommended to reduce local recurrence or metastasis.

Antiestrogens, such as tamoxifen, have been tested both in vitro for antiproliferative activity in canine mammary tumor cell lines[25] and to a limited degree in clinical cases.[31,32] In one study, tamoxifen was administered in dosages ranging from 2.5 to 10 mg PO BID. (0.18–1.0 mg/kg, median 0.42 mg/kg) to seven dogs with inoperable or metastatic tumor. Five of 7 dogs had objective tumor responses. The mean survival time was reported to be 4 months.[31] Clinical toxicities noted were vulvar swelling, vaginal discharge, incontinence, urinary tract infection, stump pyometra, and signs of estrus.[31] In another recently published study, 18 dogs were treated with tamoxifen following mastectomy and ovariohysterectomy. Only 6 of 18 had malignant tumors. In 10 of 18 dogs (56%) treatment resulted in estrogenlike signs related to tamoxifen side effects (vulva swelling, vulva discharge, behavior changes, and nesting).[32] No antitumor activity could be documented. At this time, tamoxifen therapy is not advised in dogs.

## Prognosis

In canine mammary tumors the significant prognostic factors have been the following: histologic type, degree of invasion, degree of nuclear differentiation (grade), evidence of lymphoid cellular

**Table 23–3**　Summary of Canine Mammary Tumor Prognostic Factors*

| Good | Poor | Indifferent |
|---|---|---|
| < 3 cm | > 3 cm | Age |
| Well circumscribed | Invasive | Breed |
| Lymph node (–) | Lymph node (+) | OHE status |
| Lymphoid cellular reactivity(+) | Lymphoid cellular reactivity (–) | Weight |
| | Inflammatory carcinoma | Type of surgery (simple vs. radical) |
| ER or PR (+) | Ulceration | Number of tumors |
| | Sarcomas | Gland(s) involved |
| | ER (–) | |

*These factors should serve as relative indicators of prognosis. Individual variation will be found.

reactivity in the tumor vicinity, tumor size, increasing age at diagnosis, lymph node involvement, hormone receptor activity, ulceration, S-phase rate, and DNA aneuploidy.[6,21,22,33–36] Factors that do not seem to be associated with prognosis are tumor location, type of surgery (as long as histologically adequate resection is achieved), ovariohysterectomy at surgery, and the number of tumors present.[26,33–38] A summary of canine prognostic factors is provided in Table 23–3.

In one study, histologic grade was correlated with disease-free interval after mastectomy in 158 dogs with mammary cancer (Table 23–4).[18] In that study, only 19% of the dogs with Grade 0 (malignant proliferation limited to the anatomic borders of the mammary duct system) had recurrence or metastasis within 2 years after the initial mastectomy, compared to 60% in dogs with Grade I disease (malignant proliferations extending beyond the anatomic borders of the mammary duct system into the surrounding stroma) and 97% recurrence or metastasis in dogs with Grade II disease (invasion into vascular or lymphatic vessels). Thus, the prognosis is very good for dogs with noninvasive carcinoma (Fig. 23–3). Another factor evaluated that has been shown to be important for prognosis is the degree of nuclear differentiation.[18] The nuclear differentiation of a tumor can be categorized as poorly differentiated, moderately differentiated, and well differentiated. The degree of differentiation is usually inversely related to tumor aggressiveness. Dogs with poorly differentiated tumors have a greater than fourfold increased risk of developing recurrent or metastatic carcinoma in less than 2 years after mastectomy, with an overall 90% rate, compared to 68% for those with moderately differentiated tumors. Dogs with well-differentiated tumors have only a 24% local or systemic recur-

rence rate within 2 years of their mastectomy. Another factor that has been shown to correlate with prognosis is lymphoid cellular reactions observed in the tumor vicinity.[18] Lymphoid cellular activity may indicate morphologic evidence of an antitumor immune response. Dogs with mammary cancer that did not have evidence of lymphoid cellular activity at the time of initial mas-

**Table 23–4**　Prognosis Related to Clinical and Histologic Features in Canine Mammary Tumors[18,33]

| | % Local or Distant Recurrence at | |
|---|---|---|
| | 12 months | 24 months |
| *Tumor Size* | | |
| < 3 cm | 30 | 40 |
| > 3 cm | 70 | 80 |
| *Histologic Grade* | | |
| Grade 0 | 10 | 19 |
| Grade I | 40 | 60 |
| 　Well differentiated | NA[a] | 40 |
| 　Moderately differentiated | NA[a] | 63 |
| 　Poorly differentiated | NA[a] | 77 |
| Grade II | 85 | 97 |
| *Lymph Node Status* | | |
| Negative | 20 | 30 |
| Positive | 90 | 100 |
| *Lymphoid Cellular Reactivity* (Histologic Grade I) | | |
| Positive | NA[a] | 45 |
| Negative | NA[a] | 83 |

[a]NA = Data not available.

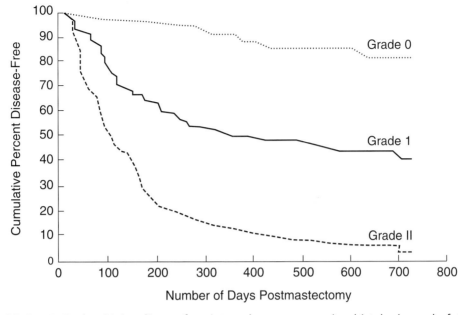

**Figure 23–3.** A Kaplan-Meier disease-free interval curve comparing histologic grade following mastectomy in 158 dogs with malignant mammary tumors. Grade 0, $n = 35$; Grade I, $n = 76$; Grade II, $n = 47$. The three stages are significantly different; $p < 0.0001$.[33]

tectomy had a threefold increased risk of developing recurrence within 2 years, compared to those with such reactivity. Dogs with histologic grade I tumors showing lymphoid cellular reactivity had a 45% recurrence rate within 2 years, and dogs without cellular reactivity had an 83% recurrence rate within 2 years.

Sarcomas are considered to have a very poor prognosis.[35,36] Most dogs with sarcomas will be dead of their disease within 9 to 12 months. Inflammatory carcinomas also have a very poor prognosis.[19] Most of these cannot be resected surgically and, if they are resected, they tend to recur within weeks to a month after surgery. In addition, these dogs also can have a low-grade, disseminated, intravascular coagulation (DIC), and we have observed a localized DIC that will manifest itself by excessive bleeding at the time of surgery.

Tumor size is also a very important prognostic factor (Fig. 23–4). The most recent WHO clinical staging system categorizes dogs according to the diameter of the largest tumor. $T_1$ is a tumor less than 3 cm in diameter, $T_2$ is a tumor 3 to 5 cm in diameter, and $T_3$ is a tumor greater than 5 cm in diameter. In dogs with locally invasive disease, significant differences have been found between $T_1$ and $T_2$, and $T_1$ and $T_3$ tumors, but not between $T_2$ and $T_3$ tumors. Thus, dogs with histologic

invasive cancer having malignant tumors of a diameter of less than 3 cm have a significantly better prognosis than dogs with malignant tumors of 3 cm or greater in diameter[33] (Fig. 23–4). In a recent study in dogs that have invasion of lymphatic vessels or lymph node metastasis, no significant differences were found between $T_1$, $T_2$, and $T_3$ size tumors.[33] In another study, dogs with a $T_3$ carcinoma (> 5 cm diameter) had a median survival time of 40 weeks compared to 112 weeks for animals with smaller tumors.[39]

There has been some controversy in the literature regarding the influence of lymph node metastases on survival. In one study, lymph node involvement was not associated with significant differences in survival.[34] In more recent studies, there was a significant difference in disease-free interval between dogs with lymph node involvement and dogs without lymph node involvement.[33,35] In one study, 80% of the dogs with lymph node involvement had recurrence within 6 months,[33] whereas dogs with negative lymph nodes will usually have a 30% recurrence rate by 2 years postsurgery (Fig. 23–5).

It has been shown that dogs with either estrogen or progesterone receptors will have a better prognosis following surgery.[6,10] The presence of these receptors has been correlated with well-dif-

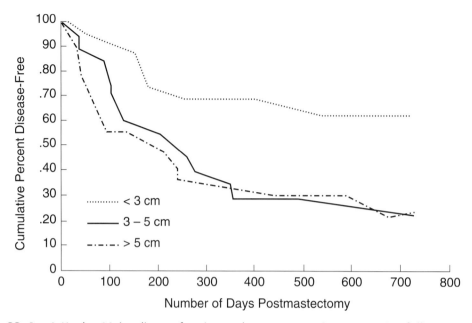

**Figure 23–4.**   A Kaplan-Meier disease free-interval curve comparing tumor size following mastectomy in 54 dogs with locally invasive, malignant mammary tumors. Dogs with tumors < 3 cm (*n* = 16) had significantly longer disease-free intervals than dogs with tumors of either 3 to 5 cm (*n* = 20) or > 5 cm (*n* = 18); *p* < .04.[33]

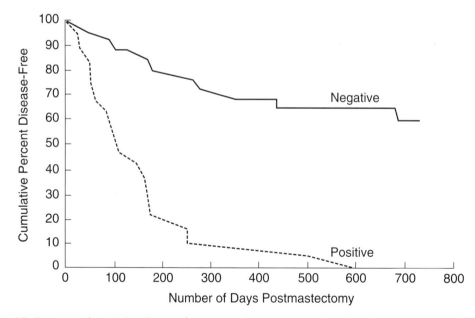

**Figure 23–5.**   A Kaplan-Meier disease-free interval curve comparing lymph node metastasis following mastectomy in 45 dogs with malignant mammary tumors. Dogs with negative lymph node states (*n* = 26) had a significantly longer disease-free interval than those with positive lymph nodes (*n* = 19); p < .001.[33]

ferentiated tumors. Unfortunately, the availability of receptor laboratory analysis for canine tumors is very limited.

## FELINE MAMMARY TUMORS

When a cat with a mammary mass is presented, a malignancy must be considered. At least 80% of feline mammary tumors are malignant.[1,39–41] Mammary tumors are known to be at least the third most frequently occurring tumor in the cat, following hematopoietic neoplasms and skin tumors.[1,41–43] The incidence of mammary tumors in the cat is less than half that of humans and dogs.[1,41–43] However, this tumor accounts for 17% of neoplasms in female cats.

Although there is no proven breed-associated predilection for mammary tumors, some investigators have suggested that domestic short-haired and Siamese cats have higher incidence rates than other cats.[41,44,45] Siamese cats may have twice the risk of any other breed of developing mammary tumors.[41]

Mammary neoplasia has been reported to occur in cats from 9 months to 23 years of age, with a mean age of occurrence of 10 to 12 years.[41–47] One study suggests that the disease occurs at an earlier age in Siamese cats and the incidence reaches a plateau at about 9 years of age.[41] The majority of affected cats are intact females; however, the disease is occasionally seen in oophorectomized females and rarely in male cats.[41,44,45]

Hormonal influences may be involved in the pathogenesis of mammary tumors in the cat. Although the association between ovariohysterectomy and incidence is not as strong as in the dog, most studies show that intact cats are more likely to develop mammary tumors than oophorectomized cats.[1,41,48] Studies have been done to determine the role of progesterone, testosterone, and estrogen in causing feline mammary tumors. Low levels of progesterone receptors have been found in the cytoplasm of some feline mammary tumors.[49–51] Several reports have also documented a strong association between the prior use of progesteronelike drugs and the development of benign or malignant mammary masses in cats.[41,52–54] Dihydrotestosterone receptors have not been found in mammary tumors in cats.[49] Only 10% of the feline tumors assayed were positive for estrogen receptors; a much higher percentage of positive tests is seen in dogs and humans.[55]

## Pathology and Natural Behavior

**Mammary Tumors**   Between 80 and 85% of the feline mammary tumors will be malignant. Many of the tumors, especially the large, more invasive neoplasms, adhere to the skin and are ulcerated. Lymphatic and lymph node invasion is frequently present and visible at necropsy.[43,44,47] In several studies, more than 80% of the cats with a mammary malignancy had metastases to one or more of the following organs at the time of euthanasia: lymph nodes, lungs, pleura, liver, diaphragm, adrenal glands, and kidneys.[41,43,44,46,56]

More than 80% of the feline mammary tumors are histologically classified as adenocarcinomas.[42–44] The frequency of diagnosis of the specific types of adenocarcinomas differs slightly among pathologists, but most agree that tubular, papillary, and solid carcinomas are the most common. The majority of adenocarcinomas have a combination of tissue types in each tumor. Sarcomas, mucinous carcinomas, duct papillomas, adenosquamous carcinomas, and adenomas are rarely seen.[40,43,44,46,56] The benign mammary gland dysplasias are infrequently reported by the pathologist, but they are an important part of a differential diagnosis.

**Mammary Hyperplasia**   There are two basic types of noninflammatory hyperplasia of the feline mammary gland: lobular hyperplasia and fibroepithelial hyperplasia.[57-59]

*Lobular Hyperplasia.*[40] Lobular hyperplasia occurs as palpable masses in one or more glands. It has been reported in cats from 1 to 14 years of age and most were 8 years. Most cats were intact females. The most common type of lobular hyperplasia involves one or more enlarged lobules with a cystic or dilated ductal component.

*Fibroepithelial Hyperplasia.*[40] (Fibroepithelial hyperplasia) will usually occur in young, cycling, or pregnant female cats and has even been seen in litters prior to their first estrus. Old, unspayed females and males given megestrol acetate have developed this condition. Most affected cats exhibit hyperplasia 1 or 2 weeks after their first estrus. The tremendously enlarged glands may appear erythematous and some of the skin may be necrotic. Edema of the skin, subcutis, and both rear legs is common. This condition can be easily confused with an acute mastitis.

These conditions are thought to be associated with hormonal stimulation of the glandular tissue. Diuretics, corticosteroids, and testosterone have been advocated but the results are variable. Necrosis and ulceration may be associated with bleeding and localized infection. Systemic infection and pulmonary embolism have been reported.

If an ovariohysterectomy is to be performed and the glands are still greatly enlarged, then a flank incision should be used. In time, the glands will regress and the ovariohysterectomy should prevent recurrence.

## History and Signs

Feline mammary tumors are often presented to the veterinarian 5 months after they are initially noted.[45] Thus, the tumors are usually in an advanced state of development when they are handled clinically. The neoplasm may adhere to the overlying skin but rarely adheres to the underlying abdominal wall. The tumor is usually firm and nodular. At least one quarter of affected patients have ulcerated masses. The involved nipples may be red and swollen and may exudate a tan or yellow fluid. The tumor can involve any or all mammary glands and is noted equally in the left and right sides.[44,45,47,56,59] More than half of the affected cats have multiple gland involvement.[44-46] Metastatic lung and thorax involvement may be extensive and may cause respiratory insufficiency because of a pleural carcinomatosis with an effusion, often containing malignant cells.

## Diagnostic Techniques and Workup

Before any diagnostic or therapeutic steps are taken, the health status of the cat must be fully assessed. A serum chemical profile, urinalysis, and complete blood count should be done to identify any presurgical abnormalities. Thoracic radiographs in both the right and left lateral and ventrodorsal planes should be made to search for pulmonary, lymph node, and pleural metastases. Mammary tumor pulmonary metastases appear radiographically as interstitial densities. They range from those that are faintly seen, to those that are several centimeters in diameter, to miliary pleural lesions than can produce significant effusion. Sternal lymphadenopathy is occasionally seen. Changes due to aging in the lungs and pleura, as well as inactive inflammatory lesions, may simulate metastatic disease. Treatment should not be withheld because of equivocal radiographic findings.

Because of the high frequency of malignancy,

an aggressive approach should be taken to confirm the diagnosis. A preliminary biopsy is usually not recommended because 80 to 85% of the masses in a mammary gland will be malignant. However, cytology may be helpful to rule out possible skin or subcutaneous nonmammary malignancies. Tissue for histopathology is taken at the time of mastectomy. If pleural fluid is removed from a cat with a mammary gland lesion, cytology should be done on the fluid to search for malignant cells.

## Clinical Staging

The most important features of staging are to (a) evaluate the primary tumor and regional lymph nodes and (b) identify any metastatic sites. The most important features to note are the number of tumors, size (very important), location, and clinical evidence of invasiveness (fixation to skin or fascia). Regional lymph nodes should be examined carefully and fine-needle aspiration or surgical removal may be necessary to determine metastasis. Table 23-5 summarizes a modified WHO clinical staging system for cats.

## Therapy

Mammary neoplasms in the cat have been treated in a variety of ways. Surgery is the most

---

**Table 23-5    Feline Mammary Tumor Staging Modified**

T: Primary
  $T_1$   < 2 cm maximum diameter
  $T_2$   2-3 cm maximum diameter
  $T_3$   > 3 cm maximum diameter

N: Regional lymph nodes
  $N_0$   No histologic metastasis
  $N_1$   Histologic metastasis

M: Distant metastasis
  $M_0$   No evidence of metastasis
  $M_1$   Evidence of metastasis

*Stage Grouping*
Stage

| Stage | T | N | M |
|---|---|---|---|
| I | $T_1$ | $N_0$ | $M_0$ |
| II | $T_2$ | $N_0$ | $M_0$ |
| III | $T_3$ | $N_0$ or $N_1$ | $M_0$ |
| IV | Any T | Any N | $M_1$ |

widely used treatment. It may be used alone or in combination with chemotherapy or other modes of cancer therapy.

**Surgery**   The success of surgery is hindered by the invasive nature of the disease and its tendency for early metastasis. Radical mastectomy (i.e., removal of all glands on the affected side) is the surgical method of choice because it significantly reduces the chance of local tumor recurrence.[45,60-62] This procedure is frequently utilized, regardless of the size of the tumor.

The surgeon's knowledge of the anatomy of the area is critical for local control of the tumor. The cat, unlike the dog, usually has four pairs of mammary glands. The two cranial glands on each side have a common lymphatic system and drain into the axillary lymph nodes and then to sternal nodes. The two caudal glands tend to drain to inguinal lymph nodes.

Several surgical principles are observed when performing a mastectomy on feline mammary tumor patients. As opposed to the dog, in which more conservative resections may be appropriate in carefully selected cases, most cats require a complete unilateral or bilateral mastectomy. Tumor fixation to the skin or abdominal fascia necessitates en bloc removal of these structures. Complete unilateral mastectomy is usually performed if the tumor or tumors are confined to one side. Staged mastectomy (2 weeks apart) or simultaneous bilateral mastectomy is done when the tumors are bilateral. The inguinal lymph node is virtually always removed with gland 4, while the axillary lymph nodes are removed only if enlarged and cytologically positive for tumor. Aggressive or prophylactic removal of axillary nodes, whether positive or negative, probably has little therapeutic benefit.[45,60-62]

Although ovariohysterectomy has been shown not to decrease the incidence of recurrence, some believe that it is warranted because of the occasionally seen coexisting ovarian and uterine disease.[41,45,63] If the mammary mass is due to a benign condition such as fibroepithelial hyperplasia, ovariohysterectomy often results in regression of the hyperplastic tissue. This condition often resolves spontaneously within a few weeks of diagnosis; in some cases without performing an ovariohysterectomy.

**Radiation Therapy**   Radiation therapy is not used routinely to treat feline mammary tumors.

Presently, there are no major claims that radiation increases the survival rate of feline mammary tumor patients.

**Chemotherapy**   Combination chemotherapy using doxorubicin (25–30 mg/M$^2$ IV slowly) and cyclophosphamide (50–100 mg/M$^2$ per os days 3, 4, 5, and 6 following doxorubicin) has been shown to induce short-term responses in about half of the cats with metastatic or nonresectable local disease.[64,65] In one study, 7 of 14 (50%) had a partial response (> 50% regression). The median survival time for those cats responding was 5 months versus 2.5 months for the 7 cats that did not respond to doxorubicin and cyclophosphamide.[65] The chemotherapy protocol can be repeated every 3 to 4 weeks. We have found that the major side effect with this protocol has been profound anorexia and mild myelosuppression. Reducing the dose of doxorubicin to 20 to 25 mg/M$^2$ or 1 mg/kg or substituting mitoxantrone (5 mg/M$^2$ q 3 weeks) may limit toxicity to an acceptable level. In addition, it has been reported that doxorubicin can be nephrotoxic to the cat, although this is considered uncommon.[66] Prospective studies using combined adjuvant chemotherapy and mastectomy in the cat have yet to be performed.

**Biologic Response Modifiers**   Studies using nonspecific biologic response therapy such as levamisole[61] and bacterial vaccines[62] have shown minimal effects on reducing recurrence or prolonging the survival time in cats when combined with surgery. Studies using killed *C. parvum*[27] or liposome-encapsulated muramyl tripeptide (L-MTP)[67] after mastectomy failed to show any significant reduction in local recurrence, compared to surgery alone.[27] To date, we have no effective biologic response modifier available that has been shown to be efficacious in the cat with mammary cancer.

## Prognosis

In the last 20 years, little progress has been made in extending the survival time of feline mammary tumor patients. Because stromal invasion is almost always present and metastases are frequently present at the time of surgery, a guarded-to-poor prognosis should always be given. With conservative surgery, 66% of the cats that have had their tumors surgically excised

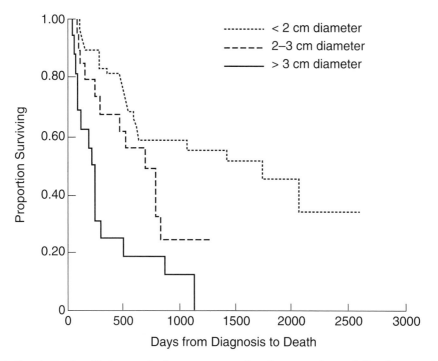

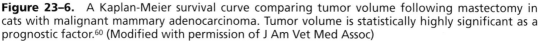

**Figure 23–6.** A Kaplan-Meier survival curve comparing tumor volume following mastectomy in cats with malignant mammary adenocarcinoma. Tumor volume is statistically highly significant as a prognostic factor.[60] (Modified with permission of J Am Vet Med Assoc)

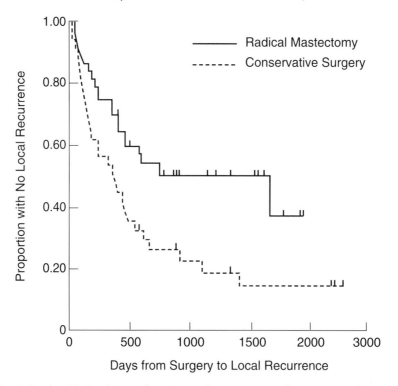

**Figure 23–7.** A Kaplan-Meier disease-free interval curve comparing conservative surgery to radical surgery in cats with malignant mammary adenocarcinoma. Cats undergoing radical mastectomy have a statistically significant reduced local recurrence rate.[60] (Modified with permission of J Am Vet Med Assoc)

have a recurrence at the surgical site.[45,60,62] Most studies state that the time from tumor detection to the death of the cat is 10 to 12 months.[41,42,45,56]

The most significant prognostic factors affecting recurrence and survival for feline malignant mammary tumors are tumor size[56,60] (Fig. 23–6), extent of surgery[60] (Fig. 23–7), and histologic grading.[56] Tumor size is the single most important prognostic factor for malignant feline mammary tumors. Cats with a tumor size of greater than 3 cm in diameter will have a median survival time of 4 to 6 months. Cats with a tumor size of 2 to 3 cm in diameter will have a significantly better survival time with a median of about 2 years, and cats with less than a 2 cm diameter tumor will have a median survival time of over 3 years. Thus, early diagnosis and treatment is a very important prognostic factor for malignant feline mammary tumors.

Few studies have reported the significance of lymph node metastasis in prognosis. In one study, 22 (49%) of 45 tumor-bearing cats had metastasis to the regional lymph node(s). Lymph nodes were clinically palpable in only 10 (21%) of these cats.[68] This provides further rationale to perform a radical mastectomy, including regional (inguinal) lymph node removal, in all cats. Because of its location, the axillary lymph node should only be removed if enlarged or cytologically positive for tumor cells.

Very few studies have been performed to evaluate the effectiveness of the extent of local therapy in malignant feline mammary tumors. One study did show that a radical mastectomy would reduce the development of local recurrence but did not increase the overall survival time (see Fig. 23–7).[60] The final prognostic factor for malignant mammary tumors is the degree of nuclear differentiation. Well-differentiated tumors with few mitotic figures have been shown to have increased survival times but, unfortunately, are rare compared to the more undifferentiated forms.[56]

## COMPARATIVE ASPECTS

Breast cancer is the most common malignant neoplasm in women. In the United States 1 out of every 9 women is likely to develop the disease, and 1 out of every 4 women with cancer will have breast cancer.[69]

The etiology of breast cancer is unknown, although there is a familial tendency, with daughters showing a higher incidence if their mothers had breast cancer. Another important factor is hormone status. Early pregnancy and early oophorectomy lower the incidence, whereas late menopause and early menarche are associated with an increased incidence. Other factors that may play a role are fat intake, obesity, body size, radiation exposure, and socioeconomic influences.[70–72]

Pathologically, the majority of breast cancers are infiltrating duct cell adenocarcinomas with varying degrees of fibrous tissue reaction. Overt metastasis occurs by local infiltration to the skin, opposite breast, and lymph nodes and by blood to the bones, lungs, liver, and brain. Bone metastases are present in more than 50% of patients with disseminated disease.[73]

Hormonal status plays an important role in the biologic behavior and treatment of breast cancer. Estrogen receptors (ERS) are present in more than 60% of the tumors, progesterone receptors (PRS) in more than 30%, and androgen receptors (ARS) in more than 20%. Receptor-positive tumors have a better prognosis with surgery and respond to hormonal therapies, such as oophorectomy and antiestrogens (tamoxifen).[74]

The management of breast cancer provides a major challenge. Treatment will usually involve a combination of mastectomy, lumpectomy, or radiation therapy to the primary site, to the axilla, or both.[75] Hormonal therapy (tamoxifen) will usually follow surgery in ER-positive tumors. Chemotherapy is usually used in patients with more advanced disease (positive lymph nodes, invasive carcinomas), and the useful agents include doxorubicin, mitoxantrone, alkylating agents, 5-fluorouracil, and methotrexate.

The prognosis for breast cancer treatment depends on the histologic tumor type, tumor size, invasiveness, lymph node status, and hormonal receptor status. The survival time for local and regional treatment of breast cancer, both of which employ partial or total breast removal, is 57% for clinically negative nodes and 38% for clinically positive nodes at 10 years.[75] The benefits of adjuvant chemotherapy for node-negative women with low ER levels, and of tamoxifen therapy for women with high ER levels, are statistically very clear. However, the clinical magnitude of these differences is small. Adjuvant chemotherapy/hormonal therapy has reduced the relapse rate from 29% to 23%.[76]

## REFERENCES

1. Dorn CR, Taylor DON, Schneider R, et al: Survey of animal neoplasms in Alameda and Contra Costa Counties, Calif.: II. Cancer morbidity in dogs and

cats from Alameda County. J Natl Cancer Inst *40*:307–318, 1968.

2. Cohen D, Reif JS, Brodey, et al: Epidemiological analysis of the most prevalent sites and types of canine neoplasia observed in a veterinary hospital. Cancer Res *34*:2859–2868, 1974.

3. Priester WA, McKay FW: The occurrence of tumors in domestic animals. NCI Monograph 54. Bethesda, MD, National Cancer Institute, 1980, p. 155.

4. Schneider R, Dorn CR, Taylor DON: Factors influencing canine mammary cancer development and postsurgical survival. J Natl Cancer Inst *43*:1249–1261, 1969.

5. MacEwen EG, Patnaik AK, Harvey HJ, et al: Estrogen receptors in canine mammary tumors. Cancer Res *42*:2255–2259, 1982.

6. Martin PM, Cotard M, Mialot JP, et al: Animal models for hormone-dependent human breast cancer. Cancer Chemothera Pharmacol *2*:13–17, 1984.

7. Hamilton JM, Else RW, Forshaw P: Oestrogen receptors in canine mammary tumors. Vet Rec *101*:258–260, 1977.

8. Inaba T, Takahashi N, Matsuda H, et al: Estrogen and progesterone receptors and progesterone metabolism in canine mammary tumors. Japanese J Vet Sci *46*:797–803, 1984.

9. Rutteman GR, Misdorp W, Blankenstein MA, et al: Oestrogen (ER) and progestin receptors (PR) in mammary tissue of the female dog: Different receptor profile in nonmalignant and malignant states. Br J Cancer *58*:594–599, 1988.

10. Sartin EA, Barnes S, Kwapien RP, et al: Estrogen and progesterone receptor status of mammary carcinomas and correlation with clinical outcome. Am J Vet Res *53*:2196–2200, 1992.

11. Rutteman GR, Willekes-Koolschijn N, Bevers MM, et al: Prolactin binding in benign and malignant mammary tissue of female dogs. Anticancer Res *6*:829–835, 1986.

12. Rutteman GR: Contraceptive steroids and the mammary gland: Is there a hazard? Breast Cancer Res Treat *23*:29–41, 1992.

13. Misdorp W: Progestogens and mammary tumors in dogs and cats. Acta Endocrinol (Kbh) *125* (Suppl):27–31, 1991.

14. Kwapien RP, Giles RC, Geil RC, et al: Malignant mammary tumors in beagle dogs dosed with investigational oral contraceptive steroids. J Natl Cancer Inst *65*:137–144, 1980.

15. Mol JA, vanGarderen E, Rutteman GR, et al: The expression of the gene encoding growth hormone in the normal and tumorous mammary gland of the dog. Proc 4th Annu Europ Soc Vet Intern Med 1994, p. 45.

16. Sonnenschein EG, Glickman LT, Goldschmidt MH, et al: Body conformation, diet and risk of breast cancer in pet dogs: A case-control study. Am J Epidemiol *133*:694–703, 1991.

17. Brodey RS, Goldschmidt MA, Roszel JR: Canine mammary gland neoplasms. J Am Anim Hosp Assoc *19*:61–90, 1983.

18. Gilbertson SR, Kurzman ID, Zachrau RE, et al: Canine mammary epithelial neoplasms: Biological implications of morphologic characteristics assessed in 232 dogs. Vet Pathol *20*:127–142, 1983.

19. Susaneck SJ, Allen TA, Hoopes J, et al: Inflammatory mammary carcinoma in the dog. J Am Anim Hosp Assoc *19*:971–976, 1983.

20. Allen SW, Prasse KW, Mahaffey EA: Cytologic differentiation of benign from malignant canine mammary tumors. Vet Pathol *23*:649–655, 1986.

21. Ferguson RH: Canine mammary gland tumors. Vet Clin North Am Small Animal Pract *15*:501–511, 1985.

22. MacEwen EG, Harvey HJ, Patnaik AK, et al: Evaluation of effects of levamisole and surgery on canine mammary cancer. J Biol Resp Mod. *4*:418–426, 1985.

23. Wilkinson GT: The treatment of mammary tumors in the bitch and a comparison with the cat. Vet Rec *89*:13–16, 1971.

24. Sautet JY, Ruberte J, Lopez C, et al: Lymphatic system of the mammary glands in the dog: An approach to the surgical treatment of malignant mammary tumors. Canine Pract *17*:30–33, 1992.

25. Sartin E, Barnes S, Toivio-Kinnucan M, et al: Heterogenic properties of clonal cell lines derived from canine mammary carcinomas and sensitivity to tamoxifen and doxorubicin. Anticancer Res *13*:229–236, 1993.

26. Parodi AL, Misdorp W, Mialot JP, et al: Intratumoral BCG and *Corynebacterium parvum* therapy of canine mammary tumors before radical mastectomy. Cancer Immunol Immunother *15*:172–177, 1983.

27. Rutten VPMG, Misdorp W, Gauthier A, et al: Immunological aspects of mammary tumors in dogs and cats: A survey including own studies and pertinent literature. Vet Immunol Immunopathol *26*:211–225, 1990.

28. Bostock DE, Gorman NT: Intravenous BCG therapy of mammary carcinoma in bitches after surgical excision of the primary tumour. Eur J Cancer *14*:879–883, 1978.

29. Sedlacek HH, Weise M, Lemmer A, et al: Immunotherapy of spontaneous mammary tumors in mongrel dogs with autologous tumor cells and neuraminidase. Cancer Immunol Immunother *6*:47–58, 1979.

30. Fowler EH, Wilson GP, Koestner AA: Biologic behavior of canine mammary neoplasms based on a histogenetic classification. Vet Pathol *11*:212–229, 1974.

31. Kitchell BE, Fidel JL: Tamoxifen as a potential therapy for canine mammary carcinoma. Proc Vet Cancer Soc 1992, p. 91.

32. Morris JS, Dobson JM, Bostock DE: Use of tamoxifen in the control of mammary neoplasia. Vet Rec *133*:539–542, 1993.

33. Kurzman ID, Gilbertson SR: Prognostic factors in canine mammary tumors. Semin Vet Med Surg 1:25–32, 1986.

34. Misdorp W, Hart AA: Canine mammary cancer: I. Prognosis. J Small Anim Pract 20:385–394, 1979.

35. Hellman E, Bergstrom R, Holmberg L, et al: Prognostic factors in canine mammary tumors: A multivariate study of 202 consecutive cases. Vet Pathol 30:20–27, 1993.

36. Misdorp W, Cotchin E, Hampe JF, et al: Canine malignant mammary tumors: I. Sarcomas. Vet Pathol 8:99–177, 1971.

37. Misdorp W, Cotchin E, Hampe JF, et al: Canine malignant mammary tumors: II. Adenocarcinomas, solid carcinomas, and spindle cell carcinomas. Vet Pathol 9:447–470, 1972.

38. Misdorp W, Cotchin EE, Hampe, JF, et al: Canine malignant mammary tumors: III. Special types of carcinomas, malignant mixed tumors. Vet Pathol 10:241–256, 1973.

39. Bostock DE: Canine and feline mammary neoplasms. British Vet J 142:506–515, 1986.

40. Carpenter JL, Andrews LK, Holzworth J, et al: Tumors and tumor-like lesions. In Holzworth J (ed): Diseases of the Cat: Medicine and Surgery, Vol. 1. Philadelphia, WB Saunders, 1987, pp. 527–538.

41. Hayes HM Jr, Milne KL, Mandell CP: Epidemiological features of feline mammary carcinomas. Vet Rec 108:476–479, 1981.

42. Schmidt RE, Langham RF: A survey of feline neoplasms. J Am Vet Med Assoc 151:1325–1328, 1967.

43. Patnaik AK, Liu SK, Hurvitz AL, et al: Non-hematopoietic neoplasms in cats. J Natl Cancer Inst 54:855–860, 1975.

44. Hayden DW, Neilsen SW: Feline mammary tumors. J Small Anim Pract 12:687–697, 1971.

45. Hayes A: Feline mammary gland tumors. Vet Clin North Am 7(1):205–212, 1977.

46. Moulton JE: Tumors in domestic animals, 2nd ed. Berkeley, University of California Press, 1978, pp. 367–369.

47. Anderson J, Jarrett WFH: Mammary neoplasia in the dog and cat: II. J Small Anim Pract 7:697–701, 1966.

48. Else RW, Wilkinson CT: Considerations for spaying. Vet Rec 94(25):600, 1974.

49. Elling H, Ungemach FR: Progesterone receptors in feline mammary cancer cytosol. J Cancer Res Clin Oncol 100(3):325–327, 1981.

50. Johnston SD, Hayden DW, Kiang DT, et al: Progesterone receptors in feline mammary adenocarcinomas. Am J Vet Res 45:379–382, 1984.

51. Rutteman GR, Blankenstein MA, Minke J, et al: Steroid receptors in mammary tumours of the cat. Acta Endocrinol 125:32–37, 1991.

52. Hernandez JF, Fernandez BB, Chertach M, et al: Feline mammary carcinomas and progestogens. Feline Pract 5:45–48, 1975.

53. Hayden DW, Johnstons JD, Kiang DT, et al: Feline mammary hypertrophy/fibroadenoma complex: Clinical and hormonal aspects. Am J Vet Res 42(10):1699–1703, 1981.

54. Hinton M, Gashell CJ: Non-neoplastic mammary hypertrophy in the cat associated with either pregnancy or with oral progestogen therapy. Vet Rec 100:277, 1977.

55. Hamilton JM, Else RW, Forshan P: Oestrogen receptors in feline mammary carcinoma. Vet Rec 99:477, 1976.

56. Weijer K, Hart AAM: Prognostic factors in feline mammary carcinoma. J Natl Cancer Inst 70:709–710, 1983.

57. Allen HL: Feline mammary hypertrophy. Vet Pathol 10:501, 1973.

58. Nommo JS, Plummer JM: Ultrastructural studies of fibroadenomatous hyperplasia of mammary glands of two cats. J Comp Pathol 91(1):41–50, 1981.

59. Graham TC, Urlson J: Mammary adenoma associated with pregnancy in the cat. VM SAC 67(1):82, 1972.

60. MacEwen EG, Hayes AA, Harvey HJ, et al: Prognostic factors for feline mammary tumors. J Am Vet Med Assoc 185:201–204, 1984.

61. MacEwen EG, Hayes AA, Mooney S, et al: Evaluation of effect of levamisole on feline mammary cancer. J Biol Response Mod 5:541–546, 1984.

62. Hayes AA, Mooney S: Feline mammary tumors. Vet Clin North Am Small Anim Pract 15:513–520, 1985.

63. Wilson GP: Mammary glands, their development and diseases. In Bojrab MJ (ed): Pathophysiology in Small Animals. Philadelphia, Lea & Febiger, 1981.

64. Jeglum KA, DeGuzman E, Young K: Chemotherapy of advanced mammary adenocarcinoma in 14 cats. J Am Vet Med Assoc 187:157–160, 1985.

65. Mauldin GN, Matus RE, Patnaik AK, et al: Efficacy and toxicity of doxorubicin and cyclophosphamide used in the treatment of selected malignant tumors in 23 cats. J Vet Intern Med 23:60–65, 1988.

66. Cotter SM, Kanki PJ, Simon M: Renal disease in five tumor-bearing cats treated with adriamycin. J Am Anim Hosp 21:405, 1985.

67. Fox L, MacEwen EG, Kurzman ID, et al: Evaluation of liposome-encapsulated muramyl tripeptide in feline mammary cancer. Cancer Biotherapy, 1995 (in press).

68. Jeglum KA, Goldschmidt MG: Serial histologic examination of feline breasts with mammary neoplasia and dysplasia. Proc Vet Can Soc 1988, p. 17.

69. Kelsey JL: A review of the epidemiology of human breast cancer. Epidemiol Rev 1:74–109, 1979.

70. MacMahon B, Cole P, Brown J: Etiology of human breast cancer: A review. J Natl Cancer Inst 50:21–42, 1973.

71. Sattin RW, Rubin GL, Webster LA, et al: Family

history and the risk of breast cancer. J Am Med Assoc *2531*:1908–1913, 1985.

72. Wynder EL, Rose DP, Cohen LA: Diet and breast cancer in causation and therapy. Cancer *58*:1804–1813, 1986.

73. Henderson IC, Harris JR, Kinne DW, et al: Cancer of the breast. *In* DeVita VT, Hellman S, Rosenberg SA (eds): Cancer: Principles and Practice of Oncology, 3rd ed. Philadelphia, JB Lippincott, 1989, pp. 1197–1268.

74. Haskell CM, Giuliano AE, Thompson RW: Breast cancer. *In* Haskell CM (ed): Cancer Treatment, 2nd ed. Philadelphia, WB Saunders, 1985, pp. 137–180.

75. Fisher B, Redmond C, Fisher ER, et al: Ten-year results of a randomized clinical trial comparing radical mastectomy and total mastectomy with or without radiation therapy. N Engl J Med *312*:674–681, 1985.

76. Margolese RG: Surgery and adjuvant chemotherapy. *In* Moossa AR, Schimpff SC, Robson MC (eds): Comprehensive Textbook of Oncology, 2nd ed. Baltimore, Williams & Wilkins, 1991, pp. 800–810.

# 24

# Tumors of the Male Reproductive Tract

Stephen J. Withrow and Nancy P. Reeves

## CANINE TESTICULAR TUMORS

Testicular tumors are the second most common tumor of the male dog.[1] These tumors are more common in the dog than any other species, including humans.[2,3] Sertoli cell tumors (SCTs), seminomas (SEMs), and interstitial cell tumors (ICTs) are the most common histologic types, occurring with approximately equal frequency in the dog[4] (Table 24–1). Combinations of several tumor types may be found in the same dog.[5] Cryptorchid males have a risk of 13.6 times greater for developing SCTs or SEMs than normal males,[1] and the average age of occurrence in cryptorchid animals is younger.[6] An increase in SEMs was detected in military working dogs after service in Vietnam but no conclusive etiologic agent was evident.[7] The right testicle is more often affected with tumors.[3,8,9]

### Incidence and Risk

**Sertoli Cell Tumor**   Approximately 50% of all SCTs occur in the abdominal or inguinal testicles.[6,9] The average age of occurrence for SCTs is nine years,[9] with no reported breed predilection.[1]

**Seminoma**   Two thirds of SEMs occur in descended testicles.[6] The average age of occurrence for SEMs is 10 years[9] and there is no reported breed predilection.[1]

**Interstitial Cell Tumor**   Virtually all ICTs occur in descended testicles.[6] ICTs are often incidental findings in older, intact male dogs and occur more often than they are clinically detected. The average age of occurrence is 11.5 years.[4] There is no apparent breed predilection for ICT.[1]

### Pathology and Natural Behavior

**Sertoli Cell Tumor**   SCTs arise from Sertoli cells and are generally slow growing. Grossly, they are smooth, lobulated, and contained within a well vascularized intact tunica. Cystic areas filled with a clear brown fluid are often found within the tumor.[4,9–11] SCTs are clinically important because of their potential for metastasis and their ability to produce excessive amounts of estrogen. SCTs have the highest rate of metastasis of all canine testicular tumors (2–15%).[9] Lymphatic spread to the regional lymph nodes is the usual route of dissemination. Metastasis to the liver, kidney, spleen, pancreas, and lung have been reported, but this is quite rare.[9]

**Seminoma**   SEMs arise from the primitive gonadal cells of the testes. They are usually homogenous, white to pinkish gray, and unencapsulated.[4,9–11] The metastatic rate is between 5 and 10%.[3,12]

**Interstitial Cell Tumor**   ICTs arise from the Leydig cells of the testicle. These tumors remain

**Table 24–1**

|                                                              | SCT   | SEM  | ICT  |
| ------------------------------------------------------------ | ----- | ---- | ---- |
| % Testicular tumors                                          | 33    | 33   | 33   |
| % Retained                                                   | 50    | 25   | < 0  |
| % Tumors in retained testicles                               | 60    | 40   | < 0  |
| Average age (years)                                          | 9     | 10   | 11.5 |
| % Functional (i.e., signs of increased hormone production)   | 25–50 | < 5  | < 0  |
| % Metastasis                                                 | 2–14  | < 5  | 0    |

SCT = Sertoli cell tumor; ICT = interstitial cell tumor; SEM = seminoma.

within the testicle and are usually surrounded by a dense, fibrous capsule. ICTs are pink to tan in color and tend to bulge out from the cut surface.[4,9–11] Metastasis does not occur.[8]

## History and Clinical Signs

**Sertoli Cell Tumor**   Scrotal or inguinal enlargement is the most common presenting sign of dogs with SCTs, although some affected dogs may present with abdominal distention, feminization, or hematologic abnormalities.[8] Feminization is a direct consequence of the increased production of estrogens by the tumor. The magnitude of hormone production is generally proportional to tumor size and is more often associated with a larger abdominal SCT.[9] Twenty-five to 50% of dogs with SCT show some sign of hyperestrogenism, such as anemia, bilaterally symmetrical alopecia of the ventral abdomen, thorax, caudal and lateral thigh, gynecomastia, and pendulous prepuce (Fig. 24–1).[4,8,9] These dogs may be lethargic and often exhibit a decreased libido. The prostate gland may enlarge because of squamous metaplasia secondary to increased serum estrogen concentrations.[4,8] Estrogen myelotoxicity is occasionally observed in association with SCTs.[13,14] Nonregenerative anemia, granulocytopenia, and thrombocytopenia are the hematologic signs of myelotoxicity.[13,14]

**Seminoma**   Scrotal or inguinal swellings are common signs of SEMs. These tumors have occasionally been associated with increased estrogen production,[2] but the clinical signs of excessive hormone production are rare.[8]

**Interstitial Cell Tumor**   ICTs are usually incidental clinical or necropsy findings. ICTs have been associated with increased testosterone levels, which have been thought to lead to an increased incidence of perineal hernias and perianal adenomas.[8]

## Diagnosis and Workup

Part of the preoperative workup for SCTs and SEMs should include a complete blood count (CBC) and platelet count to determine if estrogen myelotoxicity is present. This is especially true in dogs with large tumors, retained testicles, or clinical evidence of feminization. Lymph nodes should be evaluated for tumor spread (SCT or SEM), either radiographically or at the time of surgery for retained testicles. Ultrasonographic evaluation of the testicles or regional lymph nodes or bothh, may also be performed.[15,16] Thoracic radiographs to assess pulmonary metastases may not be cost effective because of the low metastatic rate of the tumors. Preoperative tissue biopsy or fine-needle aspiration cytology is rarely performed, since the results of these tests will not alter the treatment, which is castration. Thrombocytopenic patients should receive a fresh whole-blood transfusion or platelet-rich plasma prior to surgery and extreme care should be taken to attain adequate hemostasis during surgery.

## Therapy

Castration is the treatment of choice for all testicular tumors. Large descended testes with fixation to the scrotal skin are best managed with castration and scrotal ablation. Abdominal testicles can become very large and are frequently quite vascular (Fig. 24–2). They may be very friable, requiring care at surgery to avoid rupture and exfoliation of viable tumor cells into the abdomen. Enlarged regional lymph nodes due to tumor involvement can occasionally be excised. Chemotherapy for testicular tumors is rarely attempted, since surgery is curative in most

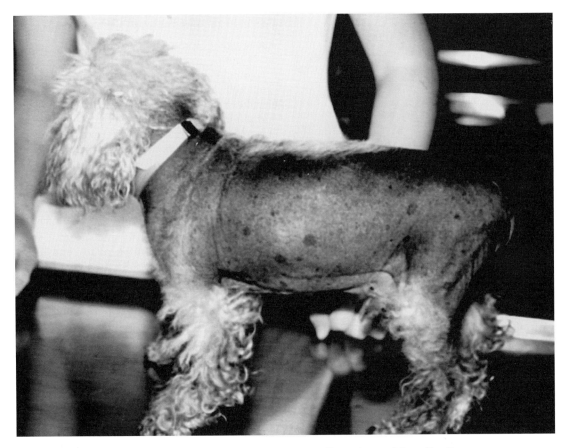

**Figure 24–1.** Dog with characteristic dermatologic manifestations of Sertoli cell tumor.

cases. There are reports of metastatic SCTs responding to drugs such as methotrexate, vinblastine, and cyclophosphamide.[10] These drugs should be considered in cases with widespread metastases. Radiation therapy was very successful in treating four dogs with metastatic seminoma to the sublumbar lymph nodes.[12]

## Prognosis

**Sertoli Cell Tumor** The prognosis for SCT without metastasis or myelotoxicity is excellent. Improvement of hematologic parameters may occur within 2 to 3 weeks of surgery.[14] Full recovery may take up to 5 months; however, myelotoxicity can prove fatal in spite of aggressive supportive care. In one study, 8 of 10 dogs died or were euthanatized because of the myelotoxic effects of estrogen secreted by their tumors.[13] Consideration should be given to use of canine bone marrow colony-stimulating factors if

available. Dogs presented with these complications should be given a very guarded prognosis.

## FELINE TESTICULAR TUMORS

Testicular tumors are rare in the cat in part because most older male cats are castrated. Several carcinomas,[17] ICTs,[17,18] a malignant SEM, and a malignant SCT have been reported.[17,19] Testicular tumors are so rare in the cat that virtually nothing can be said about their behavior. Castration is the treatment of choice for these tumors.

## Comparative Aspects

Testicular tumors account for 1% of all malignant tumors in men. They generally occur in young men and are the leading cause of cancer death in the 20- to 30 year old age group. SEMs

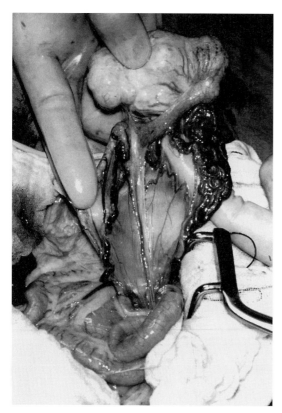

**Figure 24–2.** Intraoperative view of a Sertoli cell tumor in a retained testicle. Note the typical engorged vessels.

constitute 90% of all testicular tumors and are more frequent in the right testicle. Three other histologic types are common: embryonal carcinoma, teratoma, and choriocarcinoma. SEMs are very radiosensitive, and since they usually present at a very early stage, the prognosis is good following therapy with surgery, radiation therapy, or combination chemotherapy.[20]

## CANINE PROSTATIC TUMORS

### Incidence and Risk

Prostatic tumors are rare in the dog and most often affect older male dogs (intact or neutered), with an average age of occurrence being 10 years.[21] No particular breed is at increased risk; however, middle- to large-breed dogs seem to be over-represented.[22] Androgens are known to increase the size and weight of the normal prostate gland[23] but may not be an etiologic factor in the development of prostatic adenocarcinomas.[24,25]

## Pathology and Natural Behavior

Adenocarcinomas (ADCs) account for the majority of canine prostatic tumors.[21] Undifferentiated carcinomas, transitional cell carcinomas, squamous cell carcinomas, and leiomyosarcomas have also been reported[10] but are rare. In addition, transitional cell carcinomas of the bladder can extend into the prostate gland. There are several histologic classifications of prostatic ADCs, and complete descriptions of these categories are covered in detail elsewhere.[21] Prostatic ADCs are highly malignant tumors, with 70 to 80% of the animals having tumor spread at the time of diagnosis.[22,25] The tumors usually spread via lymphatic roots to the external and internal iliac, pelvic and sublumbar lymph nodes, and lungs and skeletal system, especially the lumbar vertebrae. Direct extension of the tumor to the bladder, colon, and surrounding tissues often occurs as well.[21] Because of the insidious onset of the disease, most tumors are quite advanced at the time of diagnosis. Benign prostatic tumors are very rare in the dog.[26]

### History and Clinical Signs

The most common clinical signs associated with prostatic ADCs are (in order of decreasing frequency): weight loss (70%), rear limb lameness or weakness (50%), tenesmus (45%), lumbar pain (30%), stranguria (30%), polyuria/polydipsia (30%), and hematuria (25%).[21] The differential diagnosis includes benign prostatic hypertrophy, prostatic cysts or abscess, and prostatitis. Of 177 dogs presented for evaluation of "prostatic disease," only 7% were confirmed to have cancer, although not all dogs had a definitive diagnosis.[27]

### Diagnosis and Workup

A complete physical examination, including a digital rectal examination of the prostate gland is essential. The malignant gland may palpate normally but is usually increased in size and irregular, with firm nodular areas. The gland may also extend into surrounding tissues, such as the colon, bladder, and pelvic structures. Laboratory evaluation should include a CBC, serum chemistry panel, and urinalysis. However, the urinalysis is rarely helpful in differentiating neoplasia from other types of prostatic disease. Thoracic and abdominal radiographs should be performed to identify metastasis to the lymph nodes, bone, or lung. Plain radiographs may demonstrate multifocal parenchymal mineral densities, which is suggestive of neoplasia.[28] Additional studies may include ultrasonography or computed tomography of the prostate and sublumbar lymph nodes.[29] Although a diagnosis of prostatic ADC can sometimes be made from the prostatic fraction of an ejaculate or a prostatic wash, false-negative results are common.[23,29–31] Diagnosis of prostatic ADC can only be made from tissue biopsy. Prostatic needle biopsy can be performed transabdominally through the perineum or transrectally (Fig. 24–3).[32] Ultrasound-guided needle biopsies may also be employed. Open biopsy (wedge or needle core) of the prostate and regional lymph nodes (for staging purposes) is the most reliable technique, however.

## Therapy

Most canine patients with prostatic ADCs are not diagnosed until late in the course of the disease, and most will have metastasis beyond the prostate. Because of this, virtually all attempts at treatment have yielded poor results. Prostatectomy may theoretically be curative; however, the high morbidity associated with the procedure as well as the high metastatic rate of these tumors often preclude this form of therapy.[33] Most prostatic cancer has spread into the trigone of the bladder or urethra by the time of diagnosis, making complete resection with preservation of the vascular and nerve supply to the bladder difficult, if not impossible. Castration may theoretically slow the growth of the tumor, but this is temporary and palliative at best. Unfortunately, most animals are euthanatized soon after the diagnosis of prostatic ADCs. Chemotherapy rarely has been attempted in the dog. Radiation therapy is used in humans with localized disease[34] and could be considered in canine patients with comparable disease. The use of intraoperative radiation therapy for localized prostatic neoplasia has had success and should be considered in dogs with disease localized to the prostate gland.[35] The use of a retained urethral catheter has been suggested for

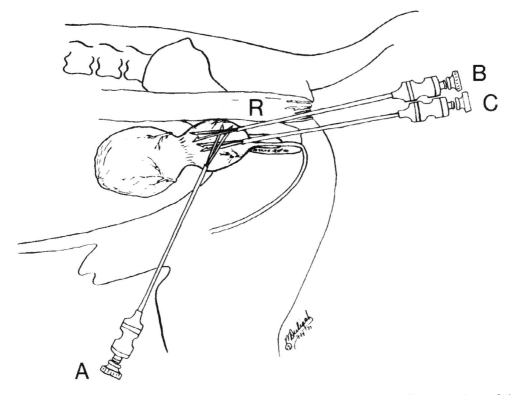

**Figure 24–3.** Various means of closed prostatic biopsy with needle punch. All penetrations of the prostate should be lateralized to avoid the urethra. The rectum is labeled R. *A*, Percutaneous punch lateral to prepuce. *B*, Transrectal route uses the punch enclosed in a glove on the index finger while the prostate is palpated rectally. *C*, Perineal approach enters the skin ventral to the rectum and travels in the pelvic canal up to the prostate.[32]

palliation in dogs with outflow obstruction and stranguria.[36]

## Prognosis

The prognosis is grave because of the high metastatic rate and aggressive nature of the local disease in dogs. Regardless of treatment, most dogs will die of local or metastatic disease 3 months of diagnosis, and effective treatment remains elusive.

## FELINE PROSTATIC TUMORS[34]

Prostatic tumors are very rare in the cat. One fibroadenoma,[19] and three carcinomas[17] have been reported. The behavior of these tumors as well as the prognosis for these cats is unknown. Aggressive surgical excision of the primary tumor and regional lymph nodes is the recommended treatment,[17] and at least one cat lived 10 months after prostatectomy and chemotherapy.[37]

## Comparative Aspects

Prostatic tumors are quite common in men over 50 years of age. ADC is the most common histologic type. Most tumors are diagnosed much earlier than in the dog and, therefore, more treatment options are available. Prostate-specific antigen is often elevated and serves as a marker for diagnosis and response to therapy. Diagnosis and treatment are often possible via transurethral resection. The treatment may also include combinations of surgery, radiation, chemotherapy, or hormonal therapy, depending on the clinical stage of the disease. Prognosis is guarded, although much better results are obtained in men than in dogs because of earlier detection and the more localized extent of the disease.[34]

## CANINE TUMORS OF THE PENIS AND EXTERNAL GENITALIA

### Canine

In the dog, the tumors that occur on the prepuce are similar to those affecting other haired regions of the body. Mast cell tumors and squamous cell carcinomas are common. Transmissible venereal tumors are the most frequently encountered type of canine penile tumor (see Chap. 29C). Penile squamous cell carcinomas have been reported[10,38,39] but are rare.

**History and Clinical Signs**    The appearance of a rapidly growing mass on the penis or prepuce is the usual presenting complaint. Drainage from the prepuce (often bloody) is also common.

**Diagnosis and Workup**    Biopsy of the lesion is necessary to arrive at a diagnosis. Ultrasonography of the caudal abdomen should be used to evaluate regional lymph nodes.

**Treatment**    Surgical excision of the lesion is the usual treatment for penile tumors, except transmissible venereal cell tumors, for which chemotherapy is superior to surgery. Extirpation of the external genitalia (prepuce and penis) with perineal urethrostomy may be required, depending on the location of the lesion. Radiation therapy may be effective therapy for sensitive tumors types, especially squamous cell carcinoma.

**Prognosis**    The prognosis is variable and depends on tumor type and stage, location of the lesion, and surgical resectability.[38,39]

### Feline Tumors

A carcinoma and a sarcoma have been reported on the external genitalia of the cat.[17]

### Comparative Aspects

Squamous cell carcinoma is the most common type of penile tumor in men but is rare, accounting for considerably less than 1% of the malignancies in the men of the United States.[40]

## REFERENCES

1. Hayes HM, Pendergrass TW: Canine testicular tumors: Epidemiologic features of 410 dogs. Int J Cancer 18:482–487, 1976.
2. Comhaire F, Matthews D, et al: Testosterone and oestradiol in dogs with testicular tumours. Acta Endocrinol 77:408–416, 1974.
3. Moulton JE: Tumors of the genital system. In Moulton JE (ed): Tumors in Domestic Animals. Berkeley, University of California Press, 1978.
4. Cotchin E: Testicular neoplasms in dogs. J Comp Pathol 70:232–247, 1960.
5. Patnaik AK, Mostofi FK: A clinicopathologic, histologic, and immunohistochemical study of mixed germ cell-stromal tumors of the testis in 16 dogs. Vet Pathol 30:287–295, 1993.
6. Reif JS, Maguire TG, et al: A cohort study of canine testicular neoplasia. J Am Vet Med Assoc 175:719–723, 1979.
7. Hayes HM, Tarone RE, Casey HW, Huxsoll DL:

Excess of seminomas observed in Vietnam service U.S. military working dogs. J Natl Cancer Inst 82:1042–1046, 1990.

8. Lipowitz AJ, Schwartz A, et al: Testicular neoplasms and concomitant clinical changes in the dog. J Am Vet Med Assoc 163:1364–1368, 1973.

9. Pulley LT: Sertoli cell tumor. Vet Clin North Am 9:145–150, 1979.

10. Theilen GH, Madewell BR: Tumors of the urogenital tract. In Theilen GH, Madewell BR (eds): Veterinary Cancer Medicine. Philadelphia, Lea & Febiger, 1979.

11. Dow C: Testicular tumours in the dog. J Comp Pathol 72:247–265, 1962.

12. McDonald RK, Walker M, Legendre AM, vanEe RT, Gompf RE: Radiotherapy of metastatic seminoma in the dog. J Vet Intern Med 2:103–107, 1988.

13. Morgan RV: Blood dyscrasias associated with testicular tumors in the dog. J Am Anim Hosp Assoc 18:971–975, 1982.

14. Sherding RG, Wilson GP, et al: Bone marrow hypoplasia in eight dogs with Sertoli cell tumor. J Am Vet Med Assoc 178:497–501, 1982.

15. Johnston GR, Feeney DA, Johnston SD, O'Brien TD: Ultrasonographic features of testicular neoplasia in dogs: 16 cases (1980–1988). J Am Vet Med Assoc 198:1779–1784, 1991.

16. Pugh CR, Konde LJ: Sonographic evaluation of canine testicular and scrotal abnormalities: A review of 26 case histories. Vet Radiol 32: 243–250, 1991.

17. Carpenter JL, Andrews LK, Holzworth J: Tumors and tumor-like lesions. In Holzworth J (ed): Diseases of the Cat. Philadelphia, WB Saunders, 1987.

18. Rosen DK, Carpenter JL: Functional ectopic interstitial cell tumor in a castrated male cat. J Am Vet Med Assoc 202:1865–1866, 1993.

19. Cotchen E: Neoplasia. In Wilkinson GT (ed): Diseases of the cat and their management. Melbourne, Blackwell, 1983.

20. Einhorn LH, Richie JP, Shipley WU: Cancer of the testis. In DeVita et al (eds): Cancer: Principles and Practice of Oncology. Philadelphia, JB Lippincott, 1993, pp. 1126–1151.

21. Leav I, Ling GV: Adenocarcinoma of the canine prostate. Cancer 22: 1329–1345, 1968.

22. Hargis AM, Miller LM: Prostatic carcinoma in dogs. Compend Contin Educ Pract Vet 5:647–653, 1983.

23. Thrall MA, Olson PN: Cytologic diagnosis of canine prostatic disease. J Am Anim Hosp Assoc 21:95–102, 1985.

24. Obradovich J, Walshaw R, Goullaud E: The influence of castration on the development of prostatic carcinoma in the dog. Vet Intern Med 1:183–187, 1987.

25. Bell FW, Klausner JS, Hayden DW, et al: Clinical and pathologic features of prostatic adenocarcinoma in sexually intact and castrated dogs: 31 cases (1970–1987). J Am Vet Med Assoc 199:1623–1630.

26. Gilson SD, Miller RT, Hardie EM, Spaulding KA: Unusual prostatic mass in a dog. J Am Vet Med Assoc 200:702–704, 1992.

27. Krawiec DR, Heflin D: Study of prostatic disease in dogs: 177 cases (1981–1986). J Am Vet Med Assoc 200:1119–1122, 1992.

28. Feeney DA, Johnston GR, Klausner JS, et al: Canine prostatic disease—comparison of radiographic appearance with morphologic and microbiologic findings: 30 cases (1981–1985). J Am Vet Med Assoc 190:1018–1026, 1987.

29. Rogers KS, Wantschek L, Lees GE: Diagnostic evaluation of the canine prostate. Compend Contin Educ Pract Vet 8:11, 1986.

30. Barsanti JA, Finco DR: Evaluation of techniques for diagnosis of canine prostatic diseases. J Am Vet Med Assoc 185:2, 1984.

31. Kay ND, Ling GV, Nyland TG, et al: Cytological diagnosis of canine prostatic disease using a urethral brush technique. J Am Anim Hosp Assoc 25:517–526, 1989.

32. Withrow SJ, Lowes N: Biopsy techniques for use in small animal oncology. J Am Anim Hosp Assoc 17:889–902, 1981.

33. Hardie EM, Barsanti JA, Rawlings CA: Complications of prostatic surgery. J Am Vet Med Assoc 20:50, 1984.

34. Hanks GE, Meyers CE, Scardino PT: Cancer of the prostate. In De Vita VT et al (eds): Cancer: Principles and Practice of Oncology. Philadelphia, JB Lippincott, 1993.

35. Turrel JM: Intraoperative radiotherapy of carcinoma of the prostate gland in ten dogs. J Am Vet Med Assoc 190:1, 1987.

36. Mann FA, Barrett RJ, Henderson RA: Use of a retained urethral catheter in three dogs with prostatic neoplasia. Vet Surg 21:342–347, 1992.

37. Hubbard BS, Vulgamott JC, Liska WD: Prostatic adenocarcinoma in a cat. J Am Vet Med Assoc 197:1493–1494, 1990.

38. Patnaik AK, Matthiesen DT, Zawie DA: Two cases of canine penile neoplasm: Squamous cell carcinoma and mesenchymal chondrosarcoma. J Am Anim Hosp Assoc 24:403–406, 1988.

39. Wakui S, Furusato M, Nomura Y, et al: Testicular epidermoid cyst and penile squamous cell carcinoma in a dog. Vet Pathol 29:543–545, 1992.

40. Fair WR, Fuks ZY, Scher HI: Cancer of the urethra and penis. In DeVita VT et al (eds): Cancer: Principles and Practice of Oncology. Philadelphia, JB Lippincott, 1993, pp. 1114–1125.

# 25

# Tumors of the Urinary System

Stephen J. Withrow

# A. Renal Cancer

## INCIDENCE AND RISK FACTORS

Primary renal cancer accounts for approximately 1% of all cancers, while metastatic cancer to the kidney is common (presumably because of the high blood flow and rich capillary network). Epithelial malignancies are most common and are seen in older patients with a mean age of 9 years.[1] Male dogs are more commonly affected with epithelial tumors than females, with a ratio of 1.5:1. Embryonal neoplasms may be seen in younger patients and even puppies, with a mean age of 4 years.[2]

A syndrome of dermal fibrosis, uterine polyps, and concomitant renal cystadenocarcinoma is seen almost exclusively in the German shepherd and may be heritable.[3,4]

## PATHOLOGY AND NATURAL BEHAVIOR

More than 90% of primary renal tumors in the dog and cat are malignant. The rarely reported benign tumors include fibroma,[5] hemangioma,[6] adenoma,[7] papilloma,[1] leiomyoma,[8] and interstitial cell tumor.[9] Over half of malignancies are epithelial (tubular adenocarcinoma and transitional cell carcinoma), 20% are mesenchymal (fibrosarcoma, chondrosarcoma, etc.), and 10% are derived from embryonal pluripotential blastema (Wilm's tumor, nephroblastoma, embryonal nephroma).[10] Some tumors, especially adenocarcinoma and lymphoma, are often bilateral. Lymphoma is the most common tumor affecting the feline kidney but is only occasionally localized to the kidney. The mean age of affected cats is 6 years.[11]

Renal adenocarcinomas usually arise in the cortex or one pole. They can be highly invasive to regional structures and may invade the vena cava. Metastasis to the regional lymph nodes, lung, liver, and bone occurs in more than half the cases.[1]

Transitional cell carcinoma of the kidney usually arises in the renal pelvis but may be very locally invasive. The metastatic rate appears to be less than that of renal tubular adenocarcinoma.[1]

Nephroblastoma is usually not metastatic but often attains a large size and may implant the peritoneal cavity if it ruptures.

## HISTORY AND CLINICAL SIGNS

The onset of symptoms is generally slow and nonspecific over weeks to months. The signs may include weight loss, depression, fever, abdominal distention, lameness, and pain. Gross hematuria is an uncommon finding except with hemangioma[12] and renal pelvic locations (transitional cell carcinoma). Hypertrophic osteopathy has been described in association with renal tumors.[13,14]

Slow-growing firm skin and subcutaneous fibrous nodules in German shepherds should

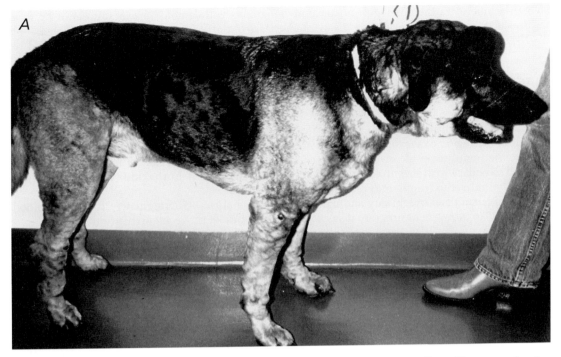

**Figure 25–1A.** Middle-aged German shepherd dog exhibiting numerous, firm, fibrous, and painless nodules in the skin and subcutaneous tissues. Note the large lesion over the frontal sinus area.

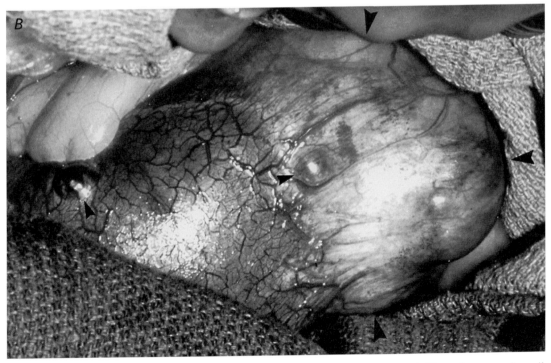

**Figure 25–1B.** Operative view of a kidney from the patient in Figure 25–1A. Note the several small cystic masses (small arrows) and larger mass (large arrows) on the right pole. The diagnosis was confirmed as bilateral renal cystadenocarcinoma. No treatment was performed. This patient survived 18 months after the first detection of skin and subcutaneous fibrosis.

alert the clinician to the possibility of concomitant renal cystadenocarcinoma (Figs. 25–1A and 25–1B).[3,4]

## DIAGNOSTIC TECHNIQUES AND WORKUP

Careful abdominal palpation may reveal a mass or pain in the region of the kidneys (presumably from tension on the capsule or ureteral obstruction and secondary hydronephrosis).

Abdominal radiographs may demonstrate renal enlargement and irregularity and should be followed by an intravenous urogram if suspicious (Figs. 25–2A and 25–2B).[1] Further tests such as arteriography and ultrasound may be needed to demonstrate subtle lesions.[9,15] Thoracic radi-

ographs will demonstrate metastasis in up to a third of the cases, especially adenocarcinoma.

Hematologic changes may include a mild to moderate anemia secondary to hematuria. Polycythemia, presumably due to increased erythropoietin production, has been documented on rare occasions in several dogs and at least one cat.[16–18] A profound neutrophilic leukocytosis has also been associated with canine renal tubular carcinoma.[19,20]

Serum chemistries are usually normal but may reveal signs of renal failure (primary or obstructive) if both kidneys or ureters are involved.

Urinalysis will frequently reveal red blood cells but definite identification of exfoliated tumor cells is rare. Proteinuria is a common but nonspecific finding.[1]

Transabdominal or "closed" renal biopsy has been described[21] but is usually reserved for

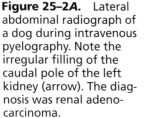

**Figure 25–2A.**  Lateral abdominal radiograph of a dog during intravenous pyelography. Note the irregular filling of the caudal pole of the left kidney (arrow). The diagnosis was renal adenocarcinoma.

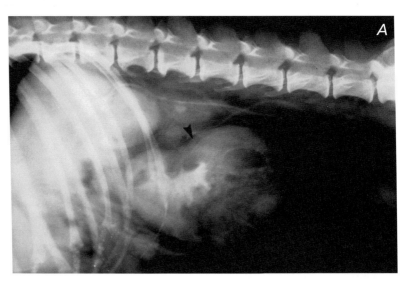

**Figure 25–2B.**  Gross photo of kidneys from the dog in Figure 25–2A. No treatment was offered because of metastasis to several bones and the lung.

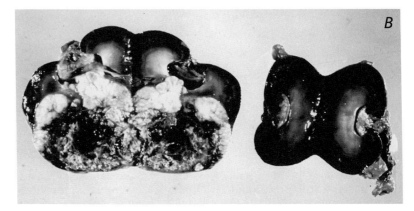

patients with bilateral involvement (precluding surgical treatment) or suspect lymphoma when medical treatment would be employed. Ultrasound guided biopsies may improve the accuracy and safety of renal biopsy.

Surgical exploration for biopsy, staging, or treatment is preferred for patients with only one kidney involved.

## THERAPY

Unilateral renal cancer is best treated by complete nephrectomy. This includes removal of the ureter and possibly retroperitoneal muscle and tissue if extension through the capsule has occurred. Early ligation of the renal vein is advisable to prevent tumor emboli from leaving the kidney. Partial nephrectomy is rarely possible or desired except in cases with bilateral renal involvement. Regional lymph nodes (para-aortic) should be biopsied if visible or enlarged. Some tumors (especially nephroblastoma) can attain a very large size (Figs. 25–3A, 25–3B, 25–3C) and still be easily operable.

Actinomycin D has been advocated as therapeutic or adjuvant treatment for nephroblastomas in dogs, but unequivocal proof of its efficacy is lacking.[14]

Lymphoma can be effectively treated with

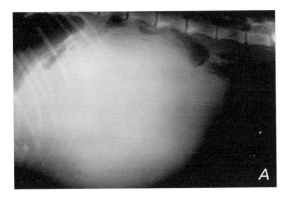

**Figure 25–3A.** Lateral radiograph of a dog with a large midabdominal mass. The mass could have arisen from several intra-abdominal structures but was confirmed as nephroblastoma.

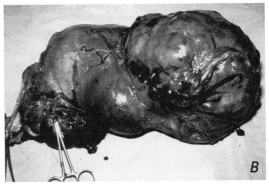

**Figure 25–3B.** Renal tumor weighing 8 kg that was removed from the patient in Figure 25–3A.

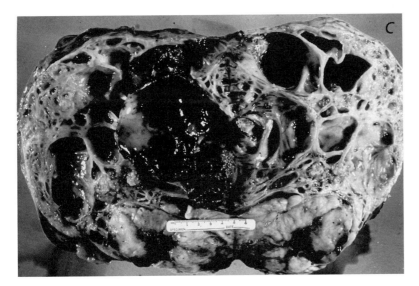

**Figure 25–3C.** Note the multiple cystic areas, which make accuracy of closed biopsy difficult. Surgical removal resulted in 16-month survival, following which the patient was lost to further follow-up.

chemotherapy, but the prognosis is poor if renal failure or central nervous system involvement is present (Chap. 28C).[11,22]

Radiation therapy has rarely been attempted for renal cancer.

## PROGNOSIS

Few treated cases with long-term follow-up exist in the veterinary literature.[1,23] Carcinomas will be metastatic, bilateral, or locally invasive in more than half the cases.[24] Mean survival is 6 to 10 months for canine patients, who are deemed operable and who live at least 21 days postoperatively.[1] However, survivals of up to 4 years have been reported.[23,25,26] Nephroblastoma is less metastatic, and complete nephrectomy has the potential to be curative.[1,27]

Renal lymphoma will respond to chemotherapy but is usually not curable and will often progress to the generalized form. Central nervous system metastasis is a common sequela in cats with renal lymphoma.[22] Signs of renal failure denote a poor prognosis even with the use of chemotherapy.[11,22]

The German shepherd syndrome of bilateral cystadenocarcinomas is rarely amenable to surgery but survival may be many months or more without treatment.[28]

## COMPARATIVE ASPECTS[29]

Benign and cystic lesions comprise more than 85% of the space-occupying lesions of the human kidney. Malignant primary cancer is generally adenocarcinoma (hypernephroma), renal pelvic transitional cell carcinoma, or Wilm's tumor (nephroblastoma).

The experimental and clinical carcinogens and risk factors for hypernephroma include radiation, hormones (especially estrogen), excess body weight, dietary protein, and tobacco products.[30] Transitional cell carcinoma of the renal pelvis is associated with an almost 50% incidence of other urinary cancer that is felt to be due to a common exposure to carcinogens (field defect) rather than tumor cell reimplantation. Treatment for the above two tumors is generally complete nephroureterectomy. Radiation, chemotherapy, immunotherapy, or hormonal treatment play lesser roles. Five-year survivals are 30 to 40%.

Wilm's tumor generally affects children under 7 years of age (30% < 1 year). A dramatic improvement in prognosis, with combinations of surgery, radiation, and chemotherapy (vincristine and actinomycin D), has resulted in 5-year survival rates of 80% or better.

## REFERENCES

1. Klein MK, Cockerell GL, Withrow SJ, et al: Canine primary renal neoplasms: A retrospective review of 54 cases. J Am Anim Hosp Assoc 24:443–452, 1988.
2. Hayes HM, Fraumeni JF: Epidemiological features of canine renal neoplasms. Cancer Res 37:2553–2556, 1977.
3. Suter M, Lott-Stolz G, Wild P: Generalized nodular dermatofibrosis in six Alsatians. Vet Pathol 20:632–634, 1983.
4. Lium B, Moe L: Hereditary multifocal renal cystadenocarcinomas and nodular dermatofibrosis in the German shepherd dog: Macroscopic and histopathologic changes. Vet Pathol 22:447–455, 1985.
5. Picut CA, Valentine BA: Renal fibroma in four dogs. Vet Pathol 22:422–423, 1985.
6. Widmer WR, Carlton WW: Persistent hematuria in a dog with renal hemangioma. J Am Vet Med Assoc 197:237–239, 1990.
7. Clark WR, Wilson RB: Renal adenoma in a cat. J Am Vet Med Assoc 193:1557–1559, 1988.
8. Mills JHL, Moore JT, Orr JP: Canine renal leiomyoma—An unusual tumour. Can Vet J 18:76–78, 1977.
9. Diters RW, Wells M: Renal interstitial cell tumors in the dog. Vet Pathol 23:74–76, 1986.
10. Caywood DD, Osborne CA: Oncology section: Urinary system. In Slatter DH (ed): Textbook of Small Animal Surgery. Philadelphia, WB Saunders, 1985, pp. 2561–2574.
11. Weller RE, Stann SE: Renal lymphosarcoma in the cat. J Am Anim Hosp Assoc 19:363–367, 1983.
12. Cadwallader JA, Goulden BE, Wyburn RS, Jolly RD: Renal hemangioma in a dog. New Z Vet J 21:48–51, 1973.
13. Nafe LA, Herron AJ, Burk RL: Hypertrophic osteopathy in a cat associated with renal papillary adenoma. J Am Anim Hosp Assoc 17:659–662, 1981.
14. Caywood DD, Osborne CA, Stevens JB, Jessen CR, O'Leary TP: Hypertrophic osteoarthropathy associated with an atypical nephroblastoma in a dog. J Am Anim Hosp Assoc 16:855–865, 1980.
15. Konde LJ, Park RD, Wrigley RH, Lebel JL: Comparison of radiography and ultrasonography in the evaluation of renal lesions in the dog. J Am Vet Med Assoc 188:1420–1425, 1986.
16. Peterson ME, Zanjani ED: Inappropriate erythropoietin production from a renal carcinoma in a dog with polycythemia. J Am Vet Med Assoc 179:995–996, 1981.

17. Scott RC, Patnaik AK: Renal carcinoma with secondary polycythemia in the dog. J Am Anim Hosp Assoc 8:275–283, 1972.

18. Gorse MJ: Polycythemia associated with renal fibrosarcoma in a dog. J Am Vet Med Assoc 192:793–794, 1988.

19. Madewell BR, Wilson DW, Hornof WJ, Gregory CR: Leukemoid blood response and bone infarcts in a dog with renal tubular adenocarcinoma. J Am Vet Med Assoc 197:1623–1625, 1990.

20. Lappin MR, Latimer KS: Hematuria and extreme neutrophilic leukocytosis in a dog with renal tubular carcinoma. J Am Vet Med Assoc 192:1289–1292, 1988.

21. Jeraj K, Osborne CA, Stevens JB: Evaluation of renal biopsy in 197 dogs and cats. J Am Vet Med Assoc 181:367–369, 1982.

22. Mooney SC, Hayes AA, MacEwen EG, et al: Treatment and prognostic factors in feline lymphomas: 103 cases. (1977–1981). J Am Vet Med Assoc 194:696–699, 1989.

23. Lucke VM, Kelly DF: Renal carcinoma in the dog. Vet Pathol 13:264–276, 1976.

24. Baskin GB, DePaoli A: Primary renal neoplasms of the dog. Vet Pathol 14:591–605, 1977.

25. Burger GT, Moe JB, White JD, Whitney GD: Renal carcinoma in a dog. J Am Vet Med Assoc 171:282–283, 1977.

26. Waters DJ, Prueter JC: Secondary polycythemia associated with renal disease in the dog: Two case reports and review of literature. J Am Anim Hosp Assoc 24:109–114, 1988.

27. Sukhiani HR, Holmberg DL, Atilola MAO: What is your diagnosis? J Am Vet Med Assoc 203(2):221–222, 1993.

28. Cosenza SF, Seely JC: Generalized nodular dermatofibrosis and renal cystadenocarcinomas in a German shepherd dog. J Am Vet Med Assoc 189:1587–1590, 1986.

29. Linehan WM, Shipley WU, Parkinson DR: Cancer of the kidney and ureter. In DeVita VT, et al (eds): Cancer: Principles of Practice of Oncology. Philadelphia, JB Lippincott, 1993, pp. 1023–1051.

30. Chow WH, Gridley G, McLaughlin JR, et al: Protein intake and risk of renal cell cancer. J Natl Cancer Inst 86:1131–1139, 1994.

# B. Cancer of the Ureter

Primary cancer of the ureter is extremely rare. Reported cases have included leiomyoma, leiomyosarcoma, fibropapilloma, and transitional cell carcinoma.[1-4] More commonly, the ureter is involved secondary to cancer of the kidney, bladder, or retroperitoneal space. Treatment is generally with nephroureterectomy, although very distal lesions could have the proximal ureter reimplanted in the bladder or anastomosed to the contralateral ureter. Tension-free end-to-end anastomosis, after resection of a segment, is difficult. Benign lesions carry an excellent prognosis with resection.[1,2]

## REFERENCES

1. Liska WD, Patnaik AK: Leiomyoma of the ureter of a dog. J Am Anim Hosp Assoc 13:83–84, 1977.

2. Berzon JL: Primary leiomyosarcoma of the ureter in a dog. Clinical reports. J Am Vet Med Assoc 175(4):374–376, 1979.

3. Hattel AL, Diters RW, Snavely DA: Ureteral fibropapilloma in a dog. J Am Vet Med Assoc 188(8):873, 1986.

4. Hanika C, Rebar AH: Ureteral transitional cell carcinoma in the dog. Vet Pathol 17:643–646, 1980.

# C. Urinary Bladder Cancer

## INCIDENCE AND RISK FACTORS

Bladder cancer is the most common urinary tract cancer but accounts for less than 1% of all cancer. It is more common in the dog than the cat. Experimentally, many chemicals are carcinogenic[1] and, clinically, cyclophosphamide has caused transitional cell carcinoma in the dog.[2,3] One report has suggested that topical insecticides, especially in obese dogs, increases the likelihood of developing bladder cancer.[4] That metabolites of tryptophan (a proposed carcinogen) are excreted in higher concentrations in the urine of the dog versus the cat may account for the higher incidence in the canine.[5] The average age of affected dogs is 10 years and affected cats 9.7 years. Female dogs and male cats are at higher risk for the development of bladder cancer.[6,7]

## PATHOLOGY AND NATURAL BEHAVIOR

Malignant cancers are more common clinically than are benign lesions. Transitional cell carcinoma is the most common histologic type, followed by squamous cell carcinoma and adenocarcinoma.[8,9] Primary sarcomas (fibrosarcoma, leiomyosarcoma, and hemangiosarcoma) of the bladder are uncommon. A rare cancer of the younger dog is botryoid or embryonal rhabdomyosarcoma.[10,11] Fibromas, leiomyomas, and papillomas are the most common benign lesions.[12] Pyogranulomatous or diffuse polypoid cystitis may mimic diffuse uroepithelial cancer.[13]

Malignant carcinomas, especially transitional cell carcinomas, are very locally invasive and will metastasize to the regional lymph nodes and lung in more than half the cases.[14]

## HISTORY AND SIGNS

Most animals present with signs similar to cystitis (hematuria, dysuria, and increased frequency of urination). The signs may be present for weeks to several months, and apparent short-term response to antibiotics may be observed. Hematuria may be more pronounced than with other bladder disorders. Occasionally hypertrophic osteopathy may be observed secondary to bladder cancer, especially in association with botryoid rhabdomyosarcoma.[10,15] Cystitis or hematuria that is refractory to conservative medical treatment warrants further diagnostic evaluation.

## DIAGNOSTIC TECHNIQUES AND WORKUP

Routine blood tests and physical examination rarely help diagnose these tumors. Occasional patients have renal failure secondary to obstruction. Most bladder cancer is not detectable by abdominal palpation.

A urinalysis will often reveal white blood cells, red blood cells, and protein compatible with routine cystitis. Secondary bacteriuria may also be noted. Neoplastic cells may be exfoliated into the urine[8] but are often difficult to distinguish from reactive transitional cells. Flow cytometric techniques may be more sensitive for neoplasia than cytology in evaluating urine samples and warrants further investigation.[16]

Radiography is a valuable tool in the diagnosis and localization of bladder lesions. Positive or

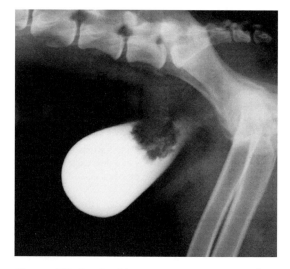

**Figure 25–4.** Positive contrast cystogram of an 8-year-old male dog with a large filling defect in the area of the trigone. A diagnosis of transitional cell carcinoma was confirmed by excisional biopsy. A partial cystectomy with transplantation of one ureter resulted in cessation of signs for 5 months, at which time local recurrence and metastasis to regional lymph nodes was evident.

negative contrast cystograms will usually reveal a mucosal mass lesion. Diffuse trigonal involvement often denotes transitional cell carcinoma (Fig. 25–4). Polypoid lesions away from the trigone have a higher likelihood of being benign (Fig. 25–5). An intravenous urogram to evaluate the bladder lumen may be done if a urethral catheter cannot be passed or if ureteral obstruc-

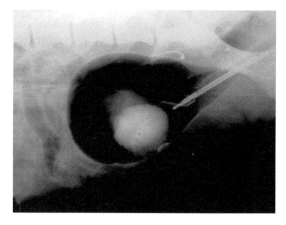

**Figure 25–5.** Double contrast cystogram of an 11-year-old dog with a circular mass visible on the floor of the bladder. This was a fibroma.

tion is suspected. Hydronephrosis or hydroureter associated with bladder tumors is a poor prognostic sign, since involvement of the trigone is likely. Sublumbar lymph nodes and the lumbar vertebrae and pelvis should be examined radiographically for metastasis. Thoracic radiographs are generally performed but will only occasionally be positive at the time of initial diagnosis.[17] Ultrasound has also been proposed as a diagnostic tool to detect bladder masses and may be more accurate than cystograms.[18,19]

Bladder tumors may be biopsied via cystoscopy,[20–23] catheter biopsy,[24,25] or more commonly at laparotomy.

## TREATMENT

Surgery is generally the treatment of choice, especially for tumors not involving the trigone. Before opening the bladder, a careful inspection of the abdominal cavity should be made for metastatic disease. Particular attention should be paid to the sublumbar lymph nodes, and any palpable nodes should be removed or biopsied for staging purposes. The ureters should also be inspected for increased size and tumor invasion. The bladder is then carefully palpated and a cystotomy incision made at least 1 cm away from the suspect tumor. Transitional cell carcinoma is usually red and friable (Fig. 25–6). Benign lesions (usually small, well circumscribed, and pedunculated) can be excised with a conservative, full-thickness bladder wall removal (Fig. 25–7). Malignant lesions pose a greater surgical problem because most patients will have advanced-stage disease in a critical location. The ureters and trigone are frequently involved, making resection and reconstruction of a continent lower urinary tract difficult, if not impossible. Transposition of ureters to the body of the bladder is possible but unlikely to be curative. If the cancer is in the apex of the bladder, a very wide full-thickness partial cystectomy may be attempted. More than 80% of the bladder may be removed, with eventual return to normal or near normal volume capacity.

Attempts at complete cystectomy with rerouting of urine into the bowel have yielded only short-term success and must be considered experimental in animals. In a series of 10 dogs that underwent complete cystectomy (± prostatectomy or urethrectomy) and ureterocolostomy, mean survival was only 4 months.[26] Complications such as pyelonephritis, ureteral obstruction, and hyperchloremic acidosis were common.[26] The

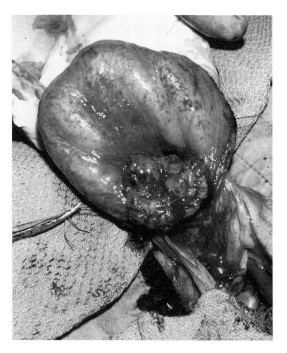

**Figure 25–6.** Operative view of a cauliflower-like and friable transitional cell carcinoma of the bladder. Partial cystectomy is usually palliative but rarely curative.

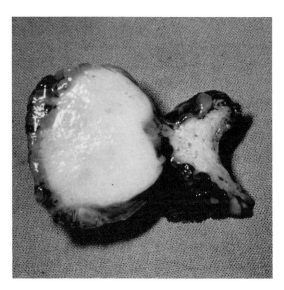

**Figure 25–7.** Cross section of the tumor depicted in Figure 25–5, with a section of the removed bladder wall. Note the homogeneous white density and the narrow stalk compatible with a benign lesion. Recovery was uneventful, and the patient is free of disease 3 years postoperatively.

morbidity of the procedure, coupled with a high metastatic rate, makes this procedure undesirable. Ureterostomy to the skin, bowel, or to the uterus,[27] has been rarely reported in the dog,[27-31] although it is commonly performed in humans.

Intraoperative irradiation (delivery of large doses of radiation [20–30 Gy] during operative exposure) followed by fractionated external beam irradiation (30 Gy) resulted in poor local control and serious bladder fibrosis with resultant incontinence in dogs.[32,33] Fractionated external beam irradiation alone is generally not recommended because of the high doses required to eradicate advanced cancer and subsequent serious risk of bowel injury.

Systemic chemotherapy with cisplatin may have some antitumor activity but large case series are lacking. Combination treatment with cisplatin and radiation is a reasonable idea and needs further evaluations in large case studies.[34-36] Local infusion of chemotherapy is an attractive idea[37,38] but will usually not penetrate beyond the submucosa and, unfortunately, most animal tumors have infiltrated to muscularis or serosa.[38,39] Hyperthermic chemotherapy infusions or infusions of immuno- therapy are being investigated in humans.[40] One report of dogs with transitional cell carcinoma of the bladder suggests that the median survival of dogs treated with doxorubicin and cyclophosphamide have a median survival of 259 days (11 dogs), compared to surgery (86 days, 14 dogs), or intravesicular thiotepa (57 days, 6 dogs).[41]

Attempts at using intralesional BCG-cell wall preparations at the time of partial excision have yielded variable results. Two of seven dogs treated this way seemed to benefit from the intralesional therapy, but two dogs developed severe granulomatous reactions that resulted in a complete obstruction.[42] The appropriate use of antibiotics and anti-flammatory drugs such as piroxicam may result in several months of palliation in some dogs. In a recent study,[44] dogs with transitional cell carcinoma were treated with piroxicam (0.3 mg/kg PO SID) and six had measured responses. The median survival for all dogs was 181 days.[44]

Appropriate combinations of surgery, chemotherapy, and radiation need further investigation for bladder cancer in the dog and cat.

## PROGNOSIS

The prognosis for malignant cancer of the urinary bladder (especially transitional cell carcinoma) is poor because of the usual advanced stage at diagnosis. Even if resection is possible, most patients will suffer local recurrence or metastasis within 1 year.[35,41,43] Dogs with cancer apparently confined to the apex of the bladder (without metastases) that undergo subtotal cystectomy have a mean survival of 1 year.[35] Unfortunately, this group of patients represents only 15 to 20% of all cancers of the lower urinary tract. However, palliation of symptoms with surgery can be attained for several months or longer. One dog with botryoid rhabdomyosarcoma was free of disease 21 months after surgery and adjuvant chemotherapy with doxorubicin and cyclophosphamide.[11]

Benign lesions may be cured with surgical resection.[12]

## COMPARATIVE ASPECTS[45]

Numerous chemical carcinogens, often associated with industrial exposure, have been implicated in the development of human bladder cancer. Naturally occurring substances in urine may also be growth-promoting factors (urea and glycoprotein).

Ninety percent of epithelial cancers are transitional cell carcinoma. Multicentric tumors are common, presumably because of diffuse exposure and alteration of the bladder mucosa to carcinogens (probably true in animals as well).

Carcinoma in situ may be treated with transurethral resection while more advanced stages are often treated with complete cystectomy and urinary diversion. Radiation may be employed curatively or adjuvantly. Chemotherapy may be systemic (cisplatin) or via intravesicular routes (thiotepa, doxorubicin, etc). Intravesicular chemotherapy is usually reserved for superficial lesions.

Tumor size, stage, and histologic grade are important prognostic variables.

## REFERENCES

1. Okajima E, Hiramatsu T, Hirao K, Ijuin M, et al: Urinary bladder tumors induced by n-butyl-n-(4-hydroxybutyl) nitrosamine in dogs. Cancer Res 41:1958–1966, 1981.
2. Macy DW, Withrow SJ, Hoopes J: Transitional cell carcinoma of the bladder associated with cyclophosphamide administration. J Am Anim Hosp Assoc 19:965–969, 1983.
3. Weller RE, Wolf AM, Oyejide A: Transitional cell carcinoma of the bladder associated with cyclophosphamide therapy in a dog. J Am Anim Hosp Assoc 15:733–736, 1979.
4. Glickman LT, Schofer FS, McKee LJ: Epidemiologic study of insecticide exposures, obesity, and risk of

bladder cancer in household dogs. J Toxicol Environ Health 28:407–414, 1989.

5. Osborne CA, Low DG, et al: Neoplasms of the canine and feline urinary bladder: Incidence, etiologic factors, occurrence and pathologic features. Am J Vet Res 29:2041, 1968.

6. Schwarz PD, Greene RW, Patnaik AK: Urinary bladder tumors in the cat: A review of 27 cases. J Am Anim Hosp Assoc 21:237–245, 1985.

7. Crow SE: Urinary tract neoplasms in dogs and cats. Comp Contin Educ Pract Vet 7:607–618, 1985.

8. Caywood DD, Osborne CA, Johnston GR: Neoplasms of the canine and feline urinary tracts. Current Vet Therapy 7: 1203–1212, 1980.

9. Patnaik AK, Schwarz PD, Greene RW: A histopathologic study of twenty urinary bladder neoplasms in the cat. J Small Anim Pract 27:433–445, 1986.

10. Halliwell WH, Ackerman N: Botryoid rhabdomyosarcoma of the urinary bladder and hypertrophic osteoarthropathy in a young dog. J Am Vet Med Assoc 165:911–913, 1974.

11. Senior DF, Lawrence DT, Gunson C, Fox LE, et al: Successful treatment of botryoid rhabdomyosarcoma in the bladder of a dog. J Am Anim Hosp Assoc 29:386–390, 1993.

12. Esplin DG: Urinary bladder fibromas in dogs: 51 cases (1981–1985). J Am Vet Med Assoc 190:440–444, 1987.

13. Johnston SD, Osborne CA, Stevens JB: Canine polypoid cystitis. J Am Vet Med Assoc 166:1155–1160, 1975.

14. Stone EA: Urogenital tumors. Vet Clin North Am 15:597–608, 1985.

15. Brodey RS, Riser WH, Allen H: Hypertrophic pulmonary osteoarthropathy in a dog with carcinoma of the urinary bladder. J Am Vet Med Assoc 162:474–477, 1971.

16. Badalament RA, Hermansen DK, Kimmel M, Gay H, et al: The sensitivity of bladder wash flow cytometry, bladder wash cytology, and voided cytology in the detection of bladder carcinoma. Cancer 60:1423–1427, 1987.

17. Walter PA, Haynes JS, Feeney DA, Johnston GR: Radiographic appearance of pulmonary metastases from transitional cell carcinoma of the bladder and urethra of the dog. J Am Vet Med Assoc 185:411–418, 1984.

18. Leveille R, Biller DS, Kantrowitz B, Partington BP, Miyabayashi T: Sonographic investigation of transitional cell carcinoma of the urinary bladder in small animals. Vet Radiol Ultrasound 33:103–107, 1992.

19. Biller DS, Kantrowitz B, Partington BP, Miyabayashi T: Diagnostic ultrasound of the urinary bladder. J Amer Anim Hosp Assoc 26:397–402, 1990.

20. McCarthy TC, McDermaid SL: Prepubic percutaneous cystoscopy in the dog and cat. J Am Anim Hosp Assoc 22:213–219, 1986.

21. Cooper JE, Milroy JG, Turton JA, Wedderburn N, Hicks RM: Cystoscopic examination of male and female dogs. Vet Rec 115:571–574, 1984.

22. Brearley MJ, Cooper JE: The diagnosis of bladder disease in dogs by cystoscopy. J Small Anim Pract 28:75–85, 1987.

23. Senior DF, Sundstrom DA: Cystoscopy in female dogs. Compend Contin Educ Pract Vet 10:890–895, 1988.

24. Holt PE, Lucke VM, Brown PJ: Evaluation of a catheter biopsy technique as a diagnostic aid in lower urinary tract disease. Vet Rec 118:681–684, 1986.

25. Melhoff T, Osborne CA: Bladder biopsy. In Kirk RW (ed): Current Veterinary Therapy: Small Animal Practice. Philadelphia, WB Saunders, 1977, p. 1173.

26. Stone EA, Withrow SJ, Page RL, Ureterocolonic anastomosis in ten dogs with transitional cell carcinoma. Vet Surg 17:147–153, 1988.

27. Anderson SM, Lippincott CL: Ureterohysterostomy in the dog. Proc Am Coll Vet Surg, 1990, p. 55.

28. Bjorling DE, Mahaffey MB, Crowell WA: Bilateral ureteroileostomy and perineal urinary diversion in dogs. Vet Surg 14:204–212, 1985.

29. Schwarz PD, Egger EL, Klause SE: Modified "cup-patch" ileocystoplasty for urinary bladder reconstruction in a dog. J Am Vet Med Assoc 198:273–277, 1991.

30. Fries CL, Binnington AG, Valli VE, Connolly JG, et al: Enterocystoplasty with cystectomy and subtotal intracapsular prostatectomy in the male dog. Vet Surg 20:104–112, 1991.

31. Montgomery RD, Hankes GH: Ureterocolonic anastomosis in a dog with transitional cell carcinoma of the urinary bladder. J Am Vet Med Assoc 190:1427–1429, 1987.

32. Withrow SJ, Gillette EL, Hoopes PJ, McChesney SL: Intraoperative irradiation of 16 spontaneously occurring canine neoplasms. Vet Surg 18:7–11, 1989.

33. Walker M, Breider M: Intraoperative radiotherapy of canine bladder cancer. Vet Radiol 28:200–204, 1987.

34. Shapiro W, Kitchell BE, Fossum TW, Couto CG, Theilen G: Cisplatin for treatment of transitional cell and squamous cell carcinomas in dogs. J Am Vet Med Assoc 193:1530–1533, 1988.

35. Norris AM, Laing EJ, Valli VE, Withrow SJ, et al: Canine bladder and urethral tumors: A retrospective study of 115 cases (1980–1985). J Vet Intern Med 6:145–153, 1992.

36. Moore AS, Cardona A, Shapiro W, Madewell BR: Cisplatin (cisdiamminedichloroplatinum) for treatment of transitional cell carcinoma of the urinary bladder or urethra. J Vet Intern Med 4:148–152, 1990.

37. Blumenreich MS, Needles B, Yagoda A, et al: Intravesical cisplatin for superficial bladder tumors. Cancer 50:863–865, 1982.

38. Wientjes MG, Dalton JT, Badalament RA, et al: Bladder wall penetration of intravesical mitomycin C in dogs. Cancer Res 51:4347–4354, 1991.

39. Chai M, Wientjes MG, Badalament RA, Bladder wall penetration of intravesical doxorubicin in dogs and patients. J Urol Pharmacokinetics, in press.

40. Kubota Y, Shuin T, Miura T, Nishimura R, et al:
    Treatment of bladder cancer with a combination of
    hyperthermia, radiation and bleomycin. Cancer
    53:199–202, 1984.
41. Helfand SC, Hamilton TA, Hungerford LL, et al:
    Comparison of three treatments for transitional
    cell carcinoma of the bladder in the dog. J Am
    Anim Hosp Assoc 30:270–275, 1994.
42. MacEwen EG, Matus R: Personal communication,
    New York, Animal Medical Center, 1983.
43. Burnie AG, Weaver AD: Urinary bladder neoplasia

in the dog: A review of seventy cases. J Small
    Anim Pract 24:129–143, 1983.
44. Knapp DW, Richardson RC, Chan TCK, et al:
    Piroxicam therapy in 34 dogs with transitional cell
    carcinoma of the urinary bladder. J Vet Intern Med
    8:273–278, 1994..
45. Fair WR, Fuks ZY, Scher HI: Cancer of the bladder.
    In DeVita VT, et al (eds): Cancer: Principles and
    Practice of Oncology. Philadelphia, JB Lippincott,
    1993, pp. 1052–1072.

# D. Urethral Tumors

## INCIDENCE AND RISK FACTORS

Urethral tumors are less common than bladder tumors. The same etiologic factors that induce bladder tumors probably influence the urethra. Older female dogs are most commonly affected.[1,2] Cats are very rarely affected.

## PATHOLOGY AND NORMAL BEHAVIOR

The most common histologic types of cancer are transitional cell carcinoma and squamous cell carcinoma. Theoretically, the proximal one third of the uretha should develop transitional cell carcinomas and the distal two thirds squamous cell carcinoma. Since most of these tumors involve the entire length of the urethra and biologic differences have not been identified, some authors prefer the more general term of urethral carcinoma.[3] Benign lesions are very rare but granulo-

matous urethritis (resembling cancer) and leiomyomas have been reported.[4]

Metastasis to regional lymph nodes and further is seen in over half the cases evaluated.[1,5]

## HISTORY AND SIGNS

The history and signs such as stranguria, hematuria, pollakiuria, vaginal discharge, and complete obstruction are essentially the same as for bladder tumors.

## DIAGNOSTIC TECHNIQUES AND WORKUP

The approach is similar to bladder tumors. Only rarely will tumor cells be detected in the urine.[4] In male dogs, the most common site is the prostatic urethra which may be palpated as a firm,

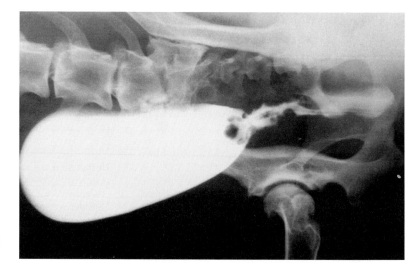

**Figure 25–8.** Urethrogram that reveals filling defects in the urethra and trigone, which was confirmed as transitional cell carcinoma.

slightly enlarged, irregular prostate by digital rectal examination and may mimic prostatic adenocarcinoma. Females will often have a small mass palpable near the urethral papilla on the floor of the vagina. A vaginal smear may reveal transitional cells which are suggestive of neoplasia.[3]

A contrast urethrogram will usually reveal an irregular and narrowed urethral lumen (Fig. 25–8). If the urethra cannot be catheterized, an intravenous pyelogram or direct injection cystogram may be performed to evaluate the bladder trigone. The male dog will often have involvement of the proximal prostatic urethra and trigone while females will have involvement of the entire length of the urethra including the trigone (Fig. 25–9).[6]

Histopathologic confirmation may be attained via biopsy through a vaginoscope or episiotomy approach in the female or by open abdominal biopsy of lymph nodes and urethra in the male or female. The use of urethral catheter with side ports for acquisition of tumor cells or even clumps of tissue has been described[7] but results may not be diagnostic in as many as a third of the cases.[4]

Radiographs of the caudal abdomen are generally indicated to evaluate for enlarged sublumbar lymph nodes or metastasis to the spine or pelvis. Ultrasound may also help visualize the urethra. Thoracic radiographs will only rarely be positive for metastasis at the time of diagnosis.

## TREATMENT

Treatment is generally ineffective due to extensive involvement of the urethra and frequent proximity to the trigone, ureters, and blood supply to the bladder. Successful resection of carefully selected urethral tumors has been reported via a sagittal pubic osteotomy, which allows exposure of the urethra. Approximately one third of all cases were deemed resectable and successful local control was achieved for up to 22 months in these dogs.[8,9] As with bladder cancer, complete urethrectomy, cystectomy, and urinary diversion must be considered experimental.

Trigonal colonic anastomosis or antepubic urethrostomy, after partial urethrectomy, has been suggested but is rarely if ever possible due to the frequent involvement of the trigone.[1,10] A permanent cystostomy can be attempted palliatively for relief of bladder obstruction but is associated with skin scalding from urine and is usually

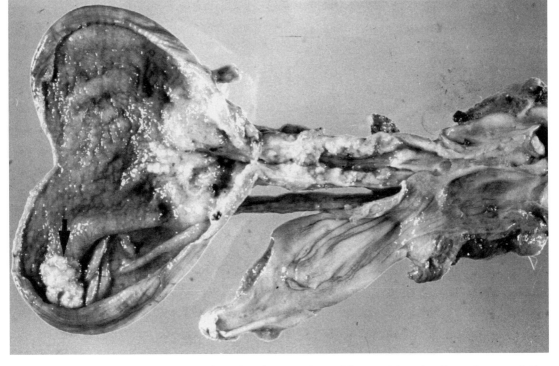

**Figure 25–9.** Bladder, urethra, and vagina from a dog with transitional cell carcinoma of the trigone and entire length of urethra. Note separate bladder lesion in lower left corner (arrow).

rapidly followed by ureteral obstruction. Permanent catheterization of the bladder, through the abdomen or via the urethra, can also be palliative for dogs with obstruction.

Intraoperative radiation therapy was unsuccessful in controlling this disease in one study.[11] The anti-inflammatory drug piroxicam has been recommended for treatment of transitional cell carcinoma of the bladder and may be of benefit for urethal tumors as well. Chemotherapy using cisplatin has been recommended but unequivocal proof of efficacy is lacking.[12]

## PROGNOSIS

The prognosis for cure or significant palliation of malignant urethral cancer is very poor. Untreated cases have lived as long as six months after diagnosis but will have a gradual progression of symptoms ending in complete occlusion of the urethra or metastatic symptoms.

## COMPARATIVE ASPECTS[13]

Urethral cancer in humans is rare. It is often preceded with a history of chronic urethritis. The disease is twice as common in females as it is in males. Proximal lesions are more likely to be transitional cell carcinoma and distal lesions squamous cell carcinoma. Adenocarcinoma has also been reported. Surgery with or without radiation therapy is the treatment of choice.

## REFERENCES

1. Tarvin G, Patnaik A, Greene R: Primary urethral tumors in dogs. J Am Vet Med Assoc 172:931–933, 1978.
2. Wilson GP, Hayes HM, Casey HW: Canine urethral cancer. J Am Anim Hosp Assoc 15:741–744, 1979.
3. Magne ML, Hoopes PJ, Kainer RA, et al: Urinary tract carcinomas involving the canine vagina and vestibule. J Am Anim Hosp Assoc 21:767–772, 1985.
4. Moroff SD, Brown BA, Matthiesen DT, Scott RC: Infiltrative urethral disease in female dogs: 41 cases (1980–1987). J Am Vet Med Assoc 199:247–251, 1991.
5. Szymanski C, Boyce R, Wyman M: Transitional cell carcinoma of the urethra metastatic to the eyes in a dog. J Am Vet Med Assoc 185:1003–1006, 1984.
6. Ticer JW, Spencer CP, Ackerman N: Transitional cell carcinoma of the urethra in four female dogs: Its urethrographic appearance. Vet Radiol 21:12–17, 1980.
7. Melhoff T, Osborne CA: Catheter biopsy of the urethra, urinary bladder and prostate gland. In Kirk RW (ed), Current Veterinary Therapy VI, Philadelphia, WB Saunders, 1977, pp. 1173–1175.
8. Davies JV, Read HM: Urethral tumors in dogs. J Small Anim Pract 31:131–136, 1990.
9. Davies JV, Read HM: Sagittal pubic osteotomy in the investigation and treatment of intrapelvic neoplasia in the dog. J Small Anim Pract 31:123–130, 1990.
10. Yoshioka MM, Carb A: Antepubic urethrostomy in the dog. J Am Anim Hosp Assoc 18:290–294, 1982.
11. Withrow SJ, Gillette EL, Hoopes PJ, McChesney SL: Intraoperative irradiation of 16 spontaneously occurring canine neoplasms. Vet Surg 18:7–11, 1989.
12. Moore AS, Cardona A, Shapiro W, Madewell BR: Cisplatin (cisdiamminedichloroplatinum) for treatment of transitional cell carcinoma of the urinary bladder or urethra. J Vet Intern Med 4:148–152, 1990.
13. Fair WR, Fuks ZY, Scher HI: Cancer of the urethra and penis. In DeVita VT, et al (eds): Cancer: Principles and Practice of Oncology. Philadelphia, JB Lippincott, 1993, pp. 1114–1125.

# 26

# Tumors of the Nervous System

Richard A. LeCouteur

## INTRACRANIAL NEOPLASIA

### Incidence and Risk Factors

Intracranial neoplasia appears to be more common in dogs than in other domestic species.[1–3] An incidence of brain tumors in dogs of 14.5 per 100,000 of the population at risk has been reported.[4] The results of a recent retrospective study of immature dogs (younger than 6 months of age) indicate that the most common sites for neoplasia, in decreasing order, were the hematopoietic system, brain, and skin.[5]

A broad spectrum of tumor types occurs in dogs.[1,2,6] Historically, gliomas (e.g., astrocytomas and oligodendrogliomas) have been reported to be the most frequently occurring primary brain tumors of dogs. More recently, however, meningiomas have been shown to be the most commonly recognized intracranial neoplasms of dogs.[1,2] This apparent alteration in prevalence may be due to the use of advanced diagnostic imaging, the longer life expectancy of dogs, or changes in breed popularity. Primary brain tumors other than gliomas or meningiomas occur infrequently in dogs.

Canine primary brain tumors usually are solitary; however, multiple primary brain tumors have been reported. Multiple meningiomas, [7,8] and cerebrospinal fluid (CSF) metastases of medulloblastoma[6] or choroid plexus carcinoma[9] occur in dogs. Multiple tumors of different histologic type rarely may occur in the brain of a dog (e.g., pituitary carcinoma and multiple meningiomas). Also, extracranial metastases of primary brain meningioma have been reported.[10]

Of secondary tumors, local extension of nasal adenocarcinoma; metastases from mammary, prostatic, or pulmonary adenocarcinoma; metastases from hemangiosarcoma, and extension of pituitary adenoma or carcinoma, are seen most frequently.[1,2,6,11] Skull tumors that affect the brain by local extension include osteosarcoma, chondrosarcoma, and multilobular osteochondrosarcoma.[12]

Brain tumors occur in dogs of any age, all breeds, and of either sex.[1,2,6] Brain tumors occur most frequently in older dogs, with the greatest incidence in dogs over 5 years of age.[1,2] The median age of 86 dogs with brain tumors was 9 years in one study.[13] Younger dogs may be affected.[2] The tumors commonly seen in young dogs include medulloblastoma, ventricular tumors (e.g. ependymoma, choroid plexus papilloma), or tumors of congenital maldevelopment (e.g., craniopharyngioma).[2] Certain breeds have a higher incidence of some tumor types. Glial cell tumors and pituitary tumors occur commonly in brachycephalic breeds, whereas meningiomas occur most frequently in dolichocephalic breeds.[1] Canine breeds that are over-represented include the boxer, golden retriever, Doberman pinscher, Scottish terrier, and Old English sheepdog.[13]

Brain tumors occur less commonly in cats than in dogs. An incidence in cats of approximately 3.5 per 100,000 population has been reported.[4] Zaki and Hurvitz reported 87 central nervous system (CNS) neoplasms in 75 of 3,915 cats necropsied over a 12-year period.[14] There does not appear to be a breed predisposition for the development of intracranial tumors in cats.[1]

Meningioma is the most common primary brain tumor of cats.[2,15] Of 48 cats with intracranial tumors in one study, 42 had meningiomas.[14] Older male cats appear to be most susceptible to meningiomas. Meningiomas in cats may occur in the absence of neurologic signs. In one series, only 25 of 36 cats with meningiomas had neurologic signs, and most tumors were located over the cerebral convexities.[15] Seventeen of 18 CNS tumors were meningiomas in a retrospective survey spanning 15 years at a large veterinary teaching hospital; 8 of these 17 cats had no related clinical signs.[16] In another study of 155 cats without neurologic signs, 8 had meningiomas on critical necropsy evaluation.[17] The meningiomas in 7 of these cats arose from the tela choroidea and were located in the third ventricle.[17] Third-ventricle meningiomas have also been described by others.[2,18,19] Meningiomas involving multiple intracranial sites occur relatively commonly in cats. In one study there were multiple tumors in 11 of 23 cats with intracranial meningiomas.[20] An unusually high incidence of meningiomas has been reported in cats with mucopolysaccharidosis type I.[21]

Primary brain tumors other than meningiomas rarely occur in cats.[18] One review of 216 primary brain tumors of cats found 10 neuroectodermal tumors (including 3 astrocytomas and 3 oligodendrogliomas) and 148 mesenchymal tumors (including 117 meningiomas).[4] Tumors that have been reported include astrocytoma, ependymoma, oligodendroglioma, choroid plexus papilloma, medulloblastoma, lymphoma, olfactory neuroblastoma, and gangliocytoma.[2,18,19] Lymphoma of the brain may be primary or secondary, or it may be one aspect of multicentric lymphoma in cats.

Secondary tumors that have been reported to occur in the brain of cats include pituitary macroadenomas and macrocarcinomas, and metastatic carcinomas. Local extension may occur either from squamous cell carcinoma of the middle ear cavity or from nasal adenocarcinoma.

The cause of intracranial neoplasia in dogs and cats is not known. Studies of dogs and cats indicating particular factors that may cause brain tumors do not exist. Genetic, chemical, viral, traumatic, and immunologic factors should be considered. For example, while the significance of a high incidence of meningiomas in the brain of young cats affected by mucopolysaccharidosis type I is unknown, genetic factors may play a role in tumor development (e.g., a specific chromosomal deletion).[22]

## Pathology

The classification of brain tumors in animals has followed the criteria used for tumors in humans.[2,23,24] Classification is primarily based on the characteristics of the constituent cell type, its pathologic behavior, its topographic pattern, and secondary changes seen within and surrounding the tumor.[3] A classification based on that of Escourolle and Poirer often is used (Fig. 26–1).[25] Fifteen to 20% of animal neuroectodermal tumors remain unclassified using this system.[23]

The intracranial neoplasms of cats or dogs may be classified as either primary or secondary, depending on their cell of origin.[2,24–26] Primary brain tumors originate from cells normally found within the brain and meninges, including the neuroepithelium, lymphoid tissues, germ cells, endothelial cells, and malformed tissues. Secondary tumors comprise either neoplasms that have reached the brain by hematogenous metastasis from a primary tumor located outside the nervous system, or neoplasms that have reached the brain by hematogenous mestastasis from a primary tumor located outside the nervous system, or neoplasms that affect the brain by local invasion, or extension, from adjacent non-neural tissues such as bone.[3,11] Pituitary gland neoplasms (adenomas or carcinomas) and tumors arising from cranial nerves (e.g., nerve sheath tumor of the oculomotor or vestibulocochlear nerves) are considered secondary brain tumors, as they affect the brain by means of local extension.

The classification of intracranial lymphoid neoplasms of dogs is controversial.[23,27–29] Such tumors generally have been grouped under a heading of either neoplastic reticulosis (or focal granulomatous meningoencephalitis), or histiocytic lymphoma (Fig. 26–2). The cells of origin of these tumors remain undetermined at this time. It is likely that both histiocytic lymphoma and neoplastic reticulosis in dogs are primary brain neoplasms.

Care must be exercised in the application of the terms *benign* and *malignant* to a brain neoplasm. In assessing the malignant potential of a brain tumor, the difference between cytologic and biologic malignancy should be emphasized.[1] Cytologic malignancy is a morphologic assessment of anaplasia, based on cytologic and nuclear pleomorphism, cellularity, necrosis, mitoses, and invasiveness. Biologic malignancy is the likelihood that a tumor will kill the animal. Most cytologically malignant brain tumors are also biologically malignant, despite the treatments presently available. Cytologically benign tumors of the brain may also be biologically malignant because of various secondary effects such as increased intracranial pressure (ICP). Particular care must be exercised in the use of the term *benign* when discussing the meningiomas of dogs and cats. Canine menin-

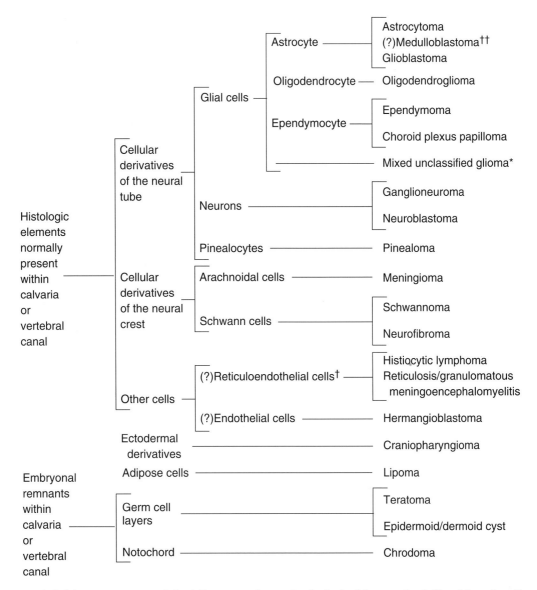

*Up to 20% of all glial tumors are composed of variable amounts of astrocytic, oligodendroglial, or ependymal differentiation, often with mixtures of poorly differentiated glial cells.[23]

†The cells of origin of primary histiocytic lymphoma and reticulosis of the brain are unknown. A resistant mononuclear phagocyte population is present in the normal canine brain, and it is suspected that neoplastic transformation of these cells may give rise to a histiocytic tumor or reticulosis.[27]

††The neuroglial precursor cell of the origin of the medulloblastoma is unknown. Likely candidates are the cells that populate the external granule cell layer of the fetal neonatal cerebellum and the cells of the medullary vela.[3,6]

**Figure 26-1.** Simplified histologic classification of primary central nervous system tumors of dogs and cats. (Modified from Escourolle R, Poirier J: Manual of Basic Neuropathology, 2nd ed., p. 21. Philadelphia, WB Saunders, 1978.[25])

gioma is characterized as "benign," yet it locally infiltrates along the Virchow-Robin space and invariably lacks demarcation from normal brain tissue.[30] In cats, meningiomas are almost always well defined and have a clear demarcation between the tumor and normal brain.[30] The growth rate of meningiomas in cats appears to be slow when compared to that of canine meningiomas.

Brain tumors result in cerebral dysfunction by causing both primary effects, such as infiltration of nervous tissue or compression of adjacent anatomic structures, and secondary effects, such

**Figure 26–2.** Transverse section of the brain of an 8-year-old spayed Airedale terrier at the level of the midbrain. The dog had a 2-month history of progressive loss of balance and a tendency to circle toward the left side. Skull radiographs and CT images of the brain were normal. There is a well-circumscribed space-occupying lesion on the left side of the midbrain and medulla (arrows). The histologic diagnosis was reticulosis.

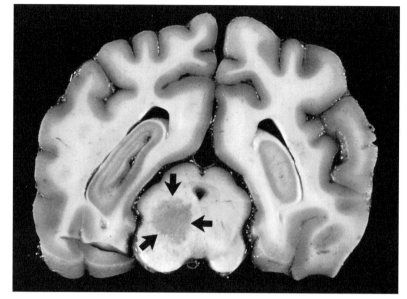

as hydrocephalus. Additional primary effects include disruption of cerebral circulation, or local necrosis, which may result in further damage to neural tissue. The most important secondary effects of a primary brain tumor include disturbance of CSF flow dynamics, elevated ICP, cerebral edema, or brain herniation.[31] Secondary effects usually are more diffuse or generalized in their clinical manifestations, and may "mask" the precise location of a focal intracranial lesion.

Primary brain tumors often are slow growing; however, because the brain is contained within the confines of the calvaria, even a slow-growing tumor may have devastating effects. In slow-growing lesions of the brain, gradual compression permits surrounding structures to adapt to increasing pressure. This occurs through a process termed *compensation*. During the time the brain is able to compensate, there may be a prolonged history of vague signs (e.g., subtle behavior alterations). However, even with a very slowly progressive tumor, clinical signs may progress rapidly when compensatory mechanisms have been exhausted. Rapidly growing tumors may not permit the process of compensation to occur to the same degree as with a slow-growing tumor, and in such cases a sudden onset of severe neurologic dysfunction may occur in the absence of premonitory signs. Should a neoplasm erode or obstruct a major blood vessel, causing hemorrhage or infarction, an acute onset of neurologic deficits may ensue. Secondary brain tumors, particularly metastases, often demonstrate an acute progression of signs.

An aspect of the pathogenesis of brain tumors that is of practical concern is the method by which a brain tumor may spread. The patterns of spread of brain tumors are quite distinct from those of other tumors because of several factors, including lack of a well-developed lymphatic system within the brain. The major patterns of spread involve local invasion and CSF seeding. Brain tumors, particularly astrocytomas, have cells that are capable of invading the normal brain to a remarkable degree. Seeding may occur by spread along the surface of the brain to local sites, or by so-called drop metastases, which spread by way of CSF to the spinal subarachnoid space and then form secondary tumors. Systemic spread by means of the hematogenous route may also occur, though extracranial metastasis rarely is seen.[10,18] As the treatment of primary brain tumors becomes more widespread, the subject of tumor spread will become more important. It is likely that an increase in various patterns of spread will be evident in association with the increased life expectancy that accompanies the successful therapy of dogs or cats with a primary brain tumor.[1]

## History and Clinical Signs

History and neurologic examination are the first steps to a definitive diagnosis in the evaluation of a dog or cat suspected of having a brain tumor. The nature and course of neurologic signs resulting from a brain tumor depend primarily on the location, extent, and rate of growth of the neoplasm.[2,32]

Many dogs or cats with a brain tumor will have a long history of "vague" signs that often are overlooked by an owner or veterinarian until the signs of brain dysfunction are well developed. These signs include subtle behavior alterations that may progress slowly over many months. While the exact cause of these "vague" signs may never be understood, it is interesting to compare this situation with experience in humans. In the majority of humans with a brain tumor, the initial symptom is headache, which is often persistent, severe, and may be worse in the morning. Because headache is a "verbalized" phenomenon in humans, it is impossible to recognize this sign of dysfunction with certainty in dogs or cats. However, cats and dogs may exhibit abnormal behavior that is consistent with the presence of a "headache," such as not wishing to be handled, or hiding during the day. In a series of cats with meningiomas examined by the author, subtle alterations in behavior, such as decreased frequency of purring or diminished activity levels, were noted by the owners for more than 1 year prior to the onset of focal neurologic signs.

The most frequently recognized clinical sign associated with a brain neoplasm of a dog or cat is seizures. This may take the form of a generalized seizure, or it may be a focal seizure. Focal seizures may aid in localizing a neoplasm.

Focal neurologic signs usually occur in association with the primary effects of a fairly well-developed mass lesion. Should a neoplasm involve the brain stem, cranial nerve deficits may be recognized. Weakness, sensory loss, or deficits in vision, hearing, or smell, may occur in association with tumors at specific sites.[2] Weakness and sensory abnormalities usually denote a lesion in the cerebral frontoparietal sensorimotor regions or their deeper pathways. Visual deficits involve the visual pathways from the occipital lobe of the cerebrum to the optic nerve.[33] Hearing loss involves the cerebellomedullary region, the brain stem, or temporal lobes of the cerebrum. Problems with the ability to smell are seen in association with lesions of the cribriform plate, olfactory or temporal lobes of the cerebrum, or other rhinencephalic connections. Difficulties with balance or gait suggest cerebellar or vestibular involvement.

The secondary effects of brain tumors, such as increased ICP, represent further advancement of tumor growth.[32] By the time these effects occur, either a large tumor or significant cerebral edema is present. The signs include alterations in behavior (e.g., lethargy, irritability), circling, head pressing, compulsive walking, altered states of consciousness, or associated locomotor disturbances.

The majority of cats or dogs with a brain tumor will be presented to a veterinarian with problems that relate to the secondary effects of a tumor. This in turn suggests that brain tumors of cats and dogs usually have reached a large size by the time an owner seeks veterinary attention. This is especially true with frontal lobe neoplasms of dogs, which may reach a very large size before causing clinical signs (Fig. 26–3).[34,35] In one study of 43 dogs with brain tumors affecting the rostral cerebrum, those animals with seizures or behavior abnormalities, or both, developed demonstrable neurologic deficits within 3 months.[34] In the same study, the clinical course from detection of demonstrable neurologic deficits to death (or euthanasia) was less than 2 weeks in the absence of therapeutic intervention.[34]

## Diagnostic Techniques and Workup

On the basis of signalment, history, and the results of complete physical and neurologic examinations, it is possible to localize a problem to the brain and, in some cases, to determine the approximate location. However, it must be remembered that the signs that result from a disease in a given location in the nervous system will be similar, regardless of the precise cause.[36] The categories of disease that may result in clinical signs similar to those of a brain tumor include congenital disorders, infections, immunologic and metabolic disorders, toxicities, nutritional disorders, trauma, vascular disorders, degeneration, and idiopathic disorders. These other categories of disease must be eliminated before a diagnosis of brain tumor may be made. For this reason it is essential to follow a logical diagnostic plan for a dog or cat that has signs of brain dysfunction.[1]

A minimum data base for a dog or cat with signs of a brain lesion should include a hemogram, serum chemistry panel, and urinalysis. Survey radiographs of the thorax and abdomen help to rule out a primary malignancy elsewhere in the body. The major objective in the completion of these tests is to eliminate extracranial causes for the signs of cerebral dysfunction.

Plain skull radiographs are of limited value in the diagnosis of a primary brain tumor; however, they may be helpful in the detection of neoplasms of the skull or nasal cavity that have involved the brain by local extension. Occasionally, lysis or hyperostosis of the skull may accompany a primary brain tumor (e.g., meningioma of cats), or there may be radiographically visible mineralization within a neoplasm (Fig. 26–4).[2,37] General anesthesia is required for pre-

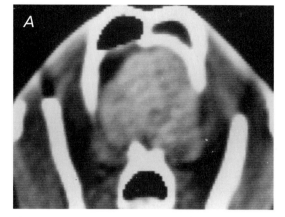

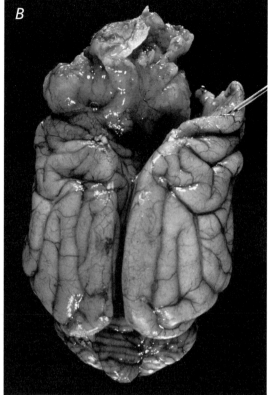

**Figure 26–3.** *A*, Transverse postcontrast CT image of the head of a 9-year-old spayed Shetland sheepdog with a history of six seizures that had occurred during the previous 4 months. The image is at the level of the frontal sinuses. There is a large space-occupying lesion that obliterates the frontal lobes of the cerebrum and extends laterally to erode the frontal bone of the skull. The histologic diagnosis was malignant meningioma. *B*, Dorsal view of the brain of the dog in *A*. A large malignant meningioma is seen arising from the left frontal lobe of the cerebrum. Although this tumor has grown to a large size in this location, the clinical signs were mild.

cise positioning of the skull for radiographs, and various projections have been recommended to identify abnormalities.[2]

Analysis of CSF is recommended as an aid in the diagnosis of a brain tumor.[38] The results of CSF analysis may help to rule out inflammatory causes of cerebral dysfunction, and in some cases may support a diagnosis of a brain tumor. Care should be used in the collection of CSF, because frequently an increased ICP may be present in association with a brain tumor, and pressure alterations associated with CSF drainage may lead to brain herniation.[31] Because CSF pressure measurements are of limited usefulness, it is often desirable to utilize techniques such as hyperventilation to decrease intracranial pressure prior to CSF collection.

In general, increased CSF protein content and a normal to increased CSF white blood cell count have been considered "typical" of a brain neoplasm.[39–43] In one study, only 39.6% of dogs with a primary brain tumor exhibited "typical" CSF alterations.[39] The results of CSF analysis were normal in 10% of the dogs in this study, while the remaining 50.4% of dogs had a variety of nonspecific CSF changes.[39] The CSF from dogs

with a meningioma often may have an elevated white blood cell count (> 50/$\mu$l), with more than 50% of these cells being polymorphonuclear leukocytes.[39] In another study, glial cell tumors predominated among those that resulted in CNS inflammation.[34] Neoplastic cells may be present in CSF, particularly when sedimentation techniques are used for analysis.[13,40,41] The use of CSF protein electrophoresis,[44] and IgG index of CSF,[45] may aid in the determination of the presence of a brain neoplasm. Little information is available regarding CSF alterations seen in association with feline brain tumors; however, changes are similar to those described for dogs.[46]

Numerous brain imaging techniques such as ventriculography, cerebral angiography, cavernous sinus venography, cisternography,[47,48] and scientigraphy[49,50] are available for use in dogs or cats.[51] However, each of these techniques has severe limitations in that they fail, in most instances, to define the exact extent of a neoplasm and its precise relationship to surrounding structures. This information is essential for the accurate treatment planning of a cerebral neoplasm.

Consequently, despite the availability of these imaging techniques, significant advances in ther-

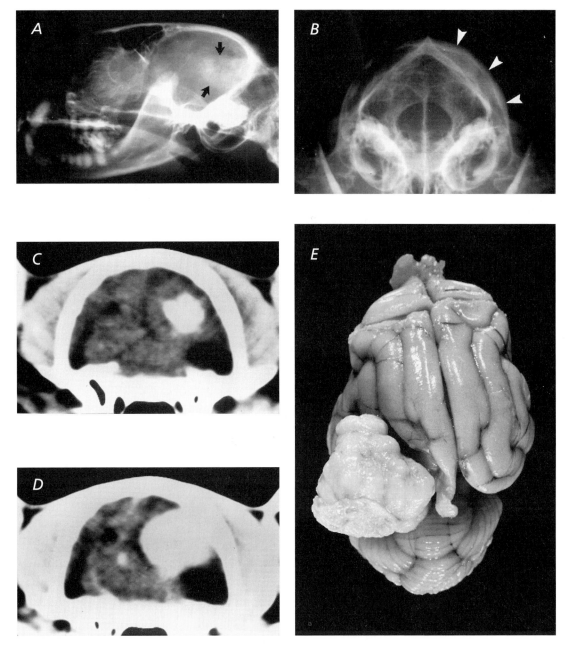

**Figure 26–4.** *A*, Lateral radiograph of the skull of an 8-year-old castrated domestic shorthair cat. The cat had a 2-month history of abnormal behavior that consisted of vocalizing and hiding from its owner. The cat had a tendency to circle toward its left side. Note the region of mineralization within the cranial vault (arrows). *B*, Rostrocaudal projection of the cranial vault of the cat in *A*. Note the mineralized opacity in the region of the left parietal bone and the increased thickness of the left parietal bone. *C*, Transverse precontrast CT image of the head of the cat in *A*. Note the focal area of calcification within the left occipital lobe of the cerebrum. *D*, Transverse postcontrast CT image of the head of the cat in *A* at a similar level to that of the CT image in *C*. There is a well-demarcated region of uniform contrast uptake in the region of the focal area of calcification that was seen in the precontrast image. In addition, there are areas of lucency around the periphery of the enhanced region that are consistent with peritumoral edema. The contrast enhancement pattern is typical of that seen with meningioma. *E*, Dorsal view of the brain of the cat in *A*. There is a large space-occupying lesion in the left occipital lobe of the cerebrum. The histologic diagnosis was meningioma. (Photographs courtesy of Dr. Allen F. Sisson.)

apy for intracranial neoplasms did not occur until techniques were developed that provided precise information regarding location and extent. With the availability of computed tomography (CT), a basis for the development of therapeutic plans for dogs and cats with a brain tumor was available.[2,9,52–59] CT provides accurate determination of the presence, location, size, and anatomic relationships of intracranial neoplasms. More recently, magnetic resonance imaging (MRI) has allowed these principles to be advanced even further.[2,57,58,60] Images obtained by means of MRI are superior to those of CT in certain brain regions (e.g. the brainstem), and the diagnostic specificity of MRI may eventually render the biopsy of tumors prior to treatment unnecessary.

While the major tumor types in dogs are reported to have characteristic CT or MRI features,[54,57] it must be remembered that non-neoplastic space-occupying lesions may mimic the CT or MRI appearance of a neoplasm (Fig. 26–5),[53] and that occasionally a metastasis may resemble a primary brain tumor on CT or MRI images (Fig. 26–6).

At the present time, biopsy is the sole method available for the diagnosis of brain tumor type in cats or dogs. Several biopsy methods have been described, including ultrasound-guided biopsy,[61] and CT-guided biopsy.[62] Ideally, an intracranial lesion should be biopsied prior to the institution of therapy of any type; however, biposy is not always attempted because of practical considerations, such as cost and morbidity. Often a needle biopsy may be as difficult and dangerous as an excisional biopsy for brain lesions.

## Therapy

The major goals of therapy for a brain tumor are to control secondary effects, such as increased ICP or cerebral edema, and to eradicate the tumor or reduce its size.[51] Beyond general efforts to maintain homeostasis, palliative therapy for dogs or cats with a brain tumor consists of glucocorticoids for edema reduction and, in some cases (e.g., lymphoma), for retardation of tumor growth.[63] Some animals with a brain tumor will demonstrate dramatic improvement in clinical signs for weeks or months with sustained glucocorticoid therapy. Should seizure therapy be needed, phenobarbital is the drug best suited for the control of generalized seizures.[36]

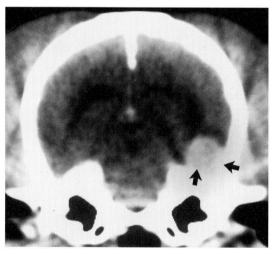

**Figure 26–6.** Transverse postcontrast CT image of the head of a 12-year-old spayed miniature schnauzer dog. The image is at the level of the tympanic cavities. The dog had a history of seizures. There is a well-circumscribed, uniformly enhancing space-occupying lesion located superficially in the right temporal lobe of the cerebrum (arrows). The lesion has a broad meningeal attachment and has all the CT characteristics of a meningioma. The tumor was removed surgically and the histologic diagnosis was metastatic chemodectoma. The dog died 7 months following surgery, at which time chemodectoma and hemangiosarcoma metastases were found in all the organs examined except the brain, which was free of tumor.

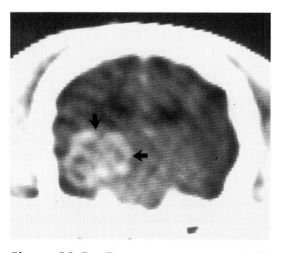

**Figure 26–5.** Transverse postcontrast CT image of the head of a 6-year-old cocker spaniel dog at the level of the thalamus. Note the well-circumscribed space-occupying lesion to the left of the thalamus (arrows). This lesion has many of the characteristics of a primary brain tumor; however, it was confirmed to be an encapsulated hematoma following surgical removal.

Four methods of therapy for a brain tumor are available at this time for use in dogs and cats: surgery, irradiation, chemotherapy, and immunotherapy (or biologic response modification).[51,64]

**Surgery**  In association with the availability of CT and the development of advanced neurosurgical and anesthetic techniques, complete or partial surgical removal of intracranial neoplasms has been practiced with increasing frequency during the past few years.[65,66] Neurosurgical intervention is now an essential consideration in the management of the intracranial neoplasms of cats or dogs, whether for complete excision, partial removal, or biopsy (Fig. 26–7).[30]

The precise location, size, and extent of a neoplasm, combined with the invasiveness of the tumor, determine the possibility of complete surgical removal. The possibility of complete excision is also affected by tumor type.[30] Meningiomas, particularly those located over the

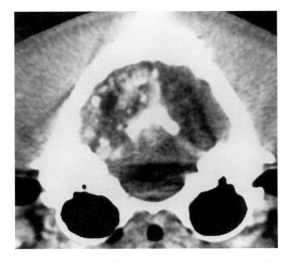

**Figure 26–7.** Transverse postcontrast CT image of the head of a 9-year-old castrated black Labrador retriever. The image is at the level of the tympanic cavities. The dog had a history of generalized seizures, blindness in the right eye, and mild right-sided postural reaction deficits. Note the irregularly enhancing space-occupying lesion in the left occipital lobe of the cerebrum. There are areas of calcification within the lesion. The tumor was partially excised surgically by means of lateral craniotomy. Surgery was followed by irradiation of the brain (45 Gy in 15 fractions over 3 weeks). The dog is alive 1 year following completion of therapy, and clinical signs other than infrequent seizures have resolved. The histologic diagnosis was chondrosarcoma.

cerebral convexities or in the frontal lobes of the cerebrum, often may be completely (or almost completely) removed by means of surgery, especially in cats. In contrast, there is a significant morbidity and mortality associated with the surgical removal of neoplasms located in the caudal fossa and brainstem of cats and dogs.[13,30,64,67,68]

In addition to providing a tissue diagnosis of tumor type, partial removal of a brain neoplasm may relieve signs of cerebral dysfunction and, in turn, may render an animal a better candidate for other forms of therapy. Cytoreduction also lessens the volume of tumor available for therapy using other treatment regimes, such as radiation therapy. However, surgical biopsy or cytoreduction of a tumor must be approached with care, as seeding of a tumor to previously uninvolved tissue may result in some cases.

Few data are available concerning the surgical management of secondary brain tumors. Calvarial tumors such as osteosarcomas, chondrosarcomas, and multilobular osteochondrosarcomas have been removed successfully, and in the author's experience, it appears that the prognosis for tumor-free survival after the removal of a calvarial osteosarcoma may be better than that for osteosarcomas of long bones. Intracalvarial primary bone tumors may also be removed surgically prior to other types of therapy. Surgical removal of focal metastases may also be considered in certain cases.

**Radiation Therapy**  The use of radiation therapy for the treatment of primary brain tumors of dogs and cats is well established.[13,51,69–75] Irradiation may be used either alone or in combination with other treatments (Fig 26–8). Radiation therapy also is recommended for the treatment of secondary brain tumors. Metastases, pituitary macroadenomas or macrocarcinomas, and skull tumors have been successfully managed by means of either radiation therapy alone or as an adjunct to surgery.[72] Lymphoma or granulomatous meningoencephalomyelitis may also be sensitive to radiation therapy.[73]

The objective of radiation therapy is to destroy a neoplasm, while at the same time minimizing damage to any normal tissue that must be included in the irradiated volume. External beam, megavoltage irradiation currently is recommended for the therapy of brain tumors in dogs or cats.[1,13] Orthovoltage radiation has been used for the treatment of canine brain tumors (total dose of 45 Gy in 3.75 Gy fractions over 28 days) without adverse effects.[75] It should be stressed, however, that orthovoltage radiation is

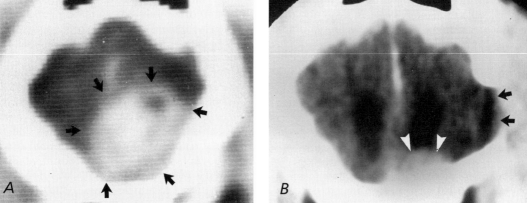

**Figure 26–8.**   *A,* Transverse postcontrast CT image of the head of a 13-year-old spayed miniature poodle at the level of the frontal lobes of the cerebrum. The dog had a history of seizures. There is a large space-occupying lesion to the right of the midline (arrows). *B,* Transverse postcontrast CT image of the head of the dog in *A* completed 436 days after partial surgical removal of the space-occupying lesion and postsurgical irradiation (4,000 Gy in 10 fractions over 22 days). The diagnosis was meningioma. Note the craniotomy site in the right frontal bone (black arrows). There is apparent recurrence of the tumor on the floor of the calvaria (white arrows). The dog was reoperated and meningioma was removed from this site. The dog was free of signs 2 years after the second surgery.

not optimal because of poor beam penetration, profile, and limited field configuration.[75]

Careful treatment planning by a qualified and experienced radiation therapist is essential to the success of radiation therapy. The selection of a radiation dose is based partly on considerations such as tumor type and location, and partly on tolerance of the tissues that surround the tumor (tumor bed) and that have not been invaded by the tumor. The response of tissues in the tumor bed may be altered by proximity to the tumor through indirect effects such as pressure, altered vascular supply, or impaired CSF drainage. In the author's experience, total doses of radiation in excess of 46.5 Gy in 15 fractions over 19 days may result in late, delayed reactions, including brain necrosis. It appears that a total dose of 45 Gy given in 15 equal fractions over 3 weeks is well tolerated by the tumor bed of cats and dogs. Further studies are needed to determine the optimal dose and number of fractions that should be given, and the time over which radiation therapy should extend.

Numerous techniques have been developed to improve the effectiveness of irradiation; however, these techniques have received only superficial attention in veterinary medicine up to the present time. Superfractionation (using two or more fractions each day) has several advantages over the protocol outlined above for the treatment of brain tumors. However, at this time the logistics

of twice-daily fractions are difficult to organize, and as each treatment requires anesthesia of the animal, these protocols would stress a dog or cat considerably. Radiation enhancers (sensitizers) such as misonidazole may also be considered. These drugs substitute for oxygen in the hypoxic areas of a brain tumor and may render them more radiation sensitive. Boron neutron capture therapy is another radiation-associated therapy that is currently under investigation.[76] Hyperthermia (local or whole body) and photoradiation therapy may also be used to potentiate the effects of radiation therapy.

Brachytherapy, or interstial radiation therapy, is a method of implantation of radioisotope seeds (e.g.,[125] I) into the center of a tumor to deliver high doses of radiation. This technique has been used in dogs with limited success.[6,13]

A recent report[77] introduces the use of a modified CT scanner to diagnose and, immediately after, to deliver accurately, multi-arc rotational irradiation to 25 dogs with (CT-diagnosed) intracranial masses. Initial results indicate marked clinical improvement in irradiated dogs, and a significant reduction in mass size, without adverse effects from irradiation.[77]

**Chemotherapy**   Several factors affect the use of chemotherapeutic agents for the treatment of brain tumors in dogs or cats.[1,78] The first, unique to the brain, is that the blood-brain barrier may prevent exposure of all or some of the tumor to a chemotherapeutic agent injected parenterally. Second, tumor cell heterogeneity may be such that only certain cells within a tumor are sensitive to a given agent. Third, a tumor may be sensitive only at dosages that are toxic to the normal brain or other organs. Methods for increasing drug delivery to the CNS are under investigation for use in humans. Intra-arterial administration of drugs, high-dose systemic therapy, and blood-brain barrier disruption are all currently under investigation in animal models.[79]

Cytosine arabinoside (ARA-C) has been used intrathecally in dogs to treat CNS lymphoma.[80] Recent investigation has shown that ARA-C penetrates the intact canine blood-brain barrier and that cytotoxic concentrations may be achieved in the CNS following intravenous administration.[81] Carmustine (BCNU) or lomustine (CCNU) have resulted in a significant reduction in tumor size, and in the improvement of clinical signs, in dogs with glial cell tumors.[64,78,82,83]

**Immunotherapy**  An approach that mobilizes cell-mediated immunity against a brain tumor by stimulating and culturing autologous lymphocytes, and then returning them to the tumor bed following tumor resection, has been utilized in dogs.[84] Reduction in tumor size and clinical improvement occurred in five dogs with cerebral gliomas.[84] The treatment of dogs with meningiomas using repeated intracisternal injections of stimulated lymphocytes also resulted in clinical improvement and reduction in tumor size.[84]

## Prognosis

There are few data concerning the survival times of dogs or cats with a brain tumor that have received only palliative therapy (i.e., therapy to control the secondary effects of a tumor without an attempt to eradicate the tumor). The results of one study indicate a mean and median survival of 81 days and 56 days, respectively, following CT diagnosis of a primary brain tumor in each of 8 dogs.[69] Six of the 8 dogs in this study died or were euthanatized within 64 days of brain tumor diagnosis, though 1 dog survived for 307 days, indicating that survival times are difficult to predict.[69] In another study that included 13 dogs with intracranial meningiomas, survival times from initial clinical signs to necropsy varied from 1 day to 405 days, with a mean survival time of 75 days.[34] In the same study, the survival times for 7 dogs with astrocytoma were from 7 days to 150 days, with a mean survival time of 77 days.[34]

In a report of 86 dogs with either primary or secondary brain tumors, the median survival time for 45 dogs receiving either no treatment (7 dogs) or symptomatic treatment (38 dogs) was 6 days.[13]

The results from several studies confirm that the prognosis for a dog or cat with a primary brain tumor may be significantly improved by surgical removal, irradiation, chemotherapy, or immunotherapy, used either alone or in combination.[13,30,64,75] In a retrospective study in which 41 dogs, with either primary or secondary brain tumors, received some form of definitive treatment (i.e., surgery, Cobalt-60 irradiation, whole-body hyperthermia,[125] I implants, and chemotherapy, alone or in combination), the factor most associated with survival time was mode of therapy.[13] Dogs that were treated with irradiation, with or without other combinations of therapy, lived significantly longer than those that received surgery (with or without[125] I implants), or those that received symptomatic therapy.[13] In this same study, the main indicators for poor prognosis, after adjusting for treatment, were involvement of multiple brain regions and moderate-to-severe neurologic signs.[13] Other factors that negatively influenced survival in this study included increased white blood cell count in CSF, a rapid and progressive clinical course, tumor types other than meningioma, and secondary brain tumors.[13]

The reports concerning surgical removal alone for the treatment of the primary brain tumors of dogs have dealt primarily with superficial, rostro-tentorial meningiomas. In one study of 4 dogs that had surgical removal of olfactory lobe meningiomas, postoperative survival times were 63 days to 203 days, with a mean survival time of 138 days.[85] In another study, 10 dogs treated surgically for intracranial meningiomas had a median survival time of 198 days, with a 1-year survival rate of 30%.[30] It appears that dogs have an excellent prognosis for long-term survival following complete surgical excision of a solitary cerebral meningioma. "Complete" removal should be confirmed following careful histologic examination of tumor margins by a pathologist. The prognosis for dogs or cats after surgery alone for removal of a meningioma is affected by the occurrence of postoperative complications, such as infection, cerebral edema, or hemorrhage.

Megavoltage irradiation, alone or in combination with surgery, has been used frequently for the treatment of canine brain tumors. In a review of four reports[13,69,74,86] of megavoltage irradiation, alone or with surgery, used as a treatment for canine brain masses (i.e., both primary and secondary brain tumors), the mean and median survival times ranged from 160 days to 433 days, and 160 days to 360 days, respectively. A median survival time of 345 days was reported for 14 dogs with a variety of brain masses that received orthovoltage irradiation.[34] In most animals, radiation therapy should commence within several days of the completion of surgery if the animal is clinically stable and can survive anesthesia.

Dogs that have been treated for a brain tumor may develop a second type of tumor elsewhere in the body. For example, in six dogs with pituitary macrocarcinomas or macroadenomas treated by means of irradiation, three developed second tumors outside the original treatment field within 2 years of the completion of therapy.[72]

There are a number of reports concerning surgical removal of feline meningiomas.[30,37,67,68,87] All the reports confirm that surgical removal of a solitary meningioma in cats results in excellent long-term survival. In a series of 10 cats treated by surgical removal of a meningioma, 1 cat died immediately after surgery, and 3 cats died of concurrent disease unrelated to cerebral neoplasia 2 to 30 months after surgery.[37] In another study, 4 cats that had surgical removal of a solitary meningioma had a mean survival time of 485 days, with 2 cats surviving more than 2 years after surgery (50% survival at 2 years).[30] A report of 17 cats with meningioma treated by surgical removal indicates that 3 died in the immediate postoperative period, 3 cats died with tumor recurrence at 3 months, 9 months, or 72 months after surgery, and the remaining 11 cats survived without tumor recurrence for 18 months to 47 months (median 27 months) postoperatively.[67] The results of craniotomy for the treatment of cerebral meningioma in 42 cats indicate an overall survival of 71% at 6 months, 66% at 1 year, and 50% at 2 years.[68]

At this time there are few published reports concerning surgery or radiation therapy of dogs and cats for the treatment of tumor types other than meningioma. Radiation therapy alone has been used by the author for the treatment of caudal fossa neoplasms of dogs, granulomatous meningoencephalomyelitis of dogs, and ACTH-secreting pituitary neoplasms of dogs. The preliminary results of these groups of animals confirm that the prognosis for these animals is greatly improved following radiation therapy.

## Comparative Aspects

New brain tumors develop in approximately 35,000 adult Americans each year.[88] In children,

astrocytomas and medulloblastomas are the most common tumors; in adults, the most common are metastatic tumors, astroglial neoplasms (including glioblastoma multiforme), meningiomas, and pituitary adenomas. Recent evidence suggests that the incidence of primary tumors among the elderly is increasing. Malignant gliomas account for 2.5% of the deaths due to cancer and are the third leading cause of death from cancer in persons 15 to 34 years of age.

There is little information about the relationship of environmental factors to primary brain tumors. Cranial irradiation and exposure to certain chemicals may lead to an increased incidence of both astrocytomas and meningiomas. Head injury may potentiate meningiomas but does not appear to cause astrocytomas. Sixteen percent of patients with primary brain tumors have a family history of some type of cancer.[88,89]

The morbidity and mortality associated with brain tumors in humans vary with the histologic type. Only 10% of patients with malignant astrocytoma or glioblastoma multiforme are alive 18 to 24 months after therapy, regardless of the type of therapy used. Some combination of surgery and irradiation is required to achieve 50% to 70% 5-year survival rates in virtually all the adult cases of low-grade astrocytoma, oligodendroglioma, or ependymoma. Approximately 80% of patients are free of recurrence at 5 years after the excision of a meningioma, and 50% are free of tumor at 20 years after an operation. The only factor significantly associated with recurrence-free survival following resection of a meningioma is the completeness of surgical excision. Irradiation is successful in improving the survival of patients that have had incomplete surgical resection of a meningioma.[1]

## SPINAL CORD NEOPLASIA

### Incidence and Risk Factors

Tumors affecting the spinal cord may be considered as extradural, intradural-extramedullary, and intramedullary.[2] Extradural neoplasms comprise approximately 50% of all spinal neoplasms, while intradural-extramedullary tumors and intramedullary tumors comprise 30% and 15%, respectively.[2] The reported series are not sufficiently large to yield reliable data concerning age, breed, or sex predilections.[90] In one study, 8 of 29 dogs or cats (27.6%) were 3 years of age or less, and 90% of the tumors occurred in large breeds of dog.[91]

Primary spinal cord neoplasms occur infrequently in dogs. Meningiomas appear to be the most frequently diagnosed primary spinal neoplasm of dogs.[2] Such tumors have a high incidence in the cervical spinal cord.[2] A primary spinal cord neoplasm with a high incidence in young dogs (6 months to 3 years of age) is neuroepithelioma (or spinal cord blastoma).[92-98] Hemangiosarcoma is the most common secondary tumor affecting the canine spinal cord.[99]

Primary spinal cord neoplasia, with the exception of lymphoma, is relatively rare in cats.[19] Lymphoma was diagnosed in 214 of 1,897 necropsies done on cats in one study.[19,100] Of these 214 cats, there was CNS involvement in 26 (21.1%).[100] Twenty-three of these 26 tumors involved the spinal cord, and 22 of the 23 were solitary.[100] A predilection for the thoracic and lumbar vertebral canal was noted.[100] Most cats with spinal lymphoma were young (median age 24 months).[100] In another series of 150 cats with lymphoreticular malignancies, 8 (5.3%) had gross CNS involvement.[101] Signs of neurologic dysfunction were recognized in 10 (10.9%) of 92 cats with lymphoma in another report.[19]

Etiologic factors of spinal tumors are poorly defined in cats and dogs. In cats, feline leukemia virus (FeLV) is frequently associated with lymphoma and therefore must be considered a risk factor in the development of spinal lymphoma.[100,102,103] However, a cat with spinal lymphoma may test negative for FeLV. Spinal lymphoma has also been identified in association with feline immunodeficiency virus infection.[104]

## Pathology

In dogs, the most frequently reported extradural tumors are primary malignant bone tumors (osteosarcoma, chondrosarcoma, fibrosarcoma, hemangiosarcoma, hemangioendothelioma, and myeloma), and tumors metastatic to bone and soft tissue.[3,91,105] Secondary tumors affecting the canine vertebrae arise from numerous primary tumor types.[3,91,105,106] Metastatic extradural neoplasms are unusual in dogs; however, extradural lymphomas and liposarcomas have been reported.[1,2,107,108]

Meningiomas and peripheral nerve sheath tumors are the most frequently occurring intradural-extramedullary neoplasms of dogs.[90] These tumors are reported to occur most frequently in older dogs of either gender.[90] In one report, approximately 14% of CNS meningiomas involved the spinal cord in dogs (27% cervical, 47% thoracic, and 27% lumbar spinal cord).[8] In another study of spinal meningiomas in 13 dogs, three were in the lumbar region, and 10 were located in the cervical region.[90] A review of nerve sheath tumors revealed that 39 of 60 tumors compromised the spinal cord.[8] Peripheral nerve sheath tumor was the second most common tumor (after vertebral tumors) in another review of 29 tumors affecting the spinal cord.[105]

A less frequently reported intradural-extramedullary tumor of dogs is neuroepithelioma, also classified as ependymoma, medulloepithelioma, nephroblastoma, and spinal cord blastoma.[98] This neoplasm has a predilection for the T10 through L2 spinal cord segments of young dogs, especially German shepherds and retrievers.[92-98]

Intramedullary spinal tumors of dogs occur infrequently.[3] They are predominantly of glial cell origin; astrocytoma, oligodendroglioma, undifferentiated sarcoma, ependymoma, and choroid plexus papilloma have been reported.[3] Granulomatous meningoencephalomyelitis may also occur as a primary spinal cord neoplasm. Intramedullary spinal cord metastases may occur in dogs with systemic malignancy, in the absence of tumor metastasis in the epidural space or vertebral bone, and as the first clinical manifestation of cancer.[3,99,109] It appears that hemangiosarcoma and lymphoma have a propensity for intramedullary spinal cord involvement.[99] Intramedullary metastases have also been reported in association with mammary gland adenocarcinoma and malignant melanoma.[2] Occasionally, malformation tumors may affect the spinal cord (e.g., epidermoid cyst).[3]

Extradural lymphoma, either primary or secondary, occurs frequently in cats.[100,103] Of feline extradural tumors, osteosarcoma is the most common primary vertebral neoplasm. Single or multiple osteochondromas have been identified in several cats.[19] Of the intradural-extramedullary tumors, meningiomas have been infrequently reported in the spinal cord of cats.[19] Intramedullary tumors of cats are extremely rare.[19]

## History and Clinical Signs

Extramedullary spinal cord neoplasms typically are slow growing and result in gradual spinal cord compression. The signs of spinal cord dysfunction usually worsen over weeks or months. Occasionally, an acute onset of signs may accompany hemorrhage or ischemia associated with a neoplasm. Intramedullary tumors, which may grow more rapidly, are characterized by a higher incidence of ischemia, necrosis, and hemorrhage.

The clinical signs seen in association with a spinal cord tumor usually reflect the location of the neoplasm and often are indistinguishable from the signs caused by other transverse myelopathies at the same location.[105] The presence of certain signs should cause suspicion of a spinal cord neoplasm. Extradural tumors may involve the meninges, spinal nerves, or nerve roots, resulting in discomfort that may may progress to extreme spinal hyperesthesia.[105] Neurologic deficits (e.g., paresis) may not be seen initially and, when present, may be intermittent (i.e., worsen with exercise). There is usually a progressive worsening of neurologic function caudal to the lesion. Intradural-extramedullary tumors may also result in a prolonged, intermittent expression of clinical signs and hyperesthesia; however, the signs may be alleviated by exercise.[90] Brachial or lumbar intumescence involvement may be evidenced by lameness, holding up of a limb, neurogenic muscular atrophy, and depressed spinal reflexes. Rarely, unilateral spinal cord compression may cause deficits in the contralateral limb. In contrast, intramedullary spinal cord tumors usually cause rapid progression of neurologic dysfunction.[91] Hyperesthesia rarely is associated with such tumors.[110]

## Diagnostic Techniques and Workup

The diagnosis of a neoplasm affecting the spinal cord requires a systematic approach.[111] The procedure is based on the collection and interpretation of a minimum data base that includes appropriate serologic tests (hemogram, biochemical profile), and thoracic radiographs for primary or metastatic neoplasia. Following this, survey radiographs of the vertebral column, CSF collection and analysis, and myelography may be completed during a single period of anesthesia.

General anesthesia permits accurate positioning of a dog or cat for survey radiographs of the vertebral column and allows stressed or oblique projections to be done. Primary or secondary vertebral tumors may produce bone lysis or new bone production, or both. The vertebral body and arch are more frequently affected by a neoplasm than the dorsal spinal processes or transverse processes. Plain radiographic abnormalities are uncommon with primary nervous system neoplasms. Expansion of a spinal tumor may result in the enlargement of an intervertebral foramen, widening of the vertebral canal, or thinning of surrounding bone (Fig. 26–9).

Cerebrospinal fluid collection and analysis are indicated when plain radiographs do not provide a complete diagnosis. A lumbar puncture is recommended for CSF collection, and the needle may be left in place for myelography, pending the results of the cytologic examination of CSF. The alterations in CSF caused by spinal tumors should be interpreted according to the same criteria discussed for brain tumor diagnosis; however, it must be remembered that the protein content of CSF collected from a lumbar location is normally higher than that of CSF collected from the cerebellomedullary cistern.[43] Lymphoma affecting the spinal cord often results in an elevated white cell count, predominantly abnormal lymphocytes.[100,103]

Myelography is essential for the accurate determination of the location and extent of a spinal cord neoplasm. On the basis of myelography, the tumors may be classified as extradural (Fig. 26–10), intradural-extramedullary (Fig. 26–11), or intramedullary (Fig. 26–12), although this distinction cannot always be made. For example, it is not always possible to distinguish between an intramedullary and an intradural-extramedullary lesion on the basis of myelographic findings. In such cases, CT or MRI may provide more exact localizing information (Fig. 26–13).[57,60]

## Treatment

A limited number of therapeutic options exist for a dog or cat with a spinal cord neoplasm.[112] Appropriate therapy depends on tumor location, extent, and histologic type. An immediate goal of therapy is to relieve the deleterious effects of sustained spinal cord compression. This may be achieved medically (e.g., glucocorticoids) or surgically.[111] Surgery may permit the complete removal or cytoreduction and biopsy of a neoplasm.[90,113–115] In cases in which complete removal is not possible, recurrence is to be expected, and adjunctive therapy such as irradiation is recommended.[107,114,116] The development of advanced neurosurgical techniques and the introduction of new biopsy methods has improved the outcome in many cases.[103,117–118]

Accurate biopsy diagnosis of lymphoma is essential, because lymphoma of the spinal cord may be successfully treated with chemotherapy or irradiation alone, or in combination.[80,100,103] In

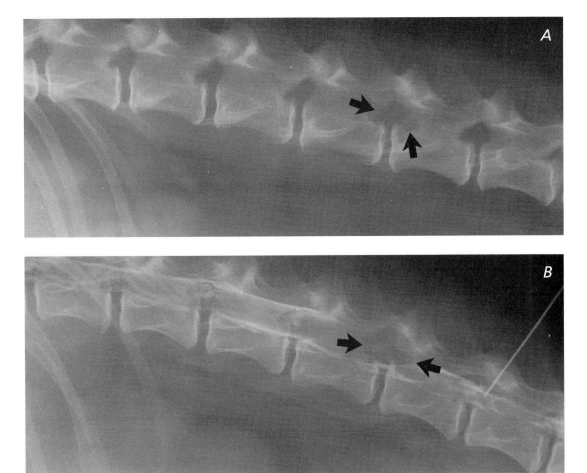

**Figure 26–9.** *A,* Lateral radiograph of the lumbar vertebral column of a 10-year-old spayed Australian shepherd dog with a 3-week history of progressive lameness in the left pelvic limb. Severe atrophy of the left quadriceps muscle was seen in association with an absent left patellar reflex. A diagnosis of left femoral neuropathy was made. Note the lysis surrounding the L4 to L5 intervertebral foramen (arrows). *B,* Myelogram of the lumbar vertebral column of the dog in *A.* There is a filling defect at the level of the L4 to L5 intervertebral foramen consistent with a space-occupying lesion (arrows). The histologic diagnosis was schwannoma. Note the positioning of the spinal needle for CSF collection and injection of contrast material.

certain cases, radiation therapy may be done prior to chemotherapy in order to effect a rapid reduction in tumor mass.[80]

## Prognosis

There are few reports in the veterinary literature concerning the long-term follow-up of dogs and cats with spinal neoplasia.[112] The prognosis depends on the resectability, histologic type, location, and severity of clinical signs. Generally, dogs or cats with an extradural metastatic neo-

plasm or vertebral neoplasm have a poor prognosis, and palliative therapy only is attempted.[112] Removal of an affected vertebra (spondylectomy), particularly in the cranial lumbar region, may be attempted in selected cases. Occasionally, intradural-extramedullary tumors may be completely resected, and in such cases the prognosis must be considered good. In one study, 5 of 13 dogs survived for longer than 6 months following the surgical resection of a meningioma.[90] Of the 5 dogs 1 was alive 5 years after surgery.[90] Few data exist concerning irradiation or chemother-

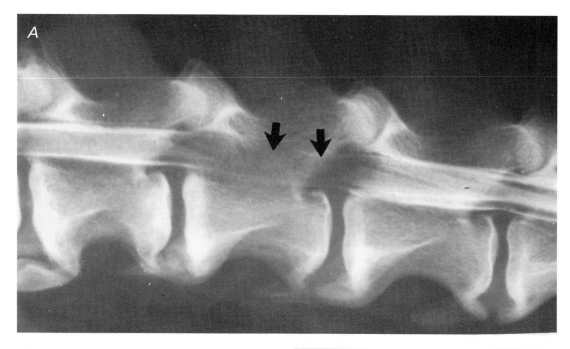

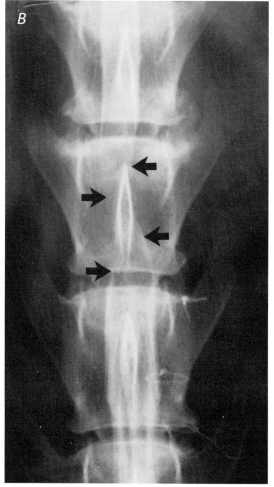

**Figure 26–10.**   Lateral (*A*) and ventrodorsal (*B*) myelogram of the midlumbar region of the vertebral column of a 12-year-old spayed Bouvier des Flandres dog with progressive paraparesis that had started 72 hours previously. Noncontrast vertebral radiographs were normal. There is a severe extradural spinal cord compression centered over the body of L4 vertebra. The spinal cord is severely compressed from the dorsal direction and from the left and right sides (arrows). The histologic diagnosis was metastatic thyroid carcinoma within the L4 vertebra.

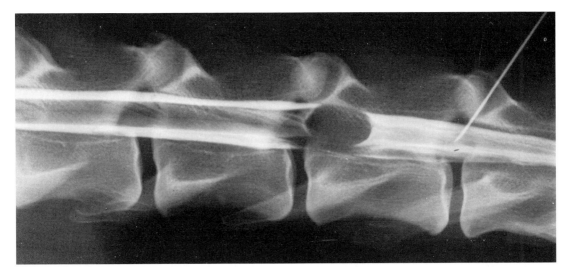

**Figure 26–11.** Lateral myelogram of the lumbar region of the vertebral column of a 10-year-old spayed Labrador retriever. The dog had progressive paraparesis of several months' duration. Non-contrast vertebral radiographs were normal. Note the well-defined intradural-extramedullary lesion at the level of L5 to L6 vertebrae. The mass was removed surgically and the histologic diagnosis was meningioma. The dog made a complete recovery and was normal 6 months following surgery.

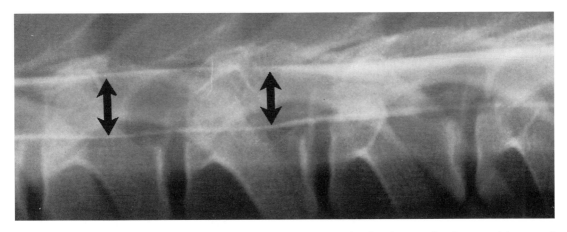

**Figure 26–12.** Lateral myelogram of the thoracic vertebral column of a 3-year-old spayed Labrador retriever with progressive paraparesis of 6 month, duration. Plain radiographs of this region were normal. The lateral myelogram outlined an expansile intramedullary lesion at the level of T5 to T6 vertebrae (arrows). The dog's signs continued to worsen, and 2 months following this study, the dog was euthanized. An astrocytoma of the spinal cord was confirmed at the level of the T5 to T6 vertebrae.

apy of spinal cord neoplasms in animals; however, such therapies should be considered.[100,103] The author has treated several intramedullary tumors of dogs (including ependymoma and lymphoma) by means of irradiation. The results in these cases indicate that the canine spinal cord tolerates irradiation well and that the clinical signs of spinal cord tumors may be alleviated for more than 1 year.

## Comparative Aspects

Intradural spinal cord neoplasms are uncommon in humans; their incidence is from 3 to 10 per

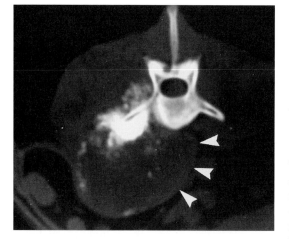

**Figure 26–13.** Transverse precontrast CT image of the vertebral column of a 7-year-old spayed Australian shepherd dog at the level of the L4 vertebra. There is a large tumor arising from the right transverse process of the L4 vertebra. The tumor involves the body of this vertebra. Note the soft tissue mass crossing the midline ventrally (arrows). The histologic diagnosis was osteosarcoma.

100,000 population.[119] The ratio of intradural to extradural tumors is approximately 3 : 2. These tumors occur predominantly in the middle decades of life, and except for an unusually high incidence of meningiomas in females, the sex incidence is approximately equal. Of the intradural-extramedullary tumors, peripheral nerve sheath tumors comprise about 30%, and meningiomas comprise about 25%.

Astrocytoma and ependymoma, each with a similar incidence, are the most common intramedullary tumors. Approximately 90% of all intradural spinal cord tumors in humans are benign and potentially resectable. Therefore, in contrast to animals, humans may have an excellent prognosis following surgical therapy.

In humans the majority of extradural spinal cord tumors are metastases. Approximately 5% of cancer patients develop spinal epidural tumors, although not all of these become clinically evident. Primary CNS tumors such as neurofibromas or meningiomas occasionally may be limited to the extradural space. The prognosis for humans with extradural spinal neoplasms depends on the histologic type, rate of onset, and severity of symptoms. A correlation between pretreatment motor status and functional outcome emphasizes the value of early diagnosis and treatment of such neoplasms. In humans, palliation is the goal in the management of patients with spinal metastasis. Radiation therapy and surgical decompression individually or in combination may be used for this purpose.[119]

## TUMORS OF PERIPHERAL NERVES

### Incidence and Risk Factors

The primary neoplasms of the peripheral nerves occur relatively infrequently in domestic animals, although they have been reported in dogs, cats, cattle, goats, sheep, and pigs.[120,121] The primary tumors of the cranial and spinal nerves and nerve roots are common in dogs.[122] Peripheral nerve sheath tumors represented 26.6% of canine nervous system tumors in one report.[1] Neurofibromatosis has been reported in dogs.[121] Of 60 peripheral nerve sheath tumors of dogs of 23 breeds reported in one study, 4 involved cranial, 39 involved spinal, and 17 involved the peripheral nerves.[8] The age distribution was from 2 to 17 years, with 43 tumors occurring between 5 and 12 years of age.[8] Forty-two dogs were male and 18 were female.[8] In the same study, 4 dogs with intraparenchymal schwannomas (one of the brain, three of the spinal cord) were reported.[8] In a review of 42 brachial plexus tumors of dogs described in the literature, 20 (48%) dogs had evidence of spinal cord invasion, and in 4 of these dogs, the tumor appeared to arise primarily in the dorsal root, within the vertebral canal.[123] The remaining 16 dogs in this review appeared to have brachial plexus tumors that originated peripheral to the vertebral canal and that only invaded the spinal cord as a terminal event.[123]

Primary nerve sheath tumors appear to be extremely rare in cats.[123] A solitary nerve sheath tumor has been described in the skin of a cat and in a thoracic vertebra in another cat.[14,18]

Neuronal and nerve cell tumors arise most frequently from the sympathetic and paraganglionic components of the autonomic nervous system. Those arising from the sympathoblasts of the sympathetic system are neuroblastomas, while the paraganglionic system gives rise to paragangliomas, the best known being pheochromcytoma and chemodectoma.[124] Such tumors occur infrequently in dogs and cats.[18,118,125]

Of secondary tumors that involve the cranial and spinal nerves and nerve roots of dogs or cats, lymphoma is the most common. Lymphoma has been reported frequently in the cranial and peripheral nerves of cats (Fig. 26–14).[14,19,126–129]

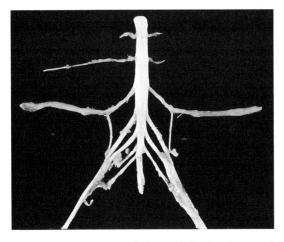

**Figure 26–14.** Dorsal view of the lumbosacral plexus of a 7-year-old spayed domestic shorthair cat with a chronic history of progressive paraparesis. Note thickening of multiple nerve roots and peripheral nerves that has resulted from infiltration by lymphoma.

## Pathology and Natural Behavior

The primary peripheral nerve tumors may affect the cranial nerves, peripheral nerves, sympathetic nerves and ganglia, and adrenal gland nerves. Most tumors of the peripheral nerves, excluding those of the sympathetic nervous system, result from neoplastic transformation (usually benign) of periaxonal Schwann cells. Such tumors are called schwannomas.[130] They have also been called neurilemmomas or neurinomas, because they arise in a nerve or nerve sheath. The terms *neurofibroma* and *neurofibrosarcoma* have been used to describe tumors thought to be derived form endo- or epineurally located fibroblasts within the nerve sheath. Peripheral nerve sheath tumors have also been called perineural fibroblastomas, based on a theory that they arise from perineural fibroblasts.[130] Other less frequently used terms include Schwann cell tumor, lemmoma, and lemnocytoma.[131]

The classification of nerve sheath tumors has been widely disputed.[23,132,133] A controversy concerning nomenclature hinges on whether such tumors arise from Schwann cells, which produce myelin, or the fibroblasts that are responsible for producing the endo-, peri-, and epineurium. The most reliable classification is based on a combination of ultrastructural features and immunocytochemical demonstration of cell-specific marker proteins.[131] On this basis, evidence has not been found for an endo-, peri-, or epineural derivation of nerve sheath tumors; therefore it is recommended that the terms *schwannoma* or *nerve sheath tumor* be used.[134,135]

For each benign form of peripheral nerve sheath tumor, there is a corresponding rare but distinct malignant form in which the cells of origin become anaplastic and on occasion may invade neighboring structures or metastasize.[135] Invasion and metastases are most common with tumors of the sympathetic nervous system.[135] Malignant nerve sheath tumors, which are infrequent, are characterized by mitosis, cellularity, anaplasia, and rarely, metastasis to the lymph nodes or lung.[134]

Nerve sheath tumors of dogs most frequently occur in brachial plexus nerves (C6–T2), although other nerves occasionally are affected.[123] Secondary extension by means of nerve roots into the spinal canal may result in spinal cord compression. These tumors also commonly affect cranial nerves;[3,133] the vestibulocochlear nerve is frequently affected.[136] Occasionally the trigeminal nerve, oculomotor nerve, or other cranial nerves, may be affected. Nerve sheath tumors occur as nodular or varicose thickenings of large nerves, and usually are firm, white to gray in color, and well circumscribed (Fig. 26–15).

Granular cell myoblastoma has been described in the peripheral nerves as a growth of Schwann cells.[23,137] It is not clear whether this tumor is a true neoplasm or a lipid disturbance of Schwann cells. Such tumors have been reported in the tongue of dogs, and may also occur in the CNS as primary tumors.[23]

## History and Clinical Signs

The signs of peripheral nerve sheath neoplasia reflect the location of the neoplasm, which may involve a solitary cranial or peripheral nerve, spinal nerve or nerve root, several cranial or peripheral nerves, a plexus, or multiple spinal nerves or nerve roots. Peripheral nerve sheath neoplasms are slow growing, and the signs usually progress over weeks to months. Occasionally, signs may develop rapidly.[138]

The brachial plexus, or C6 through T2 spinal nerves and nerve roots, are the most common sites for peripheral nerve sheath tumors.[139] This tumor always should be suspected in adult dogs with unilateral thoracic limb lameness of obscure cause.[123] With progression of the neoplasm, paresis of the affected limb and atrophy of muscles innervated

**Figure 26–15.** Surgical exposure of the brachial plexus of a 5-year-old male Airedale terrier with a 3-month history of progressive right thoracic limb lameness and right axillary pain. Note the thickening of the nerve (arrows). The histologic diagnosis was schwannoma.

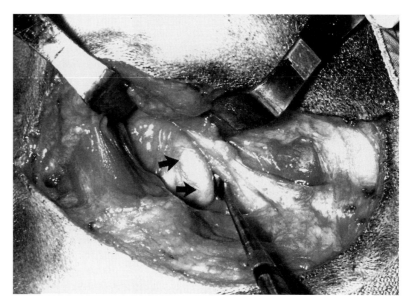

by the involved nerves may develop. An animal may hold an affected limb off the ground. The passive movement of the limb or neck may cause apparent pain to the animal, and a pain response can be elicited by deep palpation cranial to the first rib. Occasionally, a palpable enlargement of a nerve or plexus is apparent. Ipsilateral Horner's syndrome, either partial (miosis only) or complete (miosis, ptosis, enophthalmos, third-eyelid prolapse), may occur, whereby the T1 or T2 nerve roots are involved.[140] Ipsilateral loss of the panniculus reflex also may be detected. The brachial plexus nerve sheath neoplasms frequently extend proximally through an intervertebral foramen to compress the spinal cord.[120,141] The signs of spinal cord involvement usually follow a chronic period of thoracic limb lameness and progressive muscle atrophy, although they may precede, or occur concurrently with, thoracic limb lameness and atrophy. The myelopathy usually results in asymmetric pelvic limb paresis. The contralateral thoracic limb may or may not be affected.

Nerve sheath tumors of the lumbosacral plexus most often cause progressive lameness of a single pelvic limb.[120] The progression of signs is similar to that described for nerve sheath tumor of the brachial plexus; however, apparent pain is less consistently seen in association with lumbosacral plexus nerve sheath neoplasms. Urinary or fecal incontinence may be present in those dogs when the tumor invades the spinal canal. Contralateral limb involvement may also be seen late in the course of the disease.

Involvement by a nerve sheath tumor of a solitary nerve root, spinal nerve, or cranial nerve results in neurologic deficits that reflect the structure involved. Should a nerve sheath tumor of a nerve root or spinal nerve extend proximally to involve the spinal cord, then myelopathy may be the only clinical sign.

Lymphoma affecting the peripheral nervous system may be indistinguishable from nerve sheath tumor, based on clinical signs.

## Diagnostic Techniques and Workup

A neoplasm affecting a peripheral nerve should be suspected when a complete physical and neurologic examination reveals the signs described in the previous section. Single-limb paresis and muscle atrophy in association with pain on manipulation of the affected limb are the most commonly recognized signs of a plexus neoplasm.

Electrophysiologic testing may define the location and extent of peripheral nerve involvement. Electromyography (EMG) may distinguish between atrophy resulting from either disuse or denervation, or may confirm the involvement of muscles not yet atrophied. Determinations of motor and sensory nerve conduction velocity may also provide information regarding nerve involvement. Evoked spinal cord potentials in combination with these determinations may be used to provide functional evidence of sensory nerve fiber connections with the spinal cord.[140,142]

Mapping of atrophied muscles and regions of decreased cutaneous sensation in an affected limb may help to localize a peripheral nerve sheath neoplasm to a specific sensory or motor nerve, to a plexus, or to a group of spinal nerves or nerve roots.[140]

Plain radiographs of the vertebral column, CSF analysis, and myelography are essential in cases in which secondary spinal cord involvement is suspected. The most frequently observed plain radiographic abnormality seen with a nerve sheath neoplasm is the widening of an intervertebral foramen or remodeling around an enlarged nerve root,[120] although plain radiographs frequently are normal.[139] Lymphoma seldom results in alterations visible on plain radiographs. Myelography is essential in cases in which neoplasia of spinal nerves or nerve roots is suspected, in order to detect invasion of the vertebral canal that may not be clinically apparent. At the time a myelogram is done, CSF collection and analysis may be completed; however, CSF analysis rarely aids in a more definitive diagnosis. The most commonly observed CSF alteration is an elevation of protein in the absence of a cellular response.

Surgical exploration for the biopsy of a cranial or peripheral nerve, nerve root, or plexus is essential for diagnosis. The use of CT and MRI to confirm the location and extent of a neoplasm prior to biopsy may be helpful in some cases.[143] In many dogs, surgical exploration may be the only method that permits confirmation of the presence of a neoplasm.

## Therapy

Presently, the treatment of peripheral nerve sheath tumors is limited to surgical excision. Early detection and diagnosis of such tumors allow complete excision in only a few, unusual cases.[123,144] In the majority of animals, complete excision is impossible because of the proximal extension of the tumor into the vertebral canal or spinal cord.[145] Because a nerve sheath tumor generally involves several spinal nerves or nerve roots, the excision of spinal nerves as far proximally as possible, either at the level of the intervertebral foramen or at the level of the spinal cord following laminectomy and durotomy, is most commonly accompanied by amputation of the affected limb.[123] Postoperative irradiation may be attempted but has not yet been adequately investigated.

Chemotherapy for nerve sheath neoplasms may be of palliative benefit. A combination of vincristine, doxorubicin, and cyclophosphamide has been recommended.[23] Lymphoma of the peripheral nerves is treated in the same way as lymphoma is treated in other locations.

## Prognosis

Survival following surgical excision of schwannomas has been reported to range from 2 months to 2 years.[120] In one report,[146] a dog survived more than 3 years following excision of a solitary schwannoma of the sixth cervical spinal nerve; however, in most cases recurrence is common.[120] Postsurgical metastases to the lung have been reported.[123] The high rate of local recurrence following surgical excision of a peripheral nerve sheath neoplasm may reflect the proximal extension of a tumor within a nerve trunk. Grossly visible margins of a tumor at the time of operative resection may not accurately demarcate the extent of tumor invasion.

## Comparative Aspects

The types of nerve sheath tumors of dogs are very similar to those of humans. The controversy concerning classification of peripheral nerve sheath tumors in humans is similar to that discussed in dogs.[147] The goals of treatment for a benign peripheral nerve sheath neoplasm in humans are tumor resection and the preservation of nerve function. Most benign schwannomas in humans may be totally removed without nerve damage, and recurrences are quite rare.[147] Malignant nerve sheath neoplasms in humans have a high tendency to recur after local excision. A recurrence rate of over 40% following local excision has been reported. Radical excision, often in combination with amputation, is therefore recommended for the treatment of malignant nerve sheath tumors. Although the benefit of postoperative irradiation has not been proven, it has been recommended in humans.[147]

Multiple cutaneous and peripheral neurofibromas are the hallmark of von Recklinghausen's neurofibromatosis.[147] The peripheral nerve tumors associated with this disease may be benign or malignant in behavior, although a tendency exists toward malignant transformation. The similarity between this disease and neurofibromatosis in cattle and dogs has been noted; however, the disease as it occurs in humans has not been confirmed in dogs at this time.[122]

## NEUROLOGIC COMPLICATIONS OF SYSTEMIC CANCER

The incidence of neurologic complications of systemic cancer in dogs and cats is unknown; however, direct and indirect effects on the nervous system of cancer originating outside the nervous system are known to occur.[148–154]

More than 20% of humans with systemic cancer develop neurologic symptoms either as direct or indirect effects of their underlying disease.[155,156] These are summarized in Table 26–1. Metastasis to the brain is the most common complication of systemic cancer. Autopsy studies confirm that 25% of patients who die from cancer have intracranial metastases at the time of death. Metastasis to the spinal cord and nerve roots is the second most common neurologic complication of systemic cancer; it occurs in 5 to 10% of human cancer patients.[155]

Nonmetastatic nervous system complications of systemic cancer in humans occur less commonly than metastatic disease. Frequently, nonmetastatic complications develop acutely. They are often fully reversible, but they may be fatal if they are not recognized and treated.[155] Metabolic encephalopathy is a common nonmetastatic complication. It is a behavioral change that results from the failure of cerebral metabolism because of a systemic illness such as electrolyte imbalance, hepatic or renal failure, hypoxia, or sepsis.

Cancer patients may be susceptible to CNS infections because of altered immune mechanisms or neutropenia. Neutropenia is common in patients with hematogenous malignancies, in those with bone marrow depletion caused by a metastatic tumor, and in those receiving chemotherapy.

A high incidence of thrombocytopenia or coagulation deficits results in the increased risk of cerebrovascular complications. Embolic infarction may occur secondary to endocarditis or sepsis.

Neurologic complications may also result from cancer treatment.[155] Although permanent damage to the nervous system from irradiation is rare, it is known to occur. Several chemotherapeutic agents (e.g., methotrexate, cisplatin, vinca alkaloids, fluorouracil) may produce neurotoxicity in the central or peripheral nervous system, either directly or indirectly by toxicity to other organs such as the liver or kidney.[157]

Paraneoplastic syndromes or "remote effects" are nervous system abnormalities that occur in patients with malignant systemic tumors but that are not caused by metastatic invasion of the nervous system or by any identifiable effect of cancer on the nervous sytem, such as infection or chemotherapy.[154,156,158,159] In about 50% of cases, nervous system symptoms precede the diagnosis of cancer. The cause and pathogenesis of paraneoplastic syndromes are not known, although possible mechanisms include autoimmune reactions, viral infections, toxins secreted by a tumor, and nutritional deprivation. Commonly recognized paraneoplastic effects are sensorimotor polyneuropathy, myasthenia gravis (associated with thymoma), and polymyositis.[153]

## REFERENCES

1. LeCouteur RA: Tumors of the nervous system. *In* Withrow SJ, MacEwen EG (eds): Clinical Veterinary Oncology. Philadelphia, JB Lippincott, 1989, p. 325.
2. Bagley RS, Kornegay JN, Page RL, et al: Central nervous system. *In* Slatter DD (ed): Textbook of Small Animal Surgery, 2nd ed. Philadelphia, WB Saunders, 1993, p. 2137.
3. Braund KG: Clinical Syndromes in Veterinary Neurology, 2nd ed. St. Louis, MO, Mosby, 1994, p. 198.
4. Vandevelde M: Brain tumors in domestic animals: An overview. Proceedings of the Conference on Brain Tumors in Man and Animals, Research Triangle Park, NC, September 5–6, 1984.
5. Keller ET, Madewell BR: Locations and types of neoplasms in immature dogs: 69 cases (1964–1989). J Am Vet Med Assoc *200*:1530, 1992.
6. Kornegay JN: Central nervous system neoplasia. *In* Kornegay JN (ed): Neurologic Disorders: Con-

---

**Table 26–1** Neurologic Complications of Systemic Cancer

---

*Metastasis to the Nervous System*
  Intracranial neoplasia
  Spinal neoplasia
  Leptomeningeal neoplasia
  Cranial/peripheral nerve neoplasia

*Nonmetastatic Neurologic Complications*
  Metabolic encephalopathy
  Central nervous system infections
  Cerebrovascular disorders
  Adverse effects of treatment
  Paraneoplastic effects

---

temporary Issues in Small Animal Practice, Vol. 5. New York, Churchill-Livingstone, 1986, p. 78.

7. Patnaik AK, Kay WJ, Hurvitz AI: Intracranial meningioma: A comparative pathologic study of 28 dogs. Vet Pathol 23:369, 1986.

8. McGrath JT: Morphology and classification of brain tumors in domestic animals. Proceedings of the Conference on Brain Tumors in Man and Animals, Research Triangle Park, NC, September 5–6, 1984.

9. LeCouteur RA, Fike JR, Cann CE, et al: Computed tomography of brain tumors in the caudal fossa of the dog. Vet Radiol 22:244, 1981.

10. Schulman FY, Ribas JL, Carpenter JL, et al: Intracranial meningioma with pulmonary metastasis in three dogs. Vet Pathol 29:196, 1992.

11. Fenner WR: Metastatic neoplasms of the central nervous system. Sem Vet Med Surg 5:253, 1990.

12. Straw RC, LeCouteur RA, Powers BE, et al: Multilobular osteochondrosarcoma of the canine skull: 16 cases (1978–1988). J Am Vet Med Assoc 195:1764, 1989.

13. Heidner GL, Kornegay JN, Page RL, et al: Analysis of survival in a retrospective study of 86 dogs with brain tumors. J Vet Intern Med 5:219, 1991.

14. Zaki FA, Hurvitz AI: Spontaneous neoplasms of the central nervous system of the cat. J Small Anim Pract 17:773, 1976.

15. Nafe LA: Meningiomas in cats: A retrospective clinical study of 36 cases. J Am Vet Med Assoc 174:1224, 1979.

16. Engle GC, Brodey RS: A retrospective study of 395 feline neoplasms. J Am Anim Hosp Assoc 5:21, 1969.

17. Luginbuhl H: Studies on meningiomas in cats. Am J Vet Res 22:1030, 1961.

18. Averill DR: Tumors of the nervous system. In Holzworth J (ed): Diseases of the Cat. Philadelphia, WB Saunders, 1987, p. 554.

19. Kornegay JN: Feline neurology. Prob Vet Med 3:391, 1991.

20. McGrath JT: Meningiomas in animals. J Neuropathol Exp Neurol 21:327, 1962.

21. Haskins ME, McGrath JT: Meningiomas in young cats with mucopolysaccharidosis. J Neuropathol Exp Neurol 42:664, 1983.

22. LeCouteur RA: Brain tumors of dogs and cats. Vet Med Rep 2:332, 1990.

23. Holliday TA, Higgins RJ, Turrel JM: Tumors of the nervous system. In Theilen GH, Madewell BR (eds): Veterinary Cancer Medicine, 2nd ed. Philadelphia, Lea & Febiger, 1987, p. 601.

24. Johnson GC: Genesis and pathology of tumors of the nervous system. Sem Vet Med Surg 5:210, 1990.

25. Escourolle R, Poirier J: Manual of Basic Neuropathology, 2nd ed. Philadelphia, WB Saunders, 1978, p. 21.

26. Braund KG: Neoplasia of the nervous system. Compend Contin Educ Pract Vet 6:717, 1984.

27. Vandevelde M: Morphological and histological characteristics of GME and reticulosis: One disease or two? The Bern perspective. Proc 4th ACVIM Forum, Washington, DC, 1986, p. 11/81.

28. Fankhauser R, Fatzer R, Luginbuhl H, et al: Reticulosis of the central nervous system in dogs. Adv Vet Sci Comp Sci 16:35, 1972.

29. Vandevelde M, Fatzer R, Fankhauser R: Immunohistological studies on primary reticulosis of the canine brain. Vet Pathol 18:577, 1981.

30. Niebauer GW, Dayrell-Hart BL, Speciale J: Evaluation of craniotomy in dogs and cats. J Am Vet Med Assoc 198:89, 1991.

31. Kornegay JN, Oliver JE, Gorgacz EJ: Clinicopathologic features of brain herniation in animals. J Am Vet Med Assoc 182:1111, 1983.

32. Kornegay JN: Pathogenesis of diseases of the central nervous system. In Slatter D (ed): Textbook of Small Animal Surgery, 2nd ed. Philadelphia, WB Saunders, 1993, p. 1022.

33. Davidson MG, Nasisse MP, Breitschwerdt EB, et al: Acute blindness associated with intracranial tumors in dogs and cats: Eight cases (1984–1989). J Am Vet Med Assoc 199:755, 1991.

34. Foster ES, Carrillo JM, Patnaik AK: Clinical signs of tumors affecting the rostral cerebrum in 43 dogs. J Vet Intern Med 2:71, 1988.

35. Moore MP, Gavin PR, Kraft SL, et al: MR, CT and clinical features from four dogs with nasal tumors involving the rostral cerebrum. Vet Radiol 32:19, 1991.

36. LeCouteur RA, Child G: Clinical management of epilepsy of dogs and cats. In Indrieri RJ (ed): Epilepsy, Problems in Veterinary Medicine, Vol. 1. Philadelphia, JB Lippincott, 1989, p. 578.

37. Lawson DC, Burk RL, Prata RG: Cerebral meningioma in the cat: Diagnosis and surgical treatment of ten cases. J Am Anim Hosp Assoc 20:333, 1984.

38. Nafe LA: The clinical presentation and diagnosis of intracranial neoplasia. Sem Vet Med Surg 5:223, 1990.

39. Bailey CS, Higgins RJ: Characteristics of cisternal cerebrospinal fluid associated with primary brain tumors in the dog: A retrospective study. J Am Vet Med Assoc 188:414, 1986.

40. Vandevelde M, Fankhauser RR: Liquoruntersuchungen bei neurologisch kranken Hunden und Katzen. Schweiz Arch Tierheilk 129:443, 1987.

41. Grevel V, Machus B: Diagnosing brain tumors with a CSF sedimentation technique. Vet Med Rep 2:403, 1990.

42. Moore MP, Gavin PR, Bagley RS, et al: Cerebrospinal fluid analysis in dogs with intracranial tumors. Proc 12th ACVIM Forum, San Francisco, CA, 1994, p. 917.

43. Thomson CE, Kornegay JN, Stevens JB: Analysis of cerebrospinal fluid from the cerebellomedullary and lumbar cisterns of dogs with

focal neurologic disease: 145 cases (1985–1987). J Am Vet Med Assoc 196:1841, 1990.

44. Sorjonen DC, Golden DL, Levesque DC, et al: Cerebrospinal fluid protein electrophoresis. A clinical evaluation of a previously reported diagnostic technique. Prog Vet Neurol 2:261, 1991.

45. Tipold A, Pfister H, Vandevelde M: Determination of the IgG index for the detection of intrathecal immunoglobulin synthesis in dogs using an ELISA. Res Vet Sci 54:40, 1993.

46. Rand JS, Parent J, Percy D, et al: Clinical, cerebrospinal fluid, and histological data from thirty-four cats with primary noninflammatory disease of the central nervous system. Can Vet J 35:174, 1994.

47. Voorhout G: Cisternography combined with linear tomography for visualization of the pituitary gland in healthy dogs. A comparison with computed tomography. Vet Radiol 31:68, 1990.

48. Voorhout G, Rijnberk A: Cisternography combined with linear tomography for visualization of pituitary lesions in dogs with pituitary-dependent hyperadrenocorticism. Vet Radiol 31:74, 1990.

49. Daniel BD, Twardock AR, Yucker RL, et al: Brain scintigraphy. Prog Vet Neurol 3:25, 1992.

50. Dykes NL, Warnick LD, Summers BA, et al: Retrospective analysis of brain scintigraphy in 116 dogs and cats. Vet Radiol Ultrasound 35:59, 1994.

51. LeCouteur RA, Turrel JM: Brain tumors in dogs and cats. In Current Veterinary Therapy IX: Small Animal Practice. Philadelphia, WB Saunders Co, 1986, p. 820

52. Fike JR, LeCouteur RA, Cann CE, et al: Computerized tomography of brain tumors of the rostral and middle fossas in the dog. Am J Vet Res 42:275, 1981.

53. Plummer SB, Wheeler SJ, Thrall DE, et al: Computed tomography of primary inflammatory brain disorders in dogs and cats. Vet Radiol Ultrasound 33307, 1992.

54. Turrel JM, Fike JR, LeCouteur RA, et al: Computed tomography characteristics of primary brain tumors in 50 dogs. J Am Vet Med Assoc 188:851, 1986.

55. LeCouteur RA, Fike JR, Cann CE, et al: X-ray computed tomography of brain tumors in cats. J Am Vet Med Assoc 183:301, 1983.

56. Jeffery ND, Thakkar CH, Yarrow TG: Introduction to computed tomography of the canine brain. J Small Anim Pract 33:2, 1992.

57. Kornegay JN: Imaging brain neoplasms. Computed tomography and magnetic resonance imaging. Vet Med Rep 2:372, 1990.

58. Bailey MQ: Diagnostic imaging of intracranial lesions. Sem Vet Med Surg 5:232, 1990.

59. LeCouteur RA, Cann CE, Fike JR: Computed tomography. In Gourley IG, Vasseur PB (eds): Textbook of Small Animal Soft Tissue Surgery. Philadelphia, JB Lippincott, 1985, p. 989.

60. Thomson CE, Kornegay JN, Burn RA, et al: Magnetic resonance imaging—A general overview of principles and examples in veterinary neurodiagnosis. Vet Radiol Ultrasound 34:2, 1993.

61. Thomas WB, Sorjonen DC, Hudson JA, et al: Ultrasound-guided brain biopsy in dogs. Am J Vet Res 54:1942, 1993.

62. Harari J, Moore MM, Leathers CW, et al: Computed tomographic-guided, free-hand needle biopsy of brain tumors in dogs. Prog Vet Neurol 4:41, 1993.

63. Speciale J, Koffman BM, Bashirelahi N, et al: Identification of gonadal steroid receptors in meningiomas from dogs and cats. Am J Vet Res 51:833, 1990.

64. Jeffery N, Brearley MJ: Brain tumours in the dog: Treatment of 10 cases and review of recent literature. J Small Anim Pract 34:367, 1993.

65. Feder BM, Fry TR, Kostolich M, et al: Nd:YAG laser cytoreduction of an invasive intracranial meningioma in a dog. Prog Vet Neurol 4:3, 1993.

66. Shores A: Intracranial surgery. In Slatter D (ed): Textbook of Small Animal Surgery, 2nd ed. Philadelphia, WB Saunders, 1993, p. 1122.

67. Gallagher JG, Berg J, Knowles KE, et al: Prognosis after surgical excision of cerebral meningiomas in cats: 17 cases (1986–1992). J Am Vet Med Assoc 203:1437, 1993.

68. Gordon LE, Thacher C, Matthiesen DT, et al: Results of craniotomy for the treatment of cerebral meningioma in 42 cats. Vet Surg 23:94, 1994.

69. Turrel JM, Fike JR, LeCouteur RA, et al: Radiotherapy of brain tumors in dogs. J Am Vet Med Assoc 184:82, 1981.

70. Turrel JM, Higgins RJ, Child G: Prognostic factors associated with irradiation of canine brain tumors. Vet Cancer Soc 6th Annu Conf. West Lafayette, IN, 1986.

71. LeCouteur RA, Sisson AF, Dow SW, et al: Combined surgical debulking and irradiation for the treatment of a large frontal meningioma in 8 dogs. Vet Cancer Soc 7th Annu Conf. Madison, WI, 1987.

72. Dow SW, LeCouteur RA, Gillette EL, et al: Response of dogs with functional pituitary macroadenomas and macrocarcinomas to radiation therapy: Results of a prospective study. J Small Anim Pract 31:287, 1990.

73. Sisson AF, LeCouteur RA, Dow SW, et al: Radiation therapy of granulomatous meningoencephalomyelitis of dogs. Proc 7th ACVIM Forum, San Diego, CA, 1989, p. 1031.

74. LeCouteur RA, Gillette EL, Dow SW, et al: Radiation response of autochthonous canine brain tumors. Int J Radiat Biol Oncol Biol Phys 13:166, 1987.

75. Evans SM, Dayrell-Hart B, Powlis W, et al: Radiation therapy of canine brain masses. J Vet Intern Med 7:216, 1993.

76. Moore MP, Gavin PR, Weidner JP, et al: Boron

neutron capture therapy for brain tumors. Proc 11th ACVIM Forum, Washington, DC, 1993, p. 725.

77. Iwamoto KS, Norman A, Freshwater DB, et al: Diagnosis and treatment of spontaneous canine brain tumors with a CT scanner. Radiother Oncol 26:76, 1993.

78. Cook JR: Chemotherapy for brain tumors. Vet Med Rep 2:391, 1990.

79. Neuwelt EA: Blood-brain barrier manipulation: Current status of laboratory and clinical studies. Proc 12th ACVIM Forum, San Francisco, CA, 1994, p. 908.

80. Couto CG, Cullen J, Pedroia V, et al: Central nervous system lymphosarcoma in the dog. J Am Vet Med Assoc 184:809, 1984.

81. Scott-Moncrieff JCM: Plasma and cerebrospinal fluid pharmacokinetics of intravenous ARA-C (cytosine arabinoside) in the dog (thesis). West Lafayette, IN, Purdue University, 1989.

82. Dimski DS, Cook JR: Carmustine-induced partial remission of an astrocytoma in a dog. J Am Anim Hosp Assoc 26:179, 1990.

83. Fulton LM, Steinberg HS: Preliminary study of lomustine in the treatment of intracranial masses in dogs following localization by imaging techniques. Semin Vet Med Surg 5:241, 1990.

84. Ingram M, Jacques DB, Freshwater DB, et al: Adoptive immunotherapy of brain tumors in dogs. Vet Med Rep 2:398, 1990.

85. Kostolich M, Duliisch ML: A surgical approach to the canine olfactory bulb for meningioma removal. Vet Surg 16:273, 1987.

86. Gavin PR, Kraft SL, DeHaan CE, et al: Magnetic resonance and computed tomographic features of canine brain tumors following boron neutron capture therapy. 32nd Annu Mtg Am Soc Ther Rad Oncol, Miami, FL, 1990 (Abstract).

87. Shell L, Colter SB, Blass CE, et al: Surgical removal of a meningioma in a cat after detection by computerized axial tomography. J Am Anim Hosp Assoc 21:439, 1985.

88. Black P McL: Brain tumors (first of two parts). New Engl J Med 324:1471, 1991.

89. Levin VA, Gutin PH, Leibel S: Neoplasms of the central nervous system. In DeVita VT, Hellman S, Rosenberg SA (eds): Cancer: Principles and Practice of Oncology, 4th ed. Philadelphia, JB Lippincott, 1993, p. 1679.

90. Fingeroth JM, Prata RG, Patnaik AK: Spinal meningiomas in dogs: 13 cases (1972–1987). J Am Vet Med Assoc 191:720, 1987.

91. Luttgen PJ, Braund KG, Brauner WR, et al: A retrospective study of twenty-nine spinal tumors in the dog and cat. J Small Anim Pract 21:213, 1980.

92. Summers BA, deLahunta A: Unusual intradural extramedullary spinal cord tumors in twelve dogs. J Neuropathol Exp Neurol 45:322, 1986.

93. Summers BA, deLahunta A, McEntee M, et al: A novel intradural extramedullary spinal cord

tumor in young dogs. Acta Neuropathol 75:402, 1988.

94. Tamke PG, Foley GL: Neuroepithelioma in a dog. Can Vet J 28:606, 1987.

95. Blass CE, Kirby BM, Kreege JM, et al: Teratomatous medulloepithelioma in the spinal cord of a dog. J Am Anim Hosp Assoc 24:51, 1988.

96. Moissonnier P, Abbott DP: Canine neuroepithelioma: Case report and literature review. J Am Anim Hosp Assoc 29:397, 1993.

97. Ferretti A, Scanziani E, Colombo S: Surgical treatment of a spinal cord tumor resembling nephroblastoma in a young dog. Prog Vet Neurol 4:84, 1993.

98. Ribas JL: Thoracolumbar spinal cord blastoma: A unique tumor of young dogs. Proc 8th ACVIM Forum, Washington, DC, 1990, p. 1129.

99. Waters DJ, Hayden DW: Intramedullary spinal cord metastasis in the dog. J Vet Intern Med 4:207, 1990.

100. Lane SB, Kornegay JN, Duncan JR, et al: Feline spinal lymphosarcoma: A retrospective evaluation of 23 cats. J Vet Intern Med 8:99, 1994.

101. Meincke JE, Hobbie WV, Hardy WD: Lymphoreticular malignancies in the cat: Clinical findings. J Am Vet Med Assoc 160:1093, 1972.

102. Kornegay JN: Feline neurology. Compend Contin Ed Pract Vet 3:203, 1981.

103. Spodnick GJ, Berg J, Moore FM, et al: Spinal lymphoma in cats: 21 cases (1976–1989). J Am Vet Med Assoc 200:373, 1992.

104. Barr MC, Butt MT, Anderson KL, et al: Spinal lymphosarcoma and disseminated mastocytoma associated with feline immunodeficiency virus infection in a cat. J Am Vet Med Assoc 202:1978, 1993.

105. Wright JA, Bell DA, Clayton-Jones DG: The clinical and radiological features associated with spinal tumors in thirty dogs. J Small Anim Pract 20:461, 1979.

106. Morgan JP, Ackerman N, Bailey CS, et al: Vertebral tumors in the dog: A clinical, radiologic, and pathologic study of 61 primary and secondary lesions. Vet Radiol 21:197, 1980.

107. Lewis DD, Kim DY, Paulsen DB, et al: Extradural spinal liposarcoma in a dog. J Am Vet Med Assoc 199:1606, 1991.

108. Turner JL, Luttgen PJ, VanGundy TE, et al: Multicentric osseous lymphoma with spinal extradural involvement in a dog. J Am Vet Med Assoc 200:196, 1992.

109. Macpherson GC, Chadwick BJ, Robbins PD: Intramedullary spinal cord metastasis of a primary lung tumour in a dog. J Small Anim Pract 34:242, 1993.

110. Neer TM, Kreeger JM: Cervical spinal cord asrocytoma in a dog. J Am Vet Med Assoc 191:84, 1987.

111. Luttgen PJ: Neoplasms of the spine. Vet Clin North Am 22:973, 1992.

112. Gilmore DR: Neoplasia of the cervical spinal cord and vertebrae in the dog. J Am Anim Hosp Assoc 19:1009, 1983.

113. Schueler RO, Roush JK, Oyster RA: Spinal ganglioneuroma in a dog. J Am Vet Med Assoc 203:539, 1993.

114. Jeffery ND: Treatment of epidural haemangiosarcoma in a dog. J Small Anim Pract 32:359, 1991.

115. Bentley JF, Simpson ST, Hathcock JT, et al: Metastatic thyroid follicular carcinoma in the cervical portion of the spine of a dog. J Am Vet Med Assoc 197:1498, 1990.

116. Bell FW, Feeney DA, O'Brien TJ, et al: External beam radiation therapy for recurrent intraspinal meningioma in a dog. J Am Anim Hosp Assoc 28:318, 1992.

117. Irving G, McMillan MC: Fluoroscopically guided percutaneous fine-needle aspiration biopsy of thoracolumbar spinal lesions in cats. Prog Vet Neurol 1:473, 1990.

118. Poncelet L, Snaps F, Jacobovitz D, et al: Successful removal of an intramedullary spinal paraganglioma from a dog. J Am Anim Hosp Assoc 30:213, 1994.

119. Wara WM, Sheline GE: Radiation therapy of tumors of the spinal cord. In Youmans JR (ed): Neurological Surgery, 2nd ed. Vol. 5. Philadelphia, WB Saunders, 1982, p. 3222.

120. Bradley RL, Withrow SJ, Snyder SP: Nerve sheath tumors in the dog. J Am Anim Hosp Assoc 18:915, 1982.

121. Innes JRH, Saunders LZ: Neoplastic diseases. In Innes JRH, Saunders LZ (eds): Comparative Neuropathology. New York, Academic Press, 1962, p. 721.

122. Goedegebuure SA: A case of neurofibromatosis in the dog. J Small Anim Pract 16:329, 1975.

123. Sharp NJH: Neurological deficits in one limb. In Wheeler SK (ed): Manual of Small Animal Neurology. Cheltenham, British Small Animal Veterinary Association, 1989, p. 183.

124. Lewis JC, Reardon MJ, Montgomery A Jr: Paraganglioma involving the spinal cord of a dog. J Am Vet Med Assoc 168:864, 1976.

125. Speciale J, Hendrick MJ, Steinberg SA: Paraganglioma cell tumors of nonbranchiomeric origin in three dogs. J Am Anim Hosp Assoc 29:49, 1993.

126. Allen JG, Amis T: Lymphosarcoma involving cranial nerves in a cat. Aust Vet J 51:155, 1975.

127. Luginbuhl H, Fankhauser R, McGrath JT: Spontaneous neoplasms of the nervous system in animals. Prog Neurol Surg 2:85, 1968.

128. Schaer M, Zaki FA, Harvey HJ, et al: Laryngeal hemiplegia due to neoplasia of the vagus nerve in a cat. J Am Vet Med Assoc 174:513, 1979.

129. Hobbs SL, Cobb MA: A cranial neuropathy associated with lymphosarcoma in a dog. Vet Rec 127:525, 1990.

130. Russel DS, Rubinstein LJ: Pathology of Tumors of the Nervous System, 4th ed. Baltimore, Williams & Wilkins, 1977, p. 372.

131. Dahme E, Bilzer T, Stavrou D: Classification of canine PNS-tumors based on EM- and PAP-techniques. Proc Joint Mtg, World Assoc of Vet Pathologists, Utrecht, the Netherlands, 1984.

132. Lusk MD, Kline DG, Garcia CA: Tumors of the brachial plexus. Neurosurgery 21:439, 1987.

133. Zachary JF, O'Brien DP, Ingles BW, et al: Multicentric nerve sheath fibrosarcomas of multiple cranial nerve roots in two dogs. J Am Vet Med Assoc 188:723, 1986.

134. Cordy DR: Tumors of the nervous system and eye. In Moulton JE (ed): Tumors of Domestic Animals, 2nd ed. Berkeley, University of California Press, 1978, p. 430.

135. Cravioto H: Neoplasms of peripheral nerves. In Wilkins RH, Rengachary SS (eds): Neurosurgery. New York, McGraw-Hill, 1985, p. 1894.

136. deLahunta A: Veterinary Neuroanatomy and Clinical Neurology, 2nd ed. Philadelphia, WB Saunders Co, 1983, p. 249.

137. Budzilovich GN: Granular cell "myoblastoma" of vagus nerve. Acta Neuropathol 10:162, 1968.

138. Targett MP, Dyce J, Houlton JEF: Tumors involving the nerve sheaths of the forelimb in dogs. J Small Anim Pract 34:221, 1993.

139. Carmichael S, Griffiths IR: Tumors involving the brachial plexus in seven dogs. Vet Rec 108:435, 1981.

140. Bailey CS: Patterns of cutaneous anesthesia associated with brachial plexus avulsions in the dog. J Am Vet Med Assoc 185:889, 1984.

141. Boring JG, Swaim SF: Malignant schwannoma (neurilemmoma): An extramedullary intradural tumor causing cervical cord compression in a dog. J Am Anim Hosp Assoc 9:342, 1973.

142. Holliday TA: Electrodiagnostic examination: Somatosensory evoked potentials and electromyography. Vet Clin North Am 22:833, 1992.

143. McCarthy RJ, Feeney DA, Lipowitz AJ: Preoperative diagnosis of tumors of the brachial plexus by use of computed tomography in three dogs. J Am Vet Med Assoc 202:291, 1993.

144. Troy GC, Hurov LI, King GK: Successful surgical removal of a cervical subdural neurofibrosarcoma. J Am Anim Hosp Assoc 15:477. 1979.

145. Bradney IW, Forsyth WM: A schwannoma causing cervical spinal cord compression in a dog. Aust Vet J 63:374, 1986.

146. Bailey CS: Long-term survival after surgical excision of a schwannoma of the sixth cervical spinal nerve in a dog. J Am Vet Med Assoc 196:754, 1990.

147. Youmans JR, Ishida WY: Tumors of peripheral and sympathetic nerves. In Youmans JR (ed): Neurological Surgery. Philadelphia, WB Saunders, 1982, p. 3299.

148. Braund KG, McGuire JA, Amling KA, et al: Peripheral neuropathy associated with malignant neoplasms in dogs. Vet Pathol 24:16, 1987.

149. Braund KG, Steiss JE, Amling KA, et al: Insulinoma and subclinical peripheral neuropathy in two dogs. J Vet Intern Med 1:86, 1987.

150. Griffiths IR, Duncan ID, Swallow JS: Peripheral polyneuropathies in dogs: A study of five cases. J Small Anim Pract 18:101, 1977.

151. Presthus J, Teige J Jr: Peripheral neuropathy associated with lymphosarcoma in a dog. J Small Anim Pract 27:463, 1986.

152. Sorjonen DC, Braund KG, Hoff EJ: Paraplegia and subclinical neuromyopathy associated with a primary lung tumor in a dog. J Am Vet Med Assoc 180:1209, 1982.

153. Braund KG: Remote effects of cancer on the nervous system. Sem Vet Med Surg 5:262, 1990.

154. Duran ME, Ezquerra J, Roncero V, et al: Acute necrotizing myelopathy associated with a hepatocarcinoma. Prog Vet Neurol 3:35, 1992.

155. Patchell RA, Posner JB: Neurologic complications of systemic cancer. Neurol Clin 3:729, 1985.

156. Silverstein SR, Marx JA: Neurologic emergencies in patients with cancer. Top Emerg Med 8:1, 1986.

157. Kaplan RS, Wernik PH: Neurotoxicity of antitumor agents. In Perry MC, Yarbro J (eds): Toxicity of Chemotherapy. New York, Grune & Stratton, 1984.

158. Posner JB: Neurological complications of systemic cancer. Med Clin North Am 63:783, 1979.

159. Kornblith PL, Walker MD, Cassady JR: Neurologic Oncology. Philadelphia, JB Lippincott, 1987, p. 38.

# 27

# Ocular Tumors

Paul E. Miller and Richard R. Dubielzig

Tumors of the eye, orbit, or adnexa can have devastating consequences for vision and the comfort of the animal and may be harbingers of potentially life-threatening diseases. By virtue of their location, even benign ocular tumors may cause blindness and loss of the eye. Although these tumors affected only 0.87% of all dogs and 0.34% of all cats recorded in the Veterinary Medical Data Base in the last 10 years, their actual frequency is undoubtedly greater because many presumably benign ocular tumors are not histologically examined. This chapter describes the more common ocular tumors in small animals.

## TUMORS OF THE EYELIDS, THIRD EYELID, AND OCULAR SURFACE

### Incidence and Risk Factors

Ocular papillomas tend to occur in young dogs and are believed to have a papovavirus etiology. Histiocytomas affect the eyelid skin of young to middle-aged dogs.[1,2] Benign adenomas and melanomas typically occur in older dogs, whereas sebaceous adenocarcinomas and malignant melanomas tend to affect very old dogs.[1,2] One study cites boxers, collies, weimaraners, cocker spaniels, and springer spaniels at greater risk of eyelid neoplasia than the general hospital population;[1] and another suggests that beagles, Siberian huskies, and English setters have greater risk than mixed-breed dogs.[2]

Squamous cell carcinoma (SCC) comprises up to two thirds of feline eyelid and third-eyelid tumors[3] and has a predilection for the lower eyelid and medial canthus of white cats (Fig. 27–1). Ocu-

lar SCC is less frequent in dogs,[1,4] but in both species increased exposure to solar radiation and lack of adnexal pigmentation are believed to be predisposing factors. Canine conjunctival melanomas may have an older age (mean = 11 years), female, weimaraner, and possibly German shepherd/large-breed dog predisposition.[5] Melanomas also have a propensity for the nictitating membrane and superior palpebral conjunctiva.[5] Corneal tumors have a predilection for the limbus.

### Pathology and Natural Behavior

A substantial majority (75–90%) of canine eyelid tumors are histologically benign, and sebaceous

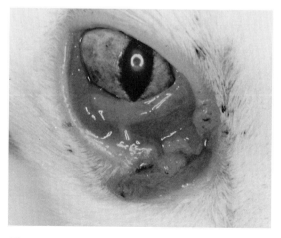

**Figure 27–1.** Squamous cell carcinoma has a predilection for the medial canthus of elderly white cats. (Photograph courtesy of Dr. Christopher J. Murphy.)

gland adenomas and adenocarcinomas, papillomas, and melanomas comprise more than 80% of canine eyelid neoplasms.[1,2] Even histologically malignant eyelid tumors in dogs rarely metastasize, although they are more likely to be locally invasive and recur following surgery.[1,2] In contrast, most feline eyelid and ocular surface tumors are malignant.

Papillomas tend to be well demarcated and superficial and minimally alter the dermis or deeper tissues. Surgical manipulation has occasionally been associated with dispersal of papillomas throughout the ocular surface.[6,7] Papillomas, like histiocytomas, often spontaneously resolve in young dogs, although they may persist in the older dog. SCC may also develop superficially but, following transformation, the preinvasive actinic plaque becomes capable of local tissue invasion. Late in the course of the disease, SCC may spread to regional lymph nodes and, uncommonly, distantly metastasize. SCC of the third eyelid may more readily invade the orbit than corneal or eyelid SCC.

Adenocarcinomas of the gland of the third eyelid are generally well differentiated with infrequent mitotic figures and infiltrative growth.[8] They may mimic prolapse of the gland of the nictitans ("cherry eye") by appearing as localized, firm, smooth, pink swellings on the posterior surface of the nictitans, but a key differentiating feature is their occurrence in much older dogs (10–16 years). Although excision of the grossly visible tumor may initially appear adequate, recurrence is common if the entire gland is not removed.[8] Local lymph node and orbital involvement was reported in 1 of 7 dogs.[8]

The natural behavior of conjunctival vascular, melanocytic, and mast cell tumors is very poorly understood, in part because they are uncommon. Conjunctival hemangiomas and hemangiosarcomas tend to remain relatively superficial but recur following incomplete excision.[9] Hemangiosarcomas may exhibit a more aggressive course and must be differentiated from metastasis, but metastasis of primary conjunctival vascular tumors appears to be rare.[9] Feline conjunctival melanomas originate on the bulbar conjunctiva and invade the eyelid.[10] They may locally recur, involve regional lymph nodes, metastasize, and lead to death within 4 months.[10] Similarly, canine conjunctival melanomas were reported to recur locally following surgical excision in 55% of cases, and at least 17% of the dogs experienced orbital invasion or spread to the regional lymph nodes or lungs.[5] Melanomas originating from the palpebral conjunctiva may more readily metastasize.[5] Mitotic index, cell type, and degree of pigmentation are not useful predictors of malignancy for canine conjunctival melanomas.[5] Two cases of apparently benign subconjunctival mast cell tumors have been reported in dogs.[11]

## History and Clinical Signs

Vascular tumors are often focal, raised, soft, red masses with visible feeder vessels. SCC of the eyelid, third eyelid, or ocular surface may appear as a focally thickened, roughened, usually reddened lesion in older animals or, more commonly, as an ulcerated lesion with a protracted course. In contrast, papillomas in young dogs appear verrucous and usually progress rapidly over weeks to a few months. Fibrous histiocytomas are also relatively rapidly growing, smooth, raised, pink lesions originating from the limbus, sclera, third eyelid, or eyelid. The degree of pigmentation, however, does not reliably predict the histologic nature of eyelid tumors.[1]

Other clinical signs of eyelid or ocular surface tumors in addition to a mass lesion may include epiphora, conjunctival injection, mucopurulent ocular discharge, protrusion of the third eyelid, conjunctival/corneal roughening or ulceration, and corneal neovascularization or pigmentation. Occasionally, palpebral conjunctival masses protrude only when their bulk no longer can be accommodated by the space between the eyelid and globe, and very advanced tumors may create exophthalmia or enophthalmia if the orbit is invaded. Large tumors and sebaceous adenomas often have a substantial inflammatory component or are secondarily infected.

## Diagnostic Techniques and Workup

In addition to fluorescein staining and examination with a cobalt filter or blacklight, the extent of involvement of the bulbar and palpebral conjunctiva should be determined by everting the eyelid (and third eyelid if affected). Nasolacrimal lavage and possibly positive contrast dacryocystorhinography may help characterize medial canthal masses. In general, small eyelid and ocular surface tumors are best diagnosed and treated by excisional biopsy. Fine-needle aspirates or incisional biopsies of larger tumors aid in prognostication and in planning definitive therapy. Occasionally, skull radiographs or computed tomography, regional lymph node cytology, and thoracic radiographs are required to stage potentially malignant tumors such as SCC, mast cell tumors, adenocarcinomas of the third eyelid, and conjunctival melanomas.

## Therapy

All eyelid tumors, whether benign or malignant, should be regarded as having the potential to affect vision or ocular comfort. Indications for tumor removal include (a) any tumor of the feline eyelid, (b) rapid growth, (c) irritation of the ocular surface or interference with eyelid function, (d) owner concern or unappealing appearance. In young dogs, observation of nonirritating papillomas or histiocytomas may be appropriate, as spontaneous regression is common.

Tumors involving less than one fourth to one third of the length of the eyelid are best treated by a V-Plasty (wedge) or 4-sided excision.[12] The latter technique affords superior apposition of the eyelid margins and wound stability, especially in tumors approaching the one-fourth to one-third limit, because the initial incision is made perpendicular to the eyelid margin rather than obliquely. In general, only one fourth of the feline eyelid can be removed with these techniques. Antibiotic or anti-inflammatory therapy may reduce large infected tumors or sebaceous adenomas with a substantial granulomatous inflammation so that a wedge or 4-sided excision becomes possible. Electrosurgical excision should be avoided.

Tumors greater than one fourth to one third of the eyelid usually require advanced reconstructive blepharoplasty or an alternative therapy. Some may be responsive to chemotherapy (e.g., lymphoma, mast cell tumors) or local radiation therapy (SCC). An attractive alternative to extensive blepharoplasty, cryosurgery has been reported to be effective in several canine eyelid tumor types (see Chapter 8).[2,13] It is quick, less technically demanding than blepharoplasty, and usually permits preservation of the nasolacrimal puncta and canaliculus. In many old or debilitated patients cryosurgery can be accomplished with only sedation or local/topical anesthesia. Following pretreatment with dexamethasone (0.1mg/kg IV), the mass is isolated with a chalazion forceps (if possible) and debulked flush with the lid margins. Using liquid nitrogen and a closed probe that approximates the diameter of the mass as much as possible, a double freeze-thaw is performed so that the iceball extends 3 to 5 mm beyond the visible margins of the mass. Iceballs should overlap in large tumors. Freezing may be repeated a second or third time if complete regression is not achieved following the first ses-

sion. Substantial postoperative swelling and usually transient depigmentation of the frozen tissue are to be expected. Reconstructive blepharoplasty is usually performed only if cryosurgery is likely to fail, or has failed.

Wide surgical excision is the most effective therapy for the majority of tumors involving the conjunctiva and third eyelid (especially conjunctival melanomas and nictitans adenocarcinomas), but excision of the entire nictitans should not be taken lightly, because significant undesirable sequelae such as ocular drying and chronic keratitis frequently result. Bulbar conjunctival tumors move freely and, if small, are generally amenable to excision with topical anesthesia and perhaps sedation. Cryosurgery may permit the nictitans to be spared in the cases of papillomas and early SCC, or can be used as an adjunct to excision in advanced canine conjunctival melanomas and SCC.[5]

Superficial keratectomy/sclerectomy is preferred for many corneal and scleral tumors, although some tumors require a full-thickness resection of the cornea or sclera. In the latter case, donor cornea, sclera, or autologous tissue grafts should be used to maintain ocular structural integrity. Limbal SCC and epibulbar melanoma may also be amenable to cryosurgery, although the iceball should be carefully monitored to avoid unnecessary freezing of intraocular structures.

## Prognosis

The prognosis for most canine primary eyelid tumors is excellent, whether treated by excision or cryosurgery. Metastasis is rare, even in histologically malignant primary lid tumors, and recurrence rates are low (approximately 10–15%).[2] New primary eyelid tumors are not uncommon and must be distinguished from recurrence. Because most eyelid tumors in cats are malignant, the prognosis is not as good as that for dogs, and it is unclear how prognosis correlates with the histologic features. Conjunctival melanomas and nictitans adenocarcinomas frequently recur following only partial excision of the nictitans, even if all the clinically visible tumor was removed.[5]

## LIMBAL (EPIBULBAR) MELANOMAS

Limbal melanomas in dogs and cats are benign, slightly raised, heavily pigmented masses originating from the sclera or subconjunctival connec-

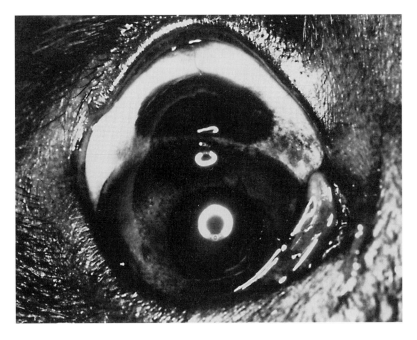

**Figure 27–2.** Epibulbar melanomas typically originate from the superior limbal region of the globe.

tive tissue (Fig. 27–2).[14–16] The vast majority of these slowly growing tumors originate in the superior limbal region, suggesting exposure to solar radiation may be a risk factor.[9] Affected dogs average 5 to 6 years old (cats are 8+ years), and a female/German shepherd predilection has been inconsistently reported.[14–17] Metastasis has not been described in dogs or cats, and mitotic figures are rarely encountered, although two of four cats also had FeLV-associated lymphoma or leukemia, and a third cat had a second intraocular pigmented mass unassociated with the limbal tumor.[7] Lightly pigmented spindle cells capable of division are seen histologically, but the dominant cell is presumably a hypermature spindle cell that is large, round, pigment laden, and benign.[4]

The clinical signs are typically minimal, because the mass is often incidentally noted, although local corneal invasion, epiphora, and mild conjunctival irritation may be seen.[15,16] Differential diagnoses include conjunctival melanoma, invasive uveal melanoma, metastatic melanoma, and staphyloma or coloboma. Gonioscopy aids in differentiating invasive intraocular tumors from limbal melanomas.

Therapy should be considered in young to middle-aged animals, if the tumor has invaded the eye, or if growth is rapid. Given its benign nature and usually slow growth rate (imperceptible growth over 18 months has been described), observation alone may be appropriate in older dogs. If intervention is required, lamellar keratec-

tomy/sclerectomy with graft placement is often curative. Beta-irradiation and cryosurgery have been used as adjuncts to surgery. Cryosurgery alone may also be effective. Regrowth following local surgical excision occurs in approximately 30% of patients, but 2 to 3 years may pass before the anterior chamber is invaded and enucleation is required.[14,16] Enucleation is curative, and is indicated if painful intraocular disease is present.[14]

## PRIMARY OCULAR TUMORS

### Canine Anterior Uveal Melanomas

**Incidence and Risk Factors** In the Armed Forces Institute of Pathology collection of tumors from the canine eye, orbit, and adnexa, intraocular melanomas comprised 12%, other primary intraocular tumors 14%, and metastatic intraocular neoplasms 9%.[18] Any age is at risk, but most dogs are older than 7 years of age, and breed or sex predilections are inconsistent.[14] Ocular melanomas have been induced experimentally by exposing dogs to radium and by intraocular injections of feline sarcoma virus in kittens.[19]

**Pathology and Natural Behavior** The majority of canine intraocular melanomas are benign, and arise from the iris or ciliary body (Fig. 27–3).[14,15,20] Several classification schemes based on cell type and growth pattern have been

**Figure 27–3.** Most anterior uveal melanomas originate from the iris or ciliary body and are benign.

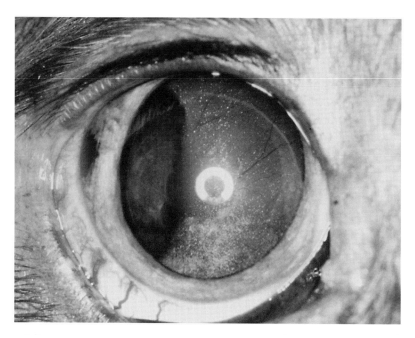

proposed, generally with little correlation to clinical outcome or natural behavior. The most clinically useful scheme classifies these tumors simply as melanocytoma (benign) and melanoma (potentially malignant).[14] Benign tumors have <2 mitotic figures/10 high power fields (mitotic index), and malignant tumors demonstrate nuclear pleomorphism and a mitotic index of at least 4, and often >30. Destruction of the eye is not, by itself, sufficient for a diagnosis of malignancy.[14] The overall rate of metastasis of intraocular melanomas is approximately 4%[20] and is usually via the hematogenous route. Local spread along ocular vessels and nerves or via direct penetration of the sclera or cornea also occurs. Malignant tumors tend to not be as darkly pigmented as benign tumors.[14]

Circumscribed, nevus-like pigmented iridal growths have been described in young dogs (7 months to 2 years old).[15] The natural history of these lesions is variable, as enlargement may not occur over several years.[15,18] Some, however, are capable of rapid growth, but all to date are clinically and histologically benign.

**History and Clinical Signs**  Common presentations of intraocular tumors include a visible intraocular or scleral mass, glaucoma, hyphema, anterior uveitis, extrabulbar spread, or their emergence as an incidental finding during ophthalmic examination.[14,20] Because glaucoma or hyphema are often the only overtly visible clinical signs,[14,20] intraocular neoplasia should always be considered in animals with hyphema or glaucoma or both, that lack a history of trauma or coagulopathy. Small masses frequently create few symptoms other than pupillary distortion. Pigmentation is variable and not a reliable indicator of tumor type.

**Diagnostic Techniques and Workup**  Usually the clinical or ultrasonographic appearance (if the media are opaque) is strongly suggestive of intraocular neoplasia, although it is difficult to arrive at a definitive diagnosis without invading the eye or removing it. Because most anterior uveal brown or black masses are cystic and not neoplastic, transillumination should be attempted before more invasive procedures. Uveal cysts typically permit bright light to pass, are roughly spherical, and may be free-floating. Once suspected, most primary canine intraocular tumors are followed for progression, although occasionally fine-needle aspiration (with its risks of inflammation, infection, and hemorrhage) or attempts at intraocular resection or enucleation are used for diagnostic purposes. The possibility of metastasis from another primary site (i.e., oral cavity or nail bed) to the eye, or from the eye to other organs, should also be eliminated.

**Therapy**  Canine primary intraocular tumors are generally observed. Enucleation is advised if there is concern about malignancy, or if complications such as intractable uveitis or secondary glaucoma occur.[21] The low risk of metastasis and unproven efficacy of enucleation at preventing metastasis in the few malignant tumors that have been reported, however, makes it difficult to enucleate automatically normotensive, noninflamed, visual eyes.[14] Isolated primary masses involving only the iris or a portion of the ciliary body may be amenable to local resection by sector iridectomy/cyclectomy in order to preserve the eye and vision.[15,18] These intraocular procedures, however, require an accomplished ophthalmic surgeon and often have unsatisfactory long-term results. Recently, trans-scleral and transcorneal Nd:YAG laser therapy has induced remission in some small to moderate-sized primary intraocular tumors.[21] Although the results were variable, perhaps because the tumors were not characterized histologically prior to therapy, this new method holds promise for the palliation or potential cure of a number of intraocular tumor types while also preserving vision. Metastasis was not observed in 15 cases following this procedure.[21]

**Prognosis**  Although the data in most studies are heavily "censored," the prognosis for histologically benign melanomas appears to be excellent. Enucleation is curative, but attempts at local excision or laser photoablation may be only palliative, especially if the ciliary body or trabecular meshwork is involved. The presence of black, nonsolid material within the orbit following the enucleation of benign melanomas with scleral invasion apparently does not affect prognosis, because these cells appear incapable of continued growth.[15] Approximately 25% of histologically malignant melanomas demonstrate metastasis, typically within 3 months of enucleation, and most dogs with metastasis are euthanatized within 6 months of enucleation.[14]

## Choroidal Melanomas

Choroidal melanomas are rare intraocular melanocytic tumors, comprising only 4% of canine uveal melanomas, with no clear breed or sex predisposition.[22] Middle-aged (6–7 years), medium- to large-breed dogs predominate.[22] Generally, these tumors are well delineated, raised subretinal pigmented masses with tapering margins, bulging centers, and a propensity for the peripapillary region and optic nerve.[22,23] In some cases the tumor may remain virtually static for many years, whereas others exhibit infiltration into the overlying retina, through the sclera, up the optic nerve, and into the orbit.[22] Nuclear anaplasia is minimal and generally mitotic figures are absent.[23] Metastasis has not been reported to date, although follow-up in most studies is incomplete. Most dogs with tumors involving a limited portion of the choroid are asymptomatic and the mass is incidentally noted on ophthalmoscopy. Larger tumors frequently present with chronic uveitis, secondary glau-

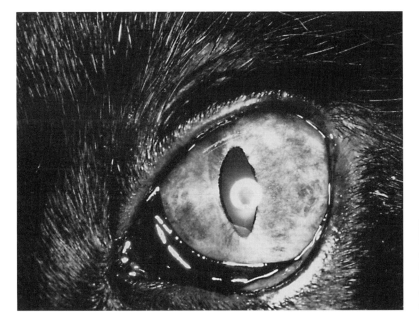

**Figure 27–4.**  Diffuse iris melanomas may first appear as multifocal to diffuse pigmentary changes, as seen in the coalescing darker regions of the iris in this cat.

coma, retinal detachment, intraocular hemorrhage, or blindness.[22,23] Ocular ultrasonography may demonstrate mass lesions if anterior segment changes or retinal detachment obscures an underlying mass. Therapy consists of enucleation once progression has been documented, or if the eye is painful. Optic nerve involvement may warrant a more cautious prognosis.

## Feline Primary Intraocular Melanomas

**Incidence and Risk Factors**   Infrequent, anterior uveal melanomas are suggested to be the most common primary intraocular tumor in cats (Fig. 27–4).[24] There appears to be no breed or sex predisposition, and most cats are more than 10 years of age at the time of diagnosis,[24] although the prodromal period for many of these tumors may be quite long.

**Pathology and Natural Behavior**   In the malignant form of uveal melanoma, the rate of metastasis (frequently to the liver and lungs) is generally regarded to be as high as 55 to 66%.[24–26] Iridal hyperpigmentation, however, frequently takes months to years to progress to the extent to which the eye is enucleated, and an additional 1 to 3 years after enucleation are required before metastatic disease may become evident.[24,26,27] No single morphologic feature is predictive of outcome, but metastasis has been linked to a greater mitotic index, larger tumors, those with extensive iris stroma infiltration, and scleral venous plexus invasion.[24]

A poorly characterized benign form may also exist, however, as many ophthalmologists have noted unilateral or occasionally bilateral progressive iridal pigmentary changes (especially in older orange cats) that apparently do not lead to metastatic disease over many years to a decade or more. It is possible, in some cats, that these initially benign-appearing accumulations of small angular pigmented cells on the anterior iridal surface undergo transformation to the larger, rounded cells typical of the potentially malignant diffuse iris melanoma. Of concern to the clinician waiting to document progression before advising treatment, however, is that transformation is not readily observable clinically and that these cells, once transformed, appear to be capable of quickly dropping off into the anterior chamber and entering the drainage apparatus and vasculature.

**History, Clinical Signs, Diagnostic Techniques, and Workup**   Slowly progressive, diffuse iridal hyperpigmentation is the most common clinical sign, although occasionally a pigmented iridal nodule or amelanotic mass is seen. Secondary glaucoma is common, and the diffuse form may be mistaken for chronic anterior uveitis with iridal hyperpigmentation.[24,26]

The diagnosis of melanoma, generally made clinically, requires demonstration of progression and iridal thickening or irregularity of the iris surface or pupil. The prognostic and diagnostic value of fine-needle aspirates of the iridal surface or iridal biopsies is unclear and worthy of further study.

**Therapy**   The treatment of feline uveal melanomas is controversial. Enucleation is commonly performed if iridal pigment changes have been demonstrated to increase progressively in size or number, or if intractable uveitis or glaucoma occurs. It seems logical that early enucleation would optimize survival but this is unproven, and enucleation markedly enhances the metastatic rate in feline sarcoma virus-induced uveal melanomas in cats.[19] The applicability of this experimental model to spontaneous disease, however, is unclear. Finally, we have monitored select, slowly progressing cases for many years without apparent metastasis.

**Prognosis**   The metastatic potential of feline uveal melanomas is believed to be high. There is some suggestion that enucleation of small tumors may warrant a better prognosis than when gross distortion of the eye has occurred. Because the tumor is relatively slow growing, the period until metastatic disease becomes apparent may be measured in years, and, even then, substantial additional time may be required before metastasis is life-threatening.

## Feline Primary Ocular Sarcomas

Sarcomas following ocular trauma may be second only to melanomas in frequency as a primary ocular tumor of cats.[28,29] Cats 7 to 15 years of age are most commonly affected, and the latency period following trauma averages 5 years.[29] Damage to the lens and chronic uveitis may be risk factors.[28,29] Although the cell of origin and the role of feline sarcoma virus is unclear, it is likely that chronic inflammation may eventually lead to neoplastic transformation of a pluripotent cell.[28,29] These tumors, often within the same eye, exhibit a spectrum of changes from granulation tissue, to fibrosarcoma, osteosarcoma, and anaplastic spindle cell sarcoma.[29] They tend to circumferentially line the choroid, quickly infiltrating the retina and optic nerve.[29] White or pinkish discoloration of the affected eye or change in the shape or consistency of the globe are the most common presenting signs. Skull radiographs may demonstrate bony involvement or metallic foreign bodies.[30]

Because this tumor is uncommon, many ophthalmologists will not remove a comfortable phthisical feline eye unless it changes appearance. The advanced stage at which many of these tumors are first identified and the propensity for early optic nerve involvement, however, indicate that enucleation at this point may be only palliative and not prolong life. This has led some authors to advocate prophylactic enucleation of phthisical feline eyes or of feline eyes that are blind and have been severely traumatized or are chronically inflamed.[28,30] As much of the optic nerve as possible should be removed during enucleation of an ocular sarcoma so that the extent of infiltrative disease and prognosis may be accurately determined. To date, there have been no reports of treatment by radiation or chemotherapy.

Extraocular extension is common, as is recurrence following orbital exenteration.[28,30] Continued growth up the remainder of the optic nerve into the chiasm/brain, with vision loss or other neurologic signs, involvement of regional lymph nodes, and distant metastasis, has been reported.[28,29] The vast majority of animals die from neoplasia-related causes, typically within several months of enucleation.[28–30]

## Ciliary Body Epithelial Tumors

Primary ciliary body tumors (ciliary body adenomas and adenocarcinomas and, less commonly, medulloepitheliomas and astrocytomas) are infrequent in dogs and rare in cats. In the authors' experience, these tumors usually are nonpigmented, but pigmented tumors may be grossly indistinguishable from anterior uveal melanomas. Breed or sex predilection, biologic behavior, or the significance of variations in morphology have not been well defined, but middle-aged to older dogs are the most commonly affected.[31] Most appear to be benign, fairly well-delineated, slow-growing tumors originating in the pars plicata of the ciliary body, and they seldom penetrate the sclera.[31] Adenocarcinomas tend to be more locally invasive, but metastasis is uncommon and occurs late in the course of the disease, if at all.[31,32]

Clinical signs include a retro-iridal mass that may displace the iris or lens by expansive growth; if the tumor is large, secondary glaucoma, ocular pain, and intraocular hemorrhage may be noted.[32] The diagnostic workup and differential diagnosis are similar to that of anterior uveal melanomas. Early enucleation has been recommended, although benign adenomas may remain static for years,[32] making enucleation controversial for small tumors unassociated with secondary ocular disease.[14,21] Local intraocular resection or Nd:YAG laser photoablation may permit vision and ocular comfort to be maintained.[21]

## Secondary Uveal Neoplasms

Numerous malignant tumors, especially adenocarcinomas, have been reported to metastasize to the highly vascular uveal tract. Lymphoma is the most common secondary intraocular tumor in the dog and cat, and ocular lesions are present in approximately one third of dogs with the disease.[32–34] It often appears as bilateral inflammatory disease. Common presentations include severe uveitis, retinal hemorrhages, hyphema, conjunctivitis, and keratitis characterized by corneal infiltrates, edema, vascularization, and intrastromal hemorrhage.[32,34] Glaucoma may also occur. Posterior segment lesions may include retinal vascular tortuosity, papilledema, multiple intraretinal hemorrhages, retinal detachment, and optic nerve or central blindness or exophthalmia. In one study, the life span of dogs with intraocular lymphoma was only 60 to 70% as long as dogs without ocular involvement when treated with cyclophosphamide, vincristine and prednisolone (COP), or doxorubicin.[34] Topical or systemic corticosteroid therapy or enucleation is palliative. (See Chap. 28*B,C* for the definitive therapy of lymphoma.)

## Tumors of the Orbit and Optic Nerve

**Incidence and Risk Factors** Risk factors other than middle to old age, and possibly sex (female dogs), have not been described.[35,36] Tumors involving the optic nerve are rare, although secondary invasion occurs in feline post-traumatic sarcomas and canine choroidal melanomas. Intraorbital meningiomas, the most common tumor of the optic nerve, comprise only 3% of all meningiomas in dogs.[37]

**Pathology and Natural Behavior** Orbital neoplasia may be primary (most common in dogs), secondary to extension of adjacent tumors into the orbit (most common in cats), or the result of distant metastasis. In cats and dogs, more than 90% of orbital tumors are malignant, and regional infiltration (including into the CNS) or distant metastasis is common.[35,36] At least 26 types of orbital tumors, roughly equally divided between connective tissue, bone, epithelial, and hemolymphatic origins, have been reported in dogs.[36] Osteosarcomas, mast cell tumors, reticulum cell sarcomas, fibrosarcomas, and neurofibrosarcomas are the most common canine primary orbital tumors.[36] More than two thirds of feline orbital tumors are epithelial in origin, with SCC being the most common,[35] but at least 15 other tumor types have been described in cats.

Optic nerve sheath meningiomas exhibit unpredictable biologic behavior. Although they rarely distantly metastasize, they may be osteolytic and invade surrounding tissues, including the CNS.[38,39] Primary optic nerve tumors in dogs include neurofibrosarcoma, glioma, and meningioma.[39]

**History and Clinical Signs**   Slowly progressive exophthalmia, no pain to minimal pain on opening the mouth, difficulty in retropulsing the eye, and deviation of the globe typify orbital neoplasia. Sudden erosion of nasal or sinus tumors into the orbit occasionally results in acute exophthalmia and substantial orbital pain. Enophthalmia may occur if the mass is anterior to the equator of the globe. Chronic epiphora secondary to obstruction of the nasolacrimal duct, exposure keratoconjunctivitis, palpable orbital masses following enucleation, or unexplained orbital pain also suggest orbital neoplasia.[35] Intraocular pressure measurement differentiates glaucomatous ocular enlargement from exophthalmia.

Optic nerve lesions may result in unilateral or bilateral blindness (the latter if the optic chiasm is affected); optic nerve head pallor, papilledema, or marked protrusion and congestion on ophthalmoscopy. A relatively mild degree of exophthalmia with vision loss suggests optic nerve neoplasia, because tumors of other orbital tissues typically cause profound exophthalmos before visual loss. Tumors affecting the retrobulbar, intracanalicular, or chiasmal portions of the optic nerve may not result in exophthalmia or visible change in the optic nerve head.

**Diagnostic Techniques and Workup**   It is essential to differentiate non-neoplastic orbital inflammatory diseases (granulomas, cellulitis, abscesses, myositis of the extraocular and mastica-

tory muscles) and orbital emphysema from neoplasia. Animals with inflammatory disease typically exhibit significant pain on opening the mouth. The location of an orbital mass can usually be determined by careful physical examination, including retropulsion of the globe, oral examination caudal to the last molar, and determination of the direction of malposition of the eye.

In addition to physical examination, cytology of regional lymph nodes, orbital ultrasound, and skull and thoracic radiographs should be performed. In one study of cats with orbital neoplasia, 59% had radiographic signs of orbital bone lesions, and 15% had evidence of metastasis on thoracic radiographs.[35] Computed tomography or magnetic resonance imaging offer superior imaging of the orbit, and facilitate planning of either radiation or surgical therapy (Fig. 27–5). Histologic characterization by fine-needle aspirates or needle-core biopsies (performed via the mouth or through the orbital skin), with ultrasound guidance if necessary, are helpful in arriving at a definitive diagnosis. The globe, major orbital

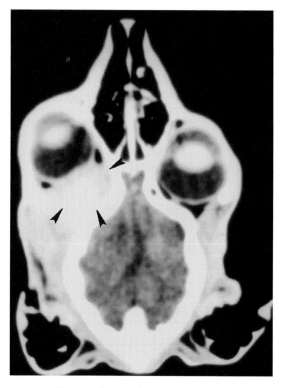

**Figure 27–5.**   Computed tomography (dorsal view) provides detailed information about the location and extent of orbital tumors, as in this 17-year-old cat with orbital osteosarcoma.

blood vessels, and optic nerve should be avoided. Because 50% of orbital tumors may have a non-diagnostic fine-needle aspirate, especially in cases of SCC,[35] exploratory orbitotomy via a number of approaches[40,41] or exenteration may be required to characterize the mass and resect it if possible. Cerebrospinal fluid taps may aid in distinguishing optic nerve neoplasia from optic neuritis.

**Therapy** Primary orbital and optic nerve tumors that lack metastasis or regional lymph node involvement may be amenable to surgical excision.[38] If bony involvement is not present, orbital exenteration by widely dissecting around the mass (stripping periorbita if necessary) is usually the preferred procedure, as the advanced stage of the tumor at the time of diagnosis typically makes it impossible to excise the mass completely and preserve a functional or comfortable eye. If periorbital bones are involved, radical "orbitectomy," which resects the affected orbital tissues and surrounding bones, should be considered.[42] When treating optic nerve tumors, as much of the ipsilateral optic nerve as possible should be removed in an attempt to obtain complete excision.[37]

If preservation of a comfortable eye and vision appears possible, a variety of orbitotomy techniques, ranging from small incisions through the eyelid or mouth to reflection of the zygomatic arch, have been described.[40,41] Postoperative complications are common and may include secondary enophthalmia with entropion and possibly diplopia (double vision). Surgical debulking can be palliative, and some dogs may survive a year or more with minimal therapy.

The role of chemotherapy and radiation therapy, either alone or as an adjunct to surgery, is yet to be defined in the treatment of orbital tumors, although chemotherapy for orbital lymphoma may be effective. Systemic corticosteroids may permit some patients with optic nerve meningioma to maintain vision for several weeks to months. Radiation therapy may be helpful in the case of nasal tumors with orbital extension,[35,36] in subtotally excised or recurrent meningiomas,[38] and in other select cases.

**Prognosis** With conservative treatment the prognosis for most tumors involving the orbit and optic nerve is poor,[35,36] especially if there is bony involvement on skull radiographs. Recurrence at the primary site and involvement of adjacent or distant sites are common, often occurring within weeks to a few months. Even benign-appearing tumors may be locally invasive and have a propensity for recurrence following wide excision.[36,42] In one study, however, radical orbitectomy (with or without chemotherapy or radiation therapy) provided a median survival time of 281 days, and 75% of the animals had apparent permanent local disease control.[42] In another study, the mean survival time for cats with orbital tumors treated by radiation therapy, chemotherapy, or surgery that included resection of affected orbital bones was only 4.3 months.[35] In a study of 23 dogs with orbital tumors, most of whom were treated by exenteration with or without adjunct therapy, only 3 survived 3 years or longer.[36] The majority of these animals died as a direct result of the tumor, or were euthanized at the time of diagnosis.[35,36]

## OCULAR EFFECTS OF CANCER THERAPEUTIC MODALITIES

The ocular effect of external beam radiation therapy for nasal and periocular tumors can have a substantial impact on an animal's quality of life. Common complications include chronic keratoconjunctivitis, corneal ulceration, "dry eye," enophthalmia, entropion, cataracts, retinal hemorrhages, retinal detachments, and blindness (Fig. 27–6). Many of these conditions respond poorly to treatment, and vigorous attempts at prevention should be made in order to avoid chronic ocular pain and blindness. In humans, blurred vision, partial visual field defects, loss of color vision, and diplopia have been associated with several antineoplastic drugs.[43] Similar effects probably occur in animals, but would be difficult to detect. Additionally, in humans, the bacillus Calmette-Gérin, or BCG, has been associated with uveitis; cyclophosphamide with dry eye; cisplatin with neuroretinal toxicity; doxorubicin with excessive lacrimation and conjunctivitis; 5-fluorouracil with blurred vision, excessive lacrimation, blepharitis, conjunctivitis, and keratitis; and vincristine with cranial nerve palsies, optic neuropathy, and cortical and night blindness.[43]

## COMPARATIVE ASPECTS

Malignant melanoma of the choroid and ciliary body is the most common primary ocular malignancy in adult humans. It is unclear whether enucleation prolongs survival or enhances the risk of metastasis, and a large, multicenter study

**Figure 27–6.** Radiation therapy for periocular tumors can cause significant ocular complications such as keratonconjunctivitis and cataract formation, as in this dog.

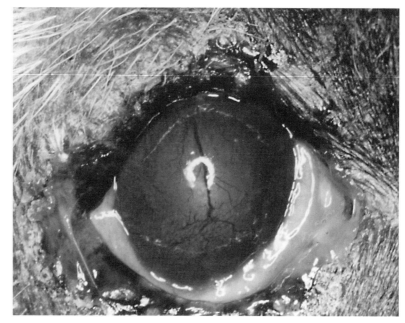

comparing enucleation to local radiation therapy is under way.[44] Retinoblastoma is the most common malignant intraocular tumor of children, and a genetic basis has been well described for it. With therapy, long-term survival is over 85%, but many patients develop second tumors, especially osteosarcoma.[45] Cancer-associated retinopathy is an uncommon, possibly immune-mediated paraneoplastic phenomenon in humans.[46] In this condition, patients with small cell lung carcinoma and other tumors may develop blurred vision, impaired color vision, substantial visual field defects, or complete blindness as tumor antigens cross-react with specific retinal components.[46]

## REFERENCES

1. Krehbiel JD, Langham RF: Eyelid neoplasms in dogs. Am J Vet Res 36:115–119, 1975.
2. Roberts SM, Severin GA, Lavach JD: Prevalence and treatment of palpebral neoplasms in the dog: 200 cases (1975–1983). J Am Vet Med Assoc 189:1355–1359, 1986.
3. McLaughlin SA, Whitley RD, Gilger BC, et al: Eyelid neoplasms in cats: A review of demographic data (1979 to 1989). J Am Anim Hosp Assoc 29:63–67, 1983.
4. Barrie KP, Gelatt KN, Parshall CP: Eyelid squamous cell carcinoma in four dogs. J Am Anim Hosp Assoc 18:123–127, 1982.
5. Collins BK, Collier LL, Miller MA, et al: Biologic behavior and histologic characteristics of canine conjunctival melanoma. Prog Vet Compar Ophthalmol 3:135–140, 1993.
6. Bonney CH, Koch SA, Dice PF, et al: Papillomatosis of conjunctiva and adnexa in dogs. J Am Vet Med Assoc 176:48–51, 1980.
7. Collier LL, Collins BK: Excision and cryosurgical ablation of severe periocular papillomatosis in a dog. J Am Vet Med Assoc 204:881–885, 1994.
8. Wilcock B, Peiffer R: Adenocarcinoma of the gland of the third eyelid in seven dogs. J Am Vet Med Assoc 193:1549–1550, 1988.
9. Hargis AM, Lee AC, Thomassen RW: Tumor and tumor-like lesions of perilimbal conjunctiva in laboratory dogs. J Am Vet Med Assoc 173:1185–1190, 1978.
10. Patnaik AK, Mooney S: Feline melanoma: A comparative study of ocular, oral and dermal neoplasms. Vet Pathol 25:105–112, 1988.
11. Johnson BW, Brightman, Whiteley HE: Conjunctival mast cell tumor in two dogs. J Am Anim Hosp Assoc 24:439–442, 1988.
12. Gelatt KN: The canine eyelids. In Gelatt KN (ed): Veterinary Ophthalmology, 2nd ed. Philadelphia, Lea & Febiger, 1991, pp. 256–275.
13. Holmberg DL, Withrow SJ: Cryosurgical treatment of palpebral neoplasms: Clinical and experimental results. Vet Surg 8:68–73, 1979.
14. Wilcock BP, Peiffer RL: Morphology and behavior of primary ocular melanomas in 91 dogs. Vet Pathol 23:418–424, 1986.
15. Diters RW, Dubielzig RR, Aquirre GD, et al: Primary ocular melanoma in dogs. Vet Pathol 20:379–395, 1983.

16. Diters RW, Ryan AM: Canine limbal melanoma. Vet Med Small Anim Clin 78:1529–1534, 1983.

17. Harling DE, Peiffer RL, Cook CS, et al: Feline limbal melanoma: Four cases. J Am Anim Hosp Assoc 22:795–802, 1986.

18. Gelatt KN, Johnson KA, Peiffer RL: Primary iridal pigmented masses in three dogs. J Am Anim Hosp Assoc 15:339–344, 1979.

19. Niederkorn JY, Shadduck JA, Albert DM: Enucleation and the appearance of second primary tumors in cats bearing virally induced intraocular tumors. Invest Ophthalmol Vis Sci 23:719–725, 1982.

20. Bussanich NM, Dolman PJ, Rootman J, et al: Canine uveal melanomas: Series and literature review. J Am Anim Hosp Assoc 23:415–422, 1987.

21. Nasisse MP, Davidson MG, Olivero DK, et al: Neodymium: YAG laser treatment of primary canine intraocular tumors. Prog Vet Compar Ophthalmol 3:152–157, 1993.

22. Collinson PN, Peiffer RL: Clinical presentation, morphology, and behavior of primary choroidal melanomas in eight dogs. Prog Vet Compar Ophthalmol 3: 158–164, 1993.

23. Dubielzig RR, Aquirre GD, Gross SL, et al: Choroidal melanomas in dogs. Vet Pathol 22:582–585, 1985.

24. Duncan DE, Peiffer RL: Morphology and prognostic indicators of anterior uveal melanomas in cats. Prog Vet Compar Ophthalmol 1:25–32, 1991.

25. Bellhorn RW, Henkind P: Intraocular malignant melanoma in domestic cats. J Small Anim Pract 10: 631–637, 1970.

26. Patnaik AK, Mooney S: Feline melanoma: A comparative study of ocular, oral and dermal neoplasms. Vet Pathol 25: 105–112, 1988.

27. Acland GM, McLean IW, Aquirre GD, et al: Diffuse iris melanoma in cats. J Am Vet Med Assoc 176: 52–56, 1980.

28. Peiffer RL, Monticello T, Bouldin TW: Primary ocular sarcomas in the cat. J Small Anim Pract 29: 105–116, 1988.

29. Dubielzig RR, Everitt J, Shadduck JA, et al: Clinical and morphologic features of post-traumatic ocular sarcomas in cats. Vet Pathol 27: 62–65, 1990.

30. Hakanson N, Shively JN, Reed RE, et al: Intraocular spindle cell sarcoma following ocular trauma in a cat: Case report and literature review. J Am Anim Hosp Assoc 26: 63–66, 1990.

31. Peiffer RL: Ciliary body epithelial tumours in the dog and cat: A report of thirteen cases. J Small Anim Pract 24: 347–370, 1983.

32. Gwin RM, Gelatt KN, Williams LW: Ophthalmic neoplasms in the dog. J Am Anim Hosp Assoc 18: 853–866, 1982.

33. Williams LW, Gelatt KN, Gwin RM: Ophthalmic neoplasms in the cat. J Am Anim Hosp Assoc 17: 999–1008, 1981.

34. Krohne SG, Henderson NM, Richardson RC, et al: Prevalence of ocular involvement in dogs with multicentric lymphoma: Prospective evaluation of 94 cases. Vet and Compar Ophthalmol 4:127– 135, 1994.

35. Gilger BC, McLaughlin SA, Whitley RD, et al: Orbital neoplasms in cats: 21 cases (1974–1990). J Am Vet Med Assoc 201: 1083–1086, 1992.

36. Kern TJ: Orbital neoplasia in 23 dogs. J Am Vet Med Assoc 186: 489–491, 1985.

37. Braund KG, Ribas JL: Central nervous system meningiomas. Compend Contin Educ Pract Vet 8: 241–248, 1986.

38. Dugan SJ, Schwarz PD, Roberts SM, et al: Primary optic nerve meningioma and pulmonary metastasis in a dog. J Am Anim Hosp Assoc 29:11–16, 1993.

39. Spiess BM, Wilcock BP: Glioma of the optic nerve with intraocular and intracranial involvement in a dog. J Comp Pathol 97: 79–84, 1987.

40. Slatter DH: Orbit. In Slatter DH (ed): Fundamentals of Veterinary Ophthalmology, 2nd ed. Philadelphia, WB Saunders, 1990, pp. 478–511.

41. Gilger BC, Whitley RD, McLaughlin SA: Modified lateral orbitotomy for removal of orbital neoplasms in two dogs. Vet Surg 23: 53–58, 1994.

42. Withrow SJ, O'Brien MG, Straw RC, et al: Orbitectomy in the dog and cat: 21 cases. Vet Cancer Soc, 13th Annu Conf, Columbus, OH, 1993.

43. Imperia PS, Lazarus HM, Lass JH: Ocular complications of systemic cancer chemotherapy. Surv Ophthalmol 34: 209–230, 1989.

44. Olsen KR, Curtin VT: Enucleation and plaque treatment. In Albert DM, Jokabiec FA (eds): Principles and Practice of Ophthalmology. Philadelphia, WB Saunders, 1994, pp. 3217–3233.

45. Petersen RA: Retinoblastoma: Diagnosis and non-radiation therapies. In Albert DM, Jokabiec FA (eds): Principles and Practice of Ophthalmology. Philadelphia, WB Saunders, 1994, pp. 3279–3285.

46. Wiggs JL: Ocular syndromes associated with systemic malignancy. In Albert DM, Jokabiec FA (eds): Principles and Practice of Ophthalmology. Philadelphia, WB Saunders, 1994, pp. 3350–3355.

# 28

# Hematopoietic Tumors

## A. FELINE RETROVIRUSES

## Dennis W. Macy

The cat has the largest number of different retroviruses of any companion animal. Retroviral infections in the cat produce a wide spectrum of disease, including cancer.[1-3] Retroviruses are considered the number one infectious cause of morbidity and mortality in the feline population; thus they are the most important infectious agents in clinical veterinary medicine.

The cat has both endogenous and exogenous retroviruses. The endogenous retroviruses are generally considered nonpathogenic, are present in the host DNA, and are passed from generation to generation genetically like other chromosomal genes through the genome. Three families of endogenous retroviruses have been identified in the cat, including the RD-114 virus and the MAC-1 sequences and DNA sequences associated with the endogenous feline leukemia virus (FeLV). Molecular studies indicate that the endogenous virus RD-114 originated from the ancestral baboon 3 to 10 million years ago.[3] RD-114 is a xenotropic virus; i.e., it does not infect or replicate in cat cells but replicates in noncat cells such as those of human or dog.[4,5] The endogenous feline MAC-1 sequences appear to be similar to the MAC-1 endogenous primate oncoviruses originally isolated from a macaque cell line.[6,7] The endogenous FeLV-related sequences are believed to have come from an ancestral rat some 10 million years ago, probably via exogenous FeLV integration events.[8]

The exogenous retroviruses contain both pathogenic and nonpathogenic viruses that are passed horizontally and vertically between cats.

Pathogenic exogenous retroviruses include FeLV and the feline immunodeficiency virus (FIV). An additional pathogenic retrovirus, the feline sarcoma virus (FeSV), arises from the combination of the exogenous FeLV and proto-oncogenes contained within the cat's genome. The feline syncytium-forming virus (FeSFV), or feline foamy virus, a nonpathogenic exogenous retrovirus, is also found in cats.

The exogenous FeLV is believed to have been first contracted from the ancestral rat approximately 10 million years ago.[9] The ancestral source of FIV and FeSFV are unknown.

The three pathogenic retroviruses of clinical importance are FeLV, FIV, and FeSV.

### FELINE LEUKEMIA VIRUS

FeLV is a retrovirus belonging to the subfamily oncornavirus or tumor-producing RNA viruses. Like other retroviruses, it has a single strand of ribonucleic acid (RNA), and an enzyme called reverse transcriptase (RT). RT is an enzyme used for the synthesis of DNA from the virus RNA template. FeLV contains a variety of proteins, several of which are important clinically. The basic groups of FeLV proteins are the envelope proteins and core proteins, several of which are important clinically. The basic groups of FeLV proteins are the envelope proteins and core proteins. Two envelope proteins have particular clinical significance: P15E (Transmembrane [TM15]) and the Gp 70 glycoproteins (surface glycoprotein [SU70]).[10–12] P15E is an envelope protein that is thought to be one of the mediators of FeLV-induced immunosuppression in FeLV-infected cats.[12] The glycoprotein of the envelope GP70 may contain subgroup antigens A, B, C. Combinations of these subgroup viruses may exist in an individual cat.[13,14] There is considerable antigenic variation within each subgroup that can affect the biologic properties of the individual isolates or strains of FeLV. These subgroup antigens are responsible for binding of the virion to receptors on the surface of cells. The specific characteristics of these proteins also predict the pathogenicity, host range, infectivity, and other biologic properties of the virus.[3,15] The antibodies produced against envelope proteins can be neutralizing and thus can prevent infection. Envelope proteins are very important components of FeLV vaccines. Core proteins (capsid) include P15-C, P12, P10, and P27. P27 (capsid 27 [CA27]) is present in large amounts in infected cats and is quite soluble and can be found in the cytoplasm of cells and body fluids such as tears and serum.[10–12] P27 is the antigen that is detected in the immunofluorescence test (IFA) and the enzyme-linked immunoabsorbent assay (ELISA) test commonly used in the diagnosis of FeLV infections.[15–21]

## Feline Genome

The FeLV genome consists from left to right (5 prime to 3 prime) of the genes LTR-GAG-POL-ENV-LTR.[11,15] The LTR gene does not produce a protein like other genes; rather the LTR, or long terminal repeat gene sequence, has a regulatory function and thus controls expression of other viral genes (i.e., the LTR gene sequence will determine the replication of the virus in various tissues, and plays an important role in determining the pathogenicity of individual virus isolates). The GAG gene (group-associated antigen) codes for internal proteins of the virus P15C, P12, P10, P27. The POL gene, or polymerase gene, encodes an RT enzyme. The ENV (envelope gene) encodes for the transmembrane protein P15E and the envelope protein GP70.[11,15]

## Transmission of FeLV

FeLV is very fragile and is easily killed. Desiccation rapidly reduces the amount of viable virus in saliva, inactivating virus in 1 to 3 hours. In moist environments such as exudates or blood, the virus remains viable for only 48 hours at 37° C or 1 week at 22° C.[22] Like most retroviruses, FeLV is rapidly inactivated by heating.[22,23] Similar to other envelope viruses, FeLV is readily inactivated by disinfectants. Given these charateristics of FeLV, it is unlikely that environmental contaminants such as examination tables, cages, and waiting rooms can be considered potential sources for contracting FeLV infections.[3] Housing of susceptible cats adjacent to FeLV-positive cats has failed to result in the spread of infection, indicating that aerosolization is also an unlikely source of this virus.[24,25] Although saliva may contain up to $10^5$ virus particles/ml, prolonged intimate contact with infected cats is required for transmission. The most frequently incriminated activities associated with transmission of FeLV are licking, biting, grooming, and shared litter pan, food, and water dishes. Intimate contact is enhanced in catteries and multiple-cat households, where infection rates can be very high.[3] Although as little as 0.01 ml of blood from a viremic cat has been shown to transmit FeLV, the role of biting insects in the transmission of FeLV remains undocumented. All bodily fluids of infected cats contain infected white blood cells (WBCs) and free virus, but the role of semen, for example, in the transmission of FeLV is still unknown.[26]

Although cats may be infected with FeLV subgroups A,B, or C, only A has been found to be present in cell-free fluids and is thought to be associated with the natural transmission of FeLV. Subgroups B and C are more cell associated and are not thought to be transmitted in nature.[27,28] The cell-associated nature of FeLV subgroups B and C are similar to the cell-associated nature of FIV and FeSFV.[27–30] To put the relative risk of transmission of these retroviruses in a multiple-cat household in perspective, one should consider this example. If an FeLV-positive cat, an FIV-positive cat, and an FeSFV cat were gang-housed with 100 susceptible negative cats, one would expect 60 to 75% of the cats to have evidence of exposure to FeLV. Thirty percent of these cats would be eventually persistently viremic for FeLV, and only 1 to 3% of these cats would be positive for FIV or FeSFV.[29,30] The low FIV and FeSFV infection rate observed in these animals not only reflects the difficulty in transmitting a cell-associated virus but also the importance of social relationships of cats in the transmission of feline retroviruses. Cats that do not fight among themselves because of the social structure that develops within groups of cats are going to have a decreased chance of transmitting FIV and FeSFV. However, in a large group of cats, intimate social behavioral activities such as communal grooming develop that facilitate the transmission of FeLV. The overall prevalence of FeLV in the United States is between 1 to 3%.[1,2,3,30,31] The prevalence in singlecat households is less than 1% and as much as 30% in multiplecat households.[1,2,3,32] The incidence in sick cats is 11.5%.

Cats may be infected with subgroups A, B or C, or combinations of these subgroups. These subgroups are characterized by their ability for crossinterference with homologous but not heterologous subgroups of FeLV, as well as host range and other characteristics of the virus.[13,14] All naturally infected FeLV cats contain subgroup A. Fifty percent of infected cats contain a combination of subgroups A and B, and 1% of infected cats in nature contain a mixture of subgroup C, either as AC or ABC.[1,33,34]

The clinical relevance of FeLV subgroups and strains is essential in the understanding of the diversity of clinical disease caused by FeLV infection. Although subgroups A, B, and C maintain 85% of genomic homology, cats infected with various combinations of these subgroups may produce vastly different diseases. A variety of strains of subgroup A exist, from nonpathogenic to the very pathogenic.[35] Although most strains of subgroup A alone have limited pathogenicity, if combined with other subgroups, this pathogenicity increases dramatically. Subgroup B is created when subgroup A recombines with endogenous FeLV envelope sequences already in the feline genome.[36–39] Each recombination is unique, and thus there are many strains of FeLV-B.[40] The combination of subgroups A and B are more contagious and pathogenic then subgroup A is alone.[33,34,41,42] Cats infected with subgroups A and B often develop thymic lymphoma and myeloproliferative diseases.[37,43] Subgroup C arises from a mutation of subgroup A.[44] Cats may have a combination of A and C or A, B, and C. These combinations are uncommon and are found in only 1% of naturally infected cats with FeLV infections. FeLV-C is antigenically similar to the feline oncovirus-associated membrane antigen (FOCMA), and cats carrying FeLV-C develop severe erythroid aplasia and anemia, and usually die within 1 to 2 months of infection.[27]

## Feline Oncovirus-Associated Antigen

FOCMA is a protein found on the surface of FeLV- and FeSV-induced neoplasms but not on nonneoplastic feline cells.[45–47] The presence of FOCMA is determined serologically by the ability of cells to react to immunoglobulins produced in cats that have regressed FeSV-induced fibrosarcoma or FeLV infections. The presence of FOCMA antibody is determined by the ability of the serum to react with FL74 cells, a transformed cultured infected lymphocyte.[47] FOCMA appears to be closely related to FeLV-C GP70 antigens. Antibodies to FOCMA protect against neoplastic and myeloproliferative disease development in cats. Some FeLV vaccines contain FOCMA and elicit an anti-FOCMA response.[48] The relative importance of this in preventing disease in vaccinates is yet to be proven.[48]

## Pathogenesis

Most cats contract FeLV through contact with infectious saliva via the oronasal route. Following replication in the epithelial and lymphoid tissues in the pharyngeal region, infected lymphocytes and other cells drain to mandibular lymph nodes and replicate in these sites, subsequently entering the blood stream and spreading systemically.[49] The bone marrow then becomes infected as a sequel to the amplification of the virus in these regional lymph nodes.[49] The high mitotic index of the bone marrow cells is ideal for FeLV replication and the further amplification of FeLV that is necessary to continue the pathogenesis of the FeLV infection.[50] It is here in the bone marrow where infection is frequently stopped through a successful host immune response. It is at this point that cats may eliminate the infection, develop latency, or sequester the FeLV infection. If the viral burden is too great, the infected bone marrow cells eventually circulate throughout the body, spreading the viral infection to epithelial cells throughout the body, including salivary tissue, urinary tract, etc.[49,50] Once salivary tissues are infected, the saliva becomes heavily laden with virus, thus completing the infectious cycle.[49,51,52] The time of exposure to the presence of infectious virus in the saliva may be as short as 3 weeks or as long as months to years.

## Consequences of FeLV Exposure

After exposure to FeLV, there are three possible outcomes: lack of infection, persistent viremia, and transient infection. Approximately 28% of cats exposed to FeLV do not acquire the infection (Table 28–1). There are a number of explanations for this phenomenon, including natural resistance, age resistance, or insufficient exposure.

Persistent viremia results in 30% of the cats after exposure to FeLV. This results in a high

**Table 28–1**   Consequences of Exposure to FeLV

| Permanent FeLV Status | Exposure to FeLV | FeLV Immune Response | Cats (%) |
|---|---|---|---|
| Never infected | None | Not immune | 30 |
| Not infected (nonviremic) | Exposed | Immune | 42[a] |
| Infected (viremic) | Exposed | Not immune | 28 |

[a]Transiently infected.

likelihood of developing either lymphoma or other FeLV-related diseases.

Transient infections occur in approximately 42% of cats exposed to FeLV.[49,52] In these cats, the virus enters the blood and replicates for a period of 4 to 6 weeks before being rejected by the host immune response.[49,51,52] After this brief period of infection, cats usually go through a period of viral latency for 4 to 9 months.[53–55] In about 10% of cats, viral latency will persist indefinitely. In latently infected cats, nonreplicating provirus remains within the DNA of some of the cat's tissues, usually the bone marrow or lymphoid tissues.[54] Viral latency is not detected using routine FeLV diagnostic tests and requires either polymerase chain reaction (PCR) or a bone marrow co-culturing technique to demonstrate its presence. Cats that are latently infected are not contagious to other cats. Before latently infected cats eliminate the virus, cats may have recrudescence of their infection by the administration of steroids or possibly following periods of stress.[54] Cats with recrudescence of the infections may become persistently viremic. Still other cats—5 to 10% of exposed cats—will develop what is termed *sequestered infection*. These infection sites are confined to local tissues such as mammary tissues or salivary gland tissues.[18,21] In these cats, viremia does not exist, but there is enough viral replication to produce detectable levels of soluble P27 in the blood. Cats with sequestered infections are ELISA positive and IFA negative and are often referred to as "discordant" cats.[18,21,56] Studies indicate that 50% of these discordant cats will eventually become negative, 25% will become viremic, and another 25% will remain discordant indefinitely.

## FeLV Disease Manifestations

The wide spectrum of disease manifestations associated with persistent FeLV infections corresponds to the many different strains and subgroup combinations of this virus found in cats. Despite its name, only 20% of cats persistently infected with the FeLV develop lymphoma or lymphoid leukemia.[57–59] Cytopathic and immunosuppressive effects of this virus are responsible for 80% of the deaths attributed to this virus.[3,59,60] The degenerative effects of certain strains of FeLV on a variety of bone marrow elements result in anemia, neutropenia, thrombocytopenia, and lymphoid depletions. Similar degenerative cytopathic effects are noted on rapidly dividing intestinal epithelial cells, resulting in enteritis, and when these cytopathic effects involve the placenta or developing fetus, the results are fetal death, resorption, abortion, or stillbirths. The lymphoid depletion, neutropenia, and other functional immune aberrations result in severe immunosuppression, culminating in the acquisition of opportunistic infections. In addition to these opportunistic infections, persistently infected cats are subject to the development of immune-mediated diseases.

A variety of lymphoid and nonlymphoid proliferative diseases develop in cats infected with FeLV. Both FeLV-positive and FeLV-negative lymphomas have been linked to FeLV infection. Although not all lymphomas are caused by FeLV and lymphoma and myeloproliferative diseases have been described in SPF cats, 70% of lymphomas are IFA positive for FeLV at the time of diagnosis. (Table 28–2). Lymphomas develop earlier in viremic cats, mean between 2 to 5 years of age, when compared to nonviremic cats, mean between 4 to 9 years of age.[61–63] In addition, the (prodromal) period between viremia to tumor development is shorter in younger cats.[64] The number of FeLV-positive lymphomas varies with the anatomic location of the disease. Approximately 80% of the mediastinal lymphomas, spinal lymphomas, and multicentric lymphomas are positive by IFA. A lesser percentage (30%) of extranodal sites such as ocular, cutaneous, or renal, are positive for FeLV. The alimentary form of lymphoma occurs in older cats and is often negative for feline leukemia; only 23% of alimentary lymphomas are found to be FeLV positive by IFA. However, epidemiologic studies have

**Table 28–2**   Classification of Feline Lymphomas

| Anatomic Site[b] | Total (%) | FeLV Status[b] (Percentage Positive) |
|---|---|---|
| Multicentric | 44 | 80 |
| Mediastinal (thymic) | 38 | 77 |
| Alimentary | 13 | 23 |
| Miscellaneous | 5 | 38 |

[a]Classification according to World Health Organization.
[b]Determined by IFA against peripheral blood smears.

shown that many cats that develop FeLV-negative lymphomas have the same degree of exposure to FeLV as do cats that develop FeLV-positive lymphomas. Recent studies using the more sensitive PCR procedure have found that 13% of the IFA FeLV-negative lymphomas contain the exogenous FeLV provirus.[64a] The anatomic distribution of lymphomas in the cat is known to vary depending on geography.[65–67] Some geographic locations have a higher incidence of thymic lymphomas, for example. These geographic variations in disease probably reflect virus strains present in a particular locality or differences in cats.[68]

**Myeloproliferative Diseases**   Myeloproliferative diseases are disorders of the bone marrow characterized by the proliferation of one or more cell lines in the bone marrow at the expense of other cell lines. Eventually this proliferation crowds out other bone marrow cell lines. The particular cell line that proliferates is probably dependent on the strain and subgroup of FeLV infecting the cat. The mechanism of the enhanced progenitor cell proliferation is thought to be due to the viral induction of growth-promoting substances acting on bone marrow stroma. This first results in overstimulation and proliferation, followed by exhaustion and eventual atrophy of bone marrow elements.[69]

**Anemias**   Anemia is a common clinical finding in FeLV-positive cats.[70,71] FeLV-related anemias may be classified into three types: aplastic, myelodysplastic, and regenerative anemias. Aplastic anemia is the most common form in the FeLV-positive cat and is thought to be the etiology in two thirds of all nonregenerative anemias in cats.[31,72,73] The anemia is either normochromic/normocytic, or normochromic/ macrocytic in character.[74] Macrocytosis is an important clinical finding, since mean corpuscular volumes (MCVS) of greater than 50 fentoliters/μl are most often observed in FeLV-positive cats. FeLV subgroup C is the most consistent isolate from

cats with aplastic anemias.[33] Affected cats are usually younger than 3 years of age and clinical signs of onset are usually gradual. Cats may not become symptomatic until packed cell volumes (PCVs) are less than 10%. The exact mechanism of the anemia is unknown; however, it appears to be associated with loss of erythroid progenitor cells and the inability of the residual progenitor cells to respond to normal physiologic stimuli such as erythropoietin, which is usually in high concentration in these cats.[74,75]

Myelodysplastic anemias are uncommon and develop an association with myeloproliferative disease.[74,76,77] Medullary fibrosis or medullary osteosclerosis is a frequent finding. Clinically, the anemias are characterized as nonregenerative and red blood cells (RBCs) may also have megablastic changes despite normal serum levels of vitamin B12 and folic acid.[78] These findings have been most often associated in cats infected with the subgroups A and B.[43,77] It is thought that the pathogenesis of this osteosclerosis is due to depressed bone growth and remodeling and not to excessive bone production. Over time, decreased osteoclastic activity in bone results in excessive unreabsorbed bone, and dramatic filling of the medullary cavity with trabecular network of cancellous bone.[79]

Ten percent of the anemias associated with FeLV infections are classified as regenerative and may be attributed to hemolysis. Bone marrows of these cats are hypercellular and a peripheral reticulocytosis and RBC macrocytosis is usually present.[76] Nucleated RBCs may also be present as a result of extramedullary hematopoiesis in the spleen and liver. Cats with FeLV-associated regenerative anemias commonly have immune-mediated hemolysis or haemobartonellosis.[16,80] FeLV subgroup A is most often isolated from cats with regenerative anemia, and the pathogenesis of these changes is thought to be associated with the concurrent immunosuppression produced by the persistent FeLV infection.[74,81]

**Neutropenia**   Neutrophils and their myeloid precursors are often affected by FeLV. The neutropenias may be persistent, transient, or cyclic in character.[49,82] A transient neutropenia of 3 to 5 weeks in duration following initial FeLV infection of bone marrow is common.[49,83,84] Cyclic neutropenia of 10 to 14 days' duration may be seen in cats that are either viremic or latently infected with FeLV.[82] Persistent neutropenia may be a preneoplastic condition that eventually progresses into a full-blown myeloproliferative disease process.[85] A panleukopenia-like syndrome or myeloblastopenia is observed in some FeLV cats that are well vaccinated against panleukopenia. This condition is characterized by a profound leukopenia with white cell counts less than 3,000, acute enterocolitis, fever, and vomiting.[85] The intestinal epithelium of these infected cats contains large amounts of P27, indicating a large virus load in this target tissue. The mechanism of the neutropenia is unknown but is most often associated with subgroup A FeLV isolates.[44] Neutropenias associated with FeLV must be differentiated from neutropenias caused by FIV and panleukopenia virus infections.

**Platelet Disorders** Platelets in FeLV-infected cats are usually larger than normal, abnormal in morphology, and frequently reduced in numbers.[86,87] These changes may be seen in acutely and persistently infected cats and are the most severe in the profoundly anemic cat. Platelets may become so large (> than 30 fentoliters), that they may be counted as RBCs by electronic counters.[88] Although platelet dysfunction can often be demonstrated in FeLV-positive cats, in the laboratory they are though to be of little clinical significance.

**Immunodeficiency** Although there are many proposed mechanisms for the immunosuppression associated with FeLV infections, it is clear that it is caused in part by marked lymphoid atrophy and T-cell suppression.[31,64,89] The degree of suppression appears to be FeLV-strain dependent.[90,91] It is believed that suppression increases the susceptibility of FeLV-infected cats to a variety of chronic and recurrent infections. These infections are important and often lead to the demise of the patient. Several types of opportunistic infections are frequently found in FeLV-positive cats and include viral (feline infections peritonitis and herpesviruses), fungal (cryptococcosis, aspergillus), rickettsial (haemobartonellosis), protozoal (toxoplasmosis, crytosporidiosis), bacterial (oral cavity), and respiratory infections. Whether these infections occur more frequently or are just more severe in FeLV-infected cats is unknown.

**Congenital Infections** Several studies have indicated that approximately 70% of infertile queens and 60% of queens that abort are positive for FeLV, and fetal reabsorption has been demonstrated in experimental FeLV infections.[72,73] Sequestered infected queens will sometimes give birth to congenitally infected kittens.[73] Young FeLV-positive kittens have a high neonatal mortality rate, whose clinical course is characterized by thymic atrophy, cachexia, and other signs. The clinical condition is often referred to as the fading-kitten syndrome.[72]

**Multicentric Osteochondromatosis** Osteochondromatosis or multiple cartilaginous exostosis has been described in the flat bones of several mature FeLV-positive cats.[3,92] In other species, osteochondromatosis is a condition of long bones in the young animals that usually stop growing when the physes closes and bone undergoes remodeling. Despite the presence of retroviral particles within the lesions of the two cases described with osteochondromatosis, the definitive association between this disease entity and FeLV infections is yet to be proven.

**Anisocoria and Other Ocular Manifestations** Ocular disease occurs in approximately 2% of FeLV-positive cats.[93] The common nonneoplastic abnormalities are associated with FeLV-induced pupillary motility abnormalities.[94] In addition, idiopathic, lymphoplasmacytic anterior uveitis appears to occur with the more common lesions associated with lymphomatous changes within the eye.[67]

**Neurologic Disease** Certain strains of FeLV have a tropism for the central nervous system. While FIV appears to produce most of its pathology in the brain, FeLV appears to produce most of its pathology in the spinal cord and peripheral nerves.[95]

Lower motor neuron paralysis, locomotion and behavioral abnormalities, and sensory and motor polyneuropathies may occur in FeLV viremic cats.[95,96] Urinary incontinence is thought to be secondary to spinal or peripheral nerve involvement and has also been described. Paraparesis or tetraparesis has been associated with focal lymphomatous masses that directly compress the cord, while in some cases no evidence of lymphoma could be found in these viremic cats. A small study involving 21 cats with spinal lymphoma found that 81% had hind limb paralysis, 84% were determined to have FeLV, and 69% had leukemic cells within the bone marrow.[97] Hence, bone marrow examination and/or FeLV status determination should be considered in cats when paraparesis or tetraparesis is present.

**Multiple Cutaneous Horns** Multiple cutaneous horns have been described in association with budding retrovirus particles on the footpads of a cat.[98] Whether this condition is caused by FeLV or is a coincidental finding remains unknown.

## Feline Sarcoma Virus

FeSVs are recombinant viruses that are generated de novo when FeLV DNA provirus recombines with cat cellular genomes called proto-oncogenes present in the cells of all cats. FeSVs are generated when the FeLV DNA provirus inserts near a protooncogene and transduces (takes up and includes) the proto-oncogene into the FeLV provirus.

The continued replication of FeLV for prolonged periods of time in cats increases the chances of the virus combining with one of 30 proto-oncogenes thought to exist in the cat. Twenty-five unique isolates of FeSV exist. About half have been well characterized. There is no evidence that FeSV can be transmitted between cats or to humans naturally.[99] Only 2% of fibrosarcomas in cats are thought to be caused by FeSV.[100] The FeSV fibrosarcomas present as multicentric subcutaneous masses in young cats, usually under 3 years of age. All FeSV cats are positive for FeLV. In contrast to the fibrosarcomas of older cats, the virus-induced fibrosarcomas are rapid-growing and frequently ulcerate.[101] Many occur on limbs, but others may start on the thorax and about one third of the FeSV-induced fibrosarcomas will metastasize to the lung or peritoneum. The FeSV-induced tumors are extremely anaplastic but may partially differentiate to chondrosarcomas or osteosarcomas. The doubling times of these tumors has been found to be as short as 12 hours.[98a] FeSV-induced tumors must be differentiated from nonvirally induced fibrosarcomas of older cats and vaccine-induced fibrosarcomas, the latter often also occurring in young cats. FeSV-caused fibrosarcomas are most like vaccine-induced fibrosarcomas in terms of their growth characteristics and histopathologic features but may be differentiated by the cat's FeLV status.[99] A number of tumors may be produced experimentally with FeSV, and the reader is referred to other sources for their description.[102–106]

## Detecting the Presence of FeLV

Testing for FeLV is becoming a routine clinical procedure and is often a part of feline health programs. It has been suggested that wide use of FeLV testing has been credited with a greater reduction in FeLV in the population than FeLV vaccination.[107] Indeed in the cattery population, the use of a test and removal program has been shown to eliminate FeLV from some catteries.

The basis of most testing procedures is detection of the FeLV group-specific core protein, P27. The two tests that are used for routine clinical testing are the IFA and the ELISA.[108] The IFA test is not an in-clinic test and specimens must be mailed out to specialized commercial laboratories. The IFA test is performed on smears made from peripheral blood or bone marrow. The IFA detects the presence of P27 in nucleated cells, neutrophils and platelets, or in bone marrow cells. A positive IFA correlates well with the presence of virus and viral shedding and indicates the advanced stages of FeLV infection. Despite its correlation with advanced stages of infection, a very small percentage of IFA-positive cats (3%) will be only transiently infected and thus should be retested in 3 months to increase the certainty that the infection is indeed persistent.[3,31] False positives can occur from lack of expertise, nonspecific fluorescence associated with thick blood smears, contaminated slides, platelet clumping, and eosinophilia. False negatives may occur when the number of nucleated cells on the smear are too few to evaluate in disease conditions commonly associated with FeLV infections that produce neutropenia and thrombocytopenia. IFAs depend upon advanced stages of infection to detect the presence of antigen and thus will not usually pick up early infections or sequestered infections that do not involve the bone marrow. IFA will not detect viral latency, a condition in which P27 is not being produced.

The ELISA test is commonly used in the detection of FeLV antigen and is 100 times more sensitive than the IFA for the detection of P27. It may be performed on a variety of substrates, including serum, plasma, whole blood, saliva and tears, or other body fluids.[108,109] Two ELISA formats exist: the microwell and the membrane filter format. Both perform well in the clinical setting. A positive ELISA indicates FeLV antigenemia but not necessarily viremia.[110] The increased sensitivity of the ELISA technique allows the detection of early infections, transient infections, and sequestered infections that may not be picked up by the IFA procedure. The ELISA does not detect FeLV viral latency. Thus, a negative ELISA does not necessarily assure that the cat does not contain an exogenous FeLV genome.

When testing substrates other than serum (i.e., tears or saliva), both the sensitivity and specificity of the ELISA test decline about 10 to 15%.[108,109] Healthy cats should be retested at monthly intervals for 3 months to eliminate the chances of false positives and to determine if the infection is transient or persistent in nature. False positives are most frequently seen in the microwell format and are due to technical errors associated with washing steps or magnification of specificity limitations when testing a low-risk population.[111] In the washing step, if washing is incomplete or there is splashing of conjugant between the wells, or conjugant is trapped in microdefects in the plastic microwells, or in chew marks on the plastic wand used to collect saliva, it may result in false positives.[112] Likewise, the biologic material such as bacterium, dental plaque, fibrin, etc., may trap conjugant and result in false positives. False negatives are rare, but it is important to remember that neither the ELISA or the IFA technique will detect viral latency.[110]

Although much has been written regarding the discordancy between the IFA and ELISA procedures, it is probably less than 10% using today's technologies.[113] The 10% discordancy may be explained in part by several biologic phenomena. The two most common situations responsible for discordancy (i.e. IFA negative, ELISA positive) are early infections and sequestered infections.[56,114] Most discordant cats that are repeatedly tested are found to change their testing pattern: 50% become negative on both the ELISA and IFA, 25% become positive on both, and 25% remain discordant indefinitely.[109,113,115]

## Other Tests for FeLV

Detection of FeLV latency may be valuable in the diagnosis of the neutropenic patient in ELISA-negative cats or when trying to ensure that a population of cats is completely free of FeLV. Bone marrow co-culturing has been used for the detection of FeLV latency but is limited to research laboratories.[54] The PCR has also been used by research labs and detects a provirus in infected cells and may soon become commercially available. The PCR is the most sensitive of the diagnostic tools used in medicine today and is capable of detecting FeLV latency. Samples, however, must be obtained by bone marrow biopsy in order to be the most valuable. Antibody titers against FOCMA have been used to detect previous FeLV exposure, but are thought to be unreliable in predicting viral latency.[116]

## Treatments of FeLV

Although no effective treatment exists for the elimination of FeLV from persistently infected cats, a variety of antiviral and biologic response modifiers have been used in the management of retroviral infections of cats and humans.

Specific therapies aside, the mainstay of therapy for cats infected with FeLV or other retroviruses is supportive care.[117–119] Maintaining the patient's hydration and nutritional status not only prolongs life but the quality of life of the patient. The cat should be maintained in a humid environment to reduce the chances of water losses. Appetite stimulants and placement of gastrostomy tubes may facilitate nutritional therapy. Cat requirements for B vitamins are 8 times that of dogs and must be maintained in order to maintain appetite. Semimoist cat foods often contain propylene glycol, which can shorten red cell survivals. These diets should not be used in the nutritional management of cats infected with FeLV.[118] Many FeLV-infected cats are anemic, and the tendency is to supply them with exogenous erythropoietin, however, this is of no value in the management of these cats, since erythropoietin levels are usually greater than 20 times normal in anemic cats.[120]

Blood transfusions supply RBCs and cats benefit from a variety of antileukemic factors in addition to the RBCs. One of these antileukemic factors is fibronectin.[121] Fibronectin appears to work by activating macrophages.[121] Fibronectin has also been used in the treatment of lymphomas and leukoid leukemias and erythroid leukemias. In 43 lymphoma cats treated with blood constituents or fibronectin, three cats underwent complete remission and 13 partial remissions, and one became virus negative.[122] Preventing FeLV-positive cats from contact with other cats may prevent respiratory infections or other secondary opportunistic infections, which are devastating in FeLV-positive cats. Cats previously vaccinated for the usual feline viral diseases are likely to be protected, and vaccination of sick cats is not recommended.

Extracorporeal immunoadsorption with staph protein A for removal of circulating immune complexes that are immunosuppressive has been used in the treatment of cats with lymphoma.[123] Reversal of viremia and partial and complete lymphoma remissions have been observed in about 15% of cats treated with extracorporeal immunoadsorption. One study reported a complete viral clearance and long-term remissions of lymphomas in 9 of 16 cats treated in this manner.[124] The parenteral administration of soluble protein A used in the extracorporeal system has been less successful in the treatment of lymphoma or FeLV viremia.[121]

**Bone Marrow Transplantation**   Allogenic bone marrow transplantation performed in 33 viremic cats has resulted in transient reduction in viremia in all cats.[125] The best combination is bone marrow transplantation of FeLV-immunized donors with concurrent AZT therapy whereby viremia has been shown to be reversed in several cases.[126]

**Whole-Body Hyperthermia**   Whole-body hyperthermia has been investigated in the treatment of retroviral infections. When cats were heated to 42°C for a period of 2 hours, a marked increase in endogenous interferon was noted concurrently with a decrease in virus infectivity, as measured by reverse transcriptase activity. Although whole-body hyperthermia in the production of endogenous interferon is insufficient to eliminate viremia itself, it may play an adjunctive role in a multimodality approach to the management of retroviral diseases in the future.[126]

**Diethylcarbamazine**   (Diethylcarbamazine (DEC) is used as an antifilarial drug but has immunomodulatory properties and has been shown to delay the development of lymphopenia in FeLV infections and prolong survival in viremic cats.[127] It has not, however, been shown to eliminate viremia in cats that are persistently infected.[128]

**Biologic Response Modifiers**   Imuvert, a biologic response modifier extracted from *Serratia marcescens* and *Streptococcus pyogenes,* has caused increased released of Interleukin-6 (IL-6), tumor necrosis factor (TNF), and Interleukin-1 (IL-1). In normal cats, weekly injections of Imuvert neither prevented or resulted in the reversal of FeLV viremia in experimental cats.[129]

Corynebacterium parvum, levamisole, and vitamin C have all been used in the management of FeSV or FeLV viremia. None of these have demonstrated efficacy against any retroviral infections.[121,122]

**Interferons**   Interferons have been studied extensively in the management of FeLV infections, with mixed results. In one study, the viremic cats treated with oral or parenteral doses of either human interferon alpha (IFNA) or bovine interferon have failed to change the viremia or result in clinical improvement.[130] Some uncontrolled studies have shown improvement in the clinical status of cats treated with oral interferon.[131] Controlled trials with cytokines such as interferon are needed to establish the true efficacy of these products. Orally administered interferon is likely to be inactivated, since it is destroyed by gastric acid in the stomach. Parenteral administration of cytokines such as interferon from other species, for example, bovine or human, are likely to produce only temporary improvement because of the production of antibodies against these cytokines in 3 to 7 weeks in cats.

**Acemannan (carrisyn)**   Acemannan is a biologic response modifier designed to enhance macrophage phagocytosis and killing. Viremic cats treated with acemannan were reported to be clinically improved, but the study was flawed by the absence of a control arm in the trial.[132]

Cytokines or those drugs that induce cytokines have been advocated for the treatment of viremias; however, none of the studies have been well controlled and thus the observed increased clinical benefit of the administration of these drugs may be due to the natural waxing and waning clinical course commonly observed in FeLV-positive patients. The positive evaluation of many of these drugs may in fact be due to the anabolic effect sometimes observed with them and is thought to be based on endorphin release rather than on the drugs' direct effect on the viral infection.[133]

**Reverse Transcriptase Inhibitors**   The gamut of drugs that inhibit reverse transcriptase (RT) and retroviruses integration into the host cell have been evaluated for their potential use in the treatment of FeLV-positive cats. The drugs evaluated include suramin (a polyionic dye used to treat filariasis in humans), nucleoside analogs (AZT, ddc, ddA, PMEA), glucose homopolymers, dextran sulfate, phosphonoformate, and others.[134–137] The reader is referred to more detailed descriptions of these therapies elsewhere.[134–137] In general, most of these agents have shown efficacy in vitro against FeLV, HIV, and in some cases even FIV. Most of these drugs result in some reduction in viremia, but none of the agents are capable of reversing established viremia, although some may prevent viremia if administered in a prophylactic setting. Most of these drugs have significant toxicities at dosage levels necessary to produce antiviral effects, and thus have not gained a lot of popularity in veterinary medicine.

AZT or zidovudine has been the most widely studied of the RT inhibitors. AZT inhibits FeLV RT.[138] When administered at 10 to 20 mg/kg divided dose, AZT prevents viremia if given within 72 hours of exposure to FeLV. The antiviral effects of AZT appear to be synergistic with interferon.[139,140] Reversal of established experimental FeLV viremia by adoptive transfer of Lectin/Interleukin-2-activated lymphocytes, interferon-α and AZT has recently been reported. Because of the toxicity associated with RT inhibitors, they should not be used as first-line therapy in the treatment of FeLV-related disease.[140]

## Prevention and Control

The most effective means of preventing FeLV infection is to eliminate contact with viremic cats.[141] The test and removal program is the most effective means of controlling FeLV in the multiple-cat household or cattery.[141] The program consists of closing the household or cattery to new cats. The cats maintained in the facility are tested every 3 months, and FeLV-positive cats are removed from the facility. When every cat tests negative for two consecutive testings, the facility cats are determined FeLV free. New cats may enter the FeLV-free facility only after a 3-month quarantine and two negative FeLV tests. The test and removal system has been shown to reduce the incidence of FeLV in a variety of settings and geographic locations.[141,142] However, neither of the current testing methods for FeLV or ELISA is sensitive enough to detect latently infected cats and thus the test and removal program is not always 100% effective.

## Prevention by Vaccination

Vaccination has helped control or eliminate many infectious diseases in veterinary medicine. The first commercial FeLV vaccine was introduced in 1985. Since then, seven FeLV vaccine products from six companies have been licensed for sale to veterinarians in the United States. However, despite the fact that a FeLV vaccine has been available for 7 years, a survey of the U.S. veterinary teaching hospitals in early 1991 found that only two out of 22 veterinary teaching hospitals considered FeLV vaccination as part of their routine feline preventative health programs.[143] The principal concern has been the perceived lack of efficacy of FeLV vaccines. Indeed, some studies of available vaccines have reported efficacies between 0 and 100%.[144] In addition to the efficacy concerns, it has been recently shown that soft tissue sarcomas may develop after the administration of FeLV vaccines.[145]

FeLV vaccine issues have been reviewed elsewhere[48] but several comments regarding FeLV vaccines should help the reader in deciding on the use of an FeLV vaccine. Vaccines may contain one, two, or three subgroup antigens. Since only subgroup A is transmitted contagiously between cats, vaccines need only contain subgroup A. The primary means of protecting against tumor development is preventing persistent viremia. If a vaccine protects against persistent FeLV infection, then there is no need for a vaccine to contain FOCMA. Vaccines should protect against a variety of strains of subgroup A. It is unfortunate that none of the available vaccines contain more than one strain of subgroup A. It is likely that the differences in the numerous published comparative studies of vaccine efficacy relate to differences in vaccine strains as well as challenge strains used in these studies. Vaccines that contain aluminum hydroxide in their adjuvants produce local reactions. These local reactions may be preneoplastic and lead to the development of soft-tissue sarcomas. Fibrosarcomas following vaccination with either rabies or FeLV are thought to occur in 1 : 1000 to 1 : 10,000 vaccinates.[48] Nonadjuvanted vaccines or vaccines that do not contain aluminum hydroxide have little or no reactions 21 days after their administration.[146]

FeLV vaccines should be targeted to those at greatest risk of contracting FeLV infection, i.e., the young and those where exposure is likely. The cats that are most at risk are neonates and animals; those up to 14 years of age should probably be targeted for FeLV immunization. It is clear, given the uncertain efficacy issues, and the risk of fibrosarcoma development following vaccination, that not all cats should be vaccinated for FeLV. Cats that need not be vaccinated for FeLV are those determined to be at reduced risk: A strictly indoor cat of a single-cat household, for example, whether FeLV positive or negative, should not be vaccinated. The FeLV-negative strictly indoor cats in multiple-cat households should not be vaccinated. Finally, no FeLV vaccines should be considered even close to delivering 100% protection in vaccinates. Thus FeLV vaccine should only be used as an adjunct to FeLV disease control along with the FeLV testing and the limiting of potential exposure.

## Prognosis for Positive Cats

The mean survival of cats persistently viremic with FeLV is 2 years.[1] Studies indicate that 83% of FeLV-positive cats will die in 3.5 years from the time of diagnosis, while only 14% of FeLV-negative cats will die in the same time period.[1] Kittens affected at birth have a significantly shorter survival than adults contracting this infection. The risk of cats living in households with FeLV-positive cats is variable, depending on the age and degree of contact.[1] Adult cats that have been living with a known positive cat for several months only have approximately a 10 to 15% chance of acquiring persistent infection over time.[1] This is in contrast to young kittens that may be brought into an FeLV-positive household and may have up to an 85% chance of contracting a persistent infection.[52]

## FELINE IMMUNODEFICIENCY VIRUS

FIV, classified as a member of the retroviruses, is in the subfamily *lentivirinae* and is distinct from other retroviruses infecting cats. Like other retroviruses, FIV is an enveloped, single-stranded RNA virus in which the RNA is copied into the DNA within infected host cells by the enzyme reverse transcriptase (RT) contained within the virus. The FIV RT differs from FeLV by having a trace element requirement for cation magnesium rather than manganese. The genome of FIV is more complex than FeLV and is composed of an LTR-gag pol-env-LTR. The nucleoside sequence of several FIV isolates has been determined in the genomic homology to fall between the isolates ranging from 97% to 86%. Despite the homology between the strains, significant differences in pathogenicity and infectivity exist between FIV strains.[147] The protein structure of FIV has been identified by immunoblotting and found to contain protein 120, 24, 17, and 10 kd, of which the most prominent is P24 (major core protein) and P17 (small core protein).[148] Two glycoproteins have been identified from infected cells as GP120 (major envelope protein) and GP41 (transmembrane protein).[148] The glycoproteins are important in the development of protective antibodies, and antibodies to glycoproteins and core proteins found in infected cats are important in the ELISA and Western Blot diagnostic test to identify infected cats. Cell tropism of HIV has been associated with a CD4 surface antigen marker found on helper T-lymphocytes.[149–152] Although FIV infects cells containing feline CD4 markers, it also infects CD4-negative cells and has been shown to infect CD8-lymphocytes and B-lymphocytes.[149–152]

## Transmission

FIV is present in all body fluids of infected cats (similar to FeLV) but at a much lower concentration. It is mainly cell associated and is relatively low in concentration in the blood, although high amounts are found in the saliva.[153–155] Feline immunodeficiency virus is thought not to be very infectious and is thought to be transmitted primarily through biting during cat fights.[156,157] However, on occasion, transmission through prolonged contact with infected cats has been documented.[158] Venereal transmission has not been documented and in utero transmission as well as transmission through nursing is uncommon.[154,159] Transfusions are potential sources of infections, and donor cats should always be tested for FeLV and FIV.[154]

## Epidemiology

Epidemiologic studies indicate that FIV prevalence varies in different geographic locations, but the virus has a worldwide distribution. Unlike HIV, FIV apparently is not a new virus to the United States, and antibodies to FIV have been found in the cat serum collected as early as 1968 in the United States.[160] The prevalence of FIV in a population varies dependent upon the density of free-roaming cats, the density of feral cats, and the age, sex, and housing environments of cats.[161,162] The highest prevalence of FIV is observed in populations with high densities of free-roaming, older male feral cats. These cats frequently defend territorial turf by fighting, which is thought to be the main mode of transmission of this virus.[159,161,162]

The age of cats infected with FIV ranges from a few months to over 18 years of age.[162] The median age of clinically healthy FIV-infected cats is 3 years, in contrast to sick cats, whose median age is 10 years.[163] This apparent age disparity between clinically healthy and sick cats infected with FIV reflects the relative long latency period of FIV infection, which is thought to be between 2 and 5 years.[153] The long latency period from the time of infection acquisition to the time of chronic disease development is characterized by relatively low morbidity and mortality; thus infected cats tend to accumulate in the population over time.[153]

In the United States, the prevalence of FIV is between 7 and 12% of sick cats and only 1 to 2% in healthy cats.[155] In general, the prevalence of

FIV is about one half that of FeLV in the same population, sick or healthy.[162] It is not surprising that between 70 and 90% of FIV-infected cats are also infected with the feline syncytial-forming virus, probably because of the common mode of transmission through cat bites.[155] In contrast, FIV and FeLV appear to be transmitted independently of each other.[155,162,164] FIV appears to be species specific, although serum from multiple species of wild felids such as the African lion have been found to have antibodies to FIV.[165,166] However, attempts to transmit the virus from wild felids to domestic cats has failed. These findings suggest that wild felids probably have their own species-specific lentivirus.[165,166]

## Clinical Stages of Infection

The pathogenesis and clinical course may be summarized:[153,167] Following the body's initial encounter with FIV, there is a prolonged period of sustained low-level virus replication, during which the pathogenesis involves the development of defects in the immune system. During this period, most cats are asymptomatic for many years. The progressive crippling nature of the immune dysfunction and the associated clinical course of FIV infection has been staged similarly to that of HIV infections in humans.[168,169]

The clinical course of FIV has been divided into five clinical stages similar to those used to classify HIV-positive people. These five clinical stages are as follows:[153,168,169]

1. Acute
2. Asymptomatic
3. Persistent generalized lymphadenopathy (nonneoplastic)
4. AIDS-related complex (ARC); clinical disease that does not need AIDS criteria
5. AIDS opportunistic infections, involving more than 20% weight loss, neurologic disease, malignancy[153,168]

## FIV-Associated Clinical Manifestations

The prevalence of neoplasms in FIV-positive cats ranges from 1 to 62%.[154,155,164,167,170–172] Lymphomas and myeloid tumors (myelogenous leukemia, myeloproliferative disease), and a few carcinomas and sarcomas are the neoplasms most commonly linked with FIV infections. One study found that cats infected with FIV alone are 5.6 times more likely to develop lymphoma or leukemia and that if they were infected with both FIV and FeLV, they had a 77.3 times greater likelihood of developing lymphoma or leukemia than noninfected cats.[167] Lymphoreticular neoplasms have been linked to HIV infection in people and SIV infections in nonhuman primates. In contrast to FeLV-associated lymphomas, FIV-associated lymphomas most frequently develop in extranodal sites and occur in older cats, mean age 8.7 years.[167]

Myeloproliferative diseases have been observed in naturally and experimentally FIV-infected cats.[154,155,158,173] Although lentiviruses such as FIV have not been thought to be oncogenic in themselves, they are markedly immunosuppressive and thus impair the body's normal ability to remove cancerous cells. Squamous cell carcinoma of the skin has been linked to FIV infections in two geographic areas, California and Colorado, but this association is believed to be due to a co-risk behavior (outdoor cats) rather than to any viral contribution to the tumor development.[174,175] Other reports have linked FIV infection to oral squamous cell carcinomas, mammary carcinomas, fibrosarcomas, myeloproliferative disease, and histiocytic mast cells.[153,155,164,176] The nature of these associations awaits further investigation.

Ocular manifestations of disease associated with FIV infection usually involve the anterior chamber.[177] Some have been linked to opportunistic infections such as toxoplasmosis, while others have not been associated with any specific primary etiology and may be virally induced.[177,178]

The central nervous system may also manifest clinical signs in cats infected with FIV. Neurologic disorders with FIV infection may be due to viral infection of the central nervous system, products of toxins, and virus-infected cells such as macrophages, or, less commonly, opportunistic infections such as toxoplasmosis.[179–181] In general, FIV tends to produce clinical disease in the brain, while FeLV clinical manifestations involve the spinal cord.[155,163] Clinical manifestations of the urinary tract have been reported to involve both the upper and lower urinary system.[164] Polyuric chronic renal failure in young cats and a recurrent bacterial or idiopathic cystitis are most commonly reported associated with FIV infections in cats.[155,163,182] A variety of immune-mediated disease including Coombs' positive anemia and immune-mediated arthritis have all been reported in FIV-infected cats.[155,163] Skin disease characterized by chronic abscessations, mange, or other parasitic infections have been reported in approximately 15% of FIV-positive cats.[151,154,164,183,184] Oral cavity disease is observed in 50% of cats infected with FIV. The lesions most commonly reported are chronic stomatitis and gingivitis, characterized by ulceration or proliferative lesions of the gingiva fauces and sometimes buccal mucosa. The lesions may be associated with bacterial overgrowth, other viruses such as calici viruses or herpesvirus, or may represent an aberrant immune response to FIV or other agents resulting in infiltrations of lymphocytes and plasmacytes, and are commonly referred to lymphocytic/plasmacytic stomatitis. Chronic respiratory disease and chronic diarrhea have also been commonly reported in cats with FIV, the pathogenesis of which is unknown.[154]

## Diagnosis

The most common abnormalities found in routine laboratory tests in FIV-infected cats are various cytopenias: leukopenia or thrombocytopenia, and hypergammaglobulinemia.[185] Although none of these abnormalities are considered diagnostic of FIV, their presence should alert the clinician to the possibility of FIV and the need to perform more specific confirmatory serology.[161] A clinical diagnosis of FIV infection is based on demonstration of the presence of FIV-specific antibodies in the blood of suspected cats.[154] The presence of these antibodies is an indicator of infection, and they usually appear within 2 to 4 weeks following infection and remain detectable throughout the course of infection, although they may dissipate in the terminal stage of the disease.[154]

Unlike FeLV, once infected with FIV, the cat is infected for life. There are three methods—IFA, ELISA and Western Blot—used in the clinical confirmation of the diagnosis of FIV infections.[55,158,186] The ELISA is considered the most effective and the Western Blot the most specific of the three tests used clinically. Diagnosis of FIV and FeLV differ in that the diagnosis of FIV is based on the presence of antibody, while the diagnosis of FeLV is based on detection of viral antigens.[187] The clinical signs of FeLV and FIV are so similar that clinicians should test for both FIV and FeLV if retroviral infection is suspected. The ELISA is the most frequently used diagnostic test for FIV; however, it may be associated with both false positives and false negatives.

False-negative results are uncommon but may occur as a result of testing patients too early (during the 2- to 4-week viral incubation period).[154,188]

False positives are more common when detecting antibodies to an organism than when testing for an antigen associated with the organism in a patient. False-positive tests are most frequently observed in the ELISA-based assays. It is reported that 22.5 to 35% of the positives obtained on in-house ELISA tests are considered negative when compared with the standard Western Blot.[148,189,190] False-positive tests may result from repeated routine immunization in which antibodies to small amounts of tissue culture antigens contained within the vaccine react with the cell culture antigen containing the viral antigen preparation used as targets in the ELISA test for FIV.[191] In addition, testing before 12 weeks of age may result in false-positive results, since kittens born to FIV-positive queens, although they seldom have the virus, will have maternally acquired antibodies. Fortunately, these maternal antibodies dissipate in 5 to 12 weeks, and testing of kittens over 12 weeks of age should be reliable.[192]

It is generally recommended that ELISA-positive tests from clinically healthy cats, especially from cats coming from low-risk populations, be confirmed by Western Blot (Immnoblot).[153] The minimum criteria for Western Blot positivities have been established and are the presence of antibodies to envelope proteins GP120 or because of the reactivity of nonviral antigens to some internal viral proteins/antibodies to at least three viral core proteins.[148]

## Treatment

The same treatment considerations used in the management of FeLV are used in the treatment of FIV-positive cats, and the reader is referred to the FeLV treatment section for a discussion of these issues.

## Prognosis

The mortality rate in asymptomatic FIV-infected cats is better than in cats infected with FeLV. Because of the prolonged latency period, asymptomatic FIV-positive cats may live many years prior to developing chronic disease associated with advanced stages of infection and immunosuppression. However, when cats reach the advanced stage (stage 5) and manifest clinical signs of ARC or AIDS-like disease, the prognosis is grave and survival is short—1 to 6 months. The reported 1-year survival rate of FIV-infected cats (presumably symptomatic) ranges from 13.5 to 24.5%.[157] The 6-month mortality rate has been reported to range from 14 to 48%.[157] Cats coinfected with FeLV, however, have a shorter survival and die at a younger age than do cats infected with FIV alone.

## Prevention

Because of the low transmissibility, a test and removal program similar to that recommended for more contagious FeLV is not applicable.[193] However, if an owner of a multiple-cat household or cattery wishes to reduce all chances of transmission, he or she may institute the test and removal program. As with FeLV, all blood donors should be screened for antibodies against FIV prior to donating for transfusion. At this time, though, no commercially available FIV vaccine exists. Experimental evidence suggests that FIV vaccines can be produced; however, cross-protection against the many varieties of strains of FIV in nature is unlikely.[193]

## REFERENCES

1. Hardy WD JR, Hess PW, MacEwen EG, et al: Biology of feline leukemia virus in the natural environment. Cancer Res 36:582–584, 1976.
2. Essex M: Feline leukemia and sarcoma viruses. In Klein G (ed): Viral Oncology. New York, Raven Press, 1980, p. 205.
3. Hardy WD Jr: The feline leukemia virus. J Am Anim Hosp Assoc 17:951, 1981.
4. McAllister RM, Nicolson M, Gardner MB, et al: C type virus released from cultured human rhabdomyosarcoma cells. Nature New Biol 235:3, 1972.
5. Livingston DM, Todaro GJ: Endogenous type C virus from a cat cell clone with properties distinct from previously described feline type C virus. Virology 53:142, 1973.
6. Bonner TI, Todaro GJ: Carnivores have sequences in their cellular DNA distantly related to the primate endogenous virus. Virology 94:224, 1979.
7. Todaro GJ, Benveniste RE, Sherwin SA, Sherr EJ: MAC-1, a new genetically transmitted type C virus of primates: Low frequency activation from stumptail monkey cell cultures. Cell 3:775, 1978.
8. Mullins JI: Evolution of feline retroviruses. In UCLA Molecular Symposium on Viruses and Human Cancer, Park City, UT, February 1986.
9. Benveniste RE, Sherr CJ, Todaro GJ: Evolution of type C viral genes: Origin of feline leukemia virus. Science 190:886, 1975.
10. Schafer W, Bolognesi DP: Mammalian type C oncornaviruses: Relationships between viral structure and cell surface antigens and their possible significance in immunological defense mechanisms. Contemp Top Immunobiol 6:127, 1977.
11. Bolognesi DP, Montelaro RC, Frank H, et al: Assembly of type C oncornaviruses: A model. Science 199:183, 1978.
12. Hardy WD Jr: Immunology of oncornaviruses. Vet Clin North Am Small Anim Pract 4:133, 1974.
13. Sarma PS, Log T: Subgroup classification of feline leukemia and sarcoma viruses by viral interference and neutralization tests. Virology 54:160, 1973.
14. Sarma PS, Log T, Jain D, et al: Differential host range of viruses of feline leukemia-sarcoma complex. Virology 64:438, 1975.
15. Velicer LF, Graves DC: Properties of feline leukemia virus. II. In vitro labeling of the polypeptides. J Virol 14:700, 1974.
16. Hardy WD Jr, Hirshaut Y, Hess P: Detection of the feline leukemia virus and other mammalian oncornaviruses by immunofluorescence. In Dutcher RM, Chieco-Bianchi L (eds): Unifying Concepts of Leukemia. Karger, Basel, 1973, p. 778.
17. Saxinger C, Essex M, Hardy W, Gallo R: Detection of antigen related to feline leukemia virus in the sera of "virus-negative" cats. Dev Cancer Res 4:489, 1980.
18. Lutz H, Pedersen NC, Higgins J, et al: Quantitation of P27 in the serum of cats during natural infection with feline leukemia virus. Dev Cancer Res 4:497, 1980.
19. Kahn DE, Mia AS, Tierney MM: Field evaluation of Leukassay F, an FeLV detection test kit. Feline Pract 10:41, 1980.
20. Mia AS, Kahn De, Tierney MM, et al: A microenzyme-linked immunosorbent assay (ELISA) test for detection of feline leukemia virus in cats. Comp Immunol Microbiol Infect Dis 4:111, 1981.
21. Lutz H, Pedersen NC, Theilen GH: Course of feline leukemia virus infection and its detection by enzyme-linked immunosorbent assay and monoclonal antibodies. Am J Vet Res 44:2054, 1983.
22. Francis DP, Essex M, Gayzagian D: Feline leukemia virus: Survival under home and laboratory conditions. J Clin Microbiol 9:154, 1979.
23. Heding LD, Schaller JP, Blakeslee JR, et al: Inactivation of tumor cell-associated feline oncornavirus for preparation of an infectious virus-free tumor cell immunogen. Cancer Res 36:1647, 1976.
24. Francis DP, Essex M, Hardy WD Jr: Excretion of feline leukemia virus by naturally infected pet cats. Nature 269:252, 1977.
25. Hoover EA, Olsen RG, Hardy WD Jr: Horizontal transmission of feline leukemia virus under experimental conditions. J Natl Cancer Inst 58:443, 1977.
26. Hoover EA, Mullins JI: Feline leukemia virus infection and diseases. J Am Vet Med Assoc 199:1287, 1991.

27. Dornsife RE, Gasper PW, Mullins JI: Induction of aplastic anemia by intrabone marrow inoculation of a molecularly cloned feline retrovirus. Leuk Res 13:745, 1989.

28. Dornsife RE, Gasper PW, Mullins JI, et al: In vitro erythrocytopathic activity of an aplastic anemia-inducing feline retrovirus. Exp Hematol 17:138, 1989.

29. Yamamoto JK, Hansen H, Ho EW, et al: Epidemiological and clinical aspects of feline immunodeficiency virus infection in cats from the continental United States and Canada and possible mode of transmission. J Am Vet Med Assoc 194:213, 1989.

30. Shelton GH, Waltier RM, Connor SC, et al: Prevalence of feline immunodeficiency virus and feline leukemia virus infections in pet cats. J Am Anim Hosp Assoc 25:7, 1989.

31. Hardy WD Jr, Old LJ, Hess PW, et al: Horizontal transmission of feline leukaemia virus. Nature 24:266, 1973.

32. Essex M, Cotter SM, Sliski AH, et al: Horizontal transmission of feline leukaemia under natural conditions in a feline leukaemia cluster household. Int J Cancer 19:90, 1977.

33. Jarrett O, Hardy WD Jr, Golder MC, et al: The frequency of occurrence of feline leukaemia virus subgroups in cats. Int J Cancer 21:334, 1978.

34. Jarrett O, Russell PH: Differential growth + transmission in cats of feline leukaemia viruses of subgroups A and B. Int J Cancer 21:466, 1978.

35. Rosenburg Z, Pederson FF, Haseltine WA: Comparative analysis of the genome of feline leukemia virus. J Virol 35:542, 1980.

36. Sarma PS, Log T, Skuntz S, et al: Experimental horizontal transmission of feline leukemia viruses of subgroups A, B and C. J Natl Cancer Inst 60:871, 1978.

37. Tzavaras T, Stewart M, McDougall A, et al: Molecular cloning and characterization of a defective recombinant feline leukaemia virus associated with myeloid leukaemia. J Gen Virol 71:343, 1990.

38. Stewart MA, Warnock M, Wheeler A, et al: Nucleotide sequences of a feline leukemia virus subgroup: An envelope gene and long terminal repeat and evidence for the recombinational origin of subgroup B viruses. J Virol 58:825, 1986.

39. Elder JM, Mullins JI: Nucleotide sequence of the envelope gene of Gardner-Arnstein feline leukemia virus B reveals unique sequence homologies with a murine mink cell focus-forming virus. J Virol 46:871, 1983.

40. Nunberg JH, Williams ME, Innis MA: Nucleotide sequences of the envelope genes of two isolates of feline leukemia virus subgroup B. J Virol 49:629, 1984.

41. Neil JC, Fulton R, Rigby M, et al: Evolution of pathogenic and oncogenic variants of FeLV. Curr Top Microbiol Immunol 171:67, 1991.

42. Jarrett O: Pathogenicity of feline leukemia virus is commonly associated with variant viruses. Leukemia 6 (Suppl 3):153S, 1992.

43. Tzavara T, Testa N, Neil JC, et al: Isolation and characterization of a myeloid leukemia inducing strain of feline leukemia virus. Hematol Bluttransfus Mod Trends Hum Leuke 8:347, 1989.

44. Rigby MA, Rojko JL, Stewart MA, et al: Partial dissociation of subgroup C phenotype and in vivo behaviour in feline leukaemia viruses with chimeric envelope genes. J Gen Virol 73:2839, 1992.

45. Essex M, Klein G, Snyder SP, et al: Feline sarcoma virus (FSV)-induced tumors: Correlation between humoral antibody and tumor regression. Nature 233:195, 1971.

46. Vedbrat S, Rasheed S, Lutz H, et al: Feline oncornavirus-associated cell membrane antigen: A viral and not a cellularly coded transformation-specific antigen of cat lymphomas. Virology 124:445, 1983.

47. Snyder HW, Singhal MC, Zuckerman EE, et al: The feline oncornavirus-associated cell membrane antigen (FOCMA) is related to, but distinguishable from, FeL V-C gp70. Virology 131:315, 1983.

48. Macy DW: Vaccination against feline retroviruses. In August J (ed): Consultations in Feline Internal Medicine. Philadelphia, WB Saunders, 1994, pp. 33–39.

49. Rojko JL, Hoover EA, Mathes LE, et al: Pathogenesis of experimental feline leukemia virus infection. J Natl Cancer Inst 63:759, 1979.

50. Rojko JL, Hoover EA, Matnes LE, et al: Detection of feline leukemia virus in tissues of cats by a paraffin embedding immunofluorescence procedure. J Natl Cancer Inst 61:1315, 1978.

51. Hoover EA, Rojko JL, Olsen RG: Host-virus interactions in progressive versus regressive feline leukemia virus infection in cats. In Essex M, Todaro G, zur Hausen H (eds): Viruses in Naturally Occurring Cancer. Cold Spring Harbor, NY, Cold Spring Harbor Laboratory Press, 1980, p. 635.

52. Hoover EA, Olsen RG, Hardy WD Jr, et al: Feline leukemia virus infection: Age-related variation in response of cats to experimental infection. J Natl Cancer Inst 57:365, 1976.

53. Madewell BR, Jarrett O: Recovery of feline leukemia virus from non-viremic cats. Vet Rec 112:339, 1983.

54. Rojko JL, Hoover EA, Quakenbush SL, Olsen RG: Reactivation of latent feline leukemia virus infection. Nature 198:385, 1982.

55. Post J, Warren L: Reactivation of latent feline leukemia virus. Dev Cancer Res 4:151, 1980.

56. Hayes KA, Rojko JL, Tarr MJ, et al: Atypical localized viral expression in a feline leukemia virus-infected cat. Vet Rec 124:344, 1989.

57. Dorn CR, Taylor DON, Schneider R, et al: Survey of animal neoplasms in Alameda and Contra Cost counties, California. II. Cancer morbidity in dogs and cats from Alameda county. J Natl Cancer Inst 40:307, 1968.

58. Schneider R: Comparison and age- and sex-specific incidence rate patterns of the leukemia complex in the cat and the dog. J Natl Cancer Inst 70:971, 1983.

59. Reinacher M: Diseases associated with spontaneous feline leukemia virus (FeL V) infection in cats. Vet Immunol Immunopathol 21:85, 1989.

60. Hardy WD Jr: Feline leukemia and sarcoma viruses. Dev Oncol 28:289, 1985.

61. Hardy WD Jr, Zuckerman EE, Essex M, et al: Feline oncornavirus-associated cell membrane antigen: An FeLV- and FeSV-induced tumor-specific antigen. In Clarkson B, Marks PA, Till JE (eds): Differentiation of Normal and Neoplastic Hematopoietic Cells. Cold Spring Harbor, NY, Cold Spring Harbor Laboratory Press, 1978, p. 601.

62. Snyder HW JR, Hardy WD Jr, Zuckerman EE, Fleissner E: Characterization of a tumor-specific antigen on the surface of feline lymphosarcoma cells. Nature 275:657, 1978.

63. Hardy WD Jr, McClelland AJ, Zuckerman EE, et al: Development of virus nonproducer lymphosarcomas in pet cats exposed to FeLV. Nature 288:90, 1980.

64. Hoover EA, Perryman LE, Kociba GJ: Early lesions in cats inoculated with feline leukemia virus. Cancer Res 33:145, 1973.

64a. Jackson ML, Haines DM, Meric SM, Misra V: Feline leukemia virus detection in paraffin-embedded, formalin-fixed tissues by polymerase chain reaction and immunohisto chemistry[10]. ACVIM Forum Proceedings, San Diego, 1992, p. 804.

65. Gruffyd-Jones TJ, Gaskell CJ: Clinical and radiological features of anterior mediastinal lymphosarcoma in the cat: A review of 30 cases. Vet Rec 104:304, 1979.

66. Essex M, Cotter SM, Hardy WJ Jr, et al: Feline oncornavirus-associated cell membrane antigen. IV. Antibody titers in cats with naturally occurring leukemia, lymphoma and other diseases. J Natl Cancer Inst 55:463, 1975.

67. Hardy WD Jr: Hematopoietic tumors of cats. J Am Anim Hosp Assoc 17:921, 1981.

68. Schneider R: Feline malignant lymphoma: Environmental factors and the occurence of this viral cancer in cats. Int J Cancer 10:345, 1972.

69. Linenberger ML, Abkowitz JL: In vivo infection of marrow stromal fibroblasts by feline leukemia virus. Exp Hematol 20:1022, 1992.

70. Essex M. Cotter SM, Stephenson JR, et al: Leukemia, lymphoma and fibrosarcoma of cats as models for similar diseases of man. In Hiatt HH, Watson JD (eds): Origins of Human Cancer. Cold Spring Harbor, NY, Cold Spring Harbor Laboratory Press, 1977, p. 1191.

71. Cotter SM, Essex ME: Animal model of human disease: Feline acute lymphoblastic leukemia and aplastic anemia. Am J Pathol 87:265, 1977.

72. Cotter SM, Hardy WD Jr, Essex ME: Association of feline leukemia virus with lymphosarcoma and other disorders in the cat. J Am Vet Med Assoc 166:449, 1975.

73. Hardy WD Jr: Feline leukemia virus nonneoplastic disorders. J Am Anim Hosp Assoc 17:941, 1981.

74. Kociba GJ: Hematologic consequences of feline leukemia virus infection. In Kirk RW (ed): Current Veterinary Therapy. Philadelphia, WB Saunders, 1986, p. 488.

75. Wardrop KJ, Kramer JW, Abkowitz JL, et al: Quantitative studies of erythropoiesis in the clinically normal, phlebotomized, and feline leukemia virus-infected cat. Am J Vet Res 478:2274, 1986.

76. Mackey L: Feline leukaemia virus and its clinical effects in cats. Vet Rec 96:5, 1975.

77. Testa NG, Onions DE, Lord BI: A feline model for the myelodysplastic syndrome: Preleukaemic abnormalities caused in cats by infections with a new isolate of feline leukaemia virus (FeLV). AB/GM1. Haematologica 73:371, 1988.

78. Dunn JK, Searcy GP, Hirsch VM: The diagnostic significance of a positive direct antiglobulin test in anemic cats. Can J Comp Med 48:349, 1984.

79. Hoover EA, Kociba GJ: Bone lesions in cats with anemia induced by feline leukemia virus. J Natl Cancer Inst 53:1277, 1984.

80. Kociba GJ, Weiser MG, Olsen RG: Enhanced susceptibility to feline leukemia virus in cats with Haemobartonella felis infection. Leuk Rev Int 1:88 (Abstract); Vet Bull 55:1021, 1985.

81. McKey LJ, Jarrett WFH, Jarrett O, Laird H: Anemia associated with feline leukemia virus infection in cats. J Natl Cancer Inst 54:1, 1975.

82. Swenson C, Kociba GJ, O'Keefe D, et al: Cyclic hematopoiesis in feline leukemia virus-infected cats. J Am Vet Med Assoc 191:93, 1987.

83. Pedersen NC, Theilen G, Keane MA, et al: Studies of naturally transmitted feline leukemia virus infection. Am J Vet Res 38:1523, 1977.

84. Lester SJ, Searcy GP: Hematologic abnormalities preceding apparent recovery from feline leukemia virus infection. J Am Vet Med Assoc 178:471, 1981.

85. Hardy WD Jr: Immunopathology induced by the feline leukemia virus. Springer Semin Immunopathol 5:75, 1982.

86. Boyce JT, Kociba GJ, Jacobs RM, Weiser RG: Feline leukemia virus-induced thrombocytopenia and macrothrombocytosis in cats. Vet Pathol 23:16, 1986.

87. Jacobs RM, Boyce JT, Kociba GJ: Flow cytometric and radioisotopic determination of platelet survival time in normal cats and feline leukemia virus-infected cats. Cytometry 7:64, 1986.

88. Laird HM, Jarrett O, Anderson LJ, Jarrett WFH: Electron microscopic detection of viruses in feline lymphosarcoma. J Am Vet Med Assoc 155:1109, 1971.

89. Hoover EA, McCullough CB, Griesemer RA: Intranasal transmission of feline leukemia. J Natl Cancer Inst 48:973, 1972.

90. Overbaugh J, Donahue PR, Quackenbush SL, et al: Molecular cloning of a feline leukemia virus that induces fatal immunodeficiency disease in cats. Science 239:906, 1988.

91. Mullins JI, Chen CS, Hoover EA: Disease-specific

and tissue-specific production of unintegrated feline leukemia virus variant DNA in feline AIDS. Nature 319:332, 1986.

92. Hardy WD Jr: The virology, immunology and epidemiology of the feline leukemia virus. Dev Cancer Res 4:33, 1980.

93. Brightman AH II, Macy DW, Gosselin Y: Pupillary abnormalities associated with the feline leukemia complex. Feline Pract 5:23, 1977.

94. Brightman AH II, Ogilvie GK, Tompkins M: Ocular disease in FeLV-positive cats: 11 cases (1981–1986). J Am Vet Med Assoc 98:1049–1051, 1991.

95. Gasper GW, Whalen LR, Overbaugh J, et al: Isolation and preliminary characterization of a neurotropic strain of feline leukemia virus. In Proc Fifth Int AIDS Conf, Montreal, 1989.

96. Dow SW, Hoover EA: Neurologic disease associated with feline retroviral infection. In Kirk RW, Bonagura JD (eds): Current Veterinary Therapy, Vol. XI. Philadelphia, WB Saunders, 1992, p. 1010.

97. Spodnick GJ, Berg J, Moore FM, Cotter SM: Spinal lymphoma in cats: 21 cases (1977–1989). J Am Vet Med Assoc 200:373, 1992.

98. Center SA, Scott DW, Scott FW: Multiple cutaneous horns on the footpads of a cat. Feline Pract 12:26, 1982.

98a. Rojko JL, Hardy WD Jr: Feline leukemia virus and other retroviruses. In Sherding RG (ed): The Cat Diseases and Clinical Management. New York, Churchill Livingston, 1989, pp. 229–333.

99. Rojko JL, Hardy WD Jr: Feline leukemia virus and other retroviruses. In Sherding RG (ed): The Cat Diseases and Clinical Management, 2nd ed, New York, Churchill Livingston, 1994, pp. 263–432.

100. Hardy WD Jr: The feline sarcoma viruses. J Am Anim Hosp Assoc 17:981, 1981.

101. Patnaik AK, Liu SK, Hurvitz AI, McClelland AJ: Nonhematopoietic neoplasms in cats. J Natl Cancer Inst 54:855, 1975.

102. Naharro G, Robbins KC, Reddy EP: Gene product of v-fgr onc: Hybrid protein containing a portion of actin and tyrosine-specific protein kinase. Science 223:63, 1984.

103. Stephens LC, King GK, Jardine JH: Attempted transmission of a feline virus-associated liposarcoma to newborn kittens. Vet Pathol 21:614, 1984.

104. McCullough B, Schaller J, Shadduck JA, Yohn DS: Induction of malignant melanomas associated with fibrosarcomas in gnotobiotic cats inoculated with Gardner feline fibrosarcoma virus. J Natl Cancer Inst 48:1893, 1972.

105. Schaller JP, Essex M, Yohn DS, Olsen RG: Feline oncornavirus-associated cell membrane antigen. V. Humoral immune response to virus and cell membrane antigens in cats inoculated with Gardner-Arnstein feline sarcoma virus. J Natl Cancer Inst 55:1373, 1975.

106. Shadduck JA, Albert DM, Niederkorn JY: Feline uveal melanomas induced with feline sarcoma

virus: Potential model of the human counterpart. J Natl Cancer Inst 67:619, 1982.

107. Neils Pedersen: Personal communication.

108. Panel Report on the Colloquium on Feline Leukemia Virus/Feline Immunodeficiency Virus: Tests and Vaccination. J Am Vet Med Assoc 199:1273, 1991.

109. Hawkins EC, Johnson K, Pedersen NC, Winston S: Use of tears for diagnosis of feline leukemia virus infection. J Am Vet Med Assoc 188:1031, 1986.

110. Hardy WD Jr, Zuckerman EE: Ten-year study comparing enzyme-linked immunosorbent assays with the immunofluorescent antibody test for detection of feline leukemia virus infection in cats. J Am Vet Med Assoc 199:1365, 1991.

111. Jacobson RH, Lopez NA: Comparative study of diagnostic testing for feline leukemia virus infection. J Am Vet Med Assoc 199:1389, 1991.

112. Tonelli QJ: Enzyme-linked immunosorbent assay methods for detection of feline leukemia virus and feline immunodeficiency virus. J Am Vet Med Assoc 199:1336, 1991.

113. Jarrett O, Pacitti AM, Hosie MJ, Reid G: Comparison of diagnostic methods for feline leukemia virus and feline immunodeficiency virus. J Am Vet Med Assoc 199:1362, 1991.

114. Jarrett O, Golder MC, Stewart MF: Detection of transient and persistent feline leukaemia virus infections. Vet Rec 110:381, 1982.

115. Pacitti AM, Jarrett O, Hay D: Transmission of feline leukaemia virus in the mild of a non-viremic cat. Vet Rec 118:381, 1986.

116. Essex M, Klein G, Snyder SP, Harrold JB: Antibody to feline oncornavirus-associated cell membrane antigen in neonatal cats. Int J Cancer 8:384, 1971.

117. Cotter SM: Feline leukemia virus: Pathophysiology, prevention and treatment. Cancer Invest 10:173, 1992.

118. Cotter SM: Management of health feline leukemia virus-positive cats. J Am Vet Med Assoc 199:1470, 1991.

119. August JR: Husbandry practices for cats infected with feline leukemia virus or feline immunodeficiency virus. J Am Vet Med Assoc 199:1474, 1991.

120. Kociba GJ, Lange RD, Dunn CD, Hoover EA: Serum erythropoietin changes in cats with feline leukemia virus-induced erythroid aplasia. Vet Pathol 20:548, 1983.

121. MacEwen EG: Current immunotherapeutic approaches in small animals. In Proceedings of the Kal Kan Symposium on Oncology, Columbus, Ohio, 1986, p. 47.

122. MacEwen EG: Current concepts in cancer therapy: Biologic therapy and chemotherapy. Semin Vet Med Surg 1:5, 1986.

123. Snyder HW Jr, Singhal MC, Hardy WD Jr, Jones FR: Clearance of feline leukemia virus from persistently infected pet cats treated by extracorporeal immunoadsorption is correlated with an

enhanced antibody response to FeLV gp70. J Immunol *132:1538, 1984.*

124. Snyder HW Jr, Reed DE, Jones FR: Remission of FeLV-associated lymphosarcoma and persistent viral infection after extracorporeal immunoadsorption of plasma using staphylococcal protein A columns: Details of immune response. Semin Hematol *26* (Suppl. 1):25, 1989.

125. Gasper PW, Fulton R, Thrall MA: Bone marrow transplantation: Update and current considerations. *In* Kirk RW, Bonagura JD (eds): Current Veterinary Therapy, Vol XI. Philadelphia, WB Saunders, 1992, p. 493.

126. Macy DW: Unpublished data.

127. Kitchen LW, Mather FJ: Hematologic effects of short-term oral diethylcarbamazine treatment given to chronically feline leukemia virus infected cats. Cancer Lett *45:*183, 1989.

128. Kitchen LW, Cotter SM: Effect of diethylcarbamazine on serum antibody to feline oncornavirus-associated cell membrane antigen in feline leukemia virus-infected cats. J Clin Lab Immunol *25:*101, 1988.

129. Elmslie RE, Ogilvie GK, Dow SW, et al: Evaluation of a biologic response modifier derived from *Serratia marcescens:* Effects on feline macrophages and usefulness for the prevention and treatment of viremia in feline leukemia virus-infected cats. Mol Biother *3:*231, 1991.

130. Beck ER: Clinical and experimental interferon therapy in the cat. Proc Vet Cancer Soc *21,* 1985.

131. Tompkins MB, Cummins JM: Response of feline leukemia virus-induced nonregenerative anemia to oral administration of an interferon-containing preparation. Feline Pract *12:*6, 1982.

132. Tizard I: Use of immunomodulators as an aid to clinical management of feline leukemia virus-infected cats. J Am Vet Med Assoc *199:*1482, 1991.

133. Koech DR, Obel AO, Minowada J, et al: Low dose oral α-interferon therapy for patients seropositive for human immunodeficiency virus type-1 (HIV-1). Mol Biother *2:*91, 1990.

134. Polas PV, Swenson CL, Sams R, et al: In vitro and in vivo evidence that the antiviral activity of 2'3'-dideoxycytidine is target cell-dependent in a feline retrovirus animal model. Antimicrob Agents Chemother *34:*1414, 1990.

135. Zeidner NS, Strobel JD, Perigo NA, et al: Treatment of FeLV-induced immunodeficiency syndrome (FeLV-FAIDS) with controlled release capsular implantation of 2',3'-dideoxycytidine. Antiviral Res *11:*147, 1989.

136. DeClerq E, Sakuma T, Baba M, et al: Antiviral activity of phosphonymethoxyalkyl derivatives of purines and pyrimidines. Antiviral Res *8:*261, 1987.

137. Hoover EA, Ebner JP, Zeidner NS, Mullins JI: Early therapy of feline leukemia virus infection (FeLV-FAIDS) with 9-(2-phosphonylmethoxyethyl) adenine (PMEA). Antiviral Res *16:*77, 1991.

138. Hoover EA, Zeidner NS, Mullins JI: Therapy of presymptomatic FeLV-induced immunodeficiency syndrome with AZT in combination with α-interferon. Ann NY Acad Sci *616:*258, 1990.

139. Zeidner NS, Myles MH, Mathiason-DuBard CK, et al: α-Interferon (2b) in combination with zidovudine for the treatment of presymptomatic feline leukemia virus-induced immunodeficiency syndrome. Antimicrob Agents Chemother *34:*1749, 1990.

140. Zeidner NS, Mathiason-DuBard CK, Hoover EA: Reversal of feline leukemia virus infection by adoptive transfer of lectin/interleukin-2-activated lymphocytes, interferon-α and zidovudine. J of Immunother *14:*22-32, 1993.

141. Hardy WD Jr, McClelland AJ, Zuckerman EE, et al: Prevention of the contagious spread of feline leukaemia virus and the development of leukemia in pet cats. Nature *263:*326, 1976.

142. Weijer K, UytdeHaag FG, Osterhaus AD: Control of feline leukaemia virus. Vet Immunol Immunopathol *21:*69, 1989.

143. Macy DW: Unpublished data, 1992.

144. Legendre AM, Hawks DM and Sebring R: Comparison of the efficacy of three commercial FeLV vaccines in a natural challenge. J Am Vet Med Assoc *199:*1446–1452, 1991.

145. Hendrick WH, Kass PH, McGill LD, Tizarol IR: Postvaccinal sarcomas in cats. J Natl Cancer Inst *86:*5,341–343, 1994.

146. Macy DW: Unpublished data, 1994.

147. Sieblink HJ, Chu I, Rimmelzwaan GF, et al: Isolation and partial characterization of infectious molecular clones of feline immunodeficiency virus directly obtained from bone marrow DNA of a naturally infected cat. Proc First Int Conf Feline Immunodefic Virus Researchers, Sept. 4–7, University of California, Davis, California, 1990, p. 39.

148. Hoise MJ, Jarrett O: Serological responses of cats to feline immunodeficiency virus. AIDS *4:*215, 1990.

149. Pedersen NC: Feline immunodeficiency virus. *In* Schellekens LT, Horzinek MC (eds): Animal Models in AIDS. Amsterdam, Esevier, 1990, p. 165.

150. Pedersen NC, Torten M, Ridewout B, et al: Feline leukemia virus infection as a potentiating cofactor for the primary and secondary stages of experimentally-induced feline immunodeficiency virus infection. J Virol *64:*598, 1990.

151. Novotney C, English RV, Houseman V, et al: Lymphocyte population changes in cats naturally infected with feline immunodeficiency virus. J Acquir Immune Defic Syndr *4:*1213, 1990.

152. Ackley CD, Yamamoto JK, Levy N, et al: Immunologic abnormalities in pathogen-free cats experimentally infected with feline immunodeficiency virus. J Acquir Immune Defic Syndr *4:*1213, 1990.

153. Pedersen NC, Barlough JE: Clinical overview of feline immunodeficiency virus. J Am Vet Med Assoc *199:*1298, 1991.

154. Yamamoto JK, Sparger E, Ho EW, et al: Pathogenesis of experimentally-induced feline immunodeficiency virus infection in cats. Am J Vet Res 49:1246, 1988.

155. Yamamoto JK, Hansen H, Ho EW, et al: Epidemiologic and clinical aspects of feline immunodeficiency virus infection in cats from the continental United States and Canada and possible mode of transmission. J Am Vet Med Assoc 194:213, 1989.

156. North TW, North GLT, Pedersen NC: Feline immunodeficiency virus, a model for reverse transcriptase-targeted chemotherapy for acquired immune deficiency syndrome. Antimicrob Agents Chemother 33:915, 1989.

157. Fleming EJ, McCaw DL, Smith JA, et al: Clinical hematologic and survival data from cats infected with feline immunodeficiency virus: 42 cases (1983–1988). J Am Vet Med Assoc 199:913, 1991.

158. Pedersen NC, Ho EW, Brown ML, et al: Isolation of a T-lymphotropic virus from domestic cats with an immunodeficiency-like syndrome. Science 235:790, 1987.

159. Wasmoen T, Armiger-Luhman S, Egan C, et al: Transmission of feline immunodeficiency virus from infected queens to kittens. Vet Immunol Immunopathol 35:83, 1992.

160. Shelton GH, Grant CK, Cotter SM, et al: Feline immunodeficiency virus (FIV) and feline leukemia virus (FeLV) infections and their relationships to lymphoid malignancies in cats: a retrospective study. J Acquir Immune Defic Syndr 3:623, 1990.

161. Pedersen NC: Feline immunodeficiency virus infection. In Pratt PW (ed): Feline infectious diseases. Goleta, CA, American Veterinary Publications, 1988, p. 115.

162. O'Connor TP, Quentin JT, Scarlett JM: Report of the national FeLV/FIV awareness project. J Am Vet Med Assoc 199:1348, 1991.

163. Shelton GH, Waltier RM, Connor SC, et al: Prevalence of feline immunodeficiency virus infections in pet cats. J Am Anim Hosp Assoc 25:7, 1989.

164. Ishida T, Wahiza T, Toriyabe K, et al: Feline immunodeficiency virus infection in cats in Japan. J Am Vet Med Assoc 194:221, 1989.

165. Lutz H, Ishenbugel E, Lehmann R, et al: Retrovirus serology in nondomestic felids. Proc First Int Conf Feline Immunodefici Virus Researchers, University of California, Davis, 1991, p. 18.

166. Barr MC, Calle PP, Roelke ME, et al: Feline immunodeficiency virus infection in nondomestic felids. J Zoo Wild Med 20:265, 1989.

167. Ishida T, Tomoda I: Clinical staging of feline immunodeficiency virus infection. Jpn J Vet Sci 52:645, 1990.

168. Cooper DA, Gold J, Maclean P, et al: Acute AIDS retrovirus infection: Definition of a clinical illness associated with seroconversion. Lancet 1:537, 1985.

169. Ishida T, Taniguchi A, Matsamura S, et al: Long-term clinical observations on feline immunodeficiency virus-infected asymptomatic carriers. Vet Immunol Immunopathol 35:15, 1992.

170. Shelton GH, Grant CK, Cotter SM, et al: Feline immunodeficiency virus and feline leukemia virus infections and their relationships to lymphoid malignancies in cats: A retrospective study (1968–1988). J Aquir Immune Defic Syndr 3:623, 1990.

171. Sabine M, Michelsen J, Thomas F, et al: Feline AIDS. Aust Vet Pract 18:105, 1988.

172. Zenger E: Clinical findings in cats with feline immunodeficiency virus. Feline Pract 18:25, 1990.

173. Swinney GR, Pauli JV, Hones BE, et al: Feline T-lymphotrophic virus (FTLV) in cats in New Zealand. NZ Vet J 37:41, 1989.

174. Hutson CA, Rideout BA, Pedersen NC: Neoplasia associated with feline immunodeficiency virus infection in cats of Southern California. J Am Vet Med Assoc 199:1357, 1991.

175. Macy DW, Podolsiki CL, Collins J: Prevalence of FeLV and FIV high risk cats in Northeastern Colorado. Proc 10th Annu Vet Cancer Soc Conf 1990, p. 38.

176. Neu H: FIV (FTLV)-infektion der Katze: II Falle Beitrag zur epidemiologic, klinischen symptomatologie undzum krankheitsverlauf. Kleintierpraxis 34:373, 1989.

177. English RV, Davidson MG, Maisse MP, et al: Intraocular disease associated with feline immunodeficiency virus infection in cats. J Am Vet Med Assoc 196:1116, 1990.

178. Lappin MR, Greene CE, Winston S, et al: Clinical feline toxoplasmosis. J Vet Intern Med 3:139, 1990.

179. Dow SW, Poss ML, Hoover EA: Feline immunodeficiency virus: A neurotropic lentivirus. J Acquir Immune Defic Syndr 3:658, 1990.

180. Podell M, Oglesbee M, Mathes L, et al: AIDS-associated encephalopathy with experimental feline immunodeficiency virus infection. J Acquir Immune Defic Syndr 6:758, 1993.

181. Heidel JR, Dubey JP, Blythe LL, et al: Myelitis in a cat infected with Toxoplasma gondii and feline immunodeficiency virus. J Am Vet Med Assoc 196:316, 1990.

182. Thomas JB, Robinson WF, Chadwick BJ, et al: Association of renal disease indicators with feline immunodeficiency virus infection. Proc Int Conf Feline Immunodefic Virus Researchers, University of California, Davis, 1991, p. 3.

183. Chalmers S, Schick RO, Jeffers J: Demodicosis in two cats seropositive for feline immunodeficiency virus. J Am Vet Med Assoc 194:256, 1989.

184. Pedersen NC: Feline syncytium-forming virus infection. In Holzworth J (ed): Diseases of the cat. Philadelphia, WB Saunders, 1987, p. 268.

185. Shelton GH, Linenberger ML, Abkowitz JC: Hematologic abnormalities in cats seropositive

for feline immunodeficiency virus. J Am Vet Med Assoc 199:1353, 1991.

186. O'Connor TP, Tanguay S, Seinman R, et al: Development and evaluation of immunoassay of detection of antibodies to the feline T-lymphotropic lentivirus (feline immunodeficiency virus). J Clin Microbiol 27:474, 1989.

187. Hardy WD Jr: General principles of retroviral immunodetection tests. J Am Vet Med Assoc 199:1282, 1991.

188. Sparger EE: Feline immuno-deficiency virus. In August JR (ed): Consultations in Feline Internal Medicine, Philadelphia, WB Saunders, 1991, p. 543.

189. Barr MC, Pough MB, Jacobson RH, et al: C101: Comparison and interpretation of diagnostic tests for feline immunodeficiency virus infection. J Am Vet Med Assoc 199:1377, 1991.

190. Hardy WD Jr, Zuckerman EE: Comparison of ELISA, IFA and immunoblot tests for detection of feline immunodeficiency virus infection. Proc First Int Conf Feline Immunodefic Virus Researchers, University of California, Davis, 1991, p. 55.

191. Barlough JE, Scott FW: Feline infectious peritonitis. In Barlough J (ed): Manual of Small Animal Infectious Disease. New York, Churchill-Livingston, 1988, p. 68.

192. Macy DW: Feline immunodeficiency virus. In Sherding RG (ed): The Cat Diseases and Clinical Management, 2nd ed. New York, Churchill-Livingston, 1994, pp. 433–445.

193. August JR: Husbandry practices for cats infected with feline leukemia virus or feline immunodeficiency virus. J Am Vet Med Assoc 199:1474, 1991.

# B. Canine Lymphoma and Lymphoid Leukemias

## E. Gregory MacEwen and Karen M. Young

## LYMPHOMA

### Introduction

The lymphomas (malignant lymphoma or lymphosarcoma) are a diverse group of neoplasms that have in common their origin from lymphoreticular cells. They usually arise or present in lymphoid tissues such as lymph nodes, spleen, and bone marrow; however, they may arise in almost any tissue in the body. Lymphoma is one of the most common neoplasms seen in the dog. The annual incidence has been estimated to range between 13 and 24/100,000 dogs at risk.[1,2] The annual incidence rates at specific ages are estimated to be 1.5/100,000 for dogs less than 1.0 year of age and 84/100,000 in the 10- to 11-year-old group.[3] Lymphoma comprises approximately 7 to 24% of all canine neoplasia and 83% of all canine hematopoietic malignancies.[4,5] Middle-aged to older (median age of 6 to 9 years) dogs are primarily affected.[1,6] A decrease risk for lymphoma was reported for intact females,[7] although most reports show that gender is not an important risk factor.[6,8] The breeds of dogs reported to have a higher incidence include boxers, basset hounds, St. Bernards, Scottish terriers, airedales, and bulldogs, whereas the breeds with lower risk include dachshunds and Pomeranians.[7] Genetic predisposition has been previously reported for a pedigree of bull mastiffs,[9] a group of related otterhounds, a family of rottweilers, and a breeding pair of unrelated Scottish terriers.[10]

### Etiology

The etiology of canine lymphoma is unknown. The hypothesis that a retrovirus may be involved in the pathogenesis of canine lymphoma has not been confirmed.[11] However, viral particles with properties similar to those of retroviruses have been identified in short-term cultures of canine lymphoma tissue.[12–15]

In people, evidence continues to accumulate implicating phenoxyacetic acid herbicides, in particular 2, 4-dichlorophenoxyacetic acid (2, 4-D), in the development of non-Hodgkin's lymphoma.[16,17] A population case control study of non-Hodgkin's lymphoma in Kansas farmers reported a 2- to 6-fold excess risk for those who frequently mixed or applied herbicides (specifically 2, 4-D).[18] A recently published hospital-based case controlled study of dogs indicated that owners in households with dogs that develop malignant lymphoma applied 2, 4-D herbicides to their lawn and/or employed commercial lawn care companies to treat their yard more frequently than owners of dogs without lymphoma.[19] The risk of canine lymphoma was reported to rise to a 2-fold excess (odds ratio = 1.3) with 4 or more yearly owner applications of 2, 4-D.[19] The results of this study have since come under criticism and question.[20] In another study, dogs exposed to lawn treatment within 7 days of application were more then 50 times as likely to have urine levels of 2, 4-D at ≥ 50 µg/L. The highest concentration was noted 2 days after application.[21] In a recent study of 28 dogs with lymphoma, the tumors of 20 dogs with known exposure to 2, 4-D were analyzed using PCR technology for cellular N-ras oncogene mutations. The ras genes influence cell proliferation and may induce differentiation through signal transduction pathways. Mutation in the ras genes results in ras proteins that promote cell growth. One dog in the series showed a mutation of N-ras. These findings show that cellular N-ras mutations are infrequent in canine lymphoma, similar to what has been found in people with lymphoma.[22]

In people, characteristic chromosome abnormalities are being described more frequently as more precise banding and other high-resolution techniques have been applied. Chromosomal aberrations are nonrandom in human lymphoma, and several aberrations serve as markers for various subtypes of lymphoma. In addition, several oncogenes that may play a role in the pathogenesis of lymphoma have been detected based on the identification of cytogenetic abnormalities.[23–25] Chromosomal aberrations have been reported in canine lymphoma, but no consistent abnormalities have been found.[26] A recent study of 61 dogs with lymphoma demonstrated a treatment advantage in dogs having trisomy of chromosome 13 (25% of the dogs studied) as evidenced by increase in duration of first remission and overall survival time.[26]

Impaired immune function has been identified in dogs with lymphoma.[27,28] Immune system alterations in the dog such as immune-mediated thrombocytopenia, independent of age and gender, have been associated with a higher risk of subsequently developing lymphoma when compared to the normal population.[29] Additional evidence for the role of the immune system in the development of lymphoma comes from observation in human transplantation patients. The risk of developing lymphoreticular cancer is increased in people with immunosuppression,[30,31] and organ transplant patients have a higher incidence of non-Hodgkin's lymphoma.[32]

## Pathology and Natural Behavior

The classification of malignant lymphoma in dogs can be distinguished on the basis of anatomic location and histologic criteria. The most common anatomic forms of lymphoma include the multicentric, cranial mediastinal, gastrointestinal, and cutaneous forms. Primary extra-nodal forms such as those occurring in the eye, central nervous system, bone, testis and nasal cavity are less commonly observed.

Eighty percent of dogs with the *multicentric form* are presented with superficial lymphadenopathy.[33] Lymph node enlargement is usually painless, rubbery, and discrete and may be localized initially to the submandibular and prescapular nodes. Many animals are asymptomatic at the time of presentation, but approximately 40% will have a history of weight loss, lethargy, anorexia, and febrile episodes.[34] Diffuse pulmonary infiltration can also be seen in 27% to 34% of affected dogs as detected by radiographic changes.[35,36] Based on bronchoalveolar lavage, the actual incidence of lung involvement may be higher.[36,37] Hepatosplenomegaly is the most common manifestation of abdominal involvement and is usually associated with an advanced stage of multicentric disease.

The *alimentary form* is much less common and usually represents 5 to 7% of all canine lymphomas.[33] This form is reported to be more common in male dogs than female dogs[7], similar to observations in people.[38] Dogs with infiltrative disease of the intestinal tract will show weight loss, anorexia, panhypoproteinemia, and evidence of malabsorption.[39,40] Primary gastrointestinal lymphoma in dogs usually occurs multifocally and diffusely throughout the submucosa and lamina propria of the small intestine, with frequent superficial ulceration and occasional transmural infiltration of the serosa. Lymphocytic-plasmacytic inflammation can be seen adjacent to, or distant from, the primary tumor.[39] Pathologically, some of these neoplasms may resemble plasma cell tumors, and aberrant production of immunoglobulins may occur. From a histopathologic standpoint, it may be difficult to differentiate gastrointestinal lymphoma from lymphocytic plasmacytic enteritis (LPE).[39] It has been suggested that LPE may be a prelymphomatous change in the GI tract. A syndrome of immunoproliferative intestinal disease characterized by lymphocytic plasmacytic enteritis has been described in Basenji dogs that subsequently develop gastrointestinal lymphoma.[41] In addition, plasma cell-rich areas with heterogeneous lymphomatous infiltration may resemble lesions of LPE. Only a few reports specifically identify the immunophenotype of the lymphocyte subpopulations in alimentary lymphoma. It is usually presumed that they are most likely B-cell in origin. However, recently 4 cases (3 Shar-Pei, 1 boxer dog) were reported to have morphologic evidence (epitheliotropism) consistent with T-cell lymphoma. The tumors of two of these dogs were T-cell positive by immunophenotyping.[42]

The *mediastinal form* occurs in approximately 5% of the cases.[33] This form is characterized by enlargement of the cranial mediastinal lymph nodes and/or thymus. Hypercalcemia is reported to occur in 10 to 40% of dogs with lymphoma and is most common in the mediastinal form.[43,44] In a recent study of 37 dogs with lymphoma and hypercalcemia, 16 (43%) had mediastinal lymphoma.[45]

*Cutaneous lymphoma* can be solitary or more generalized and is usually classified as epitheliotrophic (mycosis fungoides) or nonepitheliotrophic.[46–54] Cutaneous lymphoma may also involve the oral mucosa,[46] and extracutaneous involvement can occur, with common sites including lymph nodes, spleen, liver, and bone marrow. Canine epitheliotrophic cutaneous lymphoma is the common form and is usually of T-cell origin,[55] similar to people. In dogs the T-cells are CD8-positive, whereas in humans they are mostly CD4+

cells.[56] A rare form of cutaneous T-cell lymphoma is characterized by generalized skin involvement with evidence of circulating malignant T-cells in the peripheral blood. These lymphocytes are usually large (15–20 µm) in diameter with folded and grooved nuclei. In people, this is referred to as Sézary Syndrome,[57] which also has been reported in dogs and cats.[49,50,58] B-lymphocyte cutaneous lymphomas usually spare the epidermis and papillary dermis, affecting the mid- and deep portions of the dermis.

## Histologic Classification Systems

Many histologic classifications have been used to describe lymphoma in the dog. Two systems used to classify human lymphomas, the Working Formulation of the National Institutes of Health and the Kiel system, appear to be most readily adapted to canine tumors.[43,59–62] (Tables 28–3 and 28–4). The Working Formulation categorizes tumors based both on pattern (diffuse vs. follicular) and cell type (e.g., small cleaved cell, large cell, immunoblastic). An algorithm for this system is presented in Figure 28–1. The updated Kiel classification accounts for both the morphology of the cells (centroblastic, centrocytic, immunoblastic) and the immunophenotype (B- vs. T-cell). In both systems, the tumors can then be categorized as low-, intermediate- (Working Formulation only), or high-grade malignancies.

The most striking difference between the morphologic classifications of canine and human lymphomas is the paucity of follicular lymphomas in the dog. It is possible that some diffuse lym-

**Table 28–3** Canine Lymphomas Classified by the Working Formulation

| | | Percent | | |
|---|---|---|---|---|
| Grade | Category | Greenlee[43] (*n* = 176) | Carter/Valli[59] (*n* 285) | Teske[62] (*n* = 116) |
| Low-Grade | | **11.0** | **5.3** | **16.3** |
| | Small lymphocytic | 10.0 | 4.9 | — |
| | Follicular small cleaved | — | 0.0 | 12.0 |
| | Follicular mixed small cleaved | 1.0 | 0.4 | 4.3 |
| Intermediate | | **59.9** | **28.4** | **74.6** |
| | Follicular large cell | 3.4 | 0.4 | 31.0 |
| | Diffuse small cleaved cell | 3.4 | 5.9 | 8.6 |
| | Diffuse mix small and large | 5.1 | 2.1 | 5.0 |
| | Diffuse large cell | 48.0 | 20.0 | 30.0 |
| High | | **29.4** | **66.3** | **6.0** |
| | Diffuse immunoblastic | 25.6 | 24.9 | 6.0 |
| | Diffuse lymphoblastic | 0.6 | 17.2 | — |
| | Diffuse small noncleaved | 3.2 | 24.2 | — |

**Table 28–4**  Canine Lymphomas Classified by
the Kiel Classification

| Category | Percent Greenlee[43] ($n = 176$) | Percent Teske[62] ($n = 95$) |
|---|---|---|
| **Low-Grade** | **24.4** | **29.5** |
| Lymphocytic | 6.8 | — |
| Lymphoplasmacytic | 3.4 | 7.3 |
| Centrocytic | 4.0 | 19.0 |
| Centroblastic-centrocytic | 10.2 | 3.2 |
| **High-Grade** | **75.6** | **70.5** |
| Centroblastic | 47.2 | 65.2 |
| Lymphoblastic T | 0.6 | — |
| Lymphoblastic B | 2.2 | — |
| Immunoblastic | 25.6 | 5.3 |

phomas in the dog are initially follicular but have progressed to the more aggressive diffuse tumors by the time of diagnostic biopsy. In both the Working Formulation and Kiel systems, only a small percentage of canine lymphomas are considered to be low-grade tumors —5 to 29%.[43,59,62] Using the Working Formulation, most canine lymphomas are reported to be intermediate- to high-grade and large cell tumors. Canine lymphoblastic lymphomas represent a small percentage (0–17%) of cases.[43,59] In the Kiel classification, the majority of canine tumors are classified as high-grade malignancies of the centroblastic type. Using currently available reagents, most canine lymphomas have a B-cell phenotype. The percentage of T-cell lymphomas reported ranges from 10 to 38%.[43,62,63] The relative unavailability of monoclonal antibodies to detect specific markers on canine lymphocytes has made immunophenotyping of tumors in dogs a challenge, and development of these tools will undoubtedly result in more accurate profiles of B- and T-cells.

To be considered useful, these classification systems must in the end yield information about response to therapy, maintenance of remission, and survival. One study suggests that the subtypes within the Working Formulation can be correlated with survival, and the Kiel system may be useful in prognosticating relapse.[62] In most studies, high-grade lymphomas have significantly higher frequencies of complete response to chemotherapy than do low-grade tumors. However, dogs with low-grade tumors may live a long time without aggressive chemotherapy. Dogs with T-cell lymphomas have been shown to have a lower complete response to chemotherapy as well as shorter remission and survival times than dogs with B-cell

tumors. Furthermore, T-cell lymphomas tend to be associated with hypercalcemia.[64] In people, hypercalcemia associated with non-Hodgkin's lymphoma is most common in retrovirus-associated T-cell lymphomas and leukemia.[65–67]

Some lymphomas may still be classified as histiocytic, derived from the Rappaport classification system.[61] The term *histiocytic* comprises a heterogeneous group of tumors with larger diameters, more vesicular nuclei, and more prominent nucleoli than those of lymphocytic or undifferentiated lymphomas. These neoplasms were originally termed histiocytic by Rappaport because the malignant cells have some morphologic features of benign histiocytes.[61] However, immunophenotyping has failed to document a biologic relationship between these cells and true histiocytes, so the term is largely considered a misnomer now. Furthermore, the Rappaport classification fails to account for different morphologic subtypes and, more important, provides no information about prognosis in dogs. Most of these tumors are better classified as large cell lymphomas.[5]

To summarize, it is important to determine the histologic grade of canine lymphomas as low (small lymphocytic or centrocytic lymphomas) or intermediate to high (diffuse large cell, centroblastic, and immunoblastic lymphomas). Furthermore, determining the immunophenotype of the tumor provides useful information. Response rates to chemotherapy are better in animals with B-cell tumors and intermediate- to high-grade lymphomas. Dogs with low-grade lymphomas can have long survivals without aggressive therapy.

## History and Clinical Signs

The clinical signs associated with canine lymphoma are variable and depend on the extent and location of the tumor. *Multicentric lymphoma* is the most common form, and generalized painless lymphadenopathy is the most consistent finding. In addition, hepatosplenomegaly and bone marrow involvement occur commonly. A large array of nonspecific signs, such as anorexia, weight loss, vomiting, diarrhea, emaciation, ascites, dyspnea, polydipsia, polyuria, and fever can occur. Thoracic radiographs may reveal enlargement of the sternal and tracheobronchial lymph nodes, widening of the cranial mediastinum, and infiltration of the lung parenchyma (Fig. 28–2). Hepatosplenomegaly and mesenteric or sublumbar lymphadenopathy are the most common abnormalities found on abdominal radiographs. Dogs with *gastrointestinal or alimentary lymphoma* are usually presented

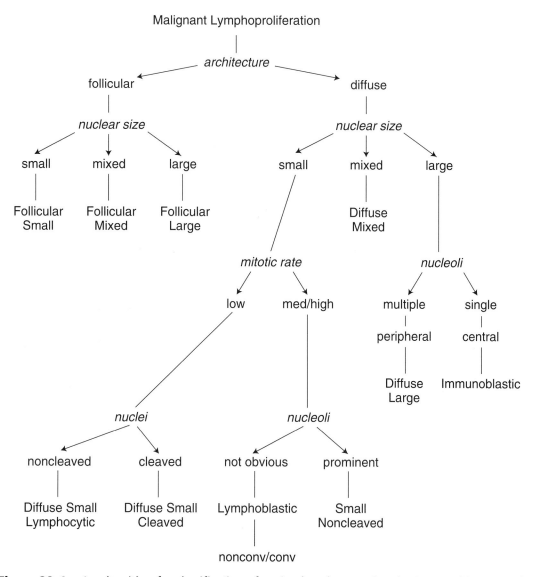

**Figure 28–1.** An algorithm for classification of canine lymphoma using the NIH Working Formulation. (Reprinted with permission Carter RF et al.[59])

with nonspecific gastrointestinal signs such as vomiting, diarrhea, weight loss, and malabsorption.[38–40] Mesenteric lymph nodes, spleen, and liver may be involved. The *mediastinal form* of lymphoma is characterized by enlargement of the cranial mediastinal structures or thymus or both, and clinical signs will be associated with the extent of disease or polydipsia/polyuria from hypercalcemia (Fig. 28–3). Commonly, dogs are presented with respiratory distress caused by a space-occupying mass and pleural effusion, exercise intolerance, and possibly regurgitation.

Signs in dogs with extranodal lymphoma depend on the specific organ involved. *Cutaneous lymphoma* is usually generalized or multifocal.[46–54] Tumors occur as nodules, plaques, ulcers, and erythremic or exfoliative dermatitis. Mycosis fungoides has a chronic clinical course with three apparent clinical stages. Initially, the skin will show scaling, alopecia, and pruritus. As the disease progresses, the skin becomes more erythematous, thickened, ulcerated, and exudative. (Fig. 28–4). The final stage is characterized by proliferative plaques and nodules with progressive ulceration (Fig. 28–5). Oral involvement may also occur, and this can appear as multicentric erythe-

**Figure 28–2.** *A,* Radiograph showing diffuse lung infiltration of lymphoma in a dog. *B,* Radiographs of the same dog following complete remission using chemotherapy.

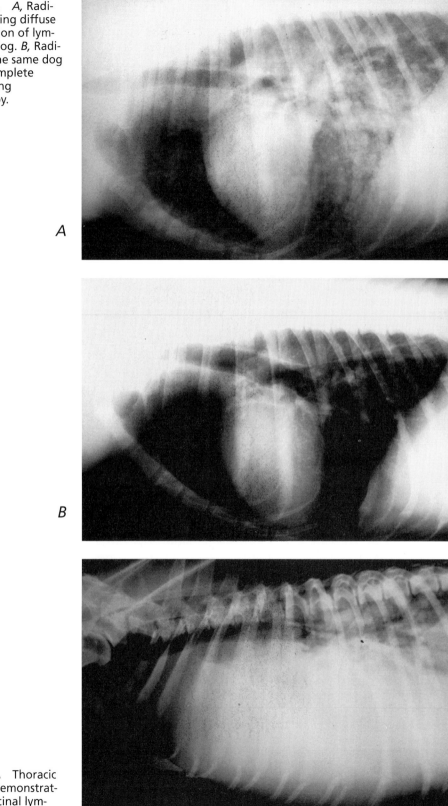

*A*

*B*

**Figure 28–3.** Thoracic radiograph demonstrating a mediastinal lymphoma.

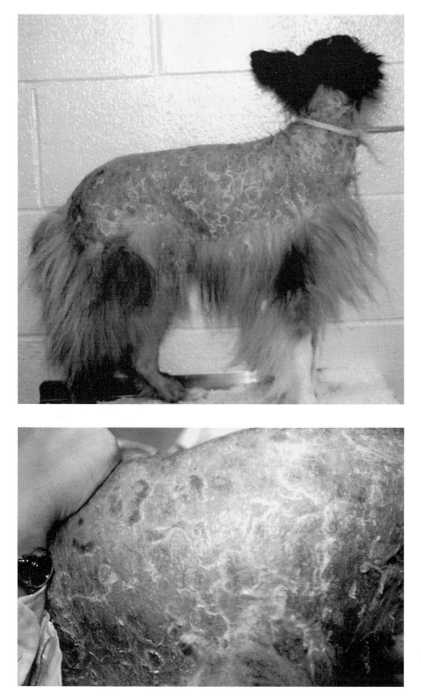

**Figure 28–4.** *A, B,* Marked scaling and erythroderma in a Shetland sheepdog with epitheliotropic T-cell lymphoma. The hair loss is caused partly by pruritus and self-trauma and is partly due to invasion of the hair follicle epithelium with atypical lymphocytes. (Courtesy of Dr. Karen A. Moriello, University of Wisconsin, School of Veterinary Medicine)

*A*

*B*

matous plaquelike lesions or nodules associated with the gum and lips[46] (Fig. 28–6). Dogs with *primary central nervous system lymphoma* (PCNSL) may be presented with either multifocal or solitary involvement.[68–70] Seizures, paralysis, and paresis may be noted. *Ocular lymphoma* is characterized by infiltration and thickening of the iris, uveitis, hypopyon, hyphema, posterior synechia, and glaucoma[71] (Fig. 28–7). In one study of 94 cases of canine multicentric lymphoma, 37% had ocular changes consistent with lymphoma.[72] Anterior uveitis was most commonly seen in the advanced stage of disease (stage V).[72]

The differential diagnosis of lymphadenopathy depends on the dog's travel history and the size, consistency, and location of the affected lymph

**Figure 28–5.** *A, B,* Cutaneous T-cell lymphoma in the plaque and nodule stage. Often generalized lymphadenopathy is present. (Courtesy of Dr. Karen A. Moriello, University of Wisconsin, School of Veterinary Medicine)

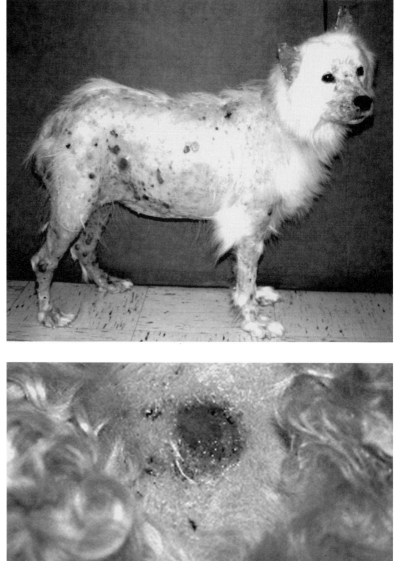

*A*

*B*

nodes. Other causes of lymphadenopathy include bacterial and viral infections, parasites (*Toxoplasma* species, *Leishmania* species), rickettsial organisms (salmon-poisoning, *Ehrlichia* species) and fungal agents (blastomycoses and *Histoplasma* species). Discrete, hard, asymmetrical lymph nodes, particularly if they are fixed to underlying tissues, may indicate metastatic tumors such as mast cell sarcoma or carcinoma. Immune-mediated diseases may also result in mildly to moderately enlarged lymph nodes. The various diseases or conditions that can be misdiagnosed as canine lymphoma are listed in Table 28–5.

Canine lymphoma may also be associated with paraneoplastic syndromes. Anemia, the most common lymphoma-related paraneoplastic syndrome,[73,74] is usually normochromic, normocytic, and nonregenerative, referred to as the anemia of chronic disease. However, hemolytic anemia may also occur. Neutrophilia can be seen in 25 to 40% of dogs with lymphoma.[74,75] Lymphocytosis is uncommon and occurs in approximately 20% of the affected dogs.[74] Thrombocytopenia may be seen in 30 to 50% of cases, but bleeding is seldom a clinical problem.[74–76]

Paraneoplastic hypercalcemia is also common in dogs with lymphoma. Hypercalcemia is characterized clinically by anorexia, weight loss, muscle weakness, lethargy, polyuria, polydipsia, and rarely central nervous system depression and

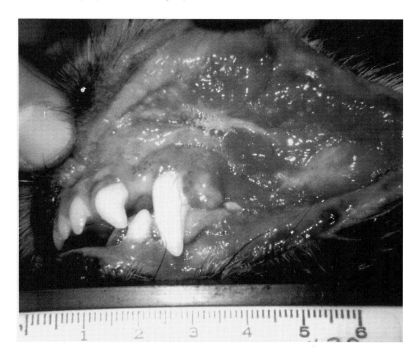

**Figure 28–6.** Lymphoma involving the gum and mucosal surface of the lips.

coma.[64,77,78] Hypercalcemia is thought to be related to the presence of a hormonelike substance, parathyroid hormone-related peptide (PTHrP), elicited by neoplastic cells.[79–81] Recently, Weir and others reported that hypercalcemia in dogs with lymphoma is most commonly associated with T-cell lymphoma.[62,64] Other paraneoplastic syndromes that may be encountered include monoclonal gammopathies and cancer cachexia.[82,83] (See Chapter 12.)

## Diagnostics and Clinical Staging

For most animals suspected of having lymphoma, the diagnostic evaluation should include a complete blood count (CBC with a differential cell count), platelet count, and a serum biochemistry profile. A bone marrow aspiration or biopsy (from proximal humerus or iliac crest) is indicated in dogs with anemia, lymphocytosis, or typical lymphocytes. To permit accurate histopathologic evaluation, a lymph node should be removed. While needle core biopsies may be satisfactory, it is important to avoid crush artifact or inadequate sample size. Most pathologists prefer whole node biopsies because they provide the maximum amount of information. Therefore, when a lymph node biopsy is performed, the entire lymph node should be removed, leaving the capsule intact to maintain nodal architecture. Care should be taken to avoid lymph nodes from reactive areas, such as submandibular lymph nodes; the prescapular or popliteal lymph nodes are preferable. Aspiration cytology can also be diagnostic; however, this method does not permit differentiation of low-, intermediate-, or high-grade lymphomas. Fine-needle aspiration is usually successful in making a definitive diagnosis of lymphoma.

Bone marrow aspiration or biopsy is very important in clinical staging of the patient with lymphoma. In one study of 53 dogs with lymphoma, 28% had circulating malignant cells and were considered leukemic, whereas bone marrow examination indicated involvement in 57% of the dogs.[84] The presence of a few prolymphocytes and lymphoblasts in the circulation of dogs with

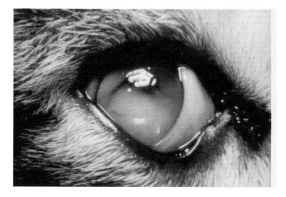

**Figure 28–7.** Ocular lymphoma involving the anterior chamber.

**Table 28–5**   Various Disorders Potentially Misdiagnosed as Canine Lymphomas

| Form of Lymphoma | Other Disorders |
|---|---|
| Multicentric | Systemic mycosis, salmon poisoning, *Ehrlichia canis* infection, lymph node hyperplasia (viral, immune, bacterial), dermatopathic lymphadenopathy |
| Mediastinal | Thymoma, ultimobranchial cyst, ectopic thyroid carcinoma, pleural carcinomatosis, congestive heart failure, pyothorax, chylothorax, hemothorax |
| Alimentary | Other gastrointestinal tumors, foreign body, lymphangiectasia, lymphocytic-plasmacytic enteritis, systemic mycosis, gastroduodenal ulceration |
| Extra-nodal | Variable, depending on organ/system involved |

*Source:* From Couto CG: Canine lymphomas: Something old, something new. Compend Contin Educ Pract Vet 7:291–301, 1985. Reprinted with permission.

lymphoma may indicate bone marrow involvement. It is important to remember these cells can also be seen with gastrointestinal parasitism, immune-mediated hemolytic anemia, and other immune-mediated diseases.

Thoracic and abdominal radiographs may be important in determining the extent of internal involvement. Diagnostic ultrasonography, including ultrasound-guided biopsy, has been very useful in evaluating involvement of the liver, spleen, or mesenteric lymph nodes.[85–88] If possible, the diagnosis should be made by sampling peripheral nodes, avoiding percutaneous biopsies of the liver or spleen. However, if there is no peripheral node involvement, it is appropriate to biopsy affected tissues in the abdominal cavity.

For alimentary lymphoma, it is extremely important to obtain a wedge biopsy without entering the intestinal lumen, and to obtain enough tissue because of the difficulty in differentiating lymphoma from LPE. Endoscopic biopsies may be inadequate because of the superficial specimen obtained. In many dogs with primary GI lymphoma, an inflammatory, nonneoplastic infiltrate (LPE) may be misdiagnosed through interpretation of biopsies that are too superficial.

Cytologic examination of cerebral spinal fluid (CSF), thoracic fluid, or aspirates from an intra-cavitary mass, is indicated in animals with CNS disease, pleural effusion or an intrathoracic mass, respectively. In one study of dogs with CNS involvement, CSF analysis was diagnostic in seven of eight dogs.[68] The characteristics of the CSF included high WBC counts in all seven dogs; 95%–100% of the cells were abnormal lymphoid cells. The CSF protein was high in five of seven dogs, ranging from 34 to 310 mg/dl (normal < 20 mg/dl).[68]

In animals with anemia or evidence of bleeding, a reticulocyte count, platelet count, and coagulation studies may also be indicated. Dogs with a high total protein, or evidence of an increased globulin fraction on a chemistry profile, should be evaluated by serum electrophoresis. Monoclonal gammopathies have been reported to occur in approximately 6% of the dogs with lymphoma.[82]

After a diagnosis has been established, the extent of disease should be determined and correlated to the clinical stage of disease. A WHO staging system is routinely used to stage dogs with lymphoma (Table 28–6). Most dogs are presented in advanced stages (III and IV).

For cutaneous lymphoma, punch biopsies (3–4 mm) should be taken from the most representative and infiltrative, but not infected, skin lesions.

**Table 28–6.**   World Health Organization's Clinical Staging System for Lymphosarcoma in Domestic Animals

1. Anatomic Site
   A. Generalized.
   B. Alimentary.
   C. Thymic.
   D. Skin.
   E. Leukemia (true)[a]
   F. Others (including solitary renal).
2. Stage (to include anatomic site)
   I. Involvement limited to a single node or lymphoid tissue in a single organ.[b]
   II. Involvement of many lymph nodes in a regional area (± tonsils).
   III. Generalized lymph node involvement.
   IV. Liver and/or spleen involvement (± Stage III).
   V. Manifestation in the blood and involvement of bone marrow and/or other organ systems (± Stage I–IV).
   Each stage is subclassified into:
   a. Without systemic signs.
   b. With systemic signs.

[a]Only blood and bone marrow involved.
[b]Excluding bone marrow.

No clinical staging system has been established for cutaneous lymphoma in dogs; however, a staging system has been developed for people with T-cell cutaneous lymphoma.[89] Table 28–7 presents a staging system modified for the dog. The recommended staging procedures for cutaneous lymphoma are presented in Table 28–8.

## Treatment of Multicentric Lymphoma

The therapeutic approach to a particular patient with lymphoma is determined by the stage of disease, the presence or absence of paraneoplastic disease, the overall physiologic status of the patient, and financial considerations. Since the majority of canine lymphomas are intermediate to high grade, histopathologic characterization has played a less important role in determining the optimal treatment.

Without treatment, most dogs with lymphoma will die of their disease in 4 to 6 weeks.[82] With few exceptions, canine lymphoma is considered a systemic disease and therefore requires systemic therapy in order to achieve remission and prolonged survival. Systemic chemotherapy

**Table 28–8** Staging Procedures for Cutaneous Lymphoma

1. Complete history and physical examination.
2. Whole-body mapping of skin lesions.
3. CBC, differential cell count, platelet count, and close examination of blood for atypical lymphocytes. A buffy coat smear to evaluate lymphocytes may be considered.
4. Serum chemistry profile.
5. Thoracic radiographs.
6. Skin biopsy and lymph node aspiration or biopsy if enlarged.
7. Bone marrow aspiration or biopsy.
8. Radiographs or ultrasound of abdomen if internal organ involvement is suspected.

continues to be the therapy of choice for canine lymphoma. Single-agent chemotherapy, except for doxorubicin, results in a lower response rate and is not as effective as combination chemotherapy.[82] Therefore, most dogs' lymphomas are best managed by combination chemotherapy. In rare cases in which lymphoma is limited to one site (especially an extranodal site) the animal is treated with radiation therapy or surgery.

Many chemotherapeutic protocols for dogs with lymphoma have been developed over the past 15 to 20 years (Table 28–9).[34,43,90–96] Conventional chemotherapy induces approximately 60 to 90% of the dogs into complete response (CR) with median survival times of 6 to 12 months, depending on the protocol used. Dogs responding to chemotherapy and undergoing complete remission are usually free of the clinical signs associated with lymphoma and subsequently return to a very good quality of life. Treating dogs with lymphoma is gratifying, since a high percentage have a complete response. Most dogs tolerate chemotherapy well, and in our experience only a minority of dogs develop significant toxicity associated with one or more chemotherapeutic drugs. Details of specific protocols are presented in (Tables 28–10 and 28–11). A CBC should be performed prior to each chemotherapy treatment. At least 2,500 neutrophils/μl should be maintained prior to the administration of chemotherapy. If the neutrophil count is < 2,500 μl it is best to wait 5 to 7 days and repeat the CBC. If the count has increased to > 2,500 cells/μl, the drug can be administered.

The fundamental goals of chemotherapy are to induce a complete remission, maintain a durable remission, and reinduce remission (rescue) after a relapse. Maintaining a first remission

**Table 28–7** TNM Classification of Cutaneous T-Cell Lymphoma

| Classification | Description |
|---|---|
| T-Skin | |
| $T_1$ | Scaling or abnormalities found only on skin biopsy. |
| $T_2$ | Erythroderma with or without scaling, or nasal lesion, or mucocutaneous lesions. |
| $T_3$ | Plaques or nodules. |
| N-Lymph Nodes | |
| $N_0$ | Nodes not palpable and not biopsied. |
| $N_1$ | Clinically enlarged nodes without malignant histopathology. |
| $N_2$ | Pathologically involved lymph nodes. |
| M Visceral Organs | |
| $M_0$ | No visceral involvement, no atypical cells in blood or bone marrow. |
| $M_1$ | Visceral involvement or atypical cells in blood or bone marrow. |

| Stage | T | N | M |
|---|---|---|---|
| IA | 1 | 0 | 0 |
| IB | 2 | 0 | 0 |
| IIA | 3 | 0,1 | 0 |
| IIB | 1–3 | 1 | 0 |
| IIIA | 1–3 | 2 | 0 |
| IIIB | 1–3 | 0–2 | 1 |

**Table 28–9.** Summary of Lymphoma Chemotherapy Protocols

| Protocol | Number of Dogs | Remission Rate (R) | Median Remission (Months) | Median Survival (Months) | % 1-Year Survival | References |
|---|---|---|---|---|---|---|
| COP | 20 | 70% | 3.3 | 7.5 | <10% | 92 |
| COP | 77 | 75% | 6.0 | NR | 19% | 91 |
| A | 22 | 77% | 6.3 | 6.3 | NR | 171 |
| A | 21 | 76% | 6.8 | 9.0 | NR | 92 |
| A | 37 | 59% | 4.4 | 7.7 | NR | 93 |
| VMC-L-ASP | 59 | 90% | 4.4 | 7.3 | 25% | 90 |
| VMC-L-ASP | 147 | 77% | 4.7 | 9.7 | 25% | 94 |
| VCA-L-ASP | 112 | 73% | 7.9 | 11.5 | 50% | 43 |
| L-ASP-COPA | 41 | 76% | 11.0 | NR | 48% | 95 |
| L-ASP-VCAM (University of Wisconsin, Madison) | 55 | 84% | 8.4 | 11.9 | 50% (24% @ 2 years) | 34 |

| | |
|---|---|
| C | = Cyclophosphamide. |
| O | = Oncovin (vincristine). |
| P | = Prednisone. |
| A | = Adriamycin (doxorubicin). |
| V | = Vincristine. |
| M | = Methotrexate. |
| L-ASP | = L-Asparaginase. |
| NR | = Not reported. |

is much easier than inducing a second remission. Dogs will relapse following chemotherapy for the following reasons: (a) inadequate dosing and frequency of administration of chemotherapy; (b) development of multidrug resistance (MDR) following exposure to selected chemotherapy agents;[97,98] (c) failure to achieve high-concentration chemotherapeutic drugs in certain sites, such as the central nervous system; and (d) insufficient monitoring of lymph node size and clinically detectable disease, thus preventing early detection of relapse.

The response to chemotherapy depends on the location of disease; the extent of disease (clinical stage); the histologic grade; the immunophenotype (T-cell vs. B-cell); the previous chemotherapy; the presence of concurrent medical problems or paraneoplastic conditions such as hypercalcemia, weight loss, and liver insufficiency; and possibly gender.[34,43,45,62,90–96] The cost to the owner depends on the drug(s) selected, the frequency of administration, and the laboratory tests needed to monitor toxicity. Currently, the most effective chemotherapy agents include doxorubicin, L-asparaginase, polyethylene glycol (PEG)-L-asparaginase,[99,100] vincristine, cyclophosphamide, and prednisone. Other drugs that also have activity and are considered second-line agents include vinblastine, cytosine arabinoside, actinomycin-D, mitoxantrone, chlorambucil, methotrexate, and DTIC.[101–106]

An unanswered question in the treatment of lymphoma is whether maintenance chemotherapy is useful following an initial course of aggressive chemotherapy lasting 6 to 9 months. No randomized studies have been performed to address the therapeutic benefit of long-term maintenance chemotherapy. Maintenance chemotherapy has been shown to be ineffective in people with Hodgkin's disease, non-Hodgkin's lymphoma, and multiple myeloma. However, in people, the initial induction course of chemotherapy is much more aggressive than that used in veterinary patients.

## Treatment Recommendations

It is difficult to provide precise treatment recommendations for the wide variety of clinical settings of dogs with lymphoma. Since 80% of the dogs with lymphoma are presented with multicentric disease (stages III and IV) and have intermediate- to high-grade tumors, we will limit our recommendations to this group of patients. Single-agent chemotherapy (i.e., doxorubicin) is the least complicated protocol. The expected complete response rate will range from 50 to 75% with an anticipated median survival of 6 to 8 months. In

**Table 28–10.** Protocols for Canine Lymphoma

| Protocol | Week 1 | 2 | 3 | 4 | 5 | 6 | 7 | 8 | 9 | 10 | 11 | 12 | 13 | 14 | 15 | 16 | 17 | 18 | 19 | 20 | 21 | 22 |
|---|---|---|---|---|---|---|---|---|---|---|---|---|---|---|---|---|---|---|---|---|---|---|
| **I. COP[91]** | | | | | | | | | | | | | | | | | | | | | | |
| Vincristine 0.75 mg/m² | • | • | • | | | | • | | | • | | | • | | | • | | | • | | | • |
| Cyclophosphamide 300 mg/m² | | | • | | | | • | | | • | | | • | | | • | | | • | | | • |
| Prednisone 1 mg/kg × 7 days then QOD PO — continuously | | | | | | | | | | | | | | | | | | | | | | |

*Comments:* Continue at 3-week intervals to week 52, then stop all chemotherapy.

| Protocol | Week 1 | 2 | 3 | 4 | 5 | 6 | 7 | 8 | 9 | 10 | 11 | 12 | 13 | 14 | 15 | 16 | 17 | 18 | 19 | 20 | 21 | 22 |
|---|---|---|---|---|---|---|---|---|---|---|---|---|---|---|---|---|---|---|---|---|---|---|
| **II. L-Asp COPA[95]** | | | | | | | | | | | | | | | | | | | | | | |
| Vincristine 0.75 mg/m² IV | • | • | • | • | | | • | | | | | | • | | | • | | | • | | | • |
| L-asparaginase 10,000 IU/m² IM | • | | • | • | | | | | | | | | | | | | | | | | | |
| Cyclophosphamide 250 mg/m² PO | | | | | | | • | | | | | | • | | | • | | | | | | |
| Doxorubicin 30 mg/m² IV | | | | | | | | | | • | | | | | | | | • | | | | |
| Prednisone 40 mg/m² × 7 days then QOD PO — continuously | | | | | | | | | | | | | | | | | | | | | | |

*Comments:* Repeat weeks 10 to 16 every 9 weeks until week 75, then stop all chemotherapy.

| Protocol | Week 1 | 2 | 3 | 4 | 5 | 6 | 7 | 8 | 9 | 10 | 11 | 12 | 13 | 14 | 15 | 16 | 17 | 18 | 19 | 20 | 21 | 22 |
|---|---|---|---|---|---|---|---|---|---|---|---|---|---|---|---|---|---|---|---|---|---|---|
| **III. VMC-L-ASP[90,94]** | | | | | | | | | | | | | | | | | | | | | | |
| L-asparaginase* 400 IU/kg IP | • | | | | | | | | | | | | | | | | | | | | | |
| Vincristine 0.7 mg/m² IV | • | | • | | • | | • | | • | | • | | • | | • | | • | | • | | • | |
| Cyclophosphamide 200–250 mg/m² IV | | • | | | | • | | | | • | | | | • | | | | • | | | | • |
| Methotrexate 0.6–0.8 mg/kg IV | | | | • | | | | • | | | | • | | | | • | | | | • | | |

*Comments:* Continue at weekly intervals to week 26, then every other week; at week 10 substitute chlorambucil 1.4 mg/kg PO (once) for cyclophosphamide if dog in CR. Stop at week 104. *Current recommendations administer L-asparaginase IM.

| Protocol | Week 1 | 2 | 3 | 4 | 5 | 6 | 7 | 8 | 9 | 10 | 11 | 12 | 13 | 14 | 15 | 16 | 17 | 18 | 19 | 20 | 21 | 22 |
|---|---|---|---|---|---|---|---|---|---|---|---|---|---|---|---|---|---|---|---|---|---|---|
| **IV. AMC (VCA-L-ASP)[43]** | | | | | | | | | | | | | | | | | | | | | | |
| L-asparaginase* 400 IU/kg IP | • | | | | | | | | | | | | | | | | | | | | | |
| Vincristine 0.7 mg/m² IV | • | | | | | | | • | | | | | | | • | | | | | | | • |
| Cyclophosphamide 200 mg/m² IV | | | | • | | | | | | | • | | | | | | | • | | | | |
| Doxorubicin 30 mg/m² IV | | | | | | • | | | | | | | • | | | | | | | • | | |
| Prednisone: 30 mg/m² PO × 7 days | • | | | | | | | | | | | | | | | | | | | | | |
| 20 mg/m² PO × 7 days | | • | | | | | | | | | | | | | | | | | | | | |
| 10 mg/m² PO × 7 days | | | • | | | | | | | | | | | | | | | | | | | |

*Comments:* Continue sequence of vincristine, cyclophosphamide, and doxorubicin at 3-week intervals after week 21 to week 36. Consolidation at week 39, vincristine (0.7 mg/m² IV) and prednisone (30 mg/m² × 7 days), week 40 cyclophosphamide (200 mg/m² IV) and prednisone (20 mg/m² × 7 days), week 41 vincristine (0.7 mg/m² IV) and prednisone (10 mg/m² × 7 days), week 42 cyclophosphamide (200 mg/m² IV). Then stop all chemotherapy. *Administer L-asparaginase IM.

**Table 28–11** University of Wisconsin–Madison School of Veterinary Medicine Canine Lymphoma Protocol[34] (L-ASP-VCAM)

| | |
|---|---|
| Week 1 | Vincristine 0.7 mg/m² IV<br>Asparaginase, 400 IU/kg, IM<br>Prednisone, 2 mg/kg, PO, SID |
| Week 2 | Cytoxan 200mg/m² IV<br>Prednisone, 1.5 mg/kg, PO, SID |
| Week 3 | Vincristine 0.7 mg/m² IV<br>Prednisone, 1.0 mg/kg, PO, SID |
| Week 4 | Adriamycin, 30 mg/m² IV<br>Prednisone, 0.5 mg/kg, PO, SID |
| Week 6 | Vincristine 0.7 mg/M² IV |
| Week 7 | Cytoxan 200 mg/m² IV |
| Week 8 | Vincristine 0.7 mg/m² IV |
| Week 9 | Adriamycin 30 mg/m² IV |
| Week 11 | Vincristine 0.7 mg/m² IV |
| Week 13 | Leukeran 1.4 mg/kg PO—one dose<br>　　or<br>Cytoxan 200 mg/m² IV (if not in CR) |
| Week 15 | Vincristine 0.7 mb/m² IV |
| Week 17 | Methotrexate 0.8 mg/kg IV |
| Week 19 | Vincristine 0.7 mg/m² IV |
| Week 21 | Leukeran 1.4 mg/kg PO—one dose<br>　　or<br>Cytoxan 200 mg/m² IV (if not in CR) |
| Week 23 | Vincristine 0.7 mg/m² IV |
| Week 25 | Adriamycin 30 mg/m² IV |

1. Continue as above (weeks 11–25) treatment with 2–3 week interval between treatments for 104 weeks.
2. Maximal dose of doxorubicin 180-200 mg/m². Then stop doxorubicin and continue methotrexate or substitute actinomycin-D at 1.1 mg/m² IV in place of doxorubicin.
3. A CBC should be performed prior to each chemotherapy. If neutrophil count < 2,500–3,000, wait 5–7 days and repeat CBC.
4. Although length of treatment has not been determined, currently we stop at week 104.
5. Expected CR rate 84%, median survival time 12 months with a 24% survival at 2 years.[34]
6. For acute lymphoblastic leukemia (ALL): administer L-asparaginase 400 IU/kg IM with each vincristine injection, until a CR is achieved.

contrast, prednisone alone may induce a 40% CR rate and a median survival of 2 to 3 months. Non-doxorubicin-based combination chemotherapy (i.e., cyclophosphamide, vincristine, and prednisone) is a relatively simple and easy protocol that is well tolerated and results in a 60 to 70%

CR rate with a median survival of 6 to 7 months. The more complicated and aggressive doxorubicin-based combination chemotherapy protocols result in an 80 to 90% CR rate, with median survival times of 12 months. In addition, 10 to 15% of the dogs are long-term survivors (> 3 years) and some are cured. Our current University of Wisconsin lymphoma protocol (see Table 28–11) is an example of one doxorubicin-based protocol in use today and it is well tolerated by dogs.

The type and aggressiveness of treatment will depend on the veterinarian's experience with chemotherapy, the philosophy of the owner and the treatment protocol, financial considerations, the time commitment and availability of the owner for follow-up, etc. It is important that clients be given all available information, such as cost, toxicity, response rates, and duration of response, so that the owner can make an informed decision.

## Rescue Chemotherapy

Rescue therapy is defined as attempting to obtain a second or possible third remission following a complete remission with an aggressive course of chemotherapy.[101,107–110] Unfortunately, most rescue approaches yield only a 10 to 40% CR rate with a duration of response of 1 to 5 months. Table 28–12 provides a summary of recent canine rescue drugs and protocols.

## Strategies to Enhance Effectiveness of Chemotherapy

To increase the therapeutic effectiveness of chemotherapy the following issues need to be considered:

1. *Drug Dosing:* Studies in animal models have indicated that maximal doses of drugs should be administered in order to achieve optimal therapeutic activity. In one model, the Ridgeway osteosarcoma (ROS) in rodents, optimal dosing increases the complete response (CR) rate to 100% with a cure rate of 60%. If the dose is reduced by 20%, the CR rate remains at 100%, but there is a dramatic reduction in cure rate (see Table 28–13).[111] Therefore, CR rate does not necessarily correlate with overall survival time. Maximal doses of drugs should be used to treat canine lymphoma.
2. *Dose intensity:* Dose intensity not only refers to the dose of the individual drugs but to the frequency and duration of treatment for all

**Table 28–12** Summary of Response for Rescue Protocols

| Protocol | Number of Animals | Overall Response % | Complete Response % | Median Response Duration (Days) | Median Duration of Complete Response (Days) | References |
|---|---|---|---|---|---|---|
| Actinomycin-D | 12 | 83 | 42 | 42 | 63 | 104 |
| Actinomycin-D | 25 | 0 | 0 | 0 | 0 | 105 |
| Mitoxantrone | 44 | 41 | 30 | Not reported | 127 | 106 |
| Doxorubicin | 12 | 42 | 33 | 145 | 152 | 107 |
| Doxorubicin-dacarbazine | 15 | 53 | 33 | < 42 | Not reported | 108 |
| MOPP (mechlorethamine, vincristine, procarbazine, prednisone) | 17 | 88 | 35 | 28 | Not reported | 109 |
| Cisplatin-cytosine arabinoside | 10 | 30 | 10 | 56 | Not reported | 110 |
| VP-16 (etoposide) | 13 | 15 | 7 | — | — | 172 |

*Source:* Table adapted from Vail DM, 1993.[101]

the drugs in a given protocol. It has been suggested that to compare different protocols and outcomes, all doses of drugs should be converted to milligrams per square meter of body surface area per week, regardless of schedule used.[112] Such an approach takes into account the impact of intervals between cycles or dose intensity. A number of human clinical studies have shown a strong link between dose intensity and outcome.[113] Studies on the treatment of Hodgkin's disease in people have shown that reduction in dose intensity by 30% results in a 30% decline in long-term survival, without changing the complete response rate.[113–115] With the use of colony-stimulating factors (G-CSF or GM-CSF) and autologous bone marrow transplantation, dose intensification is more clinically feasible.

3. *Drug resistance:* Drug resistance can develop in cancer patients following exposure to

**Table 28–13** Ridgeway Osteogenic Sarcoma, 2- to 3-g Tumors: Response to Different Relative Dose Intensities of Cyclophosphamide and L-Phenylalanine Mustard

| Relative Dose CTX | Intensities (RDIs) L-PAM | Average RDI | Percent Complete Response | Percent Cures |
|---|---|---|---|---|
| 0.38 | 0.82 | 0.60 | 100 | 60 |
| 0.75 | 0.18 | 0.47 | 100 | 44 |
| 0.25 | 0.55 | 0.44 | 100 | 10 |
| 0.50 | 0.12 | 0.31 | 10 | 0 |
| 0.17 | 0.36 | 0.27 | 0 | 0 |

*Source:* Modified from Skipper HS, 1986.[111]

selected chemotherapeutic agents and is often associated with expression of P-glycoprotein. P-glycoprotein acts as a drug efflux pump that actively extrudes drugs from tumor cells, preventing a cytotoxic drug from reaching the cellular site of action. Multiple drug resistance (MDR) and P-glycoprotein are under the control of the MDR-1 gene.[97,98,116] MDR-1 overexpression has been reported in canine lymphoma following exposure to chemotherapy.[117] In one recent study, 11 of 28 dogs with lymphoma were treated with glucocorticoids prior to the administration of chemotherapy (doxorubicin and cyclophosphamide). Those dogs pretreated with glucocorticoids had a significantly shorter remission duration (134 days) compared to those dogs that did not receive glucocorticoids (267 days).[118] Whenever possible, pretreatment with glucocorticoids should be avoided if additional chemotherapy is contemplated.

Another cause of drug resistance has been termed the Goldie-Coleman hypothesis.[119] Simply stated, cancer cells have a tendency to mutate spontaneously to a drug-resistant phenotype. Strategies such as combination chemotherapy and dose intensification are most effective in overcoming drug resistance. New treatment strategies employ the use of drugs to reverse MDR.[116]

## Treatment Approaches Using Immunologic or Biologic Agents

Results to date using immunologic procedures or biologic agents have been mixed. A study using the chemical immunomodulator levamisole, in combination with chemotherapy, proved to be unrewarding.[120] A study using a mixed bacterial vaccine (*Serratia marcescens* and *Streptococcus pyogenes*) combined with cyclophosphamide resulted in improved remission time, but had no survival advantage compared to using cyclophosphamide alone.[121]

Autologous vaccines have been shown to have some positive effects in dogs when combined with chemotherapy. A tumor vaccine extract using lymphoma cells combined with Freund's adjuvant was administered to dogs after remission induction with combination chemotherapy. The median survival time was 336 days (11 dogs) for the vaccine-treated group versus 196 days (9 dogs) for the chemotherapy alone group.[122] A subsequent study by the same investigators reported that the prolonged survival was due to the Freund's adjuvant.[123]

Intralymphatic (IL) administration of an autologous lymphoma tumor cell vaccine has been administered to dogs placed in remission using a combination chemotherapy protocol. In a study comparing 28 dogs receiving chemotherapy followed by IL-vaccination to 30 dogs receiving chemotherapy alone, the median remission times were 98 days and 28 days, respectively (*p* < .024).[124] Unfortunately, the survival times for the two groups (305 days and 184 days for chemotherapy plus IL vaccine and chemotherapy alone, respectively) were not significantly different.[124] Dogs that responded had significant increases in specific antibody to lymphoma antigens compared to those that did not respond.

More recently, another immunotherapy approach has shown more promise. MAb-231 is a murine-derived anticanine monoclonal antibody (IgG2a). It mediates antibody-dependent cellular cytotoxicity (ADCC) and complement-mediated cellular cytotoxicity (CMCC).[125,126] It also prevents outgrowth of canine lymphoma xenogrowths in nude mice.[127] A phase-I clinical trial in dogs with lymphoma given MAb-231 has not revealed any significant toxicity.[128] In a recent noncontrolled clinical study, 215 dogs were treated with chemotherapy (L-asparaginase, vincristine, cyclophosphamide, and doxorubicin). Following two cycles of chemotherapy 174 dogs achieved complete remission and were treated with intravenous infusion of MAb-231 daily for 5 days. The median survival time of the dogs treated with MAb-231 was 493 days. The 2-year survival rate was 15.6%. The median number of chemotherapy cycles in the first year was 3 and the median number of MAb-231 cycles was 1.5.[129]

Another form of immunotherapy under evaluation is the use of anti-idiotypic vaccines. In dogs with B-cell lymphoma, cell membrane preparations are used as a source of idiotypic antibody. This membrane/idiotypic antibody combination is mixed with an adjuvant (alum) and administered as a vaccine.[130] The rationale is to develop anti-idiotypic antibodies that recognize idiotypic antibody on the lymphoma cells. This mode of immunotherapy is used following chemotherapy and has shown promise in clinical trials in human lymphoma patients.[131]

## Surgery

Most dogs with lymphoma have the multicentric form and will need systemic chemotherapy to treat the disease effectively. However, surgery has been used to treat solitary lymphoma (early stage I). Careful staging is necessary in such cases to rule out multicentric involvement prior to treating local disease.

The benefit of surgical removal of the spleen in dogs with massive splenomegaly remains unclear.[132,133] In a recent report, 16 dogs with lymphoma underwent splenectomy to remove a massive spleen and were subsequently treated with chemotherapy. Within 6 weeks of splenectomy, five of the 16 dogs died of disseminated intravascular coagulation (DIC) and sepsis. The remaining 11 dogs had a complete response rate of 66%, and seven of these followed until their death had a median survival time of 14 months.[133] Splenectomy should be considered only if the lymphoma is in remission in other sites and if the splenic enlargement is from lymphoma that is not responsive to chemotherapy. In dogs with lymphoma, splenectomy can also be considered with uncontrolled hemolytic anemia and persistent thrombocytopenia.

## Radiation Therapy

The role of radiotherapy is relatively limited in the curative management of lymphoma. Using whole-body radiation without bone marrow transplantation has yielded poor results. However, there can be indications for the use of radiation therapy in selected cases.[134] The indications are:

1. Local stage I or II disease (i.e., nasal lymphoma, CNS lymphoma).
2. Palliation for local disease (i.e., submandibular lymphadenopathy, rectal lymphoma, bone involvement, etc.).
3. Total body radiation combined with bone mar-

row transplantation (see Chap. 14 on new developments in cancer therapy).

## Nonmulticentric Lymphoma

**Alimentary Lymphoma** Most dogs with alimentary lymphomas are presented with diffuse involvement in the intestinal tract. Solitary alimentary lymphomas are rare in the dog and more common in the cat. Involvement of local lymph nodes and liver is common. Chemotherapy in the dogs with diffuse involvement has been unrewarding.[39] However, if the tumor is localized and can be surgically removed, results using follow-up chemotherapy can be very encouraging.

**Primary Central Nervous System Lymphoma**
The majority of CNS lymphomas in dogs results from metastasis of multicentric lymphoma. However, primary central nervous system lymphoma (PCNSL) has been reported.[68,69] If tumors are localized, then local radiation therapy should be considered. Few studies have reported on the use of chemotherapy. In one study cytosine arabinoside (Ara-C) at a dosage of 20 mg/m$^2$ was given intrathecally by bolus injection after withdrawal of an equal volume of cerebrospinal fluid. The dose was diluted in 2 to 4 ml of lactated Ringer's solution and was injected twice weekly for a total of six treatments. This treatment was combined with systemic chemotherapy and CNS radiation.[68] Overall, the response rates were low and of short duration (several weeks to months).

**Cutaneous Lymphoma** The treatment of cutaneous lymphoma depends on the extent of disease and histologic subtype (B-cell vs. T-cell-mycosis fungoides). Solitary lesions may be treated with surgical excision or radiation therapy. Fractional radiation therapy (to a total dose of 30 to 45 Gy) has been associated with long-term control. Diffuse non-T-cell lymphoma is best managed with chemotherapy (see Tables 28–10 and 28–11), although the response rate is less than in multicentric lymphoma. Some investigators have reported that combination chemotherapy with COAP (cyclophosphamide, vincristine, cytosine arabinoside, and prednisone) will induce some long-term remissions. Five of six dogs with diffuse non-T-cell cutaneous lymphoma attained a complete or partial remission, with a median remission duration of > 250 days and a median survival of > 399 days.[135] However, in our experience, chemotherapy has generally been unrewarding.

Retinoids, such as isotretinoin (Accutane) and etretinate (Tegison) have been used successfully in canine and human T-cell cutaneous lymphomas.[52,136] In one study, 12 dogs with cutaneous lymphoma were treated with isotretinoin (3–4 mg/kg PO daily) and two were treated with etretinate (1.25–1.45 mg/kg PO daily). Eleven of these 14 dogs had T-cell cutaneous lymphoma and six of the 14 dogs achieved remission. In another study four dogs with T-cell lymphoma were treated successfully with isotretinoin for 13, 11, 10, and 5 months.[52] In our experience with retinoids, treatment must be given for a number of months, and responses have not been impressive. PEG-L-asparaginase (30 mg/kg IM weekly) induces responses in dogs with cutaneous T-cell lymphomas, although remissions are not durable and no cures have been noted.[137] Prednisone may also be necessary to control pruritus.

Topical chemotherapy is another strategy to treat cutaneous T-cell lymphoma. Mechlorethamine (Mustargen) is applied topically as an aqueous solution or an ointment base. The aqueous solution is prepared by combining 10 mg of mechlorethamine with 50 ml of tap water. The ointment is prepared by mixing 90 mg mechlorethamine with 10 ml of absolute alcohol and further combining enough xipamide (Aquaphor) to prepare 900 g of ointment. Hair must be removed prior to application. Gloves must be used when applying the drug, since mechlorethamine is carcinogenic and can induce contact hypersensitivity in people. Response to therapy is variable and often only palliative.[138]

## Prognosis

The prognosis for canine lymphoma is variable and depends on a number of factors, such as clinical stage, histologic grade, immunophenotype, anatomic location, and possibly gender. Although rarely curable (<10%), complete remission and quality survival can be achieved. Factors that have been shown to influence survival are shown in Table 28–14.

Dogs with stage I and II disease have a better prognosis than those dogs in more advanced stages (stages III, IV, and V).[90,91] Substage "a" (no clinical signs of illness) has been shown to be a positive prognostic factor (Fig. 28–8).[34] In some studies, elevated serum calcium (> 11.9 mg/dl) has been shown to be a negative prognostic factor.[43,139] This may be associated with the T-cell phenotype or the presence of concurrent renal failure.

The histologic grade (subtype) has been found

**Table 28–14**   Prognostic Factors for Canine Lymphoma

| Factor | Strongly Accepted | Possibly Accepted | Comments |
|---|---|---|---|
| WHO clinical stage | | X | Stage I/II—favorable<br>Stage V with significant bone marrow involvement—unfavorable. |
| WHO clinical substage | X | | Substage b—associated with decrease survival. |
| Histopathology | X | | High-grade/medium-grade—associated with high response rate but reduced survival. |
| Immunophenotype | X | | T-cells phenotype associated with reduced survival. |
| Hypercalcemia | | X | Negative factor if associated with T-cell subtype and reduced renal function. |
| Sex | | X | Some studies suggest females have a favorable prognosis. |
| Proliferative index | | X | Highly proliferative tumors based on AgNOR number have a more favorable prognosis. |
| Anatomic location | X | | Leukemia, diffuse cutaneous and alimentary associated with unfavorable prognosis. |

to influence prognosis. Dogs with lymphoma classified as intermediate or high grade (large cell, centroblastic, and immunoblastic) tend to respond to chemotherapy but can relapse early. Dogs with low-grade lymphomas (small lymphocytic or centrocytic) have a lower response rate to chemotherapy, yet have a survival advantage over dogs with intermediate- and high-grade lymphomas (Fig. 28–9).[62] Using the Working Formulation, low-grade lymphomas have a survival advantage when compared to intermediate and high grade (Fig. 28–10).[62] In addition to tumor grade, immunophenotype (T-cell vs. B-cell) has been shown to influence response to treatment and survival time (Fig. 28–11).[62] The T-cell phenotype is associated with a poorer prog-

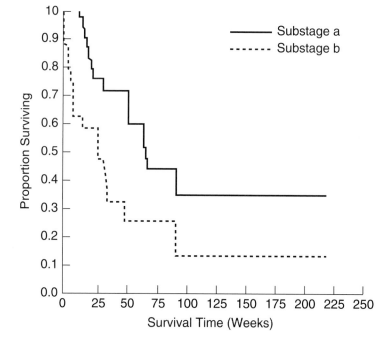

**Figure 28–8.** Kaplan-Meier curves illustrating survival according to WHO substage, for 55 dogs with lymphoma treated with chemotherapy. Substage a, *n* = 31, substage b, *n* = 24. (Reprinted with permission Keller ET et al.[34])

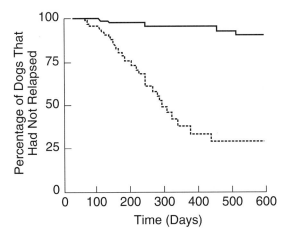

**Figure 28–9.** Kaplan-Meier curves illustrating time to relapse adjusted for clinical stage and immunophenotype among dogs treated for low-grade (———), n = 17, or high-grade (– – – –), n = 51, Kiel classification. (Reprinted with permission Teske E et al.[62])

nosis. Recently, proliferative assays using bromodeoxyuridine (BrdU) to measure tumor doubling time and argyrophilic nucleolar organizer regions (Ag-NORs) to measure proliferative activity of the tumor cells have been shown to provide significant prognostic conformation in

dogs treated with combination chemotherapy.[140,141] Dogs having tumors with short doubling times or high AgNOR frequencies have a better prognosis than those dogs with long doubling times or low AgNOR frequencies.[140]

The anatomic site of disease is also of considerable prognostic importance. Primary cutaneous, diffuse gastrointestinal, and primary central nervous lymphomas tend to be associated with a poor prognosis. Cutaneous lymphomas tend to progress slowly and in our experience have short-term responses to systemic chemotherapy. Localized lymphomas in the skin can be managed with radiation therapy or surgery or both, and these have a better prognosis. In some dogs with lymphoma there may be significant involvement in the bone marrow (tumor cells > 50% of all nucleated cells) and circulating malignant lymphoblasts in the peripheral blood. These dogs tend to have an overall poor prognosis. In some cases, it is difficult to determine whether or not the disease is arising from the bone marrow, such as in acute lymphoblastic leukemia (ALL), or is a diffuse lymphoma with extensive involvement in the marrow.

Gender has been shown to influence prognosis in some studies.[34,94] Neutered females tend to have a better prognosis. There is some suggestion that males may have a higher incidence of the T-cell phenotype, which may account for the poorer prognosis.[140]

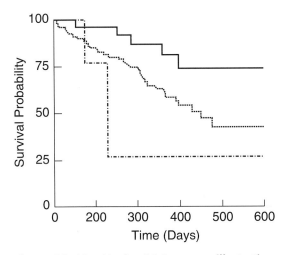

**Figure 28–10.** Kaplan-Meier curves illustrating survival times adjusted for clinical stage and immunophenotype among dogs treated for low-grade (———), n = 9, intermediate-grade (– – – –), n = 57, or high-grade (– · – · – · ), n = 3, using the working formulation for lymphoma. (Reprinted with permission Teske E et al.[62])

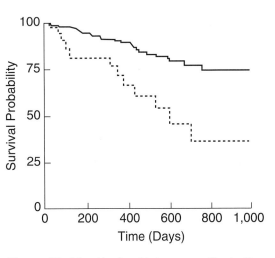

**Figure 28–11.** Kaplan-Meier curves illustrating survival times adjusted for clinical stage and histologic malignancy grade among dogs treated for B-cell type (———), n = 41, or T-cell type (– – – –), n = 14, lymphoma. (Reprinted with permission Teske E et al.[62])

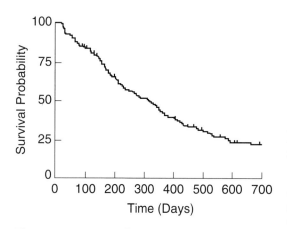

**Figure 28–12.** Kaplan-Meier survival curve for 138 dogs with malignant lymphoma treated with combination chemotherapy. (Reprinted with permission Teske E et al.[62])

In conclusion, treating canine lymphoma can be a very rewarding experience for the dog, owner, and veterinarian. In most dogs with lymphoma, doxorubicin-based combination chemotherapy can induce an 80 to 90% CR rate and a median survival time of approximately 12 months, with a 25% 2-year survival time (Fig. 28–12).[62] The advances made in the past 20 years have greatly improved the management of this disease.

## LYMPHOID LEUKEMIA

Leukemia is defined as the proliferation of neoplastic hematopoietic cells in the bone marrow; these cells may or not be circulating in the peripheral hood.

## Incidence and Risk Factors

Lymphocytic leukemia is more common than nonlymphocytic leukemia and other myeloproliferative disorders (MPDs). The true incidence is not known. In a series of 30 cases of acute lymphoblastic leukemia (ALL), the median age was 5.5 years, with a range of 1 to 12 years.[142] Eight dogs were less than 4 years old. German shepherd dogs accounted for 27% of the cases seen. The male-to-female (M:F) ratio was 3:2.[142] Welldifferentiated or chromic lymphocytic leukemia (CLL) is seen less frequently than ALL but more commonly than MPD. The median age is 10 to 12 years, and in one study of 22 dogs the M:F ratio was 1.8:1.[143]

## Etiology

As with lymphoma, the etiology is unknown. Retroviruses have been implicated in diverse animal species such as cats, cattle, fish, snakes, birds, rodents, and nonhuman primates. There is no proven evidence implicating a retroviral cause in dogs. However, recently, a retrovirus with a morphology typical of lentiviruses was isolated from mononuclear cells obtained from the peripheral blood of a dog with ALL.[144]

In people, leukemia has been associated with exposure to radiation, benzene, phenylbutazone, and antineoplastic agents.[145–149] The alkylating agents can cause chromosomal damage and are clearly carcinogenic.[149] HTLV-1 is a proven cause of leukemia in a large cohort of human patients from the southern islands of Japan.[150,151]

## Pathology and Natural Behavior

In acute lymphoblastic leukemia (ALL) the blast cells always infiltrate the bone marrow, resulting in variable degrees of anemia, thrombocytopenia, and neutropenia. Infiltration of the spleen and liver are common, and extramedullary sites, such as the nervous system, bone, and gastrointestinal tract, may be involved as well. Some animals may have lymph node involvement and develop generalized lymphadenopathy.[142]

The lymphocytes of CCL are virtually indistinguishable morphologically from normal small lymphocytes. In CCL the marrow is infiltrated with mature lymphocytes. The extent of marrow infiltration is less than that seen with ALL or MPD. Dogs tend to have a mild anemia, and the granulocytes and platelets are also only mildly reduced. Splenomegaly is common, and lymph nodes can be mild to moderately enlarged.[143] Despite the well-differentiated appearance of the lymphocytes in CLL, these cells may function abnormally. Some animals with CLL have an accompanying monoclonal gammopathy. In one study of 22 dogs with CLL, 60% were hyperglobulinemic and 68% had monoclonal gammopathies.[143] This immunoglobulin spike in the serum is associated with production of immunoglobulins by the leukemic cells (B-cells). The immunoglobulin is usually IgM or IgA. The term *macrogammaglobulinemia* is used (see Chap. 28E) to describe IgM gammopathy. Dogs with CLL and an IgM monoclonal gammopathy are referred to as having Waldenström's macroglobulinemia. Dogs can also develop hyperviscosity syndrome (see Chapter 28E).

## History and Clinical Signs

Dogs with ALL usually have a history of anorexia, weight loss, polyuria/polydipsia and lethargy. Splenomegaly is common and other physical abnormalities may include hemorrhages, lymphadenopathy, and hepatomegaly. Anemia, thrombocytopenia, and an elevated white blood cell (WBC) count are common. The anemia may be severe and is usually characterized as normocytic and normochromic (nonregenerative). WBC counts are usually elevated despite neutropenia, owing to an increased number of circulating lymphoblasts (> 14,000 cells/µl). Some dogs, however, may be leukopenic.[142] Infiltration of bone marrow by neoplastic lymphoblasts may be extensive with resultant depression of normal hematopoietic elements.

In CLL, mild lymphadenopathy and splenomegaly may be present. Most dogs tend to be anemic (PCV < 35%) and mildly thrombocytopenic (110,000 to 190,000 platelets/µl) The WBC count is usually greater than 30,000 cells/µl but can vary from normal to greater than 100,000 cells/µl, owing to an increase in circulating mature lymphocytes.[143] Lymphocytosis is usually persistent and granulocytes are usually present in normal numbers. In some dogs the disease is identified incidentally while the patient is undergoing routine evaluation.

## Diagnostics and Clinical Staging

Infiltration of neoplastic lymphoid cells in the bone marrow is the hallmark of both ALL and CLL, and careful examination of peripheral blood and bone marrow by experienced cytopathologists is essential in establishing a diagnosis of lymphocytic leukemia. If diagnostic bone marrow cannot be adequately obtained by aspiration, a bone marrow core biopsy should be performed. In ALL, lymphoblasts predominate in the bone marrow and are also present in peripheral blood. In most cases, these cells cannot be easily distinguished from blast cells of other hematopoietic lineages without the use of special cytochemical or immunologic markers.[152] Immature and differentiating lymphocytes may stain strongly for alkaline phosphatase activity, suggesting that this cytochemical staining procedure is not specific for myeloid leukemia.[152-154] Perhaps the most distinguishing feature of lymphoblasts is the nuclear chromatin pattern, which is more condensed than the chromatin in myeloblasts.[154] Lymphoblasts are larger than neutrophils, have a high nuclear-to- cytoplasmic ratio, and blue cytoplasm that in some cases is very basophilic. Nucleoli, although present, are less prominent in lymphoblasts than in myeloblasts. The infiltration of bone marrow by lymphoblasts is accompanied by a concomitant decrease in the myeloid, erythroid, and megakaryocytic cell lines.

The lymphocytes in CLL are small mature cells that occur in excessive numbers in bone marrow (≥ 30% of all nucleated cells) early in the disease.[143] Infiltration becomes more extensive as the disease slowly progresses, and eventually the neoplastic cells replace normal marrow.

A separate clinical staging system has not been developed for lymphocytic leukemia. Currently, all dogs with leukemia are classified as stage V, based in the WHO Staging System for lymphoma as presented in Table 28–6. However, a specific clinical staging system for CLL has been used in human patients and could easily be adapted for the dog.[155]

Extent of Disease

Stage O: Lymphocytosis only. Absolute lymphocyte count is 15,000/mm³ or greater and the proportion of lymphocytes in the marrow is less than 40% in a normocellular or hypercellular marrow.

Stage I: Lymphocytosis plus enlarged lymph nodes.

Stage II: Lymphocytosis plus enlarged spleen and/or liver.

Stage III: Lymphocytosis plus anemia (hemoglobin ≤ 7 g/dl).

Stage IV: Lymphocytosis plus thrombocytopenia (platelets < 100,000/mm³). Lymph node enlargement or enlargement of spleen or liver may or may not be present.

This system has been shown to provide very significant prognostic information in people.[156]

### Treatment of the Acute Lymphoblastic Leukemia
Acute lymphoblastic leukemia (ALL), similar to other infiltrative bone marrow malignancies, causes morbidity by suppressing bone marrow function. Neutropenia, thrombocytopenia, and anemia may be severe. Therapy must be aggressive: for restoration of hematopoiesis to occur 1.5 to 2.0 logarithm reduction in leukemic cell numbers (< 10^8 cells) must be achieved. Patients need supportive therapy such as fresh whole blood, broad-spectrum antibiotics, fluid therapy, and nutritional support. Patients must be carefully monitored for bleeding and thrombosis that may signal the development of disseminated intravascular coagulation.

The treatment of ALL requires aggressive chemotherapy. Table 28–11 presents an accepted treatment protocol for dogs with ALL. The cornerstone of remission induction for ALL is the combination of vincristine and prednisone with or without L-asparaginase. In one report on the use of vincristine and prednisone in dogs with acute lymphoblastic leukemia, 40% of the dogs responded to vincristine and prednisone, 20% with a complete remission and 20% with a partial remission.[142] As shown in Table 28–11, with the addition of doxorubicin and L-asparaginase it is anticipated that response rates will increase over those previously reported using vincristine and prednisone alone.

The maintenance phase of treatment begins after the animal has achieved complete remission. Complete remission is defined as 100% regression of disease based on bone marrow and peripheral blood evaluation. Chemotherapeutic treatments should be continued on a weekly basis except when doxorubicin is administered and then a 2-week rest interval is indicated before the administration of other drugs. This protocol has not been adequately evaluated in large numbers of animals with ALL, but based on one author's (EGM) experience this protocol is superior to vincristine and prednisone alone.

**Treatment of Chronic Lymphocytic Leukemia**   Because of the indolent nature of chronic lymphocytic leukemia (CLL) in many animals, it is controversial whether or not all dogs with this disease should be treated.[157,158] The clinician may elect to observe the patient if the discovery of CLL is incidental, and there are no accompanying physical or clinical signs and no significant hematologic abnormalities (stage O, as above). If the animal is anemic or thrombocytopenic, is showing evidence of lymphadenopathy or hepatosplenomegaly, or has an excessively high white blood cell count (greater than 60,000 lymphocytes/μl), therapy should be instituted. The most effective drug evaluated thus far is chlorambucil.[143] Chlorambucil is given orally at a

dose of 0.2 mg/kg or 6 mg/m$^2$ PO once daily for 7 to 14 days. The dose can then be reduced to 0.1 mg/kg or 3 mg/m$^2$ PO daily. For long-term maintenance a dose 2.0 mg/m$^2$ every other day can be used. The dose needs to be adjusted based on clinical response and bone marrow tolerance. Chlorambucil should be administered without food to increase the rate of absorption.[159] Table 28–15 presents the details on two protocols for treating CLL.

Corticosteroids are lymphocytolytic and lead to cell death by apoptosis. Studies in people have shown that the antitumor activity of chlorambucil combined with prednisone is better than that with chlorambucil alone.[160] When the bone marrow is heavily infiltrated with CLL cells and neutropenia, thrombocytopenia, and anemia occur, more aggressive use of an alkalizing agent, usually the platelet-sparing drug cyclophosphamide (50 mg/m$^2$ SID × 4 days repeat weekly), in combination with prednisone (20 mg/m$^2$ PO QOD) can be considered. When chlorambucil or cyclophosphamide with or without prednisone fail, the choice of treatment would be combination chemotherapy similar to that presented in Table 28–11. The treatment of CLL is primarily palliative, with rare complete remissions. Owing to the indolent nature of this disease, however, survival times have been in the range of 1 to 3 years with a good quality of life.

In people, splenectomy has been shown to increase survival significantly with aggressive forms of CLL.[161] The phenotypic expression of CLL is usually stable over months to years. However, the disease may evolve into an acute phase, and some dogs will develop a rapidly progressive pleomorphic (immunoblasts) lymphoma.[143] In people, this is termed Richter's Syndrome.[162] The prognosis for response to treatment is poor for this form.

### Prognosis

In general, the prognosis of ALL in the dog is very poor. In a study of 21 dogs treated with vin-

---

**Table 28–15**   Treatment of Chronic Lymphocytic Leukemia

| | |
|---|---|
| 1. Chlorambucil[a] | 0.2 mg/kg PO Day 7–14 then 0.1 mg/kg PO continuously or 2 mg/m$^2$ PO QOD. |
| Prednisone | 30 mg/m$^2$ PO SID for 7 days, then 20 mg/m$^2$ PO SID for 7 days, then 10 mg/m$^2$ PO QOD. |
| 2. Vincristine | 0.02 mg/kg IV week 1,2,3. |
| Chlorambucil[a] | 0.2 mg/kg SID PO for 7 days, then 0.1 mg/kg SID PO continuously or 2 mg/m2 PO QOD. |
| Prednisone | 30 mg/m$^2$ SID PO × 7 days, then 20 mg/m2 SID PO × 7 days, then 10 mg/m2 QOD PO continuously. |

[a]If no response, substitute cyclophosphamide 50 mg/m2 PO SID × 4, repeat weekly.

cristine and prednisone, the dogs achieving complete or partial remission had a median survival time of 120 days, and few dogs survived longer than 8 months with that protocol.[142] In one case report, a dog with ALL was treated with infusion of a large volume of fresh canine plasma and whole blood, and a complete remission was maintained for 19 months without additional therapy. This is a very unusual response and indicates that normal blood contains some antileukemic factor(s).[163]

The authors have seen several dogs with lymphocytic leukemia in which the lymphoblasts appear to be more differentiated (prolymphocytic) than in most cases of ALL. Clinically, these dogs appear to have a better prognosis, and this may represent a subtype of canine ALL. Further studies are needed to define this subpopulation, if it exists at all.

As stated before, CLL is a slowly progressive disease, and some animals will not require therapy. One dog was observed for almost 2 years without treatment.[157] For those dogs treated, normalization of white blood cell counts can be expected in 70% of cases. In one report of 17 dogs treated with vincristine, chlorambucil, and prednisone, the median survival time was approximately 12 months with an expected 30% survival at 2 years.[143] In other studies dogs treated intermittently with chlorambucil and prednisone have reported remissions of 10 to 30 months.[158,164,165]

**Comparative Features** The non-Hodgkin's lymphomas may present as "nodal" or "extra-nodal" disease. Approximately 64% of people present with peripheral lymphadenopathy, with the cervical nodes being the primary site in 60%. Most patients with non-Hodgkin's lymphoma tend to have disseminated disease.[166]

Treatment must take into consideration such factors as histologic type, stage of disease, age, and "extra-nodal" involvement. For the older patient with a good prognosis histologically (low-grade lymphoma) the treatment may be palliative. This may involve low-dose radiation and single-agent chemotherapy (chlorambucil and prednisone). Patients with more aggressive histologic cell types may be treated with combination chemotherapy (cyclophosphamide, vincristine, doxorubicin, etoposide (VP-16), bleomycin, methotrexate, and prednisone).[167]

The prognosis varies enormously with histologic grade and clinical stage. A recent analysis of 43 human patients with non-Hodgkin's lymphoma demonstrated that the most significant prognostic indicator is low-grade lymphoma. Within that subtype another important variable is the presence of a specific chromosomal translocation [T 14, 18]. In intermediate- to high-grade lymphomas, age and the presence of a different cytogenetic abnormality (1 q) are significant prognostic variables.[25] For those with localized disease and intermediate- to high-grade lymphomas, survival rates of 60 to 85% are possible; for individuals with widespread disease treated with chemotherapy, the survival is about 50 to 60% at 5 years.[167]

Cutaneous lymphoma (T-cell) can be treated with total skin electron radiation (TSE) as described in a recent review.[168] Modern TSE delivers at least 2,400 Cgy at a depth of 3 mm in the skin, and this cures about 30 to 50% of stage 1A patients. Topical mechlorethamine (nitrogen mustard) will cure approximately 25% of patients with stage 1A disease. Chemotherapy with single agents such as prednisone, chlorambucil, methotrexate, cyclophosphamide, and doxorubicin achieve remissions in about 33% of cases. Combination chemotherapy only improves the response rate by 5%. Interferon-alpha has resulted in response rates of 25 to 40% with long-term treatment. The retinoids produce response in less than 20% of patients.[168]

The treatment of ALL has seen major advances over the past 20 years. The first principle of management is to reduce the population of malignant cells to as near zero as possible by intensive combination chemotherapy. Remission is induced by a combination of cytotoxic agents (for example, prednisone, vincristine, daunorubicin, and L-asparaginase). Once remission is induced, consolidation and maintenance treatment with drugs such as 6-mercaptopurine, methotrexate, and cyclophosphamide are continued for up to 2 years or more. The central nervous system is treated with irradiation and intrathecal cytotoxic chemotherapy, usually methotrexate.[169] The overall cure rate is greater than 80% in childhood ALL versus 20 to 30% in adult ALL.

The treatment of CLL in people depends on the extent of disease and the nature of the clinical symptoms. Treatment is usually initiated if there is lymphadenopathy, anemia, or thrombocytopenia (stages I–IV). Radiation therapy may reduce the size of the lymph nodes or spleen, but the usual treatment is continuous oral chlorambucil with or without prednisone. The prognosis of CLL is generally good, despite the broad spectrum of the disorder, with a median survival time of 4 to 5 years, depending on the clinical stage of disease. Based on the clinical stage, the median survival times are: for stage 0, greater than 150 months; for stage I, 101 months; for stage II, 71 months; and for stage III/IV, 19 months.[170]

## REFERENCES

1. Backgren AW: Lymphatic leukemia in dogs. An epizootiological clinical and haematological study. Acta Vet Scand 6 (Suppl 1), 1965.
2. Dorn CR, Taylor DON, Schneider R, et al: Survey of animal neoplasms in Alameda Contra Costa counties, California II. Cancer morbidity in dogs and cats from Alameda County. J Natl Cancer Inst 40:307–318, 1968.
3. Dorn CR, Taylor DON, Schneider R: The epidemiology of canine leukemia and lymphoma In Dutcher RM, (ed): Comparative Leukemia Research Proceedings, 4th International Symposium in Comparative Leukemia Research, Cherry Hill, NJ. Bibl Haematol 36:403–415, 1970.
4. Kaiser HE: Animal neoplasms: A systemic review. In Kaiser HE (ed): Neoplasms—Comparative pathology in animals, plants and man. Baltimore, Williams and Wilkins, 1981, pp. 747–812.
5. Moulton JE, Harvey JW: Tumors of lymphoid and hematopoetic tissue. In Moulton JE (ed): Tumors of Domestic Animals, 3rd ed. University of California Press 1990, pp. 231–307.
6. Parodi A, Wyers M, Paris J: Incidence of canine lymphoid leukosis. Age, breed and sex distribution; results of a necropsy survey. Bibl Haematol 30:263, 1968.
7. Priester WA, McKay FW: The occurrence of tumors in domestic animals. National Cancer Institute, Monograph 54:1–210, 1980.
8. Jarrett WFH, Crighton GW, Dalton RE: Leukemia and lymphosarcoma in animal and man. Vet Res 79:693–699, 1966.
9. Onions DE: A prospective survey of familial canine lymphosarcoma. J Natl Cancer Inst 72:909– 912, 1984.
10. Teske E, DeVos JP, Egberin KHF, et al: Clustering of canine lymphoma. In:Non-Hodgkin's lymphoma in the dog. Characterization and experimental therapy. Chapter VIII Thesis, University of Utrecht, 1993, pp. 101–107.
11. Chapman AL, Bopp WJ, Brightwell AS, et al: A preliminary report on virus-like particles in canine leukemia and derived cell cultures. Cancer Res 27:18–25, 1967.
12. Strandstrom HV, Rimaila-Parnanen E: Canine atypical malignant lymphoma. Am J Vet Res 40:1033–1034, 1979.
13. Onions D: RNA dependent DNA polymerase activity in canine lymphosarcoma. Eur J Cancer, 16:345–350, 1980.
14. Armstrong SJ, Thomley FM, Nunes DeSouza PA,

15. Tomley FM, Armstrong SJ, Mahy BW, et al: Reverse transcriptase activity and particles of retroviral density in cultured canine lymphosarcoma supernatants. Br J Cancer 47:277–284, 1983.
16. Blair A: Herbicides and non-Hodgkin's lymphoma: new evidence from a study of Saskatchewan farmers. J Natl Cancer Inst 82:544–545, 1990.
17. Hardell L, Erickson M, Lenner P, Lundgren E: Malignant lymphoma and exposure to chemicals, especially organic solvents, chlorophenols and phenoxy acids: A case-control study. Br J Cancer 43:169–176, 1981.
18. Hoar SK, Blair A, Holmes FF, et al: Agricultural herbicide use and risk of lymphoma and soft tissue sarcoma. J Am Med Assoc 256:1141–1147, 1986.
19. Hayes HM, Tarone RE, Cantor KP, et al: Case-control study of canine malignant lymphoma: Positive association with dog owner's use of 2, 4-dichlorophenoxyacetic acid herbicides. J Natl Cancer Inst 83:1226–1231, 1991.
20. Carlo GL, Cole P, Miller AB, et al: Review of a study reporting an association between 2, 4-dichlorophenoxyacetic acid and canine malignant lymphoma: Report of an expert panel. Regul Toxicol Pharmacol 16:245–252, 1992.
21. Reynolds PM, Reif JS, Ramsdell HS. Canine exposure to herbicide treated lawns and urinary excretion of 2, 4-dichlorophenoxyacetic acid. Cancer Epidemol Biomarkers Prev 3:233–237, 1994.
22. Edward MD, Pazzi KA, Gumerlock PH: c-N-ras is activated infrequently in canine malignant lymphoma. Toxicol Pathol 21:288–291, 1993.
23. Yunis JJ, Oken MM, Theologides A, et al: Recurrent chromosomal defects found in most patients with non-Hodgkin's lymphoma. Cancer Genet Cytogenet 13:17–28, 1984.
24. Rowley JD: Chromosome studies in the non-Hodgkin's lymphomas. The role of the 14-18 translocation. J Clin Oncol 6:919–925, 1988.
25. Whang-Peng J, Knutsen T, Jaffe ES, et al: Sequential analysis of 43 patients with non-Hodgkin's lymphoma: Clinical correlations with cytogenetics, histologic, immunophenotyping and molecular studies. Blood 85:203–216, 1995.
26. Hahn KA, Richardson RC, Hahn EA, et al: Diagnostic and prognostic importance of chromosomal aberrations identified in 61 dogs with lymphosarcoma. Vet Pathol 31:528–540, 1994.
27. Weiden PL, Storb R, Kolb HJ, et al: Immune reactivity in dogs with spontaneous malignancy. J Natl Cancer Inst 53:1049–1056, 1974.

28. Owen LN, Bostock DE, Halliwell REW: Cell-mediated and humoral immunity in dogs with spontaneous lymphosarcoma. Eur J Cancer 11:187–191, 1975.

29. Keller ET: Immune-mediated disease as a risk factor for canine lymphoma. Cancer, 70:2334–2337, 1992.

30. Kersey JH, Spector BD, Good RA: Immunodeficiency and Cancer. Adv Cancer Res, 18:211–230, 1973.

31. Penn I: Cancer in immunosuppressed patients. Transplant Procedure 16:492–494, 1984.

32. Janowska-Wieczorek A, Andrews EJ, Khaliq A, et al: Deficiency of mature B and T-lymphocytes subsets in the blood of non-Hodgkin's lymphoma patients. Am J Hematol, 26:125–134, 1987.

33. Madewell BR, Thesen GH. Hematopoietic neoplasms, sarcomas and related conditions. Part IV: Canine. In Theilen GH, Madewell BR (eds): Veterinary Cancer Medicine, 2nd ed. Philadelphia, Lea and Febiger, 1987, pp. 392–407.

34. Keller ET, MacEwen EG, Rosenthal RC: Evaluation of prognostic factors and sequential combination chemotherapy with doxorubicin for canine lymphoma. J Vet Intern Med 7:289–295, 1993.

35. MacEwen EG, Brown NO, Patnaik AK, et al: Cyclic combination chemotherapy of canine lymphosarcoma. J Am Vet Med Assoc 178:1178–1181, 1981.

36. Hawkins EG, Morrison WB, DeNicola DB, et al: Cytologic analysis of bronchoalveolar lavage fluid from 47 dogs with multicentric malignant lymphoma. J Am Vet Med Assoc 203:1418–1425, 1993.

37. Yohn SE, Hawkins EC, Morrison WB, et al: Confirmation of a pulmonary component of multicentric lymphosarcoma with bronchoalveolar lavage in two dogs. J Am Vet Med Assoc 204:97–101, 1994.

38. Skudder PA Jr, Schwartz SI: Primary lymphoma of the gastrointestinal tract. Surg Gynecol Obstet 160:5–8, 1985.

39. Couto CG, Rutgers HC, Sherding RG, et al: Gastrointestinal lymphoma in 20 dogs: A retrospective study. J Vet Intern Med 3:73–78, 1989.

40. Leib MS, Bradley, RL: Alimentary lymphosarcoma in a dog. Compend Contin Educ Pract Vet 9:809–815, 1987.

41. Breitschwerdt EB, Waltman C, Hagastad HV, et al: Clinical and epidemiological characterization of a diarrheal syndrome in Basenji dog. J Am Vet Med Assoc, 180:914–920, 1982.

42. Steinberg H, Dubielzig RR, Thomson J, et al: Primary gastrointestinal lymphosarcoma with epitheliotropism in three Shar-Pei and one Boxer dog. Vet Pathol (in press).

43. Greenlee PG, Filippa DA, Quimby FW, et al: Lymphoma in dogs: A morphologic, immunologic, and clinical study. Cancer 66:480–490, 1990.

44. Chew DJ, Meuten DJ: Disorders of calcium and phosphorus metabolism. Vet Clin North Am Small Anim Pract 12:411–438, 1982.

45. Rosenberg MP, Matus RE, Patnaik AK: Prognostic factors in dogs with lymphoma and associated hypercalcemia. J Vet Intern Med 5:268–271, 1991.

46. Muller GH, Kirk RW, Scott DW: Cutaneous lymphosarcoma. In Small Animal Dermatology, 4th ed. Philadelphia, WB Saunders, pp. 918–927. 1989,

47. Kelly DF, Halliwell REW, Schwartzman RM: Generalized cutaneous eruption in a dog, with histological similarity to human mycosis fungoides. Br J Dermatol 86:164–171, 1972.

48. Shadduck JA, Reedy L, Lawton G, et al: A canine cutaneous lymphoproliferative disease resembling mycosis fungoides in man. Vet Pathol 15:716–724, 1978.

49. Thrall MA, Macy DW, Snyder SP, et al: Cutaneous lymphosarcoma and leukemia in a dog resembling Sézary's syndrome in man. Vet Pathol 21:182–186, 1984.

50. DeBoer DJ, Turrel JM, Moore PF: Mycosis fungoides in a dog: Demonstration of T-cell specificity and response to radiotherapy. J Am Anim Hosp Assoc 26:566–572, 1990.

51. Johnson JA, Patterson JM: Canine epidermotropic lymphoproliferative disease resembling pagetoid reticulosis in man. Vet Pathol 18:487–493, 1981.

52. White SD, Rosychuk RAW, Scott KV, et al: Use of isotretinoin and etretinate for the treatment of benign cutaneous neoplasia and cutaneous lymphoma in dogs. J Am Vet Med Assoc 202:387–391, 1993.

53. McKeever PJ, Grindem CB, Stevens JB, et al: Canine cutaneous lymphoma. J Am Vet Med Assoc 180:531–536, 1982.

54. Brown NO, Nesbitt GH, Patnaik AK, et al: Cutaneous lymphosarcoma in the dog: A disease with variable clinical and histologic manifestations. J Am Anim Hosp Assoc 16:565–572, 1980.

55. Moore PF, Olivry T, Naydan D: Canine cutaneous epitheliotrophic lymphoma (mycosis fungoides) is a proliferative disorder of CD8+ T-cells. Am J Pathol, 144:421–429, 1994.

56. Broder S, Muul L, Marshall S, et al: Neoplasms of immunoregulatory T-cells in clinical investigation. J Invest Dermatol 74:267–271, 1980.

57. Wieselthier JS, Koh WK: Sézary syndrome. Diagnosis, prognosis, and critical review of treatment options. J Amer Acad Dermatol 22:381–401, 1990.

58. Schick RO, Murphy GF, Goldschmidt MH: Cutaneous lymphosarcoma and leukemia in a cat. J Am Vet Med Assoc 203:1155–1158, 1993.

59. Carter RF, Valli VEO, Lumsden JH: The cytology, histology and prevalence of cell types in canine lymphoma classified according to the National Cancer Institute Working Formulation. Can J Vet Res 50:154–164, 1986.

60. Lennert K, Stein H, Kaiserling E: Cytologic and functional criteria for the classification of malig-

nant lymphomata. Br J Cancer *31* (Suppl 2): 29–43, 1975.

61. Rappaport H: Tumors of the hematopoietic system. *In* Atlas of Tumor Pathology, Section 3, Fascicle 8. Washington DC, Armed Forces Inst of Pathology, 1966.

62. Teske E, van Heerde P, Rutteman GR, et al: Prognostic factors for treatment of malignant lymphoma in dogs. J Am Vet Med Assoc *205:* 1722–1728, 1994.

63. Appelbaum FR, Sale GE, Storb R, et al: Phenotyping of canine lymphoma with monoclonal antibodies directed at cell surface antigens: Classification, morphology, clinical presentation and response to chemotherapy. Hematol Oncol *2:*151–168, 1984.

64. Weir EC, Greelee P, Matus R, et al: Hypercalcemia in canine lymphosarcoma is associated with the T-cell subtype and with secretion of a PTH-like factor. J Bone Miner Res *3,*S106, 1988 (Abstract).

65. Grossman B, Schechter GP, Horton JE, et al: Hypercalcemia associated with T-cell lymphoma-leukemia. Am J Clin Pathol *75:*149–155, 1981.

66. Kinoshita K, Kamihira S, Ikeda S, et al: Clinical, hematologic, and pathologic features of leukemic T-cell lymphoma. Cancer *50:*1554–1562, 1982.

67. Stewart AF, Horst R, Deftos LJ, et al: Biochemical evaluation of patients with cancer-associated hypercalcemia. N Engl J Med *303:*1377–1383, 1980.

68. Couto CG, Cullen J, Pedroia V, et al: Central nervous system lymphosarcoma in the dog. J Am Vet Med Assoc *184:*809–813, 1984.

69. Dallman MJ, Saunders GK: Primary spinal cord lymphosarcoma in a dog. J Am Vet Med Assoc *189:*1348–1349, 1986.

70. Rosin A: Neurologic diseases associated with lymphosarcoma in ten dogs. J Am Vet Med Assoc *181:*50–53, 1982.

71. Swanson JF: Ocular manifestations of systemic disease in the dog and cat: Recent developments. Vet Clin North Am Small Anim Pract *20:*849–867, 1990.

72. Krohne SDG, Vestre WA, Richardson RC, et al: Ocular involvement in canine lymphosarcoma: A retrospective study of 94 cases. Proc Am Coll Vet Ophth, 1987, pp. 68–84.

73. Madewell BR, Feldman BF: Characterization of anemias associated with neoplasia in small animals. J Am Vet Med Assoc *176:*419–425, 1980.

74. Jain WC: The leukemia complex. *In* Schalm's Veterinary Hematology, 4th ed. Philadelphia, Lea and Febiger, 1986, pp. 838–908.

75. Madewell BR: Hematological and bone marrow cytological abnormalities in 75 dogs with malignant lymphoma. J Am Anim Hosp Assoc *22:*235–240, 1986.

76. Grindem CB, Breitschwadt, EB, Corbett WT, et al: Thrombocytopenia associated with neoplasia in dogs. J Vet Intern Med *8:*400–405, 1994.

77. Weller RE: Paraneoplastic disorders in dogs with hematopoietic tumors. Vet Clin North Am Small Anim Pract *15:*805–816, 1985.

78. Weller RE: Holmberg CA, Theilen GH, et al: Canine lymphosarcoma and hypercalcemia: Clinical, laboratory and pathologic evaluation of twenty-four cases. J Small Anim Pract *23:*649–658, 1982.

79. Weir EC, Norrdin RW, Matus RE, et al: Humoral hypercalcemia of malignancy in canine lymphosarcoma. Endocrinology *122:*602–608, 1988.

80. Weller RE, Hoffman WE: Renal function in dogs with lymphosarcoma and associated hypercalcemia. J Small Anim Pract *33:*61–66, 1992.

81. Rosol TJ, Nagode LA, Couto CG, et al: Parathyroid hormone (PTH)-related protein, PTH, and α-25, dehydroxyvitamin-D in dogs with cancer-associated hypercalcemia. Endocrinology *131:* 1157–1164, 1992.

82. MacEwen, EG, Patnaik AK, Wilkins RJ: Diagnosis and treatment of canine hematopoietic neoplasms. Vet Clin North Am Small Anim Pract *7:*105–118, 1977.

83. Vail DM, Ogilvie GK, Wheeler SL, et al: Alterations in carbohydrate metabolism in canine lymphoma. J Vet Intern Med *4:*8–11, 1990.

84. Raskin RE, Krehbiel JD: Prevalence of leukemic blood and bone marrow in dogs with multicentric lymphoma. J Am Vet Med Assoc *194:*1427–1429, 1989.

85. Nyland TG, Park RD: Hepatic ultrasonography in the dog. Vet Radiol *24:*74–84, 1983.

86. Nyland TG: Ultrasonic pattern of canine hepatic lymphosarcoma. Vet Radiol *25:*167–172, 1984.

87. Wrigley RH, Konde LJ, Park RD, et al: Ultrasonographic features of splenic lymphosarcoma in dogs: 12 cases (1980–1986) J Am Vet Med Assoc *193:*1565–1568, 1988.

88. Feeney DA, Johnston GR, Hardy RM: Two-dimensional, gray-scale ultrasonography for assessment of hepatic and splenic neoplasia in the dog and cat. J Am Vet Med Assoc *184:*68–81, 1984.

89. Carney DN, Bunn PA Jr: Manifestations of cutaneous T-cell lymphoma. J Dermatol Surg Oncol *6:*369–377, 1980.

90. MacEwen EG, Brown NO, Patnaik AK, et al: Cyclic combination chemotherapy of canine lymphosarcoma. J Am Vet Med Assoc *178:*1178–1181, 1981.

91. Cotter SM, Goldstein MA: Treatment of lymphoma and leukemia with cyclophosphamide, vincristine, and prednisone: I. Treatment of dog. J Am Anim Hosp Assoc *19:*159–165, 1983.

92. Carter RF, Harris CK, Withrow SJ, et al: Chemotherapy of canine lymphoma with histopathological correlation: Doxorubicin alone compared to COP as first treatment regimen. J Am Anim Hosp Assoc *23:*587–596, 1987.

93. Postorino NC, Susaneck SJ, Withrow SJ, et al: Single agent therapy with adriamycin for canine

lymphosarcoma. J Am Anim Hosp Assoc 25:221–225, 1989.

94. MacEwen EG, Hayes AA, Matus RE, et al: Evaluation of some prognostic factors for advanced multicentric lymphosarcoma in the dog: 147 cases (1978–1981). J Am Vet Med Assoc 190:564–568, 1987.

95. Stone MS, Goldstein MA, Cotter SM: Comparison of two protocols for induction of remission in dogs with lymphoma. J Am Anim Hosp Assoc 27:315–3 21, 1991.

96. Madewell BR: Chemotherapy for canine lymphosarcoma. Am J Vet Res 36:1525–1528, 1975.

97. Kartner N, Riordan JR, Ling V: Cell surface P-glycoprotein associated with multidrug resistance in mammalian cell liver. Science 221:1285–1288, 1983.

98. Miller TP, Grogan TM, Dalton WS, et al: P-glycoprotein expression in malignant lymphoma and reversal of clinical drug resistance with chemotherapy plus high dose verapamil. J Clin Oncol 9:17–24, 1991.

99. MacEwen EG, Rosenthal RC, Fox LE, et al: Evaluation of L-asparaginase: Polyethylene glycol conjugate versus native L-asparaginase combined with chemotherapy. A randomized double blind study in canine lymphoma. J Vet Intern Med 6:230–234, 1992.

100. Teske E, Rutteman GR, vanHeerde P, et al: Polyethylene glycol-L-asparaginase versus native L-asparaginase in canine non-Hodgkin's lymphoma. Eur J Cancer 26:891–895, 1990.

101. Vail DM: Recent advances in chemotherapy for lymphoma of dogs and cats. Compend Small Anim 15:1031–1037, 1993.

102. Ogilvie GK, Obradovich JE, Elmslie RE, et al: Toxicoses associated with administration of mitoxantrone to dogs with malignant tumors. J Am Vet Med Assoc 198:1613–1617, 1991.

103. Ogilvie GK, Obradovich JE, Elmslie RE, et al: Efficacy of mitoxantrone against various neoplasms in dogs. J Am Vet Med Assoc 198:1618–1621, 1991.

104. Hammer AS, Couto CG, Ayl RD, et al: Treatment of tumor-bearing dogs and cats with actinomycin D. J Vet Intern Med 8:236–239, 1994.

105. Moore AS, Ogilvie GK, Vail DM: Actinomycin D for reinduction of remission in dogs with resistant lymphoma. J Vet Intern Med 8:343–344, 1994.

106. Moore AS, Ogilvie GK, Ruslander D, et al: Mitoxantrone for the therapy of canine lymphoma. Proc Vet Cancer Soc 11: 3–4, 1991.

107. Calvert CA, Leifer CE: Doxorubicin for treatment of canine lymphosarcoma after development of resistance to combination chemotherapy. J Am Vet Med Assoc 179:1011–1012, 1981.

108. Van Vechten M, Helfand SC, Jeglum KA: Treatment of relapsed canine lymphoma with doxorubicin and dacarbazine. J Vet Intern Med 4:187–191, 1990.

109. Rosenberg MP, Matus RE: The use of MOPP as rescue treatment for dogs with lymphoma. Proc 11th Annu Conf Vet Cancer Soc 56, 1991.

110. Ruslander D, Moore AS, Cotter SM, et al: Cytosine arabinoside in the treatment of canine lymphoma. Proc 11th Annu Conf Vet Cancer Soc, 61–62, 1991,

111. Skipper HS: Analysis of 42 arms of four multi-armed trials in which animals bearing 2-3 gram ROS tumors were treated with simultaneous combination of cyclophosphamide plus L-PAM with systemic variations of the relative dose intensity of each drug, and the average relative dose intensity (Booklet 5). Birmingham, AL, Southern Research Institute, 1986.

112. Hryniuk WM: Average relative dose intensity and the impact on design of clinical trials. Semin Oncol 14:65–74, 1987.

113. DeVita VT Jr: Is alternating cyclic chemotherapy better than standard four-drug chemotherapy for Hodgkin's disease? No. In DeVita VT Jr, Hellman S, Rosenberg SA (eds): Important Advances in Oncology 1993. Philadelphia, JB Lippincott, 1993, pp. 197–208.

114. Gobbi PG, Cavalli C, Rossi A, et al: The role of dose and rate of administration of MOPP drugs in 97 retrospective Hodgkin's patients. Haematologica 72:523–528, 1987.

115. LaGarde P, Bonichon H, Eghbali I, et al: Influence of dose intensity and density on therapeutic and toxic effects in Hodgkin's disease. Br J Cancer, 59:645–649, 1989.

116. Dalton WS: Overcoming the multidrug-resistant phenotype. In DeVita VT Jr, Hellman S, Rosenberg SA (eds) Cancer: Principles and Practices of Oncology, 4th ed. Philadelphia, JB Lippincott, 1995, pp. 2655–2666.

117. Bergman PJ, Ogilvie GK, Powers BE: P-glycoprotein immunohistochemistry in canine lymphoma. Proc Vet Cancer Soc 13:33–34, 1993.

118. Price SG, Page RL, Fischer BM, et al: Efficacy and toxicity of doxorubicin/cyclophosphamide maintenance therapy in dogs with multicentric lymphosarcoma. J Vet Intern Med 5:259–262, 1991.

119. Goldie JH, Coldman AJ: A mathematic model for relating the drug sensitivity of tumors to their spontaneous mutation rate. Cancer Treat Rep 63:1727–1733, 1979.

120. MacEwen EG, Hayes AA, Mooney S, et al: Levamisole as adjuvant to chemotherapy for canine lymphosarcoma. J Biol Response Mod 4:427–433, 1985.

121. MacEwen EG, Hess PW, Hayes AA, et al: A clinical evaluation of the effectiveness of immunotherapy combined with chemotherapy for canine lymphosarcoma in the 8th symposium on comparative research on leukemia and related disease. Amsterdam, 1977, p. 162 (Abstract).

122. Crow SE, Theilen GH, Benjaminini E, et al: Chemoimmunotherapy for canine lymphosarcoma. Cancer 40:2102–2108, 1977.

123. Weller RE, Theilen GH, Madewell BR, et al: Chemoimmunotherapy for canine lymphosarcoma: A prospective evaluation of specific and nonspecific immunomodulation. Am J Vet Res 41:516–521, 1980.

124. Jeglum KA, Young KM, Barnsley K, et al: Chemotherapy versus chemotherapy with intralymphatic tumor cell vaccine in canine lymphoma. Cancer 61:2042–2050, 1988.

125. Steplewski Z, Jeglum KA, Rosales C, et al: Canine lymphoma-associated antigens defined by murine monoclonal antibodies. Cancer Immunol Immunother 24:197–201, 1987.

126. Rosales C, Jeglum KA, Obrocka M, et al: Cytolytic activity of murine anti-dog lymphoma monoclonal antibodies with canine effector cells and complement. Cell Immunol 115:420–428, 1988.

127. Steplewski Z, Rosales C, Jeglum KA, et al: In vivo destruction of canine lymphoma mediated by murine monoclonal antibodies. In vivo 4:231–234, 1990.

128. Jeglum KA, Steplewski Z: A phase I clinical trial of murine anti-dog lymphoma monoclonal antibody. Proc Vet Cancer Soc 7:24, 1987.

129. Jeglum KA, Reese LP, Shephard K, Callahan JD: The efficacy of monoclonal antibody 231 in the treatment of canine lymphoma 1995 (submitted).

130. Richter K: Personal communications.

131. Meeker T, Lowder J, Cleary ML, et al: Emergence of idiotype variants during treatment of B-cell lymphoma with anti-idiotype antibodies. N Engl J Med 312: 1658–1665, 1985.

132. Moldovanu G, Friedman M, Miller DG: Treatment of canine malignant lymphoma with surgery and chemotherapy. J Am Vet Med Assoc 148:153–156, 1966.

133. Brooks MB, Matus RE, Leifer CE, et al: Use of splenectomy in the management of lymphoma in dogs: 16 cases (1976–1985). J Am Vet Med Assoc 191:1008–1010, 1987.

134. Thrall DE, Dewhirst MH: Use of radiation and/or hyperthermia for treatment of mast cell tumors and lymphosarcoma in dogs. Vet Clin North Am Small Anim Pract 15:835–843, 1985.

135. Couto CG: Cutaneous lymphosarcoma. Proc Kal Kan Symp 11:17–77, 1987.

136. Bunn PA, Hoffman SJ, Norris D, et al: Systemic therapy of cutaneous T-cell lymphoma (Mycosis fungoides and the Sézary Syndrome). Ann Intern Med 121:592–602, 1994.

137. Moriello KA, MacEwen EG, Schultz KT: PEG-asparaginase in the treatment of canine epitheliotrophic lymphoma and histiocytic proliferative dermatitis In Ihrke PJ, Mason IS, White SD (eds): New York, Advances in Veterinary Dermatology. Pergamon Press, 1993 pp. 293–300.

138. MacDonald JM: Nasal depigmentation. In Griffin CE, Kwochka KW, MacDonald JM (eds): Current Veterinary Dermatology. Mosby Yearbook. St. Louis, 1993, pp. 223–233.

139. Weller RE, Theilen GH, Madewell BR: Chemotherapeutic responses in dogs with lymphosarcoma and hypercalcemia. J Am Vet Med Assoc 181:891–893, 1982.

140. Vail DM, Ritter MA, Kisseberth WC, et al: Potential doubling time is prognostic for dogs with lymphoma. Proc Vet Cancer Soc 14:77–78, 1994.

141. Crocker J, Nar P: Nucleolar organizer regions in lymphomas. J Pathol 151:111–118, 1987.

142. Matus RE, Leifer CE, MacEwen EG: Acute lymphoblastic leukemia in the dog: A review of 30 cases. J Am Vet Med Assoc 183:859–862, 1983.

143. Leifer CE, Matus RE: Chronic lymphocytic leukemia in the dog: 22 cases (1974–1984). J Am Vet Med Assoc 189:214–217, 1986.

144. Perk K, Safran N, Dahlberg JE: Propagation and characterization of novel canine lentivirus isolated from a dog. Leukemia 6:1555–1575, 1992.

145. Farber E: Chemical carcinogenesis. N Engl J Med 305:1379–1789, 1981.

146. Rinsky RA, Smith AB, Hornung R, et al: Benzene and leukemia. N Engl J Med 316:1044–1050, 1987.

147. Rosner F, Grunwald HW: Chemicals and leukemia. In Henderson ES, Lister AT (eds): Leukemia, 5th ed. Toronto, WB Saunders, 1990, pp. 271–287.

148. Whitehouse JM: Risk of leukemia associated with cancer chemotherapy (Editorial). Br Med J Clin Res Ed 290:261–263, 1985.

149. Sieber SM, Adamson RH: Toxicity of antineoplastic agents in man, chromosomal aberrations, and antifertility effects, congenital malformations, and carcinogenic potential. Adv Cancer Res 22:57–155, 1975.

150. Finch SC: Leukemia and lymphoma in atomic bomb survivors. In Boice JD, Fraumeni JF (eds): Radiation carcinogenesis: Epidemiology and biological significance. New York, Raven Press, 1980, p. 37.

151. Blattner WA, Blayney DW, Robert-Guroff M, et al: Epidemiology of human T-cell leukemia/lymphoma virus. J Infect Dis 147:406–416, 1983.

152. Raskin RE, Nipper MN: Cytochemical staining characteristics of lymph nodes from normal and lymphoma-affected dogs. Vet Clin Pathol 21:62–67, 1992.

153. Wellman ML, Couto CG, Starkey RJ, et al: Lymphocytosis of large granular lymphocytes in three dogs. Vet Pathol 26:158–163, 1989.

154. Chapman AL, Bopp WJ, Torres J, et al: An electron microscopic study of the cell types in canine lymphoma and leukemia. J Comp Pathol 91:331–340, 1981.

155. Rai KR, Sawitsky A, Cronkite EP, et al: Clinical staging of chronic lymphocytic leukemia. Blood 46:219–234, 1975.

156. Skinnider LF, Tan L, Schmidt J, et al: Chronic lymphocytic leukemia. A review of 745 cases and assessment of clinical staging. Cancer 50:2951–2955, 1982.

157. Harvey JW, Terrell TG, Hyde DM, et al: Well-differentiated lymphocytic leukemia in a dog: Long-term survival without therapy. Vet Pathol 18:37–47, 1981.

158. Hodgkins EM, Zinkl JG, Madewell BR: Chronic lymphocytic leukemia in the dog. J Am Vet Med Assoc 117:704–707, 1980.

159. Adair CG, Bridges JM, Desai ZR: Can food affect the bioavailability of chlorambucil in patients with haematological malignancies? Cancer Chemother Pharmacol 17:99–102, 1986.

160. Han T, Ezdinli EZ, Shimaoka K, et al: Chlorambucil vs combined chlorambucil-corticosteroid therapy in chronic lymphocytic leukemia. Cancer 31:502–508, 1973.

161. Pegourie B, Sotto J, Hollard D, et al: Splenectomy during chronic lymphocytic leukemia. Cancer 59:1626–1630, 1987.

162. Januszewicz E, Cooper IA, Pelkington G, et al: Blastic transformation of chronic lymphocytic leukemia. Am J Hematol 15:399–402, 1983.

163. MacEwen EG, Patnaik AK, Hayes AA, et al: Temporary plasma-induced remission of lymphoblastic leukemia in a dog. Am J Vet Res 42:1450–1452, 1981.

164. Kristensen AT, Klausner JS, Weiss DJ, et al: Spurious hyperphosphatemia in a dog with chronic lymphocytic leukemia and an IgM monoclonal gammopathy. Vet Clin Pathol 20:45–48, 1991.

165. Couto GC, Sousa C: Chronic lymphocytic leukemia with cutaneous involvement in a dog. J Am Anim Hosp Assoc 22:374–379, 1986.

166. Urba WJ, Longo DL: Lymphocytic lymphoma: Epidemiology, etiology, pathology, and staging. In Moossa AR, Schimpff SC, Robson MC (eds): Comprehensive Textbook of Oncology. Baltimore, Williams and Wilkins. 1991, pp. 1268–1276.

167. Urba WJ, Longo DL: Lymphocytic lymphoma: Clinical course and management: In Moossa AR, Schimpff SC, Robson MC (eds): Comprehensive Textbook of Oncology. Baltimore, Williams and Wilkins. 1991, pp. 1277–1295.

168. Jones GW: Mycosis fungoides issues and management in 1995. Cancer J 7:214–219, 1994.

169. Linker CA, Levitt LJ, O'Donnell M, et al: Treatment of adult acute lymphoblastic leukemia with intensive cyclical chemotherapy: A follow-up report. Blood 78:2814–2822, 1991.

170. Disseroth AB, Andreeff M, Champlin, R, et al: Chronic leukemia. In: DeVita VT Jr, Hellman S, Rosenberg SA (eds): Cancer: Principles and Practice of Oncology, 4th ed. Philadelphia, JB Lippincott, 1995, pp. 1965–1971.

171. Page RL, Macy DW, Ogilvie GK, et al: Phase III evaluation of doxorubicin and whole-body hyperthermia in dogs with lymphoma. Int J Hyperthermia 8:187–197, 1992.

172. Hohenhaus AE, Matus RE: Etoposide (VP-16) Retrospective analysis of treatment in 13 dogs with lymphoma. J Vet Intern Med 4:239–241, 1990.

# C. Feline Lymphoma and Leukemias

## E. Gregory MacEwen

### INCIDENCE AND RISK FACTORS

Lymphoma is a proliferative disease arising from lymphoid tissues involving any organ or tissue and accounts for 50 to 90% of all hematopoietic tumors in the cat.[1,2] Since hematopoietic tumors (lymphoid and myeloid) account for approximately one-third of all feline tumors, it is estimated lymphoid neoplasia accounts for an incidence of 200 per 100,000 cats at risk.[3] In one series of 400 cats with hematopoietic tumors, 61% had lymphoma, 39% had leukemias and myeloproliferative disorders, of which 21% were categorized as undifferential leukemias, which were most likely myeloid in origin.[4]

The mean age neoplastic development is reported to range from 2 to 6 years.[5,6] In one study, males were at greater risk, and in another study females were reported to have a greater risk.[7,8]

The feline leukemia virus (FeLV) is the most common cause of hematopoietic tumors in the cat (see Chapter 28A). The incidence of FeLV (positive), based on indirect immunofluorescent antibody (IFA), will range from 30 to 80%, depending on the location of the tumor and the age of the cat (Table 28–16).[5,9] Younger cats tend to be FeLV positive and have leukemia or mediastinal lymphoma. Older cats tend to be FeLV negative and alimentary lymphoma are usually FeLV negative.[6]

There is mounting evidence that feline immunodeficiency virus (FIV) infection will increase the incidence of lymphoma in cats.[10,11] Shelton et al. determined that FIV infection alone in cats was associated with a fivefold increased

**Table 28–16**   Anatomic Forms of Feline Lymphomas

| Form | Frequency (%) | Age Average | FeLV + % |
|---|---|---|---|
| Mediastinal | 20–50% | 2–3 years | 80% |
| Alimentary | 15–45% | 8 years | 30% |
| Multicentric | 20–40% | 4 years | 80% |
| Leukemia | 25–30% | 3 years | 80% |
| Extra-nodal | | | |
| CNS | 5–10% | 3–4 years | 80% |
| Cutaneous | < 5 | 8–10 years | < 10% |

risk for development of lymphomas.[10] Coinfection with FeLV will further potentiate the development of lymphoproliferative disorders.[10] Experimentally, cats infected with FIV have developed lymphoma in the kidney and liver of B-lymphocyte origin.[12,13] It has been suggested that FIV infection may be associated with alimentary lymphoma of B-cell origin, and this may be related to chronic dysregulation of the immune system or the activation of oncogenic pathways.[14,15]

## PATHOLOGY AND NATURAL BEHAVIOR

The classification of lymphoma and leukemias can be correlated with anatomic location and histologic criteria. Anatomic classification for lymphoma has been categorized as mediastinal, alimentary, multicentric, leukemic, and extranodal form.[2] The frequency of anatomic form will vary with geographic distribution and may be related to FeLV strain as well as prevalence of FeLV vaccine use.

### Mediastinal Form

This form involves the thymus, mediastinal, and sternal lymph nodes. More commonly the disease involves the anterior and posterior lymph nodes in the mediastinum. Pleural effusion is common. Occasionally the tumor will extend out of the thoracic inlet and can be palpated in the ventral neck region. Hypercalcemia occurs frequently with mediastinal lymphoma in dogs and is very rare in cats.[16,17] The majority of cats with mediastinal lymphoma are young and FeLV positive.[2]

### Alimentary Form

Alimentary lymphoma usually consists of gastrointestinal, mesenteric lymph nodes and liver involvement. Some reports will limit the alimentary form to gastrointestinal involvement with or without extension to the liver. The low prevalence of FeLV infection in cats with gastrointestinal involvement is because most of these tumors are from B-lymphocytes in gut-associated lymphoid tissue.[18] Although recent evidence suggests some FeLV-negative tumors may be derived from transformation of multipotent lymphoid or monocyte precursors[19] or FIV transformed B-lymphocytes.[12,13] The most common site of involvement is the small intestines (50%), then the stomach (25%), followed by ileocecocolic junction and colon. The tumor can be solitary or diffuse throughout the intestines, muscle layers, and intestinal submucosa, resulting in annular thickening, leading to partial or completed intestinal obstruction. There is a report describing chronic lymphocytic-plasmacytic enteritis in cats progressing to overt lymphoma, following 6 to 18 months of conservative therapy.[20]

### Multicentric Form

The multicentric form will usually involve peripheral lymph nodes with or without simultaneous abdominal (spleen/liver) involvement. Peripheral lymphadenopathy alone is very unusual. Cats with generalized peripheral lymphadenopathy due to lymphoma may have minimal signs of illness. As the lymphoma progresses, bone marrow infiltration with malignant cells and hepatosplenomegaly may develop.

There have been reports of nonneoplastic peripheral lymphadenopathy in cats, which clinically resembles lymphoma and histologically has features that may also resemble lymphoma.[21-23] These lymph nodes may be two to three times normal size. In one report, this syndrome was termed distinctive peripheral lymph node hyperplasia (DPLH) of young cats.[22] These cats tend to be young (2–4 years), many have had episodes of fever, previous viral infections, may have hypergammaglobulinemia (polyclonal gammopathy) and most are negative for FeLV.[21] Histopathologically the nodal architecture is severely distorted with loss of subcapsular and medullary sinuses. The cell population shows an admixture of histiocytes, lymphocytes, plasma cells, and immunoblasts, and occasionally effaced lymphoid follicles. The lymph nodes will regress spontaneously in most of these cats.[21] The histologic changes noted in these lymph nodes resemble the histologic features of AIDS-related lymphadenopathy in humans.[22]

## Extranodal Lymphoma

The most common extranodal sites for lymphoma include the kidneys, eyes, retrobulbar, central nervous system (CNS), nasal cavity, and skin. *Renal lymphoma* can be primary or associated with alimentary lymphoma. In a study of 28 cases of renal lymphoma the mean age was 7 years and 50% were FeLV positive.[24] Metastasis to the CNS is a frequent sequela to renal lymphoma and occurs in 40 to 50% of treated cats.

*Primary CNS lymphoma (PCNSL)* is most commonly seen extradural in the spinal canal and most cats are FeLV (positive) (80%).[25,26] Following meningioma, lymphoma is reported to be the second most common tumor involving the CNS in cats. The mean age is 3 to 4 years with some suggestion of a male predilection.[25–27] Most cats present with paresis of the hindlegs and thoracolumbar spine and epidural space are most commonly involved. The predilection for thoracolumbar spine in cats is unknown. Feline PCNSL may be primary or secondary to multicentric involvement (especially renal or bone marrow).[28] Bone involvement is rarely seen radiographically.[29] In necropsy findings, renal involvement and bone marrow are the common sites in cats presenting with spinal lymphoma.[25,26]

*Cutaneous lymphoma* is usually primary but can rarely be seen secondary to multicentric involvement. It is commonly seen in older cats (5–14 years) with an average age of 10 to 12 years.[30–34] No sex or breed predominance has been found. Uniformly, cats with cutaneous lymphoma test FeLV negative. However, one recent case report using polymerase chain reaction (PCR) technology found evidence of FeLV provirus in tumor DNA.[34] Cutaneous lymphoma can be solitary or generalized. Two forms of cutaneous lymphoma have been distinguished histologically and immunohistochemically.[30–34] The epitheliotrophic form, also called mycosis fungoides, is associated with T-lymphocytes. Non-epitheliotrophic form is usually composed of B-lymphocytes. Neoplastic T-lymphocytes are characterized as large with abundant cytoplasm and convoluted nuclei (mycosis cells). These cells usually form intraepidermal nests of 5 to 10 cells, separated from surrounding keratinocytes by a clear space (Pautrier's microabscesses). The B-cell lymphomas show lymphocytes deep in the epidermis, with sparing of the papillary dermis and epidermis. Confirmation, using immunohistophenotyping of B-cell lymphoma in cats with cutaneous lymphoma is lacking.

Recently, a cat with cutaneous T-cell lymphoma with circulating atypical lymphocytes was diagnosed.[33] The circulating cells were lymphocytes with large, hyperchromatic, grooved nuclei. In humans, cutaneous T-cell lymphoma with circulating malignant cells is called Sézary syndrome.[35] This syndrome has also been reported in dogs.[36–38]

## Histologic Classification of Lymphomas

A number of histopathologic staging systems have been developed and used to classify human non-Hodgkin's lymphoma. Recently, the morphologic criteria of the NIH Working Formulation (See Chapter 28B) was used to classify more than 600 cases of feline lymphoma.[39] Low-grade lymphoma was found in 8.6%, intermediate-grade in 35.1%, and high-grade in 55.2% of the cases. The remaining 1.1% were plasmacytomas. More than one-third of the tumors were of the immunoblastic type. Lymphoblastic lymphoma, a subtype of the high-grade tumor, constituted less than 3%. There was considerable variation in age of the animals with various subtypes, but in general, low-grade tumors tended to develop in older cats (>10 years) and high-grade tumors developed in younger cats (<6 years).

The majority of lymphomas in the cats are composed of T-cells transformed by FeLV.[40–41] Lymphomas arising from the gastrointestinal tract are usually B-lymphocytes and most of these test FeLV negative.[2,5]

A rare reported form of alimentary lymphoma is classified as *large granular lymphoma*.[42,43] Large granular lymphocytes are characterized by abundant cytoplasm with prominent azurophilic granules. This population of cells includes natural killer cells and cytotoxic T-cells. These tumors commonly originate in the small intestine, especially the jejunum or mesenteric lymph nodes. All cats reported with this type of tumor have been FeLV negative. Large granular lymphocytes must be differentiated from several other granular cell types that may be found in the small intestine, including globule leukocytes, enterochromaffin cells, mast cells, and eosinophils.

## Leukemias

The classification of leukemias in cats is difficult because of the similarity of clinical and pathological features and the transition, overlap, or mixture of cell types involved.[44–51]

Leukemia is defined as a neoplastic proliferation of hematopoietic cells originating within the bone marrow. Cell lineage includes myeloid, neutrophils, basophils, eosinophils, monocytes, lymphoid, megakaryocytes, and erythrocytes. Table 28–17 shows a classification scheme for the leukemias identified in the cats. Leukemias also need to be classified based on the degree of differentiation.[44] Well-differentiated leukemias are usually called "chronic" leukemia. The poorly differentiated leukemias are usually referred to as "acute." This distinction has been very important in the therapeutic management and prognosis of human and canine leukemias.

### Granulocytic Leukemia (Myeloid, Neutrophilic)[45–48]

The total leukocyte count is variable, and may range from leukopenia to marked leukocytosis. Chronic granulocytic leukemia (GL) must be distinguished from leukemoid reactions associated with infections. Acute GL is characterized by a large percentage of myeloblasts or progranulocytes, or both, in blood and bone marrow. The myeloblast can be difficult to distinguish from the lymphoblast but has a finer chromatin pattern, a smaller nucleus-to-cytoplasmic ratio, more prominent or multiple nucleoli, and sometimes cytoplasmic granules. It is not uncommon

---

**Table 28–17**   Classification of Leukemia

*Myeloproliferative Disorders*
  Granulocytes
    Granulocytic (myeloid, neutrophilic) leukemia
    Eosinophilic leukemia
    Basophilic leukemia
  Monocytes
    Monocytic leukemia
  Erythrocytes
    Erythremic myelosis
    Primary erythrocytosis
  Megakaryocytes
    Megakaryocytic leukemia (myelosis)
    Primary thrombocythemia
  Miscellaneous
    Mast cell leukemia
    Myelofibrosis
    Malignant histiocytosis
    Undifferentiated leukemia
  Mixed Cell Lines
    Myelomonocytic leukemia (neutrophils and
      monocytes)
    Erythroleukemia (erythrocytes and granulocytes)
    Myelodysplastic syndrome
*Lymphoproliferative Disorders*
  Lymphocytes
    Acute lymphoblastic leukemia
    Chronic lymphocytic leukemia

---

in cats with GL to have no recognizable neoplastic cells in the peripheral blood. The bone marrow is hypercellular because of granulocytic leukemia cells.

### Myelomonocytic Leukemia[45,49,50]

Myelomonocytic leukemia (MML) results from malignant transformation of both neutrophils and monocytes. This form of leukemia is one of the most common forms of leukemia reported.

### Monocytic Leukemia[47,50]

Monocytic leukemia (ML) is a rarely reported leukemia. ML is generally considered to be an acute leukemia, regardless of the morphologic appearance of the cells.

### Eosinophilic Leukemia (EL)

Eosinophilic Leukemia (EL) is rarely diagnosed in cats and is considered a variant of chronic granulocytic or myeloid leukemia.[51,52] EL has been induced experimentally by FeLV.[52] Mature eosinophils will outnumber immature stages and anemia is uncommon in cats associated with EL. Cats will usually have an eosinophil count of 15,000 cells/$\mu$l or greater with or without immature cells in the peripheral blood. The bone marrow will show hyperplasia of eosinophilic precursors and the M:E ratio will be significantly increased. Organ infiltration, such as lymph nodes, spleen, and liver can be seen.[53] It is important to rule out eosinophilic enteritis, parasitism, eosinophilic granuloma complex, and allergic disorders in establishing a diagnosis of EL. The diagnosis of EL can be very difficult because of the hypereosinophilic syndrome (HES) seen with other disease conditions in cats.[53–55] HES is characterized by marked increase in eosinophilic count, bone marrow hyperplasia of eosinophilic precursors, and multiple organ infiltration by mature eosinophilis. Most cats have signs related to gastrointestinal involvement.[53]

### Basophilic Leukemia[56]

Basophilic leukemia (BL) is considered a variant of chronic granulocytic leukemia. Only one confirmed case of BL has been reported in the cat. It is important to differentiate BL from systemic mastocytosis with mast cell leukemia. Mast cells have numerous cytoplasmic granules and round nuclei. Basophils have segmented nuclei and cytoplasmic granules that superimpose on the nucleus, giving it a "moth-eaten" appearance.

### Erythremic Myelosis[57–60]

Erythemic myelosis (EM) is a myeloproliferative disorder characterized by excessive proliferation of erythroid elements, resulting in an increase in nucleated erythrocytes (rubriblasts to metarubricytes), and is common in cats. Severe anemia is common and within the peripheral blood numerous nucleated erythrocytes, moderate to marked anisocytosis, and increased erythrocyte mean cell volume will be seen. The bone marrow contains a preponderance of normal-appearing erythrocytic precursors. Some cats will undergo blast transformation to myeloblastic, granulocytic, or a poorly differentiated leukemia (previously referred to as reticuloendotheliosis). The transition from EM to erythroleukemia to acute granulocytic leukemia is well recognized in humans.[61]

## Erythroleukemia (Reticuloendotheliosis)[44,47,50]

Erythroleukemia or acute erythremic myelosis can develop from blast transformation of erythremic myelosis. Primitive erythroid precursors in blood and bone marrow predominate. Primitive cells resembling myeloblasts are often present in low numbers.

## Primary Erythrocytosis[62-65]

Primary erythrocytosis is rarely reported in cats and the diagnosis is based on increased packed cell volume (65–80%) with low to normal serum erythropoietin activity. Most clinical signs are associated with increased RBC volume, which increases blood volume and viscosity, causing impaired blood flow, stasis, and tissue hypoxia. Neurologic signs such as seizures, blindness, and mental depression are common.[64] The oral mucous membranes may appear brick red. It is important to differentiate this from secondary polycythemia, caused by renal tumors, chronic hypoxia, and right-to-left cardiac shunts.

## Megakaryocytic Leukemia[66-68]

Megakaryocytic leukemia is characterized by abnormal megakaryocytic hyperplasia in the bone marrow. The megakaryocytes are morphologically abnormal and some are small (dwarf megakaryocytes) and have few or no nuclear lobulations. Thrombocytopenia or thrombocytosis may be present. In people, this form of leukemia is often associated with extensive marrow fibrosis, with an increase in reticulum or collagen.[61]

## Primary Thrombocythemia[69]

Primary throbocythemia is a very rare chronic myeloproliferative disease characterized by proliferation of megakaryocytes and elevated platelet counts of > 1 million. Giant platelets and platelets with abnormal morphology may be seen in the peripheral blood. One case has been reported in the cat.

## Malignant Histiocytosis[70-72]

Malignant histiocytosis is a rare condition in cats and is characterized by systemic proliferation of malignant macrophages (histiocytes) and their precursors. A distinguishing characteristic of this disease is erythrophagocytosis. Hepatosplenomegaly with progressive anemia, sometimes Coomb's (+), and thrombocytopenia are characteristic. The erythrophagocytosis may be confused with a possible immune-mediated anemia. Bone marrow biopsy, as opposed to aspiration, as well as splenic biopsy, may be necessary to establish a diagnosis. Special stains using acid phosphatase and nonspecific esterase with fluoride inhibition (naphtol butyrate substrate) may be necessary to indicate macrophage origin.

## Myelofibrosis and Myeloid Metaplasia[73-6]

Myelofibrosis and myeloid hyperplasia are characterized by abnormal growth and differentiation of erythroid, myeloid, and megakaryocytic cell types with varying proliferation of fibroblasts in the marrow. Anemia, leukopenia, or thrombocytopenia or varying combinations are common. Myelofibrosis has been diagnosed in FeLV-positive cats and is directly associated with the virus rather than a consequence of myeloproliferative disorders. Myeloid metaplasia may terminate in acute leukemia and thus may be considered a *preleukemic event.*

## Lymphoid Leukemia

Lymphoid leukemia is the most common leukemia in cats. Approximately 25% of the cats with lymphoma will also have a leukemic blood picture.[77] Acute lymphoblastic leukemia (ALL) is the most common of the lymphoid leukemias.[78] ALL is characterized by poorly differentiated lymphoblasts and prolymphocytes in blood and bone marrow.[79] The majority of cats with ALL have normal to low white blood cell counts. A few cats will have leucocytosis with circulating blasts. A moderate to marked anemia is common. A bone marrow usually reveals extensive infiltration with lymphoblasts. Approximately 60 to 80% of cats with ALL are FeLV positive and most malignant cells have T-cell phenotypes.[80]

Chronic lymphocytic leukemia (CLL) is rarely reported in cats and is characterized by well-differentiated small, mature lymphocytes in peripheral blood and bone marrow.[79,80] Most cats have elevated white blood cell counts greater than 50,000/µl. Most cats will be FeLV negative.

## HISTORY AND CLINICAL SIGNS

The clinical signs associated with feline lymphoma and leukemia are variable and depend on location as well as extent of disease. The clinical signs of the *mediastinal form* include dyspnea, tachypnea, noncompressible anterior mediastinum with dull heart and lung sounds.[81–83] Rarely a Horner's syndrome will be seen due to pressure on the sympathetic nerve as it ascends around the first rib, and edema of the head from pressure on the cranial vena cava.[84] Pleural effusion is common and the pleural fluid is characterized by serohemorrhagic to chylous effusion.[83]

The *alimentary form* is most commonly associated with an abdominal mass originating from the gastrointestinal tract and may commonly be associated with enlarged mesenteric lymph nodes, or other organ involvement. In a minority of cats, diffuse thickening of the small bowel or localized gastric involvement will be present. Clinical signs consist of vomiting, diarrhea, anorexia, and weight loss.[84]

Cats with the *multicentric form* present with variable clinical signs, depending on the location and extent of disease. Peripheral lymphadenopathy, as the only physical finding, is a very uncommon presentation for cats with the multicentric form. Peripheral lymphadenopathy, without organomegaly, seen in cats is mostly hyperplastic or reactive.[23]

The *extranodal sites* include the kidneys, skin, eye, and CNS. *Renal lymphoma* is most consistently bilateral, even in cats that appear to have unilateral disease.[24] In general, the kidneys are uniformly enlarged; however, they may also palpate lumpy. More than 50% cats will present with evidence of renal insufficiency.[24]

*Cutaneous lymphoma* may be solitary or diffuse, with alopecia, erythema, and crusted papules. Minimal peripheral lymphadenopathy may also be present. In most cats the duration of signs will be prolonged, lasting months.[30–34]

Cats with *primary CNS lymphoma* (PCNSL) most commonly present with signs associated with thoracolumbar involvement.[25,26] The most common sites are between the second thoracic and fourth lumbar vertebrae and most are extradural.[25,26] Signs include gradual or sudden onset of weakness, upper motor neuron paralysis to bladder, tail flaccidity, hyperpathia in the region of the lesion, and progressing ataxia. The neurologic dysfunction may be insidious or progress rapidly.[26] Cats with cervical spinal cord or nerve root involvement generally show peracute tetraparesis, and diminished sensation in the thoracic limbs. Cervical root involvement may show root lesions (root signature), such as lameness and hyperesthesia upon shoulder extension. Bone marrow involvement is common in cats with PCNSL and most are FeLV positive.

All cats with lymphoma, regardless of site, may have secondary bone marrow infiltration leading to anemia and a leukemic blood profile. Cats with *acute leukemia* will usually show signs of severe anemia (pale mucous membranes), splenomegaly, and febrile episodes. Anemia is a common condition in cats with lymphoma, with at least 50% of them having moderate to severe anemia, most nonregenerative. Cats with *chronic leukemia* may have a longer duration of signs and mild anemia, with or without splenomegaly.

A number of disease conditions can be con-

**Table 28–18**   Various Disorders Potentially Misdiagnosed as Feline Lymphoma

| Form of Lymphoma | Other Disorders |
| --- | --- |
| Thymic/Mediastinal | Thymoma, chylothorax, cardiomyopathy, pyothorax, FIP, mesothelioma, diaphragmatic hernia |
| Alimentary | Inflammatory bowel disease, FIP, intestinal carcinoma, foreign body, other intestinal tumors, hyperthyroidism |
| Peripheral lymph nodes | Distinctive lymphadenopathy, reactive or hyperplasia, infection, FIV infection |
| Renal | Polycystic disease, FIP, acute renal failure, other renal tumors |
| Spinal/CNS | Trauma, other tumors, FIP, discospondylitis, aortic embolism, IV disk herniation, mycotic infection, non-neoplastic FeLV-associated myelopathy |
| Nasal | Rhinitis, inflammatory polyps, cryptococcosis, other tumors |

fused with lymphoma in cats. The various diseases or conditions that can be misdiagnosed as lymphoma are listed in Table 28–18.

## DIAGNOSTICS AND CLINICAL STAGING

For most cats with suspect lymphoma or leukemia, the diagnostic evaluation should include a complete blood count (CBC with differential cell count), platelet count, and a serum chemistry profile and test for FeLV and feline immunodeficiency virus (FIV). A bone marrow aspiration or biopsy is indicated to evaluate for possible involvement and complete staging of the extent of disease. Bone marrow evaluation is particularly indicated if anemia, cellular atypia, and leukopenia are present. Lymph node or involved organ biopsy, via surgical incision or needle-core, to obtain tissue for histopathologic evaluation is essential for a definitive diagnosis. Lymph node aspiration, especially peripheral lymph nodes may not provide a definitive diagnosis. A misdiagnosis may occur in cats with hyperplasia or distinctive lymph node hyperplasia.[21–23]

Serum chemistry profiles can help establish the overall health and clinical staging of cats. Elevated liver enzymes may indicate hepatic infiltration with lymphoma. An elevated BUN and creatinine may indicate renal lymphoma. Hypercalcemia is rarely seen in cats but has been reported in cats with mediastinal lymphoma.[16,17] Elevated globulin levels may indicate the presence of a monoclonal gammopathy, with or without serum hyperviscosity. This is a rarely reported paraneoplastic syndrome in cats with lymphoma.[85,86]

For cats with *mediastinal lymphoma*, fine-needle aspiration of suspected mass(es) or cytologic evaluation of pleural fluid may be sufficient to establish a diagnosis. In most cats the finding of lymphoblasts will establish a diagnosis.[87,88] However, definitive diagnosis of lymphoma in cats with a mediastinal mass and concurrent chylothorax can be challenging.[83] If lymphoblasts are not identified in the pleural chylous effusion, then cholesterol and triglyceride concentrations should be measured.[89] In chylous effusions, the pleural fluid triglyceride concentration will be greater than in the serum; however, anorectic cats will have lower triglyceride levels in the pleural fluid. A major differential for mediastinal lymphoma is thymoma. The cytologic features of thymoma were recently described and found to be distinct from lymphoma.[90] Cytology of thymoma can be difficult because of the preponderance of small lymphocytes as opposed to lymphoblasts, seen with lymphoma. Mast cells can also be seen in up to 50% of the aspirations from thymomas.

For the *alimentary form*, especially if primary gastrointestinal lymphoma is suspected, a wedge-biopsy through serosa and muscularis, avoiding the mucosa, may be necessary to establish a diagnosis. Caution must be used when using endoscopically obtained tissue because of the difficulty in differentiating lymphoplasmacytic gastroenteritis from primary, diffuse, intestinal lymphoma.[91] Most gastrointestinal lymphomas have secondary mesenteric lymph node involvement and ultrasound guarded biopsy may be adequate to obtain enough tissue for a diagnosis.

In cats with suspected *spinal lymphoma*, survey radiographs of the spine will rarely reveal osseous lesions. Myelograms are indicated and in approximately 75% of the cases an extradural pattern of compression will be detected.[25,26] Fluoroscopic-guided fine-needle aspiration of the epidermal lesion may yield enough tissue for a cytologic diagnosis. In one study, cerebrospinal fluid (CSF) analysis revealed a clear and colorless fluid with a mixed pleocytosis (mean 140 cells/UL: range 0 to 1,625 cells/μl) with elevated protein content (mean of 140.7 mg/dl range of 12–405 mg/dl) was identified in most cats evaluated. Malignant lymphocytes were identified in 6 of 17 cats evaluated with CSF analysis.[26] Because of the high percentage of bone marrow involvement, a bone marrow aspiration is recommended for complete clinical staging.

For *cutaneous lymphoma*, punch biopsies (3–4 mm) should be taken from the most representative and infiltrative, but not infected, skin lesions. No clinical staging system for cutaneous lymphoma has been established; however, a staging system is presented in the chapter on canine lymphoma (see Table 28–7) as well as recommended staging procedures (see Table 28–8).

A WHO staging system routinely used to stage feline lymphoma is presented in Table 28–19. This staging system is similar to the one used for dogs; however, because of the high incidence of visceral involvement, clinical staging is difficult and another staging system has been evaluated.[92] For cats with suspected *leukemia* a bone marrow aspiration or biopsy is usually diagnostic. The preferred sites for bone marrow aspirates are the proximal humerus or iliac crest. Cats with acute leukemia are likely to have malignant cellular infiltrates in organs other than

---

**Table 28–19** World Health Organization's Classification for Lymphoma

*Stage Grouping (To Include Anatomic Type)*
  I. Involvement limited to a single node or extra-nodal site, or lymphoid tissue in a single organ, including cranial mediastinum.[a]
 II. Involvement of many lymph nodes in a regional area, a resectable GI tract tumor, extra-nodal site with regional lymph node involvement.
III. Generalized lymph node involvement, non-resectable-intra-abdominal disease or epidural tumor.
 IV. Liver and/or spleen involvement associated with stages I–III.
  V. Manifestation in the blood and involvement of bone marrow involvement with stages I–IV.
       Each stage is subclassified into:
           a. without systemic signs, or
           b. with systemic signs.

[a]Excluding bone marrow.

---

bone marrow.[48] A bone marrow aspirate with greater than 30% abnormal blast cells is necessary to make a diagnosis of an acute leukemia. In cats with suspected CLL, infiltration of the bone marrow with more than 20% mature lymphocytes helps confirm the diagnosis. All cats with leukemia should be tested for FeLV.

## TREATMENT OF MALIGNANT LYMPHOMA

Significant advances have been made in the treatment of canine lymphoma; however, the response rate and duration of response using chemotherapy to treat feline lymphoma have not been as impressive.

The chemotherapeutic agents used most commonly to treat feline lymphoma include vincristine, cyclophosphamide, methotrexate, L-asparaginase and prednisone.[24,92–95] Current protocols for treating feline lymphoma are detailed in Table 28–20. A current protocol in use at the University of Wisconsin–Madison is presented in Table 28–21. This protocol has been used in more than 25 cats with various forms of lymphoma and is tolerated well.

Doxorubicin is a very effective agent and is commonly used for treating canine lymphoma; however, in cats significant toxicity results when it is used at a dose of 30 mg/m² IV q 3 weeks. However, at lower doses, 20 mg/m² IV or 1 mg/kg IV doxorubicin can be used without significant toxicity. The major toxicity noted with doxorubicin is profound anorexia; myelosuppression; and if perivascular leaking, severe tissue damage. Doxorubicin-induced cardiac toxicity has not been documented in cats, but there is no information indicating cats are resistant to myocardial damage. Renal toxicity has been produced experimentally in rats and rabbits, and has been reported in cats.[96,97] In our experience, the incidence is low in cats at total accumulative doses of less than 50 mg doxorubicin total dose per cat.

Response and duration of response will vary depending on the stage of disease, FeLV status, and anatomic location. Most combination chemotherapy protocols will induce 60 to 70% complete response rate (CR) and median survival times of 5 to 7 months with an approximate 30% survival at 1 year.[24,92,93] In general, cats tolerate chemotherapy very well. Gastrointestinal toxicity is less common when compared to the dog.

Radiation therapy has been effectively used to treat localized lymphoma, such as epidural, mediastinal masses, and nasal lymphoma. Total doses of 10 to 15 Gy usually result in a CR.[98] Recently, 10 cats with localized lymphoma were treated with radiation alone or with chemotherapy, using doses of 8 to 40 Gy. Eight of 10 cats achieved a CR with a median response of 114 weeks.[99] Radiation therapy has also been used to treat nasal lymphoma, and in one study the disease-free survival was greater than 500 days in a small number of cats.[99]

Very little has been published regarding the treatment of cutaneous lymphoma or mycosis fungoides in cats. Cats with a solitary mass should be treated with surgical excision, although clinical staging may be necessary to rule out possible internal involvement. For cutaneous lymphoma (nonmycosis fungoides) combination chemotherapy can be considered. If the disease is localized to a small region, radiation therapy is usually effective. Mycosis fungoides may be effectively treated with retinoids, such as isotretinoin (Accutane) at 3 to 4 mg/kg PO daily or

**Table 28–20** Protocols for Feline Lymphoma

| Treatment Protocol | Tumor Location | Cases | Complete Remission Rate (%) | Median Remission (Months) | Median Survival (Months) | Ref |
|---|---|---|---|---|---|---|
| 1. **COP:** Cyclophosphamine 300 mg/m$^2$ PO q 3 wks | Thymic | 12 | 92 | 6.0 | NR | 93 |
| Vincristine 0.75 mg/m$^2$ IV q 3 wks | Alimentary | 7 | 86 | 4.5 | NR | |
| Prednisone 2 mg/kg PO continuously | Peripheral nodes | 5 | 80 | 28 | NR | |
| Treatment continued for 1 year | Multicentric disease | 4 | 100 | 5.0 | NR | |
| | *Overall* | — | 79 | 5.0 | NR | |
| 2. **VCM:** Vincristine 0.025 mg/ kg IV week 1 | Thymic | 31 | 45 | 2.0 | 1.5 | 94 |
| Cyclophosphamide 10 mg/kg IV week 2 | Alimentary | 9 | 50 | 6.0 | 9.6 | |
| Vincristine 0.025 mg/kg IV week 3 | Renal | 6 | 16 | — | 5.0 | |
| Methotrexate 0.8 mg/kg IV week 4 | Multicentric | 16 | 68 | — | 18.0 | |
| Repeat weekly treatments as above Continue prednisone at 5 mg orally Mediastinal involvement L-asparaginase 400 IU/kg IM at 1st treatment Treatment continued for 2 years | *Overall* | — | 52 | — | 2.0 | |
| 3. **VCM:** L-asparaginase: Same protocol as above except prednisone 2mg/kg PO continuously L-asparaginase 400 IU/kgIM week 1 with vincristine | *All types* | 103 | 62 | — | 7.0 | 92 |
| For renal lymphoma only—after complete remission substitute cytosine arabinoside 600 mg/ m$^2$ SQ divided 4 doses over 2 days in place of cyclophosphamide Treatment continued for 2 years | Renal | 28 | 61 | 4.0 | 5.7 | 24 |

NR = Not reported.

etretinate (Tegison) at 1.25 mg/kg PO daily. However, no clinical studies have been published demonstrating efficacy in cats.

## TREATMENT OF LEUKEMIAS

### Lymphoid Leukemia

The use of chemotherapy to treat acute lymphoblastic leukemia (ALL) has been disappointing. Using a combination of cyclophosphamide, vincristine, and prednisone (COP), a 27% complete response rate was reported.[93,97] One report described a short-term remission in a cat with lymphoid leukemia, using a low dose (10 mg/m$^2$) of cytosine arabinoside SQ twice daily.[100]

Chronic lymphoid leukemia (CLL) can be treated with chlorambucil at a dose of 0.2 mg/kg PO or 2 mg/cat QOD, and prednisone at a dose of 1 mg/kg PO daily.

**Table 28–21** University of Wisconsin-Madison School of Veterinary Medicine: Feline Lymphoma Protocol

| | | | |
|---|---|---|---|
| Week 1 | Vincristine 0.7 mg/m² IV once<br>Asparaginase, 400 IU/kg, IM once<br>Prednisone, 2 mg/kg, PO, SID daily | Week 11 | Vincristine 0.7 mg/m² IV once |
| Week 2 | Cyclophosphamide 250 mg/m² IV once<br>Prednisone, 2 mg/kg, PO, SID daily | Week 13* | Chlorambucil 1.4 mg/kg PO—once<br>or<br>Cyclophosphamide 250 mg/m² IV (if not in CR) |
| Week 3 | Vincristine 0.7 mg/m² IV once<br>Prednisone, 1.0 mg/kg, PO, SID daily | Week 15 | Vincristine 0.7 mg/m² IV once |
| Week 4 | Doxorubicin, 20 mg/m² IV once<br>Prednisone, 1.0 mg/kg, PO, SID daily | Week 17 | Methotrexate 0.8 mg/kg IV once |
| | | Week 19 | Vincristine 0.7 mg/m² IV once |
| Week 6 | Vincristine 0.7 mg/m² IV once<br>Prednisone 1 mg/kg EOD | Week 21* | Chlorambucil 1.4 mg/kg PO—once<br>or<br>Cyclophosphamide 250 mg/m² IV (if not in CR) |
| Week 7* | Cyclophosphamide 250 mg/m² IV once | | |
| Week 8 | Vincristine 0.7 mg/m² IV once | Week 23 | Vincristine 0.7 mg/m² IV once |
| Week 9 | Doxorubicin 20 mg/m² IV once | Week 25 | Doxorubicin 20 mg/m² IV once |

*Renal lymphoma-substitute cytosine arabinoside at 600 mg/m² div SC BID over 2 days.

1. A CBC should be performed prior to each chemotherapy. If granulocyte < 2,500–3,000 cell/μl, wait 5–7 days, repeat CBC, then administer the drug.
2. Continue prednisone at 1 mg/kg PO EOD starting week 5.
3. Continue as above (week 11–25) treatment with 2-week intervals to week 52. Week 52–104, continue treatments every 3–4 weeks.
4. Maximal dose of doxorubicin 180–200 mg/m² (approximately 45–50 mg total per cat). Then stop doxorubicin and continue methotrexate or substitute mitoxantrone at 5 mg/m² IV.
5. Doxorubicin cardiac toxicity has not been documented in cats, however, some cats have developed renal failure on long-term doxorubicin. Periodically, cats on treatment need to have renal function evaluated.
6. The dose of methotrexate (0.8 mg/kg IV) may be low; new data have been reported that normal cats may tolerate much higher doses.[101] However, clinical studies in cats using higher doses of methotrexate to treat lymphoma/leukemia have not been reported.

## Nonlymphoid Leukemia

A combination of cytosine arabinoside combined with cyclophosphamide, combined with multiple blood transfusions was effective in inducing a response for 3 months in a cat with acute megakaryocytic leukemia.[68] Hydroxyurea (Hydrea) can be used to treat chronic myeloid leukemia and primary erythrocytosis. Hydroxyrea is available in 500 mg capsules and the dose is 25 to 50 mg/kg PO daily. Some cats have been given 500 mg every 5 to 7 days; however, methemoglobulinemia and hemolytic anemia with Heinz bodies has been seen.[64] A better recommendation is to have the drug recapsuled into 125 mg capsules, which is a more appropriate dosage. However, care must be used in making these capsules because hydroxyurea is potentially carcinogenic. A recommended treatment schedule for hydroxyurea is 125 mg daily to every other day depending on the type of leukemia under treatment. At this dose level the drug is tolerated very well.

## GENERAL RECOMMENDATIONS

It is difficult to provide precise treatment recommendation for the wide variety of clinical settings of cats with lymphoma. Our current recommendation is to treat cats with lymphoma using the protocol as outlined in Table 28–21. If the treatment veterinarian is unfamiliar with doxorubicin, then an alternative protocol to consider the COP protocol as published by Cotter,[93] and outlined in Table 28–20.

All cats undergoing chemotherapy need to be monitored for toxicity. A CBC needs to be performed prior to each chemotherapy treatment. It is advised that at least a 2,500 to 3,000 granulocyte/μ be maintained. If the WBC count drops below the above recommended level, withhold chemotherapy for 5 to 7 days and repeat the CBC.

Hair loss is not a problem in cats on chemotherapy, although they may lose whiskers as well as guard hairs. One of the most common side effects of chemotherapy is anorexia. Diazepam has been used to stimulate appetite but has minimal benefit. Cryoheptadine at a dose of 1 to 2 mg BID to TID or megestrol acetate 2 mg BID PO may be helpful to stimulate appetite.

Nutritional support, especially for cats with alimentary lymphomas, is especially important. It may be necessary to place a feeding tube into cats undergoing chemotherapy for alimentary lymphoma, particularly if anorexia is present. (see Chap. 12).

Relapse of tumor is common following or during chemotherapy. Few studies have been performed to evaluate chemotherapy agents to be used as rescue agents in cats. Agents such as mitoxantrone, actinomycin-D, and L-asparaginase can be considered.

## PROGNOSIS

In 1987 Cotter reported on the results of treating 38 cats with lymphoma and 15 with lymphoblastic leukemia.[93] All cats were treated with COP (cyclophosphamide, vincristine and prednisone) as presented in Table 28–20. Overall 79% of the cats with lymphoma had a complete response (CR) compared to 27% with ALL. The median duration of remission was 5 months, with 9 cats (26%) remaining in remission at 1 year. Cats with primarily peripheral nodal disease had a median remission time of 28 months ($n$=5).

In another study of 75 cats with lymphoma, treated with combination chemotherapy, (vincristine, cyclophosphamide, methotrexate with or without prednisone, and L-asparaginase (see Table 28–20) of the 62 cats that had follow-up, 32 (52%) attained a CR for a median of 4 months, and the overall median survival time was 2 months for all cats treated.[94] Response and duration of response varied with tumor location. Mediastinal lymphoma ($n$=31) had a 45% response rate with a median survival time of 1.5 months. Multicentric lymphoma ($n$=16) had a 68% response rate with a median survival of 18 months; renal lymphoma ($n$=6) showed only a 16% response rate and a median survival of 5 months, and alimentary form ($n$=9) showed a 50% response rate and a median survival time of 9.6 months.

In 1989, Mooney et al. presented the results of 103 cats treated with combination chemotherapy (vincristine, L-asparaginase, cyclophosphamide, methotrexate, and prednisone; see Table 28–20).[92] Sixty-four (62%) of 103 cats had a CR with a median survival time of 7 months, with a 30% survival at 1 year. Cats with stage I and II disease (median survival time of 7.6 months) had a statistically better prognosis than stages III, IV, and V (median of 2.5–3 months) (Fig. 28–13). Another important factor related to prognosis was FeLV status. FeLV-negative cats had a median survival time of 7.0 months, compared to 3.5 months for FeLV positive cats. For cats that had a complete response, those FeLV negative had a median survival of 9 months, compared to 4.2 months for FeLV-positive cats (Fig. 28–14). The cats with the best prognosis are FeLV negative— stage I and II disease. The expected median survival time is 17 months (Fig. 28–15).

In another study by Mooney et al., 28 cats with primary renal lymphoma were treated with combination chemotherapy (Table 28–20).[24] A complete response was noted in 17 cats (61%) and 9 (33%) had a partial response (PR). The median survival time for the CR cats was 5.7 months, and 1 month for cats showing a PR. Duration of response to chemotherapy did not correlate to the degree of renal insufficiency except in those cats with a BUN> 150 mg/dl. Metastasis to the CNS developed in 40% of these treated cats. The investigators revised their chemotherapy protocol to include cytosine arabinoside, which can penetrate the blood barrier, to prevent or reduce CNS metastasis (Fig. 28–16).

In a recent study, 36 cats with lymphoma were treated with COP chemotherapy (Table 28–20), and 19 (50%) who achieved a CR were randomized at week 7 to receive maintenance COP or doxorubicin (25 mg/m$^2$ IV q 3 weeks) for another 6 months. The median remission for the 7 cats given doxorubicin was 259 days (range 123–547 days), and those on COP had a median survival of 83 days (range 45–208 days).[102]

In a study of cats with alimentary lymphoma, 28 received COP (Table 28–20) chemotherapy. Some cats also were given other drugs, including doxorubicin, L-asparaginase, chlorambucil, idarubicin, and mitoxantrone. Nine cats (32%) had a CR for a median of 213 days and four cats survived 1 year or longer. For all cats treated, the overall median survival was 50 days.[102]

**Figure 28–13.**
Kaplan-Meier survival curve correlating clinical stage of disease to survival following combination chemotherapy using VCM-L-asparaginase. Cats with stages I and II disease had a significant survival advantage compared to more advanced disease (stages III–V). (Reprinted with permission, Mooney SC et al, *J Am Vet Med Assoc 194*:696–702, 1989.)

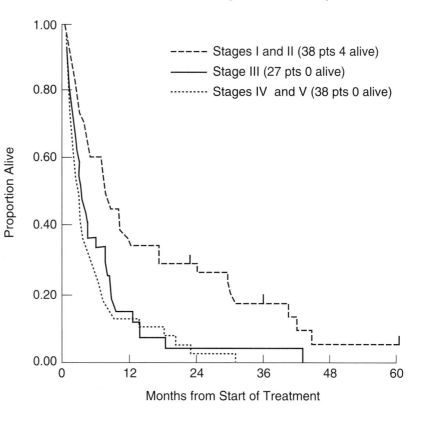

**Figure 28–14.**
Kaplan-Meier survival curve correlating FeLV status to survival following combination chemotherapy using VCM-L asparaginase. (Reprinted with permission, Mooney SC et al, *J Am Vet Med Assoc 194*:696–702, 1989.)

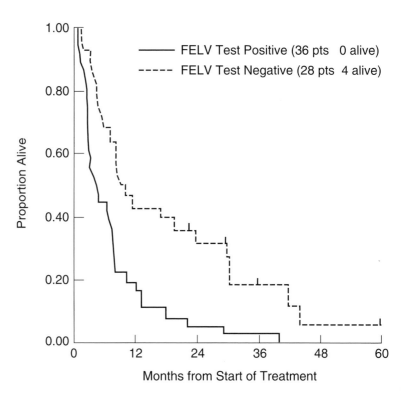

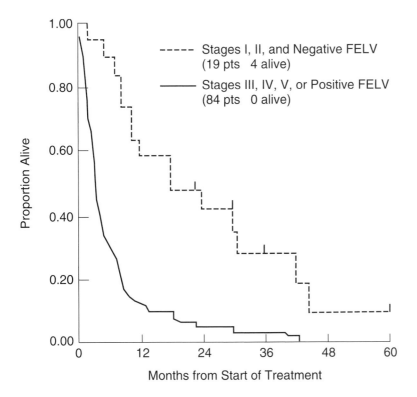

**Figure 28–15.** Kaplan-Meier survival curve correlating stage of disease, FeLV status to survival following combination chemotherapy using VCM-L-asparaginase. (Reprinted with permission, Mooney SC et al, J Am Vet Med Assoc *194*:696–702, 1989.)

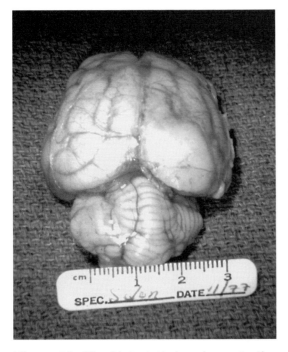

**Figure 28–16.** Metastatic lymphoma to the brain of a cat 7 months following successful remission of renal lymphoma using VCM-L-asparaginase chemotherapy.

Few studies have been reported on the results of treating cats with spinal lymphoma. In one study of four cats treated with chemotherapy (L-asparaginase, vincristine, prednisone) combined with spinal radiation (*n*=3) or surgical cytoreduction (*n*=1), most cats were euthanatized by 5 months, although one cat survived 13 months.[26] In another study of nine cats treated with chemotherapy (vincristine, cyclophosphamide, and prednisone), three cats achieved a complete response with a duration of 14 weeks, and three cats achieved a partial response with a duration of 6 weeks.[25] One cat treated with dorsal decompression laminectomy and chemotherapy survived 13 months.[25] Although the numbers are small overall, the prognosis for spinal lymphoma is poor.

In 15 cats with ALL treated with COP, four achieved a CR and six cats had a PR[93] The median remission was 7 months (range 1–24 months).

The prognosis for other acute nonlymphoblastic leukemias is very poor. However, cats with CLL have a good prognosis and survive 1 to 2 years when treated with chlorambucil. Cats with primary erythrocytosis, without treatment, are reported to survive 6 to 20+ weeks.[62,64] Phlebotomy alone every 2 to 3 months was used to treat one cat and the survival was greater than 20 months.[63] Hydroxyurea treatment for primary erythrocytosis was used in eight cats and all survived longer than 1 year.[64]

## REFERENCES

1. Couto CG: Oncology. The cat: Diseases and Clinical Management, ed. Sherding Churchill-Livingston, NY. 1989, pp. 589–647.

2. Hardy WD Jr: Hematopoietic tumors of cats. J Am Anim Hosp Assoc 17:921–940, 1981.

3. Essex M and Francis DP: The risk to humans from malignant diseases of their pets: An unsettled issue. J Am Anim Hosp Assoc 12:386–390, 1976.

4. Theilen GH; Madewell BR: Feline hematopoietic neoplasms. In Theilen GH and Madewell BR (eds): Veterinary cancer medicine, 2nd ed. Philadelphia, Lea and Febiger, 1987, pp. 354–381.

5. Hardy WD Jr, McClelland AJ, Zuckerman, EE, et al: Development of virus nonproducer lymphosarcomas in pet cats exposed to FeLV. Nature 288:90–92, 1980.

6. Francis DP, Cotter SM, Hardy WD, Jr, et al: Comparison of virus-positive and virus-negative cases of feline leukemia and lymphomas. Cancer Res 39:3866–3870, 1979.

7. Dorn CR, Taylor DO, Schneider R, Hibbard HH; Klauber, MR: Survey of animal neoplasms in Alameda and Contra Costa Counties, California. II. Cancer morbidity in dogs and cats from Alameda County. J Natl Cancer Inst 40:307–318, 1968.

8. Nielsen SW: Neoplastic diseases. In Catcott EJ (ed): Feline Medicine and Surgery. Santa Barbara CA, Am Vet Publ, 1964, p. 156.

9. Hardy WD Jr, MacEwen EG: Hematopoietic tumors: Feline retroviruses. In Withrow SJ and MacEwen EG (eds.): Clinical Veterinary Oncology. Philadelphia, JB Lippincott, 1989, pp. 362–380.

10. Shelton GH, Grant CK, Cotter SM, et al: Feline immunodeficiency virus (FIV) and feline leukemia virus (FeLV) infections and their relationship to lymphoid malignancies in cats: A retrospective study (1968–1988). J Acquir Immuno Def Synd 3:623–630, 1990.

11. Hutson CA, Rideout BA, Pederson NC: Neoplasia associated with feline immunodeficiency virus infection in cats of southern California. J Am Vet Med Assoc 199:1357–1362, 1991.

12. Poli A, Abramo F, Baldinotti F, et al: Malignant lymphoma associated with experimentally induced feline immunodeficiency virus infection. J Comp Pathol 110:319–328, 1994.

13. Callanan JJ, McCandlish IA, O'Neil B, et al: Lymphosarcoma in experimentally induce feline immunodeficiency virus infection. Vet Rec 130:293–295, 1992.

14. Rosenberg MP, Hohenhaus AE, and Matus RE: Monoclonal gammopathy and lymphoma in a cat infected with feline immunodeficiency virus. J Am Anim Hosp Assoc 27:335–337, 1991.

15. Buracco P, Guglielmino R, Abate O, et al: Large granular lymphoma in a FIV-positive and FeLV-negative cat. J Small Anim Pract 33:279–284, 1992.

16. McMillan FD: Hypercalcemia associated with lymphoid neoplasia in two cats. Feline Pract 15:31–34, 1985.

17. Chew DJ, Schaer M, Liu SK, et al: Pseudohyperparathyroidism in a cat. J Am Anim Hosp Assoc 11:46–52, 1975.

18. Hardy WD, Jr: The feline leukemia virus. J Am Anim Hosp Assoc 17:951–980, 1981.

19. Rojko JC, Kociba GJ, Abkowitz JC, et al: Feline lymphomas: Immunological and cytochemical characterization. Cancer Res. 49:345–351, 1989.

20. Davenport DJ, Lieb MS, and Roth L: Progression of lymphocytic-plasmacytic enteritis to gastrointestinal lymphosarcoma in three cats. 7th Annu Conf Vet Cancer Soc, 1987.

21. Mooney SC, Patnaik AK, Hayes AA, et al: Generalized lymphadenopathy resembling lymphoma in cats: Six cases (1972–1976). J Am Vet Med Assoc 190:897–900, 1987.

22. Moore FM, Emerson WE, Cotter SM, et al: Distinctive peripheral lymph node hyperplasia of young cats. Vet Pathol 23:386–391, 1986.

23. Cotter SM: Feline lymphoid hyperplasia. In Kirk R (ed): Current Veterinary Therapy X. Philadelphia, WB Saunders, 1989, pp. 535–537.

24. Mooney SC, Hayes AA, Matus RE, et al: Renal lymphoma in cats: 28 cases (1977–1984) J Am Vet Med Assoc 191:1473–1477, 1987.

25. Spodnick GJ, Berg J, Moore FM, et al: Spinal lymphoma in cats: 21 cases (1976–1989). J Am Vet Med Assoc 200:373–376, 1992.

26. Lane SB, Kornegay JN, Duncan JR. et al: Feline spinal lymphosarcoma: A retrospective evaluation of 23 cats. J Vet Intern Med 8:99–104, 1994.

27. Cordy DR: Tumors of the nervous system and eye. In: Moulton JE (ed): Tumors in Domestic Animals, 3rd ed. Los Angeles, University of California Press, 1990, pp. 640–665.

28. Prasse KW, Mahaffey EA, Cotter SM, et al: The hematopoietic system. In Holzworth J (ed) Diseases of the cat: Medicine and surgery. Philadelphia, WB Saunders, 1987, pp. 739–807.

29. Suess RP Jr., Martin RA, Shell LG, et al: Vertebral lymphosarcoma in a cat. J Am Vet Med Assoc 197:101–103, 1990.

30. Baker JL, Scott DW: Mycosis fungoides in two cats. J Am Anim Hosp 25:97–101, 1989.

31. Caciolo PL, Hayes AA, Patnaik AK, et al: A case of mycosis fungoides in a cat and literature review. J Am Anim Hosp Assoc 19:505–512, 1983.

32. Caciolo PL, Nesbitt GH, Patnaik AK, et al: Cutaneous lymphosarcoma in the cat: A report of nine cases. J Am Anim Hosp Assoc 20:491–496, 1984.

33. Schick RO, Murphy GF, Goldschmidt MH: Cutaneous lymphosarcoma and leukemia in a cat. J Am Vet Med Assoc 203:1155–1158, 1993.

34. Tobey JC, Houston DM, Breur GJ et al: Cutaneous T-cell lymphoma in a cat. J Am Vet Med Assoc 204:606–609, 1994.

35. Wieselthier JS, Koh HK: Sézary syndrome: diagnosis, prognosis, and critical review of treatment options. J Amer Acad Dermatol 22:381–401, 1990.

36. DeBoer DJ, Turrel JM, Moore PF: Mycosis Fungoides in a dog: Demonstration of T-cell specificity and response to radiotherapy. J Am Anim Hosp Assoc 26:566–572, 1990.

37. McKeever PJ, Grindem CB, Stevens JB, et al: Canine cutaneous lymphoma. J Am Vet Med Assoc 180:531–536, 1982.

38. Thrall MA, Macy DW, Snyder SP, et al: Cutaneous lymphosarcoma and leukemia in a dog resembling Sézary syndrome in man. Vet Pathol 21:182–186, 1984.

39. Valli VEO, Norris A, Withrow SJ, et al: Anatomical and histological classification of feline lymphoma using the National Cancer Institute Working Formulation. 9th Annul Conf Vet Cancer Soc, 1989.

40. Hardy WD Jr, Zuckerman, EE, MacEwen EG, et al: A feline leukemia virus and sarcoma virus-induced tumor-specific antigen. Nature (London) 270:249–251, 1977.

41. Cockerell GL, Krakowka S, Hoover EA, et al: Characterization of feline T- and B-lymphocytes and identification of an experimental reduced T-cell neoplasm in the cat. J Natl Cancer Inst 57:907–913, 1976.

42. Franks PT, Harvey JW, Calderwood-Mays M, et al: Feline large granular lymphoma. Vet Pathol 23:200–202, 1986.

43. Wellman ML, Hammer AS, DiBartola SP, et al: Lymphoma involving large granular lymphocytes in cats. 11 cases (1982–1991). J Am Vet Med Assoc 201:1265–1269, 1992.

44. Jain NC: Schalms' Veterinary Hematology, 7th ed. Philadelphia, Lea and Febiger, 1986.

45. Grindem CB: Ultrastructural morphology of leukemia cells in the cat. Vet Pathol 22(2):147–55, 1988.

46. Gorman NT, Evans RJ: Myeloproliferative disease in the dog and cat: Clinical presentations, diagnosis and treatment. Vet Rec 121:490–496, 1987.

47. Grindem CB et al: Morphological and clinical pathological characteristics of spontaneous leukemia in 10 cats. J Am Anim Hosp Assoc 21:227–229, 1985.

48. Blue JT, French TW, and Scarlett-Kranz J: Nonlymphoid hematopoietic neoplasia in cats: A retrospective study of 60 cases. Cornell Vet 78:21–42, 1988.

49. Raskin RE, Krehbiel JD: Myelodysplastic changes in a cat with myelomonocytic leukemia. J Am Vet Med Assoc 187:171–174, 1985.

50. Facklam NR, Kociba GJ: Cytochemical characterization of feline leukemic cells. Vet Pathol 23:155–161, 1986.

51. Finlay D: Eosinophilic leukemia in the cat: A case report. Vet Rec 116:567, 1985.

52. Lewis MG, Kociba GJ, Rojko JL, et al: Retroviral associated eosinophilic leukemia in the cat. Am J Vet Res 46:1066–1070, 1985.

53. Huibregtse BA, and Turner JL: Hypereosinophilic syndrome and eosinophilic leukemia: A comparison of 22 hypereosinophilic cats. J Am An Hosp Assoc 30:591–599, 1994.

54. McEwen SA, Valli VEO, Hullard TJ: Hypereosinophilic syndrome in cats: A report of three cases. Can J Comp Med 49(3):248–253, 1986.

55. Neer TM: Hypereosinophilic syndrome in cats. Compend Contin Educ Pract Vet 13:549–555, 1991.

56. Henness AM, Crow SE: Treatment of feline myelogenous leukemia: Four case reports. J Am Vet Med Assoc 171:263–266, 1977.

57. Zawidzka ZZ, Jansen E, and Grice HC: Erythremic myelosis in a cat. Vet Pathol 1:530–541, 1964.

58. Schalm OW: Myeloproliferative disorders in the cat. 3. Progression from erythroleukemia into granulocytic leukemia. Feline Pract 5:31–33, 1975.

59. Latimer KS: Leukocytes in health and disease. In Ettinger SJ, Feldman EC (eds): Textbook of Veterinary Internal Medicine, 4th ed. Philadelphia, WB Saunders, 1995, pp. 1892–1929.

60. Harvey JW: Myeloproliferative disorders in dogs and cats. Vet Clin North Am Small Anim Pract 11:349–381, 1981.

61. Williams WJ, Beutler E, Ersler AJ, et al: Hematology, 2nd ed. New York, McGraw-Hill, 1977, pp. 770–850.

62. Reed C, Ling GV, Gould D, et al: Polycythemia vera in a cat. J Amer Vet Med Assoc 157:85–91, 1970.

63. Foster ES, Lothrop CD Jr: Polycythemia vera in a cat with cardiac hypertrophy. J Am Vet Med Assoc 192:1736–1738, 1988.

64. Watson ADJ, Moore AS, and Helfand SC: Primary erythrocytosis in the cat: Treatment with hydroxyurea. J Small Anim Pract 35:320–325, 1994.

65. Swinney G, Jones BR, Kissling K: A review of polycythaemia vera in the cat. Aust Vet Pract 22:60–66, 1992.

66. Michel RL, O'Handley P, and Dade AW: Megakaryocytic myelosis in a cat. J Am Vet Med Assoc 168:1021–1025, 1976.

67. Colbatzky F., and Hermanns W: Acute megakaryoblastic leukemia in one cat and two dogs. Vet Pathol 30:186–194, 1993.

68. Hamilton TA, Morrison WB, and DeNicola DB: Cytosine arabinoside chemotherapy for acute megakaryocytic leukemia in a cat. J Am Vet Med Assoc 199:359–361, 1991.

69. Hammer AS, Couto CG, Getzy D, et al: Essential thrombocythemia in a cat. J Vet Intern Med 4:87–91, 1990.

70. Gafner F, and Bestetti GE: Feline malignant histiocytosis and the lysozyme detection. Schweiz Arch Tierheilkd 130:349–356, 1988.

71. Count EA, Earnest-Koons KA, Barr SC, et al: Malignant histiocytosis in a cat. J Am Vet Med Assoc 203:1300–1302, 1993.

72. Freeman L, Stevens J, Loughman C, et al: Malignant histiocytosis in a cat. J Vet Intern Med (in press).

73. Harvey JW, Shields RP, Gaskin JM: Feline myeloproliferative disease: Changing manifestations in the peripheral blood. Vet Pathol 15:437–448, 1978.

74. Hoover EA, and Kociba GJ: Bone lesions in cats with anemia induced by feline leukemia virus. J Natl Cancer Inst 53:1277–1284, 1974.

75. Flecknell PA, Gibbs C, Kelly DF: Myelosclerosis in a cat. J Comp Pathol 88:627–631, 1978.

76. Zenoble RD, Rowland GN: Hypercalcemia and proliferative, myelosclerotic bone reaction associated with feline leukovirus infection in a cat. J Am Vet Med Assoc 175:591–595, 1979.

77. Theilen GH, Madewell BR: Leukemia-sarcoma disease complex. In Theilen GH, Madewell BR (eds): Veterinary Cancer Medicine. Philadelphia, Lea and Febiger, 1979, pp. 204–288.

78. Cotter SM, Essex M: Animal model: Feline acute lymphoblastic leukemia and aplastic anemia. Am J Path 87:265–268, 1977.

79. MacKey LJ, Jarrett WFH: Pathogenesis of lymphoid neoplasia in cats and its relationship to immunologic cell pathways. I. Morphologic Aspects. J Natl Cancer Inst 49:853–865, 1972.

80. Essex ME: Feline leukemia: A naturally occurring cancer of infectious origin. Epidemiol Rev 4:189–203, 1982.

81. Holzworth J: Neoplasia of blood-forming organs in cats. Ann NY Acad Sci 108:691–701, 1963.

82. Thrall MA: Lymphoproliferative disorders. Lymphocytic leukemia and plasma cell myeloma. Vet Clin North Am Small Anim Pract. 11: 321–347, 1981.

83. Forrester SD, Fossum TW, Rogers KS, et al: Diagnosis and treatment of chylothorax associated with lymphoblastic lymphosarcoma in four cats. J Am Vet Med Assoc 198:291–294, 1991.

84. Carpenter JL, Andrews LK, and Holzworth J: Tumors and tumorlike lesions. In Holzworth J (ed): Diseases of the Cat. Philadelphia, WB Saunders, 1987, pp. 406–596.

85. Williams DA, and Goldschmidt MH: Hyperviscosity syndrome with IgM monoclonal gammopathy and hepatic plasmacytoid lymphosar-

86. Dust A, Norris AM, and Valli VEO: Cutaneous lymphosarcoma with IgG immunoglobulin monoclonal gammopathy, serum hyperviscosity and hypercalcemia in a cat. Can Vet J 23:235–239, 1982.

87. Gruffydd-Jones TJ, Gaskell CJ: Clinical and radiographical features of anterior mediastinal lymphosarcoma in the cat: A review of 30 cases. Vet Rec 104:304–307, 1979.

88. Gruffydd-Jones TJ, and Flecknell PA: The prognosis and treatment related gross appearance and laboratory characteristics of pathologic thoracic fluids in the cats. J Small Anim Pract 19:315–328, 1978.

89. Fossum TW, Jacobs RM, Birchard SJ: Evaluation of cholesterol and triglyceride concentrations in differentiating chylous and nonchylous pleural effusions in dogs and cats. J Am Vet Med Assoc 188:49–51, 1986.

90. Rae CA, Jacobs RM, Couto CG: A comparison between the cytological and histological characteristics in 13 canine and feline thymomas. Can Vet J 30:497–500, 1989.

91. Dennis JS, Kruger JM, Mullaney TP: Lymphocytic/plasmacytic gastroenteritis in cats: 14 cases (1985–1990). J Am Vet Med Assoc 200:1712–1718, 1992.

92. Mooney SC, Hayes AA, MacEwen EG, et al: Treatment and prognostic factors in lymphoma in cats: 103 cases (1977–1981). J Am Vet Med Assoc 194:696–702, 1989.

93. Cotter SM: Treatment of lymphoma and leukemia with cyclophosphamide, vincristine, and prednisone. II. Treatment of cats. J Am Anim Hosp Assoc 19:166–172, 1983.

94. Jeglum KA, Whereat A, Young K: Chemotherapy of lymphoma in 75 cats. J Am Vet Med Assoc 190:174–178, 1987.

95. Moore AS, Frimberger AE, L'Heureux DA, et al: Doxorubicin vs COP for maintenance of remission in feline lymphoma. Proc 14th Annu Vet Cancer Soc 1994, p. 42.

96. Cotter SM, Kanki PJ, and Simon M: Renal disease in five tumor-bearing cats treated with adriamycin. J Am Anim Hosp Assoc 21:405–409, 1985.

97. Cotter SM: Feline leukemia/lymphoma: Diagnosis and treatment. Feline medicine symposium. Proc North Am Vet Conf, Waltham, MA, 1994, pp. 29–35.

98. Turrel JM: Radiation therapy and hyperthermia. In Holzworth J (ed.): Diseases of the cat: Medicine and surgery. Philadelphia, WB Saunders, 1987, p. 606.

99. Elmslie RE, Ogilvie GK, Gillette EL, et al: Radiotherapy with and without chemotherapy for localized lymphoma in 10 cats. Vet Radiol 32:277–280, 1991.

100. Helfand SC: Low dose cytosine arabinoside-

induced remission of lymphoblastic leukemia in a cat. J Am Vet Med Assoc 191:707–710, 1987.

101. Marks SL, Cook AK, Griffey S, et al: Dietary alteration of methotrexate enterotoxicity in cats. Proc Vet Cancer Soc 14:25, 1994.

102. Ogilivie GK, Moore AS: Managing the veterinary cancer patient. Trenton, NJ, Veterinary Learning System, 1995, pp. 249–259.

# D.

# Canine Myeloproliferative Disorders

Karen M. Young and E. Gregory MacEwen

# and

# Malignant Histiocytosis

E. Gregory MacEwen

The main focus of this chapter is myeloproliferative diseases of dogs. At the end of the chapter, there is a short section on malignant histiocytosis in Bernese mountain dogs and other breeds.

Myeloproliferative disorders are a group of neoplastic diseases of bone marrow in which there is unregulated and senseless proliferation of clones of cells derived from defective hematopoietic stem cells.[1] These disorders are classified based on the biologic behavior, the degree of cellular differentiation, and the lineage of the neoplastic cells (granulocytic, monocytic, erythroid, megakaryocytic, or mixed). Excessive proliferation of cells with defective maturation and function leads to reduction of normal hematopoiesis and invasion of other tissues.

## Incidence and Risk Factors

Myeloproliferative disorders (MPDs) are uncommon or rare in the dog; they occur 10 times less frequently than lymphoproliferative disorders.[2] However, accurate information about incidence and other epidemiologic information awaits consistent use of a uniform classification system (see later discussion). There is no known age, breed, or sex predisposition. In dogs the etiology of spontaneously occurring leukemia is unknown; it is likely that genetic and environmental factors (including exposure to radiation, drugs, or toxic chemicals) play a role. In people, acquired chromosomal derangements lead to clonal overgrowth with arrested development.[3] Certain forms of leukemia in dogs have been produced experimentally following irradiation.[4–6] In contrast to MPDs in cats, no causative viral agent has been demonstrated in dogs, although retrovirus-like budding particles were observed in the neoplastic cells of a dog with granulocytic leukemia.[7]

## Pathology and Natural Behavior

A review of normal hematopoiesis will aid in understanding the various manifestations of MPDs. Hematopoiesis is the process of proliferation, differentiation, and maturation of stem cells into terminally differentiated blood cells. A simplified scheme is presented in Figure 28–17. Pluripotent stem cells differentiate into either lymphopoietic or hematopoietic multipotent stem cells.[8] Under the influence of specific regulatory and microenvironmental factors, multipotent stem cells in bone marrow differentiate into progenitor cells committed to a specific hematopoietic cell line, for example, erythroid, granulocytic-monocytic, or megakaryocytic. Maturation results in the production of terminally

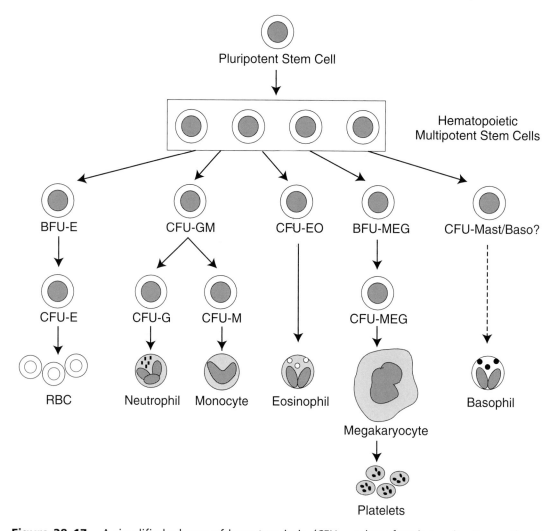

**Figure 28–17.** A simplified scheme of hematopoiesis. (CFU = colony-forming units; E = erythroid; GM = granulocytic-monocytic; EO = eosinophil; Meg = megakaryocyte.)

differentiated blood cells—erythrocytes, granulocytes, monocytes, and platelets—which are delivered to the circulation. In some cases, as in the maturation of reticulocytes to erythrocytes, final development may occur in the spleen.

Proliferation and differentiation of hematopoietic cells are controlled by a group of regulatory growth factors.[8,9] Of these, erythropoietin is the best characterized; it regulates erythroid proliferation and differentiation and is produced in the kidney, where changes in oxygen tension are detected. The myeloid compartment is dependent on a group of factors, collectively referred to as colony-stimulating factors (CSFs). These factors act at the level of the committed progenitor cells but also influence the functional capabilities of

mature cells. Some of these factors have a broad spectrum of activity; others are more restricted in their target cells and actions. CSFs are produced in vitro by a multitude of cell types, including monocytes, macrophages, lymphocytes, and endothelial cells, and these cells likely play a role in the production and regulation of these factors in vivo. The gene for thrombopoietin has recently been cloned, and it appears that this hormone alone can induce differentiation of megakaryocytes and platelet production.[10] Recombinant forms of many of these hormones are increasingly available.

The clonal disorders of bone marrow include myeloaplasia (usually referred to as aplastic anemia), myelodysplasia, and myeloproliferation. A preleukemic syndrome, characterized by peripheral pancytopenia and bone marrow hyperplasia with maturation arrest, is more correctly termed myelodysplasia because the syndrome does not always progress to overt leukemia. This syndrome has been described in cats, usually in association with feline leukemia virus infection, but has only rarely been recognized in dogs.[11-13] MPDs may be manifested by abnormalities in any or all the different cell lines, since hematopoietic cells share a common stem cell. In addition, transformation from one MPD to another may occur.[14]

MPDs are classified in several ways. The terms *acute* and *chronic* refer to the degree of cellular differentiation of the leukemic cells, but these terms also correlate with the biologic behavior of the neoplasm.[15] Disorders resulting from uncontrolled proliferation of cells incapable of maturation lead to the accumulation of poorly differentiated, or "blast," cells. These disorders are termed acute MPDs or acute nonlymphocytic leukemias. Disorders resulting from unregulated proliferation of cells that exhibit progressive, albeit incomplete and defective, maturation lead to the accumulation of differentiated cells. These disorders are termed chronic MPDs and include polycythemia vera, chronic myelogenous leukemia and its variants, essential thrombocythemia, and possibly primary myelofibrosis. MPDs are further classified by the lineage of the dominant cell type(s), defined by Romanowsky stains, special cytochemical stains, and ultrastructural features, and have recently been classified into subtypes (see later discussion).

Acute leukemias have a more sudden onset and are more aggressive. In both acute and chronic disorders, however, abnormalities in proliferation, maturation, and functional characteristics can occur in any hematopoietic cell line.[1] In addition, normal hematopoiesis is adversely affected. Animals with leukemia usually have decreased numbers of circulating normal cells. The pathogenesis of the cytopenias is complex and may result in part from production of inhibitory factors. Eventually, normal hematopoietic cells are displaced by neoplastic cells, termed myelophthisis. Anemia and thrombocytopenia are particularly common. Neutropenia and thrombocytopenia result in infection and hemorrhage, which may be more deleterious to the animal than the primary disease process. Despite the disseminated nature of the disease at the time of diagnosis, parenchymal organ dysfunction usually occurs only in very advanced cases of myeloproliferative disorders.

## ACUTE MYELOPROLIFERATIVE DISORDERS

Acute MPDs are rare and are characterized by aberrant proliferation of a clone of cells without maturation. This results in the accumulation of immature blast cells in bone marrow and peripheral blood. The white blood cell (WBC) count is variable and ranges from leukopenia to counts up to 150,000/µl. The spleen, liver, and lymph nodes are commonly involved, and other tissues, including the tonsils, kidney, heart, and central nervous system (CNS), may be infiltrated as well. There is no characteristic age, and even very young dogs may be affected.[16] The clinical course of these disorders tends to be rapid. Production of normal peripheral blood cells is usually diminished or absent, and anemia, neutropenia, and thrombocytopenia are common. Infection and hemorrhage are frequent sequelae. Occasionally, malignant blasts are present in bone marrow but not in peripheral blood. This is termed *aleukemic* leukemia, while *subleukemic* suggests a normal or decreased WBC with some neoplastic cells in circulation.

In 1985 the Animal Leukemia Study Group was formed under the auspices of the American Society for Veterinary Clinical Pathology to develop specific cytomorphologic criteria for classifying acute nonlymphocytic leukemias. Recognition of specific subtypes of leukemia is required to accumulate accurate and useful information about prognosis and response to treatment, as well as to compare studies from different sites. In 1991, this group proposed a classification system following adaptation of the French-American-British (FAB) system and criteria established by the National Cancer Institute Workshop.[17] The group members examined blood and bone marrow from 49 dogs and cats with MPDs. Romanowsky-stained specimens were examined first to identify blast cells and their percentages. Lineage specificity was then determined using cytochemical markers. The percentage of blasts and the information about lineage specificity were used in combination to classify disorders as acute undifferentiated leukemia (AUL), acute myeloid leukemia (AML, subtypes M1–M5 and M7), and erythroleukemia with or without erythroid predominance (M6 and M6Er). A description of these subtypes is presented in Table 28–22 (p. 503).

With the exception of acute promyelocytic leukemia, or M3, all of these subtypes have been described in dogs. However, since this modified FAB system has only recently been adopted, the names given to these disorders in the literature vary considerably. In addition, in the absence of special cytochemical staining and/or electron microscopy, the specific subtype of leukemia has often been uncertain, making retrospective analysis of epidemiologic information, prognosis, and response to therapy confusing at best. Although defining specific subtypes may seem to be an academic exercise owing to the uniformly poor prognosis of acute leukemias, this information is critical to improving the management of these diseases. Because of the low incidence of MPDs, national and international cooperative efforts will be required to accumulate information on the pathogenesis and response to different treatment modalities of specific subtypes. Utilization of a uniform classification system is an essential first step.

The most commonly reported acute leukemias in the dog are acute myeloblastic leukemia (M1 and M2) and acute myelomonocytic leukemia (M4).[2,18-27] Megakaryoblastic leukemia (M7) is also well recognized in dogs[28-35] and may be associated with platelet dysfunction.[33] Monocytic leukemias have likely included those with and without monocytic differentiation (M5a and M5b),[36,37] but in some cases the diagnosis may have been chronic myelomonocytic or chronic monocytic leukemia (see later discussion). There are few reports in dogs of spontaneously occurring erythroleukemia (M6) in which the leukemic cells comprise myeloblasts, monoblasts, and erythroid elements.[38,39] AULs have uncertain lineages, since they are negative for all cytochemical markers. These leukemias should be distinguished from lymphoid leukemias. Examination of blast cells by electron microscopy may reveal characteristic ultrastructural features.

## CHRONIC MYELOPROLIFERATIVE DISORDERS

Chronic MPDs are characterized by excessive production of differentiated bone marrow cells, resulting in the accumulation of erythrocytes (polycythemia vera), granulocytes and/or monocytes (chronic myelogenous leukemia and its variants), or platelets (essential thrombocythemia). Primary myelofibrosis as a clonal disorder of marrow stromal cells, characterized by proliferation of fibroblasts with accumulation of collagen in bone marrow, is not recognized in animals. Myelofibrosis is considered a response to injury and may occur secondary to MPDs.

## Polycythemia Vera

Polycythemia vera (PV) is a clonal disorder of stem cells, although whether the defect is in the pluripotent stem cell or the hematopoietic multipotent stem cell is still not clear. In people, progenitor cells have an increased sensitivity to insulin-like growth factor 1, which stimulates hematopoiesis.[40] It is not known whether this hypersensitivity is the primary defect or is secondary to another gene mutation. In any case, the result is overproduction of red blood cells. The disease is rare and must be distinguished from more common causes of polycythemia, including relative and secondary absolute polycythemia (see later discussion). In PV, there is neoplastic proliferation of the erythroid series with terminal differentiation to red blood cells. The disease has been reported in dogs that tend to be middle-aged with no breed or sex predilection[41-49] and is characterized by an increased red blood cell mass evidenced by an elevated packed cell volume (PCV), red blood cell (RBC) count, and hemoglobin concentration. The PCV is typically in the range of 65 to 85%. The bone marrow is hyperplastic, although the myeloid-erythroid ratio (M:E) tends to be normal. In contrast to the disease in people, other cell lines do not appear to be involved, and transformation to other MPDs has not been reported. The disease in dogs may be more appropriately termed primary erythrocytosis.

## Chronic Myelogenous Leukemia

Chronic myelogenous leukemia (CML) is a neoplastic proliferation of the neutrophil series, although concurrent eosinophilic and basophilic differentiation can occur. CML can occur in dogs of any age.[16,50-53] Neutrophils and neutrophilic precursors accumulate in bone marrow and peripheral blood and invade other organs. The peripheral WBC count is usually, but not always, greater than 100,000/μl. Both immature and mature neutrophils are present; mature forms are usually more numerous, but sometimes an "uneven" left shift is present. Eosinophils and basophils may also be increased. The bone marrow is characterized by granulocytic hyperplasia, and morphologic abnormalities may not be present. Erythroid and megakaryocytic lines may be affected, resulting in anemia, thrombocytopenia, or less commonly thrombocytosis. This disorder must be distinguished from severe neutrophilic leukocytosis and "leukemoid reactions" caused by inflammation or immune-mediated diseases. Leukemoid reactions can also occur as a paraneoplastic syndrome. In people with CML, characteristic cytogenetic abnormalities are present in all bone marrow cells, signifying a lesion at the level of an early multipotent stem cell. Typically these individuals have a chromosomal translocation, resulting in the Philadelphia chromosome.[54] No consistent cytogenetic abnormalities have been demonstrated in spontaneously occurring CML in dogs. Variants of CML are chronic myelomonocytic leukemia (CMML) and chronic monocytic leukemia (CMoL). These diagnoses are made based on the percentage of monocytes in the leukemic cell population.

In addition to accumulating in bone marrow and peripheral blood, leukemic cells also invade the red pulp of the spleen, the periportal and sinusoidal areas of the liver, and sometimes lymph nodes. Other organs, such as the kidney, heart, and lung, are less commonly affected. In addition, extramedullary hematopoiesis may be present in the liver and spleen. Death is usually due to complications of infection or hemorrhage secondary to neutrophil dysfunction and thrombocytopenia. In some cases, CML may terminate in "blast crisis," in which there is a transformation from a predominance of well-differentiated granulocytes to excessive numbers of poorly differentiated blast cells in peripheral blood and bone marrow. This phenomenon is well documented in the dog.[50–51,53]

## Basophilic and Eosinophilic Leukemia

Basophilic leukemia, although rare, has been reported in dogs and is characterized by an elevated WBC count with a high proportion of basophils in peripheral blood and bone marrow.[55,56] Hepatosplenomegaly, lymphadenopathy, and thrombocytosis may be present. The dogs have all been anemic. Basophilic leukemia should be distinguished from mast cell leukemia (mastocytosis). Whether dogs develop eosinophilic leukemia remains in question. Reported cases have had high blood eosinophil counts and eosinophilic infiltrates in organs.[57,58] One dog responded well to treatment with corticosteroids. The distinction between neoplastic proliferation of eosinophils and idiopathic hypereosinophilic syndrome remains elusive. Disorders associated with eosinophilia, such as parasitism, skin diseases, or diseases of the respiratory and gastrointestinal tracts, should be considered first in an animal with eosinophilia.

## Essential Thrombocythemia

In people, essential thrombocythemia, or primary thrombocytosis, is characterized by platelet counts that are persistently greater than $600,000/\mu l$. There are no blast cells in circulation, and marked megakaryocytic hyperplasia of the bone marrow without myelofibrosis is present. Thrombosis and bleeding are the most common sequelae, and most patients have splenomegaly. Other MPDs, especially PV, should be ruled out, and importantly, there should be no primary disorders associated with reactive thrombocytosis.[59] These include inflammation, hemolytic anemia, iron deficiency anemia, malignancies, recovery from severe hemorrhage, rebound from immune-mediated thrombocytopenia, and splenectomy. Recently, essential thrombocythemia has been recognized in dogs.[14,60–61] In one dog, the platelet count exceeded 4 million/$\mu l$ and bizarre giant forms with abnormal granulation were present. The bone marrow contained increased numbers of megakaryocytes and megakaryoblasts, but circulating blast cells were not seen. Other findings included splenomegaly, gastrointestinal bleeding, and increased numbers of circulating basophils. Causes of secondary or reactive thrombocytosis were ruled out.[60] In another dog, primary thrombocytosis was diagnosed and then progressed to CML.[14] In some cases reported in the literature as essential thrombocythemia, the dogs had microcytic hypochromic anemias. Since iron deficiency anemia is associated with reactive or secondary thrombocytosis, care must be taken to rule out this disorder.

## OTHER BONE MARROW DISORDERS

### Myelofibrosis

Primary myelofibrosis with clonal proliferation of marrow fibroblasts has not been reported in dogs.[62] In people, myelofibrosis is characterized by collagen deposition in bone marrow and increased numbers of megakaryocytes, many of which exhibit morphologic abnormalities. In fact, breakdown of intramedullary megakaryocytes and subsequent release of factors that promote fibroblast proliferation or inhibit collagen breakdown may be the underlying pathogenesis of the fibrosis.[63] Focal osteosclerosis is sometimes present. Anemia, thrombocytopenia, splenomegaly, and myeloid metaplasia (production of hematopoietic cells outside the bone marrow) are consistent features. The extramedullary hema-topoiesis is ineffective in maintaining or restoring normal peripheral blood counts.

In dogs, myelofibrosis occurs secondary to MPDs, radiation damage, and congenital hemo-lytic anemias.[64–67] In some cases, the inciting cause is unknown (idiopathic myelofibrosis). There may be concurrent marrow necrosis in cases of ehrlichiosis, septicemia, or drug toxicity (estrogens, cephalosporins), and there is specula-tion that fibroblasts proliferate in response to release of inflammatory mediators associated with the necrosis.[62] Myeloid metaplasia has been reported to occur in the liver, spleen, and lung.[67] Extramedullary hematopoiesis is ineffective in preventing or correcting the pancytopenia that eventually develops.

## Myelodysplastic Syndrome

Dysfunction of the hematopoietic system can be manifested by a variety of abnormalities that com-prise the myelodysplastic syndrome. In dogs, there usually are cytopenias in two or three lines in the peripheral blood (anemia, neutropenia, and/or thrombocytopenia). Other blood abnormalities can include macrocytic erythrocytes and metarubricy-tosis. The bone marrow is typically normo- or hypercellular, and dysplastic changes are evident in several cell lines. Myelodysplasia is sometimes referred to as "preleukemia" because in some cases it may progress to an acute leukemia.[11–13]

## History and Clinical Signs

Dogs with MPDs have similar presentations regardless of the specific disease entity, although animals with acute MPDs have a more acute onset of illness and a more rapid clinical course. A his-tory of lethargy, inappetence, and weight loss is common. Clinical signs include emaciation, persis-tent fever, pallor, petechiation, hepatospleno-megaly, and less commonly, lymphadenopathy and enlarged tonsils. Shifting leg lameness, ocular lesions, and recurrent infections are also seen. Vomiting, diarrhea, dyspnea, and neurologic signs are variable features. Serum chemistries may be within the reference range but can change if sig-nificant organ infiltration occurs. Animals with myelodysplastic syndrome may be lethargic and anorectic and have pallor, fever, and hepatospleno-megaly. In PV, dogs often have erythema of mucous membranes owing to the increase in red blood cell mass. Some dogs are polydipsic. In addi-tion, neurologic signs, such as disorientation, ataxia, or seizures, may be present and are thought to be the result of hyperviscosity or hyper-volemia.[45] Hepatosplenomegaly is usually absent.

Peripheral blood abnormalities are consistently found. In addition to the presence of neoplastic cells, other abnormalities, including a decrease in the numbers of normal cells of any or all hematopoietic cell lines, may be present. Occa-sional nucleated RBCs are present in the blood of about half the dogs with acute nonlymphocytic leukemia.[17] Nonregenerative anemia and throm-bocytopenia are present in most cases. The anemia is usually normocytic and normochromic, although macrocytic anemia is sometimes present. Pathogenic mechanisms include effects of inhibitory factors leading to ineffective hema-topoiesis, myelophthisis, immune-mediated ane-mia secondary to neoplasia, and hemorrhage sec-ondary to thrombocytopenia, platelet dysfunc-tion, or disseminated intravascular coagulation. Anemia is most severe in acute MPDs, although both anemia and thrombocytopenia may be milder in animals with the M5 subtype (acute monocytic leukemia). In myelofibrosis, the anemia is characterized by anisocytosis and poikilocytosis. In addition, pancytopenia and leukoerythroblasto-sis, in which immature erythroid and myeloid cells are in circulation, may be present. These phenom-ena probably result from the replacement of mar-row by fibrous tissue with resultant sheering of red cells and escape of immature cells normally confined to bone marrow. In polycythemia vera, the PCV is elevated, usually in the range of 65 to 85%. The bone marrow is hyperplastic, and the M:E is usually in the normal range.

The neoplastic cells are often defective func-tionally. Platelet dysfunction has been reported in a dog with acute megakaryoblastic leukemia (M7),[33] and in CML, the neutrophils have decreased phagocytic capacity and other abnor-malities. One exception to this was a report of CML in a dog in which the neutrophils had enhanced phagocytic capacity and superoxide pro-duction.[68] The authors hypothesized that increased synthesis of GM-CSF resulted from a lactoferrin deficiency in the neoplastic neutrophils and mediated the enhanced function of these cells.

## Diagnostic Techniques and Workup

In all cases of MPD, the diagnosis depends on the examination of peripheral blood and bone mar-row. Acute MPDs are diagnosed on the basis of finding blast cells with clearly visible nucleoli in blood and bone marrow. Most dogs with acute leukemia have circulating blasts. These cells may be present in low numbers in peripheral blood, and a careful search of the smear, especially at the feathered edge, should be made. Even if blasts are not detected in circulation, indications of bone marrow disease, such as nonregenerative anemia or thrombocytopenia, are usually present. Occasionally neoplastic cells can be found in cerebrospinal fluid in animals with invasion of the CNS. Smears of aspirates from organs such as the lymph, spleen, or liver may contain blasts but usually contribute little to the diagnostic workup.

Examination of blasts stained with standard Romanowsky stains may give clues as to the lineage of the cells. In AML, in addition to myeloblasts, some progranulocytes with their characteristic azurophilic granules may be present. In myelomonocytic leukemia, the nuclei of the blasts are usually pleomorphic, with round to lobulated forms. In some cells, the cytoplasm may contain large azurophilic granules or vacuoles. Blasts in megakaryocytic leukemia may contain vacuoles and have cytoplasmic blebs. In addition, bizarre macroplatelets may be present. While these distinguishing morphologic features may suggest a definitive diagnosis, special stains are usually required to define the lineage of the blasts. Several investigators have reported modification of diagnoses following cytochemical staining.[69,70]

The Animal Leukemia Group has recommended the following diagnostic criteria, summarized in Figure 28–18.[17] Using well-prepared Romanowsky-stained blood and bone marrow films, a minimum of 200 cells are counted to determine the leukocyte differential in blood and the percentage of blasts in bone marrow calculated both as a percentage of all nucleated cells (ANC) and nonerythroid cells (NEC). Blast cells are further characterized using cytochemical markers.[69-71] Neutrophil differentiation is identified by positive staining of blasts for peroxidase, Sudan Black B, and chloracetate esterase. Nonspecific esterases (alpha-naphthyl acetate esterase or alpha-naphthyl butyrate esterase), especially if they are inhibited by sodium fluoride, mark monocytes. Monocytes may also be positive for peroxidase activity. Acetylcholinesterase is a marker for megakaryocytes in dogs and cats. In addition, positive immunostaining for von Willebrand's factor (factor VIII-related antigen) and GPIIIa on the surface of blasts identifies them as megakaryocyte precursors.[30-35] Alkaline phosphatase (AP) only rarely marks normal cells in dogs and cats but is present in blasts cells in acute myeloblastic and myelomonocytic leukemias. However, owing to reports of AP activity in lym-

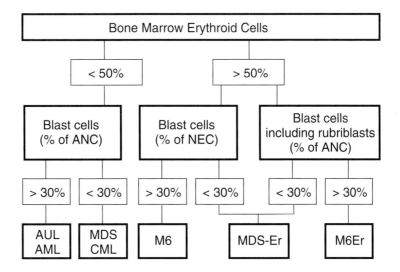

**Figure 28–18.** A scheme to classify myeloid leukemias and myelodysplastic syndromes in dogs and cats. (Blast cells = myeloblasts, monoblasts, and megakaryoblasts; ANC = all nucleated cells in bone marrow, including lymphocytes, plasma cells, macrophages, and mast cells; NEC = nonerythroid cells in bone marrow; AUL = acute undifferentiated leukemia; AML = acute myeloid leukemias M1–M5 and M7; CML = chronic myeloid leukemias, including chronic myelogenous, chronic myelomonocytic, and chronic monocytic leukemias; MDS = myelodysplastic syndrome; MDS-Er = myelodysplastic syndrome with erythroid predominance; M6 = erythroleukemia; M6Er = erythroleukemia with erythroid predominance.) From Jain NC, Blue JT, Grindem CB, et al: Proposed criteria for classification of acute myeloid leukemia in dogs and cats. Vet Clin Pathol *20*(3):63–82, 1991 (figure is from p. 71; reprinted with permission).

phoid leukemias in dogs, its specificity as a marker for myeloid cells is not certain.

Bone marrow differential counts and cytochemical staining should be performed and interpreted by experienced veterinary cytomorphologists. If erythroid cells comprise <50% of ANC and the blast cells are >30%, a diagnosis of AML or AUL is made. If erythroid cells are >50% of ANC and the blast cells are >30%, a diagnosis of erythroleukemia (M6) is made. If rubriblasts comprise a significant proportion of the blast cells, a diagnosis of M6Er, or erythroleukemia with erythroid predominance, can be made.

In some cases, electronmicroscopy is required to identify the lineage of the blast cells. For example, megakaryocyte precursors are positive for platelet peroxidase activity and contain demarcation membranes and alpha granules.[31,35] Both of these features are detected at the ultrastructural level. Immunophenotyping, used to identify cell lineages in human patients, awaits development of appropriate markers for animal species. Hematopoietic cells from people with leukemia often have abnormal chromosome patterns. Cytogenetic abnormalities have been found in leukemic cells from a small number of dogs.[72] While no consistent patterns could be correlated with the type of leukemia, cytogenetic analysis may eventually prove to be a valuable diagnostic and prognostic aid.

Owing to the degree of differentiation of cells in chronic MPDs, these disorders must be distinguished from non-neoplastic causes of increases in these cell types. In order to make a diagnosis of PV, it must first be established that the polycythemia is absolute rather than relative. In relative polycythemias, plasma volume is decreased from hemoconcentration, dehydration, or hypovolemia, and the absolute red cell mass is not increased. Splenic contraction can also result in relative polycythemia. Absolute polycythemia, in which the RBC mass is increased, is usually secondary to tissue hypoxia causing appropriate increased production of erythropoietin. Rarely, erythropoietin may be produced inappropriately by a tumor (e.g., renal cell carcinoma) or in renal disease (pyelonephritis) or localized renal hypoxia.[73–75] These causes of polycythemia should be eliminated by appropriate laboratory work, thoracic radiographs, arterial blood gas analysis, and renal ultrasonography. In people with PV, plasma erythropoietin (Epo) levels are low. Epo levels in dogs with PV tend to be low or low-normal, whereas in animals with secondary absolute polycythemia the levels are high.[76,77] Samples for determination of Epo concentrations should be taken prior to therapeutic phlebotomy used to treat hyperviscosity and, owing to fluctuations in Epo levels, should be repeated if results are incongruous with other information.

There are no pathognomonic features of CML in dogs, and other common causes for marked leukocytosis with a left shift ("leukemoid reaction") and granulocytic hyperplasia of bone marrow must be eliminated. These include infections, especially pyogenic ones, immune-mediated diseases, and other malignant neoplasms. In CML maturation sometimes appears disorderly, and there may be variation in the size and shape of neutrophils at the same level of maturation. In addition, neoplastic leukocytes may disintegrate more rapidly and appear vacuolated.[16] Because of the invasive nature of CML, biopsy of liver or spleen may also help to distinguish true leukemia from a leukemoid reaction, assuming the animal can tolerate the procedure. If characteristic cytogenetic abnormalities can be found in dogs with CML, this analysis may be helpful.

Basophilic leukemia is diagnosed by finding excessive numbers of basophils in circulation and in bone marrow. Basophilic leukemia must be differentiated from mastocytosis based on the morphology of the cell type present. Basophils have a segmented nucleus and variably sized granules, whereas mast cells have a round to oval nucleus that may be partially or totally obscured by small, round, metachromatic-staining granules. This distinction is usually easy to make; however, in basophilic leukemia, changes in the morphology of the nucleus and granules make the distinction less clear.[56]

Essential thrombocythemia has been diagnosed based on finding persistent and excessive thrombocytosis (>600,000/μl) without circulating blast cells and in the absence of another MPD (e.g., polycythemia vera), myelofibrosis, or disorders known to cause secondary thrombocytosis.[59] These include iron deficiency anemia, chronic inflammatory diseases, recovery from severe hemorrhage, rebound from immune-mediated thrombocytopenia, and absence of a spleen. Thrombocytosis is transient in these disorders or abates with resolution of the primary disease. In essential thrombocythemia, platelet morphology may be abnormal, with bizarre giant forms and abnormal granulation.[60] In the bone marrow megakaryocytic hyperplasia is a consistent feature, and dysplastic changes may be evident in megakaryocytes. Spurious hyperkalemia may be present in serum samples from dogs with thrombocytosis from any cause owing to the release of potassium from platelets during clot formation.[78] Measuring potassium in plasma is recommended in these cases and usually demonstrates a potassium concentration within reference range.

In myelodysplastic syndromes (MDSs), abnormalities in two or three cell lines are usually manifested in peripheral blood as neutropenia with or without a left shift, nonregenerative anemia, or thrombocytopenia. Other changes include macrocytosis and metarubricytosis. The bone marrow is typically normo- or hypercellular with an increased M:E ratio, and blasts cells, although increased, comprise <30% of the nucleated cells. Dysplastic changes can be detected in any cell line. Dyserythropoiesis is characterized by asynchronous maturation of erythroid cells typified by large hemoglobinized cells with immature nuclei (megaloblastic change). If the erythroid component is dominant, the MDS is called MDS-Er (Table 28–22). In dysgranulopoiesis, giant neutrophil precursors and abnormalities in nuclear segmentation and cytoplasmic granulation can be seen. Finally, dysthrombopoiesis is characterized by giant platelets and micromegakaryocytes.

Myelofibrosis should be suspected in animals with nonregenerative anemia or pancytopenia, abnormalities in erythrocyte morphology, especially shape, and leukoerythroblastosis. Bone marrow aspiration is usually unsuccessful, resulting in a "dry tap." This necessitates a bone marrow biopsy taken with a Jamshidi needle. The specimen is processed for routine histopathologic examination, and if necessary, special stains for fibrous tissue can be used. Since myelofibrosis occurs secondary to other diseases of bone marrow, such as MPD, chronic hemolytic anemia, or bone marrow necrosis, the clinician should look for a primary disease process.

## Treatment

**Acute Leukemias**  Owing to the poor response of acute nonlymphocytic leukemias, treatment has been unrewarding to date. However, we have little information on the response of specific subtypes of leukemia to uniform chemotherapeutic protocols. The veterinarian is advised to contact a veterinary oncologist for advice on new protocols and appropriate management of these cases.

The therapeutic goal is to eradicate leukemic cells and re-establish normal hematopoiesis. Currently, this is best accomplished by cytoreductive chemotherapy, and the agents most commonly utilized include a combination of cytosine arabinoside plus an anthracycline, such as doxorubicin.[11,20,79–81] In people, the introduction of cytosine arabinoside has been the single most important development in the therapy of acute nonlymphocytic leuke-

**Table 28–22**  Subtypes of Leukemias and Dysplasias Adapting the FAB System

| ACUTE LEUKEMIAS Subtype | Description |
| --- | --- |
| AUL | Acute undifferentiated leukemia (formerly called reticuloendotheliosis) |
| M1 | Myeloblastic leukemia, without differentiation |
| M2 | Myeloblastic leukemia, with some neutrophilic differentiation |
| M3 | Promyelocytic leukemia (not recognized in animals) |
| M4 | Myelomonocytic leukemia |
| M5a | Monocytic leukemia, without differentiation |
| M5b | Monocytic leukemia, with some monocytic differentiation |
| M6 | Erythroleukemia |
| M6Er | Variant of M6 with erythroblasts comprising erythroid component |
| M7 | Megakaryoblastic leukemia |

| CHRONIC MYELOID LEUKEMIAS Subtype | Description |
| --- | --- |
| CML | Chronic myelogenous leukemia |
| CMML | Chronic myelomonocytic leukemia |
| CMoL | Chronic monocytic leukemia |

| HEMATOPOIETIC DYSPLASIA Subtype | Description |
| --- | --- |
| MDS | Myelodysplastic syndrome |
| MDS-Er | Myelodysplastic syndrome with erythroid predominance |

mia.[82] In dogs, 100 to 200 mg/m$^2$ cytosine arabinoside by slow influsion (12–24 hrs) daily for 3 days and repeated weekly has been used. Doxorubicin, at 30 mg/m$^2$ IV every 2 to 3 weeks, can be administered at 2-week intervals alternating with cytosine arabinoside. If remission is achieved, as evidenced by normalization of the hemogram, the COAP protocol (cyclophosphamide, vincristine, cytosine arabinoside, and prednisone), as described for canine lymphoma, could be used as maintenance therapy.[79] Another protocol that has been used in treating acute myeloblastic leukemia is presented in Table 28–23.

Regardless of the chemotherapy protocol used, significant bone marrow suppression will develop, and intensive supportive care will be necessary. Transfusions of whole blood or platelet-rich plasma may be required to treat anemia and thrombocytopenia, and infection should be managed with aggressive antibiotic therapy. Because of the poor response, the major thrust of therapy may be just to provide palliative supportive care.

**Polycythemia Vera**    In treating PV, therapy is directed at reducing the red cell mass. The PCV should be reduced to 50 to 60% or by one-sixth of its starting value; phlebotomies should be performed as needed, administering appropriate colloid and crystalloid solutions to replace lost electrolytes; 20 ml of whole blood/kg of body weight can be removed at regular intervals.[43]

Radiophosphorus ($^{32}$P) has been shown to provide long-term control but can only be used in specialized centers.[83] The chemotherapeutic drug of choice is hydroxyurea. This drug should be administered at an initial dose of 30 mg/kg for 10 days and then reduced to 15 mg/kg PO daily.[45] The major goal of treatment is to maintain the PCV as close to normal as possible.

**Chronic Myelogenous Leukemia**    CML is best managed with chemotherapy to control the proliferation of the abnormal cell line and improve the quality of life. Hydroxyurea, an inhibitor of DNA synthesis, is the most effective agent for treating CML during the chronic phase.[84] The initial dosage is 20 to 25 mg/kg twice daily. Treatment with hydroxyurea should continue until the leukocyte count falls to 15,000 to 20,000 cells/μl.[50,55] Then the dosage of hydroxyurea can be reduced by 50% on a daily basis or to 50 mg/kg given bi- or triweekly. In people, the alkylating agent busulfan can be used as an alternative.[85] An effective dosage has not been established in the dog, but following human protocols, 0.1 mg/kg/day PO is given until the leukocyte count is reduced to 15,000 to 20,000 cells/μl.

Despite response to chemotherapy and control for many months, most dogs with CML will eventually enter a terminal phase of their disease. In one study of seven dogs with CML, four underwent terminal phase blast crisis.[50] In people, blast crisis may be lymphoid or myeloid.[86] In dogs, it is usually difficult to determine the cell of origin. These dogs have a poor prognosis and the best treatment to consider, if any, would be that listed in Table 28–23.

**Essential Thrombocythemia**    Few cases have been reported, but one dog was treated successfully with a combination chemotherapy protocol that included vincristine, cytosine arabinoside, cyclophosphamide, and prednisone.[61] Treatment is controversial in people because of the lack of evidence that asymptomatic patients benefit from chemotherapy. Patients with thrombosis or bleeding are given cytoreductive therapy. Hydroxyurea is the drug of choice for initially controlling the thrombocytosis.[59]

**Myelodysplastic Syndrome**    There is no standard therapeutic regime for the MDS. Often, people receive no treatment if the cytopenias do not cause clinical signs. Transfusions are given

**Table 28–23**   Protocol for the Treatment of Acute MPD[79]

| Drug | Dosage | Route |
|---|---|---|
| *Remission Induction:* | | |
| Cytosine arabinoside | 100 mg/m$^2$/day | IV over 60 min every 12 hours |
| 6-Thioguanine | 40 mg/m$^2$ | PO for 4 days |
| Doxorubicin | 10–15 mg/m$^2$ | IV daily for 3 days |
| *For Maintenance:* | | |
| Cytosine arabinoside | 100 mg/m$^2$ | SQ or IV once or twice weekly |
| 6-Thioguanine | 40 mg/m$^2$ | PO twice weekly |
| Doxorubicin | 30 mg/m$^2$ | IV every 3 weeks |

when necessary, and patients with fever are evaluated rapidly to detect infections. Growth factors, such as erythropoietin, GM-CSF, G-CSF, and IL-3, are sometimes used in patients who require frequent transfusions to increase their blood cell counts and enhance neutrophil function.[87,88] Other factors that induce differentiation of hematopoietic cells include retinoic acid analogues,[89] 1,25 dihydroxyvitamin D3,[90] interferon-alpha, and conventional chemotherapeutic agents, such as 6-thioguanine and cytosine arabinoside.[91] The propensity of these factors to enhance progression to leukemia is not known in many cases, but the potential risk exists.

## Prognosis

In general, the prognosis for animals with chronic MPDs is better than for dogs with acute MPDs, in which it is grave. The prognosis for PV and chronic granulocytic leukemia is guarded, but significant remissions have been achieved with certain therapeutic regimes and careful monitoring. Animals commonly survive a year or more.[50,55] Development of blast crisis portends a grave prognosis.

## Comparative Aspects

The pathophysiology and therapy of nonlymphocytic leukemia in humans is being studied intensively. The MPDs have been demonstrated to be clonal, with abnormalities evident in all hematopoietic cell lines. Leukemogenesis is likely caused by mutation or amplification of proto-oncogenes in a two-step process that initially involves a single cell and is followed by additional chromosomal alterations that may involve oncogenes.[1,3] These alterations are manifested as chromosomal abnormalities. Environmental factors known to cause leukemia are exposure to high-dose radiation, benzene (chronic exposure), and alkylating agents.[92]

Therapeutic modalities under investigation include combination chemotherapy, immunotherapy, cytokine therapy, and bone marrow transplantation. The prognosis for chronic MPDs is better than for acute MPDs. For acute nonlymphocytic leukemias, the prognosis is better for children than adults, with only 10% of adults receiving chemotherapy maintaining remissions for more than 5 years.[92] The spontaneous canine diseases probably occur too infrequently to serve as useful models. MPDs have been induced experimentally in the dog by irradiation and transplantation in an attempt to create models for study. Many similarities between human and canine MPDs exist, and veterinary medicine may benefit from any therapeutic advances made in the human field.

Malignant histiocytosis (MH) is a neoplastic dis-

# Malignant Histiocytosis

## Gregory MacEwen

order arising from cells of the mononuclear phagocytic system.[93–94] These include alveolar and peritoneal macrophages, Kupffer cells in the liver, and macrophages lining the sinusoids of the spleen and stroma of lymph nodes and bone marrow. Synonyms for mononuclear phagocytes are histiocytes and macrophages. In dogs, MH is a rare tumor reported in various breeds, especially Bernese mountain dogs, and appears to have a male predisposition.[94] MH in Bernese mountain dogs is inherited with a polygenic mode of inheritance, and in one study of 500 tumors examined from this breed, 25 to 40% were classified as MH.[95] Dogs are presented with weight loss, lethargy, coughing, pyrexia, depression, and lymphadenopathy. Bernese mountain dogs often have respiratory and CNS signs, and pulmonary and hilar lymph node involvement are common. Neoplastic infiltrates can be found in spleen, liver, and bone marrow. Anemia is a common feature of MH and is usually secondary to erythrophagocytosis by atypical histiocytes. Thrombocytopenia has also been reported and attributed to phagocytosis by malignant cells.

A variant of MH has been termed *systemic histiocytosis* and is characterized by cutaneous involvement.[96] This has been reported most commonly in Bernese mountain dogs and consists of poorly circumscribed, firm, nodular masses up to 4 cm in diameter. The overlying epidermis is either smooth or partially alopectic or ulcerated and crusted. Cutaneous lesions are commonly noted on the nasal apex, nasal planum, eyelids, and face. Some dogs have nasal mucosal swelling and associated respiratory stertor and nasal discharge.

The diagnosis of MH is usually established by finding the characteristic cells in biopsy material obtained from skin, bone marrow, lung, spleen or lymph nodes.[93,94,97] Histologically, the predominating cells are pleomorphic mononuclear cells and multinucleated giant cells. The tumors are often infiltrated by lymphocytes and neutrophils, and there is commonly phagocytosis of erythrocytes, neutrophils, and other cells. In people, some forms of lymphoma have been misdiagnosed as MH in the past. Cytochemical and ultrastructural studies are often necessary to establish whether neoplastic cells are of macrophage origin or represent a diffuse large-cell lymphoma.[98]

Ferritin may be a tumor marker for MH. In a recent case report, a dog with MH had a marked elevation in the serum ferritin concentration (6,636 ng/ml with a reference range of 80–800 ng/ml), suggesting production of ferritin by malignant cells.[99] The pathogenesis of hyperferritinemia in malignant histiocytosis is believed to be the synthesis and secretion of ferritin by neoplastic mononuclear phagocytes.

Overall, the treatment for MH has been unrewarding and few reports exist in the literature. Normal mature macrophages are nonproliferating and are relatively insensitive to ionizing radiation and most commonly used chemotherapeutic agents. Conversely, normal proliferating mononuclear phagocyte precursors in the bone marrow are very sensitive to radiation and cytotoxic drugs. This information does not necessarily predict the response of neoplastic cells to various treatment modalities, and, unfortunately, attempts to treat this rare malignancy with combination chemotherapy have yielded only palliative responses.

## REFERENCES

1. Lichtman MA: Classification and clinical manifestations of the hemopoietic stem cell disorders. *In* Beutler E, Lichtman MA, Coller BS, Kipps TJ (eds): Williams Hematology, 5th ed. New York, McGraw-Hill, 1995, pp. 229–238.
2. Nielsen SW: Myeloproliferative disorders in animals. *In* Clarke WJ, Howard EB, Hackett PL (eds): Myeloproliferative Disorders in Animals and Man. Oak Ridge, TN, USAEC Division of Technical Information Extension, 1970, pp. 297–313.
3. Jandl JH: Hematopoietic malignancies. *In* Blood: Pathophysiology. Boston, Blackwell Scientific Publications, 1991, pp. 254–275.
4. Anderson AC, Johnson RM: Erythroblastic malignancy in a beagle. J Am Vet Med Assoc *141*:944–946, 1962.
5. Seed TM, Tolle DV, Fritz TE, et al: Irradiation-induced erythroleukemia and myelogenous leukemia in the beagle dog: Hematology and ultrastructure. Blood *50*:1061–1079, 1977.
6. Tolle DV, Seed TM, Fritz TE, et al: Acute monocytic leukemia in an irradiated beagle. Vet Pathol *16*:243–254, 1979.
7. Sykes GP, King JM, Cooper BC: Retrovirus-like particles associated with myeloproliferative disease in the dog. J Comp Pathol *95*(4):559–564, 1985.
8. Quesenberry PJ: Hemopoietic stem cells, progenitor cells, and cytokines. *In* Beutler E, Lichtman MA, Coller BS, Kipps TJ (eds): Williams Hematology, 5th ed. New York, McGraw-Hill, 1995, pp. 211–228.
9. Metcalf D: The Hemopoietic Colony Stimulating Factors. New York, Elsevier, 1984, pp. 55–96.
10. Lok S, Kaushansky K, Holly RD, et al: Cloning and expression of murine thrombopoietin cDNA and stimulation of platelet production in vivo. Nature *369*:565–568, 1994.
11. Couto CG, Kallet AJ: Preleukemic syndrome in a dog. J Am Vet Med Assoc *184*:1389–1392, 1984.
12. Couto CG: Clinicopathologic aspects of acute leukemias in the dog. J Am Vet Med Assoc *186*(7):681–685, 1985.
13. Weiss DJ, Raskin R, Zerbe C: Myelodysplastic syndrome in two dogs. J Am Vet Med Assoc *187*(10):1038–1040, 1985.
14. Degen MA, Feldman BF, Turrel JM, et al: Thrombocytosis associated with a myeloproliferative disorder in a dog. J Am Vet Med Assoc *194*(10):1457–1459, 1989.
15. Evans JR, Gorman NT: Myeloproliferative disease in the dog and cat: Definition, aetiology and classification. Vet Rec *121*:437–443, 1987.
16. Jain NC: The leukemia complex. *In* Schalm's Veterinary Hematology, 4th ed. Philadelphia, Lea and Febiger, 1986, pp. 838–908.
17. Jain NC, Blue JT, Grindem CB, et al: A report of the animal leukemia study group. Proposed criteria for classification of acute myeloid leukemia in dogs and cats. Vet Clin Pathol *20*(3):63–82, 1991.
18. Barthel CH: Acute myelomonocytic leukemia in a dog. Vet Pathol *11*:79–86, 1974.
19. Green RA, Barton CL: Acute myelomonocytic leukemia in a dog. J Am Anim Hosp Assoc *13*:708–712, 1977.
20. Jain NC, Madewell BR, Weller RE, et al: Clinicalpathological findings and cytochemical characteri-

zations of myelomonocytic leukaemia in 5 dogs. J Comp Pathol 91:17–31, 1981.

21. Linnabary RD, Holscher MA, Glick AD, et al: Acute myelomonocytic leukemia in a dog. J Am Anim Hosp Assoc 14:71–75, 1978.

22. Moulton JE, Dungworth DL: Tumors of the lymphoid and hemopoietic tissues. In Moulton JE (ed): Tumors in Domestic Animals, 2nd ed. Berkeley, University of California Press, 1978, pp. 150–204.

23. Ragan HA, Hackett PL, Dagle GE: Acute myelomonocytic leukemia manifested as myelophthistic anemia in a dog. J Am Vet Med Assoc 169: 421–425, 1976.

24. Rohrig KE: Acute myelomonocytic leukemia in a dog. J Am Vet Med Assoc 182:137–141, 1983.

25. Madewell BR, Jain NC, Munn RJ: Unusual cytochemical reactivity in canine acute myeloblastic leukemia. Comp Haematol Int 1(2):117–120, 1991.

26. Christopher MM, Metz AL, Klausner J, et al: Acute myelomonocytic leukemia with neurologic manifestations in the dog. Vet Pathol 23(2):140–147, 1986.

27. Keller P, Sager P, Freudiger U, et al: Acute myeloblastic leukemia in a dog. J Comp Pathol 95(4):619–632, 1985.

28. Holscher MA, Collins RD, Glick AD, et al: Megakaryocytic leukemia in a dog. Vet Pathol 15:562–565, 1978.

29. Canfield PJ, Church DB, Russ IG: Myeloproliferative disorder involving the megakaryocytic line. J Small Anim Pract 34(6):296–301, 1993.

30. Colbatzy F, Hermanns W: Acute megakaryoblastic leukemia in one cat and two dogs. Vet Pathol 30(2):186–194, 1993.

31. Bolon B, Buergelt CD, Harvey JW et al: Megakaryoblastic leukemia in a dog. Vet Clin Pathol 18(3):69–72, 1989.

32. Shull RM, DeNovo RC, McCracken MD: Megakaryblastic leukemia in a dog. Vet Pathol 23(4):533–536, 1986.

33. Cain GR, Feldman BF, Kawakami TG, et al: Platelet dysplasia associated with megakaryoblastic leukemia in a dog. J Am Vet Med Assoc 188(5):529–530, 1986.

34. Cain GR, Kawakami TG, Jain NC: Radiation-induced megakaryoblastic leukemia in a dog. Vet Pathol 22(6):641–643, 1985.

35. Messick J, Carothers M, Wellman M: Identification and characterization of megakaryoblasts in acute megakaryoblastic leukemia in a dog. Vet Pathol 27(3):212–214, 1990.

36. Latimer KS, Dykstra MJ: Acute monocytic leukemia in a dog. J Am Vet Med Assoc 184:852–854, 1984.

37. Mackey LJ, Jarrett WFH, Lauder IM: Monocytic leukaemia in the dog. Vet Rec 96:27–30, 1975.

38. Capelli JL: Erythroleukemia in a dog. Pratique Medicale and Chirurgicale de l'Animal de Compagnie 26(4):337–340, 1990.

39. Hejlasz Z: Three cases of erythroleukemia in dogs. Medycyna Weterynaryjna 42(6):346–349, 1986.

40. Prchal J: Primary polycythemias. In Adamson JW (ed): Current Opinion in Hematology, Vol. 2. Philadelphia, Current Science, 1995, pp. 146–152.

41. Bush BM, Fankhauser R: Polycythaemia vera in a bitch. J Small Anim Prac 13:75–89, 1972.

42. Carb AV: Polycythemia vera in a dog. J Am Vet Med Assoc 154:289–297, 1969.

43. McGrath CJ: Polycythemia vera in dogs. J Am Vet Med Assoc 164:1117–1122, 1974.

44. Miller RM: Polycythemia vera in a dog. Vet Med/Small Anim Clin 63:222–223, 1968.

45. Peterson ME, Randolph JK: Diagnosis of canine primary polycythemia and management with hydroxyurea. J Am Vet Med Assoc 180:415–418, 1982.

46. Quesnal AD, Kruth SA: Polycythemia vera and glomerulonephritis in a dog. Can Vet J 33(10):671–672, 1992.

47. Meyer HP, Slappendel RJ, Greydanus-van-der-Putten SWM: Polycythaemia vera in a dog treated by repeated phlebotomies. Vet Quarterly 15(3):108–111, 1993.

48. Wysoke JM, Van Heerden J: Polycythaemia vera in a dog. J S African Vet Assoc 61(4):182–183, 1990.

49. Holden AR: Polycythaemia vera in a dog. Vet Rec 120(20):473–475, 1987.

50. Leifer CE, Matus RE, Patnaik AK, et al: Chronic myelogenous leukemia in the dog. J Am Vet Med Assoc 183:686–689, 1983.

51. Pollet L, Van Hove W, Matheeuws D: Blastic crisis in chronic myelogenous leukaemia in a dog. J Small Anim Pract 19:469–475, 1978.

52. Grindem CB, Stevens JB, Brost DR, et al: Chronic myelogenous leukaemia with meningeal infiltration in a dog. Comp Haematol Int 2(3):170–174, 1992.

53. Dunn JK, Jeffries AR, Evans RJ, et al: Chronic granulocytic leukaemia in a dog with associated bacterial endocarditis, thrombocytopenia and pre-retinal and retinal hemorrhages. J Small Anim Pract 28(11):1079–1086, 1987.

54. Lichtman MA: Chronic myelogenous leukemia and related disorders. In Beutler E, Lichtman MA, Coller BS, Kipps TJ (eds): Williams Hematology, 5th ed. New York, McGraw-Hill, 1995, pp. 298–324.

55. MacEwen EG, Drazner FH, McClellan AJ, et al: Treatment of basophilic leukemia in a dog. J Am Vet Med Assoc 166:376–380, 1975.

56. Mahaffey EA, Brown TP, Duncan JR, et al: Basophilic leukemia in a dog. J Comp Pathol 97(4)393–399, 1987.

57. Jensen AL, Nielsen OL: Eosinophilic leukemoid reaction in a dog. J Small Anim Pract 33(7):337–340, 1992.

58. Ndikuwera J, Smith DA, Obwolo MJ, et al: Chronic granulocytic leukaemia/eosinophilic leukaemia in a dog. J Small Anim Prac 33(11):553–557, 1992.

59. Schafer AI: Essential (primary) thrombocythemia. In Beutler E, Lichtman MA, Coller BS, Kipps TJ (eds): Williams Hematology, 5th ed. New York, McGraw-Hill, 1995, pp. 340–345.

60. Hopper PE, Mandell CP, Turrel JM, et al: Probable

essential thrombocythemia in a dog. J Vet Intern Med 3(2):79–85, 1989.

61. Simpson JW, Else RW, Honeyman P: Successful treatment of suspected essential thrombocythemia in the dog. J Small Anim Pract 31(7):345–348, 1990.

62. Reagan WJ: A review of myelofibrosis in dogs. Toxicol Pathol 21(2):164–169, 1993.

63. Castro-Malaspina H: Pathogenesis of myelofibrosis: Role of ineffective megakaryopoiesis and megakaryocyte components. In Berk PD, Castro-Malaspina H, Wasserman LR (eds): Myelofibrosis and the Biology of Connective Tissue. New York, Alan R. Liss, 1984, pp. 427–454.

64. Rudolph R, Huebner C: Megakaryozytenleukose beim hund. Kleintier-Praxis 17:9–13, 1972.

65. Dungworth DL, Goldman M, Switzer JW, et al: Development of a myeloproliferative disorder in beagles continuously exposed to $^{90}$Sr. Blood 34:610–632, 1969.

66. Prasse KW, Crouser D, Beutler E, et al: Pyruvate kinase deficiency anemia with terminal myelofibrosis and osteosclerosis in a beagle. J Am Vet Med Assoc 166:1170–1175, 1975.

67. Thompson JC, Johnstone AC: Myelofibrosis in the dog: Three case reports. J Small Anim Pract 24(9):589–601, 1983.

68. Thomsen MK, Jensen AL, Skak-Nielsen T, et al: Enhanced granulocyte function in a case of chronic granulocytic leukemia in a dog. Vet Immunol Immunopathol 28(2):143–165, 1991.

69. Grindem CB, Stevens JB, Perman V: Cytochemical reactions in cells from leukemic dogs. Vet Pathol 23:103–109, 1986.

70. Facklam NR, Kociba GJ: Cytochemical characterization of leukemic cells from 20 dogs. Vet Pathol 22:363–369, 1986.

71. Jain NC: Cytochemistry of normal and leukemic leukocytes. In Schalm's Veterinary Hematology, 4th ed. Philadelphia, Lea and Febiger, 1986, pp. 909–939.

72. Grindem CB, Buoen LC: Cytogenetic analysis of leukaemic cells in the dog. A report of 10 cases and a review of the literature. J Comp Pathol 96:623–635, 1986.

73. Peterson ME, Zanjani ED: Inappropriate erythropoietin production from a renal carcinoma in a dog with polycythemia. J Am Vet Med Assoc 179:995–996, 1981.

74. Scott RC, Patnaik AK: Renal carcinoma associated with secondary polycythemia in a dog. J Am Anim Hosp Assoc 8:275–283, 1972.

75. Waters DJ, Prueter JC: Secondary polycythemia associated with renal disease in the dog: Two case reports and review of literature. J Am Anim Hosp Assoc 24:109–114, 1988.

76. Cook SM, Lothrop, CD: Serum erythropoietin concentrations measured by radioimmunoassay in normal, polycythemic, and anemic dogs and cats. J Vet Intern Med 8(1):18–25, 1994.

77. Giger U: Serum erythropoietin concentrations in polycythemic and anemic dogs. Proc Ann Vet Med Forum 9:143–145, 1991.

78. Reimann KA, Knowlen CG, Tvedten HW: Factitious hyperkalemia in dogs with thrombocytosis. J Vet Intern Med 3:47–52, 1989.

79. Theilen GH, Madewell BR, Gardner MB: Hematopoietic neoplasms, sarcomas and related conditions. In Theilen GH, Madewell BR (eds): Veterinary Cancer Medicine, 2nd ed. Philadelphia, Lea and Febiger, 1987, pp. 392–407.

80. Hamlin RH, Duncan RC: Acute nonlymphocytic leukemia in a dog. J Am Vet Med Assoc 196:110–112, 1990.

81. Gorman NT, Evans RJ: Myeloproliferative disease in the dog and cat: Clinical presentations, diagnosis and treatment. Vet Rec 121:490–496, 1987.

82. Mayer RJ: Current chemotherapeutic treatment approaches to the management of previously untreated adults with de novo acute myelogenous leukemia. Semin Oncol 14:384–396, 1987.

83. Smith M, Turrel JM: Radiophosphorus ($^{32}$P) treatment of bone marrow disorders in dogs: 11 cases (1970–1987). J Am Vet Med Assoc 194:98–102, 1982.

84. Lyss, AP: Enzymes and random synthetics. In MC Perry (ed): The Chemotherapy Source Book. Baltimore, Williams and Wilkins, 1992, pp. 398–412.

85. Bolin RW, Robinson WA, Sutherland J, et al: Busulfan versus hydroxyurea in long-term therapy of chronic myelogenous leukemia. Cancer 50:1683–1686, 1982.

86. Rosenthal S, Canellos GP, Whang-Pang J, et al: Blast crisis of chronic granulocytic leukemia: Morphologic variants and therapeutic implications. Am J Med 63:542–547, 1977.

87. Lichtman MA, Brennan JK: Myelodysplastic disorders. In Beutler E, Lichtman MA, Coller BS, Kipps TJ (eds): Williams Hematology, 5th ed. New York, McGraw-Hill, 1995, pp. 257–272.

88. Ganser A, Hoelzer D: Treatment of myelodysplastic syndromes with hematopoietic growth factors. Hematol Oncol Clin North Am 6:633–653, 1992.

89. Ohno R, Noe, T, Hirano M, et al: Treatment of myelodysplastic syndromes with all-trans retinoic acid. Blood 81:1152–1154, 1993.

90. Kelsey SM, Newland AC, Cunningham J, et al: Sustained haematological response to high dose oral alfacalcidol in patients with myelodysplastic syndrome [Letter]. Lancet 340:316, 1992.

91. Jacobs A: Treatment for the myelodysplastic syndromes. Hematologica 72:477–480, 1987.

92. Lichtman MA: Acute myelogenous leukemia. In Beutler E, Lichtman MA, Coller BS, Kipps TJ (eds): Williams Hematology, 5th ed. New York, McGraw-Hill, 1995, pp. 272–278.

93. Wellman MC, Davenport DJ, Morton D, et al: Malignant histiocytosis in four dogs. J Am Vet Med Assoc 187:919–926, 1985.

94. Moore PF, Rosin A: Malignant histiocytosis of Bernese mountain dogs. Vet Pathol 23:1–10, 1986.

95. Padgett GA, Madewell BR, Keller ET, et al: Inheritance of histiocytosis in Bernese mountain dogs. J Small Anim Pract 36:93–98, 1995.

96. Moore PF: Systemic histiocytosis of Bernese mountain dogs. Vet Pathol 21:554–563, 1984.
97. Rosin A, Moore P, Dubielzig R: Malignant histiocytosis in Bernese mountain dogs. J Am Vet Med Assoc 188:1041–1045, 1986.
98. Ornvold K, Carstensen H, Junge J, et al: Tumours classified as "malignant histiocytosis" in children are T-cell neoplasms. APMIS 100:558–566, 1992.
99. Newlands CE, Houston DM, Vasconcelos DY: Hyperferritinemia associated with malignant histiocytosis in a dog. J Am Vet Med Assoc 205:849–851, 1994.

# E. Plasma Cell Neoplasms

## David M. Vail

Plasma cell neoplasms arise when a cell of the B-lymphocyte lineage proliferates to form a malignant population of similar cells. This population is believed to be monoclonal—that is, derived from a single cell—as they typically produce homogenous immunoglobulin. A wide variety of clinical syndromes are represented by plasma cell neoplasms, including multiple myeloma, IgM (Waldenstrom's) macroglobulinemia, and solitary plasmacytoma (including solitary osseous plasmacytoma and extramedullary plasmacytoma). In veterinary practice, multiple myeloma is the most important plasma cell neoplasm based on incidence and severity.

### INCIDENCE AND RISK FACTORS

While multiple myeloma (MM) represents less than 1% of all malignant tumors in animals, it is responsible for approximately 8% of all hematopoietic tumors and 3.6% of all primary and secondary tumors affecting bones in dogs.[1,2] Early studies indicated a male predisposition,[3] whereas subsequent reports do not suggest a sex predilection for the dog.[1,4] Older dogs are affected, with an average age of between 8 and 9 years.[1,3,4] In one large case series, German Shepherd dogs were over-represented based on the hospital population.[1]

The true incidence of MM in the cat is unknown. However, it is a much rarer diagnosis than in the dog, representing only 1 of 395 and 4 of 3,248 tumors in two large compilations of feline malignancies.[5,6] MM occurs in aged cats, and no breed or sex predilection has been consistently reported. MM has not been associated with either FeLV or FIV infections.

The etiology of MM is for the most part unknown. Genetic predispositions, viral infections, chronic immune stimulation, and exposure to carcinogens have all been suggested as contributing factors.[4,7–9] In rodent models, chronic immune stimulation and exposure to implanted silicone gel has been associated with development of MM[7,8] as have chronic infections and prolonged hyposensitization therapy in humans.[9] Viral Aleutian disease of mink results in monoclonal gammopathies in a small percentage of cases.[10] Exposure to the agricultural industry, petroleum products, and irradiation are known risk factors for development in humans.[11–13]

### PATHOLOGY AND NATURAL BEHAVIOR

Multiple myeloma is a systemic proliferation of malignant plasma cells or their precursors arising as a clone of a single cell that usually involves multiple bone marrow sites. Malignant plasma cells can have a varied appearance on histologic sections and cytologic preparations. The degree of differentiation ranges from those resembling normal plasma cells in late stages of differentiation to very large anaplastic round cells with a high mitotic index representing early stages of differentiation.[3,4,15]

Malignant plasma cells typically produce an overabundance of a single type of, or component of, immunoglobulin, which is referred to as the M-component. The M component can be represented by any class of immunoglobulin or by only a portion of the molecule such as the light chain (Bence Jones protein) or heavy chain ("Heavy Chain disease") of the molecule. In the dog, the M component is usually represented by either IgG or IgA immunoglobulin types in nearly equal incidence.[1,3,4] If the M component is of the IgM type, the term *macroglobulinemia* (Waldenstrom's) is applied. One case of bicional gammopathy in the dog has also been reported.[15] Occasionally, cryoglobulinemia has been reported in dogs with MM and IgM macroglobulinemia.[4,16,25] Cryoglobulins are paraproteins that are insoluble at temperatures below 37° C and require blood collection and clotting to be performed at 37° C prior to serum separation. If whole blood is allowed to clot at temperatures below this, the protein precipitates in the clot and is lost. Most cases of MM in the cat are associated with IgG immunoglobulin elevations, with only a few reports of IgA or IgM gammopathies.[4,6,17–21]

The pathology associated with MM is a result of either high levels of circulating immunoglobulins, organ infiltration with neoplastic cells, or both. Associated pathological conditions include bone disease, bleeding diatheses, hyperviscosity syndrome, renal disease, hypercalcemia, immunodeficiency (and subsequent susceptibility to infections), cytopenias, and cardiac failure.

Bone lesions can be isolated, discrete lesions (including pathological fractures) or diffuse osteopenias. Approximately one-quarter to two-thirds of dogs with MM have evidence of bony lysis or diffuse osteoporosis.[1,3,4,22] Those bones engaged in active hematopoiesis are more commonly affected, including the vertebrae, ribs, pelvis, skull, and proximal long bones.[3] Skeletal lesions are rare, however, in cats with MM, and dogs with IgM (Waldenstrom's) macroglobulinemia.[4,6,18] In macroglobulinemia, malignant cells often infiltrate the spleen, liver, and lymph tissue rather than bone.[4,23–25]

Bleeding diatheses can result from one or a combination of events. M components may interfere with coagulation by inhibiting platelet aggregation and the release of platelet factor 3; causing adsorption of minor clotting proteins; generating abnormal fibrin polymerization; and producing a functional decrease in calcium.[4,26–28] Approximately one-third of dogs have clinical evidence of hemmorhage.[1] Of these, nearly half have abnormal prothrombin (PT) and partial thromboplastin (PTT) times. Thrombocytopenia may also play a role if bone marrow infiltration is significant (i.e., myelopthesis).

Hyperviscosity syndrome (HVS) represents one or a constellation of clinicopathologic abnormalities resulting from greatly increased serum viscosity. The magnitude of viscosity changes are related to the type, size, shape, and concentration of the M component in the blood. It is more common with IgM macroglobulinemias due to the high molecular weight of this class of immunoglobulin. IgA myelomas, usually present as a dimer in the dog, may undergo polymerization resulting in increased serum viscosity.[1,4,26] IgG-associated HVS can also occur, albeit less frequently. High serum viscosity occurs in approximately 20% of dogs with MM and can result in bleeding diathesis, neurological signs (e.g., dementia, depression, seizure activity, coma), ophthalmic abnormalities (e.g., dilated and tortuous retinal vessels, retinal hemorrhage, retinal detachment), and increased cardiac workload with the potential for subsequent development of cardiomyopathy.[1,4,24,26,29,30] These consequences are thought to be a result of sludging of blood in small vessels, ineffective delivery of oxygen and nutrients, and coagulation abnormalities. HVS is less common in cats with MM but has been reported in association with IgG-, IgA-, and IgM-secreting tumors.[4,6,17,19–21]

Renal disease is present in approximately one-third to one-half of dogs with MM.[1,3] The pathogenesis of renal failure is often multifactorial and can ensue as a result of Bence Jones (light chain) proteinuria, tumor infiltration into renal tissue, hypercalcemia, amyloidosis, diminished perfusion secondary to hyperviscosity syndrome, dehydration, or ascending urinary tract infections.[1,4,26–28] Normally, heavy- and light-chain synthesis is well balanced in non-neoplastic immunoglobulin production. In the case of MM, an unbalanced excess of light-chain products may be produced.[27] Light chains are of low molecular weight and are normally filtered by the renal glomerulus; their presence in urine can result in protein precipitates and subsequent renal tubular injury. Tubules become obstructed by large laminated casts containing albumin, immunoglobulin, and light chains.[4,26–28] Bence Jones proteinuria occurs in approximately 25 to 40% of dogs with MM.[1,3] The true incidence of Bence Jones proteinuria in cats is not well established, although numerous cases have been reported.[4,6,18,20]

Hypercalcemia is reported in 15 to 20% of dogs with MM[1,4] and is thought to result primarily from the production of osteoclast-activating factor by neoplastic cells.[4,31] Other factors, including elevated levels of lymphotoxin, tumor necrosis factor, interleukin-1, and interleukin-6 have been implicated in human MM. In 2 dogs with MM and hypercalcemia, serum elevations in circulating N-terminal parathyroid hormone-related protein were noted, although its relative contribution to hypercalcemia is unknown.[32] Hypercalcemia may also be exacerbated by associated renal disease.

Susceptibility to infection and immunodeficiency have long been associated with MM and are often the ultimate cause of death in affected animals.[1,4,18] Infection rates in people with MM are 15 times higher than normal and usually represent pneumonia or urinary tract infections.[33] Response to vaccination has also been shown to be suppressed.[34] Normal immunoglobulin levels are usually severely depressed in affected animals.[4] In addition, leukopenias may be present secondary to myelopthesis.

Variable cytopenias may be observed in association with MM. A normocytic, normochromic, nonregenerative anemia is encountered in approximately two-thirds of dogs with MM.[1,3,4] This can result from marrow infiltration (myelopthesis), blood loss from coagulation disorders, anemia of chronic disease, or increased erythrocyte destruction secondary to high serum viscosity. Similar factors lead to thrombocytopenia and leukopenia in nearly one-third and one-quarter of dogs with MM, respectively.

Cardiac disease if present is usually a result of excessive cardiac workload and myocardial hypoxia secondary to hyperviscosity.[26,35] Myocardial infiltration with amyloid and anemia may be complicating factors.

Solitary collections of monoclonal plasmacytic tumors can originate in bone or soft tissues and are referred to as solitary osseous plasmacytoma (SOP) and extramedullary plasmacytoma (EMP), respectively. The majority of SOPs eventually progress to systemic MM.[36,37] SOPs have been reported in the dog involving the appendicular skeleton, zygomatic arch and ribs.[36] Cutaneous EMP in dogs is typically a benign disorder that is highly amenable to local therapy and is discussed at length in Chapter 15. The natural behavior of noncutaneous EMP appears to be more aggressive in the dog. Gastrointestinal EMPs have been reported on a number of occasions in the veterinary literature, including the esophagus,[38] stomach,[39,40] and small[40] and large intestines.[39,42,43] Metastasis to associated lymph nodes is common in these cases; however, bone marrow involvement and monoclonal gammopathies are less commonly encountered. One report exists of subcutaneous EMP in a cat with IgG gammopathy that progressed to develop lymph node disease and distant metastasis.[44]

## HISTORY AND CLINICAL SIGNS

Clinical signs of MM may be present up to a year prior to diagnosis with a median duration of one month.[1] Signs can be variable based on the wide range of pathological effects possible. Table 28–24 lists the relative frequencies of clinical signs

**Table 28–24** Frequency of Clinical Signs for Dogs with Multiple Myeloma[1]

| Clinical Sign | Frequency Reported (%) (n = 60 dogs) |
|---|---|
| Lethargy and weakness | 62 |
| Lameness | 47 |
| Bleeding | 37 |
| Funduscopic abnormalities | 35 |
| Polyuria/polydipsia | 25 |
| CNS deficits | 12 |

observed in the dog based on a compilation of 60 cases.[1] Bleeding diathesis is usually represented by epistaxis and gingival bleeding. Polyuria and polydipsia can result from hypercalcemia or renal failure. Fundoscopic abnormalities may include retinal hemorrhage, venous dilatation with sacculation and tortuosity, retinal detachment, and blindness.[1,4,26,29,30] Central nervous system signs may include dementia, seizure activity, and deficiencies in midbrain or brain stem, localizing reflexes secondary to HVS or extreme hypercalcemia. Signs reflective of transverse myelopathies secondary to vertebral column infiltration, pathologic fracture, or extradural mass compression can also occur.[1,4,16,22] One case of ataxia and seizure activity in a dog with EMP secondary to tumor-associated hypoglycemia has been reported.[45]

In the cat with MM, anorexia and weight loss are the most common clinical signs.[6,18] A history of chronic respiratory infections may be present. Skeletal lesions are uncommon; therefore bone pain or lameness is not often associated with the condition. Hepatosplenomegaly and renomegaly can occur due to organ infiltration. Bleeding diathesis due to HVS is less common in the cat; however epistaxis, pleural and peritoneal hemorrhagic effusions, retinal hemorrhage, and central neurological signs have been reported.[4,6,17–21] Polydipsia and polyuria can occur secondary to renal disease, and dehydration may develop. Hind limb paresis secondary to osteolysis of lumbar vertebral bodies has been reported in a cat.[46]

## DIAGNOSIS AND STAGING

The diagnosis of multiple myeloma usually follows the demonstration of bone marrow plasmacytosis, the presence of osteolytic bone lesions, and the demonstration of serum or urine myeloma proteins (M component). In the absence of osteolytic bone lesions, a diagnosis can also be made if marrow plasmacytosis is associated with a progressive increase in the M component.

All animals suspected of plasma cell tumors should receive a minimal diagnostic evaluation, including a CBC, platelet count, serum biochemistry profile, and urinalysis. Particular attention should be paid to renal function and serum calcium levels. Serum electrophoresis and immunoelectrophoresis are performed to determine the presence of a monoclonal spike (Figure 28–19) and to categorize the immunoglobulin class involved. Heat precipitation and electrophoresis of urine is performed to determine the presence of Bence Jones proteinuria because commercial urine dipstick methods are not capable of this determination. Definitive diagnosis usually follows the performance of a bone marrow aspirate. A bone marrow core biopsy may be necessary because of the possibility of clustering of plasma cells in the bone marrow. Normal marrow contains less than 5% plasma cells, whereas myelomatous marrow often greatly exceeds this level. Skeletal survey radiographs are recommended to determine the presence and extent of osteolytic lesions, which may have diagnostic, prognostic, and therapeutic implications. Rarely, biopsy of

osteolytic lesions (i.e., Jamshidi core biopsy) is necessary for diagnosis. In one case of MM in a dog, splenic aspirates were diagnostically helpful.[47] If clinical hemorrhage is present, a coagulation assessment (e.g., platelet count, PT, PTT) and serum viscosity measurements should be undertaken. All animals should undergo a careful fundoscopic exam.

A clinical staging system for canine multiple myeloma has been suggested;[1] however, at present no prognostic significance has been attributed to it.

The diagnosis of solitary osseous plasmacytoma and extramedullary plasmacytoma usually requires tissue biopsy for diagnosis. It is important to stage such cases thoroughly, including bone marrow aspirate, serum electrophoresis, and skeletal survey radiographs, to ensure disease is confined to a local site prior to initiation of therapy. In the case of poorly differentiated solitary plasmacytic tumors, immunohistochemical studies, directed at detecting immunoglobulin, light and heavy chains, and thioflavin T may be helpful in differentiating these tumors from other round cell tumors.[36,48–50]

Disease syndromes other than plasma cell

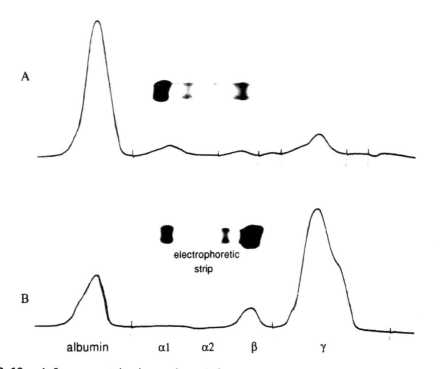

**Figure 28–19.** *A,* Serum protein electrophoresis from a normal dog. Stained cellulose acetate electrophoretic strip with accompanying densitogram. *B,* Serum protein electrophoresis from a dog with multiple myeloma. Note large M component spike (representing an IgA monoclonal gammopathy) present in the γ region.

tumors can be associated with monoclonal gammopathies and should be considered in any list of differentials. These include other lymphoreticular tumors (lymphoma, chronic and acute lymphocytic leukemia), chronic infections (e.g., Erhlichiosis, leishmaniasis, FIP), and monoclonal gammopathy of unknown significance (MGUS).[3,51–56] MGUS (i.e., "benign," "essential," or "idiopathic" monoclonal gammopathy), a benign monoclonal gammopathy, does not fit the diagnostic criteria of MM in that immunoglobulin elevations are relatively modest and nonprogressive and are not associated with osteolysis, bone marrow infiltration, or Bence Jones proteinuria.

## TREATMENT

### Initial Therapy of Multiple Myeloma

Therapy for multiple myeloma is directed at both the tumor cell mass as well as at the secondary systemic effects they elicit. Chemotherapy is highly effective in reducing myeloma cell burden, relieving bone pain, initiating skeletal healing, and reducing levels of serum immunoglobulins. Its use will greatly extend both the quality and quantity of most patients' lives.[1,4] Complete elimination of neoplastic myeloma cells is not achieved, however, with currently available chemotherapeutics, and while MM remains a gratifying disease to treat for both the clinician and the companion animal owner, eventual relapse is to be expected.

Melphalan, an alkylating agent, is the chemotherapeutic of choice for the treatment of multiple myeloma.[1,4] In the dog, an initial starting dose of 0.1 mg/kg per os, once daily for 10 days, is reduced to 0.05 mg/kg per os, once daily continuously. The addition of prednisone therapy is thought to increase the efficacy of melphalan therapy. Prednisone is initiated at a dosage of 0.5 mg/kg, per os, once daily for 10 days, then reduced to 0.5 mg/kg every other day prior to discontinuation after 60 days of therapy. Melphalan, however, is continued at 0.05 mg/kg/day until clinical relapse occurs or myelosuppression necessitates a dose reduction. The vast majority of dogs on melphalan and prednisone combination therapy tolerate the regimen well. The most clinically significant toxicity of melphalan is myelosuppression, in particular thrombocytopenia. Complete blood counts, including platelet counts, should be performed biweekly for two months of therapy and monthly thereafter. If significant myelosuppression occurs (usually

thrombocytopenia or neutropenia), reduction of the dose or treatment frequency may be necessary. An alternative pulse dosing regimen for melphalan (7mg/m$^2$ per os, daily for 5 consecutive days every 3 weeks) has been used successfully at the University of Wisconsin in a small number of cases in which myelosuppression was limiting more conventional continuous low-dose therapy. Melphalan and prednisone therapy have also been used in cats with multiple myeloma.

Cyclophosphamide has been used as an alternative alkylating agent or in combination with melphalan in dogs with multiple myeloma.[1,4,40] There is no evidence to suggest it is superior to melphalan therapy in most cases. In the author's practice, cyclophosphamide is limited to those cases presenting with severe hypercalcemia or with widespread systemic involvement where a faster-acting alkylating agent may more quickly alleviate systemic effects of the disease. Cyclophosphamide is initiated at a dosage of 200 mg/m$^2$ IV, once, at the same time oral melphalan therapy is started. Because cyclophosphamide is less likely to affect thrombocytes, it may be substituted in those patients in which thrombocytopenia has developed secondary to long-term melphalan use.

Chlorambucil, another alkylating agent, has been used successfully for the treatment of IgM macroglobulinemia in dogs at a dosage of 0.2 mg/kg, per os, once daily.[4] Few or no clinical signs of toxicity result from this dosing schedule.

### Evaluation of Response to Therapy

Evaluation of response to systemic therapy for multiple myeloma is based on improvement in clinical signs, clinicopathologic parameters, and radiographic improvement of skeletal lesions.[1,4] Subjective improvement in clinical signs of bone pain, lameness, lethargy, and anorexia should be evident within 3 to 4 weeks following initiation of therapy. Objective laboratory improvement, including reduction in serum immunoglobulin or Bence Jones proteinuria, usually is noted within 3 to 6 weeks. Radiographic improvement in osteolytic bone lesions may take months, and resolution may be only partial.

As previously discussed, complete resolution of multiple myeloma does not occur, and a good response is defined as a reduction in measured M component (i.e., immunoglobulin or Bence Jones proteins) of at least 50% of pretreatment values.[4] Reduction in serum immunoglobulin levels may lag behind reductions in Bence Jones proteinuria because the half-lives are 15 to 20 days and 8 to

12 hours respectively.[57] For routine follow-up, quantification of the elevated serum immunoglobulin or urine Bence Jones protein is performed monthly until a good response is noted and then every 2 to 3 months thereafter. Repeat bone marrow aspiration for evaluation of plasma cell infiltration may be occasionally necessary.

## Therapy Directed at Complications of Multiple Myeloma

The long-term control of complications, including hypercalcemia, hyperviscosity syndrome, bleeding diathesis, renal disease, immunosuppression, and pathological skeletal fractures, depends on controlling the primary tumor mass. Therapy directed more specifically at these complications may, however, be indicated in the short term.

If hypercalcemia is marked and significant clinical signs exist, standard therapies, including fluid diureses, with or without pharmacologic agents (e.g., calcitonin), may be indicated (see Chapter 4). Moderate hypercalcemia will typically resolve within 2 to 3 days following initiation of melphalan/prednisone chemotherapy.

Hyperviscosity syndrome is best treated in the short term by plasmaphoresis.[4,26,54] Whole blood is collected from the patient and centrifuged to separate plasma from packed cells. Packed red cells are resuspended in normal saline and reinfused into the patient. Bleeding diathesis will usually resolve along with HVS. However, platelet-rich plasma transfusions may be necessary in the face of thrombocytopenia.

Renal impairment may necessitate aggressive fluid therapy in the short term and maintenance of adequate hydration in the long term. Careful attention to secondary urinary tract infections and appropriate antimicrobial therapy is indicated. Ensuring adequate water intake at home is important, and occasionally educating owners in home subcutaneous fluid administration is indicated. Continued monitoring of renal function is recommended along with follow-up directed at tumor response.

Patients with multiple myeloma can be thought of as immunologic cripples. Some have recommended prophylactic antibiotic therapy in dogs with multiple myeloma;[4] however, in people, no benefit for this approach has been seen over diligent monitoring and aggressive antimicrobial management when indicated.[27] Cidal antimicrobials are preferred over static drugs, and avoidance of nephrotoxic antimicrobials is recommended.

Pathological fractures of weight-bearing long bones and vertebrae resulting in spinal cord compression may require immediate intervention in conjunction with systemic chemotherapy. Orthopedic stabilization of fractures should be undertaken and may be followed with external beam radiotherapy (Figure 28–20).

## Rescue Therapy

When multiple myeloma eventually relapses in dogs undergoing melphalan therapy or in the uncommon case initially resistant to alkyating agents, rescue therapy may be attempted. The author has had success with a combination of doxorubicin (30 mg/m$^2$, IV, q 21 days), vincristine (0.7 mg/m$^2$ IV, days 8 and 15), and prednisone (1.0 mg/kg PO, daily), given in 21-day cycles. While most dogs initially respond to this rescue protocol, the duration of response tends to be short, lasting only a few months. High-dose cyclophosphamide (300 mg/m$^2$ IV, q 7 days) has also been used with limited success as a rescue agent.

## Therapy for Solitary Plasmacytic Tumors

Animals with solitary forms of plasma cell tumors may be treated with local therapy in the absence of systemic chemotherapy provided thorough clinical staging, including skeletal survey radiographs and bone marrow evaluations, do not reveal systemic involvement. Treatment for cutaneous plasma cell tumors is discussed in Chapter 15.

Effective local control of solitary plasmacytomas has been achieved with surgical excision or external beam radiotherapy alone or in combination. Surgery is recommended in combination with radiotherapy for cases of solitary osseous plasmacytoma (SOP) in which the lesion results in an unstable long bone fracture, or the patient is nonambulatory from neurological compromise resulting from a vertebral body SOP. In the latter case, spinal cord decompression, mass excision, and possibly spinal stabilization may be necessary. Radiotherapy can be used alone (i.e., without surgery) in cases in which fractures are stable, or in the case of vertebral SOP, the patient is ambulatory and experiencing little or no pain. Good local control is usually achieved; however, most patients go on to develop systemic multiple myeloma. SOP of the axial skeleton can be managed by excision or radiotherapy alone. As previously discussed, the majority of SOP cases will eventually develop systemic disease.[36,37]

There is controversy among veterinary oncologists as to whether systemic chemotherapy

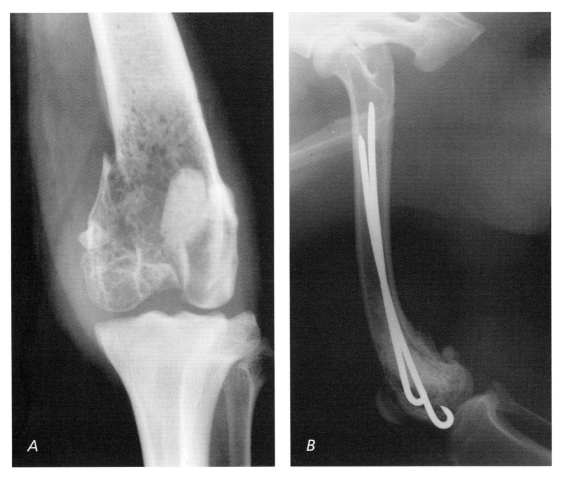

**Figure 28–20.** *A,* Radiograph of a distal femur demonstrating severe osteolysis and a pathologic fracture. *B,* Radiograph of the same pathologic fracture after surgical repair with Rush rods and bone cement. The local site was treated with adjuvant radiation. The dog was continued on chemotherapy for 2 more years and did well.

should be initiated at the time of local therapy for SOP. Systemic spread may not occur for many months to even years beyond SOP diagnosis in people, and studies in humans reveal no benefit derived from initiation of systemic chemotherapy prior to documentation of subsequent systemic spread.[27] However, because most SOP cases in dogs progress to systemic involvement within 6 months, initiation of chemotherapy at the time of SOP diagnosis is often undertaken. Other solitary sites, including EMP of the gastrointestinal tract, are treated most commonly by surgical excision and thorough staging of disease. Systemic therapy is not initiated unless systemic involvement is documented.

Long-term follow-up of patients with solitary plasmacytoma is indicated in order to recognize both recurrence of disease and systemic spread.

Careful attention is paid to serum globulin levels, bone pain, and radiographic appearance of bone healing in cases of SOP. Restaging of disease, including bone marrow evaluation, is indicated if systemic spread is suspected.

## PROGNOSIS

The prognosis for dogs with multiple myeloma is good for initial control of tumor and a return to good quality of life. In a group of 60 dogs with multiple myeloma, approximately 43% achieved a complete remission (i.e., serum immunoglobulins normalized), 49% achieved a partial remission (i.e., immunoglobulins < 50% pretreatment values), and only 8% did not respond to melphalan and prednisone chemotherapy.[1] Long-term

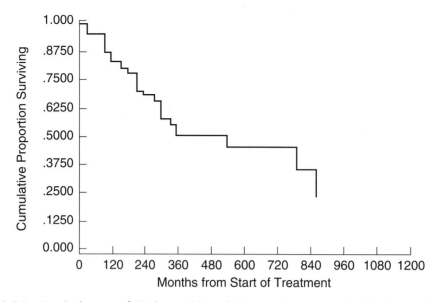

**Figure 28–21.**   Survival curve of 37 dogs with multiple myeloma treated with chemotherapy. The median survival time is 540 days. (Reprinted with permission from Matus RE, Leifer CE, MacEwen EG, et al: Prognostic factors for multiple myeloma in the dog. J Am Vet Med Assoc *188*:1288–1292, 1986).

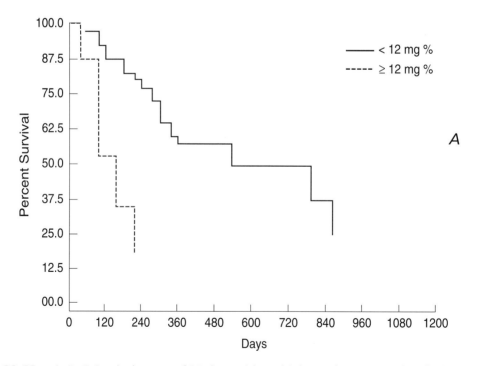

**Figure 28–22.**   *A, B, C,* Survival curves of 37 dogs with multiple myeloma treated with chemotherapy. The curves reveal that hypercalcemia, Bence Jones protein, and bony lysis are all associated with a poor prognosis (p < 0.05). (Reprinted with permission from Matus RE, Leifer CE, MacEwen EG, et al: Prognostic factors for multiple myeloma in the dog. J Am Vet Med Assoc *188*:1288–1292, 1986).

**Figure 28–22.** *(continued)*

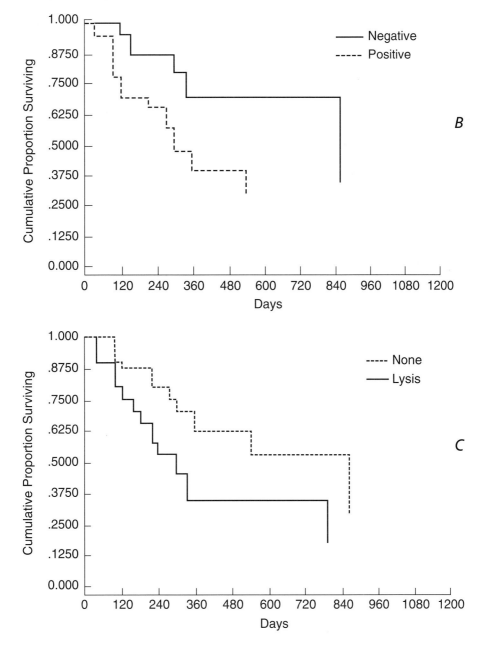

*B*

*C*

survival is the norm, with a median of 540 days reported (Fig. 28–21). The presence of hypercalcemia, Bence Jones proteinuria, and extensive bony lysis are known negative prognostic indices in the dog (Fig. 28–22).[1] The long-term prognosis for dogs with multiple myeloma is poor because recurrence of tumor mass and associated clinical signs are expected. Eventually, the tumor no longer responds to available chemotherapeutics,

and death follows from either renal failure, sepsis, or euthanasia for intractable bone or spinal pain.[1,4]

The prognosis for multiple myeloma in the cat is not as favorable as in the dog. While most cats transiently respond to melphalan/prednisone or cyclophosphamide-based protocols, responses are not durable, and most succumb to their disease within 2 to 3 months.[6,18,20,58]

Experience in dogs with IgM macroglobuline-mia is more limited. Response to chlorambucil is to be expected, and in 9 dogs treated, 77% achieved remission, with a median survival of 11 months.[4]

Prognosis for solitary plasma cell tumors is generally good. Cutaneous plasmacytomas are usually cured following surgical excision (see Chapter 15). Dogs with extramedullary plasma-cytoma (EMP) of the alimentary tract treated by surgical excision in combination with sys-temic chemotherapy (if metastasis is present) enjoy long-term survival in the majority of cases.[36,38,40,42,43,59] As previously discussed, the majority of cases of SOP will eventually develop systemic disease; however, long disease-free peri-ods usually precede the event.

## COMPARATIVE FEATURES

Plasma cell tumors are not uncommon in people and represent a similar spectrum of syndromes, including multiple myeloma, IgM macroglobu-linemia, solitary plasmacytoma, and monoclonal gammopathy of unknown significance (MGUS).

Many similarities exist between multiple myeloma in people compared with the compan-ion animal population.[27,28] In people, approxi-mately 50% of multiple myelomas produce IgG immunoglobulin, 21% IgA, 12% IgM, and 11% light chain only.[60] Interestingly, with immuno-fixation techniques, approximately half of all cases are now thought to be biclonal gammo-pathies (i.e., 33% are IgG and IgA and 24% are IgM and IgG). Males have a slightly higher inci-dence than females: 88% are proteinuric, 80% have radiographic evidence of skeletal involve-ment, 50% have Bence Jones proteinuria, and 30% are hypercalcemic.[61]

Hyperviscosity syndrome is present in approx-imately 4% and 22% of people with IgG and IgM disease, respectively. Several growth factors have been implicated in the expansion of neoplastic plasma cell clones, including interleukin-6 (IL-6), IL-1α, IL-1β, and possibly IL-3.[27] Serum IL-6 lev-els are elevated in many multiple myeloma patients. Several prognostic indices have been identified for multiple myeloma in people. A number of clinical staging systems have been developed; however, none has been found to be as prognostic as single-risk factors, in particular blood hemoglobin and serum creatinine levels.[62] Proliferation indices (e.g., Ki[67] and bromod-eoxyuridine labels) have recently been shown to have prognostic significance in people.

The gold standard for therapy of malignant melanoma in people is also melphalan and pred-nisone combinations. Approximately half of all cases will experience a good response.[63] Treat-ment is continued in responders for 2 years, then discontinued until such time as evidence of relapse is documented. There appears to be no benefit for continued maintenance therapy beyond the 2-year interval. Recently, the addition of interferon α-2b maintenance therapy along with standard chemotherapy protocols appears to prolong the duration of response.[64] New direc-tions in therapy for multiple myeloma in people include serotherapy (i.e., anti-CD-38 antibody), anti-IL-6 monoclonal antibody therapy, and immunotoxin therapy.[27]

Solitary plasmacytomas (SOP and EMP) in people are treated locally with surgery or radio-therapy, alone or in combination.[27,28] Whereas the majority of patients with SOP and approxi-mately half of those with EMP eventually progress to multiple myeloma, no benefit has, as yet, been observed for initiation of systemic chemotherapy prior to documentation of sys-temic spread of disease.

MGUS occurs in older (> 65 yrs) individuals and is associated with a mild monoclonal spike (< 4g/dL), no proteinuria, and less than 5% plasma cells in bone marrow. Approximately 22% of patients with MGUS develop classic mul-tiple myeloma.[27]

## REFERENCES

1. Matus RE, Leifer CE, MacEwen EG, Hurvitz AI: Prognostic factors for multiple myeloma in the dog. J Am Vet Med Assoc 188:1288–1291, 1986.
2. Liu SK, Dorfman HD, Hurvitz AI, et al: Primary and secondary bone tumors in the dog. J Small Anim Pract 18:313–326, 1977.
3. Osborne CA, Perman V, Sautter JH, et al: Multiple myeloma in the dog. J Am Vet Med Assoc 153:1300–1319, 1968.
4. MacEwen EG, Hurvitz AI: Diagnosis and manage-ment of monoclonal gammopathies. Vet Clin N Am Small Anim Pract 7:119–132, 1977.
5. Engle GC, Brodey RS: A retrospective study of 395 feline neoplasms. J Am Anim Hosp Assoc 5:21–31, 1969.
6. Carpenter JL, Andrews LK, Holzworth J: Tumors and tumor-like lesions. In Holzworth J (ed): Dis-eases of the Cat. Medicine and Surgery. Philadel-phia, W.B. Saunders, 1987, pp. 406–596.
7. Potter M: A résumé of the current status of the development of plasma cell tumors in mice. Can-cer Res 28:1891–1896, 1968.
8. Potter M, Morrison S, Weiner F, et al: Induction of

plasmacytomas with silicone gel in genetically susceptible strains of mice. J Natl Cancer Inst 86:1058–1065, 1994.

9. Imahori S, Moore GE: Multiple myeloma and prolonged stimulation of RES. NY State J Med 72:1625–1628, 1972.

10. Porter DD: The development of myeloma-like condition in mink with Aleutian disease. Blood 25:736–741, 1967.

11. Bourget CC, Grufferman S, Delzell E, et al. Multiple myeloma and family history of cancer. Cancer 56:2133–2139, 1985.

12. Cuzick J, DeStavola B: Multiple myeloma. A case control study. Br J Cancer 57:516–520, 1988.

13. Linet MS, Sioban DH, McLaughlin JK: A case-control study of multiple myeloma in whites: Chronic antigenic stimulation, occupation and drug use. Cancer Res 47:2978–2981, 1987.

14. Moulton JE, Harvey JW: Tumors of the lymphoid and hematopoietic tissues. In Moulton JE (ed): Tumors in Domestic Animals, 3rd ed. Berkeley, University of California Press, 1990, pp. 231–307.

15. Jacobs RM, Couto CG, Wellman ML: Biclonal gammopathy in a dog with myeloma and cutaneous lymphoma. Vet Pathol 23:211–213, 1986.

16. Braund KG, Everett RM, Bartels JE, DeBuysscher E: Neurologic complications of IgA multiple myeloma associated with cryoglobulinemia in a dog. J Am Vet Med Assoc 174:1321–1325, 1979.

17. Hawkins EC, Feldman BF, Blanchard PC: Immunoglobulin A myeloma in a cat with pleural effusion and serum hyperviscosity. J Am Vet Med Assoc 188:876–878, 1986.

18. Drazner FH: Multiple myeloma in the cat. Comp Cont Ed Pract Vet 4:206–216, 1982.

19. Williams DA, Goldschmidt MH: Hyperviscosity syndrome with IgM monoclonal gammopathy and hepatic plasmacytoid lymphosarcoma in a cat. J Small Anim Pract 23:311–323, 1982.

20. Forrester SD, Greco DS, Relford RL: Serum hyperviscosity syndrome associated with multiple myeloma in two cats. J Am Vet Med Assoc 200:79–82, 1992.

21. Hribernik TN, Barta O, Gaunt SD, Boudreaux MK: Serum hyperviscosity syndrome associated with IgG myeloma in a cat. J Am Vet Med Assoc 181:169–170, 1982.

22. Van Bree H, Pollet L, Cousemont W, et al: Cervical cord compression as a neurologic compilation in an IgG multiple myeloma in a dog. J Amer Anim Hosp Assoc 19:317–323, 1983.

23. Hill RR, Clatworthy RH: Macroglobulinemia in the dog, the canine analogue of gamma M nonoclonal gammopathy. J S Afr Vet Med Assoc 42:309–313, 1971.

24. Hurvitz AI, Haskins SC, Fischer CA: Macroglobulinemia with hyperviscosity syndrome in a dog. J Am Vet Med Assoc 157:455–460, 1970.

25. Hurvitz AI, MacEwen EG, Middaugh CR, Litman GW: Monoclonal cryoglobulinemia with macroglobulinemia in a dog. J Am Vet Med Assoc 170:511–516, 1977.

26. Shull RM, Osborne CA, Barrett RE, et al: Serum hyperviscosity syndrome associated with IgA multiple myeloma in two dogs. J Am Anim Hosp Assoc 14:58–70, 1978.

27. Anderson K: Plasma cell tumors. In Holland JF, Frei E, Bast RC, Kufe DW, Morton DL, Weichselbaum RR (eds): Cancer Medicine, 3rd ed. Philadelphia, Lea & Febiger, 1993, pp. 2075–2092.

28. Salmon SE, Cassady JR: Plasma cell neoplasms. In DeVita VT, Hellman S, Rosenberg SA (eds): Cancer: Principles and Practice of Oncology, 4th ed. Philadelphia, J. B. Lippincott, 1993, pp. 1984–2025.

29. Center SA, Smith JF: Ocular lesions in a dog with hyperviscosity secondary to an IgA myeloma. J Am Vet Med Assoc 181:811–813, 1982.

30. Kirschner SE, Niyo Y, Hill BL, Betts DM: Blindness in a dog with IgA-forming myeloma. J Am Vet Med Assoc 193:349–350, 1988.

31. Mundy GR, Bertolini DR: Bone destruction and hypercalcemia in plasma cell myeloma. Semin Oncol 13:291–297, 1986.

32. Rosol TJ, Nagode LA, Couto cg, et al: Parathyroid hormone (PTH)-related protein, PTH, and 1,25-dihydroxyvitamin D in dogs with cancer associated hypercalcemia. Endocrinology 131:1157–1164, 1992.

33. Twomey JJ: Infections complicating multiple myeloma and chronic lymphocytic leukemia. Arch Intern Med 132:562–565, 1973.

34. Fahey JL, Scoggins R, Utz JP, Szwed CF: Infection, antibody response, and gammaglobulin components in multiple myeloma and macroglobulinemia. Am J Med 35:698–702, 1963.

35. Mcbride W, Jackman JJD, Bammon RS, Willerson JT: High output cardiac failure in patients with multiple myeloma. N Engl J Med 319:1651–1653, 1988.

36. MacEwen EG, Patnaik AK, Hurvitz AI, Bradley R: Nonsecretory multiple myeloma in two dogs. Am Vet Med Assoc 184:1283–1286, 1984.

37. Meis JM, Butler JJ, Osborne BM, Ordonez NG: Solitary plasmacytomas of bone and extramedullary plasmacytomas. Cancer 59:1475–1485, 1987.

38. Hamilton TA, Carpenter JL: Esophageal plasmacytoma in a dog. J Am Vet Med Assoc 204:1210–1211, 1994.

39. MacEwen EG, Patnaik AK, Johnson GF, Hurvitz AI: Extramedullary plasmacytoma of the gastrointestinal tract in two dogs. J Am Vet Med Assoc 184:1396–1398, 1984.

40. Brunnert SR, Dee LA, Herron AJJ, Altman NH: gastric extramedullary plasmacytoma in a dog. J Am Vet Med Assoc 200:1501–1502, 1992.

41. Jackson MW, Helfand SC, Smedes SL, et al: Primary IgG secreting plasma cell tumor in the gastrointestinal tract of a dog. J Am Vet Med Assoc 204:404–406, 1994.

42. Lester SJ, Mesfin GM: A solitary plasmacytoma in a dog with progression to a disseminated myeloma. Can Vet J 21:284–286, 1980.

43. Trevor PB, Saunders GK, Waldron DR, Leib MS:

Metastatic extramedullary plasmacytoma of the colon and rectum in a dog. J Am Vet Med Assoc *203*:406–409, 1993.

44. Carothers MA, Johnson GC, DiBartola SP, et al: Extramedullary plasmacytoma and immunoglobulin-associated amyloidosis in a cat. J Am Vet Med Assoc *195*:1593–1597, 1989.

45. DiBartola SP: Hypoglycemia and polyclonal gammopathy in a dog with plasma cell dyscrasia. J Am Vet Med Assoc *180*:1345–1348, 1982.

46. Mitcham SA, McGillivray SR, Haines DM: Plasma cell sarcoma in a cat. Can Vet J *26*:98–100, 1985.

47. O'Keefe DA, Couto CG: Fine-needle aspiration of the spleen as an aid in the diagnosis of splenomegaly. J Vet Int Med *1*:102–109, 1987.

48. Breuer W, Colbatzky F, Platz S, Hermanns W: Immunoglobulin-producing tumours in dogs and cats. J Comp Path *109*:203–216, 1993.

49. Brunnert SR, Altman NH: Identification of immunoglobulin light chains in canine extramedullary plasmacytomas by thioflavine T and immunohistochemistry. J Vet Diagn Invest *3*:245–251, 1991.

50. Kyriazidou A, Brown PJ, Lucke VM: An immunohistochemical study of canine extramedullary plasma cell tumours. J Comp Path *100*:259–266, 1989.

51. Matus RE, Leifer CE, Jurvitz AI: Use of plasmapheresis and chemotherapy for treatment of monoclonal gammopathy associated with Ehrlichia canis infection in a dog. J Am Vet Med Assoc *190*:1302–1304, 1987.

52. Breitschwerdt EB, Woody BJ, Zerbe CA, et al: Monoclonal gammopathy associated with naturally occurring canine ehrlichiosis. J Vet Intern Med *1*:2–9, 1987.

53. Hoenig M, O'Brien JA: A benign hypergammaglobulinemia mimicking plasma cell myeloma. J Am Anim Hosp Assoc *24*:688–690, 1988.

54. MacEwen EG, Hurvitz AI, Hayes A: Hyperviscosity syndrome associated with lymphocytic leukemia in three dogs. J Am Vet Med Assoc *170*:1309–1312, 1977.

55. Dewhirst MW, Stamp GL, Hurvitz AI: Idiopathic monoclonal (IgA) gammopathy in a dog. J Am Vet Med Assoc *170*:1313–1316, 1977.

56. Font A, Closa JM, Mascort J: Monoclonal gammopathy in a dog with visceral leishmaniasis. J Vet Intern Med *8*:233–235, 1994.

57. Ferhangi M, Osserman EF: The treatment of multiple myeloma. Sem Hematol *10*:149–161, 1973.

58. Farrow BRH, Penny R: Multiple myeloma in a cat. J Am Vet Med Assoc *158*:606–611, 1971.

59. Geisel O, Stiglmai-Herb M, Linke RP: Myeloma associated with immunoglobulin lambda-light chain derived amyloid in a dog. Vet Pathol *27*:374–376, 1990.

60. Pruzanski W, Ogryzlo MA: Abnormal proteinuria in malignant disease. Adv Clin Chem *13*:355–382, 1970.

61. Kyle RA: Multiple myeloma. Review of 869 cases. Mayo Clin Proc *50*:29–40, 1975.

62. Gassman W, Pralle H, Haferlach T, et al: Staging systems for multiple myeloma: A comparison. Br J Haematol *59*:703–711, 1985.

63. Kyle RA: New approaches to the therapy of multiple myeloma. Blood *76*:1678–1679, 1990.

64. Cooper MR: Interferons in the management of multiple myeloma. Sem Oncol *15*:21–25, 1988.

# 29

# Miscellaneous Tumors

## A. Hemangiosarcoma

### E. Gregory MacEwen

## INCIDENCE AND RISK FACTORS

Hemangiosarcoma (HSA), also known as malignant hemangioendothelioma or angiosarcoma, is a malignant neoplasm of vascular endothelial origin. HSA occurs more frequently in the dog than any other species.[1,2] HSA has been seen in 0.3 to 2% of recorded canine necropsies, and represents about 5% of all nonskin primary malignant neoplasms in the dog.[3,4] HSA is much less common in the cat and has been reported to occur in 18 of 3,145 cats examined at autopsy in one study.[5] In five combined surveys, 20 of 1,006 tumors in cats were HSAs.[6]

Dogs with HSA are usually older and the mean age varies between 8 and 13 years of age, although there are reports of dogs 1 year or younger developing HSA.[4,7] In cats a mean age of 8 to 10 (range of 5 months to 17 years) years of age has been reported.[5,8] HSA can occur in any breed of dog or cat. In dogs, the majority are large breeds and the German shepherd is the most common breed. Most reports do not cite a sex predisposition, but several indicate a higher incidence of HSA in males.[4,9,10] In cats, males and females tend to be equally represented. Most of the HSAs have been reported in the domestic short-haired cat.[11,12] Although the etiology is unknown, reports in the human have been related to exposure to thorium dioxide, arsenicals, or vinyl chloride.[13,14] Local irradiation is also reported to be a contributory factor.[15] Methylnitrosamine is a carcinogen found in fish meal and has been shown to cause HSA in mink.[4]

Cutaneous HSAs are found more frequently in dogs with poor pigmentation and light hair and may be associated with ultraviolet light exposure. Breeds at increased risk include whippets, salukis, blood hounds, and English pointers.[16]

## PATHOLOGY AND NATURAL BEHAVIOR

In the dog the site of primary involvement is usually the spleen, although the tumor has been reported in many locations.[1–4,9,17] These other sites include the right atrium, skin, subcutaneous tissue, liver, lungs, kidneys, oral cavity, muscle, bone, urinary bladder, and peritoneum.[3,4,7,9,18–21] In the cat approximately 50% of the HSAs will occur either in the liver, spleen, or mesentery; other sites reported are the subcutis, thoracic cavity, and nasal cavity.[6,12] In two recent reports in dogs, one based on 1,480 cases of splenic disease[22] and another of 100 cases,[23] approximately 25 to 50% of the tumors in the spleen will be HSA.

HSA may be single or multiple in any organ. In an animal with multiple tumors, it may be difficult to determine which is the primary tumor site. These tumors are variable in size, pale gray to dark red, nodular, and soft. They may contain areas of hemorrhage and necrosis. They are poorly circumscribed, nonencapsulated, and often adhered to adjacent organs. Rupture and hemorrhage are frequently seen. On cut section the tumors may appear solid or may have irregular spaces formed by fragile trabeculae. The spaces may contain free or clotted blood, or pink fluid that oozes from the cut surface. There are usually pale gray fibrous strands or foci and yellow to pink friable areas of necrosis. A large mass may vary greatly with regard to hemorrhage and location of neoplastic tissue. Multiple tissue samples may be required to establish a diagnosis. Immunohistochemistry can be used to help establish a diagnosis of HSA. HSA cells are positive for factor VIII-related antigen in about 90% of the specimens.[24] Factor VIII staining differentiates HSA from other nonvascular tumors.

The differential diagnosis for splenic masses includes nonvascular malignant tumors such as leiomyosarcomas, lymphoma, osteosarcomas, fibrosarcomas, liposarcomas, undifferentiated sarcomas, and malignant fibrous histiocytomas[22,23,25,26] and nonneoplastic splenic hematoma and hemangioma.[27] It is particularly important not to confuse hematoma with HSA. Splenic hematomas are also seen in older, large-breed dogs and have a clinical appearance that resembles HSA.

The right atrium is the third most common site for HSA.[9,20,28] Most are solitary, but can be multiple within the atrium and auricle. Erosion of the endocardium may result in rupture of the atrial wall and the development of cardiac tamponade.

Cutaneous HSA are found in the dermis or extending deep into the subcutaneous tissues. The most common site is ventral-abdominal or preputial skin.[29,30] In a recent study, tumors confined to the dermis exhibit a predilection for lightly haired skin, when compared to haired skin.[31] HSA confined to dermis has a low metastatic behavior, as contrasted to those that show invasion. The invasive cutaneous HSA have a high metastatic behavior.[29]

HSAs tend to metastasize rapidly through hematogenous routes, and the most frequent reported sites are liver, omentum, mesentery, and lungs.[2,3,9,32] Approximately 25% of dogs with splenic HSA may also have right atrial HSA.[32] Other sites of metastasis reported have been the kidney, muscle, peritoneum, lymph nodes, adrenal glands, brain, and diaphragm. In dogs, HSA is considered the sarcoma most often metastatic to the brain.[33] In a study of 85 dogs with HSA, 12 (14.2%) had brain metastases.[33] The cerebrum is the most common site. Dogs with pulmonary metastases or multiple metastatic sites were more likely to have brain metastases.[33] In untreated cases with splenic HSA, death is usually due to metastases or rupture of the primary tumor.

HSAs in cats are rare tumors and arise equally in abdominal organs and subcutis. Common sites include spleen, mesentery, liver, intestines, and abdominal musculature.[6,12] Intra-abdominal HSA in cats also tends to have a very high metastatic potential. The liver appears to be the most common site of metastasis, followed by the omentum, diaphragm, pancreas, and lung.[5,12]

## HISTORY AND CLINICAL SIGNS

The clinical signs vary, depending upon the location and size of the primary tumor. The most dramatic presentation is sudden death from rupture of a critically placed tumor focus or acute blood loss into a body cavity. The clinical signs most commonly reported are weakness, distention of the abdomen, increased pulse and respirations, pale mucous membranes, and weight loss. The history may also reveal intermittent episodes of weakness or collapse, often with spontaneous recovery in 12 to 24 hours. Usually these incidents are associated with hemorrhage and subsequent blood resorption. Eventually, this trend becomes fatal, as the majority of all naturally occurring deaths in HSA are associated with hemorrhage from tumor rupture or disseminated intravascular coagulation (DIC).

Other presenting signs are related to the specific organ of involvement and may present with syncope, lameness, ataxia, seizures, or cardiac arrhythmias. Pericardial effusion or cardiac tamponade associated with right atrial HSA is also a common sequela.[19,21] Muffled heart sounds are detected with cardiac tamponade and the eventual development of acute right heart failure.[20] The skin from of HSA most often presents as discrete firm, raised, dark-red-purple papules, or nodules or subcutaneous hemorrhagic masses, usually not ulcerative. Bone and muscle forms can be presented with localized swelling, lameness, and pain. Metastasis to the brain or vertebrae can cause seizures, dementia, and paresis.

In the cat signs of HSA depend on the location and extent of the primary and metastatic tumors. Cats with visceral tumors usually have a history of lethargy, anorexia, vomiting, dyspnea, or a distended abdomen. On physical examination, pallor, pleural or peritoneal fluid, and a palpable abdominal mass are often found. Bleeding, common because vascular channels in the tumor are friable, may be intermittent—causing (episodic) weakness—or acute—causing sudden collapse—sometimes in an apparently healthy cat. Most cats with visceral HSA have mild to severe anemia.

## DIAGNOSTIC TECHNIQUES AND WORKUP

The presumptive diagnosis of HSA in the dog and the cat is usually based on clinical history, physical examination, hematologic testing, radiographic findings, and paracentesis when indicated. HSA effusions are serosanguinous (or frank blood if ruptured), and usually do not clot. The ultimate diagnosis is based on histopathologic evaluation.

The diagnosis of HSA is most reliably made by biopsy or removal of the primary or metastatic tumor. Following surgical removal of the spleen, the spleen should be sectioned like a bread loaf and multiple samples from different regions of the tumor should be submitted for histopathologic analysis. If no obvious tumor is noted in the spleen, then further sections from various areas of spleen or the entire spleen should be sent for histopathologic evaluation. Following surgical removal of the spleen, biopsy samples of liver and omentum should be submitted for histopathology to evaluate for metastatic disease.

Animals with HSA often have pleural or peritoneal effusions. The fluid may be clear or chylous or in most cases bloody. Fusiform neoplastic cells are only rarely detected in cytologic examinations of such fluids in both the dog and cat. Only 25% of effusions associated with HSA yield a cytologic diagnosis in dogs.[21,34]

In evaluating an animal with suspected HSA, particular attention should be directed at detection of metastatic disease because development of overt metastatis is extremely high (70–80%). All animals with suspected HSA should have radiographic evaluation of both the thoracic and abdominal cavity. In dogs, if cardiac involvement is suspected, echocardiography can be used to image cardiac masses, including HSA.[21,35] Abdominal ultrasonography is valuable in evaluating the primary tumor and in helping to determine the presence of metastases.[36] A mixed or nonhomogeneous echo pattern is commonly seen in dogs with splenic HSA. Hepatic metastases appear as hypoechoic or anechoic on ultrasound, but a tissue diagnosis is necessary to prove that metastatic disease is present.

Thoracic radiographs are important in the evaluation of possible lung metastasis and potential cardiac involvement. Ideally right and left lateral and ventrodorsal views should be performed. The metastatic lesions may consist of either solitary nodules or a diffuse coalescing miliary pattern. In a recent study of 77 dogs with

HSA, all had thoracic radiographs as well as a necropsy. Forty-six of 77 dogs had lung metastases based on necropsy. Radiography detected lung metastasis in 78% of the dogs with proven lung metastasis on necropsy.[37] Thoracic radiographs were only able to detect cardiac involvement in 47% of those with confirmed cardiac HSA. The most common radiographic abnormality associated with cardiac HSA was pericardial effusion.[37] HSA is the most common cardiac neoplasm in dogs and should be suspected in any dog with pericardial effusion. Cardiac ultrasonography is more accurate than survey radiographs in evaluating the heart for HSA. In one study, pneumopericardiography successfully outlined masses in the right atrium in 7 of 12 dogs.[19]

Radiographs of HSA of the bone are typical of other primary bone neoplasms with a tendency to be more lytic than productive (Fig. 29–1).[38]

In both dogs and cats intracavitary hemor-

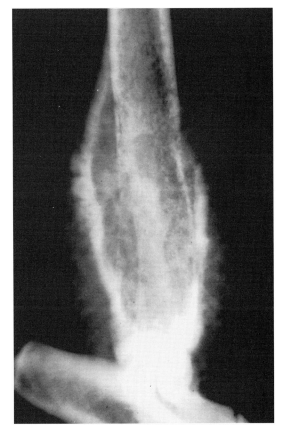

**Figure 29–1.** A primary hemangiosarcoma of the distal tibia in a dog. These tumors tend to show prominent lysis.

rhage or microangiopathic hemolysis may cause a regenerative anemia (normocytic-normochromic) characterized by polychromasia, anisocytosis, hypochromasia, reticulocytosis, and nucleated red cells in the peripheral blood. Fragmentation of red cells, which occurs in humans and dogs with HSA, has not been documented in the cat.[39] Four causes have been proposed for this fragmentation. (1) Local mechanical trauma to red cells traversing irregular vascular spaces of the tumor; (2) formation of spherocytes and destruction of older red blood cells with lower ATP when blood flow is sluggish and oxygen tension is low; (3) increased fragility of red blood cells made hypochromatic by blood loss and lower iron content; (4) altered cholesterol phospholipid ratios in red cell membranes because of altered hepatic lipoprotein metabolism, possibly accounting for acanthocytosis and schistocytes in dogs with hepatic hemangiosarcoma.[39] In dogs anemia is the most common encountered hematologic abnormality.[2,4,9,40] In addition, a neutrophilic leukocytosis may frequently be seen. Spontaneous hemorrhage, secondary to disseminated intravascular coagulation (DIC) or thrombocytopenia (from microangiopathy) may occur.[40,41,42] HSA should be considered in all dogs with DIC. Thrombocytopenia is common in dogs with HSA.[40–43] Approximately 30 to 60% of dogs with HSA will be thrombocytopenic (<200,000 cells/$\mu$l).

Another feature noted in dogs with HSA is the presence of nucleated red blood cells in the peripheral blood. This has been seen in about 15% of the reported HSA cases, and the mean is approximately 20 nucleated RBC/100 WBC. Table 29–1 demonstrates the typical hematologic findings in dogs with HSA. The physiologic causes for nucleated RBCs in the peripheral blood may include (1) bone marrow infiltration by malignant cells, (2) extramedullary hematopoiesis, (3) hypoxemia, (4) hyposplenism associated with neoplastic infiltration.

A clinical staging system for HSA is given in Table 29–2.

## THERAPY

Surgery remains the first treatment of choice for all dogs and cats with HSA. The surgery should be as radical as possible to remove all locally affected tissue. In the case of the HSA of the spleen, a splenectomy is absolutely necessary.[9] At the time of splenectomy any suspicious lesions in the liver or omentum should be submitted for biopsy. Dogs undergoing splenectomy are prone to develop ventricular arrhythmias following surgery. In a study of 59 dogs, 24% developed arrhythmias.[44] Anemia, anoxia, and hypovolemia were considered possible causes.[44]

In dogs with HSA of the heart, particularly the right atrium, exploratory thoracotomy may be performed, not only as a diagnostic procedure, but as a treatment for this tumor.[19,45] Right atrial or auricular appendage tumor may be partially removed with staples or hand suturing. Complete removal is generally not possible and the pericardectomy is probably more palliative than the mass removal. Perioperative, ventricular, and supraventricular arrhythmias are a common feature in dogs with primary cardiac HSA. Treatment of ventricular premature contractions and ventricular tachycardia may require the use of such agents as lidocaine and procainamide.

**Table 29–1**  Hematologic Abnormalities in Dogs with Hemangiosarcoma

| Hematologic Abnormalities | Normal Value | Dogs with HSA at All Locations (Total: 98 Dogs) Number of Dogs (%) | Dogs with Splenic HSA (Total: 60 Dogs) Number of Dogs (%) |
|---|---|---|---|
| Anemia | Hematocrit 37–52% Hemoglobin 12–18 gm/dl Red blood cells 5–8 × 10⁶ | 49 (50%) | 41 (69%) |
| Neutrophilic leukocytosis | 56–78% (3–10 × 10³) | 49 (50%) | 40 (67%) |
| Increase in band neutrophils | 0–2% | 55 (56%) | 42 (70%) |
| Increased reticulocyte count | 0–1% (< 800 × 10³) | 15 (16%) | 13 (22%) |
| Thrombocytopenia | 200–500 × 10³ | 35 (36%) | 31 (51%) |
| Nucleated red blood cells | 2/100 WBC seen | 13 (13%) | 10 (17%) |

*Source:* The Animal Medical Center, July 1, 1980 to January 1, 1983.[40] Reprinted with permission.

**Table 29–2** Clinical Staging System of Canine Hemangiosarcoma

T Primary Tumor
$T_0$ — no evidence of tumor
$T_1$ — tumor less than 5 cm in diameter and confined to primary site or dermis
$T_2$ — tumor 5 cm or greater or ruptured, invading subcutaneous tissues
$T_3$ — tumor invading adjacent structures, including muscle

N Regional Lymph Nodes
$N_0$ — no regional lymph node involvement
$N_1$ — regional lymph node involvement
$N_2$ — distant lymph node involvement

M Distant Metastasis
$M_0$ — no evidence of distant metastasis
$M_1$ — distant metastasis

Stages
I — $T_0$ or $T_1$, $N_0$, $M_0$
II — $T_1$ or $T_2$, $N_0$ or $N_1$, $M_0$
III — $T_2$ or $T_3$, $N_0$, $N_1$ or $N_2$, $M_1$

Paroxysmal atrial tachycardia is seen less frequently and may require treatment using digoxin and propranolol hydrochloride.[19]

In animals with primary bone HSA, a complete limb amputation is required.

## Chemotherapy

Because of the metastatic nature of nondermal HSA, other forms of therapy need to be considered in addition to surgery. Combination chemotherapy will most likely offer the best chance of controlling this disease.[46] Combination chemotherapy using cyclophosphamide, doxorubicin, and vincristine (VAC)[47,48] or doxorubicin and cyclophosphamide (AC)[49] are chemotherapeutic combinations that have shown potential in studies in the dog. In another study, doxorubicin was used to treat 46 dogs with metastatic (stage III) HSA in various sites. The mean survival time for dogs treated with surgery followed by doxorubicin was 267 days, compared to 67 days for those dogs treated with doxorubicin alone.[50] Recommended chemotherapy protocols are presented in Table 29–3. Other combinations such as vincristine, cyclophosphamide, and methotrexate (VCM) have also yielded minimal but at least some improvement in overall survival time.[9,40] Interestingly, single-agent vincristine induced a complete remission in a dog with metastatic pulmonary HSA.[51]

## Biologic Therapy

Very few studies have been done using biologic therapy. One study using a mixed bacterial vaccine showed some improvement in dogs treated with splenic HSA.[9] We have recently completed a randomized trial evaluating liposome–muramyl tripeptide–phosphatidylethanolamine (L–MTP–PE), a monocyte/macrophage activator (see Chap. 11) combined with doxorubicin and cyclophosphamide, compared to the same chemotherapy alone in dogs following splenectomy for

**Table 29–3** Adjuvant Chemotherapy Protocols for Canine Hemangiosarcoma

| | | |
|---|---|---|
| I. **VAC** | | |
| | Day 1 | Doxorubicin[a] 30 mg/m² IV. |
| | | Cyclophosphamide 100–200 mg/m² IV. |
| | Days 8 and 15 | Vincristine 0.75 mg/m² IV. |
| | Day 22 | Repeat cycle for a total of 4–6 cycles. |
| | | a. Monitor CBC prior to each chemotherapy treatment if granulocyte < 3,000 cells/μl—withhold chemotherapy for 5–7 days. |
| | | b. Prophylactic antibiotics—sulfadiazine/trimethoprim (Tribrissen) at 10–20 mg/kg orally b.i.d. days 1 to 8. |
| II. **AC** | | |
| | Day 1 | Doxorubicin[a] 30 mg/m² IV. |
| | | Cyclophosphamide 100–150 mg/m² IV or 50 mg/m² PO days 3, 4, 5, 6. |
| | Day 22 | Repeat cycle for 4–6 cycles. |
| | | a. Monitor CBC prior to each chemotherapy as above. |
| | | b. Prophylactic antibiotics may be required as above. |
| III. **A** | | Doxorubicin[a] 30 mg/m² IV q 3 weeks × 5 treatments. |
| | | a. Monitor CBC prior to each chemotherapy as above. |
| | | b. Prophylactic antibiotics may be required as above. |

[a]For cats—reduce dose of doxorubicin to 20 mg/m².

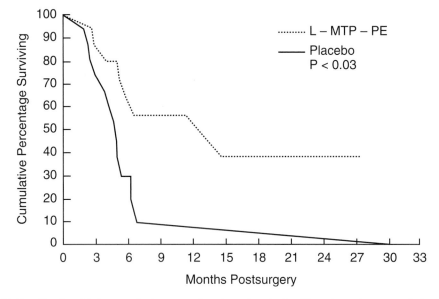

**Figure 29–2.**  Kaplan-Meier survival curves for dogs treated with splenectomy and chemotherapy (doxorubicin and cyclophosphamide) and randomized to L-MTP-PE (*n* = 16) or placebo (*n* = 16).[53]

HSA.[52,53] Thirty-two dogs were entered into this study and the median survival time for the dogs treated with chemotherapy alone was 143 days versus 277 days (p = .03) treated with L–MTP-PE combined with chemotherapy (Fig. 29–2). This study demonstrated the significant potential of combining immunotherapy with chemotherapy and surgery to treat splenic HSA.[52,53]

A summary of the results of several reports on the treatment of splenic HSA is presented in Table 29–4. Results of using radiation therapy to treat HSA have not been published.

The same chemotherapy recommendations hold for cats with visceral HSA. Chemotherapy protocols, in addition to surgery, should be considered and would generally include a combi-

**Table 29–4**  Comparison of Survival Times in Dogs with Splenic Hemangiosarcoma

| Treatment | Number of Dogs | Median Survival (Days) | References |
|---|---|---|---|
| Splenectomy | 59 | 19 | 27 |
| Splenectomy | 21 | 65 | 9 |
| Splenectomy | 19 | 56 | 23 |
| Splenectomy | 32 | 83 | 54 |
| Splenectomy + MBV[a] | 10 | 91 | 9 |
| Splenectomy + MBV[a] + VMC[b] | 10 | 117 | 9 |
| Splenectomy + VAC[c] | 6 | 145 | 47 |
| Splenectomy + AC[d] | 6 | 179 | 49 |
| Splenectomy + AC[d] | 16 | 143 | 53 |
| Splenectomy + AC[d] + L-MTP-PE[e] | 16 | 277 | 53 |

[a]MBV = Mixed bacterial vaccine.

[b]VMC = Vincristine, methotrexate, cyclophosphamide.

[c]VAC = Vincristine, doxorubicin, cyclophosphamide.

[d]AC = Doxorubicin, cyclophosphamide.

[e]L-MTP-PE = Liposome encapsulated muramyl tripeptide-phosphatidylethanolamine.

nation of doxorubicin and cyclophosphamide (AC) or VAC or doxorubicin alone. (as shown in Table 29–3).

## PROGNOSIS

Overall, dogs and cats have a poor prognosis for nondermal HSA. Results of surgery alone (splenectomy) yield median survival times ranging from 19 to 83 days.[9,22,27,54] Death is usually due to metastatic disease. Two studies have shown that dogs with nonruptured splenic tumors (stage I) had a better prognosis than those dogs with a ruptured splenic tumor (stage II) (Fig. 29–3).[9,53] With the addition of chemotherapy (VAC or AC) following splenectomy, median survival times ranging from 141 to 179 days have been reported. [47–49] Less than 10% of the dogs treated survive a year or longer. The addition of immunotherapy with chemotherapy (AC), using L–MTP-PE has increased survival to a median of 273 days.[52,53]

In a recent study of surgically treated cutaneous HSA, tumors involving the dermis (without hypodermal or deep invasion), the median survival time was 780 days for 10 treated dogs.[29] Tumors with hypodermal ($n$ = 10) and underlying muscular involvement ($n$ = 5), had a median survival time of 172 and 307 days, respectively, although there was no statistical difference between these survival times. The authors of this study concluded the surgery alone is adequate for dermal tumors but hypodermal or deep invasive tumors should be treated with adjuvant therapy.[29]

In a study of 38 dogs with primary cardiac HSA, 16 of 38 dogs underwent an exploratory thoracotomy, 7 (44%) were euthanatized at the time of surgery because of nonresectability of the primary tumor or gross metastatic disease.[19] In 9 dogs (56%) the tumor was resected by removing part of the right atrium. The mean survival time for these 9 dogs was 4 months (range 2 days to 8 months).[19] In another study in 4 dogs, right atrial appendage HSAs were removed (2 also received doxorubicin) and all dogs were dead by 3 to 5 months.[45]

Primary HSA in bone is a very rare tumor and appears to have the same highly metastatic potential as other nondermal sites. No series of treated bone cases has been published. Two dogs treated with amputation followed by doxorubicin and cyclophosphamide only survived 151 to 154 days and died of metastatic disease.[49] In another study with HSA of the rib, 2 of 3 dogs treated with surgical removal died within 5 months of surgery.[55]

In cats the prognosis for visceral HSA is also very poor. Most cats will die from recurrence of the primary lesion or metastasis and in 5 cats

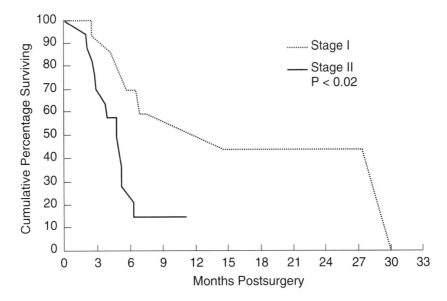

**Figure 29–3.** Kaplan-Meier survival curves for dogs with stage I, stage II splenic HSA treated with surgery, chemotherapy ± immunotherapy.[53]

undergoing splenectomy, survival ranged from 6 to 35 weeks (median 20 weeks).[12] HSA located in cutaneous and subcutaneous sites, have recurrence rates of 60 to 80% but metastasis is uncommon.[11,12] In one study of 10 cats undergoing complete excision of cutaneous HSA, recurrence occurred on the average in 4 months, 5 of these cats died within a mean of 44 weeks.[12]

In summary, surgery still offers the best approach to therapy. The value of adjuvant chemotherapy for the treatment of this neoplasm needs to be more fully defined. Too few studies have been done to evaluate the true effectiveness of adjuvant chemotherapy or biologic therapy in conjunction with surgery. More studies are needed to evaluate potential therapeutic modalities with this particular tumor.

## COMPARATIVE FEATURES[56]

In humans, HSAs or angiosarcomas are uniformly high-grade soft tissue sarcomas. They are uncommon, however, comprising only 2% of all soft tissue sarcomas. Most tumors arise in the skin or subcutaneous tissue but they can occur anywhere in the body. The female breast is a common site. These tumors are extremely aggressive and generally have a poor prognosis. With multimodality therapy, the 5-year survival rate is around 10 to 15%. Liver angiosarcoma is a rare neoplasm, with most patients dying within 6 months. Attempts to treat hepatic angiosarcomas with radiation therapy and chemotherapy have been disappointing.

## REFERENCES

1. Priester, WA, McKay FW: The Occurrence of Tumors in Domestic Animals. National Cancer Institute Monograph 54. Washington DC, U.S. Government Printing Office, 1980.
2. Madewell BR, Theilen GH: Skin tumors of mesenchymal origin. *In* Theilen GH and Madewell BR (eds): Veterinary Cancer Medcine, 2nd ed. Philadelphia, Leo and Febiger, 1987, pp. 295–297.
3. Moulton JE: Tumors in Domestic Animals, 2nd ed. Berkeley, University of California Press, 1978, pp. 35–36.
4. Oksanen A: Hemangiosarcomas in dogs. J Comp Pathol 88:585–595, 1978.
5. Patnaik AK, Liu SK: Angiosarcoma in Cats. J Small Anim Pract 18:191–198, 1977.
6. Carpenter JL, Andrews LK, Holzworth J: Tumors and Tumor-like Lesions in Diseases of the Cat, Vol.

7. Arp LH, and Grier RL: Disseminated cutaneous hemangiosarcoma in a young dog. J Am Ver Med Assoc 185:671–673, 1984.
8. Schmidt RE, and Langhan RF: A survey of feline neoplasms. J Am Vet Med Assoc 151:1325–1328, 1967.
9. Brown NO, Patnaik AR, MacEwen EG: Canine Hemangiosarcoma: Retrospective analysis of 104 cases. J Am Vet Assoc 186:56–58, 1985.
10. Pearson GR, and Head KW: Malignant Hemangioendothelioma (angiosarcoma) in the dog. J Small Anim Pract 17:737–745, 1976.
11. Miller MA, Ramos JA, Kreeger JM: Cutaneous vascular neoplasia in 15 cats: Clinical morphologic and immunohistochemical studies. Vet Pathol 29:329–336, 1992.
12. Scavelli TD, Patnaik AK, Mehlhaff CJ, et al: Hemangiosarcoma in the cat: Retrospective evaluation of 31 surgical cases. J Am Vet Med Assoc 187:817–819, 1985.
13. Adam YG, Huvos AG, Hajdu SI: Malignant vascular tumors in the liver. Ann Surg 175:375–383, 1972.
14. Ludwig J, Hoffman HN: Hemangiosarcoma of the liver: Spectrum of morphologic changes and clinical findings. Mayo Clin Proc 50:255–263, 1970.
15. Rebar A, Han FF, Halliwell WH, et al: Microangiopathic hemolytic anemia associated with radiation-induced hemangiosarcoma. Vet Pathol 17:443–454, 1980.
16. Nikula KJ, Benjamin SA, Angleton GM, et al: Ultraviolet radiation, solar dermatosis, and cutaneous neoplasia in beagle dogs. Radiat Res 129:11–18, 1992.
17. Fees DL, Withrow SJ: Canine hemangiosarcoma. Compend Contin Educ Pract Vet 3:1047–1052, 1981.
18. Martinez SA, Schulman AJ: Hemangiosarcoma of the urinary bladder in a dog. J Am Vet Med Assoc 192:655–656, 1988.
19. Aronsohn M: Cardiac Hemangiosarcoma in the dog: A review of 38 cases. J Am Vet Med Assoc 187:922–926, 1985.
20. Kline LJ, Zook BC, Munson TO: Primary Cardiac Hemangiosarcoma in Dog. J Am Vet Med Assoc 157:326–337, 1970.
21. Berg RJ, Wingfield W: Pericardial Effusion in the Dog: A review of 42 cases. J Am Anim Hosp Assoc 20:721–730, 1984.
22. Spangler WL, Culbertson MR: Prevalence, type, and importance of splenic diseases in dogs: 1,480 cases (1985–1989). J Am Vet Med Assoc 200:829–834, 1992.
23. Johnson KA., Powers BE, Withrow SJ et al: Splenomegaly in dogs. J Vet Intern Med 3:160–166, 1989.
24. Von Beust BR: Factor VIII-related antigen in canine endothelial neoplasms. An immunohistochemical study. Vet Pathol 25:251–255, 1988.
25. Weinstein MJ, Carpenter JL, Mehlhaff-Schunk CJ:

1, ed. Holzworth J. Philadelphia, WB Saunders, 1987, pp. 480–483.

Nonangiogenic and nonlymphomatous sarcomas of the canine spleen: 57 cases (1975–1987). J Am Vet Med Assoc 195:784–788, 1989.

26. Hendrick MJ, Brooks JJ, Bruce EH: Six cases of malignant fibrous histiocytoma of the canine spleen. Vet Pathol 29:351–354, 1992.

27. Prymak C, McKee LJ, Goldschmidt MH, et al: Epidemiologic, clinical, pathologic, and prognostic characteristics of splenic hemangiosarcoma and splenic hematoma in dogs: 217 cases (1985). J Am Vet Med Assoc 193:706–716, 1988.

28. Srebernik N, Appleby EG: Breed prevalence and sites of haemangioma and haemangiosarcoma in dogs. Vet Rec 129:408–409, 1991.

29. Ward H, Fox LE, and Calderwood-Mays MB, et al: Cutaneous hemangiosarcoma in 25 dogs: A retrospective study. J Vet Intern Med 8:345–348, 1994.

30. Culbertson MR: Hemangiosarcoma of the canine skin and tongue. Vet Pathol 19:556–558, 1982.

31. Hargis AM, Ihrke PJ, Spangler WL: A retrospective clinicopathologic study of 212 dogs with cutaneous hemangiomas and hemangiosarcomas. Vet Pathol 29:316–328, 1992.

32. Waters DJ, Caywood DD, Hayden DW, et al: Metastatic pattern in dogs with splenic hemangiosarcomas: Clinical implications. J Small Anim Pract 29:805–814, 1988.

33. Waters DJ, Hayden DW, Walter PA: Intracranial lesions in dogs with hemangiosarcoma. J Vet Intern Med 3:222–230, 1989.

34. Legendre AM, Krehbiel JD: Disseminated intravascular coagulation in a dog with hemothorax and hemangiosarcoma. J Am Vet Med Assoc 171:1070–1071, 1977.

35. Keene BW, Rush JE, Cooley AJ, et al: Primary left ventricular hemangiosarcoma diagnosed by endomyocardial biopsy in a dog. J Am Vet Med Assoc 197:1501–1503, 1990.

36. Wrigley RH, Park RD, Konde LJ, et al: Ultrasonographic features of splenic hemangiosarcoma in dogs: 18 cases (1980–1986). J Am Vet Med Assoc 192:1113–1117, 1988.

37. Holt D, Van Winkle T, Schelling C, et al: Correlation between thoracic radiographs and postmortem findings in dogs with hemangiosarcoma: 77 cases (1984–1989). J Am Vet Med Assoc 200:1535–1539, 1992.

38. Dueland R, Dahlin DC: Hemangioendothelioma of Canine Bone. J Am Anim Hosp Assoc 8:81–85, 1972.

39. Hirsch VM, Jacobsen J, Mills JHL: A retrospective study of canine hemangiosarcoma and its association with acanthocytosis. Can Vet J 22: 152–155, 1981.

40. Brown NO: Hemangiosarcoma. Vet Clin North Am Small Anim Pract 15:569–575, 1985.

41. Hargis AM, and Feldman BF: Evaluation of hemostatic defects secondary to vascular tumors in dogs: 11 cases (1983–1988). J Am Vet Med Assoc 198:891–894, 1991.

42. Hammer AS, Couto CG, Swardson C, et al: Hemostatic abnormalities in dogs with hemangiosarcoma. J Vet Intern Med 5:11–14, 1991.

43. Grindem CB, Breitschwerdt EB, Corbett WT, et al: Thrombocytopenia associated with neoplasia in dogs. J Vet Intern Med 8:400–405, 1994.

44. Keyes MC, Rush JE, Autran de Morais HS, et al: Ventricular arrhythmias in dogs with splenic masses. Vet Emerg Crit Care 3:33–38, 1994.

45. Wykes PM, Rouse GP, Orton EC: Removal of five canine cardiac tumors using a stapling instrument. Vet Surg 15:103–106, 1986.

46. Hammer AS, and Couto CG: Diagnosing and treating canine hemangiosarcoma. Vet Med (March): 188–201, 1992.

47. Hammer AS, Couto CG, Filppi J, et al: Efficacy and toxicity of VAC chemotherapy (vincristine, doxorubicin, and cyclophosphamide) in dogs with hemangiosarcoma. J Vet Intern Med 5:160–166, 1991.

48. De Madron E, Helfand SC, and Stebbins KE: Use of chemotherapy for treatment of cardiac hemangiosarcoma in a dog. J Am Vet Med Assoc 190: 887–891, 1987.

49. Sorenmo KU, Jeglum KA, Helfand SC: Chemotherapy of canine hemangiosarcoma with doxorubicin and cyclophosphamide. J Vet Intern Med 7:370–376, 1993.

50. Ogilvie GH, Powers BE, Mallinckrodt CH, et al: Doxorubicin chemotherapy and surgery for hemangiosarcoma in the dog. Proc Vet Cancer Soc 14:39–40, 1994.

51. Hahn KA: Vincristine sulfate as single-agent chemotherapy in a dog and a cat with malignant neoplasms. J Am Vet Med Assoc 197:504–506, 1990.

52. MacEwen EG, Kurzman ID, Helfand S, et al: Current studies of liposome muramyl tripeptide (CGP 19835A) lipid. Therapy for metastasis in spontaneous tumors: A progress review. J Drug Targeting 2:391–396, 1994.

53. Vail DM, MacEwen EG, Kurzman ID, et al: Liposome-encapsulated muramyl tripeptide phosphatidylethanolamine (L-MTP-PE) adjuvant immunotherapy for splenic hemangiosarcoma in the dog: A randomized multi-institutional clinical trial. Clin Cancer Res, 1995, in press..

54. Wood CA, Moore AS, Gliatto JG, et al: Prognosis for dogs with Stage I or Stage II splenic hemangiosarcoma treated by splenectomy alone: 32 cases (1991–1993). J Am Vet Med Assoc 1995, (in press).

55. Pirkey-Ehrhart N, Straw RC, Withrow SJ et al: Primary rib tumors in 54 dogs. J Am Anim Hosp Assoc 3:65–69, 1995.

56. Yang JC, Rosenberg SA, Glatstein EJ, and Antman KH: Sarcomas of soft tissues. In Cancer VT DeVita, Jr, S Hellman, JA Rosenberg (eds): Principles and Practice of Oncology, 4th ed. Philadelphia, JB Lippincott, 1995, pp. 1436–1488.

# B. Thymoma

## Stephen J. Withrow

## INCIDENCE AND RISK FACTORS

Thymomas are rare in the dog and even more uncommon in the cat. Even though the normal thymus is larger and more active in puppies and kittens, the disease is generally diagnosed in the older animal (dogs, 9 years; cats, 10 years). No consistent breed predilection is known; however, medium and large breed dogs may be over-represented.[1,2] One study demonstrated a female prevalence,[3] while most studies show no sex predilection.[1]

## PATHOLOGY AND NATURAL BEHAVIOR

Thymomas originate from thymic epithelium but are variably and even predominantly infiltrated with mature lymphocytes. The epithelium is the neoplastic component. Squamous cell carcinoma has been rarely documented to arise within feline thymomas.[4] Different histologic cell types can be seen (differentiated epithelial, lymphocyte rich, and clear cell) but prognostic differences between these groups are not apparent.[5] "Benign" thymomas are noninvasive and well encapsulated, while "malignant" thymomas will invade adjacent structures (precava, rib cage, and pericardium) but rarely metastasize.[6] The terms *benign* and *malignant* are derived more from their clinical features (resectability) than from histologic features. Distant metastasis is rare but has been reported.[7]

The most common anterior mediastinal tumors are lymphomas and thymomas, followed by branchial cysts, ectopic thyroid, chemodectoma, and a variety of rare neoplasms.[1,8]

## HISTORY AND CLINICAL SIGNS

Most patients present with signs of respiratory distress (coughing, tachypnea, and dyspnea). Precaval syndrome (facial, neck, and/or front leg swelling) may also occur secondary to obstruction of venous and lymphatic drainage from the head, neck, and legs. The paraneoplastic syndrome of myasthenia gravis has also been documented in up to 40% of dogs and the rare cat and is characterized by muscle weakness and megaesophagus.[1–3,9,10] In 20 to 40% of patients, nonthymic neoplasms, various autoimmune diseases, and polymyositis have also been associated with the presence of thymoma.[2,3,11]

## DIAGNOSTIC TECHNIQUES AND WORKUP

Physical exam findings may include painless, bilateral pitting edema of the head, neck, or front legs as a result of precaval syndrome. Jugular veins may be enlarged and tortuous. Auscultation of the thoracic cavity may reveal decreased lung sounds over the anterior mediastinum (mass) or ventral lung fields (pleural effusion). The heart sounds may be heard more dorsal and caudal than normal as a result of cardiac displacement. In smaller dogs and cats, decreased compressibility of the anterior chest cavity may also be detected.

Routine hematologic and biochemistry tests are usually normal although lymphocytosis has been reported.[5,7,12] Hypercalcemia is only rarely reported with thymomas but will obviously confuse the diagnosis with thymic lymphoma.[5,13] Thoracic radiographs will generally reveal a variable size mass in the anterior mediastinum, pleural effusion, and displacement of the cardiac silhouette caudally and dorsally (Fig. 29–4). Dilation of the esophagus may be seen with myasthenia gravis.

Transthoracic fine-needle aspiration for cytologic preparations is a simple and safe procedure but has been associated with unreliable results in the author's experience. Cytologic results usually reveal a preponderance of lymphocytes rather than the epithelial component of the tumor. Mast cells are also commonly seen.[5] Thymomas are commonly cystic and will frequently yield nondiagnostic material (Fig. 29–5).[2] Since the major differential diagnosis is lymphoma, which is treated differently, this distinction is important. As opposed to thymoma, feline thymic lymphoma is usually seen in young cats (mean 2

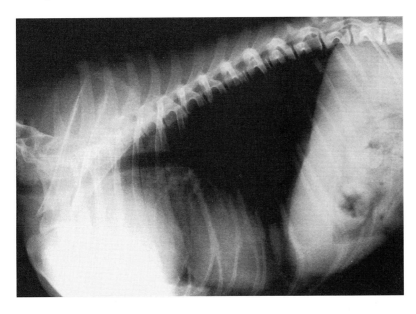

**Figure 29–4.** Anterior mediastinal mass is seen on lateral radiograph of a 13-year-old female mixed-breed dog.

years) that are feline leukemia virus positive (80%).[14] Canine thymic lymphoma is often associated with hypercalcemia (25 to 50%) or generalized lymphadenopathy.[15] Cytologic evaluation of pleural effusion in thymoma cases should yield mature lympho*cytes* as opposed to lympho*blasts* seen with lymphoma.[11,15]

Transthoracic needle core biopsy can be diagnostic but will often yield cystic and necrotic material with a preponderance of lympho*cytes,* making definitive diagnosis difficult.

Angiography, ultrasound, and computed tomographic evaluation of mediastinal masses should be further evaluated for their sensitivity in differentiating thymoma from lymphoma.[16–18] Ultrasonography of thymomas will generally suggest a pattern of mixed echogenicity with cavitation, whereas lymphoma more commonly has a homogeneous hypoechoic mass.[17]

The definitive presurgical diagnosis of thymoma is difficult and frequently rests on trying to rule out the more common diseases. Most

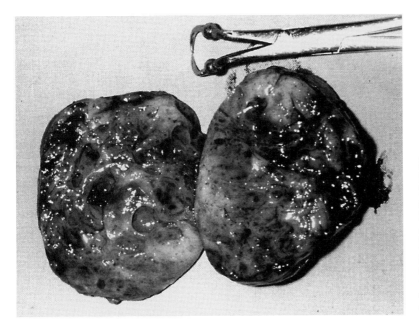

**Figure 29–5.** Cross-section of well-encapsulated thymoma surgically removed from patient in Figure 29–4. Note the cystic nature of the lesion, which may complicate cytologic diagnosis. Patient is alive and free of disease more than 3 years postoperatively.

thymic lymphoma cases respond rapidly and completely to aggressive chemotherapy. Thymoma should be suspected in patients with a partial remission or stable disease 10 to 14 days after chemotherapy administration.

## THERAPY

The definitive therapy for thymoma is surgical resection. Smaller masses may be approached via a midline thoracotomy, but the more common large masses should be approached via a midline sternotomy. Once the mass is seen, the surgeon must make a clinical judgment as to resectability. Approximately 50% of thymomas are resectable and nothing (including size) is uniformly predictive in the preoperative evaluation. Invasive and malignant thymomas will be adherent to surrounding tissues, especially major veins, the trachea, and the esophagus, making removal difficult or impossible.

Debulking of invasive thymomas can be attempted in hopes of alleviating symptoms of the physical mass or possibly enhancing potential chemotherapy treatment but will frequently be associated with extensive morbidity.

If the mass is deemed unresectable and other treatments are to be pursued, large wedge biopsies should be taken at surgery, it being kept in mind that thymomas are not homogeneous and are cystic.

Attempts at treatment with chemotherapy have been reported, but objective partial or complete remissions are very uncommon.[2,5,19,20] Chemotherapy has gained in popularity in treating humans with thymoma and should be tested more in animals, especially those with megaesophagus who are poor surgical risks.[21–23] Radiation therapy has rarely been attempted, but either chemotherapy and radiation should theoretically decrease the lymphoid component of the mass.[24]

Myasthenia gravis, if present, generally requires treatment with immunosuppression (prednisone) or anticholinesterase drugs but may not be reversible.[5,10]

## PROGNOSIS

The prognosis for surgically resectable (benign) thymomas in dogs without megaesophagus is good. Long-term remissions and cures can be expected in dogs without megaesophagus with resectable tumors.[5,7,9,19,25] Dogs without megae-

sophagus and a resectable tumor had an 83% 1-year survival.[5]

The outlook for patients with nonresectable thymomas remains poor until use of other treatments (chemotherapy or radiation therapy) can be optimized.

Myasthenia gravis may or may not improve with complete removal of the thymoma, but improvement may require many months.[1,5,10,26] Two untreated thymoma cases, followed with thoracic radiographs only, lived 6 and 36 months, implying slow growth of some thymomas.[3]

Surgical resection of thymomas in 12 cats suggests a good prognosis. Two cats died in the perioperative period, while none of the remaining 10 cats developed local recurrence or metastasis. Median survival was almost 2 years. Myasthenia gravis developed postoperatively in two cats.[27]

## COMPARATIVE ASPECTS[28]

Thymomas are very similar in animals and man. Sixty-five percent are encapsulated and noninvasive, while 35% are invasive.

Multiple paraneoplastic syndromes have been associated with thymomas (autoimmune, endocrine, infectious, and nonthymic cancer). Up to 50% of patients will have symptoms of myasthenia gravis. Only 25% of these patients will have improvement in muscle strength after removal of the thymoma.

Treatment is surgical removal with at least 80% free of disease at 5 years. Radiation therapy is indicated for invasive thymomas and they are considered moderately sensitive.[29] Corticosteroids have caused regressions of some thymomas. Other single agents with some efficacy include doxorubicin, cisplatin, and alkylating agents.[21–23]

## REFERENCES

1. Stevenson S: Thymoma. *In* Textbook of Small Animal Surgery. Philadelphia, WB Saunders, 1985, pp. 1235–1241.
2. Aronsohn M: Canine thymoma. Vet Clin North Am 15:755–767, 1985.
3. Aronsohn MG, Schunk KL, Carpenter JL, King NW: Clinical and pathologic features of thymoma in 15 dogs. J Am Vet Med Assoc 184:1355–1362, 1984.
4. Carpenter JL, Valentine BA: Brief communications and case reports. Squamous cell carcinoma arising in two feline thymomas. Vet Pathol 29:541–543, 1992.

5. Atwater SW, Powers BE, Park RD, et al: Canine thymoma: 23 cases (1980–1991). J Am Vet Med Assoc 205(7)1007–1013, 1994.

6. Robinson WC, Cantwell HD, Crawley RR, Weirich WE, Blevins WE: Invasive thymoma in a dog: A case report. J Am Anim Hosp Assoc 13:95–97, 1977.

7. Bellah JR, Stiff ME, Russell RG: Thymoma in the dog: Two case reports and review of 20 additional cases. J Am Vet Med Assoc 183:306–311, 1983.

8. Liu SK, Patnaik AK, Burk RL: Thymic branchial cysts in the dog and cat. J Am Vet Med Assoc 182:1095–1098, 1983.

9. Poffenbarger E, Klausner JS, Caywood DD: Acquired myasthenia gravis in a dog with thymoma: A case report. J Am Anim Hosp Assoc 21:119–124, 1985.

10. Scott-Moncrieff JC, Cook JR, Lantz GC: Acquired myasthenia gravis in a cat with thymoma. J Am Vet Med Assoc 196:1291–1293, 1990.

11. Carpenter JL, Holzworth J: Thymoma in 11 cats. J Am Vet Med Assoc 181:248–251, 1982.

12. Theilen GH, Madewell BR: Tumors of the respiratory tract and thorax. In Theilen GM, Madewell BR (eds): Veterinary Cancer Medicine. Philadelphia, Lea and Febiger, 1979, p. 351.

13. Harris CL, Klausner JS, Caywood DD, Leininger JR: Hypercalcemia in a dog with thymoma. J Am Anim Hosp Assoc 27:281–284, 1991.

14. Hardy WD: Hematopoietic tumors of cats. J Am Anim Hosp Assoc 17:921–940, 1981.

15. Theilen GS, Madewell BR: Leukemia-sarcoma disease complex. In Theilen GH, Madewell BR (eds), Veterinary Cancer Medicine. Philadelphia, Lea and Febiger, 1979, pp. 241–252.

16. Burk RL: Computed tomography of thoracic diseases in dogs. J Am Vet Med Assoc 199:617–621, 1991.

17. Konde LJ, Spaulding K: Sonographic evaluation of the cranial mediastinum in small animals. Vet Radiol 32:178–184, 1991.

18. Stowater JL, Lamb CR: Ultrasonography of non-cardiac thoracic diseases in small animals. J Am Vet Med Assoc 195:514–520, 1989.

19. Willard MD, Tvedten H, Walshaw R, Aronson E: Thymoma in a cat. J Am Vet Med Assoc 176:451–453, 1980.

20. Martin RA, Evans EW, August JR, Franklin JE: Surgical treatment of a thymoma in a cat. J Am Anim Hosp Assoc 22:347–354, 1986.

21. Fornasiero A, Daniel O, Ghiotto C, et al: Chemotherapy for invasive thymoma. A 13-year experience. Cancer 68:30–33, 1991.

22. Macchiarini P, Chella A, Ducci F, et al: Neoadjuvant chemotherapy, surgery and postoperative radiation therapy for invasive thymoma. Cancer 68:706–713, 1991.

23. Park HS, Shin DM, Lee JS, et al: Thymoma: A retrospective study of 87 cases. Cancer 73:2491–2498, 1994.

24. Hitt ME, Shaw DP, Hogan PM, et al: Radiation treatment for thymoma in a dog. J Am Vet Med Assoc 190:1187–1190, 1987.

25. Simpson RM, Waters DJ, Gebhard DH, Casey HW: Case report: Massive thymoma with medullary differentiation in a dog. Vet Pathol 29:416–419, 1992.

26. Klebanow ER: Thymoma and acquired myasthenia gravis in the dog: A case report and review of 13 additional cases. J Am Anim Hosp Assoc 28:63–69, 1992.

27. Gores BR, Berg J, Carpenter JL, Aronsohn MG: Surgical treatment of thymoma in cats: 12 cases (1987–1992). J Am Vet Med Assoc 204:1782–1785, 1994.

28. Rosenberg JC: Neoplasms of the mediastinum. In DeVita VT et al (ed) Cancer; Principles and Practice of Oncology. Philadelphia, JB Lippincott, pp. 759–775, 1993.

29. Jackson MA, Ball DL: Postoperative radiotherapy in invasive thymoma. Radiother Oncol 21:77–82, 1991.

# C. Transmissible Venereal Tumor

## E. Gregory MacEwen

### INCIDENCE AND RISK FACTORS

Transmissible venereal tumor, or TVT, ("Sticker" tumor) is a contagious venereal tumor and is a naturally occurring tumor in dogs. It commonly affects the external genitalia and is usually transmitted at coitus. The development of the TVT as a coitally transmitted neoplasm in the dog is probably facilitated by some unique characteristic of sexual intercourse in this species that leads to injuries of the vaginal or penile mucosa and thus provides the susceptible bed for tumor transplantation. TVTs are naturally transplanted tumors that are derived from a common origin; these tumors apparently have a cellular mode of transmission and have been maintained in the canine population of the world for many generations.[1,2] The tumor has been reported to occur in most parts of the world, but appears to be more prevalent in temperate climates. Studies have shown that the prevalence of TVT is inversely correlated to geographic latitude and positively correlated to higher mean annual temperature and increased rainfall.[3,4] It is seen most often in young, roaming, sexually active dogs.

A viral etiology has been investigated but not verified.[5] Virus particles have been observed, but the tumor has not been transmitted by cell-free filtrates.

## PATHOLOGY AND NATURAL BEHAVIOR

The TVT consists of undifferentiated round cells that are loosely packed and are regarded to be of reticuloendothelial origin. The TVT will usually maintain a relatively consistent karyotype. Special staining and evaluation of TVT cell mitotic figures has demonstrated that most cells have a stem-line chromosome number of 59 (range 57–64).[6] Of these 59 chromosomes, 16 or 17 are metacentric and 43 or 42 are acrocentric. These constant and highly specific chromosome aberrations are regarded as being suggestive of a cellular mechanism of transmission. The normal dog karyotype is 78 chromosomes. It has also been shown that the same histocompatibility complex (DL-A) antigens are expressed on the surface of TVT cells that originate from different dogs and from different geographic locations.[7]

Immunologic studies clearly demonstrate that the TVT tumor is antigenic in the dog and that the immune response against the tumor plays a major role in determining the course of disease. The TVT possesses tumor-associated antigens, as determined by both immunodiffusion and enzyme-linked immunosorbent assays (ELISA), and the immunologic response plays a major role in the inhibiting growth and spread of this neoplasm.[4,8] The anti-TVT immune response is mounted, at least in part, against DL-A, resulting in regression of the tumor and the development of immunity to subsequent reinfections. The peripheral blood lymphocytes of dogs with regressing tumors have been shown to be cytotoxic to tumor cells, whereas lymphocytes from normal dogs or from dogs with progressive venereal tumors were not.[9,10] Passive transfer of postregression sera can inhibit the growth of experimentally transplanted tumor and prevent development of the tumor if administered prior to transplantation.[4] Antibodies from regressor animals are cytotoxic to TVT cells in the presence of complement and may therefore destroy the tumor cells in vivo without the involvement of cellular effect or mechanisms.[11] The demonstration that passive transfer of immune serum can induce tumor regression indicates that antibody-dependent mechanisms are involved in the induction of tumor regression. In addition, in vitro assays suggest that suppressive serum factors may facilitate tumor growth in the initial stages of disease.[11]

One interesting observation noted in animals heavily infected with large burdens of TVT is that these animals may develop a polycythemia.[4] It has been suggested that TVT cells probably synthesize and secrete erythropoietin.

Once an animal becomes infected, the TVT may progress to a certain point or to a certain size, and then regress if there is an appropriate antitumor immunologic response. This probably happens in most of the animals that are naturally infected with TVT and it is also possible that the TVT may continue to grow and metastasize. Although metastasis has been reported, it is considered to be quite uncommon. Metastasis has been seen in the lymph nodes, skin, eye, liver, and brain.[2] The TVT may also involve extragenital sites and this may occur because of autotransplantation (licking and sniffing). This may be the way in which TVTs develop in the oral cavity and nasal cavity.[12,13] TVT can be transmitted to young puppies by subcutaneous inoculation.[14,15] Within 1 week, tumors are palpable and range in size from 3 mm to 5 mm in diameter. Nodules will enlarge and grow to 10 mm to 20 mm over a 1- to 2-month period and most will eventually regress.

## HISTORY AND CLINICAL SIGNS

Most cases of naturally occurring TVT are confined to the external genitalia. In the vagina, TVTs may range in size from 0.5 mm to more than 10 cm in diameter. They are usually cauliflower-like in appearance, friable, and red to flesh-colored (Fig. 29–6). It is not uncommon to see areas of necrosis with superficial bacterial infection. Hemorrhage is a common problem, and many animals will be presented because of persistent bleeding. In the male, a serosanguineous discharge from the prepuce is often the presenting clinical sign. TVTs are frequently

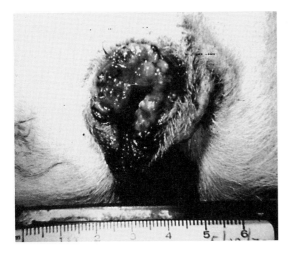

**Figure 29–6.** Vaginal TVT. Note cauliflower-like appearance.

located around the glans penis and therefore require total extension of the penis for visualization (Fig. 29–7). Extremely large masses may preclude total extension of the penis. These tumors can also be multicentric along the penis; they tend to be very friable and hemorrhage is quite possible.

TVTs can be seen in the oral cavity, the skin

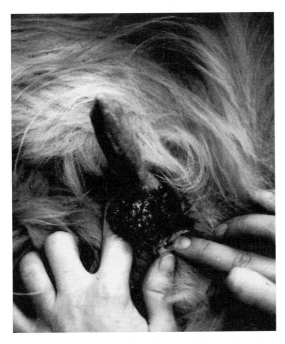

**Figure 29–7.** Proliferative TVT involving the base of the penis. The penis usually must be totally extended to visualize the tumor.

(Fig. 29–8), the sclera, and the anterior chamber. Intranasal TVTs frequently cause epistaxis and sneezing.

## DIAGNOSTIC TECHNIQUES AND WORKUP

The definitive diagnosis is based on either a histologic or cytologic evaluation of the tumor. Cytologically, the TVT has a very distinct appearance. The cells will appear round to oval, and mitotic figures are common (Fig. 29–9). Chromatin clumping and one or two prominent nuclei are obvious. Perhaps the most striking cytologic finding is the presence of multiple clear cytoplasmic vacuoles, frequently arranged in chains. The cytologic appearance of TVT is not readily confused with other neoplasms such as mast cell tumors, histiocytoma, and malignant lymphomas (see Chap. 5). Some of the oral TVTs have been misdiagnosed as an amelanotic melanoma or poorly differentiated sarcoma. In some cases it is easier to make a definitive diagnosis with cytology than with histology. If one suspects that a tumor may be a TVT, it is advisable to make impression smears of the tumor before or at the time of biopsy.

As previously mentioned, TVTs have been associated with a secondary polycythemia. A CBC should be performed during the evaluation of an animal with a TVT. Although metastasis is uncommon, regional lymph nodes should be evaluated thoroughly and for the possibility of metastasis. If there is any evidence of regional lymphadenopathy, then a fine-needle aspiration should be performed to rule out possible metastasis. Thoracic radiographs are invariably negative for metastasis.

## THERAPY

TVTs will respond to many forms of therapy. Surgery can be an effective therapy for small localized TVTs. Usually the TVT is too extensive for an adequate surgical excision, and other therapies must be considered.[16] Another problem with surgical excision has been the high recurrence rate associated with this treatment. Recurrence rates will vary from 20% to 60% depending on the location and extent of disease.[16]

Radiation therapy is also an effective method of treating TVT. Dosage recommendations range from 15 Gy (1,500 rads) divided over 5 days to 45

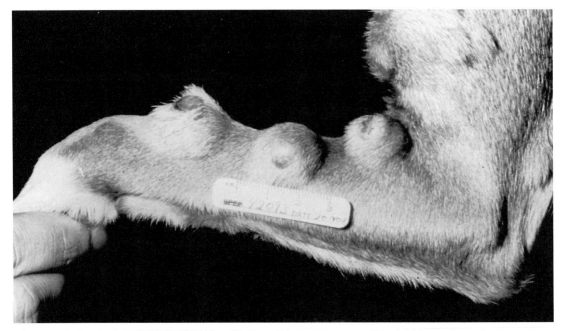

**Figure 29–8.**  TVT nodules in the skin of a dog. (Photo courtesy of Dr. Jack Broadhurst.)

Gy divided over 3 weeks. In one study, 18 TVT cases were treated with orthovoltage radiotherapy. Complete regression of the tumor in all 18 dogs was induced by radiotherapy, and no recurrence was observed within 1 year after completion of treatment. A dose of 10 Gy was applied in each treatment, and in most cases, 3 treatments were used to induce complete remission of the tumor.[17]

The most effective and efficient way to treat TVT is using chemotherapy.[18] A number of agents have been used to treat TVT. These include cyclophosphamide, vincristine, methotrexate, and doxorubicin. Vincristine has been reported to be one of the most effective agents in treating TVT.[19] Vincristine can be given at a dose of 0.5 to 0.7 mg/m$^2$ IV once weekly. An average of 4 to 6 treatments will be necessary in order to induce a complete remission. Complete cure can

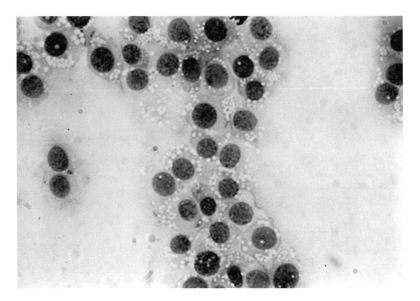

**Figure 29–9.**  A characteristic cytologic preparation of a fine-needle aspirate from a TVT. Note the prominent nuclei and multiple clear cytoplasmic vacuoles.

be expected in more than 90% of the cases treated. Doxorubicin has also been used quite effectively to treat TVT in vincristine-resistant cases. The dose commonly used is 30 mg/m² IV every 21 days. Two treatment courses are usually sufficient to induce complete and prolonged remissions.[20] In a recent study of 14 dogs infected with TVT[21] and treated with cyclophosphamide (50 mg/m² PO or IV) day 1 to 4 weekly for 6 weeks, only 2 of 14 dogs showed a partial response (<50% regression).[21] Another group of 8 dogs with TVT were treated with oral methotrexate (2.5 mg/m² PO QOD for 6 weeks) and no responses were noted.[21] Finally, 20 dogs with TVT were treated with vincristine (0.5 mg/m² IV) weekly until a response was noted.[21] All 20 dogs had a complete response and only 1 dog had recurrence within 12 months.[21] No toxicity was noted in those dogs treated with vincristine.

Biologic response modifiers have also been used experimentally to treat TVTs. Agents such as bacillus Calmette-Guérin (BCG), cell walls, and Staphylococcus Protein A have been used to treat TVTs.[22,23] Although responses have been noted with these treatments, the results are inconsistent and recurrences are frequent. To date, the use of biologic response modifiers must be considered to be investigational and certainly not as effective as chemotherapy.

## PROGNOSIS

With surgical excision alone there tends to be a high recurrence rate. Recurrence rates will vary from 20% to 60%, depending on the location and extent of disease.[24]

TVT is one neoplastic process that can be readily cured with chemotherapy. Most chemotherapy protocols will cure 90% to 95% of the animals treated.[18,19,21] The two drugs that have been shown to be most effective are vincristine and doxorubicin.

## REFERENCES

1. Stookey SL: Transmissible venereal tumors of dogs. J Natl Cancer Inst 32:315–320, 1969.
2. Richardson RC: Canine Transmissible Venereal Tumors. Compend Contin Educ Pract Vet 31:951–956, 1981.
3. Higgins DA: Observations on the canine transmissible venereal tumor as seen in the Bahamas. Vet Rec 79:67–71, 1966.
4. Cohen D: The canine transmissible venereal tumor: A unique result of tumor progression. Adv Cancer Res 43:75–112, 1985.
5. Sapp WJ, Adams EW: C-type viral particles in canine venereal tumor cell cultures. Am J Vet Res 31:1321–1323, 1970.
6. Murray M, James H, Martin WJ: A study of the cytology and karyotype of the canine transmissible venereal tumor. Res Vet Sci 10:565–568, 1969.
7. Epstein RB, Bennett BT: Histocompatibility typing and course of canine venereal tumors transplanted into unmodified random dogs. Cancer Res 34:788–793, 1974.
8. Palker TJ, Yang TJ: Identification and physiochemical characterization of a tumor-associated antigen from canine transmible venereal sarcoma. J Natl Cancer Inst 66:779–787, 1981.
9. Chandler JP, Yang TJ: Canine transmissible venereal sarcoma: Distribution of T and B lymphocytes in blood, draining lymph nodes, and tumours at different stages of growth. Br J Cancer 44:514–521, 1981.
10. Cohen D: In vitro cell mediated cytotoxicity and antibody-dependent cellular cytotoxicity to the transmissible venereal tumor of the dog. J Natl Cancer Inst 64:317–321, 1980.
11. Bennett BT, Debelak-Fehir KM, Epstein RB: Tumor blocking and inhibiting serum factors in the clinical cause of canine venereal tumor. Cancer Res 35:2942–2947, 1975.
12. Perez J, Bautista MJ, and Carrasco L, et al: Primary extragenital occurrence of transmissible venereal tumors: Three case reports. Canine Practice 19:7–10, 1994.
13. Weir EC, Pond MJ, Duncan JR, et al: Extragenital occurrence of transmissible venereal tumor in the dog: Literature review and case reports. J Am Anim Hosp Assoc 14:532–536, 1978.
14. Yang TJ, Jones JB: Canine transmissible venereal sarcoma: Transplantation studies in neonatal and adult dogs. J Natl Cancer Inst 51:1915–1918, 1973.
15. Yang TJ: Metastatic transmissible venereal sarcoma in a dog. J Am Vet Med Assoc 5:550–555, 1987.
16. Brodey RS, Roszel JF: Neoplasms of the canine uterus, vagina, and vulva. A clinicopathologic survey of 90 cases. J Am Vet Med Assoc 151:1294–1307, 1967.
17. Thrall DE: Orthovoltage radiotherapy of canine transmissible venereal tumors. Vet Rad 23:217–219, 1982.
18. Brown NO, Calvert C, MacEwen EG: Chemotherapeutic management of transmissible venereal tumors in 30 dogs. J Am Vet Med Assoc 176:983–986, 1980.
19. Calvert CA, Leifer CE, MacEwen, EG: Vincristine for treatment of transmissible venereal tumor. J Am Vet Med Assoc 181:163–164, 1982.
20. MacEwen EG: Personal observations, 1987.
21. Amber EI, Henderson RA, Adeyanju TB, et al: Single-drug chemotherapy of canine transmissible venereal tumor with cyclophosphamide, metho-

trexate, or vincristine. J Vet Intern Med 4:144–147, 1990.

22. Hess AD, Catchatourian R, et al: Intralesional Bacillus-Calmette-Guérin immunotherapy of canine venereal tumors. Cancer Res 37:3990–3994, 1977.

23. Cohen D, Fer MF, Pearson, et al: Treatment of canine transmissible venereal tumor by intravenous administration of Protein A. J Biol Resp Mod 3:271–277, 1984.

24. Amber EI, Henderson RA: Canine transmissible venereal tumor: Evaluation of surgical excision of primary and metastatic lesions in Zaria-Nigera. J Am Anim Hosp Assoc 18:350–352, 1982.

# D. Mesothelioma

## Laura D. Kravis, Richard R. Dubielzig, and E. Gregory MacEwen

### INCIDENCE AND RISK FACTORS

Mesothelioma is a rare neoplasm of dogs and cats affecting the epithelial cells lining the coelomic cavities of the body. In 1962, Geib et al. cited other reports indicating one case of mesothelioma in 1,000 dogs and three cases in 5,315 dogs.[1] In dogs, primary tumors affecting the thoracic cavity, abdominal cavity, pericardial sac, and vaginal tunics of the scrotum have been reported.[2,3] In the cat, primary mesotheliomas have been reported in the pericardium, pleura, and peritoneum.[4–7] Exposure to asbestos may be an important contributory factor to mesothelioma in pet dog populations. Affected dogs often have owners who have jobs or hobbies for which exposure to asbestos is a known risk.[8] The level of asbestos in lung tissues of affected dogs has been documented to be greater than controls.[8,9] Asbestos is a mineral that readily separates into long, flexible fibers, which are classified into chrysotile, which appears as a silky, serpentine fiber, and the amphiboles, which separate into straight, rodlike fibers. In humans, greater risk has been related to amphibole asbestos rather than chrysotile exposure.[10] Fortunately, more than 90% of asbestos used in North America is chrysotile.[10]

The underlying mechanisms of the neoplastic transformation of mesothelial cells, despite its association with asbestos, is not completely understood. There is considerable evidence to show that asbestos is a complete carcinogen, an initiator, and a tumor promoter, and causes chromosomal mutations in a variety of mammalian cells.[11,12] The neoplastic change is thought to result from repeated genetic damage to the tumor precursor cells due to oxygen-free radicals generated by macrophages as the cellular response to asbestos fiber phagocytosis. The simultaneous release of several growth factors [IL-1, fibroblast growth factor, and platelet-derived growth factor (PDGF)] from asbestos-activated macrophages contribute to the proliferative response.[13,14] In addition, the iron present in asbestos fibers may catalyze the generation of hydroxyl radicals responsible for DNA-strand breaks.[15]

Mesothelial tumors occur most often in older animals; however, in cattle and in sheep, newborn or young animals are affected.[16] A recent report of a 7-week old puppy with mesothelioma suggests a congenital form may exist for canines as well.[17]

### PATHOLOGY AND NATURAL BEHAVIOR

The normal mesothelium is a monolayer of flattened mesothelial cells. These cells are distinguished by the presence of microvilli, desmosomes, and evidence of phagocytic potential. Disease conditions associated with inflammation or irritation of the lining of the body cavity commonly result in a marked physiologic proliferation of the mesothelial cells. Fluid accumulation in a body cavity promotes exfoliation and implantation of mesothelial cells. Mesotheliomas are considered malignant because of their ability to seed the body cavity, resulting in multiple tumor growths. Distant metastasis is rare.

Mesothelial cells appear morphologically as epithelial cells; however, their derivation is from mesoderm. Mesothelioma can appear histologically as epithelial, mesenchymal, or mixed morphologic types. The epithelial form, which resembles carcinoma or adenocarcinoma, is by far the most common form in small animals. There are also several reports of a variation of the mes-

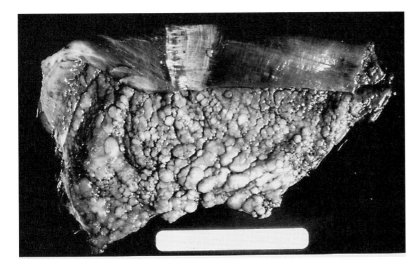

**Figure 29–10.** The diaphragm from a dog with abdominal mesothelioma is folded to show the affected side and the unaffected side.

enchymal form, which resembles sarcoma, and is referred to as sclerosing mesothelioma.[2,18–20]

## HISTORY AND SIGNS

Classical mesotheliomas occur as a diffuse nodular mass covering the surfaces of the body cavity (Fig. 29–10). Extensive effusions occur because of exudation from the tumor surface or from tumor-obstructed lymphatics; therefore, the most common presenting sign is dyspnea from pleural effusion or a distended abdomen from peritoneal effusion. Dogs with pericardial mesotheliomas can present with acute tamponade and right-sided heart failure.[21]

Sclerosing mesothelioma is a variation of mesothelial tumor seen primarily in male dogs with German shepherds being over-represented.[2,20] These tumors present as thick fibrous linings in the abdominal or pleural cavities (Fig. 29–11). Restriction occurs around organs in the affected area, and in the abdomen such changes can impinge on organs and often lead to vomiting and urinary problems.

## DIAGNOSTIC TECHNIQUE AND WORKUP

Mesothelioma should be suspected in adult dogs with evidence of chronic disease and fluid accumu-

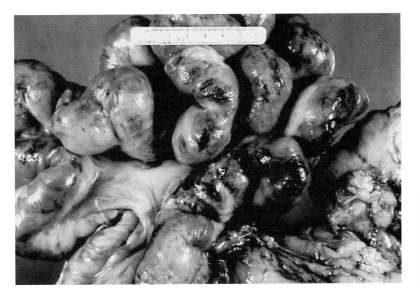

**Figure 29–11.** Loops of intestine from a dog with sclerosing mesothelioma. The thickening sclerosal surfaces must be distinguished from chronic inflammation.

lation in any of the body cavities. Cytologic evaluation of fluid can be diagnostic for other disease processes, such as infection or lymphoma, but will not conclusively diagnose mesothelioma. Mesothelial cells can be expected to proliferate under any circumstance associated with fluid accumulation in the body cavity, making the distinction between physiologic mesothelial proliferation and neoplasia difficult. Although malignant mesothelial cells easily exfoliate into effusion fluid, they are hard to distinguish from reactive hypertrophic mesothelial cells cytologically. Phagocytic transformation normally occurs in hyperplastic mesothelial reactions, thus making morphologic clues of malignancy difficult to assess.

Establishing a definitive diagnosis of malignant mesothelioma may be difficult, particularly early in the disease. The diagnosis of mesothelioma requires adequate tissue sampling, preferrably from an open, visually directed biopsy. The increasing availability of thoracoscopy and laparoscopy for small animals provides a less invasive way to evaluate these cases. In either procedure, the clinician or surgeon is cautioned to biopsy any body cavity lining when an obvious cause for fluid accumulation is not found. Sclerosing mesothelioma must be distinguished from chronic inflammatory diseases of the body cavity, such as chronic peritonitis, and histologic examination of biopsy material is essential to establish the diagnosis.

The most useful criteria in establishing a diagnosis of mesothelioma is to demonstrate that the tumor is primarily a neoplasm of the coelomic cavity lining and that the principle method of tumor spread is by transcoelomic implantation. Mesothelioma should be considered when the bulk of the neoplastic tissue exists on the coelomic surface. Histologically, mesotheliomas need to be differentiated from carcinomas, adenocarcinomas, or sarcomas, depending on the morphologic type of the mesothelioma. Unfortunately, there are no cellular markers that conclusively define the mesothelial cell. Recent advances in immunohistochemical staining has provided additional ways to examine neoplastic cells to help differentiate mesothelioma from other epithelial or mesenchymal tumors.[21–23]

## TREATMENT AND PROGNOSIS

No satisfactory treatment exists for mesothelioma. Radical excision may benefit some animals, but usually the tumors are too advanced locally and have spread by implantation early in the course of disease. Median survival without therapy is difficult to assess from reports, as the tumors are rare and animals frequently are euthanatized at the time of diagnosis.

Intracavitary cisplatin has shown good palliative potential in the dog; it was well tolerated and greatly decreased fluid accumulation in one study.[24] The treatments also appeared to arrest tumor growth for a limited time. Five of the six dogs treated had a partial response, with survivals close to one year, with one dog still alive at 807 days.[24] Unfortunately, penetration of the chemotherapy is only to a small depth (2–3 mm) and thus large masses will not be affected significantly. In such cases, combining debulking surgery or systemic chemotherapy, such as doxorubicin, vincristine, and cyclophosphamide (VAC), with intracavitary cisplatin may be of benefit.

## COMPARATIVE ASPECTS

In people, mesothelioma is closely linked to exposure to aerosolized asbestos fibers. More than 70% of cases have a history of industrial exposure to asbestos crystals in asbestos-related occupations or avocations.[25,26] Occupations such as shipbuilding, asbestos mining, auto mechanics, welding, and construction work are strong risk factors in the development of mesothelioma in people.[25] Family members of exposed industrial workers are at risk because of asbestos fiber exposure from the workers' clothing. Affected individuals routinely have greatly increased counts of asbestos fibers in parenchymal lung tissue.[25] The latency period from the time of exposure to tumor development is at least 20 years.[26]

Asbestos causes genetic damage that likely leads to a population of mesothelial cells that can secrete their own growth factors and thus begin unregulated growth.[26,27] Also, alterations in humoral and cellular immunity have been observed in individuals.[28,29] Suppression of cell-mediated immunity, especially depressed total T-cells and T-helper cells, has been found.[30,31] Thus, chronic immunosuppression may contribute to the development of the neoplasm.

In man, the median survival is 8 to 12 months after diagnosis. There is no standard therapy, as no therapies have been found to increase survival in randomized trials. In select patients with good prognostic indicators, including very confined disease, aggressive multimodality therapy, such as surgery, intracavitary cisplatin, and systemic chemotherapy, has been tried with some success in palliation and occasional long-term survival.[32] Doxorubicin either alone or in combination with other chemotherapeutic agents such as cyclophosphamide, DTIC, or mitomycin has shown some minimal responses. Aggressive surgery followed by radiation or chemotherapy, and more recently photodynamic therapy, have all been tried. Ongoing research at the molecular level of the neoplastic cells may define abnormalities that will allow for specific therapy at the biomolecular level.

## REFERENCES

1. Geib LW, DeNarvaez F, Eby CH: Pleural mesothelioma in a dog. J Am Vet Med Assoc *140*:1317–1319, 1962.
2. Dubielzig RR: Sclerosing mesothelioma in five dogs. J Am Anim Hosp Assoc *15*:745–748, 1979.
3. Thrall DE, Goldschmidt MM: Mesothelioma in the Dog: Six Case Reports. JAVRS *19*:107, 1978.
4. Tilley LP, Owens JM, Wilkins RJ, et al: Pericardial mesothelioma with effusion in a cat. J Am Anim Hosp Assoc *11*:60–65, 1978.
5. Carpenter JL, Andrews LK, Holzworth J, et al: Tumors and tumor-like lesions. *In* Holzworth J (ed): Diseases of the Cat: Medicine and Surgery. Philadelphia, WB Saunders, 1987, pp. 583–585.
6. Schaer M, Meyer DL: Benign peritoneal mesothelioma, hyperthyroidism, nonsuppurative hepatitis, and chronic disseminated intravascular coagulation in a cat: A case report. J Am Anim Hosp Assoc *24*:195–202, 1988.
7. Umphlet RC, Bertoy RW: Abdominal mesothelioma in a cat. Mod Vet Pract *69*:71–73, 1988.
8. Glickman LT, Domanski LM, Maguire TG, et al: Mesothelioma in pet dogs associated with exposure of their owners to asbestos. Environmental Res *32*:305, 1983.
9. Harbison ML, Godleski JJ: Malignant mesothelioma in urban dogs. Lab Invest *46*:34A, 1982.
10. Passeto MA, Calabresi P: Neoplasms of the mediastinum and mesothelioma. *In* Calabresi P, Schein PS, Rosenberg SA (eds): Medical Oncology. New York, Macmillian,1985, pp. 758–785.
11. Rieder CL, Sluder G, Brinkley BR: Some possible routes for asbestos-induced aneuploidy during mitosis in vertebrate cells. *In* Harris CC, Lechner JF, Brinkley BR (eds): Cellular and Molecular Aspects of Fiber Carcinogenesis. Plainview, TX, Cold Spring Harbor Lab Press, 1991, pp. 1–26.
12. Barrett JC: Role of chromosome mutations in asbestos-induced cell transformation. *In* Harris CC, Lechner JF, Brinkley BR (eds): Cellular and Molecular Aspects of Fiber Carcinogenesis. Plainview, TX Cold Spring Harbor Lab Press, 1991, pp. 27–39.
13. Betta PG: Recent advances in the biology of diffuse malignant mesothelioma. Cancer J *5*:249–253, 1992.
14. Craighead JE: Current pathogenetic concepts of diffuse malignant mesothelioma. Hum Pathol *18*:544–557, 1987.
15. Turver CJ, Brown RC: The role of catalytic iron in asbestos-induced lipid peroxidation and DNA-strand breakage in CH310T1/2 cells. Brit J Cancer *56*:133–136, 1987.
16. Head KW: Tumors of the alimentary tract. *In* Moulton JE (ed): Tumors in Domestic Animals, 3rd ed. Berkeley, University of California Press, 1990, pp. 422–427.
17. Leisewitz AL, Nesbit JW: Malignant mesothelioma in a seven-week-old puppy. J So Afr Vet Assn *63*:70–73, 1992.
18. Kannerstein M, Churg J: Desmoplastic diffuse malignant mesothelioma. Prog Surg Pathol *2*:19–29, 1979.
19. Whitaker D, Shilkin KB: Diagnosis of pleural malignant mesothelioma in life—A practical approach. J Pathol *143*:147–175, 1984.
20. Schoning P, Layton CE, Fortney WD, et al: Sclerosing peritoneal mesothelioma in a dog evaluated by electron microscopy and immunoperoxidase techniques. J Vet Diagn Invest *4*:217–220, 1992.
21. McDonough SP, MacLachlan NJ, Tobias AH: Canine pericardial mesothelioma. Vet Pathol *29*:256–260, 1992.
22. Brown RW, Clark GM, Tandon AK, et al: Multiple-marker immunohistochemical phenotypes distinguishing malignant pleural mesothelioma from pulmonary adenocarcinoma. Hum Pathol *24*:347–354, 1993.
23. Mayall FG, Goddard H, Gibbs AR: The diagnostic implications of variable cytokeratin expression in mesotheliomas. J Pathol *170*:165–168, 1993.
24. Moore AS, Kirk C, Cardona A: Intracavitary cisplatin chemotherapy experience with six dogs. J Vet Intern Med *5*:227–231, 1991.
25. McDonald JC, McDonald AD: Epidemiology of mesothelioma from estimated incidence. Prov Mod *6*:426, 1977.
26. Ramael M, Van Meerbeeck J, Van Marck E: Mesothelioma: Current insights. Cancer J *7*:174–180, 1994.
27. Pogrebniak HW, Lubensky IA, Pass HI: Differential expression of platelet-derived growth factor-beta in malignant mesothelioma: A clue to future therapies? Surg Oncol *2*(4):235–240, 1993.
28. Kagan E, Soloman A, Cochran JC, et al: Immunological studies of patients with asbestosis. I. Studies of cell-mediated immunity. Clin Exp Immunol *28*:261–267, 1977.
29. Kagan E, Soloman A, Cochran JC, et al: Immunological studies of patients with asbestosis. II. Stud-

ies of circulating lymphoid cell numbers and humoral immunity. Clin Exp Immunol 28:268–274, 1977.

30. Miller LG, Sparrow D, Ginns LC: Asbestos exposure correlates with alternations in circulating T-cells subsets. Clin Exp Immunol 51:110–116, 1983.

31. Lew F, Tsang P, Holland JF, et al: High frequency of immune dysfunctions in asbestos workers and in patients with malignant mesothelioma. J Clin Immunol 6:225–233, 1986.

32. Rice TW, Adelstein DJ, Kirby TJ, et al: Aggressive multimodality therapy for malignant pleural mesothelioma. Ann Thorac Surg 58(1):24–29, 1994.

# E. Neoplasia of the Heart

## William C. Kisseberth

## INCIDENCE AND RISK FACTORS

Cardiac tumors are rare in the dog and even more uncommon in the cat. Primary cardiac tumors were found in two of 2,500 dogs necropsied consecutively, and in one of 309 dogs evaluated with cardiac lesions.[1,2] The only primary tumors of the cardiovascular system found in a series of 4,933 feline necropsies were one case of mesothelioma of the pericardium and two cases of chemodectoma.[3] No age, sex, or breed predispositions have been reported specific for the site of these uncommon tumors. However, predisposing factors based on tumor histology are of significance. In the majority of reports, German shepherd dogs are the most commonly affected breed with hemangiosarcoma of the right atrium and auricle.[4,5] Aortic body tumors occur most commonly in older brachycephalic dogs.[6,7]

## PATHOLOGY AND NATURAL BEHAVIOR

Tumors of the heart may occur in intracavitary, intramural, or pericardial locations. Primary tumors may be benign or malignant, with most primary tumors in the dog occurring in the right atrium (Fig. 29–12). Metastatic tumors are more common than primary tumors in the heart; however, both are uncommon. Metastatic hemangiosarcoma (right auricle usually not involved), lymphoma, mammary gland carcinoma, pulmonary carcinoma, salivary gland adenocarcinoma, oral melanoma, oral squamous cell carcinoma, and mast cell tumor have been reported in the cat.[3,8,9]

The most common primary cardiac tumor in the dog is hemangiosarcoma, followed by aortic body tumors. Other primary cardiac tumors that have been reported in the dog include undifferentiated sarcoma, myxoma (Fig. 29–13), ectopic thyroid carcinoma, fibroma, fibrosarcoma, rhabdomyosarcoma, chondrosarcoma, mesothelioma, granular cell tumor, and osteosarcoma.[10–22]

## HISTORY AND CLINICAL SIGNS

The clinical signs of cardiac neoplasia are highly variable, making diagnosis difficult. Clinical signs vary, depending on the size and location of the primary tumor. Acute death from rupture of the tumor with subsequent acute blood loss, with or without cardiac tamponade, is a common sequelae of cardiac hemangiosarcoma. Sudden death due to cardiac dysrhythmia may also occur. Canine cardiac hemangiosarcoma, as well as the majority of other reported primary sarcomas of the heart in dogs, generally produce signs of right heart failure due to cardiac tamponade, and a preponderance of right-sided masses cause inflow obstruction. The clinical signs most commonly reported are dysrhythmias, ascites, exercise intolerance, dyspnea, pulse deficits, jugular pulses, muffled heart sounds, and syncope.[10–22] The clinical signs with heart-base tumors are most often associated with pericardial involvement of the tumor and an accompanying pericardial effusion.[3] Edema, ascites, cough, dyspnea, weight loss, and vomiting are the signs most commonly reported with aortic body tumors in the dog.[23] Heart-based masses are a common

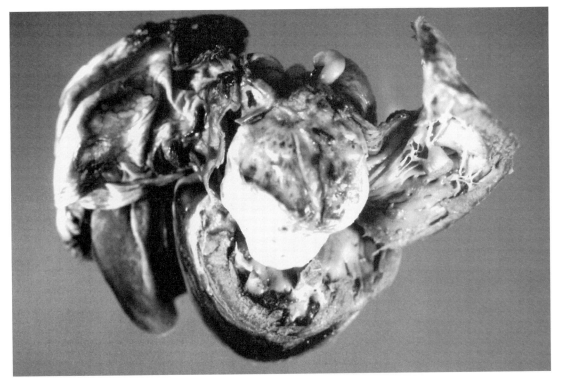

**Figure 29–12.** Right atrial mass in the heart of a dog. The histologic diagnosis was fibroma.

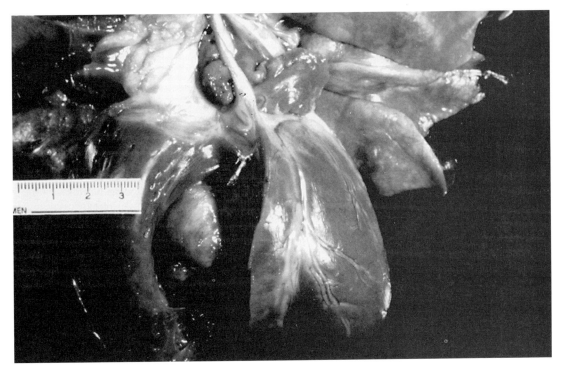

**Figure 29–13.** Intraventricular cardiac myxoma in a dog.

cause for cranial vena cava syndrome (edema of the head, neck, and forelimbs) due to tumor pressure on the cranial vena cava.

## DIAGNOSTIC TECHNIQUES AND WORKUP

The diagnosis of cardiac neoplasia in the dog and cat is usually based on clinical history, physical examination, radiographic findings, and echocardiographic findings, and is confirmed with biopsy when indicated. Electrocardiography may show any of a variety of dysrhythmias, which may correlate with the specific location of the primary or metastatic tumor, or be secondary to myocardial ischemia or hypoxia. Low-amplitude QRS complexes and electrical alternans may be seen in animals with pericardial effusion.[24] Thoracic radiographs may reveal cardiomegaly or effusions associated with cardiac tamponade. Mass lesions, if seen, are most common in the area of the right atrium and heart base. Echocardiography has become the most valuable diagnostic procedure for identifying tumors of the heart in cats and dogs.[25,26] In one canine study of histologically confirmed hemangiosarcoma of the right atrium/auricle, two-dimensional echocardiography had a positive predictive value of 92% (11/12) and a negative predictive value of 64% (9/14).[26] Tumor location (extrapericardial, noncavitary pericardial, and small right auricular masses) and size appear to be the most important factors for false negative results with echocardiography.[26] Pericardial effusions are a common finding associated with cardiac tumors in both the cat and the dog[20,26,27] Other clinical diagnostic methods for the evaluation of cardiac or pericardial masses include pneumopericardiography, selective and nonselective angiography, gated radionuclide imaging, and endomyocardial biopsy of selected patients.[28–30] Cytologic evaluation of pericardial fluid has proven to be nonspecific and of limited usefulness in the dog.[31]

Every effort should be made to determine the extent of disease and the existence of primary or metastatic sites elsewhere in the patient. A minimum data base of a CBC, serum biochemical profile, coagulation profile, thoracic radiographs, and abdominal ultrasound or radiographs should be obtained in patients identified with cardiac masses. If no other evidence of neoplastic disease is found, then surgical exploration with biopsy and attempted resection may be indicated.

Surgery may be best for palliation of clinical signs associated with the mass, particularly in cases of cardiac tamponade, which may benefit from pericardectomy.

## THERAPY

The treatment of most primary cardiac tumors is confined to medication directed at control of heart failure and dysrhythmias. Unfortunately, in many cases the hemodynamic consequences of the mass are relatively refractory to medical management. Surgical resection may be indicated in a small number of primary cardiac tumors.[4,13,32] Surgical resection of right auricular masses in dogs with cardiac hemangiosarcoma must be considered a palliative procedure because of the high probability of metastatic disease.

A mean survival time of 4 months has been reported for dogs with cardiac hemangiosarcoma undergoing surgery.[4] Doxorubicin, cyclophosphamide, vincristine combination chemotherapy has been reported for treatment of cardiac hemangiosarcoma in the dog (see Chap. 29A).[33]

## PROGNOSIS

The prognosis for primary cardiac tumors is generally poor. Most of the cases reported were poorly responsive to medical management. A mean survival time of 4 months (range 2 days to 8 months) has been reported for a small series of nine dogs with cardiac hemangiosarcoma undergoing surgery.[4] In another small series of four dogs treated with surgical excision for atrial hemangiosarcoma (two also received doxorubicin), all dogs died 3 to 5 months following surgery.[32] Tumors found at exploratory thoracotomy are commonly judged to be unresectable; however, a few cases of longer disease-free intervals following resection of tumors other than hemangiosarcoma have been reported.[13,32]

## COMPARATIVE ASPECTS

Primary tumors of the heart and pericardium are rare. In human beings they occur at a frequency of 0.001 to 0.28 % in reported or collected postmortem series.[34] Primary tumors are usually intracavitary and 75% are benign. Myxomas are the most frequent benign tumor of the heart. Seventy-five percent of myxomas occur in the left atrium; however, systemic tumor embolization occurs with high frequency.[35] Surgical resection of a myxoma is the treatment of choice, with recurrence of atrial myxomas being rare following resection.[35] Rhabdomyoma is the most frequent cardiac tumor of infants and children.[34] Other benign primary cardiac tumors that have been reported in people include fibroma, papillary fibroelastoma, lipoma, mesothelioma of the AV valve, hemangioma, lymphangioma, and intrapericardial paraganglioma.[35]

Almost all primary malignant cardiac tumors are sarcomas, most frequently, angiosarcomas. As is the case with hemangiosarcoma in the dog, angiosarcoma in people most commonly originates from the right atrium or pericardium.[35] Rhabdomyosarcoma and mesothelioma rank second and third, respectively, in frequency among primary malignant tumors of the heart and pericardium in human beings.[35] Effective palliation and local control of malignant primary tumors can be achieved with extensive resection. Adjuvant chemotherapy and radiation therapy may improve long-term prognosis. Cardiac transplantation has been utilized on occasion.[35]

Metastatic tumors involve the heart and pericardium 20 to 40 times more frequently than primary tumors.[36,37] Incidence rates of 3.4 % and 5.7 % myocardial metastases have been reported in two large autopsy studies of patients who died of cancer.[36,37] Malignant melanoma metastasizes to the myocardium most frequently, occurring in more than 50% of cases.[35] Cardiac metastases are frequent with bronchogenic carcinoma and carcinoma of the breast as well.[35]

# REFERENCES

1. Loppnow H von: Zur Kasuistik primärer Herztumoren beim Hund (2 Fälle von Häemangiomen am Rechten Herzohr). Berl Münch Tierärztl Wschr 74:214–217, 1961.
2. Luginbühl H, Detweiler DK: Cardiovascular lesions in dogs. Ann NY Acad Sci 127:517–540, 1968.
3. Tilley LP, Bond B, Patnaik AK, Liu SK: Cardiovascular tumors in the cat. J Am Anim Hosp Assoc 17:1009–1021, 1981.
4. Aronsohn M: Cardiac hemangiosarcoma in the dog: A review of 38 cases. J Am Vet Med Assoc 187:922–926, 1985.
5. Kleine W, Zook BC, Munson TO: Primary cardiac hemangiosarcoma in dogs. J Am Vet Med Assoc 157:326–337, 1970.
6. Hayes HM Jr: An hypothesis for the aetiology of canine chemoreceptor system neoplasms, based upon an epidemiological study of 73 cases among hospital patients. J Small Anim Pract 16:337–343, 1975.
7. Patnaik AK, Liu SK, Hurvitz AI, McClelland AJ: Canine chemodectoma (extra-adrenal paragangliomas)—A comparative study. J Small Anim Pract 16:785–801, 1975.
8. Klausner JS, Bell FW, Hayden DW, Hegstad RL, Johnston SD: Hypercalcemia in two cats with squamous cell carcinomas. J Am Vet Med Assoc 196:103–105, 1990.
9. Bortnowski HB, Rosenthal RC: Gastrointestinal mast cell tumors in two cats. J Am Anim Hosp Assoc 28:271–275, 1992.
10. Swartout MS, Ware WA, Bonagura JD: Intracardiac tumors in two dogs. J Am Anim Hosp Assoc 23:533–538, 1987.
11. Roberts SR: Myxoma of the heart in a dog. J Am Vet Med Assoc 134:185–188, 1959.
12. Bright JM, Toal RL, Blackford LM: Right ventricular outflow obstruction caused by primary cardiac neoplasia. J Vet Intern Med 4:12–16, 1990.
13. Ware WA, Merkley DF, Riedesel DH: Intracardiac thyroid tumor in a dog: Diagnosis and surgical removal. J Am Anim Hosp Assoc 30:20–23, 1994.
14. Lombard CW, Goldschmidt MH: Primary fibroma in the right atrium of a dog. J Am Anim Pract 21:439–448, 1980.
15. Atkins CE, Badertscher II RR, Greenlee P, Nash S: Diagnosis of an intracardiac fibrosarcoma using two-dimensional echocardiography. J Am Anim Hosp Assoc 20:131–137, 1984.
16. Vicini DS, Didier PJ, Ogilvie GK: Cardiac fibrosarcoma in a dog. J Am Vet Med Assoc 189:1486–1488, 1986.
17. Krotje LJ, Ware WA, Niyo Y: Intracardiac rhabdomyosarcoma in a dog. J Am Vet Med Assoc 197:368–371, 1990.
18. Southerland EM, Miller RT, Jones CL: Primary right atrial chondrosarcoma in a dog. J Am Vet Med Assoc 203:1697–1698, 1993.
19. Greenlee PG, Liu SK: Chondrosarcoma of the mitral leaflet in a dog. Vet Pathol 21:540–542, 1984.
20. Cobb MA, Brownlie SE: Intrapericardial neoplasia in 14 dogs. J Small Anim Pract 33:309–316, 1992.
21. Sanford SE, Hoover DM, Miller RB: Primary cardiac granular cell tumor in a dog. Vet Pathol 21:489–494, 1984.
22. Schelling SH, Moses BL: Primary intracardiac osteosarcoma in a dog. J Vet Diagn Invest 6:396–398, 1994.
23. Johnson KH: Aortic body tumors in the dog. J Am Vet Med Assoc 152:154–160, 1968.
24. Bonagura JD: Electrical alternans associated with pericardial effusion in the dog. J Am Vet Med Assoc 178:574–579, 1981.
25. Thomas WP, Sisson D, Bauer TG, Reed JR: Detection of cardiac masses in dogs by two-dimensional echocardiography. Vet Radiol 25:65–71, 1984.
26. Fruchter AM, Miller CW, O'Grady MR: Echocardiographic results and clinical considerations in

dogs with right atrial/auricular masses. Can Vet J *33:*171–174, 1992.

27. Rush JE, Keene BW, Fox PR: Pericardial disease in the cat: A retrospective evaluation of 66 cases. J Am Anim Hosp Assoc *26:*39–46, 1990.

28. Berg RJ, Wingfield W: Pericardial effusion in the dog: A review of 42 cases. J Am Anim Hosp Assoc *20:*131–137, 1984.

29. Ogilvie GK, Brunkow CS, Daniel GB, Haschek WM: Malignant lymphoma with cardiac and bone involvement in a dog. J Am Vet Med Assoc *194:*793–796, 1989.

30. Keene BW, Rush JE, Cooley AJ, Subramanian R: Primary left ventricular hemangiosarcoma diagnosed by endomyocardial biopsy in a dog. J Am Vet Med Assoc *197:*1501–1503, 1990.

31. Sisson D, Thomas WP, Ruehl WW, Zinkl JG: Diagnostic value of pericardial fluid analysis in the dog. J Am Vet Med Assoc *184:*51–55, 1984.

32. Wykes PM, Rouse GP, Orton C: Removal of five canine cardiac tumors using a stapling instrument. Vet Surg *15:*103–106, 1986.

33. De Madron E, Helfand SC, Stebbins KE: Use of chemotherapy for the treatment of cardiac hemangiosarcoma in a dog. J Am Vet Med Assoc *190:*887–891, 1987.

34. McAllister HA Jr: Primary tumors and cysts of the heart and pericardium. *In* Harvey WP (ed): Current Problems in Cardiology *4*(2):1–51, 1979. Chicago, Year Book Medical, 1979.

35. Hall RJ, Cooley DA, McAllister HA Jr, Frazier OH: Neoplastic heart disease. *In* Schlant RC et al (eds): Hurst's the Heart: Arteries and Veins. New York, McGraw-Hill, 1994, pp. 2007–2029.

36. Prichard RW: Tumors of the heart: Review of the subject and report of one hundred and fifty cases. Arch Pathol *51:*98–128, 1951.

37. DeLoach JF, Haynes JW: Secondary tumors of the heart and pericardium: Review of the subject and report of one hundred thirty-seven cases. Arch Intern Med *91:*224–249, 1953.

# 30

# Companion Animal Death and Pet Owner Grief*

Laurel Lagoni, Carolyn Butler, and Stephen J. Withrow

Cancer is the leading cause of death in dogs and cats and shows no signs of decreasing.[1] Although many animals who have cancer can be treated and even cured, patient death is an inevitable part of veterinary oncology. Companion animal death is often accompanied by grief. Therefore, helping pet owners deal with grief is also an essential aspect of contemporary veterinary oncology.

Many veterinary oncologists feel awkward and uncomfortable when attempting to help pet owners deal with grief. In fact, it is tempting for some veterinary oncologists to treat their clients' manifestations of grief the way some pet owners treat their pets' mysterious physical "lumps and bumps" that is, to silently say, "I'll just watch them and hope they will go away." The grief specific to veterinary oncology, though, does not go away and should not be side stepped. This chapter addresses many of the medical *and* emotional issues pertinent to veterinary oncology and offers suggestions about how veterinarians can effectively help pet owners attend to them.

## THE HUMAN-ANIMAL BOND

Pet owners who seek involved and often costly treatment for their companion animals' cancers are usually highly attached to their pets. Highly attached owners often think of their pets as chil-

dren, best friends, partners, confidantes, and even soul mates. One study has shown that 99% of cat and dog owners consider their pets to be full-fledged family members.[2] In another report 82% of cat owners and 73% of dog owners cite companionship as the major reason for owning their pets.[3]

The pressures of a modern, mobile society have changed the nature of traditional support systems. In today's culture, divorced, widowed, never-married, and childless people make up larger segments of Western society than ever before. Frequent moves and self-care situations for children whose parents work are common. Later in life, many men and women live by themselves and endure the hardship of loneliness in their personal lives. Without spouses, close friends, or sympathetic family members nearby, many people have grown to rely on animals for comfort and companionship. In fact, for many people, companion animals are their primary sources of emotional and social support, and their pets' devotion is often credited with pulling owners through the "rough spots" in their lives.[4]

## WHEN THE HUMAN-ANIMAL BOND IS BROKEN

Mounting evidence indicates that the grief pet owners feel when their pets die is often over-

*This chapter is based, in large part, on previously published material found in Lagoni L, Butler C, Hetts S: *The Human-Animal Bond and Grief.* Philadelphia, WB Saunders Company, 1994; and in Butler C, Lagoni L, Dickinson K,

Withrow SJ: Cancer. *In* Cohen SP, Fudin CE (eds): *Problems in Veterinary Medicine: Animal Illness and Human Emotion,* Vol. 3, No. 1, 1991, pp. 21–37. Permission has been granted by the publishers , JB Lippincott Company, Philadelphia.

whelming and that the response to pet loss often parallels the response to the loss of human companions. In one study, 75% of pet owners reported experiencing difficulties or disruptions in their lives after pets died.[5] For example, one third of the owners experienced difficulties in their relationships with others and/or needed to take time off from work because of their feelings of grief.

In this study, researchers examined the responses of 242 middle-aged couples who reported the death of a pet within the past 3 years. Couples were asked to rate the stress level associated with 48 events they had endured, including the death of a spouse, a divorce, marriage, the loss of children, the loss of a job, and the death of a pet. Researchers found that the death of a pet was the most frequently reported trauma experienced by the couples participating in the study.[5] Survey participants said the deaths of their pets were less stressful than the deaths of human members of their immediate families, but more stressful than the deaths of other relatives. Forty percent of wives and 28% of husbands reported that the loss of a pet was "quite" or "extremely" disturbing.[5]

Grief is the natural and spontaneous response to loss. It is the normal way to adjust to endings and to change. Grief is the necessary process for healing the emotional wounds caused by loss. Grief is a *process*, not an event. Normal grief may last for days, weeks, months, or even years, depending on the significance of the loss. During the process of normal grieving, the level of emotional intensity ranges on a continuum from no reactions at all to suicide ideation (e.g., thinking about suicide, but not acting on the thoughts). The intensity of a person's grief response is based on several factors. These include the nature of the loss, the circumstances surrounding the loss, the griever's emotional status before the loss, and the availability of emotional support before, during and after the loss.[4] If progressing in a healthy manner, grief lessens in intensity over time. Clinical experience shows that when the expression of grief is restricted in some way, the healing time for recovery is prolonged. Likewise, when grief is freely expressed, the healing time for recovery from loss is, in general, greatly reduced.

The grief response is unique to each individual. There is no right or wrong way to grieve. Grief is also unique to different groups, societies, and cultures. In most cases, the variables of age, gender, and developmental status greatly affect people's expressions of grief. For instance, research has conclusively confirmed that women shed more tears and cry more often when grieving than men.[6] This is probably because men are socialized to maintain their composure during emotional times, while women are socially conditioned to express their feelings more openly.

Research also confirms that children grieve just as deeply as adults, though, because of their shorter attention spans, they do so more sporatically. Children most often express their grief through behaviors rather than through words. They act out their grief through artwork, play behaviors, or expressions of anger and irritability. In large part, this is because, until children reach the age of 8 or 9 they do not possess the cognitive development and language capabilities necessary to express grief verbally.[7]

## CANCER DIAGNOSIS

Many pet owners who bring their companion animals to veterinary oncologists have been referred by their local veterinarians. Most often, they already suspect that their companion animals have cancer. So they are somewhat prepared to have their worst fears confirmed.

However, when owners receive a diagnosis of cancer from a veterinarian, it is often a startling revelation. There are few words in the English language that evoke such depth and variety of emotion as the word *cancer*. For many, the word suggests pain, suffering, and a death sentence for their pet. Believing death is imminent, many pet owners turn to their veterinary oncologist for help in coping with their emotional pain. Therefore, diagnosis should be viewed as a time for both medical consultation and emotional support.

### The Goals of Diagnosis

Veterinary oncologists often need to deliver bad news to pet owners. If veterinarians fail to win their client's trust during the delivery of bad news, effective case management is jeopardized. Therefore, the time invested in educating and reassuring clients during this crucial time pays off later. Clinical experience shows that the majority of angry, time-consuming interactions that take place later between clients and their veterinarians are traceable to previous episodes of poor communication during the delivery of bad news[1] and the details that accompany it (e.g., explanations of treatment options, possible complications, and probable outcomes). The goals when delivering diagnoses to clients, then, are to provide bad news in a sensitive manner while, at the same time, establishing trust and rapport. Both of these goals are accomplished by patiently and effectively addressing clients' fears, anxiety, and grief.

**Establishing Trust and Rapport**  Veterinarians should keep several things in mind when delivering bad news. First, one of the best techniques for establishing trust and rapport with clients and for conveying understanding and concern is making direct eye contact. Another effective technique is using a calm, quiet voice. The tone, pacing, and pitch of a veterinarin's voice is also important. To be calming and reassuring, veterinarians need to use a voice that is slightly more quiet, slow paced, and low pitched than normal. Also, instead of becoming caught up in their client's panic (often reflected in their voices by high pitch and rapid rate of speech), veterinarians can counter it with attentive, calm, and controlled speech.

It is also important for veterinarians to remember that when pet owners receive a diagnosis of cancer for their pets, the normal grief process begins, and it often begins with an emotional crisis. People in crisis drop to lower levels of functioning. This means that the typical methods they use to respond to information are altered or suspended. It also means that shock, denial, and high levels of anxiety inhibit and distort information processing.

Clients in crisis are helped by structure. Concise directions from their veterinarian help them know what steps to take next. "Please have a seat," "Follow me over here to the view box. I want to be sure you understand the X rays," and "I'm going to give you time to think about this and review what we've talked about while I see my next client. I'll be back to answer any questions you have in about 20 minutes," are examples of gentle, directive statements that provide appropriate structure during crisis.

As feelings of grief overwhelm pet owners, many of them openly display their emotions. If emotions are ignored, clients feel uncared for and if emotions are dwelled on, clients feel embarrassed. There are many nurturing ways to address clients' emotions. Many of these make use of nonverbal communication. For example, there is a nurturing and a non-nurturing way to

hand facial tissues to clients who are crying. The non-nurturing way is to avoid eye contact, pick up the tissue box, and wave it in the clients' direction as they struggle to gain composure. The nurturing way is to pull one or two tissues from the box, make direct eye contact with the clients, hand them the tissues, and touch them lightly on the arm. Saying something like, "I see how much you love Rex. I would expect you to cry in this situation," reassures pet owners and gives them permission to respond to the cancer diagnosis in whatever way feels right to them.

When pet owners feel their emotional concerns are valid and understood, they can relax and listen to more medical information. For example, at this point, pet owners can be told about treatment procedures, clinic philosophies, and staff availability. They can also be given specific information about acceptable and unacceptable activities for animals who are undergoing treatment. It is a good idea to collect handouts covering a wide range of cancer-related topics into an informational packet. Handout topics can include details on what to expect from amputation, cryosurgery, limb sparing, radiation and chemotherapy (each drug and protocol should have a separate handout), euthanasia, and grief support services.

**Providing Bad News in a Sensitive Way**
There are no strategies or methods that allow veterinarians to break bad news painlessly. No matter how carefully veterinarians handle their clients' feelings, awkward moments and various manifestations of grief always occur. When delivering bad news, veterinarians should prepare themselves to deal with shock, disbelief, anger, sadness, and even hysteria, because how clients will react to bad news is largely unpredictable. Sometimes clients react with rage, confusion, or aimless pacing. They may also direct suspicious accusations at the veterinarian or overwhelming feelings of guilt at themselves. In contrast, numbness and shock may cause some clients to appear calm, detached, stoic, and in control. In the wake of bad news, this control can seem eerie, confusing, and grossly inappropriate.

Three methods of approach can be used to deliver bad news:[8] (1) the blunt and unfeeling way; (2) the kind and sad way; and (3) the understanding and positive way. The last is probably the most effective. To convey bad news with an understanding and positive attitude, it should be delivered in stages, because it takes time for clients to realize fully the magnitude of what they have been told. In fact, many clients will remember little about the first conversation concerning the bad news about their pet. Thus, they may ask many of the same questions during their next conversation with their veterinarian.

A leading crisis intervention expert suggests a three-step process for delivering bad news to clients:[9] (1) preparing clients emotionally for what is to come, (2) predicting how clients may feel or respond when the news is given, and (3) offering clients information in brief bits of conversation. For instance, when delivering a diagnosis of cancer, a veterinarian might say, "Mrs. Brown, I have some bad news that may be upsetting for you to hear" (preparing and predicting) and then continue with, "The tests results show that Rambo has osteosarcoma or cancer of the bone (information). This is a kind of cancer we can treat but may not be able to cure (information)." After saying this much, the veterinarian should stop because, at this point, there is usually some sort of emotional reaction from the client. It might be sobbing, protests of disbelief, anger, or complete silence. It is important then to ask what the client needs next, providing the client with more detailed medical information immediately, providing it in a half-hour or so by seeing or calling again after the veterinarian has seen another patient, or setting an appointment for later in the day (perhaps with the addition of other family members or supportive friends) so medical details can be discussed at length.

When delivering a diagnosis, veterinarians need to be aware of of the effect of silence. Silence can be hard to read. Sometimes it is hard to know whether clients need time to cry or to collect their thoughts or whether they are unsure about what to say next or how to answer your question. Veterinarians sometimes feel that silence means they have offended their client somehow. The most effective way to address silence is simply to make comments such as

"I'm right here for you. Take your time."
"I can imagine how hard this is for you to talk about. Cry if you need to . . . I would cry, too, if I were facing this situation."
"All of this is pretty overwhelming."
"You've been very quiet for a while now. Do you want to continue talking with me at this time or shall we arrange a time to talk later?"

When veterinarians are uncomfortable with silences, they often repeat themselves or relay information in booming "lecture" voices. They may also "protect" themselves from the tension silence can create by placing physical and emotional barriers between them and their clients. Exam tables, chairs, and clipboards are all examples of protective barriers. When nothing else is available, open space works as one. Thus, veterinarians may position themselves at one end of an exam room while clients sit or stand at the other.

Veterinarians may also attempt to protect themselves by discussing cancer in ambiguous or evasive ways. In addition, they may rely too much on medical jargon. However, false promises, cancer euphemisms, and complicated scientific explanations do not help the average pet owner. In fact, they can be confusing and upsetting. A sympathetic, simple, and honest discussion of cancer is far more beneficial.

Another technique veterinarians can use in delivering bad news is called structuring the environment, that is, planning ahead for potentially emotional conversations by taking control of the physical parts of the interaction. Preparations may include arranging chairs for face-to-face conversation, gathering educational props and materials, or stocking the room with facial tissue before bringing clients into the room. It may even mean setting up videotape equipment so pet owners can view educational programs specific to their pet's disease or treatment.

Animal health technicians or other staff members can also be helpful to clients who receive disturbing diagnoses when they take notes or draw pictures of complicated medical information as the veterinarian talks. Sometimes they can even arrange or facilitate meetings with other clients whose pets have similar conditions.

Some veterinarians tape-record their diagnosis and descriptions of treatment options and give the audiotapes to clients so they can literally take the information home with them. Tape-recording the diagnosis allows clients to listen to the information again when they are in a more relaxed, familiar environment and to share the information with other members of their family as well. In a survey of 41 human patients whose physicians used tape recordings, 77% of them wrote extremely positive comments about the technique and no negative statements were made.[10] When delivering diagnoses, it is also helpful to make written information available for clients to read.

Well-planned diagnostic presentations greatly increase client's understanding of disease and its treatment. They also go a long way in calming clients' fears and easing their feelings of anxiety.

It cannot be overemphasized that the diagnostic encounters that take place between veterinarians and their clients set the groundwork for all the other interactions that follow.

## What to Say, What to Do during Diagnosis

In response to open displays of emotion like crying, which is a normal and natural response to loss, veterinarians can offer their clients facial tissues and then remain silent until they have had a chance to work through the wave of emotion. It is best not to leave the room. Leaving communicates embarrassment or disapproval. In some cases, veterinarians might suspect that a diagnosis of cancer is tied to another experience with cancer or death and say something like, "What is your personal experience with cancer? Has someone close to you had this disease?" Veterinarians should demonstrate genuine concern. If veterinarians are unable to spend much time with clients, they can find another staff member or a human service professional who can and then check in with the clients as often as possible.

In response to the question "How long does my pet have?" the veterinarian might say,

> How long Pepper will live depends on a variety of factors, including tumor size, tumor location, rate of growth, type of treatment, and so forth. I can and will give you "exact" figures for survival for a series of animals, but it is important to remember that Pepper is an individual and outcomes can be better or worse than the averages. For example, if I tell you that 50% of animals with this disease and treatment live 1 year, the good news is that there is a 50% chance that Pepper will live 1 year or longer. On the other hand, however, the bad news is that there is also a 50% chance that Pepper will *not* live a year. In other words, we can give you only general probabilities of survival and not absolute numbers. Whatever happens, though, we will fight this thing together and as a team.
>
> In response to the question "Should I have found the cancer sooner?" the veterinarian might say, for example,
>
>> It probably would have been hard for you to find it sooner. All cancers are relatively advanced when first detected. In one cubic centimeter, or the tip of your little finger, there are already a billion cells. For some cancers, size is important in allowing effective treatment. For others, it isn't. We've found it now and that is what is important.

Gestures (e.g. light touches on the arm), body posture (e.g., leaning toward clients), and facial expressions (e.g., reassuring smiles) should be

patient and kind and match the veterinarian's calming words.

In response to the question "Is my pet in pain?" the veterinarian might say, for example,

> Rarely does cancer cause excruciating pain. Rather it causes dull aches, loss of function, or flulike symptoms. The best form of pain relief is to treat Pepper's underlying cause of disease and that is what we will do with cancer treatment. We can give Pepper pain medication, but only rarely does it have a meaningful impact on chronic, serious discomfort.

## CANCER TREATMENT

All too often, veterinarians in private practice recommend no treatment or euthanasia when cancer is diagnosed or even suspected in companion animals. Yet owners often want and always deserve more accurate diagnostic and treatment options in addition to euthanasia for cancer in their pets. Options are easier to provide when the reasons behind the increase in the numbers of owners who seek cancer treatment for their pets are clearly understood. There are four main reasons:

1. *The increase in the prevalence of cancer in companion animals.* With modern advances in veterinary and preventative medicine, companion animals now live longer lives. Routine physical examinations, good nutrition, regular vaccinations, and stricter leash laws all play roles in the longer life spans enjoyed by today's pets. With advanced age, though, comes an increase in the likelihood that companion animals will develop cancer. In fact, cancer accounts for almost half of the deaths of pets 10 years of age or older.[1]

2. *The status many companion animals enjoy in families.* The bonds between pet owners and companion animals often intensify as traditional family structures and support systems change (e.g., couples divorce, choose not to have children, outlive their spouses). Pets are often thought of as children, best friends, partners, and confidantes and viewed as consistent sources of unconditional love and companionship. Many pet owners consider their pets to be full family members and want to care for them just as they would care for human members of their families.[2]

3. *Pet owners' personal experiences with cancer and their heightened levels of awareness about treatment possibilities.* It is most likely that many of the pet owners that veterinarians encounter have previous personal experience with the disease of cancer, since one fourth of

U.S. citizens can be expected to develop cancer in their lifetimes. Pet owners may have cancer themselves. Even clients who have not encountered cancer in their personal lives may be well informed about the disease because of the extensive exposure about advances and progress in treatment in the media.

4. *The desire to participate in the battle against cancer.* Regardless of the outcome, when two forces meet—one life-sustaining (spirit) and one life-threatening (cancer)—the result is intensely moving. Because the course of most cancer treatment is often unpredictable, the fight against it is mental and emotional as well as physical. Patients, pet owners, families, friends, and members of the veterinary treatment team all are caught up in the spirit of battle. For many owners, playing even a small role in the attempt to learn about and eradicate the disease of cancer is a satisfying accomplishment.

## The Goals of Treatment

When cancer is confirmed, some action is usually advised. Several options for treatment are offered, including palliation, cure, and sending the pet "home to die" with no further intervention. Depending on the medical status of the animal, a fourth option is euthanasia. Two further propositions much appreciated by pet owners are permission to seek second opinions from other veterinarians and referral to veterinary oncologists who are practicing at hospitals specializing in cancer treatments.

There is a widely held belief that directing clients to specialists causes them to abandon their referring veterinarians. Clinical experience indicates that clients appreciate their referring veterinarians much more when they realize how much referrals to specialists impact their pets' quality of life and survival. Timely referrals only serve to deepen pet owners' loyalty to and trust in their referring veterinarians.

The two main goals veterinary oncologists strive toward during treatment are to prolong the quality and quantity of pets' lives and to guide pet owners through the emotional ups and downs of cancer treatment. Several predictable crisis points occur during treatment: the recurrence of tumor, unexpected complications, unexpected death, and the decision to euthanatize. While treatment progresses, veterinarians must strike a balance between sustaining client hope and providing honest, realistic assessments about the status of the disease. When hope runs too high, veterinarians must offer gentle reminders about the cancer treatment's ultimate outcome.

### Prolonging Quality and Quantity of Life
Quantity of life is meaningless without quality of life. Quality of life means different things to different people. For some, it is manifested in their pets' abilities to chase balls or greet them in the evenings. For others, it is in simply knowing their pets are eating and sleeping through peaceful, painless days.

The quality-of-life issue that holds the most significance for owners is pain. Most responsible owners are loathe to treat cancer when they feel there is a significant chance of long-term or chronic pain for their pets. They are also prepared to stop treatment when the spread of the disease causes their companion animals undue discomfort. When a cure is not possible, palliative procedures (e.g., pain relief, use of anti-inflamatory drugs) improve the patient's quality of life while not necessarily improving the odds of survival. The veterinary oncologist must help clients stay clear on the difference between quantity and quality of life.

Some cancers are incurable with the current methods of treatment. When a cure is possible, treatment for cancer is often aggressive. Cures do occur for pets afflicted with cancer, but they are not guaranteed. The research data on cure rates report 1- or 2-year survival times as applied to large groupings of companion animals. These statistics do not necessarily apply to individual pets. With all of the scientific knowledge veterinarians have at their disposal, the hard fact is that medicine at large, and oncology specifically, is riddled with a degree of uncertainty.

### Guiding Owners through Treatment   Owners respond to their pets' cancer treatments in many ways. Two of the most extreme responses are fierce dedication and deep doubt. It is predictable that clients displaying either of these responses are more anxious about facing the imminent deaths of their pets.

Clients who are fiercely dedicated to their pets sometimes give up huge portions of their personal lives to care for their companion animals. Some spend several months sleeping on floors beside their pets or quit their jobs in order to be available to them full time. Clients with deep doubts about treatment often second-guess each decision and begin every day with anxiety. The question "Is today the day that Pepper will die?" is never far from their thoughts.

These kinds of clients present veterinary oncologists with unique challenges. The reassurance and support required by these clients is perhaps best met when one member of the treatment team is a professional pet-loss counselor. Veterinary oncologists are, after all, medical professionals and are not expected to attend fully to the sometimes complicated psychosocial and emotional problems of their clients.

## What to Say, What to Do during Treatment

In response to pet owners' financial concerns, the veterinarian might say,

> I will give you all of the options and support you with whichever option you feel is right for you. Cancer treatments can cost thousands of dollars and very few people can afford treatments that interfere with their basic living expenses. Every family has pressing priorities and treating pets for cancer is only one of those priorities.

The veterinarian must be aware that financial pressures arise throughout treatment and may cause clients to terminate treatment unexpectedly.

Many pet owners feel guilty after stopping cancer treatment or after euthanatizing their pets. Articles in popular magazines, television programs, or well-meaning neighbors who claim to know "miracle-working" veterinarians cause clients to second-guess their decisions. In response to expressions of guilt, the veterinarian might say something like, "You have done everything you could possibly do for Pepper. We could dream up something more to do *to* him, but that would not be doing the best thing *for* him. If you could do this all over again, would you do anything different?" Clients *usually* respond to this question by saying no and, after reviewing their decisions, are reassured that they acted in their pets' best interests every step of the way.

## When Cancer Treatment Options are Exhausted—Patient Death and Euthanasia

With modern veterinary medicine, so many conventional and experimental treatments are available for cancer that it is easy for owners to settle into a false sense of security about never-ending treatment options. When all treatment methods fail, though, helpless and hopeless feelings similar to those that overcame clients at the initial diagnosis may resurface. This is the phase during which it is appropriate to "watch and wait" as the disease takes its inevitable course.

During this phase, it is the responsibility of each member of the veterinary oncology team to continue to relay honest information about the perceived amount of discomfort the animal is experiencing and to remind clients gently about the low probability for quality life in the future. False hope at this time encourages denial and is ultimately unfair to both clients and patients.

As veterinary professionals wait and continue to watch the companion animals they have grown to love and respect, they must discuss with owners what signals to look for as death draws near. Owners are encouraged to establish personal "bottom lines" for their pet's levels of deterioration. For some, the bottom line is their pet's lack of interest in eating or in going for walks. For others, it is the agony of watching their pet struggle to breathe or to "get comfortable." For many clients, it is either their pet's inability to respond to them *or* their pet's struggle to muster even a small response that aids their final decision to euthanatize. Clinical experience shows that the majority of pet owners "know" instinctively when their pet's fight with cancer is over and that their decision to euthanatize is supported by treatment team members 99% of the time.

Even though there is agreement about timing, the euthanasia of a companion animal after intense bouts with cancer treatment is an emotionally draining experience for everyone involved in the case. The results from studies in human medicine show that deaths after long, lingering illnesses are among the hardest losses people face.[11] Survivors often feel exhausted after they have cared for loved ones who have lingered and who have needed considerable physical care during and after treatment. These findings are equally relevant to pet loss. Like human caregivers, pet owners and veterinary professionals who provide extensive medical and nursing care for pets with cancer frequently struggle with conflicting feelings of grief and relief after their pets die.

The more negative feelings associated with grief, such as guilt, doubt, regret, and anger, are greatly reduced when care is taken to provide pets and pet owners with the most sensitively conducted euthanasias possible. A great deal has been written about client-present euthanasia in recent years. Humane procedures and emotionally supportive methods are well defined.[4] Several points are unique to cancer-related euthanasias.

More and more frequently, euthanasia is viewed, by veterinarians and companion animal owners alike, as a medical privilege and as a gift that can be lovingly bestowed upon dying animals. Thus, today, many euthanasias are conducted like ceremonies, with the process itself treated with the respect and reverence it deserves. To facilitate owner-present euthanasias effectively, veterinarians must prepare owners to be present (if this is what they choose to do) during their animal's death and they must understand how to facilitate the actual euthanasia procedure with both technical efficiency and emotional sensitivity.

## The Goals When Treatment Options Are Exhausted

Because the owners of pets with cancer have invested so much in the physical care of their companion animals, their pets' bodies become symbolic to them. During treatment, they become very attuned to even the most subtle physical changes in their pets. As death approaches, owners expect their veterinarians to continue to treat their pets' bodies with respect and reverence. The goals of post-treatment interactions, then, are to facilitate sensitively the euthanasia procedure and provide effective follow-up care for both the clients and the members of the veterinary oncology team.

### Sensitively Facilitating the Euthanasia Procedure
Without question, it is emotionally painful for owners to be present when their dearly loved companion animals die. However, clinical experience with owners shows that *not* being present when their companion animals die potentially increases pet owners' feelings of pain and distress. There are several reasons owners want to be present when their companion animals die or are euthanatized:

1. Owners feel their companion animals have always "been there" for them; therefore, owners do not want to feel they have abandoned their pets at death.
2. Owners want to know for certain that their companion animals died peacefully and without pain and that their deaths actually occurred.
3. Owners want the last thing their animals hear and feel to be the owners' soothing words and the owners' loving touches. They also want the chance to say good-bye to their companion animals, not before or after death, but at the moment death occurs.

It is intimidating for some owners to ask to be present with their animals when they die. From the perspective of companion animal owners, veterinarians are authority figures. It is the veterinarian's responsibility, then, to *offer* companion animal owners the choice to be present at euthanasia.

To make educated and informed choices about this option, owners need to know what the procedure entails. Veterinary oncologists may provide this information to pet owners by saying something like the following:

> Sarah, we know that Buster is very important to you and to your family. Therefore, we are committed to making the euthanasia experience as meaningful and as positive for you as possible. In order to decide whether or not you want to be with Buster when he dies, you need accurate information about euthanasia. Would you like me to explain the procedure to you now?

With the owner's permission, the veterinarian continues:

> The first thing we may do in preparation for euthanatizing Buster is to take him back to our treatment area, shave a small area of fur, and place an intravenous catheter in a vein, most likely in one of his rear legs. The use of a catheter allows us to administer the euthanasia solution more smoothly. It also means that we can accomplish what we need to do without interfering with your desire to pet or to hold Buster's head.
>
> After this, Buster will be brought back to you and you will be given time to spend with him, if you so desire. Then, when all of us agree that it is time to proceed, we will begin the euthanasia process. The method we prefer to use involves three injections. The first is merely a saline solution flush that ensures the catheter is working. The second is a barbiturate, usually thiopental, which places Buster into a soothing state of relaxation. The third injection is the euthanasia solution, usually pentobarbitol sodium. This injection will actually stop Buster's heart, brain activity, and other bodily functions, and ultimately cause his death. Many people are surprised by how quickly death takes place because it occurs within a matter of seconds after the last injection is given.
>
> You should also know that, although humane death by euthanasia is usually peaceful, Buster may urinate, have a bowel movement, twitch, or even let out a few loud sighs. He will not be aware of any of this, though, and he will not feel any pain. In addition, Buster's eyes will probably not close. (Pause) Do you have any questions about any of this?

If the owner expresses understanding, the veterinarian concludes:

Sarah, after Buster has died, you can stay with his body as long as possible.

Altogether, this explanation need take only about 5 to 10 minutes. This explanation is greatly enhanced when the conversation is conducted in a private, quiet setting with both the owners and the veterinarian sitting or standing at the same eye level. It is also enhanced when veterinarians demonstrate their sense of compassion by offering facial tissues, supportive touches, or even hugs to owners who cry or openly express their feelings.

The second component of euthanasia preparation is planning and agreeing upon the logistical details of the procedure. For example, appropriate times and sites for the procedure must be determined. Owners must also decide who else, if anyone, they want to accompany them to the euthanasia. For example, with proper preparation, children often choose to be present when their companion animals die. It is a good idea for veterinarians to encourage owners to ask someone to attend their companion animals' euthanasias with them, because even sensitively conducted euthanasias are difficult to bear alone.

Regardless of where and when euthanasia occurs, procedural matters should be dealt with beforehand, if possible. For instance, consent forms should be signed and arrangements for payment should be made. If appropriate, the option of necropsy should be explained. If time allows, suggestions for how to memorialize a pet can also be discussed.

Whenever possible, decisions about body care (and necropsy) should be made prior to euthanasia. Owners should be offered all of the options available to them and each should be explained with honesty and sensitivity. It is helpful to use visual aids during this explanation. For example, if veterinarians make caskets or urns available for owners to purchase, samples can be shown.

Body care options can be explained by either veterinarians or technicians. Typically, the options include burial, cremation, rendering, or veterinary disposal. If pet owners choose burial and are taking their pet's body with them, they should be encouraged to bring something in which to transport the body. If they choose to have their veterinarian dispose of their pet's body for them, they should be given an honest explanation of what that means. For instance, if animals are buried in a mass grave at the landfill, owners should be told that.

Ideally, owner-present euthanasias are sched-uled during times when veterinarians feel most able to meet the wishes of their clients and the emotional demands of the procedure. This may be during the early morning, late afternoon, or even during evening hours. If all involved have agreed that the veterinary facility is the best environment for the euthanasia, owners who arrive for euthanasia appointments should never be kept waiting. Rather, they should be given first priority over everything except medical emergencies. They should also be immediately escorted to the euthanasia site.

It is highly recommended that all owner-present euthanasias be conducted by a team of at least two veterinary professionals. This allows whoever is assisting the veterinarian to focus on the owner's needs and allows the veterinarian to concentrate on the medical aspects of the procedure.

It is also highly recommended that, if an owner has elected to be present, the use of a catheter be carefully evaluated. A catheter is not always necessary and it does not always improve the *medical* procedures involved with euthanasia. However, it is often an enhancement to the *emotional* side of euthanasia for clients. The use of a catheter allows injections to be administered smoothly and quickly. It also reduces the possibility that the animal will resist, pull away, or even appear to struggle during the injection. If an owner's perception is that their animal seemed to *fight* the euthanasia procedure, their feelings of guilt and grief are often magnified.

If the veterinarian decides to use a catheter, it should be placed in a rear leg of the animal. This allows the owner free access to the face and head of the pet. After the intravenous catheter has been placed and the animal has been returned to the euthanasia site, owners should be given the opportunity to spend a short time alone with their companion animals, if they so desire. If owners are left alone to say their last good-byes, the veterinarian should state when he or she will return. For instance, the veterinarian may say, "I will be back in about 10 minutes."

If, after about 10 minutes, owners are still saying good-bye, the veterinarian can approach them and gently say, "It is time for us to proceed. May we begin?" Most owners will indicate their answer by either nodding or shaking their heads. If their answer is no, it is appropriate for the veterinarian to give them 5 or 10 minutes more. Any statement to this effect, though, must be made in a calm, quiet voice with no overtones of impatience or scolding detectable. Owners often report that they felt rushed through the euthanasia process by their veterinarian and feel the hastiness negated all of the other positive aspects of their experience.

When owners are ready to proceed, it is normal for the veterinary team members to feel somewhat awkward as they enter the environment in which the euthanasia is to be performed. Many wonder what they should say or do to comfort their grieving clients. Often, no words are necessary. A touch on an owner's arm or a hug around his or her shoulders communicates support and understanding quite well.

Before veterinarians begin the lethal injections, they should again tell the owners that they are ready to begin. Whenever possible, syringes should be kept out of sight (e.g., in the pocket of a laboratory coat or a smock) and handled very discreetly, as some people become very alarmed at the sight of syringes and needles. Once the procedure has begun, the drugs should be injected quickly, with little or no lapse of time between the injections. As the drugs are injected, each may be named so owners are kept abreast of how the procedure is progressing. Aside from these statements, it is best for veterinarians to remain silent. Most owners want to focus on saying good-bye to their animals and find comments, questions, and chatter distracting to their concentration.

With this combination of drugs, adverse side effects rarely occur. Thus, this method of facilitating euthanasia usually goes so smoothly that owners often do not realize their pets have actually died. It is very important, then, for the veterinarian to use a stethoscope to listen for a final heartbeat. When the veterinarian can do so with certainty, he or she must pronounce the animal dead. The veterinarian should do this with a clear, simple statement such as "Sarah, Buster is dead." At this time, the owners may gasp, cry, sob, or sigh with relief. They may make remarks about how quickly death came and about how peaceful the experience was.

Once death has occurred, the owners may review their pet's life by sharing special or funny stories about the pet. During this time, owners and veterinary professionals alike may feel a need to say good-bye, to comfort one another, and to express their feelings of grief. Creating opportunities to fulfill these needs is important, as support and emotional catharsis are variables known to have positive impact on people's overall experience of the grief process.[12,13]

After euthanasia, some people want to leave the euthanasia site quickly, while others need more time alone with their pets. When the owners are ready to leave, they should be escorted out a side or back door, if possible, so they don't have to exit through the busy waiting area. Also, if possible, a staff member should stay with the animal's body if the owners are not taking it with them. Almost without exception, owners take one last look back at their pet before they actually leave. When they see a friendly, familiar face next to their pet, they feel reassured that their companion animal will not be forgotten or treated with disrespect once they leave.

**Providing Effective Follow-Up Care**     Treating companion animals for cancer is often a long-term process. Surgery results in convalescence and the need for nursing care. Chemotherapy and radiation require multiple treatments. Treatments require follow-ups and rechecks. Because cancer treatments occur over such extended periods, pets and their owners establish special bonds with the veterinary professionals who treat and support them. Pet owners and veterinary professionals alike, then, often experience secondary losses when their pets die.

Secondary losses are the changes that accompany the primary loss of a pet, such as the loss of caregiving routines, the loss of a sense of purpose to life, and the loss of routine interactions with people who have come to be friends.[4] For clients with limited family or community support, the last secondary loss is a big one. Most likely, the veterinary professionals who have assisted them in their pet's battle against cancer have become an integral part of their process of anticipating, and ultimately adjusting to, the death of their pet. Many clients feel they have shared a profoundly significant process with their veterinary oncologist and thus have difficulty severing their relationships.

It is imperative that veterinary professionals understand and respect this unique aspect of oncological caregiving. It is also important for them to show their clients that their commitments extend beyond the companion animals they care for to the clients themselves.

Such feelings can be expressed through the use of routine exit interviews or follow-up telephone calls or a combination of the two. Exit interviews provide opportunities for clients to ask final questions about the disease or its course of treatment and to say good-bye and thank you to the veterinary oncologist and members of the treatment team. This time can also be used by veterinarians to settle any feelings about uncomfortable interchanges with clients that may have occurred during treatment. For example, they might comment on a time that the client seemed angry or resentful about the lack of treatment options. The goal in talking about these issues is to remove, whenever possible, any remaining barriers to the clients' full satisfaction with their veterinarians' caregiving. Follow-up telephone calls also provide opportunities for closure but may not be enough for some clients, particularly if the cancer treatment period has been either very short or very long.

Sending clients personalized condolence cards or letters is standard procedure in most veterinary practices. The time frame for sending condolences is not as important as the content of the cards or letters themselves. Along with personal comments about pets who die, veterinarians point out that the decision to euthanatize was both timely and humane and that pet owners did all that could be done to help their pets fight cancer while, at the same time, limiting their suffering. It also helpful to mention any preliminary necropsy results that serve to validate client decisions.

At the Colorado State University Veterinary Teaching Hospital (CSU-VTH), oncology staff members write an annual cancer newsletter that includes heartwarming and informative stories about pets they have treated for cancer. Owners whose pets have died are especially touched by this tribute to their beloved companion animals. It is another reminder that their pet was special and has not been forgotten.

Providing quality care for oncology patients also impacts veterinary oncologists. The same issues that impact pet owners—the "roller coaster" treatment dilemma of remission and recurrence, the grief felt at a pet's death after long-term treatment and care, and the subsequent growth of intense relationships between pet owners and members of the veterinary oncology team—affect veterinarians.

Riding the emotional roller coaster of cancer treatment is inevitable. Recurrence and metastatic disease often prevail. These realities often weight heavily on veterinarians and members of the oncological care team. Therefore, routine staff debriefings to encourage discussions about emotions are extremely helpful as a way to combat the feelings of frustration inherent in oncological veterinary medicine.

Veterinary professionals need time to process information, share memories, and express personal feelings about their patients' illnesses and deaths if they are to avoid the burnout associated with cancer caregiving. They need time to discuss how to modify treatment approaches based on what they learn from each case and to give colleagues constructive feedback and praise. Time to talk about their successes and victories is also necessary. By routinely making this time available, veterinarians help lower staff stress levels, foster team unity, and increase job satisfaction.

Case debriefing is best accomplished when weekly "bereavement rounds" are established and when all the treatment team members and clinic staff are required to attend. Half-hour sessions are generally adequate for case discussion when they occur on a regular, weekly basis. These meetings are most effective when veterinarians, technicians, receptionists, and pet loss counselors are present on a consistent basis.

Counselors from Changes: The Support for People and Pets Program at the CSU-VTH conduct bereavement rounds every Friday morning with students and members of the oncology faculty and staff. Successes, as well as losses and patient deaths, are discussed, along with effective ways to help pet owners deal with grief.

Since many animals diagnosed with cancer will eventually die from their disease, acknowledging personal grief as cases end is a vital coping tool for veterinary oncology professionals. It is important for all team members, in the final stages of the patient-client interaction, to evaluate their work individually and draw it to a close. Closure, a process of letting go or saying good-bye, can take place within structured debriefing sessions, as discussed earlier, or in private. Some methods for drawing closure privately include making donations in pets' name, to animal-related causes, conducting symbolic memorial services for special pets who have died, and keeping personal journals about feelings and experiences.

The extensive treatment protocols and continued recheck schedules inherent in cancer treatment breed familiarity, and thus relationships with clients often become friendships. Having clients as friends is a positive experience, but it is important to remember that the demands of friendships differ from the demands of professional relationships. The boundaries placed on interactions, then, differ from veterinarian to veterinarian. For example, some veterinarians enjoy social dinners with clients and others draw the line at any social involvement with clients at all.

One of the best ways to draw boundaries is to use the team approach to veterinary oncology. It is very difficult for veterinarians in busy practices to meet successfully all of the medical and emotional needs of their oncology patients and clients. It is important, therefore, to limit the time spent with any one client. Sharing time with clients with other team members helps insulate veterinarians and prevent them from becoming too involved with the clients they serve. It also helps clients not to become too dependent on any one team member.

Veterinarians, as team leaders, show emotional support for their staff members when they encourage them to take care of themselves. One of the best ways to help staff prioritize self-care is by role modeling. For instance, if veterinarians tell staff members to take stress breaks after challenging client interactions, they should also take stress breaks themselves. Actions speak louder than words, and veterinarians' exemplary behaviors promote self-care.

**What to Say, What to Do When Treatment Options Are Exhausted**　In response to indecision about euthanasia, the veterinarian might say, for example, "From this point on, you can't make a wrong decision. Buster may have a couple of good hours each day or an occasional upswing in her overall attitude and mood, but the reality is that her disease will soon kill her." This must be said very gently. Pause after this statement to allow time for reflection. Continue with,

> I see that you're struggling with the decision to help Buster die. This is a very difficult decision to make. I trust you will make the right choice for Buster *and* for you. Keep watching and communicating with Buster as you always have and, in your heart, you'll know when it's time.

In response to "Maybe I put her through too much. You said we'd get six months and we only got one!" the veterinarian might say, for example,

> Hind sight is always 20/20. As we said in the beginning, nothing was guaranteed except that we would all try as hard as we could and be there for you and Buster throughout the good times and bad. Even though Buster's survival was short, most of that time was good time with the family she loved.

In response to an oncology staff member saying, "I feel foolish and unprofessional for crying in front of a client," the veterinarian might say, for example, "Crying is a statement of compassion and shows empathy for pets and their owners. I've never had a client tell me that they disliked it when a staff member cried. In fact, it touches clients deeply when they know you care that much."

In response to pet owners' feelings of helplessness, the veterinarian might say, for example, "Even though there is nothing more we can do for Pepper medically, there is a lot we can do for him—and for you—emotionally." Turn attention to finding ways to make the last weeks or days that clients have with their pets emotionally satisfying and meaningful. Help them find special ways to say good-bye and to make decisions about body care, memorialization, and presence at euthanasia.

## CONCLUSION

As stated previously, the practice of veterinary oncology is both rewarding and frustrating. On difficult days, veterinarians feel they are fighting a futile battle against a superior force. When several patients die in the course of a week, they feel that, no matter what they do, they will never make a difference.

It is important to remember, though, that with veterinary oncology, success cannot solely be defined as cure, nor can failing be defined as recurrence or death. Success takes place every day as each patient's quality and quantity of life are extended. It takes place when the suffering of companion animals is alleviated and when clients are genuinely supported through difficult times.

When it is done well, the procedure of euthanatizing companion animals also contributes to a feeling of success. Veterinary oncology has contributed a great deal to what is known about effectively facilitating client-present euthanasias. The clinical experience of veterinary oncologists has proved that client-present euthanasia is a vital medical procedure, as worthy of a medical professional's time and attention as treatment itself. One day, veterinary oncologists may pave the way for human medicine to begin to see that euthanasia for people may also be of great value. If the trend toward legalizing human euthanasia continues, it is a procedure veterinarians will, undoubtedly, be asked to teach human health professionals about in the future.

## REFERENCES

1. Butler C, Lagoni L, Dickinson K, Withrow SJ: Cancer. Prob Vet Med Anim Illness Hum Emotion 3(1):21–37, 1991.
2. Voith, VL: Attachment of people to companion animals. Vet Clin North Am Small Anim Pract *15* (2):289–296, 1985.

3. American Pet Products Manufacturers Association: Survey of pet ownership in the USA. Pet Business *14* (4):1–4, 1988.

4. Lagoni, L, Butler, C, Hetts, S: The Human-Animal Bond and Grief. Philadelphia, WB. Saunders, 1994.

5. Gage G, Holcomb R: Couples' perceptions of the stressfulness of the death of the family pet. Family Relations *40* (1): 103–105, 1991.

6. Frey, WH, Lanseth, M: Crying: The Mystery of Tears. Minneapolis, Winston Press, 1985.

7. Cook, AS, Dworkin, DS: Helping the Bereaved: Therapeutic Interventions for Children, Adolescents, and Adults. New York, Basic Books, 1992.

8. Brewin, TR: Three ways of giving bad news. Lancet *337:* 1207–1209, 1991.

9. Slaikeu, KA: Crisis Intervention: A Handbook for Practice and Research. Newton, MA, Allyn & Bacon, 1984.

10. Hogbin, B: Getting it taped: The "bad news" consultation with cancer patients. Br J Hosp Med *41:* 330–332, 1989.

11. Sanders, CM: Effects of sudden illness versus chronic illness death on bereavement outcomes. Omega *13:* 227–241, 1982.

12. Rando, TA: Grief, Dying, and Death: Clinical Interventions for Caregivers. Champaign, IL, Research Press Company, 1984.

13. Maddison, D, Walker, WL: Factors affecting the outcome of conjugal bereavement. Br J Psychiatry *113:* 1057–1067, 1967.

# INDEX

Note: Page numbers in *italics* indicate illustrations; those followed by t refer to tables.

**561**

ISBN 0-7216-5592-0

90038